REA

OVERSIZE

REA

P9-BIL-918

HEALTH CARE STATE RANKINGS
1997

Health Care in the 50 United States

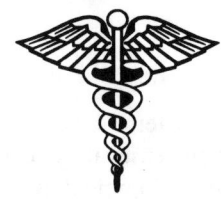

Kathleen O'Leary Morgan and Scott Morgan, Editors

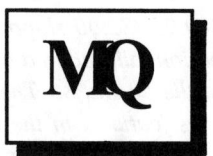

Morgan Quitno Press
© Copyright 1997, All Rights Reserved

P.O. Box 1656, Lawrence, KS 66044
800-457-0742 or 913-841-3534
http://www.morganquitno.com

Fifth Edition

© Copyright 1997 by
Morgan Quitno Corporation
512 East 9th Street, P.O. Box 1656
Lawrence, Kansas   66044-8656

800-457-0742 or 913-841-3534
http://www.morganquitno.com

ISBN: 1-56692-317-4
ISSN: 1065-1403

Health Care State Rankings 1997 sells for $49.95 ($2.00 shipping) and is only available in sewn, hardcover binding. For those who prefer ranking information tailored to a particular state, we also offer Health Care State Perspectives, state-specific reports for each of the 50 states. These individual guides provide information on a state's data and rank for each of the categories featured in the national Health Care State Rankings volume. Perspectives sell for $19.00 or $9.50 if ordered with Health Care State Rankings. If crime statistics are your interest, please ask about our annual Crime State Rankings ($49.95 hardcover). If you are interested in city and metropolitan crime data, we offer City Crime Rankings for $37.95. If you are interested in a general view of the states, please ask about our annual State Rankings ($49.95 hardcover). We also offer the data in our books on diskette (.dbf format). Shipping is $2.00 for all books up to a maximum of $6.00 per order.

Fifth Edition
Printed in the United States of America
April 1997

PREFACE

Which state has the highest percentage of primary care physicians? Which state's citizens pay the least for health care services? Which state has the highest incidence of malaria? From basic health care facts to interesting bits of trivia, *Health Care State Rankings 1997* provides a fascinating portrait of health care in the 50 United States.

This fifth edition of *Health Care State Rankings* features data from a number of government and private sector sources, pulling them together into one comprehensive health care volume. No other single source offers such a breadth of up-to-date health care statistics for states. This year's volume provides 508 tables of state health care comparisons -- our largest edition yet.

Important Notes About *Health Care State Rankings*

With each annual update of *Health Care State Rankings* we review each table to ensure that our readers have the most up-to-date, reliable information available. This fifth edition is no exception. We have updated most tables, added some and tossed a few. In some cases updated information is not available and tables are repeated. Our regular readers will note that this year's finance chapter has a number of repeat tables. This is because the Health Care Financing Administration will not have available updated state estimates of health care expenditures until later in 1997.

While our annual review process brings about many changes to our books, there are many popular features that are retained. These include source information and other pertinent footnotes clearly shown at the bottom of each page. National totals, rates and percentages are prominently displayed at the top of each table. Every other line is shaded in gray for easier reading. In addition, we provide numerous information finding tools: a thorough table of contents, table listings at the beginning of each chapter, a roster of sources with addresses and phone numbers, a detailed index and a chapter thumb index.

As in all of our reference books, the numbers shown in *Health Care State Rankings* are "complete," meaning that no additional calculations are required to convert them from millions, thousands, etc. (So put that calculator away!) All states are ranked on a high to low basis, with any ties among the states listed alphabetically for a given ranking. Negative numbers are shown in parentheses "( )." For tables with national totals (as opposed to rates, per capita's, etc.) a separate column is included showing what percent of the national total each individual state's total represents. This column is headed by "% of USA." This percentage figure is particularly interesting when compared with a state's share of the nation's population for a particular year (provided in an appendix).

If you are interested in looking for information for just one state, we once again are offering our *Health Care State Perspective* series of publications. These 21-page comb bound reports feature data and ranking information for an individual state, pulled from the national *Health Care State Rankings* book. (For example *California Health Care in Perspective* features information about the state of California only.) They serve as handy, quick reference guides for those who do not want to page through the entire *Health Care State Rankings* volume searching for information for their particular state. When purchased by themselves, *Health Care State Perspectives* sell for $19. When purchased with a copy of *Health Care State Rankings*, these handy quick reference guides are just $9.50.

Other Books From Morgan Quitno Press

In addition to *Health Care State Rankings*, our company offers three other rankings reference books. The first of these, *State Rankings*, provides a general view of the states. Statistics are featured in a wide variety of categories including agriculture, transportation, government finance, health, population, crime, education, social welfare, energy and environment. In its eighth edition for 1997, this book has received great acclaim for its ease of use and simple presentation of state data.

Our annual compilation of state crime data is featured in *Crime State Rankings*. In its fourth edition for 1997, this reference volume contains a huge collection of user friendly statistics on law enforcement personnel and expenditures, corrections, arrests and offenses. Our readers' thirst for crime statistics proved to be so voracious that we added a companion volume of crime data, *City Crime Rankings*, to our list of titles. Now available in an expanded third edition, *City Crime Rankings* compares cities with 75,000 or more population (approximately 300 cities) as well as all metropolitan areas. Numbers of crimes, crime rates, changes in crime rates over one and five years are presented for all major crime categories reported by the FBI.

City Crime Rankings sells for $37.95. The *State Rankings* and *Crime State Rankings* books each are available for $49.95. (S/H $2 per book or $6 maximum per order) All books are hardcover. The data in our books are also available on diskette (.dbf format). This electronic format allows you to put our data into your program for your own tailor-made analysis. If you would like a brochure or further information, please give us a call at 1-800-457-0742.

Finally, we want to thank the many librarians, government and health care industry officials who helped us in developing, designing and producing this book. Your suggestions and contributions of data have helped to make *Health Care State Rankings* a truly usable reference volume. We so appreciate the many comments and suggestions we receive from our readers. Please keep sending us your ideas!

THE EDITORS

WHICH STATE IS HEALTHIEST?

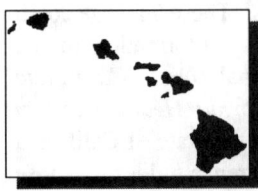

This just does not seem like a hard sell. Sometimes a state wins one of our awards and it takes a little convincing. However, naming the great state of Hawaii as the winner of our fifth annual Healthiest State Award should strike very few as odd. After all, how could paradise be unhealthy?

Each year we take a step back from our objective reporting of health statistics, throw some basic figures into our computer and determine which is the Healthiest State. Moving up from 3rd place last year, Hawaii eases into 1997's top spot. Last year's winner, Iowa, fell to 8th place.

Based on the 23 categories listed below, the Aloha State preceded Minnesota, Connecticut, New Hampshire and Utah as the top of the top five healthiest states. Ranking last for the fourth straight year (with continued apologies to the Clintons) is Arkansas, preceded by Louisiana, Alabama, West Virginia and Tennessee.

Admittedly the categories selected have a lot to do with the outcome of the award. We try to refrain from changing many of the factors so that one year is comparable to

1997 HEALTHIEST STATE AWARD

RANK	STATE	AVG	'96	RANK	STATE	AVG	'96
1	Hawaii	36.48	3	26	Kansas	26.30	8
2	Minnesota	34.13	5	27	Maine	25.43	21
3	Connecticut	33.13	6	27	New Mexico	25.43	26
4	New Hampshire	32.86	7	29	Colorado	25.13	28
5	Utah	32.09	4	30	Rhode Island	24.43	29
6	Vermont	31.70	2	31	Ohio	24.09	31
7	Washington	30.57	15	32	Delaware	23.43	33
8	Iowa	30.48	1	33	Texas	23.35	35
9	Nebraska	30.09	9	34	Oklahoma	23.30	27
10	Massachusetts	29.52	20	35	Georgia	22.87	38
11	Idaho	29.22	11	36	South Carolina	22.26	38
12	Montana	28.61	18	37	Michigan	22.17	42
13	Virginia	28.39	10	38	Pennsylvania	21.83	40
14	California	28.22	24	39	Indiana	21.39	37
15	Maryland	27.78	17	40	Arizona	20.61	34
16	Alaska	27.43	14	41	Nevada	20.04	47
17	Illinois	27.35	30	42	Mississippi	19.65	44
18	New York	27.30	32	43	Missouri	19.52	46
19	North Carolina	27.13	25	44	Florida	19.43	43
20	South Dakota	27.04	16	45	Kentucky	18.39	40
21	Oregon	27.00	22	46	Tennessee	18.13	36
22	New Jersey	26.74	22	47	Alabama	17.65	48
23	Wisconsin	26.57	18	48	Louisiana	16.04	49
24	North Dakota	26.35	13	49	West Virginia	15.87	45
25	Wyoming	26.32	12	50	Arkansas	15.04	50

another. This year we have kept the same factors but updated the data. Overall, the factors chosen reflect affordability of health care, access to health care and a generally healthy population. All factors were given equal weight.

Once the factors were determined, we averaged each state's rankings for the 23 categories. Based on these averages, states were then ranked from "healthiest" (highest average ranking) to "least healthy" (lowest average ranking). States with no data available for a given category were ranked only on the remaining factors. The tables in *Health Care State Rankings 1997* list data from highest to lowest. However, for purposes of this award, we inverted rankings for those factors we determined to be "positive." Thus the state with the highest percent of its children immunized in the book (ranking 1st) would be given a "50" for purposes of this award.

The table above shows how each state fared in the 1997 Healthiest State Award as well as its placement in 1996. We are always pleased with the level of discussion generated by this award in many state capitals and hope that the constructive dialogue will continue. Congratulations to the fine (and healthy) citizens of Hawaii!

The Editors

POSITIVE (+) AND NEGATIVE (-) FACTORS CONSIDERED:

1. Births of Low Birthweight as a Percent of All Births (Table 15) -
2. Births to Teenage Mothers as a Percent of Live Births (Table 27) -
3. Percent of Mothers Receiving Late or No Prenatal Care (Table 54) -
4. Death Rate (Table 77) -
5. Infant Mortality Rate (Table 84) -
6. Estimated Age Adjusted Death Rate by Cancer (Table 110) -
7. Death Rate by Suicide (Table 160) -
8. Percent of Population Not Covered by Health Insurance (Table 237) -
9. Change in Percent of Population Uninsured: 1991 to 1995 (Table 244) -
10. Health Care Expenditures as a Percent of Gross State Product (Table 260) -
11. Per Capita Personal Health Expenditures (Table 261) -
12. Estimated Rate of New Cancer Cases (Table 356) -

13. AIDS Rate (Table 380) -
14. Combined Notifiable Disease Rate (Tables 384-413) -
15. Percent of Population Lacking Access to Primary Care (Table 442) -
16. Percent of Adults Who Are Binge Drinkers (Table 502) -
17. Percent of Adults Who Smoke (Table 503) -
18. Percent of Adults Overweight (Table 506) -
19. Number of Days in Past Month When Physical Health was "Not Good" (Table 507) -
20. Community Hospitals per 1,000 Square Miles (Table 181) +
21. Beds in Community Hospitals per 100,000 Population (Table 192) +
22. Percent of Children Aged 19-35 Months Fully Immunized (Table 411) +
23. Safety Belt Usage Rate (Table 511) +

TABLE OF CONTENTS

I. Births and Reproductive Health

TABLE OF CONTENTS (continued)

TABLE OF CONTENTS (continued)

TABLE OF CONTENTS (continued)

III. Facilities

TABLE OF CONTENTS (continued)

TABLE OF CONTENTS (continued)

TABLE OF CONTENTS (continued)

TABLE OF CONTENTS (continued)

TABLE OF CONTENTS (continued)

VII. Physical Fitness

VIII. Appendix

IX. Sources

X. Index

I. BIRTHS AND REPRODUCTIVE HEALTH

I. BIRTHS AND REPRODUCTIVE HEALTH
(CONTINUED)

Abortions

Births in 1995

National Total = 3,900,089 Live Births*

ALPHA ORDER

RANK	STATE	BIRTHS	% of USA
23	Alabama	60,939	1.56%
47	Alaska	10,233	0.26%
18	Arizona	72,355	1.86%
34	Arkansas	35,155	0.90%
1	California	561,091	14.39%
24	Colorado	54,311	1.39%
28	Connecticut	45,141	1.16%
46	Delaware	10,258	0.26%
4	Florida	188,542	4.83%
9	Georgia	113,589	2.91%
39	Hawaii	18,598	0.48%
40	Idaho	18,012	0.46%
5	Illinois	185,425	4.75%
13	Indiana	84,304	2.16%
33	Iowa	36,611	0.94%
32	Kansas	37,644	0.97%
25	Kentucky	51,672	1.32%
21	Louisiana	67,420	1.73%
42	Maine	13,911	0.36%
19	Maryland	71,585	1.84%
15	Massachusetts	74,818	1.92%
8	Michigan	132,577	3.40%
22	Minnesota	62,911	1.61%
30	Mississippi	41,368	1.06%
16	Missouri	74,121	1.90%
44	Montana	11,113	0.28%
37	Nebraska	23,257	0.60%
36	Nevada	25,043	0.64%
41	New Hampshire	14,894	0.38%
10	New Jersey	108,637	2.79%
35	New Mexico	27,038	0.69%
3	New York	264,459	6.78%
11	North Carolina	102,029	2.62%
48	North Dakota	8,655	0.22%
6	Ohio	155,633	3.99%
27	Oklahoma	45,906	1.18%
29	Oregon	42,810	1.10%
7	Pennsylvania	151,448	3.88%
43	Rhode Island	12,386	0.32%
26	South Carolina	49,935	1.28%
45	South Dakota	10,521	0.27%
17	Tennessee	73,597	1.89%
2	Texas	328,586	8.43%
31	Utah	39,530	1.01%
49	Vermont	6,842	0.18%
12	Virginia	93,092	2.39%
14	Washington	78,302	2.01%
38	West Virginia	21,123	0.54%
20	Wisconsin	67,498	1.73%
50	Wyoming	6,335	0.16%

RANK ORDER

RANK	STATE	BIRTHS	% of USA
1	California	561,091	14.39%
2	Texas	328,586	8.43%
3	New York	264,459	6.78%
4	Florida	188,542	4.83%
5	Illinois	185,425	4.75%
6	Ohio	155,633	3.99%
7	Pennsylvania	151,448	3.88%
8	Michigan	132,577	3.40%
9	Georgia	113,589	2.91%
10	New Jersey	108,637	2.79%
11	North Carolina	102,029	2.62%
12	Virginia	93,092	2.39%
13	Indiana	84,304	2.16%
14	Washington	78,302	2.01%
15	Massachusetts	74,818	1.92%
16	Missouri	74,121	1.90%
17	Tennessee	73,597	1.89%
18	Arizona	72,355	1.86%
19	Maryland	71,585	1.84%
20	Wisconsin	67,498	1.73%
21	Louisiana	67,420	1.73%
22	Minnesota	62,911	1.61%
23	Alabama	60,939	1.56%
24	Colorado	54,311	1.39%
25	Kentucky	51,672	1.32%
26	South Carolina	49,935	1.28%
27	Oklahoma	45,906	1.18%
28	Connecticut	45,141	1.16%
29	Oregon	42,810	1.10%
30	Mississippi	41,368	1.06%
31	Utah	39,530	1.01%
32	Kansas	37,644	0.97%
33	Iowa	36,611	0.94%
34	Arkansas	35,155	0.90%
35	New Mexico	27,038	0.69%
36	Nevada	25,043	0.64%
37	Nebraska	23,257	0.60%
38	West Virginia	21,123	0.54%
39	Hawaii	18,598	0.48%
40	Idaho	18,012	0.46%
41	New Hampshire	14,894	0.38%
42	Maine	13,911	0.36%
43	Rhode Island	12,386	0.32%
44	Montana	11,113	0.28%
45	South Dakota	10,521	0.27%
46	Delaware	10,258	0.26%
47	Alaska	10,233	0.26%
48	North Dakota	8,655	0.22%
49	Vermont	6,842	0.18%
50	Wyoming	6,335	0.16%
	District of Columbia	8,831	0.23%

Source: U.S. Department of Health and Human Services, National Center for Health Statistics "Monthly Vital Statistics Report" (Vol. 45, No. 3(S)2, October 4, 1996)
*Data are preliminary estimates by state of residence.

Birth Rate in 1995

National Rate = 14.8 Live Births per 1,000 Population*

ALPHA ORDER

RANK	STATE	RATE
20	Alabama	14.3
5	Alaska	17.0
4	Arizona	17.2
22	Arkansas	14.2
2	California	17.8
16	Colorado	14.5
32	Connecticut	13.8
20	Delaware	14.3
39	Florida	13.3
8	Georgia	15.8
9	Hawaii	15.7
11	Idaho	15.5
9	Illinois	15.7
16	Indiana	14.5
43	Iowa	12.9
14	Kansas	14.7
38	Kentucky	13.4
11	Louisiana	15.5
50	Maine	11.2
22	Maryland	14.2
47	Massachusetts	12.3
30	Michigan	13.9
34	Minnesota	13.6
13	Mississippi	15.3
30	Missouri	13.9
44	Montana	12.8
22	Nebraska	14.2
6	Nevada	16.4
42	New Hampshire	13.0
33	New Jersey	13.7
7	New Mexico	16.0
15	New York	14.6
22	North Carolina	14.2
37	North Dakota	13.5
27	Ohio	14.0
27	Oklahoma	14.0
34	Oregon	13.6
45	Pennsylvania	12.5
45	Rhode Island	12.5
34	South Carolina	13.6
18	South Dakota	14.4
27	Tennessee	14.0
3	Texas	17.5
1	Utah	20.3
48	Vermont	11.7
26	Virginia	14.1
18	Washington	14.4
49	West Virginia	11.6
40	Wisconsin	13.2
40	Wyoming	13.2

RANK ORDER

RANK	STATE	RATE
1	Utah	20.3
2	California	17.8
3	Texas	17.5
4	Arizona	17.2
5	Alaska	17.0
6	Nevada	16.4
7	New Mexico	16.0
8	Georgia	15.8
9	Hawaii	15.7
9	Illinois	15.7
11	Idaho	15.5
11	Louisiana	15.5
13	Mississippi	15.3
14	Kansas	14.7
15	New York	14.6
16	Colorado	14.5
16	Indiana	14.5
18	South Dakota	14.4
18	Washington	14.4
20	Alabama	14.3
20	Delaware	14.3
22	Arkansas	14.2
22	Maryland	14.2
22	Nebraska	14.2
22	North Carolina	14.2
26	Virginia	14.1
27	Ohio	14.0
27	Oklahoma	14.0
27	Tennessee	14.0
30	Michigan	13.9
30	Missouri	13.9
32	Connecticut	13.8
33	New Jersey	13.7
34	Minnesota	13.6
34	Oregon	13.6
34	South Carolina	13.6
37	North Dakota	13.5
38	Kentucky	13.4
39	Florida	13.3
40	Wisconsin	13.2
40	Wyoming	13.2
42	New Hampshire	13.0
43	Iowa	12.9
44	Montana	12.8
45	Pennsylvania	12.5
45	Rhode Island	12.5
47	Massachusetts	12.3
48	Vermont	11.7
49	West Virginia	11.6
50	Maine	11.2
	District of Columbia	15.9

*Source: U.S. Department of Health and Human Services, National Center for Health Statistics
"Monthly Vital Statistics Report" (Vol. 45, No. 3(S)2, October 4, 1996)*
*Data are preliminary estimates by state of residence.

Births in 1994

National Total = 3,952,767 Live Births*

<u>ALPHA ORDER</u>

RANK	STATE	BIRTHS	% of USA
23	Alabama	60,939	1.54%
45	Alaska	10,678	0.27%
19	Arizona	70,846	1.79%
34	Arkansas	34,718	0.88%
1	California	567,930	14.37%
24	Colorado	54,071	1.37%
28	Connecticut	45,655	1.16%
47	Delaware	10,411	0.26%
4	Florida	190,654	4.82%
10	Georgia	111,011	2.81%
39	Hawaii	19,517	0.49%
40	Idaho	17,526	0.44%
5	Illinois	189,257	4.79%
14	Indiana	82,595	2.09%
33	Iowa	37,079	0.94%
32	Kansas	37,379	0.95%
25	Kentucky	52,983	1.34%
21	Louisiana	67,817	1.72%
42	Maine	14,441	0.37%
16	Maryland	73,971	1.87%
13	Massachusetts	83,787	2.12%
8	Michigan	138,028	3.49%
22	Minnesota	64,305	1.63%
29	Mississippi	41,954	1.06%
17	Missouri	73,543	1.86%
44	Montana	11,067	0.28%
37	Nebraska	23,156	0.59%
36	Nevada	23,911	0.60%
41	New Hampshire	15,106	0.38%
9	New Jersey	117,501	2.97%
35	New Mexico	27,591	0.70%
3	New York	278,392	7.04%
11	North Carolina	101,420	2.57%
48	North Dakota	8,584	0.22%
7	Ohio	155,944	3.95%
27	Oklahoma	45,703	1.16%
30	Oregon	41,837	1.06%
6	Pennsylvania	157,071	3.97%
43	Rhode Island	13,466	0.34%
26	South Carolina	52,043	1.32%
46	South Dakota	10,507	0.27%
18	Tennessee	73,191	1.85%
2	Texas	321,114	8.12%
31	Utah	38,279	0.97%
49	Vermont	7,377	0.19%
12	Virginia	95,039	2.40%
15	Washington	77,358	1.96%
38	West Virginia	21,375	0.54%
20	Wisconsin	68,282	1.73%
50	Wyoming	6,428	0.16%

<u>RANK ORDER</u>

RANK	STATE	BIRTHS	% of USA
1	California	567,930	14.37%
2	Texas	321,114	8.12%
3	New York	278,392	7.04%
4	Florida	190,654	4.82%
5	Illinois	189,257	4.79%
6	Pennsylvania	157,071	3.97%
7	Ohio	155,944	3.95%
8	Michigan	138,028	3.49%
9	New Jersey	117,501	2.97%
10	Georgia	111,011	2.81%
11	North Carolina	101,420	2.57%
12	Virginia	95,039	2.40%
13	Massachusetts	83,787	2.12%
14	Indiana	82,595	2.09%
15	Washington	77,358	1.96%
16	Maryland	73,971	1.87%
17	Missouri	73,543	1.86%
18	Tennessee	73,191	1.85%
19	Arizona	70,846	1.79%
20	Wisconsin	68,282	1.73%
21	Louisiana	67,817	1.72%
22	Minnesota	64,305	1.63%
23	Alabama	60,939	1.54%
24	Colorado	54,071	1.37%
25	Kentucky	52,983	1.34%
26	South Carolina	52,043	1.32%
27	Oklahoma	45,703	1.16%
28	Connecticut	45,655	1.16%
29	Mississippi	41,954	1.06%
30	Oregon	41,837	1.06%
31	Utah	38,279	0.97%
32	Kansas	37,379	0.95%
33	Iowa	37,079	0.94%
34	Arkansas	34,718	0.88%
35	New Mexico	27,591	0.70%
36	Nevada	23,911	0.60%
37	Nebraska	23,156	0.59%
38	West Virginia	21,375	0.54%
39	Hawaii	19,517	0.49%
40	Idaho	17,526	0.44%
41	New Hampshire	15,106	0.38%
42	Maine	14,441	0.37%
43	Rhode Island	13,466	0.34%
44	Montana	11,067	0.28%
45	Alaska	10,678	0.27%
46	South Dakota	10,507	0.27%
47	Delaware	10,411	0.26%
48	North Dakota	8,584	0.22%
49	Vermont	7,377	0.19%
50	Wyoming	6,428	0.16%
	District of Columbia	9,930	0.25%

Source: U.S. Department of Health and Human Services, National Center for Health Statistics
    "Monthly Vital Statistics Report" (Vol. 44, No. 11, Supplement, June 24, 1996)
*Final data by state of residence.

Birth Rate in 1994

National Rate = 15.2 Live Births per 1,000 Population*

ALPHA ORDER

RANK	STATE	RATE
24	Alabama	14.4
3	Alaska	17.6
5	Arizona	17.4
28	Arkansas	14.2
2	California	18.1
16	Colorado	14.8
34	Connecticut	13.9
18	Delaware	14.7
38	Florida	13.7
10	Georgia	15.7
7	Hawaii	16.6
13	Idaho	15.5
9	Illinois	16.1
24	Indiana	14.4
45	Iowa	13.1
19	Kansas	14.6
37	Kentucky	13.8
10	Louisiana	15.7
50	Maine	11.6
16	Maryland	14.8
34	Massachusetts	13.9
21	Michigan	14.5
30	Minnesota	14.1
10	Mississippi	15.7
34	Missouri	13.9
47	Montana	12.9
26	Nebraska	14.3
8	Nevada	16.4
44	New Hampshire	13.3
15	New Jersey	14.9
6	New Mexico	16.7
14	New York	15.3
26	North Carolina	14.3
40	North Dakota	13.5
32	Ohio	14.0
32	Oklahoma	14.0
39	Oregon	13.6
46	Pennsylvania	13.0
40	Rhode Island	13.5
28	South Carolina	14.2
19	South Dakota	14.6
30	Tennessee	14.1
4	Texas	17.5
1	Utah	20.1
48	Vermont	12.7
21	Virginia	14.5
21	Washington	14.5
49	West Virginia	11.7
43	Wisconsin	13.4
40	Wyoming	13.5

RANK ORDER

RANK	STATE	RATE
1	Utah	20.1
2	California	18.1
3	Alaska	17.6
4	Texas	17.5
5	Arizona	17.4
6	New Mexico	16.7
7	Hawaii	16.6
8	Nevada	16.4
9	Illinois	16.1
10	Georgia	15.7
10	Louisiana	15.7
10	Mississippi	15.7
13	Idaho	15.5
14	New York	15.3
15	New Jersey	14.9
16	Colorado	14.8
16	Maryland	14.8
18	Delaware	14.7
19	Kansas	14.6
19	South Dakota	14.6
21	Michigan	14.5
21	Virginia	14.5
21	Washington	14.5
24	Alabama	14.4
24	Indiana	14.4
26	Nebraska	14.3
26	North Carolina	14.3
28	Arkansas	14.2
28	South Carolina	14.2
30	Minnesota	14.1
30	Tennessee	14.1
32	Ohio	14.0
32	Oklahoma	14.0
34	Connecticut	13.9
34	Massachusetts	13.9
34	Missouri	13.9
37	Kentucky	13.8
38	Florida	13.7
39	Oregon	13.6
40	North Dakota	13.5
40	Rhode Island	13.5
40	Wyoming	13.5
43	Wisconsin	13.4
44	New Hampshire	13.3
45	Iowa	13.1
46	Pennsylvania	13.0
47	Montana	12.9
48	Vermont	12.7
49	West Virginia	11.7
50	Maine	11.6
	District of Columbia	17.4

Source: U.S. Department of Health and Human Services, National Center for Health Statistics
   "Monthly Vital Statistics Report" (Vol. 44, No. 11, Supplement, June 24, 1996)
*Final data by state of residence.

4

Births in 1990

National Total = 4,158,212 Live Births*

ALPHA ORDER

ALPHA ORDER

RANK	STATE	BIRTHS	% of USA
23	Alabama	63,487	1.53%
44	Alaska	11,902	0.29%
21	Arizona	68,995	1.66%
33	Arkansas	36,457	0.88%
1	California	612,628	14.73%
26	Colorado	53,525	1.29%
27	Connecticut	50,123	1.21%
46	Delaware	11,113	0.27%
4	Florida	199,339	4.79%
10	Georgia	112,666	2.71%
39	Hawaii	20,489	0.49%
42	Idaho	16,433	0.40%
5	Illinois	195,790	4.71%
14	Indiana	86,214	2.07%
31	Iowa	39,409	0.95%
32	Kansas	39,020	0.94%
25	Kentucky	54,362	1.31%
20	Louisiana	72,192	1.74%
41	Maine	17,359	0.42%
15	Maryland	80,245	1.93%
13	Massachusetts	92,654	2.23%
8	Michigan	153,700	3.70%
22	Minnesota	68,013	1.64%
29	Mississippi	43,563	1.05%
16	Missouri	79,260	1.91%
45	Montana	11,613	0.28%
36	Nebraska	24,380	0.59%
38	Nevada	21,599	0.52%
40	New Hampshire	17,569	0.42%
9	New Jersey	122,289	2.94%
35	New Mexico	27,402	0.66%
3	New York	297,576	7.16%
11	North Carolina	104,525	2.51%
48	North Dakota	9,250	0.22%
7	Ohio	166,913	4.01%
28	Oklahoma	47,649	1.15%
30	Oregon	42,891	1.03%
6	Pennsylvania	171,961	4.14%
43	Rhode Island	15,195	0.37%
24	South Carolina	58,610	1.41%
47	South Dakota	10,999	0.26%
18	Tennessee	74,962	1.80%
2	Texas	316,423	7.61%
34	Utah	36,277	0.87%
49	Vermont	8,273	0.20%
12	Virginia	99,352	2.39%
17	Washington	79,251	1.91%
37	West Virginia	22,585	0.54%
19	Wisconsin	72,895	1.75%
50	Wyoming	6,985	0.17%

RANK ORDER

RANK	STATE	BIRTHS	% of USA
1	California	612,628	14.73%
2	Texas	316,423	7.61%
3	New York	297,576	7.16%
4	Florida	199,339	4.79%
5	Illinois	195,790	4.71%
6	Pennsylvania	171,961	4.14%
7	Ohio	166,913	4.01%
8	Michigan	153,700	3.70%
9	New Jersey	122,289	2.94%
10	Georgia	112,666	2.71%
11	North Carolina	104,525	2.51%
12	Virginia	99,352	2.39%
13	Massachusetts	92,654	2.23%
14	Indiana	86,214	2.07%
15	Maryland	80,245	1.93%
16	Missouri	79,260	1.91%
17	Washington	79,251	1.91%
18	Tennessee	74,962	1.80%
19	Wisconsin	72,895	1.75%
20	Louisiana	72,192	1.74%
21	Arizona	68,995	1.66%
22	Minnesota	68,013	1.64%
23	Alabama	63,487	1.53%
24	South Carolina	58,610	1.41%
25	Kentucky	54,362	1.31%
26	Colorado	53,525	1.29%
27	Connecticut	50,123	1.21%
28	Oklahoma	47,649	1.15%
29	Mississippi	43,563	1.05%
30	Oregon	42,891	1.03%
31	Iowa	39,409	0.95%
32	Kansas	39,020	0.94%
33	Arkansas	36,457	0.88%
34	Utah	36,277	0.87%
35	New Mexico	27,402	0.66%
36	Nebraska	24,380	0.59%
37	West Virginia	22,585	0.54%
38	Nevada	21,599	0.52%
39	Hawaii	20,489	0.49%
40	New Hampshire	17,569	0.42%
41	Maine	17,359	0.42%
42	Idaho	16,433	0.40%
43	Rhode Island	15,195	0.37%
44	Alaska	11,902	0.29%
45	Montana	11,613	0.28%
46	Delaware	11,113	0.27%
47	South Dakota	10,999	0.26%
48	North Dakota	9,250	0.22%
49	Vermont	8,273	0.20%
50	Wyoming	6,985	0.17%
	District of Columbia	11,850	0.28%

Source: U.S. Department of Health and Human Services, National Center for Health Statistics
"Monthly Vital Statistics Report" (Vol. 41, No. 9, Supplement, February 25, 1993)
Final data by state of residence.

Birth Rate in 1990

National Rate = 16.7 Births per 1,000 Population*

ALPHA ORDER

RANK	STATE	RATE
26	Alabama	15.7
1	Alaska	21.6
4	Arizona	18.8
29	Arkansas	15.5
3	California	20.6
20	Colorado	16.2
38	Connecticut	15.2
15	Delaware	16.7
32	Florida	15.4
9	Georgia	17.4
6	Hawaii	18.5
18	Idaho	16.3
10	Illinois	17.1
28	Indiana	15.6
48	Iowa	14.2
26	Kansas	15.7
43	Kentucky	14.8
10	Louisiana	17.1
49	Maine	14.1
13	Maryland	16.8
32	Massachusetts	15.4
16	Michigan	16.5
29	Minnesota	15.5
12	Mississippi	16.9
29	Missouri	15.5
45	Montana	14.5
32	Nebraska	15.4
8	Nevada	18.0
22	New Hampshire	15.8
22	New Jersey	15.8
7	New Mexico	18.1
16	New York	16.5
22	North Carolina	15.8
45	North Dakota	14.5
32	Ohio	15.4
39	Oklahoma	15.1
39	Oregon	15.1
45	Pennsylvania	14.5
39	Rhode Island	15.1
13	South Carolina	16.8
22	South Dakota	15.8
32	Tennessee	15.4
5	Texas	18.6
2	Utah	21.1
44	Vermont	14.7
21	Virginia	16.1
18	Washington	16.3
50	West Virginia	12.6
42	Wisconsin	14.9
32	Wyoming	15.4

RANK ORDER

RANK	STATE	RATE
1	Alaska	21.6
2	Utah	21.1
3	California	20.6
4	Arizona	18.8
5	Texas	18.6
6	Hawaii	18.5
7	New Mexico	18.1
8	Nevada	18.0
9	Georgia	17.4
10	Illinois	17.1
10	Louisiana	17.1
12	Mississippi	16.9
13	Maryland	16.8
13	South Carolina	16.8
15	Delaware	16.7
16	Michigan	16.5
16	New York	16.5
18	Idaho	16.3
18	Washington	16.3
20	Colorado	16.2
21	Virginia	16.1
22	New Hampshire	15.8
22	New Jersey	15.8
22	North Carolina	15.8
22	South Dakota	15.8
26	Alabama	15.7
26	Kansas	15.7
28	Indiana	15.6
29	Arkansas	15.5
29	Minnesota	15.5
29	Missouri	15.5
32	Florida	15.4
32	Massachusetts	15.4
32	Nebraska	15.4
32	Ohio	15.4
32	Tennessee	15.4
32	Wyoming	15.4
38	Connecticut	15.2
39	Oklahoma	15.1
39	Oregon	15.1
39	Rhode Island	15.1
42	Wisconsin	14.9
43	Kentucky	14.8
44	Vermont	14.7
45	Montana	14.5
45	North Dakota	14.5
45	Pennsylvania	14.5
48	Iowa	14.2
49	Maine	14.1
50	West Virginia	12.6

| | District of Columbia | 19.5 |

Source: U.S. Department of Health and Human Services, National Center for Health Statistics "Monthly Vital Statistics Report" (Vol. 41, No. 9, Supplement, February 25, 1993)

*Final data by state of residence.

Births in 1980

National Total = 3,612,000 Births*

ALPHA ORDER					RANK ORDER			
RANK	STATE		BIRTHS	% of USA	RANK	STATE	BIRTHS	% of USA
21	Alabama		64,000	1.77%	1	California	403,000	11.16%
48	Alaska		10,000	0.28%	2	Texas	274,000	7.59%
26	Arizona		50,000	1.38%	3	New York	239,000	6.62%
34	Arkansas		37,000	1.02%	4	Illinois	190,000	5.26%
1	California		403,000	11.16%	5	Ohio	169,000	4.68%
26	Colorado		50,000	1.38%	6	Pennsylvania	159,000	4.40%
33	Connecticut		39,000	1.08%	7	Michigan	146,000	4.04%
49	Delaware		9,000	0.25%	8	Florida	132,000	3.65%
8	Florida		132,000	3.65%	9	New Jersey	97,000	2.69%
10	Georgia		92,000	2.55%	10	Georgia	92,000	2.55%
39	Hawaii		18,000	0.50%	11	Indiana	88,000	2.44%
38	Idaho		20,000	0.55%	12	North Carolina	84,000	2.33%
4	Illinois		190,000	5.26%	13	Louisiana	82,000	2.27%
11	Indiana		88,000	2.44%	14	Missouri	79,000	2.19%
28	Iowa		48,000	1.33%	15	Virginia	78,000	2.16%
32	Kansas		41,000	1.14%	16	Wisconsin	75,000	2.08%
22	Kentucky		60,000	1.66%	17	Massachusetts	73,000	2.02%
13	Louisiana		82,000	2.27%	18	Tennessee	69,000	1.91%
40	Maine		16,000	0.44%	19	Minnesota	68,000	1.88%
22	Maryland		60,000	1.66%	19	Washington	68,000	1.88%
17	Massachusetts		73,000	2.02%	21	Alabama	64,000	1.77%
7	Michigan		146,000	4.04%	22	Kentucky	60,000	1.66%
19	Minnesota		68,000	1.88%	22	Maryland	60,000	1.66%
28	Mississippi		48,000	1.33%	24	Oklahoma	52,000	1.44%
14	Missouri		79,000	2.19%	24	South Carolina	52,000	1.44%
41	Montana		14,000	0.39%	26	Arizona	50,000	1.38%
36	Nebraska		27,000	0.75%	26	Colorado	50,000	1.38%
43	Nevada		13,000	0.36%	28	Iowa	48,000	1.33%
41	New Hampshire		14,000	0.39%	28	Mississippi	48,000	1.33%
9	New Jersey		97,000	2.69%	30	Oregon	43,000	1.19%
37	New Mexico		26,000	0.72%	31	Utah	42,000	1.16%
3	New York		239,000	6.62%	32	Kansas	41,000	1.14%
12	North Carolina		84,000	2.33%	33	Connecticut	39,000	1.08%
45	North Dakota		12,000	0.33%	34	Arkansas	37,000	1.02%
5	Ohio		169,000	4.68%	35	West Virginia	29,000	0.80%
24	Oklahoma		52,000	1.44%	36	Nebraska	27,000	0.75%
30	Oregon		43,000	1.19%	37	New Mexico	26,000	0.72%
6	Pennsylvania		159,000	4.40%	38	Idaho	20,000	0.55%
45	Rhode Island		12,000	0.33%	39	Hawaii	18,000	0.50%
24	South Carolina		52,000	1.44%	40	Maine	16,000	0.44%
43	South Dakota		13,000	0.36%	41	Montana	14,000	0.39%
18	Tennessee		69,000	1.91%	41	New Hampshire	14,000	0.39%
2	Texas		274,000	7.59%	43	Nevada	13,000	0.36%
31	Utah		42,000	1.16%	43	South Dakota	13,000	0.36%
50	Vermont		8,000	0.22%	45	North Dakota	12,000	0.33%
15	Virginia		78,000	2.16%	45	Rhode Island	12,000	0.33%
19	Washington		68,000	1.88%	47	Wyoming	11,000	0.30%
35	West Virginia		29,000	0.80%	48	Alaska	10,000	0.28%
16	Wisconsin		75,000	2.08%	49	Delaware	9,000	0.25%
47	Wyoming		11,000	0.30%	50	Vermont	8,000	0.22%
						District of Columbia	9,000	0.25%

Source: U.S. Department of Health and Human Services, National Center for Health Statistics
   "Vital Statistics of the United States, 1980" and "Monthly Vital Statistics Report"
*Live births by state of residence.

Birth Rate in 1980

National Rate = 15.9 Births per 1,000 Population*

RANK	STATE	RATE	RANK	STATE	RATE
27	Alabama	16.3	1	Utah	28.6
2	Alaska	23.7	2	Alaska	23.7
11	Arizona	18.4	3	Wyoming	22.5
27	Arkansas	16.3	4	Idaho	21.4
18	California	17.0	5	New Mexico	20.0
15	Colorado	17.2	6	Louisiana	19.5
50	Connecticut	12.5	7	South Dakota	19.2
33	Delaware	15.8	7	Texas	19.2
45	Florida	13.5	9	Mississippi	19.0
19	Georgia	16.9	10	Hawaii	18.8
10	Hawaii	18.8	11	Arizona	18.4
4	Idaho	21.4	11	North Dakota	18.4
20	Illinois	16.6	13	Montana	18.1
30	Indiana	16.1	14	Nebraska	17.4
24	Iowa	16.4	15	Colorado	17.2
15	Kansas	17.2	15	Kansas	17.2
27	Kentucky	16.3	15	Oklahoma	17.2
6	Louisiana	19.5	18	California	17.0
41	Maine	14.6	19	Georgia	16.9
43	Maryland	14.2	20	Illinois	16.6
49	Massachusetts	12.7	20	Minnesota	16.6
34	Michigan	15.7	20	Nevada	16.6
20	Minnesota	16.6	20	South Carolina	16.6
9	Mississippi	19.0	24	Iowa	16.4
30	Missouri	16.1	24	Oregon	16.4
13	Montana	18.1	24	Washington	16.4
14	Nebraska	17.4	27	Alabama	16.3
20	Nevada	16.6	27	Arkansas	16.3
39	New Hampshire	14.9	27	Kentucky	16.3
47	New Jersey	13.2	30	Indiana	16.1
5	New Mexico	20.0	30	Missouri	16.1
44	New York	13.6	32	Wisconsin	15.9
42	North Carolina	14.4	33	Delaware	15.8
11	North Dakota	18.4	34	Michigan	15.7
34	Ohio	15.7	34	Ohio	15.7
15	Oklahoma	17.2	36	Vermont	15.4
24	Oregon	16.4	37	Tennessee	15.1
46	Pennsylvania	13.4	37	West Virginia	15.1
48	Rhode Island	12.9	39	New Hampshire	14.9
20	South Carolina	16.6	40	Virginia	14.7
7	South Dakota	19.2	41	Maine	14.6
37	Tennessee	15.1	42	North Carolina	14.4
7	Texas	19.2	43	Maryland	14.2
1	Utah	28.6	44	New York	13.6
36	Vermont	15.4	45	Florida	13.5
40	Virginia	14.7	46	Pennsylvania	13.4
24	Washington	16.4	47	New Jersey	13.2
37	West Virginia	15.1	48	Rhode Island	12.9
32	Wisconsin	15.9	49	Massachusetts	12.7
3	Wyoming	22.5	50	Connecticut	12.5
				District of Columbia	14.7

*Source: U.S. Department of Health and Human Services, National Center for Health Statistics
"Vital Statistics of the United States, 1980" and "Monthly Vital Statistics Report"*
Live births by state of residence.

Fertility Rate in 1995

National Rate = 65.6 Live Births per 1,000 Women 15 to 44 Years Old*

ALPHA ORDER

RANK ORDER

RANK	STATE	RATE		RANK	STATE	RATE
24	Alabama	62.5		1	Utah	86.1
6	Alaska	73.2		2	Arizona	79.4
2	Arizona	79.4		3	California	77.9
16	Arkansas	64.9		4	Texas	75.9
3	California	77.9		5	Nevada	75.2
25	Colorado	62.4		6	Alaska	73.2
28	Connecticut	62.1		7	Hawaii	72.2
32	Delaware	61.2		8	New Mexico	71.9
16	Florida	64.9		9	Idaho	70.4
15	Georgia	65.3		10	Illinois	69.2
7	Hawaii	72.2		11	South Dakota	67.2
9	Idaho	70.4		12	Louisiana	67.0
10	Illinois	69.2		13	Kansas	66.9
21	Indiana	63.3		14	Mississippi	66.6
39	Iowa	59.6		15	Georgia	65.3
13	Kansas	66.9		16	Arkansas	64.9
42	Kentucky	58.2		16	Florida	64.9
12	Louisiana	67.0		18	Oklahoma	64.6
50	Maine	49.8		19	Nebraska	64.5
38	Maryland	59.9		20	New York	64.4
47	Massachusetts	53.1		21	Indiana	63.3
34	Michigan	60.4		22	Washington	62.9
35	Minnesota	60.1		23	North Dakota	62.6
14	Mississippi	66.6		24	Alabama	62.5
25	Missouri	62.4		25	Colorado	62.4
36	Montana	60.0		25	Missouri	62.4
19	Nebraska	64.5		27	Oregon	62.2
5	Nevada	75.2		28	Connecticut	62.1
46	New Hampshire	55.0		29	North Carolina	61.9
31	New Jersey	61.3		30	Ohio	61.6
8	New Mexico	71.9		31	New Jersey	61.3
20	New York	64.4		32	Delaware	61.2
29	North Carolina	61.9		33	Tennessee	60.9
23	North Dakota	62.6		34	Michigan	60.4
30	Ohio	61.6		35	Minnesota	60.1
18	Oklahoma	64.6		36	Montana	60.0
27	Oregon	62.2		36	Wyoming	60.0
44	Pennsylvania	57.7		38	Maryland	59.9
45	Rhode Island	55.5		39	Iowa	59.6
42	South Carolina	58.2		40	Virginia	58.9
11	South Dakota	67.2		41	Wisconsin	58.8
33	Tennessee	60.9		42	Kentucky	58.2
4	Texas	75.9		42	South Carolina	58.2
1	Utah	86.1		44	Pennsylvania	57.7
49	Vermont	50.6		45	Rhode Island	55.5
40	Virginia	58.9		46	New Hampshire	55.0
22	Washington	62.9		47	Massachusetts	53.1
48	West Virginia	52.6		48	West Virginia	52.6
41	Wisconsin	58.8		49	Vermont	50.6
36	Wyoming	60.0		50	Maine	49.8
					District of Columbia	64.0

Source: U.S. Department of Health and Human Services, National Center for Health Statistics
   "Monthly Vital Statistics Report" (Vol. 45, No. 3(S)2, October 4, 1996)
*Data are preliminary estimates by state of residence.

Births to White Women in 1995

National Total = 3,105,315 Live Births to White Women*

<u>ALPHA ORDER</u>

RANK	STATE	BIRTHS	% of USA
24	Alabama	40,145	1.29%
47	Alaska	7,093	0.23%
16	Arizona	63,687	2.05%
33	Arkansas	26,979	0.87%
1	California	457,603	14.74%
21	Colorado	49,623	1.60%
26	Connecticut	38,699	1.25%
46	Delaware	7,688	0.25%
5	Florida	142,205	4.58%
11	Georgia	72,624	2.34%
50	Hawaii	4,970	0.16%
39	Idaho	17,450	0.56%
4	Illinois	142,561	4.59%
10	Indiana	74,578	2.40%
30	Iowa	34,717	1.12%
31	Kansas	33,525	1.08%
22	Kentucky	46,452	1.50%
27	Louisiana	38,319	1.23%
41	Maine	13,583	0.44%
23	Maryland	46,373	1.49%
15	Massachusetts	64,985	2.09%
8	Michigan	106,641	3.43%
19	Minnesota	56,522	1.82%
35	Mississippi	21,596	0.70%
17	Missouri	61,660	1.99%
43	Montana	9,846	0.32%
37	Nebraska	21,321	0.69%
36	Nevada	21,535	0.69%
40	New Hampshire	14,618	0.47%
9	New Jersey	83,554	2.69%
34	New Mexico	22,791	0.73%
3	New York	195,051	6.28%
12	North Carolina	71,717	2.31%
45	North Dakota	7,794	0.25%
6	Ohio	130,850	4.21%
29	Oklahoma	36,213	1.17%
25	Oregon	39,736	1.28%
7	Pennsylvania	126,690	4.08%
42	Rhode Island	11,002	0.35%
32	South Carolina	31,314	1.01%
44	South Dakota	8,707	0.28%
20	Tennessee	56,446	1.82%
2	Texas	280,089	9.02%
28	Utah	36,754	1.18%
48	Vermont	6,723	0.22%
14	Virginia	67,744	2.18%
13	Washington	68,226	2.20%
38	West Virginia	20,201	0.65%
18	Wisconsin	58,169	1.87%
49	Wyoming	5,977	0.19%

<u>RANK ORDER</u>

RANK	STATE	BIRTHS	% of USA
1	California	457,603	14.74%
2	Texas	280,089	9.02%
3	New York	195,051	6.28%
4	Illinois	142,561	4.59%
5	Florida	142,205	4.58%
6	Ohio	130,850	4.21%
7	Pennsylvania	126,690	4.08%
8	Michigan	106,641	3.43%
9	New Jersey	83,554	2.69%
10	Indiana	74,578	2.40%
11	Georgia	72,624	2.34%
12	North Carolina	71,717	2.31%
13	Washington	68,226	2.20%
14	Virginia	67,744	2.18%
15	Massachusetts	64,985	2.09%
16	Arizona	63,687	2.05%
17	Missouri	61,660	1.99%
18	Wisconsin	58,169	1.87%
19	Minnesota	56,522	1.82%
20	Tennessee	56,446	1.82%
21	Colorado	49,623	1.60%
22	Kentucky	46,452	1.50%
23	Maryland	46,373	1.49%
24	Alabama	40,145	1.29%
25	Oregon	39,736	1.28%
26	Connecticut	38,699	1.25%
27	Louisiana	38,319	1.23%
28	Utah	36,754	1.18%
29	Oklahoma	36,213	1.17%
30	Iowa	34,717	1.12%
31	Kansas	33,525	1.08%
32	South Carolina	31,314	1.01%
33	Arkansas	26,979	0.87%
34	New Mexico	22,791	0.73%
35	Mississippi	21,596	0.70%
36	Nevada	21,535	0.69%
37	Nebraska	21,321	0.69%
38	West Virginia	20,201	0.65%
39	Idaho	17,450	0.56%
40	New Hampshire	14,618	0.47%
41	Maine	13,583	0.44%
42	Rhode Island	11,002	0.35%
43	Montana	9,846	0.32%
44	South Dakota	8,707	0.28%
45	North Dakota	7,794	0.25%
46	Delaware	7,688	0.25%
47	Alaska	7,093	0.23%
48	Vermont	6,723	0.22%
49	Wyoming	5,977	0.19%
50	Hawaii	4,970	0.16%
	District of Columbia	1,967	0.06%

Source: U.S. Department of Health and Human Services, National Center for Health Statistics
   "Monthly Vital Statistics Report" (Vol. 45, No. 3(S)2, October 4, 1996)
Preliminary data by state of residence. By race of mother.

White Births as a Percent of All Births in 1995

National Percent = 79.62% of Live Births*

ALPHA ORDER

RANK	STATE	PERCENT
44	Alabama	65.88
43	Alaska	69.31
19	Arizona	88.02
36	Arkansas	76.74
31	California	81.56
11	Colorado	91.37
24	Connecticut	85.73
39	Delaware	74.95
38	Florida	75.42
46	Georgia	63.94
50	Hawaii	26.72
4	Idaho	96.88
35	Illinois	76.88
18	Indiana	88.46
6	Iowa	94.83
15	Kansas	89.06
13	Kentucky	89.90
48	Louisiana	56.84
3	Maine	97.64
45	Maryland	64.78
21	Massachusetts	86.86
32	Michigan	80.44
14	Minnesota	89.84
49	Mississippi	52.20
29	Missouri	83.19
17	Montana	88.60
10	Nebraska	91.68
23	Nevada	85.99
2	New Hampshire	98.15
34	New Jersey	76.91
26	New Mexico	84.29
40	New York	73.75
42	North Carolina	70.29
12	North Dakota	90.05
27	Ohio	84.08
33	Oklahoma	78.89
9	Oregon	92.82
28	Pennsylvania	83.65
16	Rhode Island	88.83
47	South Carolina	62.71
30	South Dakota	82.76
37	Tennessee	76.70
25	Texas	85.24
8	Utah	92.98
1	Vermont	98.26
41	Virginia	72.77
20	Washington	87.13
5	West Virginia	95.64
22	Wisconsin	86.18
7	Wyoming	94.35

RANK ORDER

RANK	STATE	PERCENT
1	Vermont	98.26
2	New Hampshire	98.15
3	Maine	97.64
4	Idaho	96.88
5	West Virginia	95.64
6	Iowa	94.83
7	Wyoming	94.35
8	Utah	92.98
9	Oregon	92.82
10	Nebraska	91.68
11	Colorado	91.37
12	North Dakota	90.05
13	Kentucky	89.90
14	Minnesota	89.84
15	Kansas	89.06
16	Rhode Island	88.83
17	Montana	88.60
18	Indiana	88.46
19	Arizona	88.02
20	Washington	87.13
21	Massachusetts	86.86
22	Wisconsin	86.18
23	Nevada	85.99
24	Connecticut	85.73
25	Texas	85.24
26	New Mexico	84.29
27	Ohio	84.08
28	Pennsylvania	83.65
29	Missouri	83.19
30	South Dakota	82.76
31	California	81.56
32	Michigan	80.44
33	Oklahoma	78.89
34	New Jersey	76.91
35	Illinois	76.88
36	Arkansas	76.74
37	Tennessee	76.70
38	Florida	75.42
39	Delaware	74.95
40	New York	73.75
41	Virginia	72.77
42	North Carolina	70.29
43	Alaska	69.31
44	Alabama	65.88
45	Maryland	64.78
46	Georgia	63.94
47	South Carolina	62.71
48	Louisiana	56.84
49	Mississippi	52.20
50	Hawaii	26.72
	District of Columbia	22.27

Source: Morgan Quitno Press using data from U.S. Dept. of Health and Human Services, Nat'l Center for Health Statistics "Monthly Vital Statistics Report" (Vol. 45, No. 3(S)2, October 4, 1996)
*Preliminary data by state of residence. By race of mother.

Births to Black Women in 1995

National Total = 598,558 Live Births to Black Women*

ALPHA ORDER

RANK	STATE	BIRTHS	% of USA
14	Alabama	20,088	3.36%
42	Alaska	433	0.07%
32	Arizona	2,233	0.37%
21	Arkansas	7,663	1.28%
3	California	40,017	6.69%
30	Colorado	2,623	0.44%
24	Connecticut	5,226	0.87%
31	Delaware	2,355	0.39%
2	Florida	42,086	7.03%
5	Georgia	38,932	6.50%
40	Hawaii	564	0.09%
45	Idaho	74	0.01%
6	Illinois	37,057	6.19%
20	Indiana	8,759	1.46%
36	Iowa	1,000	0.17%
28	Kansas	2,920	0.49%
25	Kentucky	4,768	0.80%
7	Louisiana	27,771	4.64%
46	Maine	72	0.01%
11	Maryland	22,481	3.76%
22	Massachusetts	6,580	1.10%
9	Michigan	22,897	3.83%
29	Minnesota	2,838	0.47%
15	Mississippi	19,250	3.22%
19	Missouri	11,151	1.86%
49	Montana	39	0.01%
34	Nebraska	1,219	0.20%
33	Nevada	1,918	0.32%
44	New Hampshire	91	0.02%
16	New Jersey	19,128	3.20%
41	New Mexico	511	0.09%
1	New York	55,118	9.21%
8	North Carolina	27,025	4.52%
46	North Dakota	72	0.01%
10	Ohio	22,720	3.80%
26	Oklahoma	4,523	0.76%
37	Oregon	872	0.15%
13	Pennsylvania	21,355	3.57%
38	Rhode Island	858	0.14%
17	South Carolina	18,012	3.01%
43	South Dakota	108	0.02%
18	Tennessee	16,092	2.69%
4	Texas	39,389	6.58%
35	Utah	1,049	0.18%
50	Vermont	37	0.01%
12	Virginia	21,528	3.60%
27	Washington	2,996	0.50%
39	West Virginia	804	0.13%
23	Wisconsin	6,521	1.09%
48	Wyoming	71	0.01%

RANK ORDER

RANK	STATE	BIRTHS	% of USA
1	New York	55,118	9.21%
2	Florida	42,086	7.03%
3	California	40,017	6.69%
4	Texas	39,389	6.58%
5	Georgia	38,932	6.50%
6	Illinois	37,057	6.19%
7	Louisiana	27,771	4.64%
8	North Carolina	27,025	4.52%
9	Michigan	22,897	3.83%
10	Ohio	22,720	3.80%
11	Maryland	22,481	3.76%
12	Virginia	21,528	3.60%
13	Pennsylvania	21,355	3.57%
14	Alabama	20,088	3.36%
15	Mississippi	19,250	3.22%
16	New Jersey	19,128	3.20%
17	South Carolina	18,012	3.01%
18	Tennessee	16,092	2.69%
19	Missouri	11,151	1.86%
20	Indiana	8,759	1.46%
21	Arkansas	7,663	1.28%
22	Massachusetts	6,580	1.10%
23	Wisconsin	6,521	1.09%
24	Connecticut	5,226	0.87%
25	Kentucky	4,768	0.80%
26	Oklahoma	4,523	0.76%
27	Washington	2,996	0.50%
28	Kansas	2,920	0.49%
29	Minnesota	2,838	0.47%
30	Colorado	2,623	0.44%
31	Delaware	2,355	0.39%
32	Arizona	2,233	0.37%
33	Nevada	1,918	0.32%
34	Nebraska	1,219	0.20%
35	Utah	1,049	0.18%
36	Iowa	1,000	0.17%
37	Oregon	872	0.15%
38	Rhode Island	858	0.14%
39	West Virginia	804	0.13%
40	Hawaii	564	0.09%
41	New Mexico	511	0.09%
42	Alaska	433	0.07%
43	South Dakota	108	0.02%
44	New Hampshire	91	0.02%
45	Idaho	74	0.01%
46	Maine	72	0.01%
46	North Dakota	72	0.01%
48	Wyoming	71	0.01%
49	Montana	39	0.01%
50	Vermont	37	0.01%
	District of Columbia	6,664	1.11%

Source: U.S. Department of Health and Human Services, National Center for Health Statistics
    "Monthly Vital Statistics Report" (Vol. 45, No. 3(S)2, October 4, 1996)
*Preliminary data by state of residence. By race of mother.

Black Births as a Percent of All Births in 1995

National Percent = 15.35% of Live Births*

ALPHA ORDER				RANK ORDER		
RANK	STATE	PERCENT		RANK	STATE	PERCENT
5	Alabama	32.96		1	Mississippi	46.53
34	Alaska	4.23		2	Louisiana	41.19
37	Arizona	3.09		3	South Carolina	36.07
12	Arkansas	21.80		4	Georgia	34.27
29	California	7.13		5	Alabama	32.96
32	Colorado	4.83		6	Maryland	31.40
21	Connecticut	11.58		7	North Carolina	26.49
9	Delaware	22.96		8	Virginia	23.13
10	Florida	22.32		9	Delaware	22.96
4	Georgia	34.27		10	Florida	22.32
38	Hawaii	3.03		11	Tennessee	21.87
49	Idaho	0.41		12	Arkansas	21.80
14	Illinois	19.98		13	New York	20.84
22	Indiana	10.39		14	Illinois	19.98
39	Iowa	2.73		15	New Jersey	17.61
27	Kansas	7.76		16	Michigan	17.27
25	Kentucky	9.23		17	Missouri	15.04
2	Louisiana	41.19		18	Ohio	14.60
48	Maine	0.52		19	Pennsylvania	14.10
6	Maryland	31.40		20	Texas	11.99
26	Massachusetts	8.79		21	Connecticut	11.58
16	Michigan	17.27		22	Indiana	10.39
33	Minnesota	4.51		23	Oklahoma	9.85
1	Mississippi	46.53		24	Wisconsin	9.66
17	Missouri	15.04		25	Kentucky	9.23
50	Montana	0.35		26	Massachusetts	8.79
31	Nebraska	5.24		27	Kansas	7.76
28	Nevada	7.66		28	Nevada	7.66
46	New Hampshire	0.61		29	California	7.13
15	New Jersey	17.61		30	Rhode Island	6.93
42	New Mexico	1.89		31	Nebraska	5.24
13	New York	20.84		32	Colorado	4.83
7	North Carolina	26.49		33	Minnesota	4.51
45	North Dakota	0.83		34	Alaska	4.23
18	Ohio	14.60		35	Washington	3.83
23	Oklahoma	9.85		36	West Virginia	3.81
41	Oregon	2.04		37	Arizona	3.09
19	Pennsylvania	14.10		38	Hawaii	3.03
30	Rhode Island	6.93		39	Iowa	2.73
3	South Carolina	36.07		40	Utah	2.65
44	South Dakota	1.03		41	Oregon	2.04
11	Tennessee	21.87		42	New Mexico	1.89
20	Texas	11.99		43	Wyoming	1.12
40	Utah	2.65		44	South Dakota	1.03
47	Vermont	0.54		45	North Dakota	0.83
8	Virginia	23.13		46	New Hampshire	0.61
35	Washington	3.83		47	Vermont	0.54
36	West Virginia	3.81		48	Maine	0.52
24	Wisconsin	9.66		49	Idaho	0.41
43	Wyoming	1.12		50	Montana	0.35
					District of Columbia	75.46

Source: Morgan Quitno Press using data from U.S. Dept. of Health and Human Services, Nat'l Center for Health Statistics
"Monthly Vital Statistics Report" (Vol. 45, No. 3(S)2, October 4, 1996)
*Preliminary data by state of residence. By race of mother.

Births of Low Birthweight in 1995

National Total = 284,706 Live Births*

ALPHA ORDER

RANK	STATE	BIRTHS	% of USA
18	Alabama	5,485	1.93%
47	Alaska	553	0.19%
19	Arizona	4,920	1.73%
30	Arkansas	2,883	1.01%
1	California	33,665	11.82%
21	Colorado	4,562	1.60%
29	Connecticut	3,115	1.09%
42	Delaware	862	0.30%
4	Florida	14,518	5.10%
9	Georgia	9,882	3.47%
39	Hawaii	1,302	0.46%
40	Idaho	1,063	0.37%
5	Illinois	14,463	5.08%
15	Indiana	6,323	2.22%
34	Iowa	2,197	0.77%
32	Kansas	2,409	0.85%
26	Kentucky	3,927	1.38%
13	Louisiana	6,405	2.25%
41	Maine	876	0.31%
16	Maryland	6,085	2.14%
22	Massachusetts	4,489	1.58%
8	Michigan	9,943	3.49%
27	Minnesota	3,586	1.26%
24	Mississippi	4,054	1.42%
17	Missouri	5,633	1.98%
45	Montana	645	0.23%
38	Nebraska	1,488	0.52%
36	Nevada	1,853	0.65%
44	New Hampshire	789	0.28%
11	New Jersey	8,039	2.82%
35	New Mexico	2,028	0.71%
3	New York	20,099	7.06%
10	North Carolina	8,877	3.12%
49	North Dakota	450	0.16%
6	Ohio	11,672	4.10%
28	Oklahoma	3,168	1.11%
33	Oregon	2,355	0.83%
7	Pennsylvania	11,207	3.94%
43	Rhode Island	830	0.29%
20	South Carolina	4,644	1.63%
46	South Dakota	579	0.20%
14	Tennessee	6,329	2.22%
2	Texas	23,330	8.19%
31	Utah	2,490	0.87%
50	Vermont	369	0.13%
12	Virginia	7,075	2.49%
23	Washington	4,307	1.51%
37	West Virginia	1,669	0.59%
25	Wisconsin	4,050	1.42%
48	Wyoming	469	0.16%

RANK ORDER

RANK	STATE	BIRTHS	% of USA
1	California	33,665	11.82%
2	Texas	23,330	8.19%
3	New York	20,099	7.06%
4	Florida	14,518	5.10%
5	Illinois	14,463	5.08%
6	Ohio	11,672	4.10%
7	Pennsylvania	11,207	3.94%
8	Michigan	9,943	3.49%
9	Georgia	9,882	3.47%
10	North Carolina	8,877	3.12%
11	New Jersey	8,039	2.82%
12	Virginia	7,075	2.49%
13	Louisiana	6,405	2.25%
14	Tennessee	6,329	2.22%
15	Indiana	6,323	2.22%
16	Maryland	6,085	2.14%
17	Missouri	5,633	1.98%
18	Alabama	5,485	1.93%
19	Arizona	4,920	1.73%
20	South Carolina	4,644	1.63%
21	Colorado	4,562	1.60%
22	Massachusetts	4,489	1.58%
23	Washington	4,307	1.51%
24	Mississippi	4,054	1.42%
25	Wisconsin	4,050	1.42%
26	Kentucky	3,927	1.38%
27	Minnesota	3,586	1.26%
28	Oklahoma	3,168	1.11%
29	Connecticut	3,115	1.09%
30	Arkansas	2,883	1.01%
31	Utah	2,490	0.87%
32	Kansas	2,409	0.85%
33	Oregon	2,355	0.83%
34	Iowa	2,197	0.77%
35	New Mexico	2,028	0.71%
36	Nevada	1,853	0.65%
37	West Virginia	1,669	0.59%
38	Nebraska	1,488	0.52%
39	Hawaii	1,302	0.46%
40	Idaho	1,063	0.37%
41	Maine	876	0.31%
42	Delaware	862	0.30%
43	Rhode Island	830	0.29%
44	New Hampshire	789	0.28%
45	Montana	645	0.23%
46	South Dakota	579	0.20%
47	Alaska	553	0.19%
48	Wyoming	469	0.16%
49	North Dakota	450	0.16%
50	Vermont	369	0.13%
	District of Columbia	1,166	0.41%

Source: Morgan Quitno Press using data from U.S. Dept. of Health & Human Services, Nat'l Center for Health Statistics "Monthly Vital Statistics Report" (Vol. 45, No. 3(S)2, October 4, 1996)

*Preliminary data by state of residence. Births of less than 2,500 grams (5 pounds 8 ounces).

Births of Low Birthweight as a Percent of All Births in 1995

National Percent = 7.3% of Live Births*

ALPHA ORDER

RANK ORDER

RANK	STATE	PERCENT	RANK	STATE	PERCENT
4	Alabama	9.0	1	Mississippi	9.8
47	Alaska	5.4	2	Louisiana	9.5
31	Arizona	6.8	3	South Carolina	9.3
11	Arkansas	8.2	4	Alabama	9.0
37	California	6.0	5	Georgia	8.7
9	Colorado	8.4	5	North Carolina	8.7
29	Connecticut	6.9	7	Tennessee	8.6
9	Delaware	8.4	8	Maryland	8.5
14	Florida	7.7	9	Colorado	8.4
5	Georgia	8.7	9	Delaware	8.4
28	Hawaii	7.0	11	Arkansas	8.2
41	Idaho	5.9	12	West Virginia	7.9
13	Illinois	7.8	13	Illinois	7.8
19	Indiana	7.5	14	Florida	7.7
37	Iowa	6.0	15	Kentucky	7.6
33	Kansas	6.4	15	Missouri	7.6
15	Kentucky	7.6	15	New York	7.6
2	Louisiana	9.5	15	Virginia	7.6
35	Maine	6.3	19	Indiana	7.5
8	Maryland	8.5	19	Michigan	7.5
37	Massachusetts	6.0	19	New Mexico	7.5
19	Michigan	7.5	19	Ohio	7.5
43	Minnesota	5.7	23	Nevada	7.4
1	Mississippi	9.8	23	New Jersey	7.4
15	Missouri	7.6	23	Pennsylvania	7.4
42	Montana	5.8	23	Wyoming	7.4
33	Nebraska	6.4	27	Texas	7.1
23	Nevada	7.4	28	Hawaii	7.0
49	New Hampshire	5.3	29	Connecticut	6.9
23	New Jersey	7.4	29	Oklahoma	6.9
19	New Mexico	7.5	31	Arizona	6.8
15	New York	7.6	32	Rhode Island	6.7
5	North Carolina	8.7	33	Kansas	6.4
50	North Dakota	5.2	33	Nebraska	6.4
19	Ohio	7.5	35	Maine	6.3
29	Oklahoma	6.9	35	Utah	6.3
44	Oregon	5.5	37	California	6.0
23	Pennsylvania	7.4	37	Iowa	6.0
32	Rhode Island	6.7	37	Massachusetts	6.0
3	South Carolina	9.3	37	Wisconsin	6.0
44	South Dakota	5.5	41	Idaho	5.9
7	Tennessee	8.6	42	Montana	5.8
27	Texas	7.1	43	Minnesota	5.7
35	Utah	6.3	44	Oregon	5.5
47	Vermont	5.4	44	South Dakota	5.5
15	Virginia	7.6	44	Washington	5.5
44	Washington	5.5	47	Alaska	5.4
12	West Virginia	7.9	47	Vermont	5.4
37	Wisconsin	6.0	49	New Hampshire	5.3
23	Wyoming	7.4	50	North Dakota	5.2
				District of Columbia	13.2

Source: U.S. Department of Health and Human Services, National Center for Health Statistics
"Monthly Vital Statistics Report" (Vol. 45, No. 3(S)2, October 4, 1996)
*Preliminary data by state of residence. Births of less than 2,500 grams (5 pounds 8 ounces).

Births of Low Birthweight to White Women in 1995

National Total = 192,529 Live Births*

ALPHA ORDER

RANK ORDER

RANK	STATE	BIRTHS	% of USA
23	Alabama	2,850	1.48%
47	Alaska	362	0.19%
14	Arizona	4,203	2.18%
31	Arkansas	1,835	0.95%
1	California	25,168	13.07%
18	Colorado	3,970	2.06%
50	Connecticut	39	0.02%
42	Delaware	538	0.28%
4	Florida	9,101	4.73%
12	Georgia	4,721	2.45%
48	Hawaii	263	0.14%
37	Idaho	1,012	0.53%
5	Illinois	8,696	4.52%
10	Indiana	5,071	2.63%
29	Iowa	2,014	1.05%
30	Kansas	1,978	1.03%
20	Kentucky	3,298	1.71%
24	Louisiana	2,529	1.31%
38	Maine	842	0.44%
49	Maryland	46	0.02%
13	Massachusetts	4,224	2.19%
8	Michigan	6,612	3.43%
21	Minnesota	3,052	1.59%
34	Mississippi	1,490	0.77%
17	Missouri	4,008	2.08%
41	Montana	581	0.30%
36	Nebraska	1,301	0.68%
35	Nevada	1,443	0.75%
39	New Hampshire	775	0.40%
9	New Jersey	5,097	2.65%
32	New Mexico	1,755	0.91%
3	New York	12,288	6.38%
11	North Carolina	4,877	2.53%
45	North Dakota	397	0.21%
6	Ohio	8,374	4.35%
25	Oklahoma	2,318	1.20%
27	Oregon	2,146	1.11%
7	Pennsylvania	7,855	4.08%
40	Rhode Island	693	0.36%
28	South Carolina	2,129	1.11%
43	South Dakota	479	0.25%
16	Tennessee	4,064	2.11%
2	Texas	17,646	9.17%
26	Utah	2,279	1.18%
46	Vermont	370	0.19%
15	Virginia	4,132	2.15%
19	Washington	3,548	1.84%
33	West Virginia	1,535	0.80%
22	Wisconsin	2,967	1.54%
44	Wyoming	436	0.23%

RANK	STATE	BIRTHS	% of USA
1	California	25,168	13.07%
2	Texas	17,646	9.17%
3	New York	12,288	6.38%
4	Florida	9,101	4.73%
5	Illinois	8,696	4.52%
6	Ohio	8,374	4.35%
7	Pennsylvania	7,855	4.08%
8	Michigan	6,612	3.43%
9	New Jersey	5,097	2.65%
10	Indiana	5,071	2.63%
11	North Carolina	4,877	2.53%
12	Georgia	4,721	2.45%
13	Massachusetts	4,224	2.19%
14	Arizona	4,203	2.18%
15	Virginia	4,132	2.15%
16	Tennessee	4,064	2.11%
17	Missouri	4,008	2.08%
18	Colorado	3,970	2.06%
19	Washington	3,548	1.84%
20	Kentucky	3,298	1.71%
21	Minnesota	3,052	1.59%
22	Wisconsin	2,967	1.54%
23	Alabama	2,850	1.48%
24	Louisiana	2,529	1.31%
25	Oklahoma	2,318	1.20%
26	Utah	2,279	1.18%
27	Oregon	2,146	1.11%
28	South Carolina	2,129	1.11%
29	Iowa	2,014	1.05%
30	Kansas	1,978	1.03%
31	Arkansas	1,835	0.95%
32	New Mexico	1,755	0.91%
33	West Virginia	1,535	0.80%
34	Mississippi	1,490	0.77%
35	Nevada	1,443	0.75%
36	Nebraska	1,301	0.68%
37	Idaho	1,012	0.53%
38	Maine	842	0.44%
39	New Hampshire	775	0.40%
40	Rhode Island	693	0.36%
41	Montana	581	0.30%
42	Delaware	538	0.28%
43	South Dakota	479	0.25%
44	Wyoming	436	0.23%
45	North Dakota	397	0.21%
46	Vermont	370	0.19%
47	Alaska	362	0.19%
48	Hawaii	263	0.14%
49	Maryland	46	0.02%
50	Connecticut	39	0.02%
	District of Columbia	116	0.06%

Source: Morgan Quitno Press using data from U.S. Dept. of Health and Human Services, Nat'l Center for Health Statistics "Monthly Vital Statistics Report" (Vol. 45, No. 3(S)2, October 4, 1996)

*Preliminary data by state of residence. Births of less than 2,500 grams (5 pounds 8 ounces). Calculated by the editors by multiplying total number of births to white women by percent of such births reported as being of low birthweight.

Births of Low Birthweight to White Women
As a Percent of All Births to White Women in 1995
National Percent = 6.2% of Live Births to White Women*

ALPHA ORDER

RANK	STATE	PERCENT
6	Alabama	7.1
48	Alaska	5.1
15	Arizona	6.6
10	Arkansas	6.8
39	California	5.5
1	Colorado	8.0
29	Connecticut	6.1
8	Delaware	7.0
19	Florida	6.4
17	Georgia	6.5
45	Hawaii	5.3
37	Idaho	5.8
29	Illinois	6.1
10	Indiana	6.8
37	Iowa	5.8
35	Kansas	5.9
6	Kentucky	7.1
15	Louisiana	6.6
25	Maine	6.2
29	Maryland	6.1
39	Massachusetts	5.5
25	Michigan	6.2
43	Minnesota	5.4
9	Mississippi	6.9
17	Missouri	6.5
35	Montana	5.9
29	Nebraska	6.1
14	Nevada	6.7
45	New Hampshire	5.3
29	New Jersey	6.1
2	New Mexico	7.7
22	New York	6.3
10	North Carolina	6.8
48	North Dakota	5.1
19	Ohio	6.4
19	Oklahoma	6.4
43	Oregon	5.4
25	Pennsylvania	6.2
22	Rhode Island	6.3
10	South Carolina	6.8
39	South Dakota	5.5
5	Tennessee	7.2
22	Texas	6.3
25	Utah	6.2
39	Vermont	5.5
29	Virginia	6.1
47	Washington	5.2
3	West Virginia	7.6
48	Wisconsin	5.1
4	Wyoming	7.3

RANK ORDER

RANK	STATE	PERCENT
1	Colorado	8.0
2	New Mexico	7.7
3	West Virginia	7.6
4	Wyoming	7.3
5	Tennessee	7.2
6	Alabama	7.1
6	Kentucky	7.1
8	Delaware	7.0
9	Mississippi	6.9
10	Arkansas	6.8
10	Indiana	6.8
10	North Carolina	6.8
10	South Carolina	6.8
14	Nevada	6.7
15	Arizona	6.6
15	Louisiana	6.6
17	Georgia	6.5
17	Missouri	6.5
19	Florida	6.4
19	Ohio	6.4
19	Oklahoma	6.4
22	New York	6.3
22	Rhode Island	6.3
22	Texas	6.3
25	Maine	6.2
25	Michigan	6.2
25	Pennsylvania	6.2
25	Utah	6.2
29	Connecticut	6.1
29	Illinois	6.1
29	Maryland	6.1
29	Nebraska	6.1
29	New Jersey	6.1
29	Virginia	6.1
35	Kansas	5.9
35	Montana	5.9
37	Idaho	5.8
37	Iowa	5.8
39	California	5.5
39	Massachusetts	5.5
39	South Dakota	5.5
39	Vermont	5.5
43	Minnesota	5.4
43	Oregon	5.4
45	Hawaii	5.3
45	New Hampshire	5.3
47	Washington	5.2
48	Alaska	5.1
48	North Dakota	5.1
48	Wisconsin	5.1
	District of Columbia	5.9

Source: U.S. Department of Health and Human Services, National Center for Health Statistics
"Monthly Vital Statistics Report" (Vol. 45, No. 3(S)2, October 4, 1996)
*Preliminary data by state of residence. Births of less than 2,500 grams (5 pounds 8 ounces).

Births of Low Birthweight to Black Women in 1995

National Total = 77,813 Live Births*

RANK	STATE	BIRTHS	% of USA
14	Alabama	2,611	3.36%
42	Alaska	53	0.07%
32	Arizona	295	0.38%
21	Arkansas	1,004	1.29%
6	California	4,722	6.07%
27	Colorado	414	0.53%
24	Connecticut	638	0.82%
31	Delaware	301	0.39%
3	Florida	5,092	6.54%
4	Georgia	5,061	6.50%
40	Hawaii	63	0.08%
NA	Idaho**	NA	NA
2	Illinois	5,336	6.86%
20	Indiana	1,130	1.45%
36	Iowa	111	0.14%
28	Kansas	356	0.46%
25	Kentucky	625	0.80%
7	Louisiana	3,832	4.92%
NA	Maine**	NA	NA
12	Maryland	3,012	3.87%
23	Massachusetts	691	0.89%
9	Michigan	3,160	4.06%
29	Minnesota	341	0.44%
15	Mississippi	2,503	3.22%
19	Missouri	1,561	2.01%
NA	Montana**	NA	NA
34	Nebraska	146	0.19%
33	Nevada	261	0.34%
NA	New Hampshire**	NA	NA
17	New Jersey	2,448	3.15%
41	New Mexico	54	0.07%
1	New York	6,835	8.78%
8	North Carolina	3,729	4.79%
NA	North Dakota**	NA	NA
10	Ohio	3,158	4.06%
26	Oklahoma	565	0.73%
38	Oregon	90	0.12%
11	Pennsylvania	3,032	3.90%
37	Rhode Island	97	0.12%
16	South Carolina	2,468	3.17%
NA	South Dakota**	NA	NA
18	Tennessee	2,221	2.85%
5	Texas	4,766	6.12%
39	Utah	71	0.09%
NA	Vermont**	NA	NA
13	Virginia	2,756	3.54%
30	Washington	333	0.43%
35	West Virginia	132	0.17%
22	Wisconsin	893	1.15%
NA	Wyoming**	NA	NA

RANK	STATE	BIRTHS	% of USA
1	New York	6,835	8.78%
2	Illinois	5,336	6.86%
3	Florida	5,092	6.54%
4	Georgia	5,061	6.50%
5	Texas	4,766	6.12%
6	California	4,722	6.07%
7	Louisiana	3,832	4.92%
8	North Carolina	3,729	4.79%
9	Michigan	3,160	4.06%
10	Ohio	3,158	4.06%
11	Pennsylvania	3,032	3.90%
12	Maryland	3,012	3.87%
13	Virginia	2,756	3.54%
14	Alabama	2,611	3.36%
15	Mississippi	2,503	3.22%
16	South Carolina	2,468	3.17%
17	New Jersey	2,448	3.15%
18	Tennessee	2,221	2.85%
19	Missouri	1,561	2.01%
20	Indiana	1,130	1.45%
21	Arkansas	1,004	1.29%
22	Wisconsin	893	1.15%
23	Massachusetts	691	0.89%
24	Connecticut	638	0.82%
25	Kentucky	625	0.80%
26	Oklahoma	565	0.73%
27	Colorado	414	0.53%
28	Kansas	356	0.46%
29	Minnesota	341	0.44%
30	Washington	333	0.43%
31	Delaware	301	0.39%
32	Arizona	295	0.38%
33	Nevada	261	0.34%
34	Nebraska	146	0.19%
35	West Virginia	132	0.17%
36	Iowa	111	0.14%
37	Rhode Island	97	0.12%
38	Oregon	90	0.12%
39	Utah	71	0.09%
40	Hawaii	63	0.08%
41	New Mexico	54	0.07%
42	Alaska	53	0.07%
NA	Idaho**	NA	NA
NA	Maine**	NA	NA
NA	Montana**	NA	NA
NA	New Hampshire**	NA	NA
NA	North Dakota**	NA	NA
NA	South Dakota**	NA	NA
NA	Vermont**	NA	NA
NA	Wyoming**	NA	NA
	District of Columbia	1,033	1.33%

Source: Morgan Quitno Press using data from U.S. Dept. of Health and Human Services, Nat'l Center for Health Statistics "Monthly Vital Statistics Report" (Vol. 45, No. 3(S)2, October 4, 1996)

*Preliminary data by state of residence. Births of less than 2,500 grams (5 pounds 8 ounces). Calculated by the editors by multiplying total number of births to black women by percent of such births reported as being of low birthweight.

**Not available.

Births of Low Birthweight to Black Women
As a Percent of All Births to Black Women in 1995
National Percent = 13.0% of Live Births to Black Women*

<table>
<tr><td colspan="3">ALPHA ORDER</td><td colspan="3">RANK ORDER</td></tr>
<tr><td>RANK</td><td>STATE</td><td>PERCENT</td><td>RANK</td><td>STATE</td><td>PERCENT</td></tr>
<tr><td>18</td><td>Alabama</td><td>13.0</td><td>1</td><td>West Virginia</td><td>16.4</td></tr>
<tr><td>27</td><td>Alaska</td><td>12.3</td><td>2</td><td>Colorado</td><td>15.8</td></tr>
<tr><td>15</td><td>Arizona</td><td>13.2</td><td>3</td><td>Illinois</td><td>14.4</td></tr>
<tr><td>16</td><td>Arkansas</td><td>13.1</td><td>4</td><td>Pennsylvania</td><td>14.2</td></tr>
<tr><td>34</td><td>California</td><td>11.8</td><td>5</td><td>Missouri</td><td>14.0</td></tr>
<tr><td>2</td><td>Colorado</td><td>15.8</td><td>6</td><td>Ohio</td><td>13.9</td></tr>
<tr><td>28</td><td>Connecticut</td><td>12.2</td><td>7</td><td>Louisiana</td><td>13.8</td></tr>
<tr><td>22</td><td>Delaware</td><td>12.8</td><td>7</td><td>Michigan</td><td>13.8</td></tr>
<tr><td>30</td><td>Florida</td><td>12.1</td><td>7</td><td>North Carolina</td><td>13.8</td></tr>
<tr><td>18</td><td>Georgia</td><td>13.0</td><td>7</td><td>Tennessee</td><td>13.8</td></tr>
<tr><td>36</td><td>Hawaii</td><td>11.1</td><td>11</td><td>South Carolina</td><td>13.7</td></tr>
<tr><td>NA</td><td>Idaho**</td><td>NA</td><td>11</td><td>Wisconsin</td><td>13.7</td></tr>
<tr><td>3</td><td>Illinois</td><td>14.4</td><td>13</td><td>Nevada</td><td>13.6</td></tr>
<tr><td>21</td><td>Indiana</td><td>12.9</td><td>14</td><td>Maryland</td><td>13.4</td></tr>
<tr><td>36</td><td>Iowa</td><td>11.1</td><td>15</td><td>Arizona</td><td>13.2</td></tr>
<tr><td>28</td><td>Kansas</td><td>12.2</td><td>16</td><td>Arkansas</td><td>13.1</td></tr>
<tr><td>16</td><td>Kentucky</td><td>13.1</td><td>16</td><td>Kentucky</td><td>13.1</td></tr>
<tr><td>7</td><td>Louisiana</td><td>13.8</td><td>18</td><td>Alabama</td><td>13.0</td></tr>
<tr><td>NA</td><td>Maine**</td><td>NA</td><td>18</td><td>Georgia</td><td>13.0</td></tr>
<tr><td>14</td><td>Maryland</td><td>13.4</td><td>18</td><td>Mississippi</td><td>13.0</td></tr>
<tr><td>39</td><td>Massachusetts</td><td>10.5</td><td>21</td><td>Indiana</td><td>12.9</td></tr>
<tr><td>7</td><td>Michigan</td><td>13.8</td><td>22</td><td>Delaware</td><td>12.8</td></tr>
<tr><td>32</td><td>Minnesota</td><td>12.0</td><td>22</td><td>New Jersey</td><td>12.8</td></tr>
<tr><td>18</td><td>Mississippi</td><td>13.0</td><td>22</td><td>Virginia</td><td>12.8</td></tr>
<tr><td>5</td><td>Missouri</td><td>14.0</td><td>25</td><td>Oklahoma</td><td>12.5</td></tr>
<tr><td>NA</td><td>Montana**</td><td>NA</td><td>26</td><td>New York</td><td>12.4</td></tr>
<tr><td>32</td><td>Nebraska</td><td>12.0</td><td>27</td><td>Alaska</td><td>12.3</td></tr>
<tr><td>13</td><td>Nevada</td><td>13.6</td><td>28</td><td>Connecticut</td><td>12.2</td></tr>
<tr><td>NA</td><td>New Hampshire**</td><td>NA</td><td>28</td><td>Kansas</td><td>12.2</td></tr>
<tr><td>22</td><td>New Jersey</td><td>12.8</td><td>30</td><td>Florida</td><td>12.1</td></tr>
<tr><td>39</td><td>New Mexico</td><td>10.5</td><td>30</td><td>Texas</td><td>12.1</td></tr>
<tr><td>26</td><td>New York</td><td>12.4</td><td>32</td><td>Minnesota</td><td>12.0</td></tr>
<tr><td>7</td><td>North Carolina</td><td>13.8</td><td>32</td><td>Nebraska</td><td>12.0</td></tr>
<tr><td>NA</td><td>North Dakota**</td><td>NA</td><td>34</td><td>California</td><td>11.8</td></tr>
<tr><td>6</td><td>Ohio</td><td>13.9</td><td>35</td><td>Rhode Island</td><td>11.3</td></tr>
<tr><td>25</td><td>Oklahoma</td><td>12.5</td><td>36</td><td>Hawaii</td><td>11.1</td></tr>
<tr><td>41</td><td>Oregon</td><td>10.3</td><td>36</td><td>Iowa</td><td>11.1</td></tr>
<tr><td>4</td><td>Pennsylvania</td><td>14.2</td><td>36</td><td>Washington</td><td>11.1</td></tr>
<tr><td>35</td><td>Rhode Island</td><td>11.3</td><td>39</td><td>Massachusetts</td><td>10.5</td></tr>
<tr><td>11</td><td>South Carolina</td><td>13.7</td><td>39</td><td>New Mexico</td><td>10.5</td></tr>
<tr><td>NA</td><td>South Dakota**</td><td>NA</td><td>41</td><td>Oregon</td><td>10.3</td></tr>
<tr><td>7</td><td>Tennessee</td><td>13.8</td><td>42</td><td>Utah</td><td>6.8</td></tr>
<tr><td>30</td><td>Texas</td><td>12.1</td><td>NA</td><td>Idaho**</td><td>NA</td></tr>
<tr><td>42</td><td>Utah</td><td>6.8</td><td>NA</td><td>Maine**</td><td>NA</td></tr>
<tr><td>NA</td><td>Vermont**</td><td>NA</td><td>NA</td><td>Montana**</td><td>NA</td></tr>
<tr><td>22</td><td>Virginia</td><td>12.8</td><td>NA</td><td>New Hampshire**</td><td>NA</td></tr>
<tr><td>36</td><td>Washington</td><td>11.1</td><td>NA</td><td>North Dakota**</td><td>NA</td></tr>
<tr><td>1</td><td>West Virginia</td><td>16.4</td><td>NA</td><td>South Dakota**</td><td>NA</td></tr>
<tr><td>11</td><td>Wisconsin</td><td>13.7</td><td>NA</td><td>Vermont**</td><td>NA</td></tr>
<tr><td>NA</td><td>Wyoming**</td><td>NA</td><td>NA</td><td>Wyoming**</td><td>NA</td></tr>
<tr><td></td><td></td><td></td><td></td><td>District of Columbia</td><td>15.5</td></tr>
</table>

Source: U.S. Department of Health and Human Services, National Center for Health Statistics
"Monthly Vital Statistics Report" (Vol. 45, No. 3(S)2, October 4, 1996)
*Preliminary data by state of residence. Births of less than 2,500 grams (5 pounds 8 ounces).
**Insufficient data.

Births to Unmarried Women in 1995

National Total = 1,248,028 Live Births*

ALPHA ORDER

RANK	STATE	BIRTHS	% of USA
18	Alabama	21,024	1.68%
44	Alaska	3,060	0.25%
12	Arizona	27,640	2.21%
30	Arkansas	11,566	0.93%
1	California	178,988	14.34%
27	Colorado	13,523	1.08%
28	Connecticut	13,497	1.08%
41	Delaware	3,590	0.29%
4	Florida	67,498	5.41%
8	Georgia	39,983	3.20%
38	Hawaii	5,431	0.44%
42	Idaho	3,584	0.29%
5	Illinois	62,303	4.99%
14	Indiana	26,724	2.14%
34	Iowa	9,226	0.74%
33	Kansas	9,938	0.80%
25	Kentucky	14,778	1.18%
11	Louisiana	28,721	2.30%
39	Maine	3,867	0.31%
16	Maryland	23,909	1.92%
20	Massachusetts	19,153	1.53%
NA	Michigan**	NA	NA
24	Minnesota	14,910	1.19%
21	Mississippi	18,740	1.50%
17	Missouri	23,719	1.90%
46	Montana	2,923	0.23%
37	Nebraska	5,651	0.45%
32	Nevada	10,518	0.84%
43	New Hampshire	3,336	0.27%
10	New Jersey	29,332	2.35%
31	New Mexico	11,518	0.92%
2	New York	100,230	8.03%
9	North Carolina	32,037	2.57%
47	North Dakota	2,034	0.16%
6	Ohio	51,203	4.10%
26	Oklahoma	13,955	1.12%
29	Oregon	12,372	0.99%
7	Pennsylvania	48,918	3.92%
40	Rhode Island	3,617	0.29%
22	South Carolina	18,626	1.49%
45	South Dakota	2,988	0.24%
15	Tennessee	24,140	1.93%
3	Texas	98,576	7.90%
36	Utah	6,206	0.50%
48	Vermont	1,697	0.14%
13	Virginia	27,183	2.18%
19	Washington	20,907	1.68%
35	West Virginia	6,443	0.52%
23	Wisconsin	18,427	1.48%
49	Wyoming	1,679	0.13%

RANK ORDER

RANK	STATE	BIRTHS	% of USA
1	California	178,988	14.34%
2	New York	100,230	8.03%
3	Texas	98,576	7.90%
4	Florida	67,498	5.41%
5	Illinois	62,303	4.99%
6	Ohio	51,203	4.10%
7	Pennsylvania	48,918	3.92%
8	Georgia	39,983	3.20%
9	North Carolina	32,037	2.57%
10	New Jersey	29,332	2.35%
11	Louisiana	28,721	2.30%
12	Arizona	27,640	2.21%
13	Virginia	27,183	2.18%
14	Indiana	26,724	2.14%
15	Tennessee	24,140	1.93%
16	Maryland	23,909	1.92%
17	Missouri	23,719	1.90%
18	Alabama	21,024	1.68%
19	Washington	20,907	1.68%
20	Massachusetts	19,153	1.53%
21	Mississippi	18,740	1.50%
22	South Carolina	18,626	1.49%
23	Wisconsin	18,427	1.48%
24	Minnesota	14,910	1.19%
25	Kentucky	14,778	1.18%
26	Oklahoma	13,955	1.12%
27	Colorado	13,523	1.08%
28	Connecticut	13,497	1.08%
29	Oregon	12,372	0.99%
30	Arkansas	11,566	0.93%
31	New Mexico	11,518	0.92%
32	Nevada	10,518	0.84%
33	Kansas	9,938	0.80%
34	Iowa	9,226	0.74%
35	West Virginia	6,443	0.52%
36	Utah	6,206	0.50%
37	Nebraska	5,651	0.45%
38	Hawaii	5,431	0.44%
39	Maine	3,867	0.31%
40	Rhode Island	3,617	0.29%
41	Delaware	3,590	0.29%
42	Idaho	3,584	0.29%
43	New Hampshire	3,336	0.27%
44	Alaska	3,060	0.25%
45	South Dakota	2,988	0.24%
46	Montana	2,923	0.23%
47	North Dakota	2,034	0.16%
48	Vermont	1,697	0.14%
49	Wyoming	1,679	0.13%
NA	Michigan**	NA	NA
	District of Columbia	5,828	0.47%

Source: Morgan Quitno Press using data from U.S. Dept. of Health and Human Services, Nat'l Center for Health Statistics "Monthly Vital Statistics Report" (Vol. 45, No. 3(S)2, October 4, 1996)
*Preliminary data by state of residence. Calculated by the editors by multiplying total number of births by reported percent of births to unmarried women.
**Not available.

Births to Unmarried Women as a Percent of All Births in 1995

National Percent = 32.0% of Live Births*

ALPHA ORDER			RANK ORDER		
RANK	STATE	PERCENT	RANK	STATE	PERCENT
11	Alabama	34.5	1	Mississippi	45.3
25	Alaska	29.9	2	Louisiana	42.6
5	Arizona	38.2	2	New Mexico	42.6
14	Arkansas	32.9	4	Nevada	42.0
19	California	31.9	5	Arizona	38.2
42	Colorado	24.9	6	New York	37.9
25	Connecticut	29.9	7	South Carolina	37.3
10	Delaware	35.0	8	Florida	35.8
8	Florida	35.8	9	Georgia	35.2
9	Georgia	35.2	10	Delaware	35.0
27	Hawaii	29.2	11	Alabama	34.5
48	Idaho	19.9	12	Illinois	33.6
12	Illinois	33.6	13	Maryland	33.4
20	Indiana	31.7	14	Arkansas	32.9
41	Iowa	25.2	14	Ohio	32.9
38	Kansas	26.4	16	Tennessee	32.8
31	Kentucky	28.6	17	Pennsylvania	32.3
2	Louisiana	42.6	18	Missouri	32.0
33	Maine	27.8	19	California	31.9
13	Maryland	33.4	20	Indiana	31.7
40	Massachusetts	25.6	21	North Carolina	31.4
NA	Michigan**	NA	22	West Virginia	30.5
45	Minnesota	23.7	23	Oklahoma	30.4
1	Mississippi	45.3	24	Texas	30.0
18	Missouri	32.0	25	Alaska	29.9
39	Montana	26.3	25	Connecticut	29.9
44	Nebraska	24.3	27	Hawaii	29.2
4	Nevada	42.0	27	Rhode Island	29.2
47	New Hampshire	22.4	27	Virginia	29.2
35	New Jersey	27.0	30	Oregon	28.9
2	New Mexico	42.6	31	Kentucky	28.6
6	New York	37.9	32	South Dakota	28.4
21	North Carolina	31.4	33	Maine	27.8
46	North Dakota	23.5	34	Wisconsin	27.3
14	Ohio	32.9	35	New Jersey	27.0
23	Oklahoma	30.4	36	Washington	26.7
30	Oregon	28.9	37	Wyoming	26.5
17	Pennsylvania	32.3	38	Kansas	26.4
27	Rhode Island	29.2	39	Montana	26.3
7	South Carolina	37.3	40	Massachusetts	25.6
32	South Dakota	28.4	41	Iowa	25.2
16	Tennessee	32.8	42	Colorado	24.9
24	Texas	30.0	43	Vermont	24.8
49	Utah	15.7	44	Nebraska	24.3
43	Vermont	24.8	45	Minnesota	23.7
27	Virginia	29.2	46	North Dakota	23.5
36	Washington	26.7	47	New Hampshire	22.4
22	West Virginia	30.5	48	Idaho	19.9
34	Wisconsin	27.3	49	Utah	15.7
37	Wyoming	26.5	NA	Michigan**	NA
			District of Columbia		66.0

Source: U.S. Department of Health and Human Services, National Center for Health Statistics
"Monthly Vital Statistics Report" (Vol. 45, No. 3(S)2, October 4, 1996)
*Data are preliminary estimates by state of residence.
**Not available.

Births to Unmarried White Women in 1995

National Total = 785,645 Live Births*

ALPHA ORDER

RANK	STATE	BIRTHS	% of USA
31	Alabama	6,664	0.85%
47	Alaska	1,525	0.19%
8	Arizona	22,545	2.87%
34	Arkansas	5,774	0.73%
1	California	144,603	18.41%
19	Colorado	11,562	1.47%
23	Connecticut	9,443	1.20%
43	Delaware	1,860	0.24%
4	Florida	37,827	4.81%
14	Georgia	13,435	1.71%
49	Hawaii	815	0.10%
39	Idaho	3,385	0.43%
6	Illinois	32,789	4.17%
9	Indiana	19,912	2.53%
29	Iowa	8,263	1.05%
30	Kansas	7,677	0.98%
21	Kentucky	11,288	1.44%
28	Louisiana	8,315	1.06%
38	Maine	3,735	0.48%
24	Maryland	9,275	1.18%
13	Massachusetts	14,362	1.83%
NA	Michigan**	NA	NA
20	Minnesota	11,530	1.47%
37	Mississippi	4,060	0.52%
12	Missouri	14,737	1.88%
42	Montana	2,146	0.27%
36	Nebraska	4,456	0.57%
27	Nevada	8,420	1.07%
40	New Hampshire	3,260	0.41%
11	New Jersey	16,377	2.08%
26	New Mexico	8,729	1.11%
3	New York	57,930	7.37%
16	North Carolina	12,981	1.65%
46	North Dakota	1,528	0.19%
5	Ohio	33,367	4.25%
25	Oklahoma	8,800	1.12%
22	Oregon	11,126	1.42%
7	Pennsylvania	31,673	4.03%
41	Rhode Island	2,817	0.36%
32	South Carolina	6,231	0.79%
44	South Dakota	1,785	0.23%
18	Tennessee	12,192	1.55%
2	Texas	72,543	9.23%
35	Utah	5,293	0.67%
45	Vermont	1,654	0.21%
15	Virginia	13,007	1.66%
10	Washington	17,193	2.19%
33	West Virginia	5,838	0.74%
17	Wisconsin	12,215	1.55%
48	Wyoming	1,500	0.19%

RANK ORDER

RANK	STATE	BIRTHS	% of USA
1	California	144,603	18.41%
2	Texas	72,543	9.23%
3	New York	57,930	7.37%
4	Florida	37,827	4.81%
5	Ohio	33,367	4.25%
6	Illinois	32,789	4.17%
7	Pennsylvania	31,673	4.03%
8	Arizona	22,545	2.87%
9	Indiana	19,912	2.53%
10	Washington	17,193	2.19%
11	New Jersey	16,377	2.08%
12	Missouri	14,737	1.88%
13	Massachusetts	14,362	1.83%
14	Georgia	13,435	1.71%
15	Virginia	13,007	1.66%
16	North Carolina	12,981	1.65%
17	Wisconsin	12,215	1.55%
18	Tennessee	12,192	1.55%
19	Colorado	11,562	1.47%
20	Minnesota	11,530	1.47%
21	Kentucky	11,288	1.44%
22	Oregon	11,126	1.42%
23	Connecticut	9,443	1.20%
24	Maryland	9,275	1.18%
25	Oklahoma	8,800	1.12%
26	New Mexico	8,729	1.11%
27	Nevada	8,420	1.07%
28	Louisiana	8,315	1.06%
29	Iowa	8,263	1.05%
30	Kansas	7,677	0.98%
31	Alabama	6,664	0.85%
32	South Carolina	6,231	0.79%
33	West Virginia	5,838	0.74%
34	Arkansas	5,774	0.73%
35	Utah	5,293	0.67%
36	Nebraska	4,456	0.57%
37	Mississippi	4,060	0.52%
38	Maine	3,735	0.48%
39	Idaho	3,385	0.43%
40	New Hampshire	3,260	0.41%
41	Rhode Island	2,817	0.36%
42	Montana	2,146	0.27%
43	Delaware	1,860	0.24%
44	South Dakota	1,785	0.23%
45	Vermont	1,654	0.21%
46	North Dakota	1,528	0.19%
47	Alaska	1,525	0.19%
48	Wyoming	1,500	0.19%
49	Hawaii	815	0.10%
NA	Michigan**	NA	NA
	District of Columbia	488	0.06%

Source: Morgan Quitno Press using data from U.S. Dept. of Health and Human Services, Nat'l Center for Health Statistics "Monthly Vital Statistics Report" (Vol. 45, No. 3(S)2, October 4, 1996)

Preliminary data by state of residence. Calculated by the editors by multiplying total number of births to white women by percent of such births reported as being to unmarried white women.

***Not available.**

Births to Unmarried White Women
As a Percent of All Births to White Women in 1995
National Percent = 25.3% of Live Births*

ALPHA ORDER

RANK	STATE	PERCENT
47	Alabama	16.6
32	Alaska	21.5
3	Arizona	35.4
33	Arkansas	21.4
4	California	31.6
24	Colorado	23.3
18	Connecticut	24.4
21	Delaware	24.2
10	Florida	26.6
45	Georgia	18.5
48	Hawaii	16.4
42	Idaho	19.4
25	Illinois	23.0
9	Indiana	26.7
23	Iowa	23.8
26	Kansas	22.9
19	Kentucky	24.3
30	Louisiana	21.7
8	Maine	27.5
38	Maryland	20.0
28	Massachusetts	22.1
NA	Michigan**	NA
37	Minnesota	20.4
44	Mississippi	18.8
22	Missouri	23.9
29	Montana	21.8
35	Nebraska	20.9
1	Nevada	39.1
27	New Hampshire	22.3
40	New Jersey	19.6
2	New Mexico	38.3
5	New York	29.7
46	North Carolina	18.1
40	North Dakota	19.6
13	Ohio	25.5
19	Oklahoma	24.3
7	Oregon	28.0
16	Pennsylvania	25.0
12	Rhode Island	25.6
39	South Carolina	19.9
36	South Dakota	20.5
31	Tennessee	21.6
11	Texas	25.9
49	Utah	14.4
17	Vermont	24.6
43	Virginia	19.2
14	Washington	25.2
6	West Virginia	28.9
34	Wisconsin	21.0
15	Wyoming	25.1

RANK ORDER

RANK	STATE	PERCENT
1	Nevada	39.1
2	New Mexico	38.3
3	Arizona	35.4
4	California	31.6
5	New York	29.7
6	West Virginia	28.9
7	Oregon	28.0
8	Maine	27.5
9	Indiana	26.7
10	Florida	26.6
11	Texas	25.9
12	Rhode Island	25.6
13	Ohio	25.5
14	Washington	25.2
15	Wyoming	25.1
16	Pennsylvania	25.0
17	Vermont	24.6
18	Connecticut	24.4
19	Kentucky	24.3
19	Oklahoma	24.3
21	Delaware	24.2
22	Missouri	23.9
23	Iowa	23.8
24	Colorado	23.3
25	Illinois	23.0
26	Kansas	22.9
27	New Hampshire	22.3
28	Massachusetts	22.1
29	Montana	21.8
30	Louisiana	21.7
31	Tennessee	21.6
32	Alaska	21.5
33	Arkansas	21.4
34	Wisconsin	21.0
35	Nebraska	20.9
36	South Dakota	20.5
37	Minnesota	20.4
38	Maryland	20.0
39	South Carolina	19.9
40	New Jersey	19.6
40	North Dakota	19.6
42	Idaho	19.4
43	Virginia	19.2
44	Mississippi	18.8
45	Georgia	18.5
46	North Carolina	18.1
47	Alabama	16.6
48	Hawaii	16.4
49	Utah	14.4
NA	Michigan**	NA

District of Columbia 24.8

Source: U.S. Department of Health and Human Services, National Center for Health Statistics
"Monthly Vital Statistics Report" (Vol. 45, No. 3(S)2, October 4, 1996)
*Data are preliminary estimates by state of residence. By race of mother.
**Not available.

Births to Unmarried Black Women in 1995

National Total = 415,998 Live Births*

ALPHA ORDER				RANK ORDER			
RANK	STATE	BIRTHS	% of USA	RANK	STATE	BIRTHS	% of USA
13	Alabama	14,202	3.41%	1	New York	38,472	9.25%
40	Alaska	178	0.04%	2	Illinois	29,053	6.98%
31	Arizona	1,418	0.34%	3	Florida	28,829	6.93%
20	Arkansas	5,655	1.36%	4	Georgia	26,201	6.30%
6	California	24,851	5.97%	5	Texas	24,854	5.97%
32	Colorado	1,403	0.34%	6	California	24,851	5.97%
23	Connecticut	3,606	0.87%	7	Louisiana	20,134	4.84%
28	Delaware	1,693	0.41%	8	North Carolina	18,080	4.35%
3	Florida	28,829	6.93%	9	Ohio	17,426	4.19%
4	Georgia	26,201	6.30%	10	Pennsylvania	16,678	4.01%
41	Hawaii	128	0.03%	11	Mississippi	14,495	3.48%
46	Idaho	29	0.01%	12	Maryland	14,320	3.44%
2	Illinois	29,053	6.98%	13	Alabama	14,202	3.41%
19	Indiana	6,701	1.61%	14	Virginia	13,735	3.30%
34	Iowa	725	0.17%	15	New Jersey	12,491	3.00%
27	Kansas	1,962	0.47%	16	South Carolina	12,284	2.95%
24	Kentucky	3,423	0.82%	17	Tennessee	11,779	2.83%
7	Louisiana	20,134	4.84%	18	Missouri	8,698	2.09%
43	Maine	33	0.01%	19	Indiana	6,701	1.61%
12	Maryland	14,320	3.44%	20	Arkansas	5,655	1.36%
22	Massachusetts	4,040	0.97%	21	Wisconsin	5,399	1.30%
NA	Michigan**	NA	NA	22	Massachusetts	4,040	0.97%
26	Minnesota	1,981	0.48%	23	Connecticut	3,606	0.87%
11	Mississippi	14,495	3.48%	24	Kentucky	3,423	0.82%
18	Missouri	8,698	2.09%	25	Oklahoma	3,116	0.75%
NA	Montana**	NA	NA	26	Minnesota	1,981	0.48%
33	Nebraska	897	0.22%	27	Kansas	1,962	0.47%
30	Nevada	1,423	0.34%	28	Delaware	1,693	0.41%
42	New Hampshire	38	0.01%	29	Washington	1,642	0.39%
15	New Jersey	12,491	3.00%	30	Nevada	1,423	0.34%
39	New Mexico	301	0.07%	31	Arizona	1,418	0.34%
1	New York	38,472	9.25%	32	Colorado	1,403	0.34%
8	North Carolina	18,080	4.35%	33	Nebraska	897	0.22%
47	North Dakota	23	0.01%	34	Iowa	725	0.17%
9	Ohio	17,426	4.19%	35	Oregon	616	0.15%
25	Oklahoma	3,116	0.75%	36	West Virginia	606	0.15%
35	Oregon	616	0.15%	37	Rhode Island	572	0.14%
10	Pennsylvania	16,678	4.01%	38	Utah	431	0.10%
37	Rhode Island	572	0.14%	39	New Mexico	301	0.07%
16	South Carolina	12,284	2.95%	40	Alaska	178	0.04%
44	South Dakota	32	0.01%	41	Hawaii	128	0.03%
17	Tennessee	11,779	2.83%	42	New Hampshire	38	0.01%
5	Texas	24,854	5.97%	43	Maine	33	0.01%
38	Utah	431	0.10%	44	South Dakota	32	0.01%
48	Vermont	20	0.00%	44	Wyoming	32	0.01%
14	Virginia	13,735	3.30%	46	Idaho	29	0.01%
29	Washington	1,642	0.39%	47	North Dakota	23	0.01%
36	West Virginia	606	0.15%	48	Vermont	20	0.00%
21	Wisconsin	5,399	1.30%	NA	Michigan**	NA	NA
44	Wyoming	32	0.01%	NA	Montana**	NA	NA
					District of Columbia	5,291	1.27%

Source: Morgan Quitno Press using data from U.S. Dept. of Health and Human Services, Nat'l Center for Health Statistics
    "Monthly Vital Statistics Report" (Vol. 45, No. 3(S)2, October 4, 1996)
*Preliminary data by state of residence. Calculated by the editors by multiplying total number of births to black
women by percent of such births reported as being to unmarried black women.
**Not available.

Births to Unmarried Black Women
As a Percent of All Births to Black Women in 1995
National Percent = 69.5% of Live Births*

ALPHA ORDER

RANK	STATE	PERCENT
17	Alabama	70.7
43	Alaska	41.1
32	Arizona	63.5
10	Arkansas	73.8
34	California	62.1
38	Colorado	53.5
21	Connecticut	69.0
15	Delaware	71.9
23	Florida	68.5
25	Georgia	67.3
48	Hawaii	22.7
45	Idaho	39.2
2	Illinois	78.4
6	Indiana	76.5
13	Iowa	72.5
26	Kansas	67.2
16	Kentucky	71.8
13	Louisiana	72.5
41	Maine	45.3
31	Maryland	63.7
35	Massachusetts	61.4
NA	Michigan**	NA
19	Minnesota	69.8
8	Mississippi	75.3
4	Missouri	78.0
NA	Montana**	NA
11	Nebraska	73.6
9	Nevada	74.2
42	New Hampshire	41.7
29	New Jersey	65.3
36	New Mexico	59.0
19	New York	69.8
27	North Carolina	66.9
46	North Dakota	31.4
5	Ohio	76.7
22	Oklahoma	68.9
18	Oregon	70.6
3	Pennsylvania	78.1
28	Rhode Island	66.7
24	South Carolina	68.2
47	South Dakota	29.5
12	Tennessee	73.2
33	Texas	63.1
43	Utah	41.1
39	Vermont	53.1
30	Virginia	63.8
37	Washington	54.8
7	West Virginia	75.4
1	Wisconsin	82.8
40	Wyoming	45.7

RANK ORDER

RANK	STATE	PERCENT
1	Wisconsin	82.8
2	Illinois	78.4
3	Pennsylvania	78.1
4	Missouri	78.0
5	Ohio	76.7
6	Indiana	76.5
7	West Virginia	75.4
8	Mississippi	75.3
9	Nevada	74.2
10	Arkansas	73.8
11	Nebraska	73.6
12	Tennessee	73.2
13	Iowa	72.5
13	Louisiana	72.5
15	Delaware	71.9
16	Kentucky	71.8
17	Alabama	70.7
18	Oregon	70.6
19	Minnesota	69.8
19	New York	69.8
21	Connecticut	69.0
22	Oklahoma	68.9
23	Florida	68.5
24	South Carolina	68.2
25	Georgia	67.3
26	Kansas	67.2
27	North Carolina	66.9
28	Rhode Island	66.7
29	New Jersey	65.3
30	Virginia	63.8
31	Maryland	63.7
32	Arizona	63.5
33	Texas	63.1
34	California	62.1
35	Massachusetts	61.4
36	New Mexico	59.0
37	Washington	54.8
38	Colorado	53.5
39	Vermont	53.1
40	Wyoming	45.7
41	Maine	45.3
42	New Hampshire	41.7
43	Alaska	41.1
43	Utah	41.1
45	Idaho	39.2
46	North Dakota	31.4
47	South Dakota	29.5
48	Hawaii	22.7
NA	Michigan**	NA
NA	Montana**	NA
	District of Columbia	79.4

Source: U.S. Department of Health and Human Services, National Center for Health Statistics
    "Monthly Vital Statistics Report" (Vol. 45, No. 3(S)2, October 4, 1996)
*Data are preliminary estimates by state of residence. By race of mother.
**Not available.

Births to Teenage Mothers in 1995

National Total = 514,812 Live Births*

ALPHA ORDER

RANK	STATE	BIRTHS	% of USA
14	Alabama	11,274	2.19%
46	Alaska	1,146	0.22%
15	Arizona	10,998	2.14%
26	Arkansas	6,890	1.34%
1	California	69,575	13.51%
27	Colorado	6,626	1.29%
35	Connecticut	3,837	0.75%
43	Delaware	1,354	0.26%
3	Florida	25,830	5.02%
7	Georgia	18,515	3.60%
40	Hawaii	1,878	0.36%
38	Idaho	2,540	0.49%
5	Illinois	23,734	4.61%
13	Indiana	12,308	2.39%
34	Iowa	4,027	0.78%
31	Kansas	5,007	0.97%
20	Kentucky	8,836	1.72%
11	Louisiana	12,945	2.51%
41	Maine	1,475	0.29%
24	Maryland	7,373	1.43%
28	Massachusetts	5,611	1.09%
8	Michigan	16,440	3.19%
30	Minnesota	5,285	1.03%
18	Mississippi	9,184	1.78%
16	Missouri	10,673	2.07%
42	Montana	1,400	0.27%
39	Nebraska	2,326	0.45%
37	Nevada	3,431	0.67%
47	New Hampshire	1,132	0.22%
21	New Jersey	8,691	1.69%
32	New Mexico	4,975	0.97%
4	New York	24,595	4.78%
10	North Carolina	15,508	3.01%
49	North Dakota	831	0.16%
6	Ohio	21,322	4.14%
23	Oklahoma	7,804	1.52%
29	Oregon	5,565	1.08%
9	Pennsylvania	16,356	3.18%
45	Rhode Island	1,201	0.23%
22	South Carolina	8,639	1.68%
44	South Dakota	1,252	0.24%
12	Tennessee	12,438	2.42%
2	Texas	54,545	10.60%
33	Utah	4,269	0.83%
50	Vermont	554	0.11%
17	Virginia	10,612	2.06%
19	Washington	9,005	1.75%
36	West Virginia	3,633	0.71%
25	Wisconsin	7,087	1.38%
48	Wyoming	963	0.19%

RANK ORDER

RANK	STATE	BIRTHS	% of USA
1	California	69,575	13.51%
2	Texas	54,545	10.60%
3	Florida	25,830	5.02%
4	New York	24,595	4.78%
5	Illinois	23,734	4.61%
6	Ohio	21,322	4.14%
7	Georgia	18,515	3.60%
8	Michigan	16,440	3.19%
9	Pennsylvania	16,356	3.18%
10	North Carolina	15,508	3.01%
11	Louisiana	12,945	2.51%
12	Tennessee	12,438	2.42%
13	Indiana	12,308	2.39%
14	Alabama	11,274	2.19%
15	Arizona	10,998	2.14%
16	Missouri	10,673	2.07%
17	Virginia	10,612	2.06%
18	Mississippi	9,184	1.78%
19	Washington	9,005	1.75%
20	Kentucky	8,836	1.72%
21	New Jersey	8,691	1.69%
22	South Carolina	8,639	1.68%
23	Oklahoma	7,804	1.52%
24	Maryland	7,373	1.43%
25	Wisconsin	7,087	1.38%
26	Arkansas	6,890	1.34%
27	Colorado	6,626	1.29%
28	Massachusetts	5,611	1.09%
29	Oregon	5,565	1.08%
30	Minnesota	5,285	1.03%
31	Kansas	5,007	0.97%
32	New Mexico	4,975	0.97%
33	Utah	4,269	0.83%
34	Iowa	4,027	0.78%
35	Connecticut	3,837	0.75%
36	West Virginia	3,633	0.71%
37	Nevada	3,431	0.67%
38	Idaho	2,540	0.49%
39	Nebraska	2,326	0.45%
40	Hawaii	1,878	0.36%
41	Maine	1,475	0.29%
42	Montana	1,400	0.27%
43	Delaware	1,354	0.26%
44	South Dakota	1,252	0.24%
45	Rhode Island	1,201	0.23%
46	Alaska	1,146	0.22%
47	New Hampshire	1,132	0.22%
48	Wyoming	963	0.19%
49	North Dakota	831	0.16%
50	Vermont	554	0.11%
	District of Columbia	1,431	0.28%

Source: Morgan Quitno Press using data from U.S. Dept of Health & Human Services, National Center for Health Statistics
"Monthly Vital Statistics Report" (Vol. 45, No. 3(S)2, October 4, 1996)
*Preliminary data. Live births to women under the age of 20 years old. These numbers were calculated by the editors by multiplying the percent of live births to teenage women times total births. These are rough estimates and differ from other teenage birth numbers in this book in that they include births to women under the age of 15.

Births to Teenage Mothers as a Percent of Live Births in 1995

National Percent = 13.2% of Live Births*

ALPHA ORDER

RANK	STATE	PERCENT
4	Alabama	18.5
33	Alaska	11.2
13	Arizona	15.2
2	Arkansas	19.6
27	California	12.4
29	Colorado	12.2
45	Connecticut	8.5
23	Delaware	13.2
19	Florida	13.7
12	Georgia	16.3
40	Hawaii	10.1
18	Idaho	14.1
25	Illinois	12.8
16	Indiana	14.6
34	Iowa	11.0
22	Kansas	13.3
8	Kentucky	17.1
3	Louisiana	19.2
37	Maine	10.6
39	Maryland	10.3
50	Massachusetts	7.5
27	Michigan	12.4
46	Minnesota	8.4
1	Mississippi	22.2
17	Missouri	14.4
26	Montana	12.6
41	Nebraska	10.0
19	Nevada	13.7
49	New Hampshire	7.6
48	New Jersey	8.0
5	New Mexico	18.4
44	New York	9.3
13	North Carolina	15.2
43	North Dakota	9.6
19	Ohio	13.7
9	Oklahoma	17.0
24	Oregon	13.0
35	Pennsylvania	10.8
42	Rhode Island	9.7
6	South Carolina	17.3
30	South Dakota	11.9
10	Tennessee	16.9
11	Texas	16.6
35	Utah	10.8
47	Vermont	8.1
32	Virginia	11.4
31	Washington	11.5
7	West Virginia	17.2
38	Wisconsin	10.5
13	Wyoming	15.2

RANK ORDER

RANK	STATE	PERCENT
1	Mississippi	22.2
2	Arkansas	19.6
3	Louisiana	19.2
4	Alabama	18.5
5	New Mexico	18.4
6	South Carolina	17.3
7	West Virginia	17.2
8	Kentucky	17.1
9	Oklahoma	17.0
10	Tennessee	16.9
11	Texas	16.6
12	Georgia	16.3
13	Arizona	15.2
13	North Carolina	15.2
13	Wyoming	15.2
16	Indiana	14.6
17	Missouri	14.4
18	Idaho	14.1
19	Florida	13.7
19	Nevada	13.7
19	Ohio	13.7
22	Kansas	13.3
23	Delaware	13.2
24	Oregon	13.0
25	Illinois	12.8
26	Montana	12.6
27	California	12.4
27	Michigan	12.4
29	Colorado	12.2
30	South Dakota	11.9
31	Washington	11.5
32	Virginia	11.4
33	Alaska	11.2
34	Iowa	11.0
35	Pennsylvania	10.8
35	Utah	10.8
37	Maine	10.6
38	Wisconsin	10.5
39	Maryland	10.3
40	Hawaii	10.1
41	Nebraska	10.0
42	Rhode Island	9.7
43	North Dakota	9.6
44	New York	9.3
45	Connecticut	8.5
46	Minnesota	8.4
47	Vermont	8.1
48	New Jersey	8.0
49	New Hampshire	7.6
50	Massachusetts	7.5
	District of Columbia	16.2

Source: U.S. Department of Health and Human Services, National Center for Health Statistics
    "Monthly Vital Statistics Report" (Vol. 45, No. 3(S)2, October 4, 1996)
*Preliminary data. Live births to women under the age of 20 years old. These numbers differ from other teenage birth numbers in this book in that they include births to women under the age of 15.

Births to Teenage Mothers in 1994

National Total = 505,488 Live Births*

ALPHA ORDER					RANK ORDER			
RANK	STATE	BIRTHS	% of USA		RANK	STATE	BIRTHS	% of USA
14	Alabama	10,999	2.18%		1	California	68,332	13.52%
45	Alaska	1,210	0.24%		2	Texas	51,471	10.18%
15	Arizona	10,589	2.09%		3	New York	25,729	5.09%
26	Arkansas	6,797	1.34%		4	Florida	25,435	5.03%
1	California	68,332	13.52%		5	Illinois	24,031	4.75%
27	Colorado	6,526	1.29%		6	Ohio	20,823	4.12%
35	Connecticut	3,776	0.75%		7	Georgia	17,337	3.43%
43	Delaware	1,322	0.26%		8	Michigan	17,063	3.38%
4	Florida	25,435	5.03%		9	Pennsylvania	16,476	3.26%
7	Georgia	17,337	3.43%		10	North Carolina	15,224	3.01%
40	Hawaii	2,017	0.40%		11	Louisiana	12,633	2.50%
39	Idaho	2,248	0.44%		12	Tennessee	12,350	2.44%
5	Illinois	24,031	4.75%		13	Indiana	11,739	2.32%
13	Indiana	11,739	2.32%		14	Alabama	10,999	2.18%
34	Iowa	3,991	0.79%		15	Arizona	10,589	2.09%
32	Kansas	4,741	0.94%		16	Missouri	10,584	2.09%
19	Kentucky	8,919	1.76%		17	Virginia	10,470	2.07%
11	Louisiana	12,633	2.50%		18	New Jersey	9,345	1.85%
41	Maine	1,459	0.29%		19	Kentucky	8,919	1.76%
24	Maryland	7,332	1.45%		20	Mississippi	8,897	1.76%
28	Massachusetts	6,415	1.27%		21	South Carolina	8,585	1.70%
8	Michigan	17,063	3.38%		22	Washington	8,467	1.68%
29	Minnesota	5,336	1.06%		23	Oklahoma	7,670	1.52%
20	Mississippi	8,897	1.76%		24	Maryland	7,332	1.45%
16	Missouri	10,584	2.09%		25	Wisconsin	6,876	1.36%
44	Montana	1,320	0.26%		26	Arkansas	6,797	1.34%
38	Nebraska	2,509	0.50%		27	Colorado	6,526	1.29%
37	Nevada	3,134	0.62%		28	Massachusetts	6,415	1.27%
47	New Hampshire	1,051	0.21%		29	Minnesota	5,336	1.06%
18	New Jersey	9,345	1.85%		30	Oregon	5,240	1.04%
31	New Mexico	4,841	0.96%		31	New Mexico	4,841	0.96%
3	New York	25,729	5.09%		32	Kansas	4,741	0.94%
10	North Carolina	15,224	3.01%		33	Utah	4,043	0.80%
49	North Dakota	796	0.16%		34	Iowa	3,991	0.79%
6	Ohio	20,823	4.12%		35	Connecticut	3,776	0.75%
23	Oklahoma	7,670	1.52%		36	West Virginia	3,674	0.73%
30	Oregon	5,240	1.04%		37	Nevada	3,134	0.62%
9	Pennsylvania	16,476	3.26%		38	Nebraska	2,509	0.50%
42	Rhode Island	1,389	0.27%		39	Idaho	2,248	0.44%
21	South Carolina	8,585	1.70%		40	Hawaii	2,017	0.40%
46	South Dakota	1,192	0.24%		41	Maine	1,459	0.29%
12	Tennessee	12,350	2.44%		42	Rhode Island	1,389	0.27%
2	Texas	51,471	10.18%		43	Delaware	1,322	0.26%
33	Utah	4,043	0.80%		44	Montana	1,320	0.26%
50	Vermont	617	0.12%		45	Alaska	1,210	0.24%
17	Virginia	10,470	2.07%		46	South Dakota	1,192	0.24%
22	Washington	8,467	1.68%		47	New Hampshire	1,051	0.21%
36	West Virginia	3,674	0.73%		48	Wyoming	921	0.18%
25	Wisconsin	6,876	1.36%		49	North Dakota	796	0.16%
48	Wyoming	921	0.18%		50	Vermont	617	0.12%
						District of Columbia	1,547	0.31%

Source: Morgan Quitno Press using data from U.S. Dept of Health & Human Services, National Center for Health Statistics
(unpublished data)
*Live births to women age 15 to 19 years old by state of residence.

Teenage Birth Rate in 1994

National Rate = 58.9 Births per 1,000 Teenage Women*

ALPHA ORDER

RANK	STATE	RATE
8	Alabama	72.2
21	Alaska	55.2
2	Arizona	78.7
5	Arkansas	76.3
10	California	71.3
23	Colorado	54.3
41	Connecticut	40.3
18	Delaware	60.2
16	Florida	64.4
9	Georgia	71.7
25	Hawaii	53.5
34	Idaho	46.6
17	Illinois	62.8
20	Indiana	57.9
42	Iowa	39.7
25	Kansas	53.5
15	Kentucky	64.5
6	Louisiana	74.7
46	Maine	35.5
30	Maryland	49.7
45	Massachusetts	37.2
27	Michigan	52.1
48	Minnesota	34.4
1	Mississippi	83.0
19	Missouri	59.0
40	Montana	41.2
37	Nebraska	42.8
7	Nevada	73.6
50	New Hampshire	30.1
43	New Jersey	39.3
4	New Mexico	77.4
35	New York	45.8
13	North Carolina	66.3
47	North Dakota	34.6
22	Ohio	55.0
14	Oklahoma	65.9
28	Oregon	50.7
36	Pennsylvania	43.8
33	Rhode Island	47.7
12	South Carolina	66.5
37	South Dakota	42.8
11	Tennessee	71.0
3	Texas	77.6
39	Utah	42.7
49	Vermont	33.0
28	Virginia	50.7
31	Washington	48.2
23	West Virginia	54.3
44	Wisconsin	38.8
31	Wyoming	48.2

RANK ORDER

RANK	STATE	RATE
1	Mississippi	83.0
2	Arizona	78.7
3	Texas	77.6
4	New Mexico	77.4
5	Arkansas	76.3
6	Louisiana	74.7
7	Nevada	73.6
8	Alabama	72.2
9	Georgia	71.7
10	California	71.3
11	Tennessee	71.0
12	South Carolina	66.5
13	North Carolina	66.3
14	Oklahoma	65.9
15	Kentucky	64.5
16	Florida	64.4
17	Illinois	62.8
18	Delaware	60.2
19	Missouri	59.0
20	Indiana	57.9
21	Alaska	55.2
22	Ohio	55.0
23	Colorado	54.3
23	West Virginia	54.3
25	Hawaii	53.5
25	Kansas	53.5
27	Michigan	52.1
28	Oregon	50.7
28	Virginia	50.7
30	Maryland	49.7
31	Washington	48.2
31	Wyoming	48.2
33	Rhode Island	47.7
34	Idaho	46.6
35	New York	45.8
36	Pennsylvania	43.8
37	Nebraska	42.8
37	South Dakota	42.8
39	Utah	42.7
40	Montana	41.2
41	Connecticut	40.3
42	Iowa	39.7
43	New Jersey	39.3
44	Wisconsin	38.8
45	Massachusetts	37.2
46	Maine	35.5
47	North Dakota	34.6
48	Minnesota	34.4
49	Vermont	33.0
50	New Hampshire	30.1
	District of Columbia	114.7

Source: U.S. Department of Health and Human Services, National Center for Health Statistics
"Monthly Vital Statistics Report" (Vol. 45, No. 5(S), December 19, 1996)
*Women aged 15 to 19 years old. Final data.

Births to Teenage Mothers as a Percent of Live Births in 1994

National Percent = 12.79% of Live Births*

ALPHA ORDER				RANK ORDER		
RANK	STATE	PERCENT		RANK	STATE	PERCENT
4	Alabama	18.05		1	Mississippi	21.21
31	Alaska	11.33		2	Arkansas	19.58
14	Arizona	14.95		3	Louisiana	18.63
2	Arkansas	19.58		4	Alabama	18.05
28	California	12.03		5	New Mexico	17.55
27	Colorado	12.07		6	West Virginia	17.19
47	Connecticut	8.27		7	Tennessee	16.87
22	Delaware	12.70		8	Kentucky	16.83
19	Florida	13.34		9	Oklahoma	16.78
12	Georgia	15.62		10	South Carolina	16.50
38	Hawaii	10.33		11	Texas	16.03
21	Idaho	12.83		12	Georgia	15.62
22	Illinois	12.70		13	North Carolina	15.01
17	Indiana	14.21		14	Arizona	14.95
35	Iowa	10.76		15	Missouri	14.39
24	Kansas	12.68		16	Wyoming	14.33
8	Kentucky	16.83		17	Indiana	14.21
3	Louisiana	18.63		18	Ohio	13.35
40	Maine	10.10		19	Florida	13.34
42	Maryland	9.91		20	Nevada	13.11
49	Massachusetts	7.66		21	Idaho	12.83
26	Michigan	12.36		22	Delaware	12.70
46	Minnesota	8.30		22	Illinois	12.70
1	Mississippi	21.21		24	Kansas	12.68
15	Missouri	14.39		25	Oregon	12.52
29	Montana	11.93		26	Michigan	12.36
34	Nebraska	10.84		27	Colorado	12.07
20	Nevada	13.11		28	California	12.03
50	New Hampshire	6.96		29	Montana	11.93
48	New Jersey	7.95		30	South Dakota	11.34
5	New Mexico	17.55		31	Alaska	11.33
44	New York	9.24		32	Virginia	11.02
13	North Carolina	15.01		33	Washington	10.95
43	North Dakota	9.27		34	Nebraska	10.84
18	Ohio	13.35		35	Iowa	10.76
9	Oklahoma	16.78		36	Utah	10.56
25	Oregon	12.52		37	Pennsylvania	10.49
37	Pennsylvania	10.49		38	Hawaii	10.33
39	Rhode Island	10.31		39	Rhode Island	10.31
10	South Carolina	16.50		40	Maine	10.10
30	South Dakota	11.34		41	Wisconsin	10.07
7	Tennessee	16.87		42	Maryland	9.91
11	Texas	16.03		43	North Dakota	9.27
36	Utah	10.56		44	New York	9.24
45	Vermont	8.36		45	Vermont	8.36
32	Virginia	11.02		46	Minnesota	8.30
33	Washington	10.95		47	Connecticut	8.27
6	West Virginia	17.19		48	New Jersey	7.95
41	Wisconsin	10.07		49	Massachusetts	7.66
16	Wyoming	14.33		50	New Hampshire	6.96
					District of Columbia	15.58

Source: Morgan Quitno Press using data from U.S. Dept of Health & Human Services, National Center for Health Statistics "Monthly Vital Statistics Report" (Vol. 44, No. 11, Supplement, June 24, 1996)
*Live births to women age 15 to 19 years old by state of residence.

Births to White Teenage Mothers in 1994

National Total = 348,081 Live Births*

ALPHA ORDER				RANK ORDER			
RANK	STATE	BIRTHS	% of USA	RANK	STATE	BIRTHS	% of USA
19	Alabama	5,507	1.58%	1	California	56,731	16.30%
46	Alaska	710	0.20%	2	Texas	41,757	12.00%
10	Arizona	8,891	2.55%	3	New York	16,138	4.64%
26	Arkansas	4,369	1.26%	4	Florida	15,374	4.42%
1	California	56,731	16.30%	5	Ohio	14,918	4.29%
18	Colorado	5,702	1.64%	6	Illinois	13,669	3.93%
36	Connecticut	2,624	0.75%	7	Pennsylvania	11,059	3.18%
47	Delaware	696	0.20%	8	Michigan	10,433	3.00%
4	Florida	15,374	4.42%	9	Indiana	9,323	2.68%
11	Georgia	8,338	2.40%	10	Arizona	8,891	2.55%
50	Hawaii	344	0.10%	11	Georgia	8,338	2.40%
38	Idaho	2,162	0.62%	12	North Carolina	8,230	2.36%
6	Illinois	13,669	3.93%	13	Tennessee	8,034	2.31%
9	Indiana	9,323	2.68%	14	Kentucky	7,587	2.18%
32	Iowa	3,622	1.04%	15	Missouri	7,451	2.14%
30	Kansas	3,883	1.12%	16	Washington	7,249	2.08%
14	Kentucky	7,587	2.18%	17	Virginia	6,102	1.75%
22	Louisiana	4,932	1.42%	18	Colorado	5,702	1.64%
40	Maine	1,412	0.41%	19	Alabama	5,507	1.58%
35	Maryland	3,029	0.87%	20	Oklahoma	5,391	1.55%
21	Massachusetts	4,968	1.43%	21	Massachusetts	4,968	1.43%
8	Michigan	10,433	3.00%	22	Louisiana	4,932	1.42%
27	Minnesota	4,071	1.17%	23	New Jersey	4,918	1.41%
34	Mississippi	3,224	0.93%	24	Oregon	4,759	1.37%
15	Missouri	7,451	2.14%	25	Wisconsin	4,573	1.31%
43	Montana	1,016	0.29%	26	Arkansas	4,369	1.26%
39	Nebraska	2,067	0.59%	27	Minnesota	4,071	1.17%
37	Nevada	2,546	0.73%	28	New Mexico	4,034	1.16%
42	New Hampshire	1,029	0.30%	29	South Carolina	3,891	1.12%
23	New Jersey	4,918	1.41%	30	Kansas	3,883	1.12%
28	New Mexico	4,034	1.16%	31	Utah	3,799	1.09%
3	New York	16,138	4.64%	32	Iowa	3,622	1.04%
12	North Carolina	8,230	2.36%	33	West Virginia	3,477	1.00%
48	North Dakota	622	0.18%	34	Mississippi	3,224	0.93%
5	Ohio	14,918	4.29%	35	Maryland	3,029	0.87%
20	Oklahoma	5,391	1.55%	36	Connecticut	2,624	0.75%
24	Oregon	4,759	1.37%	37	Nevada	2,546	0.73%
7	Pennsylvania	11,059	3.18%	38	Idaho	2,162	0.62%
41	Rhode Island	1,082	0.31%	39	Nebraska	2,067	0.59%
29	South Carolina	3,891	1.12%	40	Maine	1,412	0.41%
45	South Dakota	814	0.23%	41	Rhode Island	1,082	0.31%
13	Tennessee	8,034	2.31%	42	New Hampshire	1,029	0.30%
2	Texas	41,757	12.00%	43	Montana	1,016	0.29%
31	Utah	3,799	1.09%	44	Wyoming	872	0.25%
49	Vermont	609	0.17%	45	South Dakota	814	0.23%
17	Virginia	6,102	1.75%	46	Alaska	710	0.20%
16	Washington	7,249	2.08%	47	Delaware	696	0.20%
33	West Virginia	3,477	1.00%	48	North Dakota	622	0.18%
25	Wisconsin	4,573	1.31%	49	Vermont	609	0.17%
44	Wyoming	872	0.25%	50	Hawaii	344	0.10%
					District of Columbia	43	0.01%

Source: Morgan Quitno Press using data from U.S. Dept of Health & Human Services, National Center for Health Statistics
   (unpublished data)
*Births to women age 15 to 19 years old by state of residence.

Births to White Teenage Mothers as a Percent of White Births in 1994

National Percent = 11.15% of White Live Births*

ALPHA ORDER

ALPHA ORDER

RANK ORDER

RANK	STATE	PERCENT	RANK	STATE	PERCENT
11	Alabama	13.88	1	New Mexico	17.50
34	Alaska	9.54	2	West Virginia	17.00
9	Arizona	14.44	3	Arkansas	16.56
3	Arkansas	16.56	4	Kentucky	15.93
17	California	12.26	5	Texas	15.33
23	Colorado	11.57	6	Oklahoma	15.05
47	Connecticut	6.81	7	Mississippi	14.97
37	Delaware	8.95	8	Tennessee	14.45
25	Florida	10.72	9	Arizona	14.44
20	Georgia	11.97	10	Wyoming	14.29
49	Hawaii	6.33	11	Alabama	13.88
14	Idaho	12.75	12	Louisiana	13.00
33	Illinois	9.60	13	Indiana	12.82
13	Indiana	12.82	14	Idaho	12.75
29	Iowa	10.28	15	Nevada	12.46
22	Kansas	11.70	16	Missouri	12.32
4	Kentucky	15.93	17	California	12.26
12	Louisiana	13.00	17	Oregon	12.26
30	Maine	10.00	19	South Carolina	12.15
48	Maryland	6.51	20	Georgia	11.97
46	Massachusetts	6.89	21	North Carolina	11.71
32	Michigan	9.68	22	Kansas	11.70
44	Minnesota	7.07	23	Colorado	11.57
7	Mississippi	14.97	24	Ohio	11.45
16	Missouri	12.32	25	Florida	10.72
28	Montana	10.44	25	Washington	10.72
31	Nebraska	9.77	27	Utah	10.46
15	Nevada	12.46	28	Montana	10.44
45	New Hampshire	6.93	29	Iowa	10.28
50	New Jersey	5.57	30	Maine	10.00
1	New Mexico	17.50	31	Nebraska	9.77
42	New York	7.90	32	Michigan	9.68
21	North Carolina	11.71	33	Illinois	9.60
41	North Dakota	8.08	34	Alaska	9.54
24	Ohio	11.45	35	South Dakota	9.27
6	Oklahoma	15.05	36	Rhode Island	9.14
17	Oregon	12.26	37	Delaware	8.95
39	Pennsylvania	8.49	38	Virginia	8.80
36	Rhode Island	9.14	39	Pennsylvania	8.49
19	South Carolina	12.15	40	Vermont	8.38
35	South Dakota	9.27	41	North Dakota	8.08
8	Tennessee	14.45	42	New York	7.90
5	Texas	15.33	43	Wisconsin	7.78
27	Utah	10.46	44	Minnesota	7.07
40	Vermont	8.38	45	New Hampshire	6.93
38	Virginia	8.80	46	Massachusetts	6.89
25	Washington	10.72	47	Connecticut	6.81
2	West Virginia	17.00	48	Maryland	6.51
43	Wisconsin	7.78	49	Hawaii	6.33
10	Wyoming	14.29	50	New Jersey	5.57
				District of Columbia	2.90

Source: Morgan Quitno Press using data from U.S. Dept of Health & Human Services, National Center for Health Statistics
   (unpublished data)
*Births to women age 15 to 19 years old by state of residence.

Births to Black Teenage Mothers in 1994

National Total = 140,968 Live Births*

ALPHA ORDER					RANK ORDER			
RANK	STATE		BIRTHS	% of USA	RANK	STATE	BIRTHS	% of USA
12	Alabama		5,447	3.86%	1	Illinois	10,192	7.23%
40	Alaska		81	0.06%	2	Florida	9,803	6.95%
32	Arizona		563	0.40%	3	Texas	9,250	6.56%
21	Arkansas		2,368	1.68%	4	New York	9,182	6.51%
6	California		7,681	5.45%	5	Georgia	8,892	6.31%
30	Colorado		587	0.42%	6	California	7,681	5.45%
26	Connecticut		1,077	0.76%	7	Louisiana	7,569	5.37%
29	Delaware		611	0.43%	8	North Carolina	6,506	4.62%
2	Florida		9,803	6.95%	9	Michigan	6,332	4.49%
5	Georgia		8,892	6.31%	10	Ohio	5,791	4.11%
41	Hawaii		53	0.04%	11	Mississippi	5,616	3.98%
44	Idaho		10	0.01%	12	Alabama	5,447	3.86%
1	Illinois		10,192	7.23%	13	Pennsylvania	5,211	3.70%
20	Indiana		2,373	1.68%	14	South Carolina	4,645	3.30%
35	Iowa		289	0.21%	15	New Jersey	4,326	3.07%
27	Kansas		749	0.53%	16	Virginia	4,263	3.02%
23	Kentucky		1,304	0.93%	17	Tennessee	4,235	3.00%
7	Louisiana		7,569	5.37%	18	Maryland	4,223	3.00%
43	Maine		13	0.01%	19	Missouri	3,035	2.15%
18	Maryland		4,223	3.00%	20	Indiana	2,373	1.68%
24	Massachusetts		1,239	0.88%	21	Arkansas	2,368	1.68%
9	Michigan		6,332	4.49%	22	Wisconsin	1,889	1.34%
28	Minnesota		704	0.50%	23	Kentucky	1,304	0.93%
11	Mississippi		5,616	3.98%	24	Massachusetts	1,239	0.88%
19	Missouri		3,035	2.15%	25	Oklahoma	1,179	0.84%
49	Montana		5	0.00%	26	Connecticut	1,077	0.76%
34	Nebraska		318	0.23%	27	Kansas	749	0.53%
33	Nevada		438	0.31%	28	Minnesota	704	0.50%
44	New Hampshire		10	0.01%	29	Delaware	611	0.43%
15	New Jersey		4,326	3.07%	30	Colorado	587	0.42%
39	New Mexico		114	0.08%	31	Washington	567	0.40%
4	New York		9,182	6.51%	32	Arizona	563	0.40%
8	North Carolina		6,506	4.62%	33	Nevada	438	0.31%
46	North Dakota		8	0.01%	34	Nebraska	318	0.23%
10	Ohio		5,791	4.11%	35	Iowa	289	0.21%
25	Oklahoma		1,179	0.84%	36	Oregon	251	0.18%
36	Oregon		251	0.18%	37	Rhode Island	241	0.17%
13	Pennsylvania		5,211	3.70%	38	West Virginia	195	0.14%
37	Rhode Island		241	0.17%	39	New Mexico	114	0.08%
14	South Carolina		4,645	3.30%	40	Alaska	81	0.06%
47	South Dakota		7	0.00%	41	Hawaii	53	0.04%
17	Tennessee		4,235	3.00%	42	Utah	48	0.03%
3	Texas		9,250	6.56%	43	Maine	13	0.01%
42	Utah		48	0.03%	44	Idaho	10	0.01%
49	Vermont		5	0.00%	44	New Hampshire	10	0.01%
16	Virginia		4,263	3.02%	46	North Dakota	8	0.01%
31	Washington		567	0.40%	47	South Dakota	7	0.00%
38	West Virginia		195	0.14%	48	Wyoming	6	0.00%
22	Wisconsin		1,889	1.34%	49	Montana	5	0.00%
48	Wyoming		6	0.00%	49	Vermont	5	0.00%
						District of Columbia	1,467	1.04%

Source: Morgan Quitno Press using data from U.S. Dept of Health & Human Services, National Center for Health Statistics (unpublished data)
*Births to women age 15 to 19 years old by state of residence.

Births to Black Teenage Mothers as a Percent of Black Births in 1994

National Percent = 22.15% of Black Live Births*

ALPHA ORDER			RANK ORDER		
RANK	STATE	PERCENT	RANK	STATE	PERCENT
9	Alabama	26.38	1	Arkansas	30.22
41	Alaska	16.23	2	Mississippi	28.14
25	Arizona	22.66	3	Wisconsin	27.60
1	Arkansas	30.22	4	Iowa	27.39
37	California	17.94	5	Kentucky	26.64
30	Colorado	21.17	6	Oregon	26.50
33	Connecticut	18.78	7	Indiana	26.43
12	Delaware	25.50	8	Louisiana	26.42
25	Florida	22.66	9	Alabama	26.38
24	Georgia	22.76	10	Missouri	25.56
50	Hawaii	8.45	11	Tennessee	25.51
42	Idaho	16.13	12	Delaware	25.50
14	Illinois	24.88	13	Nebraska	24.98
7	Indiana	26.43	14	Illinois	24.88
4	Iowa	27.39	15	Oklahoma	24.72
19	Kansas	23.84	16	Ohio	24.52
5	Kentucky	26.64	17	West Virginia	24.44
8	Louisiana	26.42	18	South Carolina	23.93
39	Maine	16.88	19	Kansas	23.84
38	Maryland	17.16	20	Minnesota	23.35
45	Massachusetts	15.26	21	North Carolina	23.33
22	Michigan	23.30	22	Michigan	23.30
20	Minnesota	23.35	23	Texas	22.97
2	Mississippi	28.14	24	Georgia	22.76
10	Missouri	25.56	25	Arizona	22.66
43	Montana	15.63	25	Florida	22.66
13	Nebraska	24.98	27	Pennsylvania	22.27
31	Nevada	21.07	28	Rhode Island	22.21
48	New Hampshire	9.62	29	New Mexico	21.88
34	New Jersey	18.66	30	Colorado	21.17
29	New Mexico	21.88	31	Nevada	21.07
44	New York	15.59	32	Virginia	19.09
21	North Carolina	23.33	33	Connecticut	18.78
46	North Dakota	11.76	34	New Jersey	18.66
16	Ohio	24.52	35	Vermont	18.52
15	Oklahoma	24.72	36	Washington	18.50
6	Oregon	26.50	37	California	17.94
27	Pennsylvania	22.27	38	Maryland	17.16
28	Rhode Island	22.21	39	Maine	16.88
18	South Carolina	23.93	40	Utah	16.72
49	South Dakota	9.21	41	Alaska	16.23
11	Tennessee	25.51	42	Idaho	16.13
23	Texas	22.97	43	Montana	15.63
40	Utah	16.72	44	New York	15.59
35	Vermont	18.52	45	Massachusetts	15.26
32	Virginia	19.09	46	North Dakota	11.76
36	Washington	18.50	47	Wyoming	9.84
17	West Virginia	24.44	48	New Hampshire	9.62
3	Wisconsin	27.60	49	South Dakota	9.21
47	Wyoming	9.84	50	Hawaii	8.45
				District of Columbia	18.26

Source: Morgan Quitno Press using data from U.S. Dept of Health & Human Services, National Center for Health Statistics
    (unpublished data)
*Births to women age 15 to 19 years old by state of residence.

Pregnancy Rate for 15 to 19 Year Old Women in 1992

National Average = 79.7 Births and Abortions per 1,000 Women 15-19 Years Old*

ALPHA ORDER

RANK	STATE	RATE
10	Alabama	93.2
NA	Alaska**	NA
5	Arizona	103.5
12	Arkansas	90.7
NA	California**	NA
20	Colorado	79.8
NA	Connecticut**	NA
NA	Delaware**	NA
NA	Florida**	NA
1	Georgia	106.9
13	Hawaii	86.4
35	Idaho	59.7
NA	Illinois**	NA
26	Indiana	72.2
NA	Iowa**	NA
16	Kansas	87.0
18	Kentucky	81.7
11	Louisiana	92.6
38	Maine	55.2
24	Maryland	76.9
30	Massachusetts	69.5
21	Michigan	79.7
38	Minnesota	55.2
7	Mississippi	100.8
23	Missouri	78.0
28	Montana	70.2
33	Nebraska	63.4
2	Nevada	106.0
NA	New Hampshire**	NA
29	New Jersey	69.7
6	New Mexico	101.8
8	New York	96.6
3	North Carolina	104.6
40	North Dakota	54.2
25	Ohio	74.6
NA	Oklahoma**	NA
19	Oregon	81.0
27	Pennsylvania	71.7
14	Rhode Island	88.1
15	South Carolina	88.0
36	South Dakota	59.4
9	Tennessee	94.0
4	Texas	103.7
37	Utah	55.6
31	Vermont	68.7
22	Virginia	79.0
17	Washington	85.1
32	West Virginia	66.1
34	Wisconsin	60.8
41	Wyoming	53.7

RANK ORDER

RANK	STATE	RATE
1	Georgia	106.9
2	Nevada	106.0
3	North Carolina	104.6
4	Texas	103.7
5	Arizona	103.5
6	New Mexico	101.8
7	Mississippi	100.8
8	New York	96.6
9	Tennessee	94.0
10	Alabama	93.2
11	Louisiana	92.6
12	Arkansas	90.7
13	Hawaii	86.4
14	Rhode Island	88.1
15	South Carolina	88.0
16	Kansas	87.0
17	Washington	85.1
18	Kentucky	81.7
19	Oregon	81.0
20	Colorado	79.8
21	Michigan	79.7
22	Virginia	79.0
23	Missouri	78.0
24	Maryland	76.9
25	Ohio	74.6
26	Indiana	72.2
27	Pennsylvania	71.7
28	Montana	70.2
29	New Jersey	69.7
30	Massachusetts	69.5
31	Vermont	68.7
32	West Virginia	66.1
33	Nebraska	63.4
34	Wisconsin	60.8
35	Idaho	59.7
36	South Dakota	59.4
37	Utah	55.6
38	Maine	55.2
38	Minnesota	55.2
40	North Dakota	54.2
41	Wyoming	53.7
NA	Alaska**	NA
NA	California**	NA
NA	Connecticut**	NA
NA	Delaware**	NA
NA	Florida**	NA
NA	Illinois**	NA
NA	Iowa**	NA
NA	New Hampshire**	NA
NA	Oklahoma**	NA

District of Columbia	208.4

Source: U.S. Department of Health and Human Services, Centers for Disease Control and Prevention
"State-Specific Pregnancy and Birth Rates Among Teenagers" (MMWR, Vol. 44, No. 37, 9/22/95)
The sum of live births and legal induced abortions per 1,000 women aged 15-19 years old. Births by state of residence, abortions by state of occurrence. National average is simply the average of the rates of reporting states (excluding Washington, DC).
**Not available.*

Percent Change in Pregnancy Rate for 15 to 19 Year Old Women: 1991 to 1992

National Percent Change = 4.0% Decrease*

ALPHA ORDER				RANK ORDER		
RANK	STATE	PERCENT CHANGE		RANK	STATE	PERCENT CHANGE
18	Alabama	(3.9)		1	Kansas	8.7
NA	Alaska**	NA		2	West Virginia	3.4
11	Arizona	(2.5)		3	South Dakota	3.3
34	Arkansas	(7.6)		4	New York	2.3
NA	California**	NA		5	Louisiana	0.7
14	Colorado	(3.1)		6	North Dakota	(0.3)
NA	Connecticut**	NA		7	Texas	(0.7)
NA	Delaware**	NA		8	New Mexico	(1.2)
NA	Florida**	NA		9	Rhode Island	(1.4)
10	Georgia	(2.1)		10	Georgia	(2.1)
13	Hawaii	(3.0)		11	Arizona	(2.5)
27	Idaho	(6.7)		12	Nevada	(2.6)
NA	Illinois**	NA		13	Hawaii	(3.0)
19	Indiana	(4.1)		14	Colorado	(3.1)
NA	Iowa**	NA		15	Maryland	(3.5)
1	Kansas	8.7		16	Michigan	(3.8)
33	Kentucky	(7.4)		16	North Carolina	(3.8)
5	Louisiana	0.7		18	Alabama	(3.9)
41	Maine	(14.7)		19	Indiana	(4.1)
15	Maryland	(3.5)		20	Mississippi	(4.5)
23	Massachusetts	(6.0)		21	Missouri	(5.6)
16	Michigan	(3.8)		21	Pennsylvania	(5.6)
32	Minnesota	(7.3)		23	Massachusetts	(6.0)
20	Mississippi	(4.5)		24	Utah	(6.3)
21	Missouri	(5.6)		24	Wisconsin	(6.3)
30	Montana	(7.1)		26	New Jersey	(6.5)
37	Nebraska	(8.7)		27	Idaho	(6.7)
12	Nevada	(2.6)		28	Virginia	(6.8)
NA	New Hampshire**	NA		29	South Carolina	(7.0)
26	New Jersey	(6.5)		30	Montana	(7.1)
8	New Mexico	(1.2)		31	Washington	(7.2)
4	New York	2.3		32	Minnesota	(7.3)
16	North Carolina	(3.8)		33	Kentucky	(7.4)
6	North Dakota	(0.3)		34	Arkansas	(7.6)
35	Ohio	(7.7)		35	Ohio	(7.7)
NA	Oklahoma**	NA		36	Tennessee	(7.8)
38	Oregon	(9.5)		37	Nebraska	(8.7)
21	Pennsylvania	(5.6)		38	Oregon	(9.5)
9	Rhode Island	(1.4)		38	Wyoming	(9.5)
29	South Carolina	(7.0)		40	Vermont	(12.0)
3	South Dakota	3.3		41	Maine	(14.7)
36	Tennessee	(7.8)		NA	Alaska**	NA
7	Texas	(0.7)		NA	California**	NA
24	Utah	(6.3)		NA	Connecticut**	NA
40	Vermont	(12.0)		NA	Delaware**	NA
28	Virginia	(6.8)		NA	Florida**	NA
31	Washington	(7.2)		NA	Illinois**	NA
2	West Virginia	3.4		NA	Iowa**	NA
24	Wisconsin	(6.3)		NA	New Hampshire**	NA
38	Wyoming	(9.5)		NA	Oklahoma**	NA
					District of Columbia	(7.9)

Source: U.S. Department of Health and Human Services, Centers for Disease Control and Prevention
   "State-Specific Pregnancy and Birth Rates Among Teenagers" (MMWR, Vol. 44, No. 37, 9/22/95)
*The sum of live births and legal induced abortions per 1,000 women aged 15-19 years old. Births by state of residence, abortions by state of occurrence. National percent is based on the simple average of the rates of reporting states (excluding Washington, DC).
**Not available.

Births to Teenage Mothers in 1990

National Total = 521,826 Live Births*

<table>
<tr><td colspan="4">ALPHA ORDER</td><td colspan="4">RANK ORDER</td></tr>
<tr><td>RANK</td><td>STATE</td><td>BIRTHS</td><td>% of USA</td><td>RANK</td><td>STATE</td><td>BIRTHS</td><td>% of USA</td></tr>
<tr><td>15</td><td>Alabama</td><td>11,252</td><td>2.16%</td><td>1</td><td>California</td><td>69,712</td><td>13.36%</td></tr>
<tr><td>47</td><td>Alaska</td><td>1,142</td><td>0.22%</td><td>2</td><td>Texas</td><td>48,302</td><td>9.26%</td></tr>
<tr><td>19</td><td>Arizona</td><td>9,612</td><td>1.84%</td><td>3</td><td>Florida</td><td>27,017</td><td>5.18%</td></tr>
<tr><td>27</td><td>Arkansas</td><td>7,011</td><td>1.34%</td><td>4</td><td>New York</td><td>26,608</td><td>5.10%</td></tr>
<tr><td>1</td><td>California</td><td>69,712</td><td>13.36%</td><td>5</td><td>Illinois</td><td>24,967</td><td>4.78%</td></tr>
<tr><td>28</td><td>Colorado</td><td>5,975</td><td>1.15%</td><td>6</td><td>Ohio</td><td>22,690</td><td>4.35%</td></tr>
<tr><td>33</td><td>Connecticut</td><td>4,038</td><td>0.77%</td><td>7</td><td>Michigan</td><td>20,312</td><td>3.89%</td></tr>
<tr><td>44</td><td>Delaware</td><td>1,277</td><td>0.24%</td><td>8</td><td>Georgia</td><td>18,369</td><td>3.52%</td></tr>
<tr><td>3</td><td>Florida</td><td>27,017</td><td>5.18%</td><td>9</td><td>Pennsylvania</td><td>18,216</td><td>3.49%</td></tr>
<tr><td>8</td><td>Georgia</td><td>18,369</td><td>3.52%</td><td>10</td><td>North Carolina</td><td>16,506</td><td>3.16%</td></tr>
<tr><td>39</td><td>Hawaii</td><td>2,122</td><td>0.41%</td><td>11</td><td>Tennessee</td><td>12,928</td><td>2.48%</td></tr>
<tr><td>40</td><td>Idaho</td><td>2,009</td><td>0.38%</td><td>12</td><td>Indiana</td><td>12,335</td><td>2.36%</td></tr>
<tr><td>5</td><td>Illinois</td><td>24,967</td><td>4.78%</td><td>13</td><td>Louisiana</td><td>12,270</td><td>2.35%</td></tr>
<tr><td>12</td><td>Indiana</td><td>12,335</td><td>2.36%</td><td>14</td><td>Virginia</td><td>11,353</td><td>2.18%</td></tr>
<tr><td>34</td><td>Iowa</td><td>3,989</td><td>0.76%</td><td>15</td><td>Alabama</td><td>11,252</td><td>2.16%</td></tr>
<tr><td>31</td><td>Kansas</td><td>4,722</td><td>0.90%</td><td>16</td><td>Missouri</td><td>11,227</td><td>2.15%</td></tr>
<tr><td>20</td><td>Kentucky</td><td>9,349</td><td>1.79%</td><td>17</td><td>New Jersey</td><td>10,068</td><td>1.93%</td></tr>
<tr><td>13</td><td>Louisiana</td><td>12,270</td><td>2.35%</td><td>18</td><td>South Carolina</td><td>9,721</td><td>1.86%</td></tr>
<tr><td>41</td><td>Maine</td><td>1,857</td><td>0.36%</td><td>19</td><td>Arizona</td><td>9,612</td><td>1.84%</td></tr>
<tr><td>23</td><td>Maryland</td><td>8,143</td><td>1.56%</td><td>20</td><td>Kentucky</td><td>9,349</td><td>1.79%</td></tr>
<tr><td>26</td><td>Massachusetts</td><td>7,266</td><td>1.39%</td><td>21</td><td>Mississippi</td><td>8,909</td><td>1.71%</td></tr>
<tr><td>7</td><td>Michigan</td><td>20,312</td><td>3.89%</td><td>22</td><td>Washington</td><td>8,397</td><td>1.61%</td></tr>
<tr><td>29</td><td>Minnesota</td><td>5,342</td><td>1.02%</td><td>23</td><td>Maryland</td><td>8,143</td><td>1.56%</td></tr>
<tr><td>21</td><td>Mississippi</td><td>8,909</td><td>1.71%</td><td>24</td><td>Oklahoma</td><td>7,590</td><td>1.45%</td></tr>
<tr><td>16</td><td>Missouri</td><td>11,227</td><td>2.15%</td><td>25</td><td>Wisconsin</td><td>7,281</td><td>1.40%</td></tr>
<tr><td>43</td><td>Montana</td><td>1,331</td><td>0.26%</td><td>26</td><td>Massachusetts</td><td>7,266</td><td>1.39%</td></tr>
<tr><td>38</td><td>Nebraska</td><td>2,352</td><td>0.45%</td><td>27</td><td>Arkansas</td><td>7,011</td><td>1.34%</td></tr>
<tr><td>37</td><td>Nevada</td><td>2,663</td><td>0.51%</td><td>28</td><td>Colorado</td><td>5,975</td><td>1.15%</td></tr>
<tr><td>45</td><td>New Hampshire</td><td>1,258</td><td>0.24%</td><td>29</td><td>Minnesota</td><td>5,342</td><td>1.02%</td></tr>
<tr><td>17</td><td>New Jersey</td><td>10,068</td><td>1.93%</td><td>30</td><td>Oregon</td><td>5,084</td><td>0.97%</td></tr>
<tr><td>32</td><td>New Mexico</td><td>4,367</td><td>0.84%</td><td>31</td><td>Kansas</td><td>4,722</td><td>0.90%</td></tr>
<tr><td>4</td><td>New York</td><td>26,608</td><td>5.10%</td><td>32</td><td>New Mexico</td><td>4,367</td><td>0.84%</td></tr>
<tr><td>10</td><td>North Carolina</td><td>16,506</td><td>3.16%</td><td>33</td><td>Connecticut</td><td>4,038</td><td>0.77%</td></tr>
<tr><td>49</td><td>North Dakota</td><td>793</td><td>0.15%</td><td>34</td><td>Iowa</td><td>3,989</td><td>0.76%</td></tr>
<tr><td>6</td><td>Ohio</td><td>22,690</td><td>4.35%</td><td>35</td><td>West Virginia</td><td>3,976</td><td>0.76%</td></tr>
<tr><td>24</td><td>Oklahoma</td><td>7,590</td><td>1.45%</td><td>36</td><td>Utah</td><td>3,707</td><td>0.71%</td></tr>
<tr><td>30</td><td>Oregon</td><td>5,084</td><td>0.97%</td><td>37</td><td>Nevada</td><td>2,663</td><td>0.51%</td></tr>
<tr><td>9</td><td>Pennsylvania</td><td>18,216</td><td>3.49%</td><td>38</td><td>Nebraska</td><td>2,352</td><td>0.45%</td></tr>
<tr><td>42</td><td>Rhode Island</td><td>1,564</td><td>0.30%</td><td>39</td><td>Hawaii</td><td>2,122</td><td>0.41%</td></tr>
<tr><td>18</td><td>South Carolina</td><td>9,721</td><td>1.86%</td><td>40</td><td>Idaho</td><td>2,009</td><td>0.38%</td></tr>
<tr><td>46</td><td>South Dakota</td><td>1,172</td><td>0.22%</td><td>41</td><td>Maine</td><td>1,857</td><td>0.36%</td></tr>
<tr><td>11</td><td>Tennessee</td><td>12,928</td><td>2.48%</td><td>42</td><td>Rhode Island</td><td>1,564</td><td>0.30%</td></tr>
<tr><td>2</td><td>Texas</td><td>48,302</td><td>9.26%</td><td>43</td><td>Montana</td><td>1,331</td><td>0.26%</td></tr>
<tr><td>36</td><td>Utah</td><td>3,707</td><td>0.71%</td><td>44</td><td>Delaware</td><td>1,277</td><td>0.24%</td></tr>
<tr><td>50</td><td>Vermont</td><td>702</td><td>0.13%</td><td>45</td><td>New Hampshire</td><td>1,258</td><td>0.24%</td></tr>
<tr><td>14</td><td>Virginia</td><td>11,353</td><td>2.18%</td><td>46</td><td>South Dakota</td><td>1,172</td><td>0.22%</td></tr>
<tr><td>22</td><td>Washington</td><td>8,397</td><td>1.61%</td><td>47</td><td>Alaska</td><td>1,142</td><td>0.22%</td></tr>
<tr><td>35</td><td>West Virginia</td><td>3,976</td><td>0.76%</td><td>48</td><td>Wyoming</td><td>943</td><td>0.18%</td></tr>
<tr><td>25</td><td>Wisconsin</td><td>7,281</td><td>1.40%</td><td>49</td><td>North Dakota</td><td>793</td><td>0.15%</td></tr>
<tr><td>48</td><td>Wyoming</td><td>943</td><td>0.18%</td><td>50</td><td>Vermont</td><td>702</td><td>0.13%</td></tr>
<tr><td></td><td></td><td></td><td></td><td></td><td>District of Columbia</td><td>2,030</td><td>0.39%</td></tr>
</table>

Source: U.S. Department of Health and Human Services, Centers for Disease Control and Prevention
    "Surveillance for Pregnancy and Birth Rates Among Teenagers" (MMWR, Vol. 42, No. SS-6, 12/17/93)
*Women aged 15 to 19 years old.

Teenage Birth Rate in 1990

National Rate = 59.9 Live Births per 1,000 Teenage Women*

ALPHA ORDER				RANK ORDER		
RANK	STATE	RATE		RANK	STATE	RATE
11	Alabama	71.0		1	Mississippi	81.0
17	Alaska	65.3		2	Arkansas	80.1
4	Arizona	75.5		3	New Mexico	78.2
2	Arkansas	80.1		4	Arizona	75.5
12	California	70.6		4	Georgia	75.5
28	Colorado	54.5		6	Texas	75.3
45	Connecticut	38.8		7	Louisiana	74.2
28	Delaware	54.5		8	Nevada	73.3
13	Florida	69.1		9	Tennessee	72.3
4	Georgia	75.5		10	South Carolina	71.3
20	Hawaii	61.2		11	Alabama	71.0
33	Idaho	50.6		12	California	70.6
18	Illinois	62.9		13	Florida	69.1
22	Indiana	58.6		14	Kentucky	67.6
43	Iowa	40.5		14	North Carolina	67.6
26	Kansas	56.1		16	Oklahoma	66.8
14	Kentucky	67.6		17	Alaska	65.3
7	Louisiana	74.2		18	Illinois	62.9
40	Maine	43.0		19	Missouri	62.8
30	Maryland	53.2		20	Hawaii	61.2
48	Massachusetts	35.1		21	Michigan	59.0
21	Michigan	59.0		22	Indiana	58.6
46	Minnesota	36.3		23	Ohio	57.9
1	Mississippi	81.0		24	West Virginia	57.3
19	Missouri	62.8		25	Wyoming	56.3
35	Montana	48.4		26	Kansas	56.1
42	Nebraska	42.3		27	Oregon	54.6
8	Nevada	73.3		28	Colorado	54.5
50	New Hampshire	33.0		28	Delaware	54.5
43	New Jersey	40.5		30	Maryland	53.2
3	New Mexico	78.2		31	Washington	53.1
39	New York	43.6		32	Virginia	52.9
14	North Carolina	67.6		33	Idaho	50.6
47	North Dakota	35.4		34	Utah	48.5
23	Ohio	57.9		35	Montana	48.4
16	Oklahoma	66.8		36	South Dakota	46.8
27	Oregon	54.6		37	Pennsylvania	44.9
37	Pennsylvania	44.9		38	Rhode Island	43.9
38	Rhode Island	43.9		39	New York	43.6
10	South Carolina	71.3		40	Maine	43.0
36	South Dakota	46.8		41	Wisconsin	42.6
9	Tennessee	72.3		42	Nebraska	42.3
6	Texas	75.3		43	Iowa	40.5
34	Utah	48.5		43	New Jersey	40.5
49	Vermont	34.0		45	Connecticut	38.8
32	Virginia	52.9		46	Minnesota	36.3
31	Washington	53.1		47	North Dakota	35.4
24	West Virginia	57.3		48	Massachusetts	35.1
41	Wisconsin	42.6		49	Vermont	34.0
25	Wyoming	56.3		50	New Hampshire	33.0
					District of Columbia	93.1

Source: U.S. Department of Health and Human Services, Centers for Disease Control and Prevention
   "Surveillance for Pregnancy and Birth Rates Among Teenagers" (MMWR, Vol. 42, No. SS-6, 12/17/93)
Women aged 15 to 19 years old.

Percent Change in Teenage Birth Rate: 1990 to 1994

National Percent Change = 1.67% Decrease*

ALPHA ORDER

RANK	STATE	PERCENT CHANGE
9	Alabama	1.69
49	Alaska	(15.47)
5	Arizona	4.24
29	Arkansas	(4.74)
11	California	0.99
15	Colorado	(0.37)
6	Connecticut	3.87
1	Delaware	10.46
37	Florida	(6.80)
31	Georgia	(5.03)
46	Hawaii	(12.58)
39	Idaho	(7.91)
14	Illinois	(0.16)
17	Indiana	(1.19)
21	Iowa	(1.98)
28	Kansas	(4.63)
27	Kentucky	(4.59)
12	Louisiana	0.67
50	Maine	(17.44)
35	Maryland	(6.58)
3	Massachusetts	5.98
44	Michigan	(11.69)
32	Minnesota	(5.23)
8	Mississippi	2.47
34	Missouri	(6.05)
48	Montana	(14.88)
10	Nebraska	1.18
13	Nevada	0.41
41	New Hampshire	(8.79)
25	New Jersey	(2.96)
16	New Mexico	(1.02)
4	New York	5.05
20	North Carolina	(1.92)
22	North Dakota	(2.26)
30	Ohio	(5.01)
18	Oklahoma	(1.35)
38	Oregon	(7.14)
23	Pennsylvania	(2.45)
2	Rhode Island	8.66
36	South Carolina	(6.73)
40	South Dakota	(8.55)
19	Tennessee	(1.80)
7	Texas	3.05
45	Utah	(11.96)
24	Vermont	(2.94)
26	Virginia	(4.16)
43	Washington	(9.23)
33	West Virginia	(5.24)
42	Wisconsin	(8.92)
47	Wyoming	(14.39)

RANK ORDER

RANK	STATE	PERCENT CHANGE
1	Delaware	10.46
2	Rhode Island	8.66
3	Massachusetts	5.98
4	New York	5.05
5	Arizona	4.24
6	Connecticut	3.87
7	Texas	3.05
8	Mississippi	2.47
9	Alabama	1.69
10	Nebraska	1.18
11	California	0.99
12	Louisiana	0.67
13	Nevada	0.41
14	Illinois	(0.16)
15	Colorado	(0.37)
16	New Mexico	(1.02)
17	Indiana	(1.19)
18	Oklahoma	(1.35)
19	Tennessee	(1.80)
20	North Carolina	(1.92)
21	Iowa	(1.98)
22	North Dakota	(2.26)
23	Pennsylvania	(2.45)
24	Vermont	(2.94)
25	New Jersey	(2.96)
26	Virginia	(4.16)
27	Kentucky	(4.59)
28	Kansas	(4.63)
29	Arkansas	(4.74)
30	Ohio	(5.01)
31	Georgia	(5.03)
32	Minnesota	(5.23)
33	West Virginia	(5.24)
34	Missouri	(6.05)
35	Maryland	(6.58)
36	South Carolina	(6.73)
37	Florida	(6.80)
38	Oregon	(7.14)
39	Idaho	(7.91)
40	South Dakota	(8.55)
41	New Hampshire	(8.79)
42	Wisconsin	(8.92)
43	Washington	(9.23)
44	Michigan	(11.69)
45	Utah	(11.96)
46	Hawaii	(12.58)
47	Wyoming	(14.39)
48	Montana	(14.88)
49	Alaska	(15.47)
50	Maine	(17.44)

District of Columbia   23.20

Source: Morgan Quitno Press using data from U.S. Department of Health and Human Services
"Monthly Vital Statistics Report" (Vol. 45, No. 5(S), December 19, 1996) and
"Surveillance for Pregnancy and Birth Rates Among Teenagers" (MMWR, Vol. 42, No. SS-6, 12/17/93)
*Women aged 15 to 19 years old.

Births to Teenage Mothers in 1980

National Total = 562,330 Live Births*

ALPHA ORDER

RANK	STATE	BIRTHS	% of USA
15	Alabama	13,096	2.33%
49	Alaska	1,123	0.20%
25	Arizona	8,235	1.46%
26	Arkansas	8,060	1.43%
1	California	56,138	9.98%
29	Colorado	6,592	1.17%
36	Connecticut	4,408	0.78%
45	Delaware	1,572	0.28%
6	Florida	24,042	4.28%
9	Georgia	19,137	3.40%
40	Hawaii	2,085	0.37%
38	Idaho	2,645	0.47%
3	Illinois	29,798	5.30%
12	Indiana	15,331	2.73%
31	Iowa	5,962	1.06%
30	Kansas	6,090	1.08%
16	Kentucky	12,559	2.23%
10	Louisiana	16,504	2.93%
39	Maine	2,522	0.45%
23	Maryland	8,885	1.58%
27	Massachusetts	7,765	1.38%
8	Michigan	20,401	3.63%
28	Minnesota	7,048	1.25%
19	Mississippi	11,079	1.97%
14	Missouri	13,312	2.37%
43	Montana	1,761	0.31%
37	Nebraska	3,313	0.59%
41	Nevada	2,048	0.36%
47	New Hampshire	1,475	0.26%
18	New Jersey	11,904	2.12%
34	New Mexico	4,758	0.85%
4	New York	28,206	5.02%
11	North Carolina	16,192	2.88%
48	North Dakota	1,304	0.23%
5	Ohio	26,567	4.72%
21	Oklahoma	10,206	1.81%
33	Oregon	5,731	1.02%
7	Pennsylvania	22,029	3.92%
46	Rhode Island	1,502	0.27%
20	South Carolina	10,282	1.83%
42	South Dakota	1,797	0.32%
13	Tennessee	13,792	2.45%
2	Texas	50,125	8.91%
35	Utah	4,594	0.82%
50	Vermont	1,024	0.18%
17	Virginia	12,138	2.16%
24	Washington	8,495	1.51%
32	West Virginia	5,911	1.05%
22	Wisconsin	9,220	1.64%
44	Wyoming	1,634	0.29%

RANK ORDER

RANK	STATE	BIRTHS	% of USA
1	California	56,138	9.98%
2	Texas	50,125	8.91%
3	Illinois	29,798	5.30%
4	New York	28,206	5.02%
5	Ohio	26,567	4.72%
6	Florida	24,042	4.28%
7	Pennsylvania	22,029	3.92%
8	Michigan	20,401	3.63%
9	Georgia	19,137	3.40%
10	Louisiana	16,504	2.93%
11	North Carolina	16,192	2.88%
12	Indiana	15,331	2.73%
13	Tennessee	13,792	2.45%
14	Missouri	13,312	2.37%
15	Alabama	13,096	2.33%
16	Kentucky	12,559	2.23%
17	Virginia	12,138	2.16%
18	New Jersey	11,904	2.12%
19	Mississippi	11,079	1.97%
20	South Carolina	10,282	1.83%
21	Oklahoma	10,206	1.81%
22	Wisconsin	9,220	1.64%
23	Maryland	8,885	1.58%
24	Washington	8,495	1.51%
25	Arizona	8,235	1.46%
26	Arkansas	8,060	1.43%
27	Massachusetts	7,765	1.38%
28	Minnesota	7,048	1.25%
29	Colorado	6,592	1.17%
30	Kansas	6,090	1.08%
31	Iowa	5,962	1.06%
32	West Virginia	5,911	1.05%
33	Oregon	5,731	1.02%
34	New Mexico	4,758	0.85%
35	Utah	4,594	0.82%
36	Connecticut	4,408	0.78%
37	Nebraska	3,313	0.59%
38	Idaho	2,645	0.47%
39	Maine	2,522	0.45%
40	Hawaii	2,085	0.37%
41	Nevada	2,048	0.36%
42	South Dakota	1,797	0.32%
43	Montana	1,761	0.31%
44	Wyoming	1,634	0.29%
45	Delaware	1,572	0.28%
46	Rhode Island	1,502	0.27%
47	New Hampshire	1,475	0.26%
48	North Dakota	1,304	0.23%
49	Alaska	1,123	0.20%
50	Vermont	1,024	0.18%
	District of Columbia	1,933	0.34%

Source: U.S. Department of Health and Human Services, National Center for Health Statistics
"Vital Statistics of the United States, 1980" (Vol. I-Natality, issued 1984)
*Births to women age 15 to 19 years old.

Teenage Birth Rate in 1980

National Rate = 53.0 Live Births per 1,000 Teenage Women*

ALPHA ORDER

RANK	STATE	RATE
10	Alabama	68.3
15	Alaska	64.4
12	Arizona	65.5
5	Arkansas	74.5
25	California	53.3
31	Colorado	49.9
49	Connecticut	30.5
28	Delaware	51.2
18	Florida	58.5
8	Georgia	71.9
30	Hawaii	50.7
17	Idaho	59.5
24	Illinois	55.8
21	Indiana	57.5
39	Iowa	43.0
23	Kansas	56.8
7	Kentucky	72.3
3	Louisiana	76.0
34	Maine	47.4
38	Maryland	43.4
50	Massachusetts	28.1
37	Michigan	45.0
44	Minnesota	35.4
1	Mississippi	83.7
20	Missouri	57.8
32	Montana	48.5
36	Nebraska	45.1
18	Nevada	58.5
47	New Hampshire	33.6
45	New Jersey	35.2
9	New Mexico	71.8
46	New York	34.8
21	North Carolina	57.5
40	North Dakota	41.7
27	Ohio	52.5
4	Oklahoma	74.6
29	Oregon	50.9
41	Pennsylvania	40.5
48	Rhode Island	33.0
14	South Carolina	64.8
26	South Dakota	52.6
16	Tennessee	64.1
6	Texas	74.3
13	Utah	65.2
42	Vermont	39.5
33	Virginia	48.3
35	Washington	46.7
11	West Virginia	67.8
42	Wisconsin	39.5
2	Wyoming	78.7

RANK ORDER

RANK	STATE	RATE
1	Mississippi	83.7
2	Wyoming	78.7
3	Louisiana	76.0
4	Oklahoma	74.6
5	Arkansas	74.5
6	Texas	74.3
7	Kentucky	72.3
8	Georgia	71.9
9	New Mexico	71.8
10	Alabama	68.3
11	West Virginia	67.8
12	Arizona	65.5
13	Utah	65.2
14	South Carolina	64.8
15	Alaska	64.4
16	Tennessee	64.1
17	Idaho	59.5
18	Florida	58.5
18	Nevada	58.5
20	Missouri	57.8
21	Indiana	57.5
21	North Carolina	57.5
23	Kansas	56.8
24	Illinois	55.8
25	California	53.3
26	South Dakota	52.6
27	Ohio	52.5
28	Delaware	51.2
29	Oregon	50.9
30	Hawaii	50.7
31	Colorado	49.9
32	Montana	48.5
33	Virginia	48.3
34	Maine	47.4
35	Washington	46.7
36	Nebraska	45.1
37	Michigan	45.0
38	Maryland	43.4
39	Iowa	43.0
40	North Dakota	41.7
41	Pennsylvania	40.5
42	Vermont	39.5
42	Wisconsin	39.5
44	Minnesota	35.4
45	New Jersey	35.2
46	New York	34.8
47	New Hampshire	33.6
48	Rhode Island	33.0
49	Connecticut	30.5
50	Massachusetts	28.1
	District of Columbia	62.4

Source: U.S. Department of Health and Human Services, Centers for Disease Control and Prevention
   "Surveillance for Pregnancy and Birth Rates Among Teenagers" (MMWR, Vol. 42, No. SS-6, 12/17/93)
*Women aged 15 to 19 years old.

Births to Women 35 to 49 Years Old in 1994

National Total = 437,617 Live Births*

ALPHA ORDER

RANK	STATE	BIRTHS	% of USA
26	Alabama	4,374	1.00%
44	Alaska	1,318	0.30%
20	Arizona	6,876	1.57%
38	Arkansas	2,116	0.48%
1	California	72,370	16.54%
19	Colorado	7,049	1.61%
18	Connecticut	7,094	1.62%
46	Delaware	1,100	0.25%
5	Florida	21,366	4.88%
12	Georgia	10,158	2.32%
33	Hawaii	2,698	0.62%
40	Idaho	1,662	0.38%
4	Illinois	21,500	4.91%
22	Indiana	6,655	1.52%
31	Iowa	3,433	0.78%
29	Kansas	3,693	0.84%
28	Kentucky	3,872	0.88%
24	Louisiana	5,330	1.22%
43	Maine	1,475	0.34%
13	Maryland	10,061	2.30%
10	Massachusetts	13,108	3.00%
9	Michigan	13,997	3.20%
16	Minnesota	7,858	1.80%
34	Mississippi	2,656	0.61%
21	Missouri	6,721	1.54%
45	Montana	1,266	0.29%
36	Nebraska	2,366	0.54%
37	Nevada	2,354	0.54%
39	New Hampshire	2,005	0.46%
7	New Jersey	18,433	4.21%
35	New Mexico	2,615	0.60%
2	New York	40,409	9.23%
15	North Carolina	8,857	2.02%
49	North Dakota	855	0.20%
8	Ohio	15,241	3.48%
32	Oklahoma	3,360	0.77%
25	Oregon	4,722	1.08%
6	Pennsylvania	19,026	4.35%
41	Rhode Island	1,659	0.38%
27	South Carolina	4,369	1.00%
47	South Dakota	1,022	0.23%
23	Tennessee	5,616	1.28%
3	Texas	28,698	6.56%
30	Utah	3,524	0.81%
48	Vermont	1,012	0.23%
11	Virginia	11,484	2.62%
14	Washington	9,463	2.16%
42	West Virginia	1,505	0.34%
17	Wisconsin	7,288	1.67%
50	Wyoming	611	0.14%

RANK ORDER

RANK	STATE	BIRTHS	% of USA
1	California	72,370	16.54%
2	New York	40,409	9.23%
3	Texas	28,698	6.56%
4	Illinois	21,500	4.91%
5	Florida	21,366	4.88%
6	Pennsylvania	19,026	4.35%
7	New Jersey	18,433	4.21%
8	Ohio	15,241	3.48%
9	Michigan	13,997	3.20%
10	Massachusetts	13,108	3.00%
11	Virginia	11,484	2.62%
12	Georgia	10,158	2.32%
13	Maryland	10,061	2.30%
14	Washington	9,463	2.16%
15	North Carolina	8,857	2.02%
16	Minnesota	7,858	1.80%
17	Wisconsin	7,288	1.67%
18	Connecticut	7,094	1.62%
19	Colorado	7,049	1.61%
20	Arizona	6,876	1.57%
21	Missouri	6,721	1.54%
22	Indiana	6,655	1.52%
23	Tennessee	5,616	1.28%
24	Louisiana	5,330	1.22%
25	Oregon	4,722	1.08%
26	Alabama	4,374	1.00%
27	South Carolina	4,369	1.00%
28	Kentucky	3,872	0.88%
29	Kansas	3,693	0.84%
30	Utah	3,524	0.81%
31	Iowa	3,433	0.78%
32	Oklahoma	3,360	0.77%
33	Hawaii	2,698	0.62%
34	Mississippi	2,656	0.61%
35	New Mexico	2,615	0.60%
36	Nebraska	2,366	0.54%
37	Nevada	2,354	0.54%
38	Arkansas	2,116	0.48%
39	New Hampshire	2,005	0.46%
40	Idaho	1,662	0.38%
41	Rhode Island	1,659	0.38%
42	West Virginia	1,505	0.34%
43	Maine	1,475	0.34%
44	Alaska	1,318	0.30%
45	Montana	1,266	0.29%
46	Delaware	1,100	0.25%
47	South Dakota	1,022	0.23%
48	Vermont	1,012	0.23%
49	North Dakota	855	0.20%
50	Wyoming	611	0.14%
	District of Columbia	1,317	0.30%

Source: Morgan Quitno Press using data from U.S. Dept of Health & Human Services, National Center for Health Statistics
(unpublished data)
*By state of residence.

Births to Women 35 to 49 Years Old as a Percent of All Births in 1994

National Percent = 11.07% of Live Births*

RANK	STATE	PERCENT
47	Alabama	7.18
11	Alaska	12.34
31	Arizona	9.71
50	Arkansas	6.09
10	California	12.74
9	Colorado	13.04
3	Connecticut	15.54
22	Delaware	10.57
20	Florida	11.21
37	Georgia	9.15
5	Hawaii	13.82
33	Idaho	9.48
18	Illinois	11.36
42	Indiana	8.06
35	Iowa	9.26
27	Kansas	9.88
46	Kentucky	7.31
43	Louisiana	7.86
24	Maine	10.21
7	Maryland	13.60
2	Massachusetts	15.64
25	Michigan	10.14
14	Minnesota	12.22
49	Mississippi	6.33
38	Missouri	9.14
17	Montana	11.44
23	Nebraska	10.22
28	Nevada	9.84
8	New Hampshire	13.27
1	New Jersey	15.69
33	New Mexico	9.48
4	New York	14.52
40	North Carolina	8.73
26	North Dakota	9.96
29	Ohio	9.77
45	Oklahoma	7.35
19	Oregon	11.29
15	Pennsylvania	12.11
12	Rhode Island	12.32
41	South Carolina	8.39
30	South Dakota	9.73
44	Tennessee	7.67
39	Texas	8.94
36	Utah	9.21
6	Vermont	13.72
16	Virginia	12.08
13	Washington	12.23
48	West Virginia	7.04
21	Wisconsin	10.67
32	Wyoming	9.51

RANK	STATE	PERCENT
1	New Jersey	15.69
2	Massachusetts	15.64
3	Connecticut	15.54
4	New York	14.52
5	Hawaii	13.82
6	Vermont	13.72
7	Maryland	13.60
8	New Hampshire	13.27
9	Colorado	13.04
10	California	12.74
11	Alaska	12.34
12	Rhode Island	12.32
13	Washington	12.23
14	Minnesota	12.22
15	Pennsylvania	12.11
16	Virginia	12.08
17	Montana	11.44
18	Illinois	11.36
19	Oregon	11.29
20	Florida	11.21
21	Wisconsin	10.67
22	Delaware	10.57
23	Nebraska	10.22
24	Maine	10.21
25	Michigan	10.14
26	North Dakota	9.96
27	Kansas	9.88
28	Nevada	9.84
29	Ohio	9.77
30	South Dakota	9.73
31	Arizona	9.71
32	Wyoming	9.51
33	Idaho	9.48
33	New Mexico	9.48
35	Iowa	9.26
36	Utah	9.21
37	Georgia	9.15
38	Missouri	9.14
39	Texas	8.94
40	North Carolina	8.73
41	South Carolina	8.39
42	Indiana	8.06
43	Louisiana	7.86
44	Tennessee	7.67
45	Oklahoma	7.35
46	Kentucky	7.31
47	Alabama	7.18
48	West Virginia	7.04
49	Mississippi	6.33
50	Arkansas	6.09
	District of Columbia	13.26

Source: Morgan Quitno Press using data from U.S. Dept of Health & Human Services, National Center for Health Statistics (unpublished data)
By state of residence.

Births by Vaginal Delivery in 1994

National Total = 3,087,576 Live Births*

ALPHA ORDER

RANK	STATE	BIRTHS	% of USA
23	Alabama	46,709	1.51%
45	Alaska	8,900	0.29%
16	Arizona	58,742	1.90%
34	Arkansas	25,566	0.83%
1	California	449,842	14.57%
24	Colorado	45,768	1.48%
28	Connecticut	33,812	1.10%
47	Delaware	8,128	0.26%
5	Florida	147,749	4.79%
10	Georgia	87,060	2.82%
39	Hawaii	16,024	0.52%
40	Idaho	14,816	0.48%
4	Illinois	150,668	4.88%
14	Indiana	64,933	2.10%
31	Iowa	29,917	0.97%
33	Kansas	28,924	0.94%
26	Kentucky	39,527	1.28%
22	Louisiana	48,527	1.57%
42	Maine	11,348	0.37%
20	Maryland	57,076	1.85%
13	Massachusetts	66,323	2.15%
8	Michigan	108,801	3.52%
21	Minnesota	52,426	1.70%
30	Mississippi	30,887	1.00%
17	Missouri	57,984	1.88%
44	Montana	8,922	0.29%
37	Nebraska	18,792	0.61%
36	Nevada	19,214	0.62%
41	New Hampshire	12,167	0.39%
9	New Jersey	89,025	2.88%
35	New Mexico	22,696	0.74%
3	New York	209,050	6.77%
11	North Carolina	78,763	2.55%
48	North Dakota	6,836	0.22%
7	Ohio	122,659	3.97%
32	Oklahoma	29,409	0.95%
27	Oregon	34,465	1.12%
6	Pennsylvania	125,042	4.05%
43	Rhode Island	11,096	0.36%
25	South Carolina	39,899	1.29%
46	South Dakota	8,192	0.27%
19	Tennessee	57,477	1.86%
2	Texas	241,628	7.83%
29	Utah	31,050	1.01%
49	Vermont	6,111	0.20%
12	Virginia	73,883	2.39%
15	Washington	63,983	2.07%
38	West Virginia	16,232	0.53%
18	Wisconsin	57,547	1.86%
50	Wyoming	5,276	0.17%

RANK ORDER

RANK	STATE	BIRTHS	% of USA
1	California	449,842	14.57%
2	Texas	241,628	7.83%
3	New York	209,050	6.77%
4	Illinois	150,668	4.88%
5	Florida	147,749	4.79%
6	Pennsylvania	125,042	4.05%
7	Ohio	122,659	3.97%
8	Michigan	108,801	3.52%
9	New Jersey	89,025	2.88%
10	Georgia	87,060	2.82%
11	North Carolina	78,763	2.55%
12	Virginia	73,883	2.39%
13	Massachusetts	66,323	2.15%
14	Indiana	64,933	2.10%
15	Washington	63,983	2.07%
16	Arizona	58,742	1.90%
17	Missouri	57,984	1.88%
18	Wisconsin	57,547	1.86%
19	Tennessee	57,477	1.86%
20	Maryland	57,076	1.85%
21	Minnesota	52,426	1.70%
22	Louisiana	48,527	1.57%
23	Alabama	46,709	1.51%
24	Colorado	45,768	1.48%
25	South Carolina	39,899	1.29%
26	Kentucky	39,527	1.28%
27	Oregon	34,465	1.12%
28	Connecticut	33,812	1.10%
29	Utah	31,050	1.01%
30	Mississippi	30,887	1.00%
31	Iowa	29,917	0.97%
32	Oklahoma	29,409	0.95%
33	Kansas	28,924	0.94%
34	Arkansas	25,566	0.83%
35	New Mexico	22,696	0.74%
36	Nevada	19,214	0.62%
37	Nebraska	18,792	0.61%
38	West Virginia	16,232	0.53%
39	Hawaii	16,024	0.52%
40	Idaho	14,816	0.48%
41	New Hampshire	12,167	0.39%
42	Maine	11,348	0.37%
43	Rhode Island	11,096	0.36%
44	Montana	8,922	0.29%
45	Alaska	8,900	0.29%
46	South Dakota	8,192	0.27%
47	Delaware	8,128	0.26%
48	North Dakota	6,836	0.22%
49	Vermont	6,111	0.20%
50	Wyoming	5,276	0.17%
	District of Columbia	7,705	0.25%

Source: U.S. Department of Health and Human Services, National Center for Health Statistics unpublished data

Includes VBACs (vaginal births after cesarean).

Percent of Births by Vaginal Delivery in 1994

National Percent = 78.80% of Live Births*

ALPHA ORDER

RANK	STATE	PERCENT
42	Alabama	76.79
5	Alaska	83.73
7	Arizona	83.17
48	Arkansas	74.08
28	California	79.22
1	Colorado	84.75
18	Connecticut	80.88
35	Delaware	78.14
38	Florida	77.85
33	Georgia	78.73
10	Hawaii	82.77
2	Idaho	84.74
22	Illinois	79.87
31	Indiana	78.84
17	Iowa	80.96
26	Kansas	79.29
39	Kentucky	77.54
50	Louisiana	71.68
26	Maine	79.29
40	Maryland	77.37
24	Massachusetts	79.33
24	Michigan	79.33
6	Minnesota	83.48
49	Mississippi	73.77
28	Missouri	79.22
16	Montana	81.00
15	Nebraska	81.29
19	Nevada	80.78
20	New Hampshire	80.71
46	New Jersey	76.06
12	New Mexico	82.63
41	New York	77.13
37	North Carolina	77.92
21	North Dakota	79.93
30	Ohio	79.02
43	Oklahoma	76.78
13	Oregon	82.59
23	Pennsylvania	79.80
11	Rhode Island	82.66
43	South Carolina	76.78
32	South Dakota	78.82
34	Tennessee	78.72
47	Texas	75.60
4	Utah	83.80
9	Vermont	82.87
36	Virginia	78.03
8	Washington	83.11
45	West Virginia	76.15
3	Wisconsin	84.33
14	Wyoming	82.19

RANK ORDER

RANK	STATE	PERCENT
1	Colorado	84.75
2	Idaho	84.74
3	Wisconsin	84.33
4	Utah	83.80
5	Alaska	83.73
6	Minnesota	83.48
7	Arizona	83.17
8	Washington	83.11
9	Vermont	82.87
10	Hawaii	82.77
11	Rhode Island	82.66
12	New Mexico	82.63
13	Oregon	82.59
14	Wyoming	82.19
15	Nebraska	81.29
16	Montana	81.00
17	Iowa	80.96
18	Connecticut	80.88
19	Nevada	80.78
20	New Hampshire	80.71
21	North Dakota	79.93
22	Illinois	79.87
23	Pennsylvania	79.80
24	Massachusetts	79.33
24	Michigan	79.33
26	Kansas	79.29
26	Maine	79.29
28	California	79.22
28	Missouri	79.22
30	Ohio	79.02
31	Indiana	78.84
32	South Dakota	78.82
33	Georgia	78.73
34	Tennessee	78.72
35	Delaware	78.14
36	Virginia	78.03
37	North Carolina	77.92
38	Florida	77.85
39	Kentucky	77.54
40	Maryland	77.37
41	New York	77.13
42	Alabama	76.79
43	Oklahoma	76.78
43	South Carolina	76.78
45	West Virginia	76.15
46	New Jersey	76.06
47	Texas	75.60
48	Arkansas	74.08
49	Mississippi	73.77
50	Louisiana	71.68
	District of Columbia	77.62

Source: U.S. Department of Health and Human Services, National Center for Health Statistics
   unpublished data

*Of those births for which delivery data are available. Includes VBACs (vaginal births after cesarean).

Births by Cesarean Delivery in 1994

National Total = 830,517 Live Cesarean Births

ALPHA ORDER					RANK ORDER			
RANK	STATE	BIRTHS	% of USA		RANK	STATE	BIRTHS	% of USA
19	Alabama	14,115	1.70%		1	California	117,998	14.21%
47	Alaska	1,729	0.21%		2	Texas	78,003	9.39%
22	Arizona	11,888	1.43%		3	New York	62,001	7.47%
27	Arkansas	8,944	1.08%		4	Florida	42,038	5.06%
1	California	117,998	14.21%		5	Illinois	37,985	4.57%
29	Colorado	8,238	0.99%		6	Ohio	32,576	3.92%
30	Connecticut	7,991	0.96%		7	Pennsylvania	31,662	3.81%
44	Delaware	2,274	0.27%		8	Michigan	28,352	3.41%
4	Florida	42,038	5.06%		9	New Jersey	28,023	3.37%
10	Georgia	23,521	2.83%		10	Georgia	23,521	2.83%
39	Hawaii	3,335	0.40%		11	North Carolina	22,316	2.69%
42	Idaho	2,669	0.32%		12	Virginia	20,804	2.50%
5	Illinois	37,985	4.57%		13	Louisiana	19,176	2.31%
14	Indiana	17,430	2.10%		14	Indiana	17,430	2.10%
33	Iowa	7,035	0.85%		15	Massachusetts	17,280	2.08%
31	Kansas	7,555	0.91%		16	Maryland	16,695	2.01%
23	Kentucky	11,448	1.38%		17	Tennessee	15,357	1.85%
13	Louisiana	19,176	2.31%		18	Missouri	15,210	1.83%
40	Maine	2,964	0.36%		19	Alabama	14,115	1.70%
16	Maryland	16,695	2.01%		20	Washington	13,001	1.57%
15	Massachusetts	17,280	2.08%		21	South Carolina	12,066	1.45%
8	Michigan	28,352	3.41%		22	Arizona	11,888	1.43%
26	Minnesota	10,375	1.25%		23	Kentucky	11,448	1.38%
24	Mississippi	10,983	1.32%		24	Mississippi	10,983	1.32%
18	Missouri	15,210	1.83%		25	Wisconsin	10,692	1.29%
46	Montana	2,093	0.25%		26	Minnesota	10,375	1.25%
38	Nebraska	4,325	0.52%		27	Arkansas	8,944	1.08%
37	Nevada	4,573	0.55%		28	Oklahoma	8,894	1.07%
41	New Hampshire	2,908	0.35%		29	Colorado	8,238	0.99%
9	New Jersey	28,023	3.37%		30	Connecticut	7,991	0.96%
36	New Mexico	4,771	0.57%		31	Kansas	7,555	0.91%
3	New York	62,001	7.47%		32	Oregon	7,264	0.87%
11	North Carolina	22,316	2.69%		33	Iowa	7,035	0.85%
48	North Dakota	1,717	0.21%		34	Utah	6,002	0.72%
6	Ohio	32,576	3.92%		35	West Virginia	5,085	0.61%
28	Oklahoma	8,894	1.07%		36	New Mexico	4,771	0.57%
32	Oregon	7,264	0.87%		37	Nevada	4,573	0.55%
7	Pennsylvania	31,662	3.81%		38	Nebraska	4,325	0.52%
43	Rhode Island	2,327	0.28%		39	Hawaii	3,335	0.40%
21	South Carolina	12,066	1.45%		40	Maine	2,964	0.36%
45	South Dakota	2,201	0.27%		41	New Hampshire	2,908	0.35%
17	Tennessee	15,357	1.85%		42	Idaho	2,669	0.32%
2	Texas	78,003	9.39%		43	Rhode Island	2,327	0.28%
34	Utah	6,002	0.72%		44	Delaware	2,274	0.27%
49	Vermont	1,263	0.15%		45	South Dakota	2,201	0.27%
12	Virginia	20,804	2.50%		46	Montana	2,093	0.25%
20	Washington	13,001	1.57%		47	Alaska	1,729	0.21%
35	West Virginia	5,085	0.61%		48	North Dakota	1,717	0.21%
25	Wisconsin	10,692	1.29%		49	Vermont	1,263	0.15%
50	Wyoming	1,143	0.14%		50	Wyoming	1,143	0.14%
						District of Columbia	2,222	0.27%

Source: U.S. Department of Health and Human Services, National Center for Health Statistics unpublished data

Percent of Births by Cesarean Delivery in 1994

National Percent = 21.20% of Live Births*

ALPHA ORDER				RANK ORDER		
RANK	STATE	PERCENT		RANK	STATE	PERCENT
9	Alabama	23.21		1	Louisiana	28.32
46	Alaska	16.27		2	Mississippi	26.23
44	Arizona	16.83		3	Arkansas	25.92
3	Arkansas	25.92		4	Texas	24.40
22	California	20.78		5	New Jersey	23.94
50	Colorado	15.25		6	West Virginia	23.85
33	Connecticut	19.12		7	Oklahoma	23.22
16	Delaware	21.86		7	South Carolina	23.22
13	Florida	22.15		9	Alabama	23.21
17	Georgia	21.27		10	New York	22.87
41	Hawaii	17.23		11	Maryland	22.63
49	Idaho	15.26		12	Kentucky	22.46
29	Illinois	20.13		13	Florida	22.15
19	Indiana	21.16		14	North Carolina	22.08
34	Iowa	19.04		15	Virginia	21.97
24	Kansas	20.71		16	Delaware	21.86
12	Kentucky	22.46		17	Georgia	21.27
1	Louisiana	28.32		18	South Dakota	21.18
24	Maine	20.71		19	Indiana	21.16
11	Maryland	22.63		20	Tennessee	21.08
26	Massachusetts	20.67		21	Ohio	20.98
26	Michigan	20.67		22	California	20.78
45	Minnesota	16.52		22	Missouri	20.78
2	Mississippi	26.23		24	Kansas	20.71
22	Missouri	20.78		24	Maine	20.71
35	Montana	19.00		26	Massachusetts	20.67
36	Nebraska	18.71		26	Michigan	20.67
32	Nevada	19.22		28	Pennsylvania	20.20
31	New Hampshire	19.29		29	Illinois	20.13
5	New Jersey	23.94		30	North Dakota	20.07
39	New Mexico	17.37		31	New Hampshire	19.29
10	New York	22.87		32	Nevada	19.22
14	North Carolina	22.08		33	Connecticut	19.12
30	North Dakota	20.07		34	Iowa	19.04
21	Ohio	20.98		35	Montana	19.00
7	Oklahoma	23.22		36	Nebraska	18.71
38	Oregon	17.41		37	Wyoming	17.81
28	Pennsylvania	20.20		38	Oregon	17.41
40	Rhode Island	17.34		39	New Mexico	17.37
7	South Carolina	23.22		40	Rhode Island	17.34
18	South Dakota	21.18		41	Hawaii	17.23
20	Tennessee	21.08		42	Vermont	17.13
4	Texas	24.40		43	Washington	16.89
47	Utah	16.20		44	Arizona	16.83
42	Vermont	17.13		45	Minnesota	16.52
15	Virginia	21.97		46	Alaska	16.27
43	Washington	16.89		47	Utah	16.20
6	West Virginia	23.85		48	Wisconsin	15.67
48	Wisconsin	15.67		49	Idaho	15.26
37	Wyoming	17.81		50	Colorado	15.25
					District of Columbia	22.38

Source: U.S. Department of Health and Human Services, National Center for Health Statistics
    unpublished data
*Of those births for which delivery data are available.

Percent Change in Rate of Cesarean Births: 1989 to 1994

National Percent Change = 7.0% Decrease*

ALPHA ORDER				RANK ORDER		
RANK	STATE	PERCENT CHANGE		RANK	STATE	PERCENT CHANGE
24	Alabama	(9.3)		1	South Dakota	13.3
2	Alaska	7.0		2	Alaska	7.0
23	Arizona	(9.0)		3	Maine	5.7
10	Arkansas	(4.0)		4	North Dakota	2.9
19	California	(8.1)		5	South Carolina	2.3
39	Colorado	(13.4)		6	Mississippi	1.3
28	Connecticut	(9.8)		7	Indiana	1.2
22	Delaware	(8.9)		8	Texas	(2.4)
40	Florida	(13.5)		9	New York	(3.1)
18	Georgia	(7.5)		10	Arkansas	(4.0)
44	Hawaii	(17.6)		11	Iowa	(4.8)
45	Idaho	(22.1)		12	North Carolina	(5.2)
34	Illinois	(11.3)		13	West Virginia	(5.4)
7	Indiana	1.2		14	Wyoming	(5.8)
11	Iowa	(4.8)		15	Montana	(5.9)
41	Kansas	(13.7)		16	New Jersey	(6.8)
25	Kentucky	(9.4)		17	New Mexico	(7.1)
NA	Louisiana**	NA		18	Georgia	(7.5)
3	Maine	5.7		19	California	(8.1)
NA	Maryland**	NA		20	Vermont	(8.4)
26	Massachusetts	(9.7)		21	Utah	(8.5)
26	Michigan	(9.7)		22	Delaware	(8.9)
32	Minnesota	(11.2)		23	Arizona	(9.0)
6	Mississippi	1.3		24	Alabama	(9.3)
29	Missouri	(10.0)		25	Kentucky	(9.4)
15	Montana	(5.9)		26	Massachusetts	(9.7)
NA	Nebraska**	NA		26	Michigan	(9.7)
NA	Nevada**	NA		28	Connecticut	(9.8)
36	New Hampshire	(13.1)		29	Missouri	(10.0)
16	New Jersey	(6.8)		30	Pennsylvania	(10.2)
17	New Mexico	(7.1)		31	Virginia	(10.3)
9	New York	(3.1)		32	Minnesota	(11.2)
12	North Carolina	(5.2)		32	Oregon	(11.2)
4	North Dakota	2.9		34	Illinois	(11.3)
37	Ohio	(13.3)		35	Wisconsin	(11.5)
NA	Oklahoma**	NA		36	New Hampshire	(13.1)
32	Oregon	(11.2)		37	Ohio	(13.3)
30	Pennsylvania	(10.2)		37	Tennessee	(13.3)
41	Rhode Island	(13.7)		39	Colorado	(13.4)
5	South Carolina	2.3		40	Florida	(13.5)
1	South Dakota	13.3		41	Kansas	(13.7)
37	Tennessee	(13.3)		41	Rhode Island	(13.7)
8	Texas	(2.4)		43	Washington	(16.0)
21	Utah	(8.5)		44	Hawaii	(17.6)
20	Vermont	(8.4)		45	Idaho	(22.1)
31	Virginia	(10.3)		NA	Louisiana**	NA
43	Washington	(16.0)		NA	Maryland**	NA
13	West Virginia	(5.4)		NA	Nebraska**	NA
35	Wisconsin	(11.5)		NA	Nevada**	NA
14	Wyoming	(5.8)		NA	Oklahoma**	NA
					District of Columbia	(17.4)

Source: Morgan Quitno Press using data from US Dept of Health & Human Services, National Center for Health Statistics
    unpublished data

*Of those births for which delivery data are available.

**Not available.

Births by Vaginal Delivery After a Previous Cesarean Delivery (VBAC) in 1994

National Total = 110,341 Live VBAC Births

RANK	STATE	BIRTHS	% of USA
25	Alabama	1,404	1.27%
46	Alaska	359	0.33%
21	Arizona	1,900	1.72%
33	Arkansas	859	0.78%
1	California	12,965	11.75%
23	Colorado	1,608	1.46%
24	Connecticut	1,488	1.35%
45	Delaware	367	0.33%
7	Florida	5,326	4.83%
11	Georgia	2,641	2.39%
39	Hawaii	552	0.50%
37	Idaho	618	0.56%
5	Illinois	5,618	5.09%
19	Indiana	2,045	1.85%
27	Iowa	1,255	1.14%
32	Kansas	896	0.81%
26	Kentucky	1,322	1.20%
29	Louisiana	1,102	1.00%
43	Maine	427	0.39%
16	Maryland	2,432	2.20%
10	Massachusetts	2,770	2.51%
8	Michigan	3,671	3.33%
18	Minnesota	2,098	1.90%
36	Mississippi	707	0.64%
13	Missouri	2,570	2.33%
44	Montana	393	0.36%
35	Nebraska	764	0.69%
38	Nevada	586	0.53%
40	New Hampshire	550	0.50%
9	New Jersey	3,000	2.72%
34	New Mexico	802	0.73%
2	New York	9,652	8.75%
12	North Carolina	2,626	2.38%
49	North Dakota	245	0.22%
6	Ohio	5,438	4.93%
31	Oklahoma	925	0.84%
22	Oregon	1,668	1.51%
4	Pennsylvania	6,017	5.45%
42	Rhode Island	443	0.40%
28	South Carolina	1,168	1.06%
48	South Dakota	268	0.24%
20	Tennessee	1,999	1.81%
3	Texas	7,162	6.49%
30	Utah	1,032	0.94%
47	Vermont	298	0.27%
14	Virginia	2,531	2.29%
15	Washington	2,502	2.27%
41	West Virginia	451	0.41%
17	Wisconsin	2,316	2.10%
50	Wyoming	207	0.19%

RANK	STATE	BIRTHS	% of USA
1	California	12,965	11.75%
2	New York	9,652	8.75%
3	Texas	7,162	6.49%
4	Pennsylvania	6,017	5.45%
5	Illinois	5,618	5.09%
6	Ohio	5,438	4.93%
7	Florida	5,326	4.83%
8	Michigan	3,671	3.33%
9	New Jersey	3,000	2.72%
10	Massachusetts	2,770	2.51%
11	Georgia	2,641	2.39%
12	North Carolina	2,626	2.38%
13	Missouri	2,570	2.33%
14	Virginia	2,531	2.29%
15	Washington	2,502	2.27%
16	Maryland	2,432	2.20%
17	Wisconsin	2,316	2.10%
18	Minnesota	2,098	1.90%
19	Indiana	2,045	1.85%
20	Tennessee	1,999	1.81%
21	Arizona	1,900	1.72%
22	Oregon	1,668	1.51%
23	Colorado	1,608	1.46%
24	Connecticut	1,488	1.35%
25	Alabama	1,404	1.27%
26	Kentucky	1,322	1.20%
27	Iowa	1,255	1.14%
28	South Carolina	1,168	1.06%
29	Louisiana	1,102	1.00%
30	Utah	1,032	0.94%
31	Oklahoma	925	0.84%
32	Kansas	896	0.81%
33	Arkansas	859	0.78%
34	New Mexico	802	0.73%
35	Nebraska	764	0.69%
36	Mississippi	707	0.64%
37	Idaho	618	0.56%
38	Nevada	586	0.53%
39	Hawaii	552	0.50%
40	New Hampshire	550	0.50%
41	West Virginia	451	0.41%
42	Rhode Island	443	0.40%
43	Maine	427	0.39%
44	Montana	393	0.36%
45	Delaware	367	0.33%
46	Alaska	359	0.33%
47	Vermont	298	0.27%
48	South Dakota	268	0.24%
49	North Dakota	245	0.22%
50	Wyoming	207	0.19%
	District of Columbia	298	0.27%

Source: U.S. Department of Health and Human Services, National Center for Health Statistics unpublished data

Percent of Vaginal Births After a Cesarean (VBAC) in 1994

National Percent = 26.26% of Live Births to Women Who Have Had a Cesarean*

ALPHA ORDER

RANK	STATE	PERCENT
43	Alabama	21.66
4	Alaska	37.63
22	Arizona	29.88
46	Arkansas	19.75
41	California	22.27
3	Colorado	38.81
10	Connecticut	34.09
23	Delaware	29.84
33	Florida	26.30
36	Georgia	23.72
14	Hawaii	32.86
5	Idaho	36.74
29	Illinois	27.62
37	Indiana	23.66
16	Iowa	31.89
41	Kansas	22.27
38	Kentucky	23.48
50	Louisiana	12.91
27	Maine	28.45
24	Maryland	29.76
20	Massachusetts	30.22
35	Michigan	25.57
8	Minnesota	35.32
49	Mississippi	13.98
19	Missouri	31.46
15	Montana	32.83
18	Nebraska	31.61
32	Nevada	26.48
11	New Hampshire	33.62
40	New Jersey	22.59
13	New Mexico	33.00
25	New York	29.74
30	North Carolina	27.29
28	North Dakota	28.03
21	Ohio	29.94
44	Oklahoma	21.40
2	Oregon	40.13
12	Pennsylvania	33.20
9	Rhode Island	35.02
45	South Carolina	20.86
39	South Dakota	22.98
31	Tennessee	27.07
48	Texas	18.78
26	Utah	29.11
1	Vermont	41.62
34	Virginia	26.24
7	Washington	35.40
47	West Virginia	19.14
6	Wisconsin	36.51
17	Wyoming	31.75

RANK ORDER

RANK	STATE	PERCENT
1	Vermont	41.62
2	Oregon	40.13
3	Colorado	38.81
4	Alaska	37.63
5	Idaho	36.74
6	Wisconsin	36.51
7	Washington	35.40
8	Minnesota	35.32
9	Rhode Island	35.02
10	Connecticut	34.09
11	New Hampshire	33.62
12	Pennsylvania	33.20
13	New Mexico	33.00
14	Hawaii	32.86
15	Montana	32.83
16	Iowa	31.89
17	Wyoming	31.75
18	Nebraska	31.61
19	Missouri	31.46
20	Massachusetts	30.22
21	Ohio	29.94
22	Arizona	29.88
23	Delaware	29.84
24	Maryland	29.76
25	New York	29.74
26	Utah	29.11
27	Maine	28.45
28	North Dakota	28.03
29	Illinois	27.62
30	North Carolina	27.29
31	Tennessee	27.07
32	Nevada	26.48
33	Florida	26.30
34	Virginia	26.24
35	Michigan	25.57
36	Georgia	23.72
37	Indiana	23.66
38	Kentucky	23.48
39	South Dakota	22.98
40	New Jersey	22.59
41	California	22.27
41	Kansas	22.27
43	Alabama	21.66
44	Oklahoma	21.40
45	South Carolina	20.86
46	Arkansas	19.75
47	West Virginia	19.14
48	Texas	18.78
49	Mississippi	13.98
50	Louisiana	12.91
	District of Columbia	26.51

Source: U.S. Department of Health and Human Services, National Center for Health Statistics
   unpublished data

*Vaginal births after a cesarean delivery as a percent of all births to women with a previous cesarean delivery giving birth in 1994. Percent of births for which delivery data are available.

Percent of Mothers Beginning Prenatal Care in First Trimester in 1995

National Percent = 81.2% of Mothers*

ALPHA ORDER

RANK	STATE	PERCENT
32	Alabama	81.7
23	Alaska	83.4
49	Arizona	72.1
47	Arkansas	76.6
42	California	78.2
37	Colorado	80.5
6	Connecticut	87.7
10	Delaware	85.3
30	Florida	82.6
15	Georgia	84.2
21	Hawaii	83.7
39	Idaho	79.9
35	Illinois	81.0
38	Indiana	80.2
7	Iowa	87.4
9	Kansas	85.7
13	Kentucky	84.4
36	Louisiana	80.6
3	Maine	89.6
5	Maryland	87.9
4	Massachusetts	89.4
16	Michigan	84.1
20	Minnesota	83.8
46	Mississippi	77.0
10	Missouri	85.3
34	Montana	81.5
16	Nebraska	84.1
48	Nevada	75.7
1	New Hampshire	89.9
26	New Jersey	83.1
50	New Mexico	69.5
44	New York	77.6
22	North Carolina	83.5
18	North Dakota	84.0
12	Ohio	84.6
42	Oklahoma	78.2
40	Oregon	78.8
23	Pennsylvania	83.4
2	Rhode Island	89.8
41	South Carolina	78.6
33	South Dakota	81.6
28	Tennessee	82.9
45	Texas	77.3
14	Utah	84.3
7	Vermont	87.4
19	Virginia	83.9
29	Washington	82.7
31	West Virginia	82.0
23	Wisconsin	83.4
26	Wyoming	83.1

RANK ORDER

RANK	STATE	PERCENT
1	New Hampshire	89.9
2	Rhode Island	89.8
3	Maine	89.6
4	Massachusetts	89.4
5	Maryland	87.9
6	Connecticut	87.7
7	Iowa	87.4
7	Vermont	87.4
9	Kansas	85.7
10	Delaware	85.3
10	Missouri	85.3
12	Ohio	84.6
13	Kentucky	84.4
14	Utah	84.3
15	Georgia	84.2
16	Michigan	84.1
16	Nebraska	84.1
18	North Dakota	84.0
19	Virginia	83.9
20	Minnesota	83.8
21	Hawaii	83.7
22	North Carolina	83.5
23	Alaska	83.4
23	Pennsylvania	83.4
23	Wisconsin	83.4
26	New Jersey	83.1
26	Wyoming	83.1
28	Tennessee	82.9
29	Washington	82.7
30	Florida	82.6
31	West Virginia	82.0
32	Alabama	81.7
33	South Dakota	81.6
34	Montana	81.5
35	Illinois	81.0
36	Louisiana	80.6
37	Colorado	80.5
38	Indiana	80.2
39	Idaho	79.9
40	Oregon	78.8
41	South Carolina	78.6
42	California	78.2
42	Oklahoma	78.2
44	New York	77.6
45	Texas	77.3
46	Mississippi	77.0
47	Arkansas	76.6
48	Nevada	75.7
49	Arizona	72.1
50	New Mexico	69.5
	District of Columbia	59.1

Source: U.S. Department of Health and Human Services, National Center for Health Statistics
"Monthly Vital Statistics Report" (Vol. 45, No. 3(S)2, October 4, 1996)
*Preliminary data by state of residence.

Percent of White Mothers Beginning Prenatal Care in First Trimester in 1995

National Percent = 83.5% of White Mothers*

ALPHA ORDER				RANK ORDER		
RANK	STATE	PERCENT		RANK	STATE	PERCENT
14	Alabama	87.8		1	Maryland	92.4
29	Alaska	85.7		2	Rhode Island	91.2
49	Arizona	73.2		3	Massachusetts	90.9
43	Arkansas	80.8		4	New Hampshire	90.1
46	California	78.2		5	Maine	90.0
41	Colorado	81.1		6	Connecticut	89.3
6	Connecticut	89.3		7	Georgia	88.8
9	Delaware	88.6		7	Hawaii	88.8
26	Florida	85.9		9	Delaware	88.6
7	Georgia	88.8		10	Louisiana	88.3
7	Hawaii	88.8		10	North Carolina	88.3
44	Idaho	80.1		12	Iowa	87.9
34	Illinois	84.6		12	Virginia	87.9
39	Indiana	81.9		14	Alabama	87.8
12	Iowa	87.9		15	Missouri	87.7
20	Kansas	86.8		16	Vermont	87.5
26	Kentucky	85.9		17	Ohio	87.2
10	Louisiana	88.3		18	Mississippi	87.0
5	Maine	90.0		19	Michigan	86.9
1	Maryland	92.4		20	Kansas	86.8
3	Massachusetts	90.9		21	New Jersey	86.6
19	Michigan	86.9		21	Wisconsin	86.6
24	Minnesota	86.4		23	Pennsylvania	86.5
18	Mississippi	87.0		24	Minnesota	86.4
15	Missouri	87.7		25	Tennessee	86.2
37	Montana	83.5		26	Florida	85.9
32	Nebraska	85.2		26	Kentucky	85.9
48	Nevada	76.6		26	Utah	85.9
4	New Hampshire	90.1		29	Alaska	85.7
21	New Jersey	86.6		30	South Carolina	85.5
50	New Mexico	71.6		31	South Dakota	85.3
40	New York	81.2		32	Nebraska	85.2
10	North Carolina	88.3		32	North Dakota	85.2
32	North Dakota	85.2		34	Illinois	84.6
17	Ohio	87.2		35	Wyoming	83.8
42	Oklahoma	80.9		36	Washington	83.6
45	Oregon	79.2		37	Montana	83.5
23	Pennsylvania	86.5		38	West Virginia	82.6
2	Rhode Island	91.2		39	Indiana	81.9
30	South Carolina	85.5		40	New York	81.2
31	South Dakota	85.3		41	Colorado	81.1
25	Tennessee	86.2		42	Oklahoma	80.9
47	Texas	77.6		43	Arkansas	80.8
26	Utah	85.9		44	Idaho	80.1
16	Vermont	87.5		45	Oregon	79.2
12	Virginia	87.9		46	California	78.2
36	Washington	83.6		47	Texas	77.6
38	West Virginia	82.6		48	Nevada	76.6
21	Wisconsin	86.6		49	Arizona	73.2
35	Wyoming	83.8		50	New Mexico	71.6
					District of Columbia	76.6

Source: U.S. Department of Health and Human Services, National Center for Health Statistics
   "Monthly Vital Statistics Report" (Vol. 45, No. 3(S)2, October 4, 1996)
*Preliminary data by state of residence.

Percent of Black Mothers Beginning Prenatal Care in First Trimester in 1995

National Percent = 70.3% of Black Mothers*

ALPHA ORDER				RANK ORDER		
RANK	**STATE**	**PERCENT**		**RANK**	**STATE**	**PERCENT**
34	Alabama	69.5		1	Hawaii	91.9
2	Alaska	85.4		2	Alaska	85.4
35	Arizona	68.8		3	Montana	84.2
48	Arkansas	62.1		4	New Hampshire	82.5
13	California	75.5		5	Idaho	78.6
18	Colorado	72.9		6	Maryland	77.7
11	Connecticut	76.4		7	Massachusetts	77.4
16	Delaware	74.4		8	Maine	77.2
28	Florida	71.2		9	North Dakota	76.9
13	Georgia	75.5		10	Rhode Island	76.5
1	Hawaii	91.9		11	Connecticut	76.4
5	Idaho	78.6		12	Washington	75.8
37	Illinois	67.2		13	California	75.5
40	Indiana	66.3		13	Georgia	75.5
20	Iowa	72.5		15	Kansas	74.8
15	Kansas	74.8		16	Delaware	74.4
31	Kentucky	70.2		17	Texas	73.7
32	Louisiana	70.0		18	Colorado	72.9
8	Maine	77.2		18	Oregon	72.9
6	Maryland	77.7		20	Iowa	72.5
7	Massachusetts	77.4		21	Missouri	71.8
30	Michigan	70.3		21	Vermont	71.8
47	Minnesota	63.8		23	Virginia	71.7
43	Mississippi	65.8		24	Wyoming	71.6
21	Missouri	71.8		25	North Carolina	71.3
3	Montana	84.2		25	South Dakota	71.3
29	Nebraska	70.5		25	Tennessee	71.3
43	Nevada	65.8		28	Florida	71.2
4	New Hampshire	82.5		29	Nebraska	70.5
36	New Jersey	67.3		30	Michigan	70.3
49	New Mexico	60.6		31	Kentucky	70.2
41	New York	66.1		32	Louisiana	70.0
25	North Carolina	71.3		33	Ohio	69.6
9	North Dakota	76.9		34	Alabama	69.5
33	Ohio	69.6		35	Arizona	68.8
42	Oklahoma	66.0		36	New Jersey	67.3
18	Oregon	72.9		37	Illinois	67.2
46	Pennsylvania	65.3		38	West Virginia	66.7
10	Rhode Island	76.5		39	South Carolina	66.4
39	South Carolina	66.4		40	Indiana	66.3
25	South Dakota	71.3		41	New York	66.1
25	Tennessee	71.3		42	Oklahoma	66.0
17	Texas	73.7		43	Mississippi	65.8
50	Utah	59.8		43	Nevada	65.8
21	Vermont	71.8		45	Wisconsin	65.5
23	Virginia	71.7		46	Pennsylvania	65.3
12	Washington	75.8		47	Minnesota	63.8
38	West Virginia	66.7		48	Arkansas	62.1
45	Wisconsin	65.5		49	New Mexico	60.6
24	Wyoming	71.6		50	Utah	59.8
					District of Columbia	53.8

Source: U.S. Department of Health and Human Services, National Center for Health Statistics
"Monthly Vital Statistics Report" (Vol. 45, No. 3(S)2, October 4, 1996)
Preliminary data by state of residence.

Percent of Mothers Receiving Late or No Prenatal Care in 1993

National Percent = 4.8% of Mothers*

ALPHA ORDER

RANK	STATE	PERCENT
21	Alabama	4.2
40	Alaska	2.8
2	Arizona	8.5
9	Arkansas	5.7
12	California	5.0
11	Colorado	5.1
42	Connecticut	2.5
25	Delaware	3.8
22	Florida	4.0
18	Georgia	4.5
8	Hawaii	6.0
18	Idaho	4.5
17	Illinois	4.6
13	Indiana	4.8
46	Iowa	2.3
37	Kansas	3.2
31	Kentucky	3.6
13	Louisiana	4.8
48	Maine	1.7
25	Maryland	3.8
47	Massachusetts	2.0
31	Michigan	3.6
38	Minnesota	3.1
10	Mississippi	5.4
22	Missouri	4.0
28	Montana	3.7
40	Nebraska	2.8
4	Nevada	7.7
49	New Hampshire	1.6
20	New Jersey	4.4
1	New Mexico	9.3
6	New York	6.4
22	North Carolina	4.0
43	North Dakota	2.4
35	Ohio	3.5
5	Oklahoma	7.0
25	Oregon	3.8
16	Pennsylvania	4.7
49	Rhode Island	1.6
7	South Carolina	6.3
13	South Dakota	4.8
31	Tennessee	3.6
3	Texas	8.4
43	Utah	2.4
43	Vermont	2.4
36	Virginia	3.4
28	Washington	3.7
28	West Virginia	3.7
31	Wisconsin	3.6
39	Wyoming	2.9

RANK ORDER

RANK	STATE	PERCENT
1	New Mexico	9.3
2	Arizona	8.5
3	Texas	8.4
4	Nevada	7.7
5	Oklahoma	7.0
6	New York	6.4
7	South Carolina	6.3
8	Hawaii	6.0
9	Arkansas	5.7
10	Mississippi	5.4
11	Colorado	5.1
12	California	5.0
13	Indiana	4.8
13	Louisiana	4.8
13	South Dakota	4.8
16	Pennsylvania	4.7
17	Illinois	4.6
18	Georgia	4.5
18	Idaho	4.5
20	New Jersey	4.4
21	Alabama	4.2
22	Florida	4.0
22	Missouri	4.0
22	North Carolina	4.0
25	Delaware	3.8
25	Maryland	3.8
25	Oregon	3.8
28	Montana	3.7
28	Washington	3.7
28	West Virginia	3.7
31	Kentucky	3.6
31	Michigan	3.6
31	Tennessee	3.6
31	Wisconsin	3.6
35	Ohio	3.5
36	Virginia	3.4
37	Kansas	3.2
38	Minnesota	3.1
39	Wyoming	2.9
40	Alaska	2.8
40	Nebraska	2.8
42	Connecticut	2.5
43	North Dakota	2.4
43	Utah	2.4
43	Vermont	2.4
46	Iowa	2.3
47	Massachusetts	2.0
48	Maine	1.7
49	New Hampshire	1.6
49	Rhode Island	1.6
	District of Columbia	15.8

Source: U.S. Department of Health and Human Services, National Center for Health Statistics
"Monthly Vital Statistics Report" (Vol. 44, No. 3, Supplement, September 21, 1995)
*Final data by state of residence. "Late" means care begun in third trimester.

54

Percent of White Mothers Receiving Late or No Prenatal Care in 1993

National Percent = 4.8% of White Mothers*

ALPHA ORDER			RANK ORDER		
RANK	STATE	PERCENT	RANK	STATE	PERCENT
30	Alabama	2.5	1	Texas	8.2
43	Alaska	1.9	2	New Mexico	8.1
3	Arizona	8.0	3	Arizona	8.0
11	Arkansas	4.2	4	Nevada	7.0
6	California	5.2	5	Oklahoma	5.7
8	Colorado	4.7	6	California	5.2
43	Connecticut	1.9	7	New York	4.8
30	Delaware	2.5	8	Colorado	4.7
19	Florida	3.0	8	Hawaii	4.7
22	Georgia	2.9	10	Idaho	4.4
8	Hawaii	4.7	11	Arkansas	4.2
10	Idaho	4.4	12	Indiana	4.1
16	Illinois	3.3	13	Oregon	3.7
12	Indiana	4.1	14	South Carolina	3.6
38	Iowa	2.2	15	West Virginia	3.4
25	Kansas	2.7	16	Illinois	3.3
18	Kentucky	3.1	16	Washington	3.3
30	Louisiana	2.5	18	Kentucky	3.1
48	Maine	1.6	19	Florida	3.0
45	Maryland	1.8	19	Montana	3.0
47	Massachusetts	1.7	19	Pennsylvania	3.0
36	Michigan	2.3	22	Georgia	2.9
38	Minnesota	2.2	22	South Dakota	2.9
25	Mississippi	2.7	24	New Jersey	2.8
27	Missouri	2.6	25	Kansas	2.7
19	Montana	3.0	25	Mississippi	2.7
34	Nebraska	2.4	27	Missouri	2.6
4	Nevada	7.0	27	Ohio	2.6
48	New Hampshire	1.6	27	Wyoming	2.6
24	New Jersey	2.8	30	Alabama	2.5
2	New Mexico	8.1	30	Delaware	2.5
7	New York	4.8	30	Louisiana	2.5
38	North Carolina	2.2	30	Wisconsin	2.5
45	North Dakota	1.8	34	Nebraska	2.4
27	Ohio	2.6	34	Tennessee	2.4
5	Oklahoma	5.7	36	Michigan	2.3
13	Oregon	3.7	36	Vermont	2.3
19	Pennsylvania	3.0	38	Iowa	2.2
50	Rhode Island	1.3	38	Minnesota	2.2
14	South Carolina	3.6	38	North Carolina	2.2
22	South Dakota	2.9	41	Utah	2.1
34	Tennessee	2.4	41	Virginia	2.1
1	Texas	8.2	43	Alaska	1.9
41	Utah	2.1	43	Connecticut	1.9
36	Vermont	2.3	45	Maryland	1.8
41	Virginia	2.1	45	North Dakota	1.8
16	Washington	3.3	47	Massachusetts	1.7
15	West Virginia	3.4	48	Maine	1.6
30	Wisconsin	2.5	48	New Hampshire	1.6
27	Wyoming	2.6	50	Rhode Island	1.3
				District of Columbia	7.1

Source: U.S. Department of Health and Human Services, National Center for Health Statistics
"Monthly Vital Statistics Report" (Vol. 44, No. 3, Supplement, September 21, 1995)
*Final data by state of residence. "Late" means care begun in third trimester.

Percent of Black Mothers Receiving Late or No Prenatal Care in 1993

National Percent = 9.0% of Black Mothers*

ALPHA ORDER

RANK	STATE	PERCENT
27	Alabama	7.5
NA	Alaska**	NA
10	Arizona	10.8
12	Arkansas	10.7
37	California	5.8
16	Colorado	9.4
36	Connecticut	6.7
21	Delaware	8.0
30	Florida	7.2
28	Georgia	7.3
39	Hawaii	4.1
NA	Idaho**	NA
17	Illinois	9.2
15	Indiana	9.8
30	Iowa	7.2
33	Kansas	6.9
24	Kentucky	7.7
24	Louisiana	7.7
NA	Maine**	NA
23	Maryland	7.8
38	Massachusetts	4.5
18	Michigan	8.5
5	Minnesota	11.6
20	Mississippi	8.1
13	Missouri	10.4
NA	Montana**	NA
35	Nebraska	6.8
3	Nevada	13.8
NA	New Hampshire**	NA
7	New Jersey	11.3
13	New Mexico	10.4
4	New York	11.8
21	North Carolina	8.0
NA	North Dakota**	NA
18	Ohio	8.5
2	Oklahoma	14.0
28	Oregon	7.3
1	Pennsylvania	14.5
40	Rhode Island	3.7
10	South Carolina	10.8
NA	South Dakota**	NA
32	Tennessee	7.1
8	Texas	10.9
NA	Utah**	NA
NA	Vermont**	NA
33	Virginia	6.9
26	Washington	7.6
6	West Virginia	11.5
8	Wisconsin	10.9
NA	Wyoming**	NA

RANK ORDER

RANK	STATE	PERCENT
1	Pennsylvania	14.5
2	Oklahoma	14.0
3	Nevada	13.8
4	New York	11.8
5	Minnesota	11.6
6	West Virginia	11.5
7	New Jersey	11.3
8	Texas	10.9
8	Wisconsin	10.9
10	Arizona	10.8
10	South Carolina	10.8
12	Arkansas	10.7
13	Missouri	10.4
13	New Mexico	10.4
15	Indiana	9.8
16	Colorado	9.4
17	Illinois	9.2
18	Michigan	8.5
18	Ohio	8.5
20	Mississippi	8.1
21	Delaware	8.0
21	North Carolina	8.0
23	Maryland	7.8
24	Kentucky	7.7
24	Louisiana	7.7
26	Washington	7.6
27	Alabama	7.5
28	Georgia	7.3
28	Oregon	7.3
30	Florida	7.2
30	Iowa	7.2
32	Tennessee	7.1
33	Kansas	6.9
33	Virginia	6.9
35	Nebraska	6.8
36	Connecticut	6.7
37	California	5.8
38	Massachusetts	4.5
39	Hawaii	4.1
40	Rhode Island	3.7
NA	Alaska**	NA
NA	Idaho**	NA
NA	Maine**	NA
NA	Montana**	NA
NA	New Hampshire**	NA
NA	North Dakota**	NA
NA	South Dakota**	NA
NA	Utah**	NA
NA	Vermont**	NA
NA	Wyoming**	NA
	District of Columbia	17.6

Source: U.S. Department of Health and Human Services, National Center for Health Statistics
   "Monthly Vital Statistics Report" (Vol. 44, No. 3, Supplement, September 21, 1995)
Final data by state of residence. "Late" means care begun in third trimester.
**Insufficient data.*

Percent of Births to Women Who Smoked During Pregnancy in 1994

National Percent = 14.6% of Live Births*

RANK	STATE	PERCENT
33	Alabama	13.7
4	Alaska	21.6
37	Arizona	12.2
7	Arkansas	20.0
NA	California**	NA
34	Colorado	13.3
41	Connecticut	10.8
29	Delaware	14.0
31	Florida	13.8
38	Georgia	11.8
44	Hawaii	8.6
28	Idaho	14.1
34	Illinois	13.3
NA	Indiana**	NA
12	Iowa	18.6
36	Kansas	12.9
2	Kentucky	24.6
40	Louisiana	11.5
11	Maine	18.8
39	Maryland	11.7
25	Massachusetts	15.0
12	Michigan	18.6
31	Minnesota	13.8
27	Mississippi	14.3
6	Missouri	20.7
16	Montana	18.2
14	Nebraska	18.5
22	Nevada	17.8
16	New Hampshire	18.2
45	New Jersey	8.5
42	New Mexico	9.9
47	New York	6.5
23	North Carolina	17.1
9	North Dakota	19.5
5	Ohio	21.3
16	Oklahoma	18.2
16	Oregon	18.2
10	Pennsylvania	19.3
14	Rhode Island	18.5
25	South Carolina	15.0
NA	South Dakota**	NA
16	Tennessee	18.2
46	Texas	8.4
43	Utah	9.3
21	Vermont	17.9
30	Virginia	13.9
24	Washington	17.0
1	West Virginia	26.1
8	Wisconsin	19.6
3	Wyoming	21.8

RANK	STATE	PERCENT
1	West Virginia	26.1
2	Kentucky	24.6
3	Wyoming	21.8
4	Alaska	21.6
5	Ohio	21.3
6	Missouri	20.7
7	Arkansas	20.0
8	Wisconsin	19.6
9	North Dakota	19.5
10	Pennsylvania	19.3
11	Maine	18.8
12	Iowa	18.6
12	Michigan	18.6
14	Nebraska	18.5
14	Rhode Island	18.5
16	Montana	18.2
16	New Hampshire	18.2
16	Oklahoma	18.2
16	Oregon	18.2
16	Tennessee	18.2
21	Vermont	17.9
22	Nevada	17.8
23	North Carolina	17.1
24	Washington	17.0
25	Massachusetts	15.0
25	South Carolina	15.0
27	Mississippi	14.3
28	Idaho	14.1
29	Delaware	14.0
30	Virginia	13.9
31	Florida	13.8
31	Minnesota	13.8
33	Alabama	13.7
34	Colorado	13.3
34	Illinois	13.3
36	Kansas	12.9
37	Arizona	12.2
38	Georgia	11.8
39	Maryland	11.7
40	Louisiana	11.5
41	Connecticut	10.8
42	New Mexico	9.9
43	Utah	9.3
44	Hawaii	8.6
45	New Jersey	8.5
46	Texas	8.4
47	New York	6.5
NA	California**	NA
NA	Indiana**	NA
NA	South Dakota**	NA
	District of Columbia	9.7

Source: U.S. Department of Health and Human Services, National Center for Health Statistics
(unpublished data)
*HHS defines "Smoker" as averaging at least one cigarette a day.
**Not available.

Percent of Births Attended by Midwives in 1994

National Percent = 5.53% of Live Births*

ALPHA ORDER

RANK	STATE	PERCENT
29	Alabama	4.07
2	Alaska	16.24
11	Arizona	8.49
43	Arkansas	1.68
17	California	7.16
18	Colorado	7.13
20	Connecticut	6.15
6	Delaware	10.82
10	Florida	9.86
7	Georgia	10.45
32	Hawaii	3.84
28	Idaho	4.38
42	Illinois	1.87
44	Indiana	1.08
46	Iowa	0.99
49	Kansas	0.52
39	Kentucky	2.73
47	Louisiana	0.71
9	Maine	9.88
19	Maryland	6.24
8	Massachusetts	10.43
25	Michigan	4.73
21	Minnesota	6.12
44	Mississippi	1.08
50	Missouri	0.36
15	Montana	7.70
48	Nebraska	0.67
23	Nevada	5.77
3	New Hampshire	13.04
34	New Jersey	3.63
1	New Mexico	18.56
14	New York	7.96
27	North Carolina	4.47
31	North Dakota	4.02
41	Ohio	2.32
35	Oklahoma	3.58
4	Oregon	11.88
24	Pennsylvania	5.09
13	Rhode Island	8.04
22	South Carolina	6.07
30	South Dakota	4.03
38	Tennessee	3.04
33	Texas	3.71
16	Utah	7.26
5	Vermont	11.82
40	Virginia	2.63
12	Washington	8.33
26	West Virginia	4.72
37	Wisconsin	3.13
36	Wyoming	3.34

RANK ORDER

RANK	STATE	PERCENT
1	New Mexico	18.56
2	Alaska	16.24
3	New Hampshire	13.04
4	Oregon	11.88
5	Vermont	11.82
6	Delaware	10.82
7	Georgia	10.45
8	Massachusetts	10.43
9	Maine	9.88
10	Florida	9.86
11	Arizona	8.49
12	Washington	8.33
13	Rhode Island	8.04
14	New York	7.96
15	Montana	7.70
16	Utah	7.26
17	California	7.16
18	Colorado	7.13
19	Maryland	6.24
20	Connecticut	6.15
21	Minnesota	6.12
22	South Carolina	6.07
23	Nevada	5.77
24	Pennsylvania	5.09
25	Michigan	4.73
26	West Virginia	4.72
27	North Carolina	4.47
28	Idaho	4.38
29	Alabama	4.07
30	South Dakota	4.03
31	North Dakota	4.02
32	Hawaii	3.84
33	Texas	3.71
34	New Jersey	3.63
35	Oklahoma	3.58
36	Wyoming	3.34
37	Wisconsin	3.13
38	Tennessee	3.04
39	Kentucky	2.73
40	Virginia	2.63
41	Ohio	2.32
42	Illinois	1.87
43	Arkansas	1.68
44	Indiana	1.08
44	Mississippi	1.08
46	Iowa	0.99
47	Louisiana	0.71
48	Nebraska	0.67
49	Kansas	0.52
50	Missouri	0.36

District of Columbia — 6.80

Source: Morgan Quitno Press using data from U.S. Dept of Health & Human Services, National Center for Health Statistics (unpublished data)
*Includes certified nurse midwives and other midwives.

Reported Legal Abortions in 1992

National Total = 1,359,145 Reported Legal Abortions*

RANK	STATE	ABORTIONS	% of USA
22	Alabama	13,358	0.98%
46	Alaska	1,783	0.13%
20	Arizona	14,353	1.06%
36	Arkansas	5,675	0.42%
1	California	338,700	24.92%
27	Colorado	10,607	0.78%
17	Connecticut	17,762	1.31%
39	Delaware	5,601	0.41%
4	Florida	69,285	5.10%
8	Georgia	38,052	2.80%
35	Hawaii	5,954	0.44%
48	Idaho	1,378	0.10%
5	Illinois	56,552	4.16%
23	Indiana	12,983	0.96%
33	Iowa	6,759	0.50%
28	Kansas	10,385	0.76%
30	Kentucky	8,696	0.64%
25	Louisiana	12,423	0.91%
41	Maine	3,226	0.24%
15	Maryland	19,860	1.46%
11	Massachusetts	34,527	2.54%
12	Michigan	34,496	2.54%
19	Minnesota	15,546	1.14%
32	Mississippi	7,555	0.56%
21	Missouri	13,390	0.99%
43	Montana	2,869	0.21%
37	Nebraska	5,637	0.41%
31	Nevada	8,022	0.59%
42	New Hampshire	3,129	0.23%
7	New Jersey	38,168	2.81%
38	New Mexico	5,624	0.41%
2	New York	164,274	12.09%
10	North Carolina	35,253	2.59%
47	North Dakota	1,493	0.11%
9	Ohio	36,019	2.65%
29	Oklahoma	9,881	0.73%
24	Oregon	12,685	0.93%
6	Pennsylvania	49,042	3.61%
34	Rhode Island	6,667	0.49%
26	South Carolina	11,008	0.81%
49	South Dakota	1,038	0.08%
16	Tennessee	18,029	1.33%
3	Texas	91,113	6.70%
40	Utah	3,941	0.29%
45	Vermont	2,778	0.20%
13	Virginia	29,641	2.18%
14	Washington	27,573	2.03%
44	West Virginia	2,812	0.21%
18	Wisconsin	15,549	1.14%
50	Wyoming	296	0.02%

RANK	STATE	ABORTIONS	% of USA
1	California	338,700	24.92%
2	New York	164,274	12.09%
3	Texas	91,113	6.70%
4	Florida	69,285	5.10%
5	Illinois	56,552	4.16%
6	Pennsylvania	49,042	3.61%
7	New Jersey	38,168	2.81%
8	Georgia	38,052	2.80%
9	Ohio	36,019	2.65%
10	North Carolina	35,253	2.59%
11	Massachusetts	34,527	2.54%
12	Michigan	34,496	2.54%
13	Virginia	29,641	2.18%
14	Washington	27,573	2.03%
15	Maryland	19,860	1.46%
16	Tennessee	18,029	1.33%
17	Connecticut	17,762	1.31%
18	Wisconsin	15,549	1.14%
19	Minnesota	15,546	1.14%
20	Arizona	14,353	1.06%
21	Missouri	13,390	0.99%
22	Alabama	13,358	0.98%
23	Indiana	12,983	0.96%
24	Oregon	12,685	0.93%
25	Louisiana	12,423	0.91%
26	South Carolina	11,008	0.81%
27	Colorado	10,607	0.78%
28	Kansas	10,385	0.76%
29	Oklahoma	9,881	0.73%
30	Kentucky	8,696	0.64%
31	Nevada	8,022	0.59%
32	Mississippi	7,555	0.56%
33	Iowa	6,759	0.50%
34	Rhode Island	6,667	0.49%
35	Hawaii	5,954	0.44%
36	Arkansas	5,675	0.42%
37	Nebraska	5,637	0.41%
38	New Mexico	5,624	0.41%
39	Delaware	5,601	0.41%
40	Utah	3,941	0.29%
41	Maine	3,226	0.24%
42	New Hampshire	3,129	0.23%
43	Montana	2,869	0.21%
44	West Virginia	2,812	0.21%
45	Vermont	2,778	0.20%
46	Alaska	1,783	0.13%
47	North Dakota	1,493	0.11%
48	Idaho	1,378	0.10%
49	South Dakota	1,038	0.08%
50	Wyoming	296	0.02%
	District of Columbia	17,698	1.30%

Source: U.S. Department of Health and Human Services, Centers for Disease Control and Prevention
"Abortion Surveillance-United States, 1992" (Morbidity and Mortality Weekly Report, Vol. 45, No. SS-3, 5/3/96)
*By state of occurrence.

Reported Legal Abortions per 1,000 Live Births in 1992

National Rate = 335 Reported Legal Abortions per 1,000 Live Births*

ALPHA ORDER

RANK ORDER

RANK	STATE	RATE		RANK	STATE	RATE
29	Alabama	215		1	New York	582
45	Alaska	152		2	California	564
30	Arizona	209		3	Delaware	526
42	Arkansas	163		4	Rhode Island	460
2	California	564		5	Massachusetts	396
36	Colorado	195		6	Connecticut	373
6	Connecticut	373		7	Florida	362
3	Delaware	526		8	Vermont	359
7	Florida	362		9	Nevada	357
11	Georgia	343		10	Washington	347
16	Hawaii	300		11	Georgia	343
49	Idaho	80		12	North Carolina	339
18	Illinois	295		13	New Jersey	318
44	Indiana	154		14	Virginia	306
38	Iowa	176		15	Oregon	302
20	Kansas	274		16	Hawaii	300
43	Kentucky	162		16	Pennsylvania	300
38	Louisiana	176		18	Illinois	295
33	Maine	201		19	Texas	284
21	Maryland	255		20	Kansas	274
5	Massachusetts	396		21	Maryland	255
24	Michigan	242		22	Montana	250
26	Minnesota	237		23	Tennessee	245
37	Mississippi	177		24	Michigan	242
38	Missouri	176		24	Nebraska	242
22	Montana	250		26	Minnesota	237
24	Nebraska	242		27	Ohio	222
9	Nevada	357		28	Wisconsin	220
34	New Hampshire	196		29	Alabama	215
13	New Jersey	318		30	Arizona	209
32	New Mexico	202		31	Oklahoma	208
1	New York	582		32	New Mexico	202
12	North Carolina	339		33	Maine	201
41	North Dakota	169		34	New Hampshire	196
27	Ohio	222		34	South Carolina	196
31	Oklahoma	208		36	Colorado	195
15	Oregon	302		37	Mississippi	177
16	Pennsylvania	300		38	Iowa	176
4	Rhode Island	460		38	Louisiana	176
34	South Carolina	196		38	Missouri	176
48	South Dakota	94		41	North Dakota	169
23	Tennessee	245		42	Arkansas	163
19	Texas	284		43	Kentucky	162
47	Utah	106		44	Indiana	154
8	Vermont	359		45	Alaska	152
14	Virginia	306		46	West Virginia	127
10	Washington	347		47	Utah	106
46	West Virginia	127		48	South Dakota	94
28	Wisconsin	220		49	Idaho	80
50	Wyoming	44		50	Wyoming	44
					District of Columbia**	NA

Source: U.S. Department of Health and Human Services, Centers for Disease Control and Prevention
    "Abortion Surveillance-United States, 1992" (Morbidity and Mortality Weekly Report, Vol. 45, No. SS-3, 5/3/96)
By state of occurrence.
***The District of Columbia's ratio was not listed but was noted as being greater than 1,000 abortions per 1,000 live births.*

Reported Legal Abortions per 1,000 Women Ages 15 to 44 in 1992

National Rate = 23 Reported Legal Abortions per 1,000 Women Ages 15 to 44*

ALPHA ORDER

RANK ORDER

RANK	STATE	RATE		RANK	STATE	RATE
29	Alabama	14		1	California	47
35	Alaska	12		2	New York	39
21	Arizona	17		3	Delaware	34
39	Arkansas	11		4	Rhode Island	29
1	California	47		5	Nevada	26
33	Colorado	13		6	Florida	25
7	Connecticut	24		7	Connecticut	24
3	Delaware	34		7	Massachusetts	24
6	Florida	25		9	Georgia	23
9	Georgia	23		9	Hawaii	23
9	Hawaii	23		9	Washington	23
49	Idaho	6		12	North Carolina	22
14	Illinois	21		12	Texas	22
44	Indiana	10		14	Illinois	21
39	Iowa	11		14	New Jersey	21
17	Kansas	19		16	Vermont	20
44	Kentucky	10		17	Kansas	19
35	Louisiana	12		17	Oregon	19
39	Maine	11		17	Virginia	19
21	Maryland	17		20	Pennsylvania	18
7	Massachusetts	24		21	Arizona	17
23	Michigan	16		21	Maryland	17
27	Minnesota	15		23	Michigan	16
35	Mississippi	12		23	Montana	16
39	Missouri	11		23	Nebraska	16
23	Montana	16		23	New Mexico	16
23	Nebraska	16		27	Minnesota	15
5	Nevada	26		27	Tennessee	15
35	New Hampshire	12		29	Alabama	14
14	New Jersey	21		29	Ohio	14
23	New Mexico	16		29	Oklahoma	14
2	New York	39		29	Wisconsin	14
12	North Carolina	22		33	Colorado	13
39	North Dakota	11		33	South Carolina	13
29	Ohio	14		35	Alaska	12
29	Oklahoma	14		35	Louisiana	12
17	Oregon	19		35	Mississippi	12
20	Pennsylvania	18		35	New Hampshire	12
4	Rhode Island	29		39	Arkansas	11
33	South Carolina	13		39	Iowa	11
47	South Dakota	7		39	Maine	11
27	Tennessee	15		39	Missouri	11
12	Texas	22		39	North Dakota	11
46	Utah	9		44	Indiana	10
16	Vermont	20		44	Kentucky	10
17	Virginia	19		46	Utah	9
9	Washington	23		47	South Dakota	7
47	West Virginia	7		47	West Virginia	7
29	Wisconsin	14		49	Idaho	6
50	Wyoming	3		50	Wyoming	3
					District of Columbia**	NA

Source: U.S. Department of Health and Human Services, Centers for Disease Control and Prevention
   "Abortion Surveillance-United States, 1992" (Morbidity and Mortality Weekly Report, Vol. 45, No. SS-3, 5/3/96)
*By state of occurrence.
**The District of Columbia's rate was not listed but was noted as being greater than 100 abortions per 1,000 women ages 15 to 44 years.

61

Percent of Reported Legal Abortions Obtained by Out-Of-State Residents: 1992

Reporting States' Percent = 8.0% of Reported Legal Abortions*

ALPHA ORDER				RANK ORDER		
RANK	STATE	PERCENT		RANK	STATE	PERCENT
18	Alabama	9.3		1	Kansas	46.8
NA	Alaska**	NA		2	North Dakota	31.9
38	Arizona	2.8		3	Vermont	29.9
37	Arkansas	3.0		4	Kentucky	25.5
NA	California**	NA		5	South Dakota	24.9
23	Colorado	8.4		6	Mississippi	23.3
NA	Connecticut**	NA		7	Rhode Island	20.5
NA	Delaware**	NA		8	Nebraska	19.2
NA	Florida**	NA		9	Tennessee	16.1
22	Georgia	8.5		10	Montana	15.7
40	Hawaii	0.2		11	Utah	12.9
18	Idaho	9.3		12	Oregon	11.3
NA	Illinois**	NA		13	Minnesota	10.9
35	Indiana	3.7		14	Nevada	10.3
NA	Iowa**	NA		14	West Virginia	10.3
1	Kansas	46.8		16	Wyoming	9.8
4	Kentucky	25.5		17	Ohio	9.5
NA	Louisiana**	NA		18	Alabama	9.3
24	Maine	7.1		18	Idaho	9.3
24	Maryland	7.1		20	Missouri	9.1
33	Massachusetts	3.9		21	North Carolina	9.0
33	Michigan	3.9		22	Georgia	8.5
13	Minnesota	10.9		23	Colorado	8.4
6	Mississippi	23.3		24	Maine	7.1
20	Missouri	9.1		24	Maryland	7.1
10	Montana	15.7		26	Pennsylvania	6.5
8	Nebraska	19.2		27	Virginia	6.0
14	Nevada	10.3		28	South Carolina	5.7
NA	New Hampshire**	NA		29	Wisconsin	5.0
39	New Jersey	2.5		30	New Mexico	4.8
30	New Mexico	4.8		31	Texas	4.4
36	New York	3.2		32	Washington	4.2
21	North Carolina	9.0		33	Massachusetts	3.9
2	North Dakota	31.9		33	Michigan	3.9
17	Ohio	9.5		35	Indiana	3.7
NA	Oklahoma**	NA		36	New York	3.2
12	Oregon	11.3		37	Arkansas	3.0
26	Pennsylvania	6.5		38	Arizona	2.8
7	Rhode Island	20.5		39	New Jersey	2.5
28	South Carolina	5.7		40	Hawaii	0.2
5	South Dakota	24.9		NA	Alaska**	NA
9	Tennessee	16.1		NA	California**	NA
31	Texas	4.4		NA	Connecticut**	NA
11	Utah	12.9		NA	Delaware**	NA
3	Vermont	29.9		NA	Florida**	NA
27	Virginia	6.0		NA	Illinois**	NA
32	Washington	4.2		NA	Iowa**	NA
14	West Virginia	10.3		NA	Louisiana**	NA
29	Wisconsin	5.0		NA	New Hampshire**	NA
16	Wyoming	9.8		NA	Oklahoma**	NA
					District of Columbia	53.2

Source: U.S. Department of Health and Human Services, Centers for Disease Control and Prevention
    "Abortion Surveillance-United States, 1992" (Morbidity and Mortality Weekly Report, Vol. 45, No. SS-3, 5/3/96)
*By state of occurrence.
**Not reported.

Percent of Legal Abortions Obtained by White Women in 1992

Reporting States' Percent = 60.1% of Reported Legal Abortions*

ALPHA ORDER			RANK ORDER		
RANK	STATE	PERCENT	RANK	STATE	PERCENT
26	Alabama	54.9	1	Vermont	97.6
NA	Alaska**	NA	2	Idaho	95.4
13	Arizona	81.3	3	Maine	95.0
20	Arkansas	69.5	4	South Dakota	91.4
NA	California**	NA	5	North Dakota	90.1
NA	Colorado**	NA	6	Oregon	88.3
NA	Connecticut**	NA	7	New Mexico	86.0
NA	Delaware**	NA	7	West Virginia	86.0
NA	Florida**	NA	9	Utah	84.8
30	Georgia	47.5	10	Nevada	84.7
34	Hawaii	30.6	11	Minnesota	84.6
2	Idaho	95.4	12	Montana	83.1
NA	Illinois**	NA	13	Arizona	81.3
18	Indiana	74.0	14	Rhode Island	80.8
NA	Iowa**	NA	15	Kansas	78.2
15	Kansas	78.2	15	Kentucky	78.2
15	Kentucky	78.2	17	Wisconsin	74.6
28	Louisiana	50.7	18	Indiana	74.0
3	Maine	95.0	18	Texas	74.0
32	Maryland	43.8	20	Arkansas	69.5
NA	Massachusetts**	NA	21	Missouri	62.5
NA	Michigan**	NA	21	Pennsylvania	62.5
11	Minnesota	84.6	23	Tennessee	62.4
31	Mississippi	45.3	24	Virginia	60.3
21	Missouri	62.5	25	North Carolina	55.7
12	Montana	83.1	26	Alabama	54.9
NA	Nebraska**	NA	27	South Carolina	53.7
10	Nevada	84.7	28	Louisiana	50.7
NA	New Hampshire**	NA	29	New York	50.3
33	New Jersey	36.9	30	Georgia	47.5
7	New Mexico	86.0	31	Mississippi	45.3
29	New York	50.3	32	Maryland	43.8
25	North Carolina	55.7	33	New Jersey	36.9
5	North Dakota	90.1	34	Hawaii	30.6
NA	Ohio**	NA	NA	Alaska**	NA
NA	Oklahoma**	NA	NA	California**	NA
6	Oregon	88.3	NA	Colorado**	NA
21	Pennsylvania	62.5	NA	Connecticut**	NA
14	Rhode Island	80.8	NA	Delaware**	NA
27	South Carolina	53.7	NA	Florida**	NA
4	South Dakota	91.4	NA	Illinois**	NA
23	Tennessee	62.4	NA	Iowa**	NA
18	Texas	74.0	NA	Massachusetts**	NA
9	Utah	84.8	NA	Michigan**	NA
1	Vermont	97.6	NA	Nebraska**	NA
24	Virginia	60.3	NA	New Hampshire**	NA
NA	Washington**	NA	NA	Ohio**	NA
7	West Virginia	86.0	NA	Oklahoma**	NA
17	Wisconsin	74.6	NA	Washington**	NA
NA	Wyoming**	NA	NA	Wyoming**	NA
				District of Columbia	15.4

Source: U.S. Department of Health and Human Services, Centers for Disease Control and Prevention
   "Abortion Surveillance-United States, 1992" (Morbidity and Mortality Weekly Report, Vol. 45, No. SS-3, 5/3/96)
*By state of occurrence. Includes those of Hispanic ethnicity. National percent is for reporting states only.
**Not reported.

Percent of Reported Legal Abortions Obtained by Black Women in 1992

Reporting States' Percent = 33.1% of Reported Legal Abortions*

ALPHA ORDER

RANK ORDER

RANK	STATE	PERCENT		RANK	STATE	PERCENT
8	Alabama	41.7		1	Mississippi	53.9
NA	Alaska**	NA		2	Maryland	49.5
24	Arizona	5.5		3	Georgia	48.2
14	Arkansas	28.3		4	Louisiana	47.4
NA	California**	NA		5	South Carolina	44.8
NA	Colorado**	NA		6	New Jersey	43.1
NA	Connecticut**	NA		7	New York	42.3
NA	Delaware**	NA		8	Alabama	41.7
NA	Florida**	NA		9	North Carolina	39.1
3	Georgia	48.2		10	Virginia	36.2
26	Hawaii	3.0		11	Tennessee	36.0
30	Idaho	0.8		12	Missouri	34.8
NA	Illinois**	NA		12	Pennsylvania	34.8
15	Indiana	22.1		14	Arkansas	28.3
NA	Iowa**	NA		15	Indiana	22.1
19	Kansas	17.0		16	Wisconsin	21.1
18	Kentucky	18.7		17	Texas	20.0
4	Louisiana	47.4		18	Kentucky	18.7
30	Maine	0.8		19	Kansas	17.0
2	Maryland	49.5		20	Rhode Island	13.6
NA	Massachusetts**	NA		21	West Virginia	13.1
NA	Michigan**	NA		22	Nevada	8.7
23	Minnesota	8.0		23	Minnesota	8.0
1	Mississippi	53.9		24	Arizona	5.5
12	Missouri	34.8		25	Oregon	4.6
33	Montana	0.4		26	Hawaii	3.0
NA	Nebraska**	NA		27	New Mexico	2.4
22	Nevada	8.7		28	Utah	2.1
NA	New Hampshire**	NA		29	North Dakota	1.1
6	New Jersey	43.1		30	Idaho	0.8
27	New Mexico	2.4		30	Maine	0.8
7	New York	42.3		32	Vermont	0.7
9	North Carolina	39.1		33	Montana	0.4
29	North Dakota	1.1		34	South Dakota	0.0
NA	Ohio**	NA		NA	Alaska**	NA
NA	Oklahoma**	NA		NA	California**	NA
25	Oregon	4.6		NA	Colorado**	NA
12	Pennsylvania	34.8		NA	Connecticut**	NA
20	Rhode Island	13.6		NA	Delaware**	NA
5	South Carolina	44.8		NA	Florida**	NA
34	South Dakota	0.0		NA	Illinois**	NA
11	Tennessee	36.0		NA	Iowa**	NA
17	Texas	20.0		NA	Massachusetts**	NA
28	Utah	2.1		NA	Michigan**	NA
32	Vermont	0.7		NA	Nebraska**	NA
10	Virginia	36.2		NA	New Hampshire**	NA
NA	Washington**	NA		NA	Ohio**	NA
21	West Virginia	13.1		NA	Oklahoma**	NA
16	Wisconsin	21.1		NA	Washington**	NA
NA	Wyoming**	NA		NA	Wyoming**	NA
					District of Columbia	82.6

Source: U.S. Department of Health and Human Services, Centers for Disease Control and Prevention
"Abortion Surveillance-United States, 1992" (Morbidity and Mortality Weekly Report, Vol. 45, No. SS-3, 5/3/96)
*By state of occurrence. National percent is for reporting states only.
**Not reported.

Percent of Reported Legal Abortions Obtained by Married Women in 1992

Reporting States' Percent = 20.0% of Reported Legal Abortions*

ALPHA ORDER

RANK	STATE	PERCENT
26	Alabama	18.5
NA	Alaska**	NA
17	Arizona	20.6
22	Arkansas	19.8
NA	California**	NA
11	Colorado	21.6
NA	Connecticut**	NA
NA	Delaware**	NA
NA	Florida**	NA
23	Georgia	19.6
2	Hawaii	24.8
2	Idaho	24.8
NA	Illinois**	NA
30	Indiana	18.1
NA	Iowa**	NA
26	Kansas	18.5
33	Kentucky	17.3
NA	Louisiana**	NA
13	Maine	21.3
15	Maryland	21.1
14	Massachusetts	21.2
35	Michigan	16.7
36	Minnesota	15.6
37	Mississippi	14.5
9	Missouri	22.0
21	Montana	20.0
NA	Nebraska**	NA
4	Nevada	23.6
NA	New Hampshire**	NA
12	New Jersey	21.4
28	New Mexico	18.3
17	New York**	20.6
9	North Carolina	22.0
20	North Dakota	20.2
34	Ohio	16.9
NA	Oklahoma**	NA
8	Oregon	22.2
32	Pennsylvania	17.5
7	Rhode Island	22.5
19	South Carolina	20.3
24	South Dakota	19.3
16	Tennessee	20.8
5	Texas	22.9
1	Utah	41.4
6	Vermont	22.6
31	Virginia	17.8
NA	Washington**	NA
29	West Virginia	18.2
38	Wisconsin	14.2
24	Wyoming	19.3

RANK ORDER

RANK	STATE	PERCENT
1	Utah	41.4
2	Hawaii	24.8
2	Idaho	24.8
4	Nevada	23.6
5	Texas	22.9
6	Vermont	22.6
7	Rhode Island	22.5
8	Oregon	22.2
9	Missouri	22.0
9	North Carolina	22.0
11	Colorado	21.6
12	New Jersey	21.4
13	Maine	21.3
14	Massachusetts	21.2
15	Maryland	21.1
16	Tennessee	20.8
17	Arizona	20.6
17	New York**	20.6
19	South Carolina	20.3
20	North Dakota	20.2
21	Montana	20.0
22	Arkansas	19.8
23	Georgia	19.6
24	South Dakota	19.3
24	Wyoming	19.3
26	Alabama	18.5
26	Kansas	18.5
28	New Mexico	18.3
29	West Virginia	18.2
30	Indiana	18.1
31	Virginia	17.8
32	Pennsylvania	17.5
33	Kentucky	17.3
34	Ohio	16.9
35	Michigan	16.7
36	Minnesota	15.6
37	Mississippi	14.5
38	Wisconsin	14.2
NA	Alaska**	NA
NA	California**	NA
NA	Connecticut**	NA
NA	Delaware**	NA
NA	Florida**	NA
NA	Illinois**	NA
NA	Iowa**	NA
NA	Louisiana**	NA
NA	Nebraska**	NA
NA	New Hampshire**	NA
NA	Oklahoma**	NA
NA	Washington**	NA

District of Columbia 13.8

Source: U.S. Department of Health and Human Services, Centers for Disease Control and Prevention
"Abortion Surveillance-United States, 1992" (Morbidity and Mortality Weekly Report, Vol. 45, No. SS-3, 5/3/96)
*By state of occurrence. National percent is for reporting states only.
**Not reported. New York's percentage is for New York City only.

Percent of Reported Legal Abortions Obtained by Unmarried Women in 1992

Reporting States' Percent = 76.4% of Reported Legal Abortions*

ALPHA ORDER			RANK ORDER		
RANK	STATE	PERCENT	RANK	STATE	PERCENT
17	Alabama	79.0	1	Mississippi	85.4
NA	Alaska**	NA	2	Wisconsin	84.8
37	Arizona	65.0	3	Michigan	82.7
20	Arkansas	77.4	3	Minnesota	82.7
NA	California**	NA	5	Pennsylvania	82.5
22	Colorado	77.3	6	West Virginia	81.8
NA	Connecticut**	NA	7	Kansas	81.3
NA	Delaware**	NA	8	Kentucky	81.2
NA	Florida**	NA	9	Indiana	80.8
16	Georgia	79.3	10	New Mexico	80.7
27	Hawaii	74.4	10	South Dakota	80.7
26	Idaho	74.9	12	Wyoming	80.4
NA	Illinois**	NA	13	Virginia	79.8
9	Indiana	80.8	14	North Dakota	79.7
NA	Iowa**	NA	14	South Carolina	79.7
7	Kansas	81.3	16	Georgia	79.3
8	Kentucky	81.2	17	Alabama	79.0
NA	Louisiana**	NA	18	Tennessee	78.6
28	Maine	73.9	19	New Jersey	78.3
24	Maryland	76.7	20	Arkansas	77.4
36	Massachusetts	68.8	20	New York**	77.4
3	Michigan	82.7	22	Colorado	77.3
3	Minnesota	82.7	23	Missouri	77.0
1	Mississippi	85.4	24	Maryland	76.7
23	Missouri	77.0	25	Rhode Island	76.2
34	Montana	71.0	26	Idaho	74.9
NA	Nebraska**	NA	27	Hawaii	74.4
29	Nevada	73.6	28	Maine	73.9
NA	New Hampshire**	NA	29	Nevada	73.6
19	New Jersey	78.3	30	Oregon	72.5
10	New Mexico	80.7	31	North Carolina	72.2
20	New York**	77.4	32	Ohio	71.9
31	North Carolina	72.2	33	Vermont	71.6
14	North Dakota	79.7	34	Montana	71.0
32	Ohio	71.9	35	Texas	69.4
NA	Oklahoma**	NA	36	Massachusetts	68.8
30	Oregon	72.5	37	Arizona	65.0
5	Pennsylvania	82.5	38	Utah	58.6
25	Rhode Island	76.2	NA	Alaska**	NA
14	South Carolina	79.7	NA	California**	NA
10	South Dakota	80.7	NA	Connecticut**	NA
18	Tennessee	78.6	NA	Delaware**	NA
35	Texas	69.4	NA	Florida**	NA
38	Utah	58.6	NA	Illinois**	NA
33	Vermont	71.6	NA	Iowa**	NA
13	Virginia	79.8	NA	Louisiana**	NA
NA	Washington**	NA	NA	Nebraska**	NA
6	West Virginia	81.8	NA	New Hampshire**	NA
2	Wisconsin	84.8	NA	Oklahoma**	NA
12	Wyoming	80.4	NA	Washington**	NA
				District of Columbia	82.5

Source: U.S. Department of Health and Human Services, Centers for Disease Control and Prevention
    "Abortion Surveillance-United States, 1992" (Morbidity and Mortality Weekly Report, Vol. 45, No. SS-3, 5/3/96)
*By state of occurrence. National percent is for reporting states only.
**Not reported. New York's percentage is for New York City only.

Reported Legal Abortions Obtained by Teenagers in 1992

Reporting States' Total = 165,675 Legal Abortions Obtained by Teenagers*

ALPHA ORDER

RANK	STATE	ABORTIONS	% of USA
14	Alabama	3,317	2.00%
NA	Alaska**	NA	NA
21	Arizona	2,692	1.62%
27	Arkansas	1,374	0.83%
NA	California**	NA	NA
24	Colorado	2,424	1.46%
NA	Connecticut**	NA	NA
NA	Delaware**	NA	NA
NA	Florida**	NA	NA
5	Georgia	7,994	4.83%
31	Hawaii	1,260	0.76%
39	Idaho	351	0.21%
NA	Illinois**	NA	NA
17	Indiana	2,797	1.69%
NA	Iowa**	NA	NA
20	Kansas	2,697	1.63%
23	Kentucky	2,428	1.47%
18	Louisiana	2,788	1.68%
36	Maine	638	0.39%
13	Maryland	3,987	2.41%
11	Massachusetts	5,596	3.38%
6	Michigan	7,813	4.72%
16	Minnesota	2,858	1.73%
26	Mississippi	1,839	1.11%
22	Missouri	2,676	1.62%
34	Montana	729	0.44%
30	Nebraska	1,277	0.77%
28	Nevada	1,359	0.82%
NA	New Hampshire**	NA	NA
7	New Jersey	7,470	4.51%
29	New Mexico	1,282	0.77%
1	New York	29,668	17.91%
4	North Carolina	8,146	4.92%
38	North Dakota	374	0.23%
8	Ohio	5,802	3.50%
NA	Oklahoma**	NA	NA
19	Oregon	2,716	1.64%
3	Pennsylvania	10,342	6.24%
32	Rhode Island	1,220	0.74%
25	South Carolina	2,394	1.44%
40	South Dakota	292	0.18%
12	Tennessee	4,059	2.45%
2	Texas	16,051	9.69%
33	Utah	821	0.50%
37	Vermont	618	0.37%
10	Virginia	5,729	3.46%
9	Washington	5,755	3.47%
35	West Virginia	713	0.43%
15	Wisconsin	3,255	1.96%
41	Wyoming	74	0.04%

RANK ORDER

RANK	STATE	ABORTIONS	% of USA
1	New York	29,668	17.91%
2	Texas	16,051	9.69%
3	Pennsylvania	10,342	6.24%
4	North Carolina	8,146	4.92%
5	Georgia	7,994	4.83%
6	Michigan	7,813	4.72%
7	New Jersey	7,470	4.51%
8	Ohio	5,802	3.50%
9	Washington	5,755	3.47%
10	Virginia	5,729	3.46%
11	Massachusetts	5,596	3.38%
12	Tennessee	4,059	2.45%
13	Maryland	3,987	2.41%
14	Alabama	3,317	2.00%
15	Wisconsin	3,255	1.96%
16	Minnesota	2,858	1.73%
17	Indiana	2,797	1.69%
18	Louisiana	2,788	1.68%
19	Oregon	2,716	1.64%
20	Kansas	2,697	1.63%
21	Arizona	2,692	1.62%
22	Missouri	2,676	1.62%
23	Kentucky	2,428	1.47%
24	Colorado	2,424	1.46%
25	South Carolina	2,394	1.44%
26	Mississippi	1,839	1.11%
27	Arkansas	1,374	0.83%
28	Nevada	1,359	0.82%
29	New Mexico	1,282	0.77%
30	Nebraska	1,277	0.77%
31	Hawaii	1,260	0.76%
32	Rhode Island	1,220	0.74%
33	Utah	821	0.50%
34	Montana	729	0.44%
35	West Virginia	713	0.43%
36	Maine	638	0.39%
37	Vermont	618	0.37%
38	North Dakota	374	0.23%
39	Idaho	351	0.21%
40	South Dakota	292	0.18%
41	Wyoming	74	0.04%
NA	Alaska**	NA	NA
NA	California**	NA	NA
NA	Connecticut**	NA	NA
NA	Delaware**	NA	NA
NA	Florida**	NA	NA
NA	Illinois**	NA	NA
NA	Iowa**	NA	NA
NA	New Hampshire**	NA	NA
NA	Oklahoma**	NA	NA
	District of Columbia**	NA	NA

Source: U.S. Department of Health and Human Services, Centers for Disease Control and Prevention
   "Abortion Surveillance-United States, 1992" (Morbidity and Mortality Weekly Report, Vol. 45, No. SS-3, 5/3/96)
*By state of occurrence. National total is for reporting states only.
**Not reported.

Percent of Reported Legal Abortions Obtained by Teenagers in 1992

Reporting States' Percent = 19.91% of Legal Abortions Obtained by Teenagers*

<table>
<tr><td colspan="3">ALPHA ORDER</td><td colspan="3">RANK ORDER</td></tr>
<tr><td>RANK</td><td>STATE</td><td>PERCENT</td><td>RANK</td><td>STATE</td><td>PERCENT</td></tr>
<tr><td>9</td><td>Alabama</td><td>24.83</td><td>1</td><td>South Dakota</td><td>28.13</td></tr>
<tr><td>NA</td><td>Alaska**</td><td>NA</td><td>2</td><td>Kentucky</td><td>27.92</td></tr>
<tr><td>34</td><td>Arizona</td><td>18.76</td><td>3</td><td>Kansas</td><td>25.97</td></tr>
<tr><td>11</td><td>Arkansas</td><td>24.21</td><td>4</td><td>Idaho</td><td>25.47</td></tr>
<tr><td>NA</td><td>California**</td><td>NA</td><td>5</td><td>Montana</td><td>25.41</td></tr>
<tr><td>13</td><td>Colorado</td><td>22.85</td><td>6</td><td>West Virginia</td><td>25.36</td></tr>
<tr><td>NA</td><td>Connecticut**</td><td>NA</td><td>7</td><td>North Dakota</td><td>25.05</td></tr>
<tr><td>NA</td><td>Delaware**</td><td>NA</td><td>8</td><td>Wyoming</td><td>25.00</td></tr>
<tr><td>NA</td><td>Florida**</td><td>NA</td><td>9</td><td>Alabama</td><td>24.83</td></tr>
<tr><td>25</td><td>Georgia</td><td>21.01</td><td>10</td><td>Mississippi</td><td>24.34</td></tr>
<tr><td>23</td><td>Hawaii</td><td>21.16</td><td>11</td><td>Arkansas</td><td>24.21</td></tr>
<tr><td>4</td><td>Idaho</td><td>25.47</td><td>12</td><td>North Carolina</td><td>23.11</td></tr>
<tr><td>NA</td><td>Illinois**</td><td>NA</td><td>13</td><td>Colorado</td><td>22.85</td></tr>
<tr><td>21</td><td>Indiana</td><td>21.54</td><td>14</td><td>New Mexico</td><td>22.80</td></tr>
<tr><td>NA</td><td>Iowa**</td><td>NA</td><td>15</td><td>Michigan</td><td>22.65</td></tr>
<tr><td>3</td><td>Kansas</td><td>25.97</td><td>15</td><td>Nebraska</td><td>22.65</td></tr>
<tr><td>2</td><td>Kentucky</td><td>27.92</td><td>17</td><td>Tennessee</td><td>22.51</td></tr>
<tr><td>18</td><td>Louisiana</td><td>22.44</td><td>18</td><td>Louisiana</td><td>22.44</td></tr>
<tr><td>31</td><td>Maine</td><td>19.78</td><td>19</td><td>Vermont</td><td>22.25</td></tr>
<tr><td>29</td><td>Maryland</td><td>20.08</td><td>20</td><td>South Carolina</td><td>21.75</td></tr>
<tr><td>40</td><td>Massachusetts</td><td>16.21</td><td>21</td><td>Indiana</td><td>21.54</td></tr>
<tr><td>15</td><td>Michigan</td><td>22.65</td><td>22</td><td>Oregon</td><td>21.41</td></tr>
<tr><td>35</td><td>Minnesota</td><td>18.38</td><td>23</td><td>Hawaii</td><td>21.16</td></tr>
<tr><td>10</td><td>Mississippi</td><td>24.34</td><td>24</td><td>Pennsylvania</td><td>21.09</td></tr>
<tr><td>30</td><td>Missouri</td><td>19.99</td><td>25</td><td>Georgia</td><td>21.01</td></tr>
<tr><td>5</td><td>Montana</td><td>25.41</td><td>26</td><td>Wisconsin</td><td>20.93</td></tr>
<tr><td>15</td><td>Nebraska</td><td>22.65</td><td>27</td><td>Washington</td><td>20.87</td></tr>
<tr><td>39</td><td>Nevada</td><td>16.94</td><td>28</td><td>Utah</td><td>20.83</td></tr>
<tr><td>NA</td><td>New Hampshire**</td><td>NA</td><td>29</td><td>Maryland</td><td>20.08</td></tr>
<tr><td>32</td><td>New Jersey</td><td>19.57</td><td>30</td><td>Missouri</td><td>19.99</td></tr>
<tr><td>14</td><td>New Mexico</td><td>22.80</td><td>31</td><td>Maine</td><td>19.78</td></tr>
<tr><td>37</td><td>New York</td><td>18.06</td><td>32</td><td>New Jersey</td><td>19.57</td></tr>
<tr><td>12</td><td>North Carolina</td><td>23.11</td><td>33</td><td>Virginia</td><td>19.33</td></tr>
<tr><td>7</td><td>North Dakota</td><td>25.05</td><td>34</td><td>Arizona</td><td>18.76</td></tr>
<tr><td>41</td><td>Ohio</td><td>16.11</td><td>35</td><td>Minnesota</td><td>18.38</td></tr>
<tr><td>NA</td><td>Oklahoma**</td><td>NA</td><td>36</td><td>Rhode Island</td><td>18.30</td></tr>
<tr><td>22</td><td>Oregon</td><td>21.41</td><td>37</td><td>New York</td><td>18.06</td></tr>
<tr><td>24</td><td>Pennsylvania</td><td>21.09</td><td>38</td><td>Texas</td><td>17.62</td></tr>
<tr><td>36</td><td>Rhode Island</td><td>18.30</td><td>39</td><td>Nevada</td><td>16.94</td></tr>
<tr><td>20</td><td>South Carolina</td><td>21.75</td><td>40</td><td>Massachusetts</td><td>16.21</td></tr>
<tr><td>1</td><td>South Dakota</td><td>28.13</td><td>41</td><td>Ohio</td><td>16.11</td></tr>
<tr><td>17</td><td>Tennessee</td><td>22.51</td><td>NA</td><td>Alaska**</td><td>NA</td></tr>
<tr><td>38</td><td>Texas</td><td>17.62</td><td>NA</td><td>California**</td><td>NA</td></tr>
<tr><td>28</td><td>Utah</td><td>20.83</td><td>NA</td><td>Connecticut**</td><td>NA</td></tr>
<tr><td>19</td><td>Vermont</td><td>22.25</td><td>NA</td><td>Delaware**</td><td>NA</td></tr>
<tr><td>33</td><td>Virginia</td><td>19.33</td><td>NA</td><td>Florida**</td><td>NA</td></tr>
<tr><td>27</td><td>Washington</td><td>20.87</td><td>NA</td><td>Illinois**</td><td>NA</td></tr>
<tr><td>6</td><td>West Virginia</td><td>25.36</td><td>NA</td><td>Iowa**</td><td>NA</td></tr>
<tr><td>26</td><td>Wisconsin</td><td>20.93</td><td>NA</td><td>New Hampshire**</td><td>NA</td></tr>
<tr><td>8</td><td>Wyoming</td><td>25.00</td><td>NA</td><td>Oklahoma**</td><td>NA</td></tr>
<tr><td></td><td></td><td></td><td></td><td>District of Columbia**</td><td>NA</td></tr>
</table>

Source: Morgan Quitno Press using data from US Dept of Health & Human Serv's, Centers for Disease Control-Prevention "Abortion Surveillance-United States, 1992" (Morbidity and Mortality Weekly Report, Vol. 45, No. SS-3, 5/3/96)
By state of occurrence. National percent is for reporting states only.
**Not reported.*

Reported Legal Abortions Obtained by Teenagers 17 Years and Younger in 1992

Reporting States' Total = 68,297 Reported Legal Abortions*

<table>
<tr><td colspan="4">ALPHA ORDER</td><td colspan="4">RANK ORDER</td></tr>
<tr><td>RANK</td><td>STATE</td><td>ABORTIONS</td><td>% of USA</td><td>RANK</td><td>STATE</td><td>ABORTIONS</td><td>% of USA</td></tr>
<tr><td>14</td><td>Alabama</td><td>1,480</td><td>2.17%</td><td>1</td><td>New York</td><td>13,077</td><td>19.15%</td></tr>
<tr><td>NA</td><td>Alaska**</td><td>NA</td><td>NA</td><td>2</td><td>Texas</td><td>5,932</td><td>8.69%</td></tr>
<tr><td>22</td><td>Arizona</td><td>1,047</td><td>1.53%</td><td>3</td><td>Pennsylvania</td><td>4,385</td><td>6.42%</td></tr>
<tr><td>30</td><td>Arkansas</td><td>527</td><td>0.77%</td><td>4</td><td>North Carolina</td><td>3,529</td><td>5.17%</td></tr>
<tr><td>NA</td><td>California**</td><td>NA</td><td>NA</td><td>5</td><td>Georgia</td><td>3,341</td><td>4.89%</td></tr>
<tr><td>20</td><td>Colorado</td><td>1,100</td><td>1.61%</td><td>6</td><td>Michigan</td><td>3,081</td><td>4.51%</td></tr>
<tr><td>NA</td><td>Connecticut**</td><td>NA</td><td>NA</td><td>7</td><td>New Jersey</td><td>3,027</td><td>4.43%</td></tr>
<tr><td>NA</td><td>Delaware**</td><td>NA</td><td>NA</td><td>8</td><td>Washington</td><td>2,492</td><td>3.65%</td></tr>
<tr><td>NA</td><td>Florida**</td><td>NA</td><td>NA</td><td>9</td><td>Virginia</td><td>2,344</td><td>3.43%</td></tr>
<tr><td>5</td><td>Georgia</td><td>3,341</td><td>4.89%</td><td>10</td><td>Ohio</td><td>2,074</td><td>3.04%</td></tr>
<tr><td>27</td><td>Hawaii</td><td>581</td><td>0.85%</td><td>11</td><td>Massachusetts</td><td>1,951</td><td>2.86%</td></tr>
<tr><td>40</td><td>Idaho</td><td>117</td><td>0.17%</td><td>12</td><td>Maryland</td><td>1,778</td><td>2.60%</td></tr>
<tr><td>NA</td><td>Illinois**</td><td>NA</td><td>NA</td><td>13</td><td>Tennessee</td><td>1,626</td><td>2.38%</td></tr>
<tr><td>24</td><td>Indiana</td><td>1,026</td><td>1.50%</td><td>14</td><td>Alabama</td><td>1,480</td><td>2.17%</td></tr>
<tr><td>NA</td><td>Iowa**</td><td>NA</td><td>NA</td><td>15</td><td>Kansas</td><td>1,289</td><td>1.89%</td></tr>
<tr><td>15</td><td>Kansas</td><td>1,289</td><td>1.89%</td><td>16</td><td>Wisconsin</td><td>1,274</td><td>1.87%</td></tr>
<tr><td>17</td><td>Kentucky</td><td>1,206</td><td>1.77%</td><td>17</td><td>Kentucky</td><td>1,206</td><td>1.77%</td></tr>
<tr><td>19</td><td>Louisiana</td><td>1,124</td><td>1.65%</td><td>18</td><td>Oregon</td><td>1,156</td><td>1.69%</td></tr>
<tr><td>36</td><td>Maine</td><td>274</td><td>0.40%</td><td>19</td><td>Louisiana</td><td>1,124</td><td>1.65%</td></tr>
<tr><td>12</td><td>Maryland</td><td>1,778</td><td>2.60%</td><td>20</td><td>Colorado</td><td>1,100</td><td>1.61%</td></tr>
<tr><td>11</td><td>Massachusetts</td><td>1,951</td><td>2.86%</td><td>21</td><td>Minnesota</td><td>1,069</td><td>1.57%</td></tr>
<tr><td>6</td><td>Michigan</td><td>3,081</td><td>4.51%</td><td>22</td><td>Arizona</td><td>1,047</td><td>1.53%</td></tr>
<tr><td>21</td><td>Minnesota</td><td>1,069</td><td>1.57%</td><td>23</td><td>Missouri</td><td>1,042</td><td>1.53%</td></tr>
<tr><td>26</td><td>Mississippi</td><td>850</td><td>1.24%</td><td>24</td><td>Indiana</td><td>1,026</td><td>1.50%</td></tr>
<tr><td>23</td><td>Missouri</td><td>1,042</td><td>1.53%</td><td>25</td><td>South Carolina</td><td>1,013</td><td>1.48%</td></tr>
<tr><td>33</td><td>Montana</td><td>343</td><td>0.50%</td><td>26</td><td>Mississippi</td><td>850</td><td>1.24%</td></tr>
<tr><td>31</td><td>Nebraska</td><td>459</td><td>0.67%</td><td>27</td><td>Hawaii</td><td>581</td><td>0.85%</td></tr>
<tr><td>29</td><td>Nevada</td><td>572</td><td>0.84%</td><td>28</td><td>New Mexico</td><td>577</td><td>0.84%</td></tr>
<tr><td>NA</td><td>New Hampshire**</td><td>NA</td><td>NA</td><td>29</td><td>Nevada</td><td>572</td><td>0.84%</td></tr>
<tr><td>7</td><td>New Jersey</td><td>3,027</td><td>4.43%</td><td>30</td><td>Arkansas</td><td>527</td><td>0.77%</td></tr>
<tr><td>28</td><td>New Mexico</td><td>577</td><td>0.84%</td><td>31</td><td>Nebraska</td><td>459</td><td>0.67%</td></tr>
<tr><td>1</td><td>New York</td><td>13,077</td><td>19.15%</td><td>32</td><td>Rhode Island</td><td>375</td><td>0.55%</td></tr>
<tr><td>4</td><td>North Carolina</td><td>3,529</td><td>5.17%</td><td>33</td><td>Montana</td><td>343</td><td>0.50%</td></tr>
<tr><td>39</td><td>North Dakota</td><td>126</td><td>0.18%</td><td>34</td><td>Utah</td><td>321</td><td>0.47%</td></tr>
<tr><td>10</td><td>Ohio</td><td>2,074</td><td>3.04%</td><td>35</td><td>West Virginia</td><td>292</td><td>0.43%</td></tr>
<tr><td>NA</td><td>Oklahoma**</td><td>NA</td><td>NA</td><td>36</td><td>Maine</td><td>274</td><td>0.40%</td></tr>
<tr><td>18</td><td>Oregon</td><td>1,156</td><td>1.69%</td><td>37</td><td>Vermont</td><td>245</td><td>0.36%</td></tr>
<tr><td>3</td><td>Pennsylvania</td><td>4,385</td><td>6.42%</td><td>38</td><td>South Dakota</td><td>150</td><td>0.22%</td></tr>
<tr><td>32</td><td>Rhode Island</td><td>375</td><td>0.55%</td><td>39</td><td>North Dakota</td><td>126</td><td>0.18%</td></tr>
<tr><td>25</td><td>South Carolina</td><td>1,013</td><td>1.48%</td><td>40</td><td>Idaho</td><td>117</td><td>0.17%</td></tr>
<tr><td>38</td><td>South Dakota</td><td>150</td><td>0.22%</td><td>41</td><td>Wyoming</td><td>25</td><td>0.04%</td></tr>
<tr><td>13</td><td>Tennessee</td><td>1,626</td><td>2.38%</td><td>NA</td><td>Alaska**</td><td>NA</td><td>NA</td></tr>
<tr><td>2</td><td>Texas</td><td>5,932</td><td>8.69%</td><td>NA</td><td>California**</td><td>NA</td><td>NA</td></tr>
<tr><td>34</td><td>Utah</td><td>321</td><td>0.47%</td><td>NA</td><td>Connecticut**</td><td>NA</td><td>NA</td></tr>
<tr><td>37</td><td>Vermont</td><td>245</td><td>0.36%</td><td>NA</td><td>Delaware**</td><td>NA</td><td>NA</td></tr>
<tr><td>9</td><td>Virginia</td><td>2,344</td><td>3.43%</td><td>NA</td><td>Florida**</td><td>NA</td><td>NA</td></tr>
<tr><td>8</td><td>Washington</td><td>2,492</td><td>3.65%</td><td>NA</td><td>Illinois**</td><td>NA</td><td>NA</td></tr>
<tr><td>35</td><td>West Virginia</td><td>292</td><td>0.43%</td><td>NA</td><td>Iowa**</td><td>NA</td><td>NA</td></tr>
<tr><td>16</td><td>Wisconsin</td><td>1,274</td><td>1.87%</td><td>NA</td><td>New Hampshire**</td><td>NA</td><td>NA</td></tr>
<tr><td>41</td><td>Wyoming</td><td>25</td><td>0.04%</td><td>NA</td><td>Oklahoma**</td><td>NA</td><td>NA</td></tr>
<tr><td></td><td></td><td></td><td></td><td></td><td>District of Columbia**</td><td>NA</td><td>NA</td></tr>
</table>

Source: Morgan Quitno Press using data from US Dept of Health & Human Serv's, Centers for Disease Control-Prevention
"Abortion Surveillance-United States, 1992" (Morbidity and Mortality Weekly Report, Vol. 45, No. SS-3, 5/3/96)
*By state of occurrence. National total is for reporting states only.
**Not reported.

Percent of Reported Legal Abortions Obtained
By Teenagers 17 Years and Younger in 1992
Reporting States' Percent = 8.21% of Reported Legal Abortions*

ALPHA ORDER

RANK	STATE	PERCENT
6	Alabama	11.08
NA	Alaska**	NA
35	Arizona	7.29
12	Arkansas	9.29
NA	California**	NA
8	Colorado	10.37
NA	Connecticut**	NA
NA	Delaware**	NA
NA	Florida**	NA
22	Georgia	8.78
11	Hawaii	9.76
23	Idaho	8.49
NA	Illinois**	NA
33	Indiana	7.90
NA	Iowa**	NA
3	Kansas	12.41
2	Kentucky	13.87
15	Louisiana	9.05
23	Maine	8.49
18	Maryland	8.95
40	Massachusetts	5.65
20	Michigan	8.93
37	Minnesota	6.88
5	Mississippi	11.25
34	Missouri	7.78
4	Montana	11.96
29	Nebraska	8.14
36	Nevada	7.13
NA	New Hampshire**	NA
31	New Jersey	7.93
9	New Mexico	10.26
30	New York	7.96
10	North Carolina	10.01
26	North Dakota	8.44
39	Ohio	5.76
NA	Oklahoma**	NA
14	Oregon	9.11
19	Pennsylvania	8.94
41	Rhode Island	5.62
13	South Carolina	9.20
1	South Dakota	14.45
17	Tennessee	9.02
38	Texas	6.51
28	Utah	8.15
21	Vermont	8.82
32	Virginia	7.91
16	Washington	9.04
7	West Virginia	10.38
27	Wisconsin	8.19
25	Wyoming	8.45

RANK ORDER

RANK	STATE	PERCENT
1	South Dakota	14.45
2	Kentucky	13.87
3	Kansas	12.41
4	Montana	11.96
5	Mississippi	11.25
6	Alabama	11.08
7	West Virginia	10.38
8	Colorado	10.37
9	New Mexico	10.26
10	North Carolina	10.01
11	Hawaii	9.76
12	Arkansas	9.29
13	South Carolina	9.20
14	Oregon	9.11
15	Louisiana	9.05
16	Washington	9.04
17	Tennessee	9.02
18	Maryland	8.95
19	Pennsylvania	8.94
20	Michigan	8.93
21	Vermont	8.82
22	Georgia	8.78
23	Idaho	8.49
23	Maine	8.49
25	Wyoming	8.45
26	North Dakota	8.44
27	Wisconsin	8.19
28	Utah	8.15
29	Nebraska	8.14
30	New York	7.96
31	New Jersey	7.93
32	Virginia	7.91
33	Indiana	7.90
34	Missouri	7.78
35	Arizona	7.29
36	Nevada	7.13
37	Minnesota	6.88
38	Texas	6.51
39	Ohio	5.76
40	Massachusetts	5.65
41	Rhode Island	5.62
NA	Alaska**	NA
NA	California**	NA
NA	Connecticut**	NA
NA	Delaware**	NA
NA	Florida**	NA
NA	Illinois**	NA
NA	Iowa**	NA
NA	New Hampshire**	NA
NA	Oklahoma**	NA
	District of Columbia**	NA

Source: Morgan Quitno Press using data from US Dept of Health & Human Serv's, Centers for Disease Control-Prevention
"Abortion Surveillance-United States, 1992" (Morbidity and Mortality Weekly Report, Vol. 45, No. SS-3, 5/3/96)
*By state of occurrence. National percent is for reporting states only.
**Not reported.

Percent of Teenage Abortions Obtained
By Teenagers 17 Years and Younger in 1992
Reporting States' Percent = 41.22% of Teenage Abortions*

ALPHA ORDER

RANK	STATE	PERCENT
9	Alabama	44.62
NA	Alaska**	NA
30	Arizona	38.89
31	Arkansas	38.36
NA	California**	NA
7	Colorado	45.38
NA	Connecticut**	NA
NA	Delaware**	NA
NA	Florida**	NA
19	Georgia	41.79
6	Hawaii	46.11
40	Idaho	33.33
NA	Illinois**	NA
34	Indiana	36.68
NA	Iowa**	NA
3	Kansas	47.79
2	Kentucky	49.67
23	Louisiana	40.32
14	Maine	42.95
10	Maryland	44.59
37	Massachusetts	34.86
26	Michigan	39.43
32	Minnesota	37.40
5	Mississippi	46.22
29	Missouri	38.94
4	Montana	47.05
35	Nebraska	35.94
18	Nevada	42.09
NA	New Hampshire**	NA
22	New Jersey	40.52
8	New Mexico	45.01
11	New York	44.08
12	North Carolina	43.32
39	North Dakota	33.69
36	Ohio	35.75
NA	Oklahoma**	NA
15	Oregon	42.56
16	Pennsylvania	42.40
41	Rhode Island	30.74
17	South Carolina	42.31
1	South Dakota	51.37
24	Tennessee	40.06
33	Texas	36.96
28	Utah	39.10
25	Vermont	39.64
21	Virginia	40.91
13	Washington	43.30
20	West Virginia	40.95
27	Wisconsin	39.14
38	Wyoming	33.78

RANK ORDER

RANK	STATE	PERCENT
1	South Dakota	51.37
2	Kentucky	49.67
3	Kansas	47.79
4	Montana	47.05
5	Mississippi	46.22
6	Hawaii	46.11
7	Colorado	45.38
8	New Mexico	45.01
9	Alabama	44.62
10	Maryland	44.59
11	New York	44.08
12	North Carolina	43.32
13	Washington	43.30
14	Maine	42.95
15	Oregon	42.56
16	Pennsylvania	42.40
17	South Carolina	42.31
18	Nevada	42.09
19	Georgia	41.79
20	West Virginia	40.95
21	Virginia	40.91
22	New Jersey	40.52
23	Louisiana	40.32
24	Tennessee	40.06
25	Vermont	39.64
26	Michigan	39.43
27	Wisconsin	39.14
28	Utah	39.10
29	Missouri	38.94
30	Arizona	38.89
31	Arkansas	38.36
32	Minnesota	37.40
33	Texas	36.96
34	Indiana	36.68
35	Nebraska	35.94
36	Ohio	35.75
37	Massachusetts	34.86
38	Wyoming	33.78
39	North Dakota	33.69
40	Idaho	33.33
41	Rhode Island	30.74
NA	Alaska**	NA
NA	California**	NA
NA	Connecticut**	NA
NA	Delaware**	NA
NA	Florida**	NA
NA	Illinois**	NA
NA	Iowa**	NA
NA	New Hampshire**	NA
NA	Oklahoma**	NA
	District of Columbia**	NA

Source: Morgan Quitno Press using data from US Dept of Health & Human Serv's, Centers for Disease Control-Prevention "Abortion Surveillance-United States, 1992" (Morbidity and Mortality Weekly Report, Vol. 45, No. SS-3, 5/3/96)
By state of occurrence. National percent is for reporting states only.
**Not reported.*

Reported Legal Abortions Performed at 12 Weeks or Less of Gestation in 1992

Reporting States' Total = 651,059 Abortions*

ALPHA ORDER RANK	STATE	ABORTIONS	% of USA	RANK ORDER RANK	STATE	ABORTIONS	% of USA
15	Alabama	11,972	1.84%	1	New York	139,480	21.42%
NA	Alaska**	NA	NA	2	Texas	79,702	12.24%
NA	Arizona**	NA	NA	3	Pennsylvania	43,523	6.68%
27	Arkansas	4,865	0.75%	4	Michigan	30,669	4.71%
NA	California**	NA	NA	5	Georgia	30,455	4.68%
20	Colorado	9,188	1.41%	6	North Carolina	30,411	4.67%
NA	Connecticut**	NA	NA	7	New Jersey	29,664	4.56%
NA	Delaware**	NA	NA	8	Virginia	28,263	4.34%
NA	Florida**	NA	NA	9	Washington	24,490	3.76%
5	Georgia	30,455	4.68%	10	Maryland	18,112	2.78%
26	Hawaii	5,132	0.79%	11	Tennessee	16,599	2.55%
34	Idaho	1,341	0.21%	12	Minnesota	13,729	2.11%
NA	Illinois**	NA	NA	13	Wisconsin	13,051	2.00%
14	Indiana	12,565	1.93%	14	Indiana	12,565	1.93%
NA	Iowa**	NA	NA	15	Alabama	11,972	1.84%
21	Kansas	7,701	1.18%	16	Missouri	11,766	1.81%
23	Kentucky	7,000	1.08%	17	Oregon	11,412	1.75%
19	Louisiana	10,574	1.62%	18	South Carolina	10,604	1.63%
30	Maine	2,997	0.46%	19	Louisiana	10,574	1.62%
10	Maryland	18,112	2.78%	20	Colorado	9,188	1.41%
NA	Massachusetts**	NA	NA	21	Kansas	7,701	1.18%
4	Michigan	30,669	4.71%	22	Nevada	7,391	1.14%
12	Minnesota	13,729	2.11%	23	Kentucky	7,000	1.08%
24	Mississippi	6,523	1.00%	24	Mississippi	6,523	1.00%
16	Missouri	11,766	1.81%	25	Rhode Island	6,096	0.94%
32	Montana	2,569	0.39%	26	Hawaii	5,132	0.79%
NA	Nebraska**	NA	NA	27	Arkansas	4,865	0.75%
22	Nevada	7,391	1.14%	28	New Mexico	4,415	0.68%
NA	New Hampshire**	NA	NA	29	Utah	3,623	0.56%
7	New Jersey	29,664	4.56%	30	Maine	2,997	0.46%
28	New Mexico	4,415	0.68%	31	Vermont	2,668	0.41%
1	New York	139,480	21.42%	32	Montana	2,569	0.39%
6	North Carolina	30,411	4.67%	33	West Virginia	2,538	0.39%
35	North Dakota	1,334	0.20%	34	Idaho	1,341	0.21%
NA	Ohio**	NA	NA	35	North Dakota	1,334	0.20%
NA	Oklahoma**	NA	NA	36	South Dakota	1,034	0.16%
17	Oregon	11,412	1.75%	37	Wyoming	295	0.05%
3	Pennsylvania	43,523	6.68%	NA	Alaska**	NA	NA
25	Rhode Island	6,096	0.94%	NA	Arizona**	NA	NA
18	South Carolina	10,604	1.63%	NA	California**	NA	NA
36	South Dakota	1,034	0.16%	NA	Connecticut**	NA	NA
11	Tennessee	16,599	2.55%	NA	Delaware**	NA	NA
2	Texas	79,702	12.24%	NA	Florida**	NA	NA
29	Utah	3,623	0.56%	NA	Illinois**	NA	NA
31	Vermont	2,668	0.41%	NA	Iowa**	NA	NA
8	Virginia	28,263	4.34%	NA	Massachusetts**	NA	NA
9	Washington	24,490	3.76%	NA	Nebraska**	NA	NA
33	West Virginia	2,538	0.39%	NA	New Hampshire**	NA	NA
13	Wisconsin	13,051	2.00%	NA	Ohio**	NA	NA
37	Wyoming	295	0.05%	NA	Oklahoma**	NA	NA
					District of Columbia	7,308	1.12%

Source: Morgan Quitno Press using data from US Dept of Health & Human Serv's, Centers for Disease Control-Prevention "Abortion Surveillance-United States, 1992" (Morbidity and Mortality Weekly Report, Vol. 45, No. SS-3, 5/3/96)
*By state of occurrence. National total is for reporting states only.
**Not reported.

Percent of Reported Legal Abortions Performed at 12 Weeks Or Less of Gestation in 1992
Reporting States' Percent = 85.76% of Reported Legal Abortions*

ALPHA ORDER			RANK ORDER		
RANK	STATE	PERCENT	RANK	STATE	PERCENT
16	Alabama	89.62	1	Wyoming	99.66
NA	Alaska**	NA	2	South Dakota	99.61
NA	Arizona**	NA	3	Idaho	97.31
29	Arkansas	85.73	4	Indiana	96.78
NA	California**	NA	5	South Carolina	96.33
25	Colorado	86.62	6	Vermont	96.04
NA	Connecticut**	NA	7	Virginia	95.35
NA	Delaware**	NA	8	Maine	92.90
NA	Florida**	NA	9	Nevada	92.13
34	Georgia	80.04	10	Tennessee	92.07
28	Hawaii	86.19	11	Utah	91.93
3	Idaho	97.31	12	Rhode Island	91.44
NA	Illinois**	NA	13	Maryland	91.20
4	Indiana	96.78	14	West Virginia	90.26
NA	Iowa**	NA	15	Oregon	89.96
37	Kansas	74.16	16	Alabama	89.62
33	Kentucky	80.50	17	Montana	89.54
30	Louisiana	85.12	18	North Dakota	89.35
8	Maine	92.90	19	Michigan	88.91
13	Maryland	91.20	20	Washington	88.82
NA	Massachusetts**	NA	21	Pennsylvania	88.75
19	Michigan	88.91	22	Minnesota	88.31
22	Minnesota	88.31	23	Missouri	87.87
26	Mississippi	86.34	24	Texas	87.48
23	Missouri	87.87	25	Colorado	86.62
17	Montana	89.54	26	Mississippi	86.34
NA	Nebraska**	NA	27	North Carolina	86.26
9	Nevada	92.13	28	Hawaii	86.19
NA	New Hampshire**	NA	29	Arkansas	85.73
36	New Jersey	77.72	30	Louisiana	85.12
35	New Mexico	78.50	31	New York	84.91
31	New York	84.91	32	Wisconsin	83.93
27	North Carolina	86.26	33	Kentucky	80.50
18	North Dakota	89.35	34	Georgia	80.04
NA	Ohio**	NA	35	New Mexico	78.50
NA	Oklahoma**	NA	36	New Jersey	77.72
15	Oregon	89.96	37	Kansas	74.16
21	Pennsylvania	88.75	NA	Alaska**	NA
12	Rhode Island	91.44	NA	Arizona**	NA
5	South Carolina	96.33	NA	California**	NA
2	South Dakota	99.61	NA	Connecticut**	NA
10	Tennessee	92.07	NA	Delaware**	NA
24	Texas	87.48	NA	Florida**	NA
11	Utah	91.93	NA	Illinois**	NA
6	Vermont	96.04	NA	Iowa**	NA
7	Virginia	95.35	NA	Massachusetts**	NA
20	Washington	88.82	NA	Nebraska**	NA
14	West Virginia	90.26	NA	New Hampshire**	NA
32	Wisconsin	83.93	NA	Ohio**	NA
1	Wyoming	99.66	NA	Oklahoma**	NA
			District of Columbia		41.29

Source: Morgan Quitno Press using data from US Dept of Health & Human Serv's, Centers for Disease Control-Prevention "Abortion Surveillance-United States, 1992" (Morbidity and Mortality Weekly Report, Vol. 45, No. SS-3, 5/3/96)
*By state of occurrence. National percent is for reporting states only.
**Not reported.

Reported Legal Abortions Performed At or After 21 Weeks of Gestation in 1992

Reporting States' Total = 10,925 Abortions*

ALPHA ORDER

RANK	STATE	ABORTIONS	% of USA
11	Alabama	189	1.73%
NA	Alaska**	NA	NA
NA	Arizona**	NA	NA
28	Arkansas	5	0.05%
NA	California**	NA	NA
13	Colorado	129	1.18%
NA	Connecticut**	NA	NA
NA	Delaware**	NA	NA
NA	Florida**	NA	NA
5	Georgia	787	7.20%
19	Hawaii	59	0.54%
32	Idaho	2	0.02%
NA	Illinois**	NA	NA
33	Indiana	1	0.01%
NA	Iowa**	NA	NA
4	Kansas	934	8.55%
9	Kentucky	240	2.20%
10	Louisiana	205	1.88%
25	Maine	8	0.07%
28	Maryland	5	0.05%
NA	Massachusetts**	NA	NA
14	Michigan	123	1.13%
8	Minnesota	270	2.47%
20	Mississippi	54	0.49%
17	Missouri	76	0.70%
24	Montana	21	0.19%
NA	Nebraska**	NA	NA
27	Nevada	6	0.05%
NA	New Hampshire**	NA	NA
2	New Jersey	2,267	20.75%
21	New Mexico	37	0.34%
1	New York	3,306	30.26%
18	North Carolina	61	0.56%
35	North Dakota	0	0.00%
NA	Ohio**	NA	NA
NA	Oklahoma**	NA	NA
12	Oregon	165	1.51%
7	Pennsylvania	349	3.19%
25	Rhode Island	8	0.07%
22	South Carolina	24	0.22%
35	South Dakota	0	0.00%
23	Tennessee	22	0.20%
3	Texas	955	8.74%
28	Utah	5	0.05%
28	Vermont	5	0.05%
15	Virginia	120	1.10%
6	Washington	352	3.22%
33	West Virginia	1	0.01%
16	Wisconsin	115	1.05%
35	Wyoming	0	0.00%

RANK ORDER

RANK	STATE	ABORTIONS	% of USA
1	New York	3,306	30.26%
2	New Jersey	2,267	20.75%
3	Texas	955	8.74%
4	Kansas	934	8.55%
5	Georgia	787	7.20%
6	Washington	352	3.22%
7	Pennsylvania	349	3.19%
8	Minnesota	270	2.47%
9	Kentucky	240	2.20%
10	Louisiana	205	1.88%
11	Alabama	189	1.73%
12	Oregon	165	1.51%
13	Colorado	129	1.18%
14	Michigan	123	1.13%
15	Virginia	120	1.10%
16	Wisconsin	115	1.05%
17	Missouri	76	0.70%
18	North Carolina	61	0.56%
19	Hawaii	59	0.54%
20	Mississippi	54	0.49%
21	New Mexico	37	0.34%
22	South Carolina	24	0.22%
23	Tennessee	22	0.20%
24	Montana	21	0.19%
25	Maine	8	0.07%
25	Rhode Island	8	0.07%
27	Nevada	6	0.05%
28	Arkansas	5	0.05%
28	Maryland	5	0.05%
28	Utah	5	0.05%
28	Vermont	5	0.05%
32	Idaho	2	0.02%
33	Indiana	1	0.01%
33	West Virginia	1	0.01%
35	North Dakota	0	0.00%
35	South Dakota	0	0.00%
35	Wyoming	0	0.00%
NA	Alaska**	NA	NA
NA	Arizona**	NA	NA
NA	California**	NA	NA
NA	Connecticut**	NA	NA
NA	Delaware**	NA	NA
NA	Florida**	NA	NA
NA	Illinois**	NA	NA
NA	Iowa**	NA	NA
NA	Massachusetts**	NA	NA
NA	Nebraska**	NA	NA
NA	New Hampshire**	NA	NA
NA	Ohio**	NA	NA
NA	Oklahoma**	NA	NA
	District of Columbia	19	0.17%

Source: U.S. Department of Health and Human Services, Centers for Disease Control and Prevention
    "Abortion Surveillance-United States, 1992" (Morbidity and Mortality Weekly Report, Vol. 45, No. SS-3, 5/3/96)
*By state of occurrence. National total is for reporting states only.
**Not reported.

Percent of Reported Legal Abortion Performed At or After 21 Weeks of Gestation in 1992
Reporting States' Percent = 1.5% of Reported Legal Abortions*

ALPHA ORDER

RANK ORDER

RANK	STATE	PERCENT	RANK	STATE	PERCENT
8	Alabama	1.4	1	Kansas	9.0
NA	Alaska**	NA	2	New Jersey	5.9
NA	Arizona**	NA	3	Kentucky	2.8
26	Arkansas	0.1	4	Georgia	2.1
NA	California**	NA	5	New York	2.0
11	Colorado	1.2	6	Louisiana	1.7
NA	Connecticut**	NA	6	Minnesota	1.7
NA	Delaware**	NA	8	Alabama	1.4
NA	Florida**	NA	9	Oregon	1.3
4	Georgia	2.1	9	Washington	1.3
12	Hawaii	1.0	11	Colorado	1.2
26	Idaho	0.1	12	Hawaii	1.0
NA	Illinois**	NA	12	Texas	1.0
32	Indiana	0.0	14	Wisconsin	0.8
NA	Iowa**	NA	15	Mississippi	0.7
1	Kansas	9.0	15	Montana	0.7
3	Kentucky	2.8	15	New Mexico	0.7
6	Louisiana	1.7	15	Pennsylvania	0.7
22	Maine	0.2	19	Missouri	0.6
32	Maryland	0.0	20	Michigan	0.4
NA	Massachusetts**	NA	20	Virginia	0.4
20	Michigan	0.4	22	Maine	0.2
6	Minnesota	1.7	22	North Carolina	0.2
15	Mississippi	0.7	22	South Carolina	0.2
19	Missouri	0.6	22	Vermont	0.2
15	Montana	0.7	26	Arkansas	0.1
NA	Nebraska**	NA	26	Idaho	0.1
26	Nevada	0.1	26	Nevada	0.1
NA	New Hampshire**	NA	26	Rhode Island	0.1
2	New Jersey	5.9	26	Tennessee	0.1
15	New Mexico	0.7	26	Utah	0.1
5	New York	2.0	32	Indiana	0.0
22	North Carolina	0.2	32	Maryland	0.0
32	North Dakota	0.0	32	North Dakota	0.0
NA	Ohio**	NA	32	South Dakota	0.0
NA	Oklahoma**	NA	32	West Virginia	0.0
9	Oregon	1.3	32	Wyoming	0.0
15	Pennsylvania	0.7	NA	Alaska**	NA
26	Rhode Island	0.1	NA	Arizona**	NA
22	South Carolina	0.2	NA	California**	NA
32	South Dakota	0.0	NA	Connecticut**	NA
26	Tennessee	0.1	NA	Delaware**	NA
12	Texas	1.0	NA	Florida**	NA
26	Utah	0.1	NA	Illinois**	NA
22	Vermont	0.2	NA	Iowa**	NA
20	Virginia	0.4	NA	Massachusetts**	NA
9	Washington	1.3	NA	Nebraska**	NA
32	West Virginia	0.0	NA	New Hampshire**	NA
14	Wisconsin	0.8	NA	Ohio**	NA
32	Wyoming	0.0	NA	Oklahoma**	NA
				District of Columbia	0.2

Source: U.S. Department of Health and Human Services, Centers for Disease Control and Prevention
"Abortion Surveillance-United States, 1992" (Morbidity and Mortality Weekly Report, Vol. 45, No. SS-3, 5/3/96)
*By state of occurrence. National percent is for reporting states only.
**Not reported.

II. DEATHS

II. DEATHS (Continued)

Deaths in 1995

National Total = 2,312,180 Deaths*

RANK	STATE	DEATHS	% of USA
18	Alabama	42,417	1.83%
50	Alaska	2,540	0.11%
24	Arizona	35,336	1.53%
30	Arkansas	26,665	1.15%
1	California	223,227	9.65%
32	Colorado	25,003	1.08%
27	Connecticut	28,890	1.25%
46	Delaware	6,278	0.27%
3	Florida	153,641	6.64%
12	Georgia	58,364	2.52%
43	Hawaii	7,637	0.33%
42	Idaho	8,493	0.37%
6	Illinois	108,732	4.70%
15	Indiana	52,160	2.26%
31	Iowa	25,983	1.12%
33	Kansas	23,781	1.03%
22	Kentucky	38,052	1.65%
21	Louisiana	39,564	1.71%
38	Maine	11,625	0.50%
19	Maryland	41,763	1.81%
13	Massachusetts	56,041	2.42%
8	Michigan	83,513	3.61%
23	Minnesota	37,313	1.61%
29	Mississippi	26,992	1.17%
11	Missouri	58,601	2.53%
44	Montana	7,612	0.33%
35	Nebraska	15,314	0.66%
37	Nevada	12,507	0.54%
41	New Hampshire	9,268	0.40%
9	New Jersey	74,016	3.20%
36	New Mexico	12,545	0.54%
2	New York	168,081	7.27%
10	North Carolina	64,966	2.81%
47	North Dakota	6,094	0.26%
7	Ohio	106,014	4.59%
25	Oklahoma	32,757	1.42%
28	Oregon	28,240	1.22%
5	Pennsylvania	128,116	5.54%
40	Rhode Island	9,643	0.42%
26	South Carolina	32,512	1.41%
45	South Dakota	6,829	0.30%
16	Tennessee	51,027	2.21%
4	Texas	138,830	6.00%
39	Utah	10,825	0.47%
48	Vermont	5,040	0.22%
14	Virginia	52,868	2.29%
20	Washington	40,525	1.75%
34	West Virginia	20,249	0.88%
17	Wisconsin	45,088	1.95%
49	Wyoming	3,749	0.16%

RANK ORDER

RANK	STATE	DEATHS	% of USA
1	California	223,227	9.65%
2	New York	168,081	7.27%
3	Florida	153,641	6.64%
4	Texas	138,830	6.00%
5	Pennsylvania	128,116	5.54%
6	Illinois	108,732	4.70%
7	Ohio	106,014	4.59%
8	Michigan	83,513	3.61%
9	New Jersey	74,016	3.20%
10	North Carolina	64,966	2.81%
11	Missouri	58,601	2.53%
12	Georgia	58,364	2.52%
13	Massachusetts	56,041	2.42%
14	Virginia	52,868	2.29%
15	Indiana	52,160	2.26%
16	Tennessee	51,027	2.21%
17	Wisconsin	45,088	1.95%
18	Alabama	42,417	1.83%
19	Maryland	41,763	1.81%
20	Washington	40,525	1.75%
21	Louisiana	39,564	1.71%
22	Kentucky	38,052	1.65%
23	Minnesota	37,313	1.61%
24	Arizona	35,336	1.53%
25	Oklahoma	32,757	1.42%
26	South Carolina	32,512	1.41%
27	Connecticut	28,890	1.25%
28	Oregon	28,240	1.22%
29	Mississippi	26,992	1.17%
30	Arkansas	26,665	1.15%
31	Iowa	25,983	1.12%
32	Colorado	25,003	1.08%
33	Kansas	23,781	1.03%
34	West Virginia	20,249	0.88%
35	Nebraska	15,314	0.66%
36	New Mexico	12,545	0.54%
37	Nevada	12,507	0.54%
38	Maine	11,625	0.50%
39	Utah	10,825	0.47%
40	Rhode Island	9,643	0.42%
41	New Hampshire	9,268	0.40%
42	Idaho	8,493	0.37%
43	Hawaii	7,637	0.33%
44	Montana	7,612	0.33%
45	South Dakota	6,829	0.30%
46	Delaware	6,278	0.27%
47	North Dakota	6,094	0.26%
48	Vermont	5,040	0.22%
49	Wyoming	3,749	0.16%
50	Alaska	2,540	0.11%
	District of Columbia	6,852	0.30%

Source: U.S. Department of Health and Human Services, National Center for Health Statistics
    "Monthly Vital Statistics Report" (Vol. 45, No. 3(S)2, October 4, 1996)
*Preliminary data by state of residence.

Death Rate in 1995

National Rate = 880.0 Deaths per 100,000 Population*

RANK	STATE	RATE		RANK	STATE	RATE
ALPHA ORDER				RANK ORDER		
8	Alabama	997.3		1	West Virginia	1,107.6
50	Alaska	420.8		2	Missouri	1,100.8
34	Arizona	837.8		3	Florida	1,084.6
4	Arkansas	1,073.6		4	Arkansas	1,073.6
46	California	706.7		5	Pennsylvania	1,061.3
47	Colorado	667.4		6	Mississippi	1,000.7
28	Connecticut	882.2		7	Oklahoma	999.4
30	Delaware	875.4		8	Alabama	997.3
3	Florida	1,084.6		9	Kentucky	985.7
37	Georgia	810.5		10	Rhode Island	974.2
48	Hawaii	643.5		11	Tennessee	970.8
45	Idaho	730.1		12	Ohio	950.8
21	Illinois	919.1		13	North Dakota	950.2
26	Indiana	898.8		14	South Dakota	936.7
22	Iowa	914.3		15	Maine	936.5
18	Kansas	927.0		16	Nebraska	935.4
9	Kentucky	985.7		17	New Jersey	931.6
23	Louisiana	911.1		18	Kansas	927.0
15	Maine	936.5		19	New York	926.8
35	Maryland	828.2		20	Massachusetts	922.7
20	Massachusetts	922.7		21	Illinois	919.1
32	Michigan	874.5		22	Iowa	914.3
38	Minnesota	809.5		23	Louisiana	911.1
6	Mississippi	1,000.7		24	North Carolina	902.9
2	Missouri	1,100.8		25	Oregon	899.2
31	Montana	874.7		26	Indiana	898.8
16	Nebraska	935.4		27	South Carolina	885.1
36	Nevada	817.4		28	Connecticut	882.2
39	New Hampshire	807.1		29	Wisconsin	880.1
17	New Jersey	931.6		30	Delaware	875.4
43	New Mexico	744.3		31	Montana	874.7
19	New York	926.8		32	Michigan	874.5
24	North Carolina	902.9		33	Vermont	861.9
13	North Dakota	950.2		34	Arizona	837.8
12	Ohio	950.8		35	Maryland	828.2
7	Oklahoma	999.4		36	Nevada	817.4
25	Oregon	899.2		37	Georgia	810.5
5	Pennsylvania	1,061.3		38	Minnesota	809.5
10	Rhode Island	974.2		39	New Hampshire	807.1
27	South Carolina	885.1		40	Virginia	798.8
14	South Dakota	936.7		41	Wyoming	780.7
11	Tennessee	970.8		42	Washington	746.2
44	Texas	741.5		43	New Mexico	744.3
49	Utah	554.7		44	Texas	741.5
33	Vermont	861.9		45	Idaho	730.1
40	Virginia	798.8		46	California	706.7
42	Washington	746.2		47	Colorado	667.4
1	West Virginia	1,107.6		48	Hawaii	643.5
29	Wisconsin	880.1		49	Utah	554.7
41	Wyoming	780.7		50	Alaska	420.8
					District of Columbia	1,236.3

Source: U.S. Department of Health and Human Services, National Center for Health Statistics
"Monthly Vital Statistics Report" (Vol. 45, No. 3(S)2, October 4, 1996)
Preliminary data by state of residence. Not age adjusted.

Births to Deaths Ratio in 1995

National Ratio = 1.69 Births for Every Death in 1995

ALPHA ORDER

RANK	STATE	RATIO
36	Alabama	1.44
1	Alaska	4.03
9	Arizona	2.05
44	Arkansas	1.32
3	California	2.51
6	Colorado	2.17
26	Connecticut	1.56
19	Delaware	1.63
47	Florida	1.23
11	Georgia	1.95
4	Hawaii	2.44
8	Idaho	2.12
14	Illinois	1.71
20	Indiana	1.62
39	Iowa	1.41
23	Kansas	1.58
41	Kentucky	1.36
16	Louisiana	1.70
48	Maine	1.20
14	Maryland	1.71
43	Massachusetts	1.34
22	Michigan	1.59
17	Minnesota	1.69
29	Mississippi	1.53
46	Missouri	1.26
35	Montana	1.46
30	Nebraska	1.52
10	Nevada	2.00
21	New Hampshire	1.61
33	New Jersey	1.47
7	New Mexico	2.16
24	New York	1.57
24	North Carolina	1.57
38	North Dakota	1.42
33	Ohio	1.47
40	Oklahoma	1.40
30	Oregon	1.52
49	Pennsylvania	1.18
45	Rhode Island	1.28
27	South Carolina	1.54
27	South Dakota	1.54
36	Tennessee	1.44
5	Texas	2.37
2	Utah	3.65
41	Vermont	1.36
13	Virginia	1.76
12	Washington	1.93
50	West Virginia	1.04
32	Wisconsin	1.50
17	Wyoming	1.69

RANK ORDER

RANK	STATE	RATIO
1	Alaska	4.03
2	Utah	3.65
3	California	2.51
4	Hawaii	2.44
5	Texas	2.37
6	Colorado	2.17
7	New Mexico	2.16
8	Idaho	2.12
9	Arizona	2.05
10	Nevada	2.00
11	Georgia	1.95
12	Washington	1.93
13	Virginia	1.76
14	Illinois	1.71
14	Maryland	1.71
16	Louisiana	1.70
17	Minnesota	1.69
17	Wyoming	1.69
19	Delaware	1.63
20	Indiana	1.62
21	New Hampshire	1.61
22	Michigan	1.59
23	Kansas	1.58
24	New York	1.57
24	North Carolina	1.57
26	Connecticut	1.56
27	South Carolina	1.54
27	South Dakota	1.54
29	Mississippi	1.53
30	Nebraska	1.52
30	Oregon	1.52
32	Wisconsin	1.50
33	New Jersey	1.47
33	Ohio	1.47
35	Montana	1.46
36	Alabama	1.44
36	Tennessee	1.44
38	North Dakota	1.42
39	Iowa	1.41
40	Oklahoma	1.40
41	Kentucky	1.36
41	Vermont	1.36
43	Massachusetts	1.34
44	Arkansas	1.32
45	Rhode Island	1.28
46	Missouri	1.26
47	Florida	1.23
48	Maine	1.20
49	Pennsylvania	1.18
50	West Virginia	1.04
	District of Columbia	1.29

Source: Morgan Quitno Press using data from U.S. Dept. of Health & Human Services, National Center for Health Statistics "Monthly Vital Statistics Report" (Vol. 45, No. 3(S)2, October 4, 1996)
Preliminary data. By state of residence.

Deaths in 1990

National Total = 2,148,463 Deaths*

RANK	STATE	DEATHS	% of USA
18	Alabama	39,381	1.83%
50	Alaska	2,188	0.10%
26	Arizona	28,789	1.34%
31	Arkansas	24,652	1.15%
1	California	214,369	9.98%
33	Colorado	21,583	1.00%
27	Connecticut	27,607	1.28%
46	Delaware	5,764	0.27%
3	Florida	134,385	6.25%
12	Georgia	51,810	2.41%
44	Hawaii	6,782	0.32%
42	Idaho	7,452	0.35%
6	Illinois	103,006	4.79%
14	Indiana	49,569	2.31%
28	Iowa	26,884	1.25%
32	Kansas	22,279	1.04%
22	Kentucky	35,078	1.63%
20	Louisiana	37,571	1.75%
36	Maine	11,106	0.52%
19	Maryland	38,413	1.79%
11	Massachusetts	53,179	2.48%
8	Michigan	78,744	3.67%
23	Minnesota	34,776	1.62%
30	Mississippi	25,127	1.17%
13	Missouri	50,377	2.34%
43	Montana	6,861	0.32%
35	Nebraska	14,769	0.69%
39	Nevada	9,318	0.43%
41	New Hampshire	8,488	0.40%
9	New Jersey	70,383	3.28%
37	New Mexico	10,625	0.49%
2	New York	168,936	7.86%
10	North Carolina	57,315	2.67%
47	North Dakota	5,678	0.26%
7	Ohio	98,822	4.60%
24	Oklahoma	30,378	1.41%
29	Oregon	25,136	1.17%
5	Pennsylvania	121,951	5.68%
38	Rhode Island	9,576	0.45%
25	South Carolina	29,715	1.38%
45	South Dakota	6,326	0.29%
16	Tennessee	46,315	2.16%
4	Texas	125,479	5.84%
40	Utah	9,192	0.43%
48	Vermont	4,595	0.21%
15	Virginia	48,013	2.23%
21	Washington	37,087	1.73%
34	West Virginia	19,385	0.90%
17	Wisconsin	42,733	1.99%
49	Wyoming	3,203	0.15%

RANK	STATE	DEATHS	% of USA
1	California	214,369	9.98%
2	New York	168,936	7.86%
3	Florida	134,385	6.25%
4	Texas	125,479	5.84%
5	Pennsylvania	121,951	5.68%
6	Illinois	103,006	4.79%
7	Ohio	98,822	4.60%
8	Michigan	78,744	3.67%
9	New Jersey	70,383	3.28%
10	North Carolina	57,315	2.67%
11	Massachusetts	53,179	2.48%
12	Georgia	51,810	2.41%
13	Missouri	50,377	2.34%
14	Indiana	49,569	2.31%
15	Virginia	48,013	2.23%
16	Tennessee	46,315	2.16%
17	Wisconsin	42,733	1.99%
18	Alabama	39,381	1.83%
19	Maryland	38,413	1.79%
20	Louisiana	37,571	1.75%
21	Washington	37,087	1.73%
22	Kentucky	35,078	1.63%
23	Minnesota	34,776	1.62%
24	Oklahoma	30,378	1.41%
25	South Carolina	29,715	1.38%
26	Arizona	28,789	1.34%
27	Connecticut	27,607	1.28%
28	Iowa	26,884	1.25%
29	Oregon	25,136	1.17%
30	Mississippi	25,127	1.17%
31	Arkansas	24,652	1.15%
32	Kansas	22,279	1.04%
33	Colorado	21,583	1.00%
34	West Virginia	19,385	0.90%
35	Nebraska	14,769	0.69%
36	Maine	11,106	0.52%
37	New Mexico	10,625	0.49%
38	Rhode Island	9,576	0.45%
39	Nevada	9,318	0.43%
40	Utah	9,192	0.43%
41	New Hampshire	8,488	0.40%
42	Idaho	7,452	0.35%
43	Montana	6,861	0.32%
44	Hawaii	6,782	0.32%
45	South Dakota	6,326	0.29%
46	Delaware	5,764	0.27%
47	North Dakota	5,678	0.26%
48	Vermont	4,595	0.21%
49	Wyoming	3,203	0.15%
50	Alaska	2,188	0.10%
	District of Columbia	7,313	0.34%

*Source: U.S. Department of Health and Human Services, National Center for Health Statistics
"Monthly Vital Statistics Report" (Vol. 41, No. 7(S), January 7, 1993)*
Final data by state of residence.

Death Rate in 1990

National Rate = 8.63 Deaths per 1,000 Population*

ALPHA ORDER

RANK	STATE	RATE
7	Alabama	9.74
50	Alaska	3.98
37	Arizona	7.84
2	Arkansas	10.48
44	California	7.19
47	Colorado	6.55
32	Connecticut	8.40
27	Delaware	8.64
3	Florida	10.38
35	Georgia	7.99
48	Hawaii	6.11
42	Idaho	7.40
19	Illinois	9.00
21	Indiana	8.94
8	Iowa	9.68
20	Kansas	8.99
11	Kentucky	9.51
22	Louisiana	8.90
18	Maine	9.05
34	Maryland	8.03
24	Massachusetts	8.84
31	Michigan	8.47
36	Minnesota	7.95
6	Mississippi	9.76
5	Missouri	9.84
29	Montana	8.59
14	Nebraska	9.36
38	Nevada	7.75
40	New Hampshire	7.65
16	New Jersey	9.10
46	New Mexico	7.01
13	New York	9.38
27	North Carolina	8.64
22	North Dakota	8.90
15	Ohio	9.11
9	Oklahoma	9.66
24	Oregon	8.84
4	Pennsylvania	10.26
10	Rhode Island	9.54
30	South Carolina	8.52
17	South Dakota	9.09
12	Tennessee	9.49
43	Texas	7.38
49	Utah	5.33
33	Vermont	8.17
38	Virginia	7.75
41	Washington	7.62
1	West Virginia	10.80
26	Wisconsin	8.74
45	Wyoming	7.06

RANK ORDER

RANK	STATE	RATE
1	West Virginia	10.80
2	Arkansas	10.48
3	Florida	10.38
4	Pennsylvania	10.26
5	Missouri	9.84
6	Mississippi	9.76
7	Alabama	9.74
8	Iowa	9.68
9	Oklahoma	9.66
10	Rhode Island	9.54
11	Kentucky	9.51
12	Tennessee	9.49
13	New York	9.38
14	Nebraska	9.36
15	Ohio	9.11
16	New Jersey	9.10
17	South Dakota	9.09
18	Maine	9.05
19	Illinois	9.00
20	Kansas	8.99
21	Indiana	8.94
22	Louisiana	8.90
22	North Dakota	8.90
24	Massachusetts	8.84
24	Oregon	8.84
26	Wisconsin	8.74
27	Delaware	8.64
27	North Carolina	8.64
29	Montana	8.59
30	South Carolina	8.52
31	Michigan	8.47
32	Connecticut	8.40
33	Vermont	8.17
34	Maryland	8.03
35	Georgia	7.99
36	Minnesota	7.95
37	Arizona	7.84
38	Nevada	7.75
38	Virginia	7.75
40	New Hampshire	7.65
41	Washington	7.62
42	Idaho	7.40
43	Texas	7.38
44	California	7.19
45	Wyoming	7.06
46	New Mexico	7.01
47	Colorado	6.55
48	Hawaii	6.11
49	Utah	5.33
50	Alaska	3.98

District of Columbia	12.00

Source: U.S. Department of Health and Human Services, National Center for Health Statistics
"Monthly Vital Statistics Report" (Vol. 41, No. 7(S), January 7, 1993)
*Final data by state of residence. Not age adjusted.

Deaths in 1980

National Total = 1,989,841 Deaths*

<u>ALPHA ORDER</u>

RANK	STATE	DEATHS	% of USA
19	Alabama	35,542	1.79%
50	Alaska	1,714	0.09%
32	Arizona	21,367	1.07%
29	Arkansas	22,744	1.14%
1	California	186,624	9.38%
34	Colorado	18,956	0.95%
25	Connecticut	27,275	1.37%
46	Delaware	5,044	0.25%
5	Florida	104,670	5.26%
14	Georgia	44,262	2.22%
47	Hawaii	4,981	0.25%
41	Idaho	6,763	0.34%
6	Illinois	102,935	5.17%
13	Indiana	47,345	2.38%
26	Iowa	27,120	1.36%
30	Kansas	22,034	1.11%
21	Kentucky	33,796	1.70%
18	Louisiana	35,651	1.79%
36	Maine	10,800	0.54%
20	Maryland	34,016	1.71%
10	Massachusetts	55,070	2.77%
8	Michigan	75,187	3.78%
22	Minnesota	33,366	1.68%
28	Mississippi	23,656	1.19%
11	Missouri	49,660	2.50%
42	Montana	6,666	0.34%
35	Nebraska	14,474	0.73%
44	Nevada	5,896	0.30%
40	New Hampshire	7,647	0.38%
9	New Jersey	68,943	3.46%
38	New Mexico	9,093	0.46%
2	New York	172,853	8.69%
12	North Carolina	48,440	2.43%
45	North Dakota	5,596	0.28%
7	Ohio	98,421	4.95%
24	Oklahoma	28,234	1.42%
31	Oregon	21,798	1.10%
3	Pennsylvania	123,594	6.21%
37	Rhode Island	9,325	0.47%
27	South Carolina	25,154	1.26%
43	South Dakota	6,556	0.33%
17	Tennessee	40,774	2.05%
4	Texas	108,180	5.44%
39	Utah	8,120	0.41%
48	Vermont	4,582	0.23%
15	Virginia	42,506	2.14%
23	Washington	32,007	1.61%
33	West Virginia	19,237	0.97%
16	Wisconsin	40,838	2.05%
49	Wyoming	3,221	0.16%

<u>RANK ORDER</u>

RANK	STATE	DEATHS	% of USA
1	California	186,624	9.38%
2	New York	172,853	8.69%
3	Pennsylvania	123,594	6.21%
4	Texas	108,180	5.44%
5	Florida	104,670	5.26%
6	Illinois	102,935	5.17%
7	Ohio	98,421	4.95%
8	Michigan	75,187	3.78%
9	New Jersey	68,943	3.46%
10	Massachusetts	55,070	2.77%
11	Missouri	49,660	2.50%
12	North Carolina	48,440	2.43%
13	Indiana	47,345	2.38%
14	Georgia	44,262	2.22%
15	Virginia	42,506	2.14%
16	Wisconsin	40,838	2.05%
17	Tennessee	40,774	2.05%
18	Louisiana	35,651	1.79%
19	Alabama	35,542	1.79%
20	Maryland	34,016	1.71%
21	Kentucky	33,796	1.70%
22	Minnesota	33,366	1.68%
23	Washington	32,007	1.61%
24	Oklahoma	28,234	1.42%
25	Connecticut	27,275	1.37%
26	Iowa	27,120	1.36%
27	South Carolina	25,154	1.26%
28	Mississippi	23,656	1.19%
29	Arkansas	22,744	1.14%
30	Kansas	22,034	1.11%
31	Oregon	21,798	1.10%
32	Arizona	21,367	1.07%
33	West Virginia	19,237	0.97%
34	Colorado	18,956	0.95%
35	Nebraska	14,474	0.73%
36	Maine	10,800	0.54%
37	Rhode Island	9,325	0.47%
38	New Mexico	9,093	0.46%
39	Utah	8,120	0.41%
40	New Hampshire	7,647	0.38%
41	Idaho	6,763	0.34%
42	Montana	6,666	0.34%
43	South Dakota	6,556	0.33%
44	Nevada	5,896	0.30%
45	North Dakota	5,596	0.28%
46	Delaware	5,044	0.25%
47	Hawaii	4,981	0.25%
48	Vermont	4,582	0.23%
49	Wyoming	3,221	0.16%
50	Alaska	1,714	0.09%
	District of Columbia	7,108	0.36%

Source: U.S. Department of Health and Human Services, National Center for Health Statistics
"Vital Statistics of the United States 1980" and "Monthly Vital Statistics Report"
*Final data by state of residence.

Death Rate in 1980

National Rate = 8.77 Deaths per 1,000 Population*

ALPHA ORDER			RANK ORDER		
RANK	STATE	RATE	RANK	STATE	RATE
18	Alabama	9.12	1	Florida	10.72
50	Alaska	4.25	2	Pennsylvania	10.41
40	Arizona	7.84	3	Missouri	10.08
4	Arkansas	9.94	4	Arkansas	9.94
39	California	7.86	5	West Virginia	9.87
47	Colorado	6.54	6	New York	9.84
23	Connecticut	8.77	6	Rhode Island	9.84
27	Delaware	8.47	8	Maine	9.60
1	Florida	10.72	9	Massachusetts	9.59
35	Georgia	8.09	10	South Dakota	9.47
49	Hawaii	5.15	11	Mississippi	9.37
44	Idaho	7.15	12	New Jersey	9.36
20	Illinois	8.99	13	Oklahoma	9.32
25	Indiana	8.62	14	Iowa	9.30
14	Iowa	9.30	14	Kansas	9.30
14	Kansas	9.30	16	Kentucky	9.22
16	Kentucky	9.22	17	Nebraska	9.20
28	Louisiana	8.46	18	Alabama	9.12
8	Maine	9.60	19	Ohio	9.11
36	Maryland	8.06	20	Illinois	8.99
9	Massachusetts	9.59	21	Vermont	8.95
34	Michigan	8.11	22	Tennessee	8.87
33	Minnesota	8.17	23	Connecticut	8.77
11	Mississippi	9.37	24	Wisconsin	8.67
3	Missouri	10.08	25	Indiana	8.62
28	Montana	8.46	26	North Dakota	8.56
17	Nebraska	9.20	27	Delaware	8.47
43	Nevada	7.35	28	Louisiana	8.46
30	New Hampshire	8.30	28	Montana	8.46
12	New Jersey	9.36	30	New Hampshire	8.30
45	New Mexico	6.96	31	Oregon	8.27
6	New York	9.84	32	North Carolina	8.23
32	North Carolina	8.23	33	Minnesota	8.17
26	North Dakota	8.56	34	Michigan	8.11
19	Ohio	9.11	35	Georgia	8.09
13	Oklahoma	9.32	36	Maryland	8.06
31	Oregon	8.27	37	South Carolina	8.05
2	Pennsylvania	10.41	38	Virginia	7.94
6	Rhode Island	9.84	39	California	7.86
37	South Carolina	8.05	40	Arizona	7.84
10	South Dakota	9.47	41	Washington	7.73
22	Tennessee	8.87	42	Texas	7.58
42	Texas	7.58	43	Nevada	7.35
48	Utah	5.54	44	Idaho	7.15
21	Vermont	8.95	45	New Mexico	6.96
38	Virginia	7.94	46	Wyoming	6.84
41	Washington	7.73	47	Colorado	6.54
5	West Virginia	9.87	48	Utah	5.54
24	Wisconsin	8.67	49	Hawaii	5.15
46	Wyoming	6.84	50	Alaska	4.25
				District of Columbia	11.09

Source: U.S. Department of Health and Human Services, National Center for Health Statistics
"Vital Statistics of the United States 1980" and "Monthly Vital Statistics Report"
*Final data by state of residence. Not age adjusted.

Infant Deaths in 1996

National Total = 28,400 Infant Deaths*

ALPHA ORDER

RANK	STATE	DEATHS	% of USA
15	Alabama	626	2.20%
43	Alaska	76	0.27%
17	Arizona	573	2.02%
29	Arkansas	313	1.10%
1	California	3,397	11.96%
27	Colorado	341	1.20%
34	Connecticut	207	0.73%
46	Delaware	63	0.22%
5	Florida	1,442	5.08%
9	Georgia	1,086	3.82%
40	Hawaii	106	0.37%
39	Idaho	124	0.44%
4	Illinois	1,584	5.58%
13	Indiana	666	2.35%
33	Iowa	209	0.74%
28	Kansas	321	1.13%
23	Kentucky	411	1.45%
18	Louisiana	559	1.97%
47	Maine	61	0.21%
16	Maryland	591	2.08%
25	Massachusetts	392	1.38%
8	Michigan	1,097	3.86%
26	Minnesota	391	1.38%
24	Mississippi	401	1.41%
19	Missouri	557	1.96%
42	Montana	83	0.29%
35	Nebraska	185	0.65%
38	Nevada	138	0.49%
44	New Hampshire	66	0.23%
11	New Jersey	795	2.80%
36	New Mexico	170	0.60%
3	New York	1,983	6.98%
10	North Carolina	942	3.32%
50	North Dakota	37	0.13%
6	Ohio	1,249	4.40%
22	Oklahoma	412	1.45%
31	Oregon	232	0.82%
7	Pennsylvania	1,144	4.03%
41	Rhode Island	84	0.30%
21	South Carolina	414	1.46%
45	South Dakota	64	0.23%
14	Tennessee	657	2.31%
2	Texas	2,130	7.50%
32	Utah	226	0.80%
48	Vermont	58	0.20%
12	Virginia	676	2.38%
30	Washington	245	0.86%
37	West Virginia	167	0.59%
20	Wisconsin	503	1.77%
49	Wyoming	50	0.18%

RANK ORDER

RANK	STATE	DEATHS	% of USA
1	California	3,397	11.96%
2	Texas	2,130	7.50%
3	New York	1,983	6.98%
4	Illinois	1,584	5.58%
5	Florida	1,442	5.08%
6	Ohio	1,249	4.40%
7	Pennsylvania	1,144	4.03%
8	Michigan	1,097	3.86%
9	Georgia	1,086	3.82%
10	North Carolina	942	3.32%
11	New Jersey	795	2.80%
12	Virginia	676	2.38%
13	Indiana	666	2.35%
14	Tennessee	657	2.31%
15	Alabama	626	2.20%
16	Maryland	591	2.08%
17	Arizona	573	2.02%
18	Louisiana	559	1.97%
19	Missouri	557	1.96%
20	Wisconsin	503	1.77%
21	South Carolina	414	1.46%
22	Oklahoma	412	1.45%
23	Kentucky	411	1.45%
24	Mississippi	401	1.41%
25	Massachusetts	392	1.38%
26	Minnesota	391	1.38%
27	Colorado	341	1.20%
28	Kansas	321	1.13%
29	Arkansas	313	1.10%
30	Washington	245	0.86%
31	Oregon	232	0.82%
32	Utah	226	0.80%
33	Iowa	209	0.74%
34	Connecticut	207	0.73%
35	Nebraska	185	0.65%
36	New Mexico	170	0.60%
37	West Virginia	167	0.59%
38	Nevada	138	0.49%
39	Idaho	124	0.44%
40	Hawaii	106	0.37%
41	Rhode Island	84	0.30%
42	Montana	83	0.29%
43	Alaska	76	0.27%
44	New Hampshire	66	0.23%
45	South Dakota	64	0.23%
46	Delaware	63	0.22%
47	Maine	61	0.21%
48	Vermont	58	0.20%
49	Wyoming	50	0.18%
50	North Dakota	37	0.13%
	District of Columbia	136	0.48%

Source: U.S. Department of Health and Human Services, National Center for Health Statistics
        "Monthly Vital Statistics Report" (Vol. 45, No. 7, February 19, 1997)
For 12 months ending July 1996. Provisional data. Deaths under 1 year old by state of residence.

Infant Mortality Rate in 1996

National Rate = 7.3 Infant Deaths per 1,000 Live Births*

ALPHA ORDER

RANK	STATE	RATE
2	Alabama	10.3
20	Alaska	7.9
20	Arizona	7.9
8	Arkansas	8.9
37	California	6.2
30	Colorado	7.1
44	Connecticut	5.4
36	Delaware	6.3
24	Florida	7.7
3	Georgia	9.5
41	Hawaii	5.7
32	Idaho	6.6
9	Illinois	8.6
15	Indiana	8.1
41	Iowa	5.7
4	Kansas	9.3
20	Kentucky	7.9
12	Louisiana	8.4
47	Maine	4.4
12	Maryland	8.4
47	Massachusetts	4.4
18	Michigan	8.0
37	Minnesota	6.2
1	Mississippi	10.5
26	Missouri	7.5
26	Montana	7.5
18	Nebraska	8.0
40	Nevada	6.0
46	New Hampshire	4.5
31	New Jersey	6.9
37	New Mexico	6.2
29	New York	7.4
4	North Carolina	9.3
47	North Dakota	4.4
15	Ohio	8.1
4	Oklahoma	9.3
45	Oregon	5.3
25	Pennsylvania	7.6
32	Rhode Island	6.6
14	South Carolina	8.2
34	South Dakota	6.5
7	Tennessee	9.0
34	Texas	6.5
41	Utah	5.7
11	Vermont	8.5
20	Virginia	7.9
50	Washington	3.2
9	West Virginia	8.6
26	Wisconsin	7.5
15	Wyoming	8.1

RANK ORDER

RANK	STATE	RATE
1	Mississippi	10.5
2	Alabama	10.3
3	Georgia	9.5
4	Kansas	9.3
4	North Carolina	9.3
4	Oklahoma	9.3
7	Tennessee	9.0
8	Arkansas	8.9
9	Illinois	8.6
9	West Virginia	8.6
11	Vermont	8.5
12	Louisiana	8.4
12	Maryland	8.4
14	South Carolina	8.2
15	Indiana	8.1
15	Ohio	8.1
15	Wyoming	8.1
18	Michigan	8.0
18	Nebraska	8.0
20	Alaska	7.9
20	Arizona	7.9
20	Kentucky	7.9
20	Virginia	7.9
24	Florida	7.7
25	Pennsylvania	7.6
26	Missouri	7.5
26	Montana	7.5
26	Wisconsin	7.5
29	New York	7.4
30	Colorado	7.1
31	New Jersey	6.9
32	Idaho	6.6
32	Rhode Island	6.6
34	South Dakota	6.5
34	Texas	6.5
36	Delaware	6.3
37	California	6.2
37	Minnesota	6.2
37	New Mexico	6.2
40	Nevada	6.0
41	Hawaii	5.7
41	Iowa	5.7
41	Utah	5.7
44	Connecticut	5.4
45	Oregon	5.3
46	New Hampshire	4.5
47	Maine	4.4
47	Massachusetts	4.4
47	North Dakota	4.4
50	Washington	3.2

	District of Columbia	16.2

Source: U.S. Department of Health and Human Services, National Center for Health Statistics
    "Monthly Vital Statistics Report" (Vol. 45, No. 7, February 19, 1997)
*For 12 months ending July 1996. Provisional data. Deaths under 1 year old by state of residence.

Infant Deaths in 1995

National Total = 29,300 Infant Deaths*

<table>
<tr><td colspan="4">ALPHA ORDER</td><td colspan="4">RANK ORDER</td></tr>
<tr><th>RANK</th><th>STATE</th><th>DEATHS</th><th>% of USA</th><th>RANK</th><th>STATE</th><th>DEATHS</th><th>% of USA</th></tr>
<tr><td>17</td><td>Alabama</td><td>624</td><td>2.13%</td><td>1</td><td>California</td><td>3,441</td><td>11.74%</td></tr>
<tr><td>47</td><td>Alaska</td><td>68</td><td>0.23%</td><td>2</td><td>Texas</td><td>2,150</td><td>7.34%</td></tr>
<tr><td>19</td><td>Arizona</td><td>509</td><td>1.74%</td><td>3</td><td>New York</td><td>2,067</td><td>7.05%</td></tr>
<tr><td>29</td><td>Arkansas</td><td>298</td><td>1.02%</td><td>4</td><td>Illinois</td><td>1,662</td><td>5.67%</td></tr>
<tr><td>1</td><td>California</td><td>3,441</td><td>11.74%</td><td>5</td><td>Florida</td><td>1,416</td><td>4.83%</td></tr>
<tr><td>28</td><td>Colorado</td><td>356</td><td>1.22%</td><td>6</td><td>Ohio</td><td>1,310</td><td>4.47%</td></tr>
<tr><td>31</td><td>Connecticut</td><td>271</td><td>0.92%</td><td>7</td><td>Pennsylvania</td><td>1,149</td><td>3.92%</td></tr>
<tr><td>46</td><td>Delaware</td><td>72</td><td>0.25%</td><td>8</td><td>Michigan</td><td>1,129</td><td>3.85%</td></tr>
<tr><td>5</td><td>Florida</td><td>1,416</td><td>4.83%</td><td>9</td><td>Georgia</td><td>1,110</td><td>3.79%</td></tr>
<tr><td>9</td><td>Georgia</td><td>1,110</td><td>3.79%</td><td>10</td><td>North Carolina</td><td>952</td><td>3.25%</td></tr>
<tr><td>40</td><td>Hawaii</td><td>110</td><td>0.38%</td><td>11</td><td>New Jersey</td><td>790</td><td>2.70%</td></tr>
<tr><td>39</td><td>Idaho</td><td>114</td><td>0.39%</td><td>12</td><td>Indiana</td><td>756</td><td>2.58%</td></tr>
<tr><td>4</td><td>Illinois</td><td>1,662</td><td>5.67%</td><td>13</td><td>Tennessee</td><td>709</td><td>2.42%</td></tr>
<tr><td>12</td><td>Indiana</td><td>756</td><td>2.58%</td><td>14</td><td>Virginia</td><td>688</td><td>2.35%</td></tr>
<tr><td>33</td><td>Iowa</td><td>240</td><td>0.82%</td><td>15</td><td>Louisiana</td><td>645</td><td>2.20%</td></tr>
<tr><td>30</td><td>Kansas</td><td>288</td><td>0.98%</td><td>16</td><td>Maryland</td><td>629</td><td>2.15%</td></tr>
<tr><td>22</td><td>Kentucky</td><td>409</td><td>1.40%</td><td>17</td><td>Alabama</td><td>624</td><td>2.13%</td></tr>
<tr><td>15</td><td>Louisiana</td><td>645</td><td>2.20%</td><td>18</td><td>Missouri</td><td>591</td><td>2.02%</td></tr>
<tr><td>44</td><td>Maine</td><td>75</td><td>0.26%</td><td>19</td><td>Arizona</td><td>509</td><td>1.74%</td></tr>
<tr><td>16</td><td>Maryland</td><td>629</td><td>2.15%</td><td>20</td><td>Wisconsin</td><td>498</td><td>1.70%</td></tr>
<tr><td>24</td><td>Massachusetts</td><td>407</td><td>1.39%</td><td>21</td><td>South Carolina</td><td>448</td><td>1.53%</td></tr>
<tr><td>8</td><td>Michigan</td><td>1,129</td><td>3.85%</td><td>22</td><td>Kentucky</td><td>409</td><td>1.40%</td></tr>
<tr><td>25</td><td>Minnesota</td><td>401</td><td>1.37%</td><td>23</td><td>Oklahoma</td><td>408</td><td>1.39%</td></tr>
<tr><td>26</td><td>Mississippi</td><td>394</td><td>1.34%</td><td>24</td><td>Massachusetts</td><td>407</td><td>1.39%</td></tr>
<tr><td>18</td><td>Missouri</td><td>591</td><td>2.02%</td><td>25</td><td>Minnesota</td><td>401</td><td>1.37%</td></tr>
<tr><td>43</td><td>Montana</td><td>84</td><td>0.29%</td><td>26</td><td>Mississippi</td><td>394</td><td>1.34%</td></tr>
<tr><td>36</td><td>Nebraska</td><td>178</td><td>0.61%</td><td>27</td><td>Washington</td><td>367</td><td>1.25%</td></tr>
<tr><td>38</td><td>Nevada</td><td>127</td><td>0.43%</td><td>28</td><td>Colorado</td><td>356</td><td>1.22%</td></tr>
<tr><td>45</td><td>New Hampshire</td><td>73</td><td>0.25%</td><td>29</td><td>Arkansas</td><td>298</td><td>1.02%</td></tr>
<tr><td>11</td><td>New Jersey</td><td>790</td><td>2.70%</td><td>30</td><td>Kansas</td><td>288</td><td>0.98%</td></tr>
<tr><td>35</td><td>New Mexico</td><td>191</td><td>0.65%</td><td>31</td><td>Connecticut</td><td>271</td><td>0.92%</td></tr>
<tr><td>3</td><td>New York</td><td>2,067</td><td>7.05%</td><td>32</td><td>Oregon</td><td>263</td><td>0.90%</td></tr>
<tr><td>10</td><td>North Carolina</td><td>952</td><td>3.25%</td><td>33</td><td>Iowa</td><td>240</td><td>0.82%</td></tr>
<tr><td>49</td><td>North Dakota</td><td>49</td><td>0.17%</td><td>34</td><td>Utah</td><td>200</td><td>0.68%</td></tr>
<tr><td>6</td><td>Ohio</td><td>1,310</td><td>4.47%</td><td>35</td><td>New Mexico</td><td>191</td><td>0.65%</td></tr>
<tr><td>23</td><td>Oklahoma</td><td>408</td><td>1.39%</td><td>36</td><td>Nebraska</td><td>178</td><td>0.61%</td></tr>
<tr><td>32</td><td>Oregon</td><td>263</td><td>0.90%</td><td>37</td><td>West Virginia</td><td>151</td><td>0.52%</td></tr>
<tr><td>7</td><td>Pennsylvania</td><td>1,149</td><td>3.92%</td><td>38</td><td>Nevada</td><td>127</td><td>0.43%</td></tr>
<tr><td>42</td><td>Rhode Island</td><td>87</td><td>0.30%</td><td>39</td><td>Idaho</td><td>114</td><td>0.39%</td></tr>
<tr><td>21</td><td>South Carolina</td><td>448</td><td>1.53%</td><td>40</td><td>Hawaii</td><td>110</td><td>0.38%</td></tr>
<tr><td>41</td><td>South Dakota</td><td>98</td><td>0.33%</td><td>41</td><td>South Dakota</td><td>98</td><td>0.33%</td></tr>
<tr><td>13</td><td>Tennessee</td><td>709</td><td>2.42%</td><td>42</td><td>Rhode Island</td><td>87</td><td>0.30%</td></tr>
<tr><td>2</td><td>Texas</td><td>2,150</td><td>7.34%</td><td>43</td><td>Montana</td><td>84</td><td>0.29%</td></tr>
<tr><td>34</td><td>Utah</td><td>200</td><td>0.68%</td><td>44</td><td>Maine</td><td>75</td><td>0.26%</td></tr>
<tr><td>50</td><td>Vermont</td><td>39</td><td>0.13%</td><td>45</td><td>New Hampshire</td><td>73</td><td>0.25%</td></tr>
<tr><td>14</td><td>Virginia</td><td>688</td><td>2.35%</td><td>46</td><td>Delaware</td><td>72</td><td>0.25%</td></tr>
<tr><td>27</td><td>Washington</td><td>367</td><td>1.25%</td><td>47</td><td>Alaska</td><td>68</td><td>0.23%</td></tr>
<tr><td>37</td><td>West Virginia</td><td>151</td><td>0.52%</td><td>48</td><td>Wyoming</td><td>56</td><td>0.19%</td></tr>
<tr><td>20</td><td>Wisconsin</td><td>498</td><td>1.70%</td><td>49</td><td>North Dakota</td><td>49</td><td>0.17%</td></tr>
<tr><td>48</td><td>Wyoming</td><td>56</td><td>0.19%</td><td>50</td><td>Vermont</td><td>39</td><td>0.13%</td></tr>
<tr><td></td><td></td><td></td><td></td><td></td><td>District of Columbia**</td><td>159</td><td>0.54%</td></tr>
</table>

Source: U.S. Department of Health and Human Services, National Center for Health Statistics
  "Monthly Vital Statistics Report" (Vol. 44, No. 12, July 24, 1996)
*Provisional data. Deaths under 1 year old by state of residence.
**District of Columbia's total is listed as being under reported.

Infant Mortality Rate in 1995

National Rate = 7.6 Infant Deaths per 1,000 Live Births*

ALPHA ORDER

RANK	STATE	RATE
2	Alabama	10.2
34	Alaska	6.7
26	Arizona	7.4
13	Arkansas	8.7
39	California	6.1
31	Colorado	7.1
41	Connecticut	6.0
29	Delaware	7.2
24	Florida	7.5
3	Georgia	9.8
41	Hawaii	6.0
37	Idaho	6.4
8	Illinois	9.0
8	Indiana	9.0
35	Iowa	6.6
20	Kansas	7.7
17	Kentucky	8.0
4	Louisiana	9.6
47	Maine	5.4
13	Maryland	8.7
46	Massachusetts	5.5
15	Michigan	8.5
37	Minnesota	6.4
1	Mississippi	10.6
18	Missouri	7.9
24	Montana	7.5
20	Nebraska	7.7
41	Nevada	6.0
49	New Hampshire	4.8
28	New Jersey	7.3
32	New Mexico	7.0
19	New York	7.8
6	North Carolina	9.3
45	North Dakota	5.6
16	Ohio	8.4
11	Oklahoma	8.9
39	Oregon	6.1
22	Pennsylvania	7.6
33	Rhode Island	6.9
8	South Carolina	9.0
6	South Dakota	9.3
4	Tennessee	9.6
35	Texas	6.6
48	Utah	5.1
44	Vermont	5.8
22	Virginia	7.6
50	Washington	4.7
29	West Virginia	7.2
26	Wisconsin	7.4
11	Wyoming	8.9

RANK ORDER

RANK	STATE	RATE
1	Mississippi	10.6
2	Alabama	10.2
3	Georgia	9.8
4	Louisiana	9.6
4	Tennessee	9.6
6	North Carolina	9.3
6	South Dakota	9.3
8	Illinois	9.0
8	Indiana	9.0
8	South Carolina	9.0
11	Oklahoma	8.9
11	Wyoming	8.9
13	Arkansas	8.7
13	Maryland	8.7
15	Michigan	8.5
16	Ohio	8.4
17	Kentucky	8.0
18	Missouri	7.9
19	New York	7.8
20	Kansas	7.7
20	Nebraska	7.7
22	Pennsylvania	7.6
22	Virginia	7.6
24	Florida	7.5
24	Montana	7.5
26	Arizona	7.4
26	Wisconsin	7.4
28	New Jersey	7.3
29	Delaware	7.2
29	West Virginia	7.2
31	Colorado	7.1
32	New Mexico	7.0
33	Rhode Island	6.9
34	Alaska	6.7
35	Iowa	6.6
35	Texas	6.6
37	Idaho	6.4
37	Minnesota	6.4
39	California	6.1
39	Oregon	6.1
41	Connecticut	6.0
41	Hawaii	6.0
41	Nevada	6.0
44	Vermont	5.8
45	North Dakota	5.6
46	Massachusetts	5.5
47	Maine	5.4
48	Utah	5.1
49	New Hampshire	4.8
50	Washington	4.7
	District of Columbia**	NA

Source: U.S. Department of Health and Human Services, National Center for Health Statistics
"Monthly Vital Statistics Report" (Vol. 44, No. 12, July 24, 1996)
Provisional data. Deaths under 1 year old by state of residence.

Infant Deaths in 1990

National Total = 38,351 Infant Deaths*

ALPHA ORDER

RANK	STATE	DEATHS	% of USA
18	Alabama	688	1.79%
41	Alaska	125	0.33%
22	Arizona	610	1.59%
31	Arkansas	336	0.88%
1	California	4,844	12.63%
26	Colorado	472	1.23%
29	Connecticut	398	1.04%
44	Delaware	112	0.29%
5	Florida	1,918	5.00%
9	Georgia	1,392	3.63%
40	Hawaii	138	0.36%
39	Idaho	143	0.37%
4	Illinois	2,104	5.49%
13	Indiana	831	2.17%
33	Iowa	319	0.83%
32	Kansas	329	0.86%
27	Kentucky	461	1.20%
14	Louisiana	799	2.08%
46	Maine	108	0.28%
16	Maryland	766	2.00%
20	Massachusetts	650	1.69%
7	Michigan	1,641	4.28%
25	Minnesota	496	1.29%
24	Mississippi	529	1.38%
17	Missouri	748	1.95%
47	Montana	105	0.27%
37	Nebraska	202	0.53%
38	Nevada	181	0.47%
41	New Hampshire	125	0.33%
11	New Jersey	1,102	2.87%
35	New Mexico	246	0.64%
2	New York	2,851	7.43%
10	North Carolina	1,109	2.89%
48	North Dakota	74	0.19%
8	Ohio	1,640	4.28%
28	Oklahoma	438	1.14%
30	Oregon	354	0.92%
6	Pennsylvania	1,643	4.28%
43	Rhode Island	123	0.32%
19	South Carolina	683	1.78%
45	South Dakota	111	0.29%
15	Tennessee	771	2.01%
3	Texas	2,552	6.65%
34	Utah	271	0.71%
50	Vermont	53	0.14%
12	Virginia	1,013	2.64%
21	Washington	621	1.62%
36	West Virginia	223	0.58%
23	Wisconsin	598	1.56%
49	Wyoming	60	0.16%

RANK ORDER

RANK	STATE	DEATHS	% of USA
1	California	4,844	12.63%
2	New York	2,851	7.43%
3	Texas	2,552	6.65%
4	Illinois	2,104	5.49%
5	Florida	1,918	5.00%
6	Pennsylvania	1,643	4.28%
7	Michigan	1,641	4.28%
8	Ohio	1,640	4.28%
9	Georgia	1,392	3.63%
10	North Carolina	1,109	2.89%
11	New Jersey	1,102	2.87%
12	Virginia	1,013	2.64%
13	Indiana	831	2.17%
14	Louisiana	799	2.08%
15	Tennessee	771	2.01%
16	Maryland	766	2.00%
17	Missouri	748	1.95%
18	Alabama	688	1.79%
19	South Carolina	683	1.78%
20	Massachusetts	650	1.69%
21	Washington	621	1.62%
22	Arizona	610	1.59%
23	Wisconsin	598	1.56%
24	Mississippi	529	1.38%
25	Minnesota	496	1.29%
26	Colorado	472	1.23%
27	Kentucky	461	1.20%
28	Oklahoma	438	1.14%
29	Connecticut	398	1.04%
30	Oregon	354	0.92%
31	Arkansas	336	0.88%
32	Kansas	329	0.86%
33	Iowa	319	0.83%
34	Utah	271	0.71%
35	New Mexico	246	0.64%
36	West Virginia	223	0.58%
37	Nebraska	202	0.53%
38	Nevada	181	0.47%
39	Idaho	143	0.37%
40	Hawaii	138	0.36%
41	Alaska	125	0.33%
41	New Hampshire	125	0.33%
43	Rhode Island	123	0.32%
44	Delaware	112	0.29%
45	South Dakota	111	0.29%
46	Maine	108	0.28%
47	Montana	105	0.27%
48	North Dakota	74	0.19%
49	Wyoming	60	0.16%
50	Vermont	53	0.14%
	District of Columbia	245	0.64%

Source: U.S. Department of Health and Human Services, National Center for Health Statistics
"Monthly Vital Statistics Report" (Vol. 41, No. 7(S), January 7, 1993)
*Final data by state of residence. Infant deaths are those under 1 year old.

Infant Mortality Rate in 1990

National Rate = 9.22 Infant Deaths per 1,000 Live Births*

ALPHA ORDER

RANK	STATE	RATE
5	Alabama	10.84
9	Alaska	10.50
27	Arizona	8.84
22	Arkansas	9.22
42	California	7.91
28	Colorado	8.82
41	Connecticut	7.94
13	Delaware	10.08
17	Florida	9.62
1	Georgia	12.36
48	Hawaii	6.74
29	Idaho	8.70
6	Illinois	10.75
16	Indiana	9.64
37	Iowa	8.09
32	Kansas	8.43
31	Kentucky	8.48
4	Louisiana	11.07
50	Maine	6.22
19	Maryland	9.55
47	Massachusetts	7.02
7	Michigan	10.68
45	Minnesota	7.29
2	Mississippi	12.14
21	Missouri	9.44
24	Montana	9.04
34	Nebraska	8.29
33	Nevada	8.38
46	New Hampshire	7.11
25	New Jersey	9.01
26	New Mexico	8.98
18	New York	9.58
8	North Carolina	10.61
40	North Dakota	8.00
15	Ohio	9.83
23	Oklahoma	9.19
35	Oregon	8.25
19	Pennsylvania	9.55
37	Rhode Island	8.09
3	South Carolina	11.65
12	South Dakota	10.09
10	Tennessee	10.29
39	Texas	8.07
44	Utah	7.47
49	Vermont	6.41
11	Virginia	10.20
43	Washington	7.84
14	West Virginia	9.87
36	Wisconsin	8.20
30	Wyoming	8.59

RANK ORDER

RANK	STATE	RATE
1	Georgia	12.36
2	Mississippi	12.14
3	South Carolina	11.65
4	Louisiana	11.07
5	Alabama	10.84
6	Illinois	10.75
7	Michigan	10.68
8	North Carolina	10.61
9	Alaska	10.50
10	Tennessee	10.29
11	Virginia	10.20
12	South Dakota	10.09
13	Delaware	10.08
14	West Virginia	9.87
15	Ohio	9.83
16	Indiana	9.64
17	Florida	9.62
18	New York	9.58
19	Maryland	9.55
19	Pennsylvania	9.55
21	Missouri	9.44
22	Arkansas	9.22
23	Oklahoma	9.19
24	Montana	9.04
25	New Jersey	9.01
26	New Mexico	8.98
27	Arizona	8.84
28	Colorado	8.82
29	Idaho	8.70
30	Wyoming	8.59
31	Kentucky	8.48
32	Kansas	8.43
33	Nevada	8.38
34	Nebraska	8.29
35	Oregon	8.25
36	Wisconsin	8.20
37	Iowa	8.09
37	Rhode Island	8.09
39	Texas	8.07
40	North Dakota	8.00
41	Connecticut	7.94
42	California	7.91
43	Washington	7.84
44	Utah	7.47
45	Minnesota	7.29
46	New Hampshire	7.11
47	Massachusetts	7.02
48	Hawaii	6.74
49	Vermont	6.41
50	Maine	6.22
	District of Columbia	20.68

*Source: U.S. Department of Health and Human Services, National Center for Health Statistics
"Monthly Vital Statistics Report" (Vol. 41, No. 7(S), January 7, 1993)*
Final data by state of residence. Infant deaths are those under 1 year old.

Infant Deaths in 1980

National Total = 45,526 Infant Deaths*

<table>
<tr><td colspan="4">ALPHA ORDER</td><td colspan="4">RANK ORDER</td></tr>
<tr><td>RANK</td><td>STATE</td><td>DEATHS</td><td>% of USA</td><td>RANK</td><td>STATE</td><td>DEATHS</td><td>% of USA</td></tr>
<tr><td>16</td><td>Alabama</td><td>962</td><td>2.11%</td><td>1</td><td>California</td><td>4,454</td><td>9.78%</td></tr>
<tr><td>48</td><td>Alaska</td><td>117</td><td>0.26%</td><td>2</td><td>Texas</td><td>3,326</td><td>7.31%</td></tr>
<tr><td>27</td><td>Arizona</td><td>620</td><td>1.36%</td><td>3</td><td>New York</td><td>2,994</td><td>6.58%</td></tr>
<tr><td>31</td><td>Arkansas</td><td>472</td><td>1.04%</td><td>4</td><td>Illinois</td><td>2,812</td><td>6.18%</td></tr>
<tr><td>1</td><td>California</td><td>4,454</td><td>9.78%</td><td>5</td><td>Ohio</td><td>2,160</td><td>4.74%</td></tr>
<tr><td>30</td><td>Colorado</td><td>501</td><td>1.10%</td><td>6</td><td>Pennsylvania</td><td>2,101</td><td>4.61%</td></tr>
<tr><td>33</td><td>Connecticut</td><td>433</td><td>0.95%</td><td>7</td><td>Florida</td><td>1,921</td><td>4.22%</td></tr>
<tr><td>47</td><td>Delaware</td><td>131</td><td>0.29%</td><td>8</td><td>Michigan</td><td>1,862</td><td>4.09%</td></tr>
<tr><td>7</td><td>Florida</td><td>1,921</td><td>4.22%</td><td>9</td><td>Georgia</td><td>1,337</td><td>2.94%</td></tr>
<tr><td>9</td><td>Georgia</td><td>1,337</td><td>2.94%</td><td>10</td><td>North Carolina</td><td>1,224</td><td>2.69%</td></tr>
<tr><td>39</td><td>Hawaii</td><td>187</td><td>0.41%</td><td>11</td><td>New Jersey</td><td>1,215</td><td>2.67%</td></tr>
<tr><td>38</td><td>Idaho</td><td>216</td><td>0.47%</td><td>12</td><td>Louisiana</td><td>1,178</td><td>2.59%</td></tr>
<tr><td>4</td><td>Illinois</td><td>2,812</td><td>6.18%</td><td>13</td><td>Virginia</td><td>1,067</td><td>2.34%</td></tr>
<tr><td>14</td><td>Indiana</td><td>1,050</td><td>2.31%</td><td>14</td><td>Indiana</td><td>1,050</td><td>2.31%</td></tr>
<tr><td>28</td><td>Iowa</td><td>565</td><td>1.24%</td><td>15</td><td>Missouri</td><td>980</td><td>2.15%</td></tr>
<tr><td>34</td><td>Kansas</td><td>424</td><td>0.93%</td><td>16</td><td>Alabama</td><td>962</td><td>2.11%</td></tr>
<tr><td>23</td><td>Kentucky</td><td>766</td><td>1.68%</td><td>17</td><td>Tennessee</td><td>935</td><td>2.05%</td></tr>
<tr><td>12</td><td>Louisiana</td><td>1,178</td><td>2.59%</td><td>18</td><td>Maryland</td><td>842</td><td>1.85%</td></tr>
<tr><td>41</td><td>Maine</td><td>152</td><td>0.33%</td><td>19</td><td>Mississippi</td><td>814</td><td>1.79%</td></tr>
<tr><td>18</td><td>Maryland</td><td>842</td><td>1.85%</td><td>20</td><td>South Carolina</td><td>812</td><td>1.78%</td></tr>
<tr><td>24</td><td>Massachusetts</td><td>763</td><td>1.68%</td><td>21</td><td>Washington</td><td>798</td><td>1.75%</td></tr>
<tr><td>8</td><td>Michigan</td><td>1,862</td><td>4.09%</td><td>22</td><td>Wisconsin</td><td>770</td><td>1.69%</td></tr>
<tr><td>25</td><td>Minnesota</td><td>678</td><td>1.49%</td><td>23</td><td>Kentucky</td><td>766</td><td>1.68%</td></tr>
<tr><td>19</td><td>Mississippi</td><td>814</td><td>1.79%</td><td>24</td><td>Massachusetts</td><td>763</td><td>1.68%</td></tr>
<tr><td>15</td><td>Missouri</td><td>980</td><td>2.15%</td><td>25</td><td>Minnesota</td><td>678</td><td>1.49%</td></tr>
<tr><td>40</td><td>Montana</td><td>176</td><td>0.39%</td><td>26</td><td>Oklahoma</td><td>663</td><td>1.46%</td></tr>
<tr><td>36</td><td>Nebraska</td><td>314</td><td>0.69%</td><td>27</td><td>Arizona</td><td>620</td><td>1.36%</td></tr>
<tr><td>44</td><td>Nevada</td><td>143</td><td>0.31%</td><td>28</td><td>Iowa</td><td>565</td><td>1.24%</td></tr>
<tr><td>45</td><td>New Hampshire</td><td>136</td><td>0.30%</td><td>29</td><td>Oregon</td><td>525</td><td>1.15%</td></tr>
<tr><td>11</td><td>New Jersey</td><td>1,215</td><td>2.67%</td><td>30</td><td>Colorado</td><td>501</td><td>1.10%</td></tr>
<tr><td>37</td><td>New Mexico</td><td>301</td><td>0.66%</td><td>31</td><td>Arkansas</td><td>472</td><td>1.04%</td></tr>
<tr><td>3</td><td>New York</td><td>2,994</td><td>6.58%</td><td>32</td><td>Utah</td><td>436</td><td>0.96%</td></tr>
<tr><td>10</td><td>North Carolina</td><td>1,224</td><td>2.69%</td><td>33</td><td>Connecticut</td><td>433</td><td>0.95%</td></tr>
<tr><td>42</td><td>North Dakota</td><td>145</td><td>0.32%</td><td>34</td><td>Kansas</td><td>424</td><td>0.93%</td></tr>
<tr><td>5</td><td>Ohio</td><td>2,160</td><td>4.74%</td><td>35</td><td>West Virginia</td><td>348</td><td>0.76%</td></tr>
<tr><td>26</td><td>Oklahoma</td><td>663</td><td>1.46%</td><td>36</td><td>Nebraska</td><td>314</td><td>0.69%</td></tr>
<tr><td>29</td><td>Oregon</td><td>525</td><td>1.15%</td><td>37</td><td>New Mexico</td><td>301</td><td>0.66%</td></tr>
<tr><td>6</td><td>Pennsylvania</td><td>2,101</td><td>4.61%</td><td>38</td><td>Idaho</td><td>216</td><td>0.47%</td></tr>
<tr><td>46</td><td>Rhode Island</td><td>134</td><td>0.29%</td><td>39</td><td>Hawaii</td><td>187</td><td>0.41%</td></tr>
<tr><td>20</td><td>South Carolina</td><td>812</td><td>1.78%</td><td>40</td><td>Montana</td><td>176</td><td>0.39%</td></tr>
<tr><td>42</td><td>South Dakota</td><td>145</td><td>0.32%</td><td>41</td><td>Maine</td><td>152</td><td>0.33%</td></tr>
<tr><td>17</td><td>Tennessee</td><td>935</td><td>2.05%</td><td>42</td><td>North Dakota</td><td>145</td><td>0.32%</td></tr>
<tr><td>2</td><td>Texas</td><td>3,326</td><td>7.31%</td><td>42</td><td>South Dakota</td><td>145</td><td>0.32%</td></tr>
<tr><td>32</td><td>Utah</td><td>436</td><td>0.96%</td><td>44</td><td>Nevada</td><td>143</td><td>0.31%</td></tr>
<tr><td>50</td><td>Vermont</td><td>84</td><td>0.18%</td><td>45</td><td>New Hampshire</td><td>136</td><td>0.30%</td></tr>
<tr><td>13</td><td>Virginia</td><td>1,067</td><td>2.34%</td><td>46</td><td>Rhode Island</td><td>134</td><td>0.29%</td></tr>
<tr><td>21</td><td>Washington</td><td>798</td><td>1.75%</td><td>47</td><td>Delaware</td><td>131</td><td>0.29%</td></tr>
<tr><td>35</td><td>West Virginia</td><td>348</td><td>0.76%</td><td>48</td><td>Alaska</td><td>117</td><td>0.26%</td></tr>
<tr><td>22</td><td>Wisconsin</td><td>770</td><td>1.69%</td><td>49</td><td>Wyoming</td><td>103</td><td>0.23%</td></tr>
<tr><td>49</td><td>Wyoming</td><td>103</td><td>0.23%</td><td>50</td><td>Vermont</td><td>84</td><td>0.18%</td></tr>
<tr><td></td><td></td><td></td><td></td><td></td><td>District of Columbia</td><td>234</td><td>0.51%</td></tr>
</table>

Source: U.S. Department of Health and Human Services, National Center for Health Statistics
    "Monthly Vital Statistics Report"
*Final data by state of residence. Deaths under 1 year old, exclusive of fetal deaths.

Infant Mortality Rate in 1980

National Rate = 12.60 Infant Deaths per 1,000 Live Births*

ALPHA ORDER

RANK	STATE	RATE
3	Alabama	15.15
24	Alaska	12.28
22	Arizona	12.39
18	Arkansas	12.66
35	California	11.05
46	Colorado	10.07
34	Connecticut	11.17
10	Delaware	13.92
5	Florida	14.58
7	Georgia	14.48
44	Hawaii	10.30
39	Idaho	10.71
4	Illinois	14.80
28	Indiana	11.87
29	Iowa	11.82
43	Kansas	10.41
14	Kentucky	12.86
8	Louisiana	14.34
50	Maine	9.23
9	Maryland	14.05
41	Massachusetts	10.51
15	Michigan	12.80
47	Minnesota	10.00
1	Mississippi	17.01
21	Missouri	12.42
22	Montana	12.39
33	Nebraska	11.48
38	Nevada	10.74
48	New Hampshire	9.89
19	New Jersey	12.54
32	New Mexico	11.53
20	New York	12.53
6	North Carolina	14.49
27	North Dakota	12.10
16	Ohio	12.77
17	Oklahoma	12.72
25	Oregon	12.17
13	Pennsylvania	13.23
36	Rhode Island	10.99
2	South Carolina	15.62
37	South Dakota	10.92
12	Tennessee	13.51
26	Texas	12.16
42	Utah	10.43
40	Vermont	10.65
11	Virginia	13.60
31	Washington	11.76
30	West Virginia	11.81
45	Wisconsin	10.29
49	Wyoming	9.75

RANK ORDER

RANK	STATE	RATE
1	Mississippi	17.01
2	South Carolina	15.62
3	Alabama	15.15
4	Illinois	14.80
5	Florida	14.58
6	North Carolina	14.49
7	Georgia	14.48
8	Louisiana	14.34
9	Maryland	14.05
10	Delaware	13.92
11	Virginia	13.60
12	Tennessee	13.51
13	Pennsylvania	13.23
14	Kentucky	12.86
15	Michigan	12.80
16	Ohio	12.77
17	Oklahoma	12.72
18	Arkansas	12.66
19	New Jersey	12.54
20	New York	12.53
21	Missouri	12.42
22	Arizona	12.39
22	Montana	12.39
24	Alaska	12.28
25	Oregon	12.17
26	Texas	12.16
27	North Dakota	12.10
28	Indiana	11.87
29	Iowa	11.82
30	West Virginia	11.81
31	Washington	11.76
32	New Mexico	11.53
33	Nebraska	11.48
34	Connecticut	11.17
35	California	11.05
36	Rhode Island	10.99
37	South Dakota	10.92
38	Nevada	10.74
39	Idaho	10.71
40	Vermont	10.65
41	Massachusetts	10.51
42	Utah	10.43
43	Kansas	10.41
44	Hawaii	10.30
45	Wisconsin	10.29
46	Colorado	10.07
47	Minnesota	10.00
48	New Hampshire	9.89
49	Wyoming	9.75
50	Maine	9.23
	District of Columbia	25.00

Source: U.S. Department of Health and Human Services, National Center for Health Statistics
    "Monthly Vital Statistics Report"
*Final data by state of residence. Deaths under 1 year old, exclusive of fetal deaths.

Percent Change in Infant Mortality Rate: 1990 to 1995

National Percent Change = 17.57% Decrease*

ALPHA ORDER				RANK ORDER		
RANK	STATE	PERCENT CHANGE		RANK	STATE	PERCENT CHANGE
5	Alabama	(5.90)		1	Wyoming	3.61
49	Alaska	(36.19)		2	Oklahoma	(3.16)
23	Arizona	(16.29)		3	Arkansas	(5.64)
3	Arkansas	(5.64)		4	Kentucky	(5.66)
38	California	(22.88)		5	Alabama	(5.90)
30	Colorado	(19.50)		6	Indiana	(6.64)
39	Connecticut	(24.43)		7	Tennessee	(6.71)
45	Delaware	(28.57)		8	Nebraska	(7.12)
35	Florida	(22.04)		9	South Dakota	(7.83)
33	Georgia	(20.71)		10	Kansas	(8.66)
14	Hawaii	(10.98)		11	Maryland	(8.90)
42	Idaho	(26.44)		12	Vermont	(9.52)
22	Illinois	(16.28)		13	Wisconsin	(9.76)
6	Indiana	(6.64)		14	Hawaii	(10.98)
27	Iowa	(18.42)		15	Minnesota	(12.21)
10	Kansas	(8.66)		16	North Carolina	(12.35)
4	Kentucky	(5.66)		17	Mississippi	(12.69)
19	Louisiana	(13.28)		18	Maine	(13.18)
18	Maine	(13.18)		19	Louisiana	(13.28)
11	Maryland	(8.90)		20	Ohio	(14.55)
34	Massachusetts	(21.65)		21	Rhode Island	(14.71)
31	Michigan	(20.41)		22	Illinois	(16.28)
15	Minnesota	(12.21)		23	Arizona	(16.29)
17	Mississippi	(12.69)		24	Missouri	(16.31)
24	Missouri	(16.31)		25	Montana	(17.04)
25	Montana	(17.04)		26	Texas	(18.22)
8	Nebraska	(7.12)		27	Iowa	(18.42)
44	Nevada	(28.40)		28	New York	(18.58)
48	New Hampshire	(32.49)		29	New Jersey	(18.98)
29	New Jersey	(18.98)		30	Colorado	(19.50)
36	New Mexico	(22.05)		31	Michigan	(20.41)
28	New York	(18.58)		32	Pennsylvania	(20.42)
16	North Carolina	(12.35)		33	Georgia	(20.71)
46	North Dakota	(30.00)		34	Massachusetts	(21.65)
20	Ohio	(14.55)		35	Florida	(22.04)
2	Oklahoma	(3.16)		36	New Mexico	(22.05)
41	Oregon	(26.06)		37	South Carolina	(22.75)
32	Pennsylvania	(20.42)		38	California	(22.88)
21	Rhode Island	(14.71)		39	Connecticut	(24.43)
37	South Carolina	(22.75)		40	Virginia	(25.49)
9	South Dakota	(7.83)		41	Oregon	(26.06)
7	Tennessee	(6.71)		42	Idaho	(26.44)
26	Texas	(18.22)		43	West Virginia	(27.05)
47	Utah	(31.73)		44	Nevada	(28.40)
12	Vermont	(9.52)		45	Delaware	(28.57)
40	Virginia	(25.49)		46	North Dakota	(30.00)
50	Washington	(40.05)		47	Utah	(31.73)
43	West Virginia	(27.05)		48	New Hampshire	(32.49)
13	Wisconsin	(9.76)		49	Alaska	(36.19)
1	Wyoming	3.61		50	Washington	(40.05)

District of Columbia**   NA

Source: Morgan Quitno Press using data from US Dept of Health & Human Services, National Center for Health Statistics "Monthly Vital Statistics Report" (Vol. 41, No. 7(S), January 7, 1993; Vol. 44, No. 12, July 24, 1996)
*By state of residence. Infant deaths are those under 1 year old.
**Not available.

Percent Change in Infant Mortality Rate: 1980 to 1990

National Percent Change = 26.83% Decrease in Infant Mortality Rate*

ALPHA ORDER

RANK ORDER

RANK	STATE	RATE		RANK	STATE	RATE
35	Alabama	(28.45)		1	South Dakota	(7.60)
4	Alaska	(14.50)		2	Wyoming	(11.90)
37	Arizona	(28.65)		3	Colorado	(12.41)
25	Arkansas	(27.17)		4	Alaska	(14.50)
34	California	(28.42)		5	Georgia	(14.64)
3	Colorado	(12.41)		6	West Virginia	(16.43)
38	Connecticut	(28.92)		7	Michigan	(16.56)
27	Delaware	(27.59)		8	Idaho	(18.77)
47	Florida	(34.02)		9	Indiana	(18.79)
5	Georgia	(14.64)		10	Kansas	(19.02)
49	Hawaii	(34.56)		11	Wisconsin	(20.31)
8	Idaho	(18.77)		12	Nevada	(21.97)
26	Illinois	(27.36)		13	New Mexico	(22.12)
9	Indiana	(18.79)		14	Louisiana	(22.80)
39	Iowa	(31.56)		15	Ohio	(23.02)
10	Kansas	(19.02)		16	New York	(23.54)
48	Kentucky	(34.06)		17	Tennessee	(23.83)
14	Louisiana	(22.80)		18	Missouri	(23.99)
42	Maine	(32.61)		19	Virginia	(25.00)
40	Maryland	(32.03)		20	South Carolina	(25.42)
43	Massachusetts	(33.21)		21	Rhode Island	(26.39)
7	Michigan	(16.56)		22	North Carolina	(26.78)
24	Minnesota	(27.10)		23	Montana	(27.04)
36	Mississippi	(28.63)		24	Minnesota	(27.10)
18	Missouri	(23.99)		25	Arkansas	(27.17)
23	Montana	(27.04)		26	Illinois	(27.36)
29	Nebraska	(27.79)		27	Delaware	(27.59)
12	Nevada	(21.97)		28	Oklahoma	(27.75)
31	New Hampshire	(28.11)		29	Nebraska	(27.79)
32	New Jersey	(28.15)		30	Pennsylvania	(27.82)
13	New Mexico	(22.12)		31	New Hampshire	(28.11)
16	New York	(23.54)		32	New Jersey	(28.15)
22	North Carolina	(26.78)		33	Utah	(28.38)
46	North Dakota	(33.88)		34	California	(28.42)
15	Ohio	(23.02)		35	Alabama	(28.45)
28	Oklahoma	(27.75)		36	Mississippi	(28.63)
41	Oregon	(32.21)		37	Arizona	(28.65)
30	Pennsylvania	(27.82)		38	Connecticut	(28.92)
21	Rhode Island	(26.39)		39	Iowa	(31.56)
20	South Carolina	(25.42)		40	Maryland	(32.03)
1	South Dakota	(7.60)		41	Oregon	(32.21)
17	Tennessee	(23.83)		42	Maine	(32.61)
45	Texas	(33.63)		43	Massachusetts	(33.21)
33	Utah	(28.38)		44	Washington	(33.33)
50	Vermont	(39.81)		45	Texas	(33.63)
19	Virginia	(25.00)		46	North Dakota	(33.88)
44	Washington	(33.33)		47	Florida	(34.02)
6	West Virginia	(16.43)		48	Kentucky	(34.06)
11	Wisconsin	(20.31)		49	Hawaii	(34.56)
2	Wyoming	(11.90)		50	Vermont	(39.81)

District of Columbia (17.28)

Source: Morgan Quitno Press using data from US Dept of Health & Human Services, National Center for Health Statistics
"Monthly Vital Statistics Report" (Vol. 41, No. 7(S), January 7, 1993)
"Vital Statistics of the United States, 1980" (Vol. I-Natality, issued 1984) and unpublished data
*Final data by state of residence. Infant deaths are those occurring under 1 year, exclusive of fetal deaths.

White Infant Deaths in 1994

National Total = 20,504 Deaths*

ALPHA ORDER

RANK ORDER

RANK	STATE	DEATHS	% of USA
25	Alabama	276	1.35%
45	Alaska	51	0.25%
13	Arizona	453	2.21%
31	Arkansas	216	1.05%
1	California	3,004	14.65%
22	Colorado	314	1.53%
28	Connecticut	251	1.22%
48	Delaware	40	0.20%
6	Florida	935	4.56%
12	Georgia	492	2.40%
50	Hawaii	24	0.12%
39	Idaho	114	0.56%
4	Illinois	962	4.69%
9	Indiana	551	2.69%
29	Iowa	248	1.21%
30	Kansas	229	1.12%
21	Kentucky	340	1.66%
27	Louisiana	257	1.25%
41	Maine	85	0.41%
24	Maryland	287	1.40%
16	Massachusetts	401	1.96%
8	Michigan	674	3.29%
19	Minnesota	359	1.75%
35	Mississippi	158	0.77%
17	Missouri	399	1.95%
42	Montana	69	0.34%
36	Nebraska	152	0.74%
38	Nevada	127	0.62%
40	New Hampshire	91	0.44%
11	New Jersey	515	2.51%
34	New Mexico	181	0.88%
3	New York	1,227	5.98%
10	North Carolina	530	2.58%
46	North Dakota	50	0.24%
5	Ohio	937	4.57%
23	Oklahoma	299	1.46%
26	Oregon	267	1.30%
7	Pennsylvania	831	4.05%
47	Rhode Island	49	0.24%
33	South Carolina	211	1.03%
43	South Dakota	67	0.33%
20	Tennessee	352	1.72%
2	Texas	1,746	8.52%
32	Utah	212	1.03%
44	Vermont	55	0.27%
14	Virginia	444	2.17%
15	Washington	404	1.97%
37	West Virginia	134	0.65%
18	Wisconsin	382	1.86%
48	Wyoming	40	0.20%

RANK	STATE	DEATHS	% of USA
1	California	3,004	14.65%
2	Texas	1,746	8.52%
3	New York	1,227	5.98%
4	Illinois	962	4.69%
5	Ohio	937	4.57%
6	Florida	935	4.56%
7	Pennsylvania	831	4.05%
8	Michigan	674	3.29%
9	Indiana	551	2.69%
10	North Carolina	530	2.58%
11	New Jersey	515	2.51%
12	Georgia	492	2.40%
13	Arizona	453	2.21%
14	Virginia	444	2.17%
15	Washington	404	1.97%
16	Massachusetts	401	1.96%
17	Missouri	399	1.95%
18	Wisconsin	382	1.86%
19	Minnesota	359	1.75%
20	Tennessee	352	1.72%
21	Kentucky	340	1.66%
22	Colorado	314	1.53%
23	Oklahoma	299	1.46%
24	Maryland	287	1.40%
25	Alabama	276	1.35%
26	Oregon	267	1.30%
27	Louisiana	257	1.25%
28	Connecticut	251	1.22%
29	Iowa	248	1.21%
30	Kansas	229	1.12%
31	Arkansas	216	1.05%
32	Utah	212	1.03%
33	South Carolina	211	1.03%
34	New Mexico	181	0.88%
35	Mississippi	158	0.77%
36	Nebraska	152	0.74%
37	West Virginia	134	0.65%
38	Nevada	127	0.62%
39	Idaho	114	0.56%
40	New Hampshire	91	0.44%
41	Maine	85	0.41%
42	Montana	69	0.34%
43	South Dakota	67	0.33%
44	Vermont	55	0.27%
45	Alaska	51	0.25%
46	North Dakota	50	0.24%
47	Rhode Island	49	0.24%
48	Delaware	40	0.20%
48	Wyoming	40	0.20%
50	Hawaii	24	0.12%
	District of Columbia	12	0.06%

Source: U.S. Department of Health and Human Services, National Center for Health Statistics
"Monthly Vital Statistics Report" (Vol. 45, No. 3(S), September 30, 1996)

*Final data. Deaths of infants under 1 year old, exclusive of fetal deaths. Based on race of the mother.

White Infant Mortality Rate in 1994

National Rate = 6.6 White Infant Deaths per 1,000 White Live Births*

ALPHA ORDER				RANK ORDER		
RANK	STATE	RATE		RANK	STATE	RATE
15	Alabama	7.0		1	Oklahoma	8.3
17	Alaska	6.9		2	Arkansas	8.2
8	Arizona	7.4		3	New Mexico	7.9
2	Arkansas	8.2		4	Indiana	7.6
27	California	6.5		4	South Dakota	7.6
32	Colorado	6.4		4	Vermont	7.6
27	Connecticut	6.5		7	North Carolina	7.5
48	Delaware	5.1		8	Arizona	7.4
27	Florida	6.5		9	Mississippi	7.3
12	Georgia	7.1		10	Nebraska	7.2
49	Hawaii	4.4		10	Ohio	7.2
22	Idaho	6.7		12	Georgia	7.1
20	Illinois	6.8		12	Kentucky	7.1
4	Indiana	7.6		12	Montana	7.1
15	Iowa	7.0		15	Alabama	7.0
17	Kansas	6.9		15	Iowa	7.0
12	Kentucky	7.1		17	Alaska	6.9
20	Louisiana	6.8		17	Kansas	6.9
42	Maine	6.0		17	Oregon	6.9
38	Maryland	6.2		20	Illinois	6.8
47	Massachusetts	5.6		20	Louisiana	6.8
36	Michigan	6.3		22	Idaho	6.7
38	Minnesota	6.2		23	Missouri	6.6
9	Mississippi	7.3		23	South Carolina	6.6
23	Missouri	6.6		23	West Virginia	6.6
12	Montana	7.1		23	Wyoming	6.6
10	Nebraska	7.2		27	California	6.5
38	Nevada	6.2		27	Connecticut	6.5
41	New Hampshire	6.1		27	Florida	6.5
45	New Jersey	5.8		27	North Dakota	6.5
3	New Mexico	7.9		27	Wisconsin	6.5
42	New York	6.0		32	Colorado	6.4
7	North Carolina	7.5		32	Pennsylvania	6.4
27	North Dakota	6.5		32	Texas	6.4
10	Ohio	7.2		32	Virginia	6.4
1	Oklahoma	8.3		36	Michigan	6.3
17	Oregon	6.9		36	Tennessee	6.3
32	Pennsylvania	6.4		38	Maryland	6.2
50	Rhode Island	4.1		38	Minnesota	6.2
23	South Carolina	6.6		38	Nevada	6.2
4	South Dakota	7.6		41	New Hampshire	6.1
36	Tennessee	6.3		42	Maine	6.0
32	Texas	6.4		42	New York	6.0
45	Utah	5.8		42	Washington	6.0
4	Vermont	7.6		45	New Jersey	5.8
32	Virginia	6.4		45	Utah	5.8
42	Washington	6.0		47	Massachusetts	5.6
23	West Virginia	6.6		48	Delaware	5.1
27	Wisconsin	6.5		49	Hawaii	4.4
23	Wyoming	6.6		50	Rhode Island	4.1
					District of Columbia**	NA

Source: U.S. Department of Health and Human Services, National Center for Health Statistics
   "Monthly Vital Statistics Report" (Vol. 45, No. 3(S), September 30, 1996)
*Final data. Deaths of infants under 1 year old, exclusive of fetal deaths. Based on race of the mother.
**Not available, fewer than 20 white infant deaths.

Black Infant Deaths in 1994

National Total = 10,072 Deaths*

<table>
<tr><td colspan="4">ALPHA ORDER</td><td colspan="4">RANK ORDER</td></tr>
<tr><td>RANK</td><td>STATE</td><td>DEATHS</td><td>% of USA</td><td>RANK</td><td>STATE</td><td>DEATHS</td><td>% of USA</td></tr>
<tr><td>14</td><td>Alabama</td><td>339</td><td>3.37%</td><td>1</td><td>New York</td><td>851</td><td>8.45%</td></tr>
<tr><td>42</td><td>Alaska</td><td>2</td><td>0.02%</td><td>2</td><td>Illinois</td><td>767</td><td>7.62%</td></tr>
<tr><td>31</td><td>Arizona</td><td>41</td><td>0.41%</td><td>3</td><td>California</td><td>650</td><td>6.45%</td></tr>
<tr><td>23</td><td>Arkansas</td><td>102</td><td>1.01%</td><td>4</td><td>Georgia</td><td>630</td><td>6.25%</td></tr>
<tr><td>3</td><td>California</td><td>650</td><td>6.45%</td><td>5</td><td>Florida</td><td>601</td><td>5.97%</td></tr>
<tr><td>26</td><td>Colorado</td><td>56</td><td>0.56%</td><td>6</td><td>Texas</td><td>506</td><td>5.02%</td></tr>
<tr><td>22</td><td>Connecticut</td><td>105</td><td>1.04%</td><td>7</td><td>Michigan</td><td>497</td><td>4.93%</td></tr>
<tr><td>32</td><td>Delaware</td><td>28</td><td>0.28%</td><td>8</td><td>North Carolina</td><td>462</td><td>4.59%</td></tr>
<tr><td>5</td><td>Florida</td><td>601</td><td>5.97%</td><td>9</td><td>Louisiana</td><td>458</td><td>4.55%</td></tr>
<tr><td>4</td><td>Georgia</td><td>630</td><td>6.25%</td><td>10</td><td>Pennsylvania</td><td>436</td><td>4.33%</td></tr>
<tr><td>38</td><td>Hawaii</td><td>12</td><td>0.12%</td><td>11</td><td>Ohio</td><td>417</td><td>4.14%</td></tr>
<tr><td>46</td><td>Idaho</td><td>1</td><td>0.01%</td><td>12</td><td>New Jersey</td><td>378</td><td>3.75%</td></tr>
<tr><td>2</td><td>Illinois</td><td>767</td><td>7.62%</td><td>13</td><td>Maryland</td><td>361</td><td>3.58%</td></tr>
<tr><td>20</td><td>Indiana</td><td>175</td><td>1.74%</td><td>14</td><td>Alabama</td><td>339</td><td>3.37%</td></tr>
<tr><td>34</td><td>Iowa</td><td>24</td><td>0.24%</td><td>15</td><td>Virginia</td><td>337</td><td>3.35%</td></tr>
<tr><td>29</td><td>Kansas</td><td>50</td><td>0.50%</td><td>16</td><td>Tennessee</td><td>299</td><td>2.97%</td></tr>
<tr><td>25</td><td>Kentucky</td><td>72</td><td>0.71%</td><td>17</td><td>Mississippi</td><td>294</td><td>2.92%</td></tr>
<tr><td>9</td><td>Louisiana</td><td>458</td><td>4.55%</td><td>18</td><td>South Carolina</td><td>273</td><td>2.71%</td></tr>
<tr><td>42</td><td>Maine</td><td>2</td><td>0.02%</td><td>19</td><td>Missouri</td><td>193</td><td>1.92%</td></tr>
<tr><td>13</td><td>Maryland</td><td>361</td><td>3.58%</td><td>20</td><td>Indiana</td><td>175</td><td>1.74%</td></tr>
<tr><td>24</td><td>Massachusetts</td><td>89</td><td>0.88%</td><td>21</td><td>Wisconsin</td><td>138</td><td>1.37%</td></tr>
<tr><td>7</td><td>Michigan</td><td>497</td><td>4.93%</td><td>22</td><td>Connecticut</td><td>105</td><td>1.04%</td></tr>
<tr><td>26</td><td>Minnesota</td><td>56</td><td>0.56%</td><td>23</td><td>Arkansas</td><td>102</td><td>1.01%</td></tr>
<tr><td>17</td><td>Mississippi</td><td>294</td><td>2.92%</td><td>24</td><td>Massachusetts</td><td>89</td><td>0.88%</td></tr>
<tr><td>19</td><td>Missouri</td><td>193</td><td>1.92%</td><td>25</td><td>Kentucky</td><td>72</td><td>0.71%</td></tr>
<tr><td>42</td><td>Montana</td><td>2</td><td>0.02%</td><td>26</td><td>Colorado</td><td>56</td><td>0.56%</td></tr>
<tr><td>35</td><td>Nebraska</td><td>20</td><td>0.20%</td><td>26</td><td>Minnesota</td><td>56</td><td>0.56%</td></tr>
<tr><td>33</td><td>Nevada</td><td>25</td><td>0.25%</td><td>28</td><td>Oklahoma</td><td>54</td><td>0.54%</td></tr>
<tr><td>46</td><td>New Hampshire</td><td>1</td><td>0.01%</td><td>29</td><td>Kansas</td><td>50</td><td>0.50%</td></tr>
<tr><td>12</td><td>New Jersey</td><td>378</td><td>3.75%</td><td>30</td><td>Washington</td><td>45</td><td>0.45%</td></tr>
<tr><td>40</td><td>New Mexico</td><td>7</td><td>0.07%</td><td>31</td><td>Arizona</td><td>41</td><td>0.41%</td></tr>
<tr><td>1</td><td>New York</td><td>851</td><td>8.45%</td><td>32</td><td>Delaware</td><td>28</td><td>0.28%</td></tr>
<tr><td>8</td><td>North Carolina</td><td>462</td><td>4.59%</td><td>33</td><td>Nevada</td><td>25</td><td>0.25%</td></tr>
<tr><td>42</td><td>North Dakota</td><td>2</td><td>0.02%</td><td>34</td><td>Iowa</td><td>24</td><td>0.24%</td></tr>
<tr><td>11</td><td>Ohio</td><td>417</td><td>4.14%</td><td>35</td><td>Nebraska</td><td>20</td><td>0.20%</td></tr>
<tr><td>28</td><td>Oklahoma</td><td>54</td><td>0.54%</td><td>36</td><td>Oregon</td><td>17</td><td>0.17%</td></tr>
<tr><td>36</td><td>Oregon</td><td>17</td><td>0.17%</td><td>37</td><td>Rhode Island</td><td>14</td><td>0.14%</td></tr>
<tr><td>10</td><td>Pennsylvania</td><td>436</td><td>4.33%</td><td>38</td><td>Hawaii</td><td>12</td><td>0.12%</td></tr>
<tr><td>37</td><td>Rhode Island</td><td>14</td><td>0.14%</td><td>39</td><td>West Virginia</td><td>10</td><td>0.10%</td></tr>
<tr><td>18</td><td>South Carolina</td><td>273</td><td>2.71%</td><td>40</td><td>New Mexico</td><td>7</td><td>0.07%</td></tr>
<tr><td>46</td><td>South Dakota</td><td>1</td><td>0.01%</td><td>41</td><td>Utah</td><td>4</td><td>0.04%</td></tr>
<tr><td>16</td><td>Tennessee</td><td>299</td><td>2.97%</td><td>42</td><td>Alaska</td><td>2</td><td>0.02%</td></tr>
<tr><td>6</td><td>Texas</td><td>506</td><td>5.02%</td><td>42</td><td>Maine</td><td>2</td><td>0.02%</td></tr>
<tr><td>41</td><td>Utah</td><td>4</td><td>0.04%</td><td>42</td><td>Montana</td><td>2</td><td>0.02%</td></tr>
<tr><td>49</td><td>Vermont</td><td>0</td><td>0.00%</td><td>42</td><td>North Dakota</td><td>2</td><td>0.02%</td></tr>
<tr><td>15</td><td>Virginia</td><td>337</td><td>3.35%</td><td>46</td><td>Idaho</td><td>1</td><td>0.01%</td></tr>
<tr><td>30</td><td>Washington</td><td>45</td><td>0.45%</td><td>46</td><td>New Hampshire</td><td>1</td><td>0.01%</td></tr>
<tr><td>39</td><td>West Virginia</td><td>10</td><td>0.10%</td><td>46</td><td>South Dakota</td><td>1</td><td>0.01%</td></tr>
<tr><td>21</td><td>Wisconsin</td><td>138</td><td>1.37%</td><td>49</td><td>Vermont</td><td>0</td><td>0.00%</td></tr>
<tr><td>49</td><td>Wyoming</td><td>0</td><td>0.00%</td><td>49</td><td>Wyoming</td><td>0</td><td>0.00%</td></tr>
<tr><td></td><td></td><td></td><td></td><td></td><td>District of Columbia</td><td>168</td><td>1.67%</td></tr>
</table>

Source: U.S. Department of Health and Human Services, National Center for Health Statistics
   "Monthly Vital Statistics Report" (Vol. 45, No. 3(S), September 30, 1996)
*Final data. Deaths of infants under 1 year old, exclusive of fetal deaths. Based on race of the mother.

Black Infant Mortality Rate in 1994

National Rate = 15.8 Black Infant Deaths per 1,000 Black Live Births*

ALPHA ORDER

RANK ORDER

RANK	STATE	RATE		RANK	STATE	RATE
14	Alabama	16.4		1	Iowa	22.7
NA	Alaska**	NA		2	Colorado	20.2
13	Arizona	16.5		2	Wisconsin	20.2
30	Arkansas	13.0		4	Indiana	19.5
21	California	15.2		5	Illinois	18.7
2	Colorado	20.2		6	Minnesota	18.6
8	Connecticut	18.3		6	Pennsylvania	18.6
33	Delaware	11.7		8	Connecticut	18.3
29	Florida	13.9		8	Michigan	18.3
17	Georgia	16.1		10	Tennessee	18.0
NA	Hawaii**	NA		11	Ohio	17.7
NA	Idaho**	NA		12	North Carolina	16.6
5	Illinois	18.7		13	Arizona	16.5
4	Indiana	19.5		14	Alabama	16.4
1	Iowa	22.7		15	Missouri	16.3
19	Kansas	15.9		15	New Jersey	16.3
23	Kentucky	14.7		17	Georgia	16.1
18	Louisiana	16.0		18	Louisiana	16.0
NA	Maine**	NA		19	Kansas	15.9
23	Maryland	14.7		20	Nebraska	15.7
35	Massachusetts	11.0		21	California	15.2
8	Michigan	18.3		22	Virginia	15.1
6	Minnesota	18.6		23	Kentucky	14.7
23	Mississippi	14.7		23	Maryland	14.7
15	Missouri	16.3		23	Mississippi	14.7
NA	Montana**	NA		23	Washington	14.7
20	Nebraska	15.7		27	New York	14.4
32	Nevada	12.0		28	South Carolina	14.1
NA	New Hampshire**	NA		29	Florida	13.9
15	New Jersey	16.3		30	Arkansas	13.0
NA	New Mexico**	NA		31	Texas	12.6
27	New York	14.4		32	Nevada	12.0
12	North Carolina	16.6		33	Delaware	11.7
NA	North Dakota**	NA		34	Oklahoma	11.3
11	Ohio	17.7		35	Massachusetts	11.0
34	Oklahoma	11.3		NA	Alaska**	NA
NA	Oregon**	NA		NA	Hawaii**	NA
6	Pennsylvania	18.6		NA	Idaho**	NA
NA	Rhode Island**	NA		NA	Maine**	NA
28	South Carolina	14.1		NA	Montana**	NA
NA	South Dakota**	NA		NA	New Hampshire**	NA
10	Tennessee	18.0		NA	New Mexico**	NA
31	Texas	12.6		NA	North Dakota**	NA
NA	Utah**	NA		NA	Oregon**	NA
NA	Vermont**	NA		NA	Rhode Island**	NA
22	Virginia	15.1		NA	South Dakota**	NA
23	Washington	14.7		NA	Utah**	NA
NA	West Virginia**	NA		NA	Vermont**	NA
2	Wisconsin	20.2		NA	West Virginia**	NA
NA	Wyoming**	NA		NA	Wyoming**	NA
					District of Columbia	20.9

Source: U.S. Department of Health and Human Services, National Center for Health Statistics
"Monthly Vital Statistics Report" (Vol. 45, No. 3(S), September 30, 1996)
*Final data. Deaths of infants under 1 year old, exclusive of fetal deaths. Based on race of the mother.
**Not available, fewer than 20 black infant deaths.

White Infant Mortality Rate in 1990

National Rate = 7.7 White Infant Deaths per 1,000 Live Births*

ALPHA ORDER

RANK	STATE	RATE
13	Alabama	8.3
10	Alaska	8.5
17	Arizona	8.2
21	Arkansas	8.0
32	California	7.6
12	Colorado	8.4
46	Connecticut	6.6
37	Delaware	7.3
32	Florida	7.6
4	Georgia	9.1
50	Hawaii	5.1
7	Idaho	8.7
29	Illinois	7.7
5	Indiana	8.9
26	Iowa	7.8
29	Kansas	7.7
21	Kentucky	8.0
37	Louisiana	7.3
49	Maine	6.2
47	Maryland	6.5
44	Massachusetts	6.7
24	Michigan	7.9
44	Minnesota	6.7
10	Mississippi	8.5
26	Missouri	7.8
8	Montana	8.6
39	Nebraska	7.2
19	Nevada	8.1
39	New Hampshire	7.2
43	New Jersey	6.8
3	New Mexico	9.3
29	New York	7.7
13	North Carolina	8.3
24	North Dakota	7.9
17	Ohio	8.2
2	Oklahoma	9.4
19	Oregon	8.1
26	Pennsylvania	7.8
13	Rhode Island	8.3
13	South Carolina	8.3
8	South Dakota	8.6
21	Tennessee	8.0
42	Texas	7.1
36	Utah	7.4
47	Vermont	6.5
35	Virginia	7.5
32	Washington	7.6
1	West Virginia	9.6
39	Wisconsin	7.2
6	Wyoming	8.8

RANK ORDER

RANK	STATE	RATE
1	West Virginia	9.6
2	Oklahoma	9.4
3	New Mexico	9.3
4	Georgia	9.1
5	Indiana	8.9
6	Wyoming	8.8
7	Idaho	8.7
8	Montana	8.6
8	South Dakota	8.6
10	Alaska	8.5
10	Mississippi	8.5
12	Colorado	8.4
13	Alabama	8.3
13	North Carolina	8.3
13	Rhode Island	8.3
13	South Carolina	8.3
17	Arizona	8.2
17	Ohio	8.2
19	Nevada	8.1
19	Oregon	8.1
21	Arkansas	8.0
21	Kentucky	8.0
21	Tennessee	8.0
24	Michigan	7.9
24	North Dakota	7.9
26	Iowa	7.8
26	Missouri	7.8
26	Pennsylvania	7.8
29	Illinois	7.7
29	Kansas	7.7
29	New York	7.7
32	California	7.6
32	Florida	7.6
32	Washington	7.6
35	Virginia	7.5
36	Utah	7.4
37	Delaware	7.3
37	Louisiana	7.3
39	Nebraska	7.2
39	New Hampshire	7.2
39	Wisconsin	7.2
42	Texas	7.1
43	New Jersey	6.8
44	Massachusetts	6.7
44	Minnesota	6.7
46	Connecticut	6.6
47	Maryland	6.5
47	Vermont	6.5
49	Maine	6.2
50	Hawaii	5.1

	District of Columbia	12.1

Source: U.S. Department of Health and Human Services, National Center for Health Statistics,
    "Vital Statistics of the United States"
*Deaths of infants under 1 year old, exclusive of fetal deaths. Final data by state of residence.

Black Infant Mortality Rate in 1990

National Rate = 17.0 Black Infant Deaths per 1,000 Live Births*

ALPHA ORDER

RANK ORDER

RANK	STATE	RATE		RANK	STATE	RATE
27	Alabama	15.9		1	Illinois	21.5
41	Alaska	11.2		2	Michigan	21.0
17	Arizona	16.7		3	Minnesota	19.7
33	Arkansas	13.6		4	Delaware	19.4
31	California	14.2		5	Pennsylvania	18.8
19	Colorado	16.5		5	Virginia	18.8
24	Connecticut	16.0		7	Ohio	18.3
4	Delaware	19.4		8	Wisconsin	18.1
22	Florida	16.2		9	Georgia	18.0
9	Georgia	18.0		9	Iowa	18.0
40	Hawaii	11.5		11	Missouri	17.5
42	Idaho	10.9		11	Tennessee	17.5
1	Illinois	21.5		13	New Jersey	17.3
24	Indiana	16.0		13	New York	17.3
9	Iowa	18.0		15	South Carolina	17.1
28	Kansas	15.4		16	Nebraska	16.8
33	Kentucky	13.6		17	Arizona	16.7
19	Louisiana	16.5		18	West Virginia	16.6
46	Maine	6.1		19	Colorado	16.5
21	Maryland	16.3		19	Louisiana	16.5
43	Massachusetts	10.4		21	Maryland	16.3
2	Michigan	21.0		22	Florida	16.2
3	Minnesota	19.7		23	Mississippi	16.1
23	Mississippi	16.1		24	Connecticut	16.0
11	Missouri	17.5		24	Indiana	16.0
35	Montana	13.3		24	North Carolina	16.0
16	Nebraska	16.8		27	Alabama	15.9
39	Nevada	12.5		28	Kansas	15.4
47	New Hampshire	5.4		29	Oregon	15.1
13	New Jersey	17.3		30	Washington	14.5
38	New Mexico	12.8		31	California	14.2
13	New York	17.3		32	Texas	13.9
24	North Carolina	16.0		33	Arkansas	13.6
NA	North Dakota**	NA		33	Kentucky	13.6
7	Ohio	18.3		35	Montana	13.3
36	Oklahoma	13.2		36	Oklahoma	13.2
29	Oregon	15.1		37	Utah	13.0
5	Pennsylvania	18.8		38	New Mexico	12.8
44	Rhode Island	9.7		39	Nevada	12.5
15	South Carolina	17.1		40	Hawaii	11.5
45	South Dakota	7.4		41	Alaska	11.2
11	Tennessee	17.5		42	Idaho	10.9
32	Texas	13.9		43	Massachusetts	10.4
37	Utah	13.0		44	Rhode Island	9.7
NA	Vermont**	NA		45	South Dakota	7.4
5	Virginia	18.8		46	Maine	6.1
30	Washington	14.5		47	New Hampshire	5.4
18	West Virginia	16.6		NA	North Dakota**	NA
8	Wisconsin	18.1		NA	Vermont**	NA
NA	Wyoming**	NA		NA	Wyoming**	NA
				District of Columbia		24.4

Source: U.S. Department of Health and Human Services, National Center for Health Statistics,
"Vital Statistics of the United States"
*Deaths of infants under 1 year old, exclusive of fetal deaths. Final data by state of residence.
**Not available.

Neonatal Deaths in 1994

National Total = 20,250 Deaths*

ALPHA ORDER					RANK ORDER			

RANK	STATE	DEATHS	% of USA		RANK	STATE	DEATHS	% of USA
16	Alabama	395	1.95%		1	California	2,480	12.25%
48	Alaska	35	0.17%		2	New York	1,461	7.21%
21	Arizona	331	1.63%		3	Texas	1,320	6.52%
31	Arkansas	170	0.84%		4	Illinois	1,133	5.60%
1	California	2,480	12.25%		5	Florida	1,033	5.10%
29	Colorado	221	1.09%		6	Ohio	896	4.42%
26	Connecticut	260	1.28%		7	Pennsylvania	868	4.29%
45	Delaware	48	0.24%		8	Michigan	778	3.84%
5	Florida	1,033	5.10%		9	North Carolina	737	3.64%
10	Georgia	725	3.58%		10	Georgia	725	3.58%
38	Hawaii	76	0.38%		11	New Jersey	612	3.02%
38	Idaho	76	0.38%		12	Virginia	563	2.78%
4	Illinois	1,133	5.60%		13	Louisiana	477	2.36%
14	Indiana	456	2.25%		14	Indiana	456	2.25%
32	Iowa	164	0.81%		15	Maryland	455	2.25%
30	Kansas	177	0.87%		16	Alabama	395	1.95%
27	Kentucky	250	1.23%		17	Tennessee	389	1.92%
13	Louisiana	477	2.36%		18	Missouri	358	1.77%
42	Maine	58	0.29%		19	Massachusetts	351	1.73%
15	Maryland	455	2.25%		20	South Carolina	335	1.65%
19	Massachusetts	351	1.73%		21	Arizona	331	1.63%
8	Michigan	778	3.84%		22	Wisconsin	327	1.61%
23	Minnesota	297	1.47%		23	Minnesota	297	1.47%
25	Mississippi	275	1.36%		24	Washington	280	1.38%
18	Missouri	358	1.77%		25	Mississippi	275	1.36%
46	Montana	45	0.22%		26	Connecticut	260	1.28%
36	Nebraska	104	0.51%		27	Kentucky	250	1.23%
40	Nevada	75	0.37%		28	Oklahoma	241	1.19%
41	New Hampshire	62	0.31%		29	Colorado	221	1.09%
11	New Jersey	612	3.02%		30	Kansas	177	0.87%
34	New Mexico	135	0.67%		31	Arkansas	170	0.84%
2	New York	1,461	7.21%		32	Iowa	164	0.81%
9	North Carolina	737	3.64%		33	Oregon	163	0.80%
47	North Dakota	44	0.22%		34	New Mexico	135	0.67%
6	Ohio	896	4.42%		35	Utah	126	0.62%
28	Oklahoma	241	1.19%		36	Nebraska	104	0.51%
33	Oregon	163	0.80%		37	West Virginia	93	0.46%
7	Pennsylvania	868	4.29%		38	Hawaii	76	0.38%
44	Rhode Island	49	0.24%		38	Idaho	76	0.38%
20	South Carolina	335	1.65%		40	Nevada	75	0.37%
42	South Dakota	58	0.29%		41	New Hampshire	62	0.31%
17	Tennessee	389	1.92%		42	Maine	58	0.29%
3	Texas	1,320	6.52%		42	South Dakota	58	0.29%
35	Utah	126	0.62%		44	Rhode Island	49	0.24%
48	Vermont	35	0.17%		45	Delaware	48	0.24%
12	Virginia	563	2.78%		46	Montana	45	0.22%
24	Washington	280	1.38%		47	North Dakota	44	0.22%
37	West Virginia	93	0.46%		48	Alaska	35	0.17%
22	Wisconsin	327	1.61%		48	Vermont	35	0.17%
50	Wyoming	26	0.13%		50	Wyoming	26	0.13%
						District of Columbia	127	0.63%

Source: U.S. Department of Health and Human Services, National Center for Health Statistics
   "Monthly Vital Statistics Report" (Vol. 45, No. 3(S), September 30, 1996)
*Final data. Deaths of infants under 28 days, exclusive of fetal deaths.

Neonatal Death Rate in 1994

National Rate = 5.1 Neonatal Deaths per 1,000 Live Births*

ALPHA ORDER

RANK	STATE	RATE
4	Alabama	6.5
48	Alaska	3.3
26	Arizona	4.7
22	Arkansas	4.9
33	California	4.4
38	Colorado	4.1
10	Connecticut	5.7
30	Delaware	4.6
16	Florida	5.4
4	Georgia	6.5
44	Hawaii	3.9
36	Idaho	4.3
8	Illinois	6.0
13	Indiana	5.5
33	Iowa	4.4
26	Kansas	4.7
26	Kentucky	4.7
2	Louisiana	7.0
42	Maine	4.0
7	Maryland	6.2
37	Massachusetts	4.2
12	Michigan	5.6
30	Minnesota	4.6
3	Mississippi	6.6
22	Missouri	4.9
38	Montana	4.1
32	Nebraska	4.5
50	Nevada	3.1
38	New Hampshire	4.1
19	New Jersey	5.2
22	New Mexico	4.9
19	New York	5.2
1	North Carolina	7.3
21	North Dakota	5.1
10	Ohio	5.7
17	Oklahoma	5.3
44	Oregon	3.9
13	Pennsylvania	5.5
46	Rhode Island	3.6
6	South Carolina	6.4
13	South Dakota	5.5
17	Tennessee	5.3
38	Texas	4.1
48	Utah	3.3
26	Vermont	4.7
9	Virginia	5.9
46	Washington	3.6
33	West Virginia	4.4
25	Wisconsin	4.8
42	Wyoming	4.0

RANK ORDER

RANK	STATE	RATE
1	North Carolina	7.3
2	Louisiana	7.0
3	Mississippi	6.6
4	Alabama	6.5
4	Georgia	6.5
6	South Carolina	6.4
7	Maryland	6.2
8	Illinois	6.0
9	Virginia	5.9
10	Connecticut	5.7
10	Ohio	5.7
12	Michigan	5.6
13	Indiana	5.5
13	Pennsylvania	5.5
13	South Dakota	5.5
16	Florida	5.4
17	Oklahoma	5.3
17	Tennessee	5.3
19	New Jersey	5.2
19	New York	5.2
21	North Dakota	5.1
22	Arkansas	4.9
22	Missouri	4.9
22	New Mexico	4.9
25	Wisconsin	4.8
26	Arizona	4.7
26	Kansas	4.7
26	Kentucky	4.7
26	Vermont	4.7
30	Delaware	4.6
30	Minnesota	4.6
32	Nebraska	4.5
33	California	4.4
33	Iowa	4.4
33	West Virginia	4.4
36	Idaho	4.3
37	Massachusetts	4.2
38	Colorado	4.1
38	Montana	4.1
38	New Hampshire	4.1
38	Texas	4.1
42	Maine	4.0
42	Wyoming	4.0
44	Hawaii	3.9
44	Oregon	3.9
46	Rhode Island	3.6
46	Washington	3.6
48	Alaska	3.3
48	Utah	3.3
50	Nevada	3.1

	District of Columbia	12.8

Source: U.S. Department of Health and Human Services, National Center for Health Statistics
    "Monthly Vital Statistics Report" (Vol. 45, No. 3(S), September 30, 1996)
*Final data. Deaths of infants under 28 days, exclusive of fetal deaths.

White Neonatal Deaths in 1994

National Total = 13,100 Deaths*

ALPHA ORDER

RANK	STATE	DEATHS	% of USA
27	Alabama	163	1.24%
49	Alaska	20	0.15%
14	Arizona	280	2.14%
33	Arkansas	117	0.89%
1	California	1,895	14.47%
24	Colorado	182	1.39%
25	Connecticut	177	1.35%
47	Delaware	28	0.21%
5	Florida	629	4.80%
13	Georgia	302	2.31%
50	Hawaii	18	0.14%
38	Idaho	73	0.56%
4	Illinois	646	4.93%
11	Indiana	348	2.66%
28	Iowa	150	1.15%
30	Kansas	147	1.12%
20	Kentucky	203	1.55%
26	Louisiana	174	1.33%
41	Maine	56	0.43%
22	Maryland	198	1.51%
15	Massachusetts	276	2.11%
8	Michigan	430	3.28%
17	Minnesota	240	1.83%
35	Mississippi	94	0.72%
19	Missouri	237	1.81%
42	Montana	38	0.29%
36	Nebraska	91	0.69%
40	Nevada	59	0.45%
39	New Hampshire	61	0.47%
9	New Jersey	372	2.84%
34	New Mexico	113	0.86%
3	New York	864	6.60%
10	North Carolina	371	2.83%
45	North Dakota	35	0.27%
6	Ohio	612	4.67%
23	Oklahoma	187	1.43%
28	Oregon	150	1.15%
7	Pennsylvania	570	4.35%
42	Rhode Island	38	0.29%
31	South Carolina	141	1.08%
42	South Dakota	38	0.29%
20	Tennessee	203	1.55%
2	Texas	1,006	7.68%
32	Utah	122	0.93%
45	Vermont	35	0.27%
12	Virginia	311	2.37%
16	Washington	243	1.85%
37	West Virginia	89	0.68%
18	Wisconsin	239	1.82%
48	Wyoming	23	0.18%

RANK ORDER

RANK	STATE	DEATHS	% of USA
1	California	1,895	14.47%
2	Texas	1,006	7.68%
3	New York	864	6.60%
4	Illinois	646	4.93%
5	Florida	629	4.80%
6	Ohio	612	4.67%
7	Pennsylvania	570	4.35%
8	Michigan	430	3.28%
9	New Jersey	372	2.84%
10	North Carolina	371	2.83%
11	Indiana	348	2.66%
12	Virginia	311	2.37%
13	Georgia	302	2.31%
14	Arizona	280	2.14%
15	Massachusetts	276	2.11%
16	Washington	243	1.85%
17	Minnesota	240	1.83%
18	Wisconsin	239	1.82%
19	Missouri	237	1.81%
20	Kentucky	203	1.55%
20	Tennessee	203	1.55%
22	Maryland	198	1.51%
23	Oklahoma	187	1.43%
24	Colorado	182	1.39%
25	Connecticut	177	1.35%
26	Louisiana	174	1.33%
27	Alabama	163	1.24%
28	Iowa	150	1.15%
28	Oregon	150	1.15%
30	Kansas	147	1.12%
31	South Carolina	141	1.08%
32	Utah	122	0.93%
33	Arkansas	117	0.89%
34	New Mexico	113	0.86%
35	Mississippi	94	0.72%
36	Nebraska	91	0.69%
37	West Virginia	89	0.68%
38	Idaho	73	0.56%
39	New Hampshire	61	0.47%
40	Nevada	59	0.45%
41	Maine	56	0.43%
42	Montana	38	0.29%
42	Rhode Island	38	0.29%
42	South Dakota	38	0.29%
45	North Dakota	35	0.27%
45	Vermont	35	0.27%
47	Delaware	28	0.21%
48	Wyoming	23	0.18%
49	Alaska	20	0.15%
50	Hawaii	18	0.14%
	District of Columbia	6	0.05%

Source: U.S. Department of Health and Human Services, National Center for Health Statistics
"Monthly Vital Statistics Report" (Vol. 45, No. 3(S), September 30, 1996)
*Final data. Deaths of infants under 28 days, exclusive of fetal deaths. Based on race of the mother.

White Neonatal Death Rate in 1994

National Rate = 4.2 White Neonatal Deaths per 1,000 White Live Births*

ALPHA ORDER			RANK ORDER		
RANK	STATE	RATE	RANK	STATE	RATE
30	Alabama	4.1	1	North Carolina	5.3
49	Alaska	2.7	2	Oklahoma	5.2
9	Arizona	4.5	3	New Mexico	4.9
13	Arkansas	4.4	4	Indiana	4.8
30	California	4.1	4	Vermont	4.8
41	Colorado	3.7	6	Ohio	4.7
7	Connecticut	4.6	7	Connecticut	4.6
44	Delaware	3.6	7	Louisiana	4.6
13	Florida	4.4	9	Arizona	4.5
20	Georgia	4.3	9	Illinois	4.5
NA	Hawaii**	NA	9	North Dakota	4.5
20	Idaho	4.3	9	Virginia	4.5
9	Illinois	4.5	13	Arkansas	4.4
4	Indiana	4.8	13	Florida	4.4
20	Iowa	4.3	13	Kansas	4.4
13	Kansas	4.4	13	Mississippi	4.4
20	Kentucky	4.3	13	Pennsylvania	4.4
7	Louisiana	4.6	13	South Carolina	4.4
34	Maine	4.0	13	West Virginia	4.4
20	Maryland	4.3	20	Georgia	4.3
39	Massachusetts	3.8	20	Idaho	4.3
34	Michigan	4.0	20	Iowa	4.3
27	Minnesota	4.2	20	Kentucky	4.3
13	Mississippi	4.4	20	Maryland	4.3
36	Missouri	3.9	20	Nebraska	4.3
36	Montana	3.9	20	South Dakota	4.3
20	Nebraska	4.3	27	Minnesota	4.2
48	Nevada	2.9	27	New Jersey	4.2
30	New Hampshire	4.1	27	New York	4.2
27	New Jersey	4.2	30	Alabama	4.1
3	New Mexico	4.9	30	California	4.1
27	New York	4.2	30	New Hampshire	4.1
1	North Carolina	5.3	30	Wisconsin	4.1
9	North Dakota	4.5	34	Maine	4.0
6	Ohio	4.7	34	Michigan	4.0
2	Oklahoma	5.2	36	Missouri	3.9
36	Oregon	3.9	36	Montana	3.9
13	Pennsylvania	4.4	36	Oregon	3.9
47	Rhode Island	3.2	39	Massachusetts	3.8
13	South Carolina	4.4	39	Wyoming	3.8
20	South Dakota	4.3	41	Colorado	3.7
41	Tennessee	3.7	41	Tennessee	3.7
41	Texas	3.7	41	Texas	3.7
46	Utah	3.4	44	Delaware	3.6
4	Vermont	4.8	44	Washington	3.6
9	Virginia	4.5	46	Utah	3.4
44	Washington	3.6	47	Rhode Island	3.2
13	West Virginia	4.4	48	Nevada	2.9
30	Wisconsin	4.1	49	Alaska	2.7
39	Wyoming	3.8	NA	Hawaii**	NA
				District of Columbia**	NA

Source: U.S. Department of Health and Human Services, National Center for Health Statistics
    "Monthly Vital Statistics Report" (Vol. 45, No. 3(S), September 30, 1996)
*Final data. Deaths of infants under 28 days, exclusive of fetal deaths. Based on race of the mother.
**Not available. Fewer than 20 white neonatal deaths.

Black Neonatal Deaths in 1994

National Total = 6,499 Deaths*

ALPHA ORDER

ALPHA ORDER

RANK	STATE	DEATHS	% of USA
15	Alabama	231	3.55%
47	Alaska	0	0.00%
30	Arizona	24	0.37%
24	Arkansas	52	0.80%
4	California	401	6.17%
26	Colorado	35	0.54%
21	Connecticut	79	1.22%
32	Delaware	18	0.28%
5	Florida	397	6.11%
3	Georgia	417	6.42%
38	Hawaii	7	0.11%
41	Idaho	1	0.02%
2	Illinois	478	7.35%
20	Indiana	106	1.63%
34	Iowa	12	0.18%
29	Kansas	27	0.42%
25	Kentucky	46	0.71%
8	Louisiana	300	4.62%
41	Maine	1	0.02%
12	Maryland	247	3.80%
23	Massachusetts	66	1.02%
7	Michigan	334	5.14%
27	Minnesota	34	0.52%
18	Mississippi	177	2.72%
19	Missouri	118	1.82%
41	Montana	1	0.02%
35	Nebraska	11	0.17%
33	Nevada	15	0.23%
41	New Hampshire	1	0.02%
14	New Jersey	233	3.59%
41	New Mexico	1	0.02%
1	New York	532	8.19%
6	North Carolina	345	5.31%
40	North Dakota	2	0.03%
11	Ohio	278	4.28%
28	Oklahoma	33	0.51%
36	Oregon	8	0.12%
10	Pennsylvania	281	4.32%
36	Rhode Island	8	0.12%
16	South Carolina	193	2.97%
47	South Dakota	0	0.00%
17	Tennessee	185	2.85%
9	Texas	293	4.51%
41	Utah	1	0.02%
47	Vermont	0	0.00%
13	Virginia	246	3.79%
31	Washington	21	0.32%
39	West Virginia	4	0.06%
22	Wisconsin	78	1.20%
47	Wyoming	0	0.00%

RANK ORDER

RANK	STATE	DEATHS	% of USA
1	New York	532	8.19%
2	Illinois	478	7.35%
3	Georgia	417	6.42%
4	California	401	6.17%
5	Florida	397	6.11%
6	North Carolina	345	5.31%
7	Michigan	334	5.14%
8	Louisiana	300	4.62%
9	Texas	293	4.51%
10	Pennsylvania	281	4.32%
11	Ohio	278	4.28%
12	Maryland	247	3.80%
13	Virginia	246	3.79%
14	New Jersey	233	3.59%
15	Alabama	231	3.55%
16	South Carolina	193	2.97%
17	Tennessee	185	2.85%
18	Mississippi	177	2.72%
19	Missouri	118	1.82%
20	Indiana	106	1.63%
21	Connecticut	79	1.22%
22	Wisconsin	78	1.20%
23	Massachusetts	66	1.02%
24	Arkansas	52	0.80%
25	Kentucky	46	0.71%
26	Colorado	35	0.54%
27	Minnesota	34	0.52%
28	Oklahoma	33	0.51%
29	Kansas	27	0.42%
30	Arizona	24	0.37%
31	Washington	21	0.32%
32	Delaware	18	0.28%
33	Nevada	15	0.23%
34	Iowa	12	0.18%
35	Nebraska	11	0.17%
36	Oregon	8	0.12%
36	Rhode Island	8	0.12%
38	Hawaii	7	0.11%
39	West Virginia	4	0.06%
40	North Dakota	2	0.03%
41	Idaho	1	0.02%
41	Maine	1	0.02%
41	Montana	1	0.02%
41	New Hampshire	1	0.02%
41	New Mexico	1	0.02%
41	Utah	1	0.02%
47	Alaska	0	0.00%
47	South Dakota	0	0.00%
47	Vermont	0	0.00%
47	Wyoming	0	0.00%
	District of Columbia	121	1.86%

Source: U.S. Department of Health and Human Services, National Center for Health Statistics
"Monthly Vital Statistics Report" (Vol. 45, No. 3(S), September 30, 1996)
*Final data. Deaths of infants under 28 days, exclusive of fetal deaths. Based on race of the mother.

Black Neonatal Death Rate in 1994

National Rate = 10.2 Black Neonatal Deaths per 1,000 Black Live Births*

ALPHA ORDER

RANK ORDER

RANK	STATE	RATE
11	Alabama	11.2
NA	Alaska**	NA
20	Arizona	9.7
31	Arkansas	6.6
21	California	9.4
2	Colorado	12.6
1	Connecticut	13.8
NA	Delaware**	NA
23	Florida	9.2
14	Georgia	10.7
NA	Hawaii**	NA
NA	Idaho**	NA
8	Illinois	11.7
6	Indiana	11.8
NA	Iowa**	NA
26	Kansas	8.6
21	Kentucky	9.4
15	Louisiana	10.5
NA	Maine**	NA
16	Maryland	10.0
27	Massachusetts	8.1
4	Michigan	12.3
10	Minnesota	11.3
25	Mississippi	8.9
18	Missouri	9.9
NA	Montana**	NA
NA	Nebraska**	NA
NA	Nevada**	NA
NA	New Hampshire**	NA
16	New Jersey	10.0
NA	New Mexico**	NA
24	New York	9.0
3	North Carolina	12.4
NA	North Dakota**	NA
6	Ohio	11.8
29	Oklahoma	6.9
NA	Oregon**	NA
5	Pennsylvania	12.0
NA	Rhode Island**	NA
18	South Carolina	9.9
NA	South Dakota**	NA
12	Tennessee	11.1
28	Texas	7.3
NA	Utah**	NA
NA	Vermont**	NA
13	Virginia	11.0
29	Washington	6.9
NA	West Virginia**	NA
9	Wisconsin	11.4
NA	Wyoming**	NA

RANK	STATE	RATE
1	Connecticut	13.8
2	Colorado	12.6
3	North Carolina	12.4
4	Michigan	12.3
5	Pennsylvania	12.0
6	Indiana	11.8
6	Ohio	11.8
8	Illinois	11.7
9	Wisconsin	11.4
10	Minnesota	11.3
11	Alabama	11.2
12	Tennessee	11.1
13	Virginia	11.0
14	Georgia	10.7
15	Louisiana	10.5
16	Maryland	10.0
16	New Jersey	10.0
18	Missouri	9.9
18	South Carolina	9.9
20	Arizona	9.7
21	California	9.4
21	Kentucky	9.4
23	Florida	9.2
24	New York	9.0
25	Mississippi	8.9
26	Kansas	8.6
27	Massachusetts	8.1
28	Texas	7.3
29	Oklahoma	6.9
29	Washington	6.9
31	Arkansas	6.6
NA	Alaska**	NA
NA	Delaware**	NA
NA	Hawaii**	NA
NA	Idaho**	NA
NA	Iowa**	NA
NA	Maine**	NA
NA	Montana**	NA
NA	Nebraska**	NA
NA	Nevada**	NA
NA	New Hampshire**	NA
NA	New Mexico**	NA
NA	North Dakota**	NA
NA	Oregon**	NA
NA	Rhode Island**	NA
NA	South Dakota**	NA
NA	Utah**	NA
NA	Vermont**	NA
NA	West Virginia**	NA
NA	Wyoming**	NA

District of Columbia 1.0

Source: U.S. Department of Health and Human Services, National Center for Health Statistics
"Monthly Vital Statistics Report" (Vol. 45, No. 3(S), September 30, 1996)
*Final data. Deaths of infants under 28 days, exclusive of fetal deaths. Based on race of the mother.
**Not available. Fewer than 20 black neonatal deaths.

Deaths by AIDS Through 1994

National Total = 219,842 Deaths*

ALPHA ORDER

RANK	STATE	DEATHS	% of USA
23	Alabama	1,630	0.74%
46	Alaska	114	0.05%
21	Arizona	2,159	0.98%
34	Arkansas	663	0.30%
2	California	39,855	18.13%
20	Colorado	2,326	1.06%
17	Connecticut	2,722	1.24%
37	Delaware	504	0.23%
3	Florida	20,327	9.25%
7	Georgia	7,105	3.23%
33	Hawaii	708	0.32%
44	Idaho	163	0.07%
6	Illinois	7,121	3.24%
24	Indiana	1,602	0.73%
39	Iowa	417	0.19%
32	Kansas	721	0.33%
31	Kentucky	814	0.37%
15	Louisiana	3,446	1.57%
40	Maine	333	0.15%
9	Maryland	4,964	2.26%
10	Massachusetts	4,470	2.03%
14	Michigan	3,587	1.63%
26	Minnesota	1,223	0.56%
29	Mississippi	1,113	0.51%
18	Missouri	2,461	1.12%
46	Montana	114	0.05%
41	Nebraska	327	0.15%
30	Nevada	938	0.43%
43	New Hampshire	225	0.10%
5	New Jersey	13,619	6.19%
35	New Mexico	642	0.29%
1	New York	44,272	20.14%
11	North Carolina	4,069	1.85%
50	North Dakota	46	0.02%
12	Ohio	3,823	1.74%
27	Oklahoma	1,196	0.54%
25	Oregon	1,466	0.67%
8	Pennsylvania	6,492	2.95%
36	Rhode Island	569	0.26%
19	South Carolina	2,347	1.07%
49	South Dakota	50	0.02%
22	Tennessee	1,874	0.85%
4	Texas	15,221	6.92%
38	Utah	426	0.19%
45	Vermont	137	0.06%
13	Virginia	3,599	1.64%
16	Washington	2,968	1.35%
42	West Virginia	313	0.14%
28	Wisconsin	1,141	0.52%
48	Wyoming	56	0.03%

RANK ORDER

RANK	STATE	DEATHS	% of USA
1	New York	44,272	20.14%
2	California	39,855	18.13%
3	Florida	20,327	9.25%
4	Texas	15,221	6.92%
5	New Jersey	13,619	6.19%
6	Illinois	7,121	3.24%
7	Georgia	7,105	3.23%
8	Pennsylvania	6,492	2.95%
9	Maryland	4,964	2.26%
10	Massachusetts	4,470	2.03%
11	North Carolina	4,069	1.85%
12	Ohio	3,823	1.74%
13	Virginia	3,599	1.64%
14	Michigan	3,587	1.63%
15	Louisiana	3,446	1.57%
16	Washington	2,968	1.35%
17	Connecticut	2,722	1.24%
18	Missouri	2,461	1.12%
19	South Carolina	2,347	1.07%
20	Colorado	2,326	1.06%
21	Arizona	2,159	0.98%
22	Tennessee	1,874	0.85%
23	Alabama	1,630	0.74%
24	Indiana	1,602	0.73%
25	Oregon	1,466	0.67%
26	Minnesota	1,223	0.56%
27	Oklahoma	1,196	0.54%
28	Wisconsin	1,141	0.52%
29	Mississippi	1,113	0.51%
30	Nevada	938	0.43%
31	Kentucky	814	0.37%
32	Kansas	721	0.33%
33	Hawaii	708	0.32%
34	Arkansas	663	0.30%
35	New Mexico	642	0.29%
36	Rhode Island	569	0.26%
37	Delaware	504	0.23%
38	Utah	426	0.19%
39	Iowa	417	0.19%
40	Maine	333	0.15%
41	Nebraska	327	0.15%
42	West Virginia	313	0.14%
43	New Hampshire	225	0.10%
44	Idaho	163	0.07%
45	Vermont	137	0.06%
46	Alaska	114	0.05%
46	Montana	114	0.05%
48	Wyoming	56	0.03%
49	South Dakota	50	0.02%
50	North Dakota	46	0.02%
	District of Columbia	3,364	1.53%

*Source: U.S. Department of Health and Human Services, National Center for Health Statistics
(http://wonder.cdc.gov/WONDER/)*
**Cumulative deaths through 1994. However, due to reporting delays, these totals should increase. AIDS is
Acquired Immunodeficiency Syndrome. The definition of what is AIDS was expanded in 1985, 1987 and 1993.*

Deaths by AIDS in 1994

National Total = 42,114 Deaths*

ALPHA ORDER

RANK	STATE	DEATHS	% of USA
22	Alabama	395	0.94%
47	Alaska	20	0.05%
21	Arizona	433	1.03%
32	Arkansas	151	0.36%
2	California	6,752	16.03%
23	Colorado	383	0.91%
17	Connecticut	564	1.34%
33	Delaware	137	0.33%
3	Florida	4,153	9.86%
6	Georgia	1,439	3.42%
35	Hawaii	130	0.31%
45	Idaho	31	0.07%
7	Illinois	1,413	3.36%
24	Indiana	317	0.75%
38	Iowa	83	0.20%
37	Kansas	107	0.25%
31	Kentucky	187	0.44%
15	Louisiana	645	1.53%
41	Maine	73	0.17%
9	Maryland	1,210	2.87%
11	Massachusetts	941	2.23%
13	Michigan	760	1.80%
28	Minnesota	255	0.61%
26	Mississippi	270	0.64%
20	Missouri	456	1.08%
46	Montana	26	0.06%
39	Nebraska	82	0.19%
29	Nevada	223	0.53%
43	New Hampshire	43	0.10%
5	New Jersey	2,335	5.54%
33	New Mexico	137	0.33%
1	New York	8,093	19.22%
10	North Carolina	976	2.32%
49	North Dakota	10	0.02%
12	Ohio	789	1.87%
27	Oklahoma	256	0.61%
25	Oregon	303	0.72%
8	Pennsylvania	1,290	3.06%
36	Rhode Island	115	0.27%
18	South Carolina	524	1.24%
50	South Dakota	9	0.02%
19	Tennessee	457	1.09%
4	Texas	2,745	6.52%
40	Utah	80	0.19%
44	Vermont	36	0.09%
14	Virginia	729	1.73%
16	Washington	606	1.44%
42	West Virginia	61	0.14%
30	Wisconsin	205	0.49%
48	Wyoming	13	0.03%

RANK ORDER

RANK	STATE	DEATHS	% of USA
1	New York	8,093	19.22%
2	California	6,752	16.03%
3	Florida	4,153	9.86%
4	Texas	2,745	6.52%
5	New Jersey	2,335	5.54%
6	Georgia	1,439	3.42%
7	Illinois	1,413	3.36%
8	Pennsylvania	1,290	3.06%
9	Maryland	1,210	2.87%
10	North Carolina	976	2.32%
11	Massachusetts	941	2.23%
12	Ohio	789	1.87%
13	Michigan	760	1.80%
14	Virginia	729	1.73%
15	Louisiana	645	1.53%
16	Washington	606	1.44%
17	Connecticut	564	1.34%
18	South Carolina	524	1.24%
19	Tennessee	457	1.09%
20	Missouri	456	1.08%
21	Arizona	433	1.03%
22	Alabama	395	0.94%
23	Colorado	383	0.91%
24	Indiana	317	0.75%
25	Oregon	303	0.72%
26	Mississippi	270	0.64%
27	Oklahoma	256	0.61%
28	Minnesota	255	0.61%
29	Nevada	223	0.53%
30	Wisconsin	205	0.49%
31	Kentucky	187	0.44%
32	Arkansas	151	0.36%
33	Delaware	137	0.33%
33	New Mexico	137	0.33%
35	Hawaii	130	0.31%
36	Rhode Island	115	0.27%
37	Kansas	107	0.25%
38	Iowa	83	0.20%
39	Nebraska	82	0.19%
40	Utah	80	0.19%
41	Maine	73	0.17%
42	West Virginia	61	0.14%
43	New Hampshire	43	0.10%
44	Vermont	36	0.09%
45	Idaho	31	0.07%
46	Montana	26	0.06%
47	Alaska	20	0.05%
48	Wyoming	13	0.03%
49	North Dakota	10	0.02%
50	South Dakota	9	0.02%
	District of Columbia	666	1.58%

Source: U.S. Department of Health and Human Services, National Center for Health Statistics
    "Monthly Vital Statistics Report" (Vol. 45, No. 3(S), September 30, 1996)
*AIDS is Acquired Immunodeficiency Syndrome. It is a specific group of diseases or conditions which are indicative of severe immunosuppression related to infection with the Human Immunodeficiency Virus (HIV).

Death Rate by AIDS in 1994

National Rate = 16.2 Deaths per 100,000 Population*

ALPHA ORDER

RANK	STATE	RATE
25	Alabama	9.4
43	Alaska	3.3
21	Arizona	10.6
32	Arkansas	6.2
5	California	21.5
22	Colorado	10.5
8	Connecticut	17.2
7	Delaware	19.4
2	Florida	29.8
6	Georgia	20.4
19	Hawaii	11.0
47	Idaho	2.7
15	Illinois	12.0
36	Indiana	5.5
46	Iowa	2.9
39	Kansas	4.2
38	Kentucky	4.9
11	Louisiana	14.9
34	Maine	5.9
4	Maryland	24.2
9	Massachusetts	15.6
29	Michigan	8.0
35	Minnesota	5.6
23	Mississippi	10.1
27	Missouri	8.6
45	Montana	3.0
37	Nebraska	5.1
10	Nevada	15.3
42	New Hampshire	3.8
3	New Jersey	29.5
28	New Mexico	8.3
1	New York	44.5
14	North Carolina	13.8
NA	North Dakota**	NA
31	Ohio	7.1
30	Oklahoma	7.9
24	Oregon	9.8
20	Pennsylvania	10.7
16	Rhode Island	11.5
13	South Carolina	14.3
NA	South Dakota**	NA
26	Tennessee	8.8
11	Texas	14.9
39	Utah	4.2
32	Vermont	6.2
18	Virginia	11.1
17	Washington	11.3
43	West Virginia	3.3
41	Wisconsin	4.0
NA	Wyoming**	NA

RANK ORDER

RANK	STATE	RATE
1	New York	44.5
2	Florida	29.8
3	New Jersey	29.5
4	Maryland	24.2
5	California	21.5
6	Georgia	20.4
7	Delaware	19.4
8	Connecticut	17.2
9	Massachusetts	15.6
10	Nevada	15.3
11	Louisiana	14.9
11	Texas	14.9
13	South Carolina	14.3
14	North Carolina	13.8
15	Illinois	12.0
16	Rhode Island	11.5
17	Washington	11.3
18	Virginia	11.1
19	Hawaii	11.0
20	Pennsylvania	10.7
21	Arizona	10.6
22	Colorado	10.5
23	Mississippi	10.1
24	Oregon	9.8
25	Alabama	9.4
26	Tennessee	8.8
27	Missouri	8.6
28	New Mexico	8.3
29	Michigan	8.0
30	Oklahoma	7.9
31	Ohio	7.1
32	Arkansas	6.2
32	Vermont	6.2
34	Maine	5.9
35	Minnesota	5.6
36	Indiana	5.5
37	Nebraska	5.1
38	Kentucky	4.9
39	Kansas	4.2
39	Utah	4.2
41	Wisconsin	4.0
42	New Hampshire	3.8
43	Alaska	3.3
43	West Virginia	3.3
45	Montana	3.0
46	Iowa	2.9
47	Idaho	2.7
NA	North Dakota**	NA
NA	South Dakota**	NA
NA	Wyoming**	NA

District of Columbia   116.8

Source: U.S. Department of Health and Human Services, National Center for Health Statistics
"Monthly Vital Statistics Report" (Vol. 45, No. 3(S), September 30, 1996)
*AIDS is Acquired Immunodeficiency Syndrome. It is a specific group of diseases or conditions which are indicative of severe immunosuppression related to infection with the Human Immunodeficiency Virus (HIV).
**Not available as fewer than 20 deaths by AIDS, insufficient for a reliable rate.

Estimated Deaths by Cancer in 1997

National Estimated Total = 560,000 Deaths

ALPHA ORDER

RANK	STATE	DEATHS	% of USA
20	Alabama	9,400	1.68%
50	Alaska	600	0.11%
23	Arizona	8,900	1.59%
30	Arkansas	6,400	1.14%
1	California	51,700	9.23%
31	Colorado	6,000	1.07%
28	Connecticut	7,000	1.25%
45	Delaware	1,800	0.32%
2	Florida	40,100	7.16%
13	Georgia	12,900	2.30%
43	Hawaii	1,900	0.34%
42	Idaho	2,000	0.36%
6	Illinois	26,500	4.73%
14	Indiana	12,800	2.29%
29	Iowa	6,800	1.21%
33	Kansas	5,400	0.96%
20	Kentucky	9,400	1.68%
20	Louisiana	9,400	1.68%
37	Maine	3,300	0.59%
19	Maryland	10,400	1.86%
11	Massachusetts	14,400	2.57%
8	Michigan	20,500	3.66%
23	Minnesota	8,900	1.59%
31	Mississippi	6,000	1.07%
14	Missouri	12,800	2.29%
43	Montana	1,900	0.34%
36	Nebraska	3,400	0.61%
35	Nevada	3,500	0.63%
39	New Hampshire	2,600	0.46%
9	New Jersey	18,500	3.30%
38	New Mexico	2,800	0.50%
3	New York	38,100	6.80%
10	North Carolina	16,000	2.86%
47	North Dakota	1,500	0.27%
7	Ohio	25,700	4.59%
27	Oklahoma	7,100	1.27%
26	Oregon	7,200	1.29%
5	Pennsylvania	31,300	5.59%
40	Rhode Island	2,400	0.43%
25	South Carolina	8,000	1.43%
46	South Dakota	1,600	0.29%
16	Tennessee	11,800	2.11%
4	Texas	35,300	6.30%
40	Utah	2,400	0.43%
48	Vermont	1,200	0.21%
12	Virginia	13,200	2.36%
18	Washington	11,000	1.96%
34	West Virginia	4,900	0.88%
17	Wisconsin	11,200	2.00%
49	Wyoming	830	0.15%

RANK ORDER

RANK	STATE	DEATHS	% of USA
1	California	51,700	9.23%
2	Florida	40,100	7.16%
3	New York	38,100	6.80%
4	Texas	35,300	6.30%
5	Pennsylvania	31,300	5.59%
6	Illinois	26,500	4.73%
7	Ohio	25,700	4.59%
8	Michigan	20,500	3.66%
9	New Jersey	18,500	3.30%
10	North Carolina	16,000	2.86%
11	Massachusetts	14,400	2.57%
12	Virginia	13,200	2.36%
13	Georgia	12,900	2.30%
14	Indiana	12,800	2.29%
14	Missouri	12,800	2.29%
16	Tennessee	11,800	2.11%
17	Wisconsin	11,200	2.00%
18	Washington	11,000	1.96%
19	Maryland	10,400	1.86%
20	Alabama	9,400	1.68%
20	Kentucky	9,400	1.68%
20	Louisiana	9,400	1.68%
23	Arizona	8,900	1.59%
23	Minnesota	8,900	1.59%
25	South Carolina	8,000	1.43%
26	Oregon	7,200	1.29%
27	Oklahoma	7,100	1.27%
28	Connecticut	7,000	1.25%
29	Iowa	6,800	1.21%
30	Arkansas	6,400	1.14%
31	Colorado	6,000	1.07%
31	Mississippi	6,000	1.07%
33	Kansas	5,400	0.96%
34	West Virginia	4,900	0.88%
35	Nevada	3,500	0.63%
36	Nebraska	3,400	0.61%
37	Maine	3,300	0.59%
38	New Mexico	2,800	0.50%
39	New Hampshire	2,600	0.46%
40	Rhode Island	2,400	0.43%
40	Utah	2,400	0.43%
42	Idaho	2,000	0.36%
43	Hawaii	1,900	0.34%
43	Montana	1,900	0.34%
45	Delaware	1,800	0.32%
46	South Dakota	1,600	0.29%
47	North Dakota	1,500	0.27%
48	Vermont	1,200	0.21%
49	Wyoming	830	0.15%
50	Alaska	600	0.11%
	District of Columbia	1,400	0.25%

Source: American Cancer Society (http://www.cancer.org/97tabl6.html)
"Cancer Facts & Figures-1997" (Copyright 1997, Reprinted with permission from the American Cancer Society)

Estimated Death Rate by Cancer in 1997

National Estimated Rate = 211.1 Deaths by Cancer per 100,000 Population*

<table>
<tr><td colspan="3">ALPHA ORDER</td><td colspan="3">RANK ORDER</td></tr>
<tr><td>RANK</td><td>STATE</td><td>RATE</td><td>RANK</td><td>STATE</td><td>RATE</td></tr>
<tr><td>20</td><td>Alabama</td><td>220.0</td><td>1</td><td>Florida</td><td>278.5</td></tr>
<tr><td>50</td><td>Alaska</td><td>98.8</td><td>2</td><td>West Virginia</td><td>268.3</td></tr>
<tr><td>37</td><td>Arizona</td><td>201.0</td><td>3</td><td>Maine</td><td>265.5</td></tr>
<tr><td>5</td><td>Arkansas</td><td>255.0</td><td>4</td><td>Pennsylvania</td><td>259.6</td></tr>
<tr><td>46</td><td>California</td><td>162.2</td><td>5</td><td>Arkansas</td><td>255.0</td></tr>
<tr><td>48</td><td>Colorado</td><td>156.9</td><td>6</td><td>Delaware</td><td>248.3</td></tr>
<tr><td>30</td><td>Connecticut</td><td>213.8</td><td>7</td><td>Rhode Island</td><td>242.4</td></tr>
<tr><td>6</td><td>Delaware</td><td>248.3</td><td>8</td><td>Kentucky</td><td>242.0</td></tr>
<tr><td>1</td><td>Florida</td><td>278.5</td><td>9</td><td>Missouri</td><td>238.9</td></tr>
<tr><td>42</td><td>Georgia</td><td>175.4</td><td>10</td><td>Iowa</td><td>238.4</td></tr>
<tr><td>47</td><td>Hawaii</td><td>160.5</td><td>11</td><td>Massachusetts</td><td>236.4</td></tr>
<tr><td>44</td><td>Idaho</td><td>168.2</td><td>12</td><td>North Dakota</td><td>232.9</td></tr>
<tr><td>17</td><td>Illinois</td><td>223.7</td><td>13</td><td>New Jersey</td><td>231.6</td></tr>
<tr><td>21</td><td>Indiana</td><td>219.1</td><td>14</td><td>Ohio</td><td>230.0</td></tr>
<tr><td>10</td><td>Iowa</td><td>238.4</td><td>15</td><td>Oregon</td><td>224.7</td></tr>
<tr><td>32</td><td>Kansas</td><td>210.0</td><td>16</td><td>New Hampshire</td><td>223.8</td></tr>
<tr><td>8</td><td>Kentucky</td><td>242.0</td><td>17</td><td>Illinois</td><td>223.7</td></tr>
<tr><td>28</td><td>Louisiana</td><td>216.0</td><td>18</td><td>Tennessee</td><td>221.8</td></tr>
<tr><td>3</td><td>Maine</td><td>265.5</td><td>19</td><td>Mississippi</td><td>220.9</td></tr>
<tr><td>35</td><td>Maryland</td><td>205.0</td><td>20</td><td>Alabama</td><td>220.0</td></tr>
<tr><td>11</td><td>Massachusetts</td><td>236.4</td><td>21</td><td>Indiana</td><td>219.1</td></tr>
<tr><td>31</td><td>Michigan</td><td>213.7</td><td>22</td><td>South Dakota</td><td>218.6</td></tr>
<tr><td>40</td><td>Minnesota</td><td>191.1</td><td>23</td><td>North Carolina</td><td>218.5</td></tr>
<tr><td>19</td><td>Mississippi</td><td>220.9</td><td>24</td><td>Nevada</td><td>218.3</td></tr>
<tr><td>9</td><td>Missouri</td><td>238.9</td><td>25</td><td>Wisconsin</td><td>217.1</td></tr>
<tr><td>27</td><td>Montana</td><td>216.2</td><td>26</td><td>South Carolina</td><td>216.3</td></tr>
<tr><td>34</td><td>Nebraska</td><td>205.8</td><td>27</td><td>Montana</td><td>216.2</td></tr>
<tr><td>24</td><td>Nevada</td><td>218.3</td><td>28</td><td>Louisiana</td><td>216.0</td></tr>
<tr><td>16</td><td>New Hampshire</td><td>223.8</td><td>29</td><td>Oklahoma</td><td>215.1</td></tr>
<tr><td>13</td><td>New Jersey</td><td>231.6</td><td>30</td><td>Connecticut</td><td>213.8</td></tr>
<tr><td>45</td><td>New Mexico</td><td>163.5</td><td>31</td><td>Michigan</td><td>213.7</td></tr>
<tr><td>33</td><td>New York</td><td>209.5</td><td>32</td><td>Kansas</td><td>210.0</td></tr>
<tr><td>23</td><td>North Carolina</td><td>218.5</td><td>33</td><td>New York</td><td>209.5</td></tr>
<tr><td>12</td><td>North Dakota</td><td>232.9</td><td>34</td><td>Nebraska</td><td>205.8</td></tr>
<tr><td>14</td><td>Ohio</td><td>230.0</td><td>35</td><td>Maryland</td><td>205.0</td></tr>
<tr><td>29</td><td>Oklahoma</td><td>215.1</td><td>36</td><td>Vermont</td><td>203.7</td></tr>
<tr><td>15</td><td>Oregon</td><td>224.7</td><td>37</td><td>Arizona</td><td>201.0</td></tr>
<tr><td>4</td><td>Pennsylvania</td><td>259.6</td><td>38</td><td>Washington</td><td>198.8</td></tr>
<tr><td>7</td><td>Rhode Island</td><td>242.4</td><td>39</td><td>Virginia</td><td>197.8</td></tr>
<tr><td>26</td><td>South Carolina</td><td>216.3</td><td>40</td><td>Minnesota</td><td>191.1</td></tr>
<tr><td>22</td><td>South Dakota</td><td>218.6</td><td>41</td><td>Texas</td><td>184.5</td></tr>
<tr><td>18</td><td>Tennessee</td><td>221.8</td><td>42</td><td>Georgia</td><td>175.4</td></tr>
<tr><td>41</td><td>Texas</td><td>184.5</td><td>43</td><td>Wyoming</td><td>172.6</td></tr>
<tr><td>49</td><td>Utah</td><td>120.0</td><td>44</td><td>Idaho</td><td>168.2</td></tr>
<tr><td>36</td><td>Vermont</td><td>203.7</td><td>45</td><td>New Mexico</td><td>163.5</td></tr>
<tr><td>39</td><td>Virginia</td><td>197.8</td><td>46</td><td>California</td><td>162.2</td></tr>
<tr><td>38</td><td>Washington</td><td>198.8</td><td>47</td><td>Hawaii</td><td>160.5</td></tr>
<tr><td>2</td><td>West Virginia</td><td>268.3</td><td>48</td><td>Colorado</td><td>156.9</td></tr>
<tr><td>25</td><td>Wisconsin</td><td>217.1</td><td>49</td><td>Utah</td><td>120.0</td></tr>
<tr><td>43</td><td>Wyoming</td><td>172.6</td><td>50</td><td>Alaska</td><td>98.8</td></tr>
<tr><td></td><td></td><td></td><td></td><td>District of Columbia</td><td>257.8</td></tr>
</table>

Source: Morgan Quitno Press using data from American Cancer Society (http://www.cancer.org/97tabl6.html)
"Cancer Facts & Figures-1997" (Copyright 1997, Reprinted with permission from the American Cancer Society)
*Rates calculated using 1996 Census resident population estimates. Not age adjusted.

Estimated Age-Adjusted Death Rate by Cancer in 1997

National Rate = 173 Deaths per 100,000 Population*

ALPHA ORDER

RANK	STATE	RATE
15	Alabama	179
28	Alaska	171
38	Arizona	159
14	Arkansas	180
36	California	162
47	Colorado	147
33	Connecticut	166
1	Delaware	195
31	Florida	168
22	Georgia	177
49	Hawaii	137
46	Idaho	149
10	Illinois	181
20	Indiana	178
38	Iowa	159
38	Kansas	159
3	Kentucky	193
2	Louisiana	194
5	Maine	186
4	Maryland	190
10	Massachusetts	181
22	Michigan	177
43	Minnesota	156
10	Mississippi	181
22	Missouri	177
36	Montana	162
41	Nebraska	157
6	Nevada	184
9	New Hampshire	182
6	New Jersey	184
48	New Mexico	146
27	New York	172
25	North Carolina	175
41	North Dakota	157
10	Ohio	181
29	Oklahoma	170
31	Oregon	168
15	Pennsylvania	179
15	Rhode Island	179
20	South Carolina	178
44	South Dakota	155
15	Tennessee	179
29	Texas	170
50	Utah	126
25	Vermont	175
15	Virginia	179
35	Washington	165
6	West Virginia	184
33	Wisconsin	166
45	Wyoming	154

RANK ORDER

RANK	STATE	RATE
1	Delaware	195
2	Louisiana	194
3	Kentucky	193
4	Maryland	190
5	Maine	186
6	Nevada	184
6	New Jersey	184
6	West Virginia	184
9	New Hampshire	182
10	Illinois	181
10	Massachusetts	181
10	Mississippi	181
10	Ohio	181
14	Arkansas	180
15	Alabama	179
15	Pennsylvania	179
15	Rhode Island	179
15	Tennessee	179
15	Virginia	179
20	Indiana	178
20	South Carolina	178
22	Georgia	177
22	Michigan	177
22	Missouri	177
25	North Carolina	175
25	Vermont	175
27	New York	172
28	Alaska	171
29	Oklahoma	170
29	Texas	170
31	Florida	168
31	Oregon	168
33	Connecticut	166
33	Wisconsin	166
35	Washington	165
36	California	162
36	Montana	162
38	Arizona	159
38	Iowa	159
38	Kansas	159
41	Nebraska	157
41	North Dakota	157
43	Minnesota	156
44	South Dakota	155
45	Wyoming	154
46	Idaho	149
47	Colorado	147
48	New Mexico	146
49	Hawaii	137
50	Utah	126
	District of Columbia	221

Source: American Cancer Society (http://www.cancer.org/97tabl6.html)
"Cancer Facts & Figures-1997" (Copyright 1997, Reprinted with permission from the American Cancer Society)
*Age-adjusted rates eliminate the distorting effects of the aging of the population.

Estimated Deaths by Bladder Cancer in 1997

National Estimated Total = 11,700

ALPHA ORDER

RANK	STATE	DEATHS	% of USA
25	Alabama	150	1.28%
50	Alaska	5	0.04%
19	Arizona	180	1.54%
29	Arkansas	130	1.11%
1	California	1,100	9.40%
29	Colorado	130	1.11%
19	Connecticut	180	1.54%
38	Delaware	60	0.51%
2	Florida	940	8.03%
19	Georgia	180	1.54%
44	Hawaii	40	0.34%
44	Idaho	40	0.34%
7	Illinois	530	4.53%
12	Indiana	290	2.48%
19	Iowa	180	1.54%
33	Kansas	100	0.85%
24	Kentucky	160	1.37%
29	Louisiana	130	1.11%
34	Maine	70	0.60%
18	Maryland	200	1.71%
10	Massachusetts	360	3.08%
8	Michigan	490	4.19%
25	Minnesota	150	1.28%
34	Mississippi	70	0.60%
13	Missouri	250	2.14%
47	Montana	30	0.26%
38	Nebraska	60	0.51%
42	Nevada	50	0.43%
38	New Hampshire	60	0.51%
9	New Jersey	460	3.93%
34	New Mexico	70	0.60%
3	New York	910	7.78%
11	North Carolina	300	2.56%
44	North Dakota	40	0.34%
6	Ohio	560	4.79%
25	Oklahoma	150	1.28%
28	Oregon	140	1.20%
4	Pennsylvania	630	5.38%
34	Rhode Island	70	0.60%
19	South Carolina	180	1.54%
42	South Dakota	50	0.43%
16	Tennessee	230	1.97%
5	Texas	620	5.30%
38	Utah	60	0.51%
47	Vermont	30	0.26%
13	Virginia	250	2.14%
16	Washington	230	1.97%
29	West Virginia	130	1.11%
13	Wisconsin	250	2.14%
49	Wyoming	10	0.09%

RANK ORDER

RANK	STATE	DEATHS	% of USA
1	California	1,100	9.40%
2	Florida	940	8.03%
3	New York	910	7.78%
4	Pennsylvania	630	5.38%
5	Texas	620	5.30%
6	Ohio	560	4.79%
7	Illinois	530	4.53%
8	Michigan	490	4.19%
9	New Jersey	460	3.93%
10	Massachusetts	360	3.08%
11	North Carolina	300	2.56%
12	Indiana	290	2.48%
13	Missouri	250	2.14%
13	Virginia	250	2.14%
13	Wisconsin	250	2.14%
16	Tennessee	230	1.97%
16	Washington	230	1.97%
18	Maryland	200	1.71%
19	Arizona	180	1.54%
19	Connecticut	180	1.54%
19	Georgia	180	1.54%
19	Iowa	180	1.54%
19	South Carolina	180	1.54%
24	Kentucky	160	1.37%
25	Alabama	150	1.28%
25	Minnesota	150	1.28%
25	Oklahoma	150	1.28%
28	Oregon	140	1.20%
29	Arkansas	130	1.11%
29	Colorado	130	1.11%
29	Louisiana	130	1.11%
29	West Virginia	130	1.11%
33	Kansas	100	0.85%
34	Maine	70	0.60%
34	Mississippi	70	0.60%
34	New Mexico	70	0.60%
34	Rhode Island	70	0.60%
38	Delaware	60	0.51%
38	Nebraska	60	0.51%
38	New Hampshire	60	0.51%
38	Utah	60	0.51%
42	Nevada	50	0.43%
42	South Dakota	50	0.43%
44	Hawaii	40	0.34%
44	Idaho	40	0.34%
44	North Dakota	40	0.34%
47	Montana	30	0.26%
47	Vermont	30	0.26%
49	Wyoming	10	0.09%
50	Alaska	5	0.04%
	District of Columbia	30	0.26%

Source: American Cancer Society (http://www.cancer.org/97tabp6.html)
"Cancer Facts & Figures-1997" (Copyright 1997, Reprinted with permission from the American Cancer Society)

Estimated Death Rate by Bladder Cancer in 1997

National Estimated Rate = 4.4 Deaths per 100,000 Population*

ALPHA ORDER

RANK ORDER

RANK	STATE	RATE
36	Alabama	3.5
50	Alaska	0.8
28	Arizona	4.1
12	Arkansas	5.2
36	California	3.5
38	Colorado	3.4
11	Connecticut	5.5
1	Delaware	8.3
5	Florida	6.5
48	Georgia	2.4
38	Hawaii	3.4
38	Idaho	3.4
23	Illinois	4.5
17	Indiana	5.0
6	Iowa	6.3
32	Kansas	3.9
28	Kentucky	4.1
45	Louisiana	3.0
10	Maine	5.6
32	Maryland	3.9
8	Massachusetts	5.9
15	Michigan	5.1
42	Minnesota	3.2
47	Mississippi	2.6
22	Missouri	4.7
38	Montana	3.4
35	Nebraska	3.6
44	Nevada	3.1
12	New Hampshire	5.2
9	New Jersey	5.8
28	New Mexico	4.1
17	New York	5.0
28	North Carolina	4.1
7	North Dakota	6.2
17	Ohio	5.0
23	Oklahoma	4.5
25	Oregon	4.4
12	Pennsylvania	5.2
2	Rhode Island	7.1
20	South Carolina	4.9
4	South Dakota	6.8
26	Tennessee	4.3
42	Texas	3.2
45	Utah	3.0
15	Vermont	5.1
34	Virginia	3.7
27	Washington	4.2
2	West Virginia	7.1
21	Wisconsin	4.8
49	Wyoming	2.1

RANK	STATE	RATE
1	Delaware	8.3
2	Rhode Island	7.1
2	West Virginia	7.1
4	South Dakota	6.8
5	Florida	6.5
6	Iowa	6.3
7	North Dakota	6.2
8	Massachusetts	5.9
9	New Jersey	5.8
10	Maine	5.6
11	Connecticut	5.5
12	Arkansas	5.2
12	New Hampshire	5.2
12	Pennsylvania	5.2
15	Michigan	5.1
15	Vermont	5.1
17	Indiana	5.0
17	New York	5.0
17	Ohio	5.0
20	South Carolina	4.9
21	Wisconsin	4.8
22	Missouri	4.7
23	Illinois	4.5
23	Oklahoma	4.5
25	Oregon	4.4
26	Tennessee	4.3
27	Washington	4.2
28	Arizona	4.1
28	Kentucky	4.1
28	New Mexico	4.1
28	North Carolina	4.1
32	Kansas	3.9
32	Maryland	3.9
34	Virginia	3.7
35	Nebraska	3.6
36	Alabama	3.5
36	California	3.5
38	Colorado	3.4
38	Hawaii	3.4
38	Idaho	3.4
38	Montana	3.4
42	Minnesota	3.2
42	Texas	3.2
44	Nevada	3.1
45	Louisiana	3.0
45	Utah	3.0
47	Mississippi	2.6
48	Georgia	2.4
49	Wyoming	2.1
50	Alaska	0.8

| | District of Columbia | 5.5 |

Source: Morgan Quitno Press using data from American Cancer Society (http://www.cancer.org/97tabp6.html)
"Cancer Facts & Figures-1997" (Copyright 1997, Reprinted with permission from the American Cancer Society)
Rates calculated using 1996 Census resident population estimates. Not age adjusted.

Estimated Deaths by Female Breast Cancer in 1997

National Estimated Total = 43,900 Deaths

ALPHA ORDER

RANK	STATE	DEATHS	% of USA
22	Alabama	670	1.53%
50	Alaska	60	0.14%
22	Arizona	670	1.53%
31	Arkansas	470	1.07%
1	California	4,200	9.57%
27	Colorado	520	1.18%
29	Connecticut	480	1.09%
44	Delaware	140	0.32%
3	Florida	2,900	6.61%
14	Georgia	950	2.16%
47	Hawaii	110	0.25%
42	Idaho	170	0.39%
6	Illinois	2,200	5.01%
13	Indiana	960	2.19%
26	Iowa	590	1.34%
33	Kansas	380	0.87%
24	Kentucky	650	1.48%
20	Louisiana	760	1.73%
37	Maine	240	0.55%
18	Maryland	840	1.91%
11	Massachusetts	1,100	2.51%
9	Michigan	1,500	3.42%
21	Minnesota	720	1.64%
32	Mississippi	430	0.98%
18	Missouri	840	1.91%
43	Montana	150	0.34%
35	Nebraska	270	0.62%
36	Nevada	260	0.59%
39	New Hampshire	230	0.52%
8	New Jersey	1,600	3.64%
37	New Mexico	240	0.55%
2	New York	3,400	7.74%
10	North Carolina	1,200	2.73%
46	North Dakota	120	0.27%
7	Ohio	2,100	4.78%
29	Oklahoma	480	1.09%
28	Oregon	490	1.12%
5	Pennsylvania	2,700	6.15%
40	Rhode Island	200	0.46%
25	South Carolina	620	1.41%
44	South Dakota	140	0.32%
15	Tennessee	910	2.07%
4	Texas	2,800	6.38%
40	Utah	200	0.46%
48	Vermont	80	0.18%
11	Virginia	1,100	2.51%
17	Washington	850	1.94%
34	West Virginia	320	0.73%
16	Wisconsin	890	2.03%
48	Wyoming	80	0.18%

RANK ORDER

RANK	STATE	DEATHS	% of USA
1	California	4,200	9.57%
2	New York	3,400	7.74%
3	Florida	2,900	6.61%
4	Texas	2,800	6.38%
5	Pennsylvania	2,700	6.15%
6	Illinois	2,200	5.01%
7	Ohio	2,100	4.78%
8	New Jersey	1,600	3.64%
9	Michigan	1,500	3.42%
10	North Carolina	1,200	2.73%
11	Massachusetts	1,100	2.51%
11	Virginia	1,100	2.51%
13	Indiana	960	2.19%
14	Georgia	950	2.16%
15	Tennessee	910	2.07%
16	Wisconsin	890	2.03%
17	Washington	850	1.94%
18	Maryland	840	1.91%
18	Missouri	840	1.91%
20	Louisiana	760	1.73%
21	Minnesota	720	1.64%
22	Alabama	670	1.53%
22	Arizona	670	1.53%
24	Kentucky	650	1.48%
25	South Carolina	620	1.41%
26	Iowa	590	1.34%
27	Colorado	520	1.18%
28	Oregon	490	1.12%
29	Connecticut	480	1.09%
29	Oklahoma	480	1.09%
31	Arkansas	470	1.07%
32	Mississippi	430	0.98%
33	Kansas	380	0.87%
34	West Virginia	320	0.73%
35	Nebraska	270	0.62%
36	Nevada	260	0.59%
37	Maine	240	0.55%
37	New Mexico	240	0.55%
39	New Hampshire	230	0.52%
40	Rhode Island	200	0.46%
40	Utah	200	0.46%
42	Idaho	170	0.39%
43	Montana	150	0.34%
44	Delaware	140	0.32%
44	South Dakota	140	0.32%
46	North Dakota	120	0.27%
47	Hawaii	110	0.25%
48	Vermont	80	0.18%
48	Wyoming	80	0.18%
50	Alaska	60	0.14%
	District of Columbia	130	0.30%

Source: American Cancer Society (http://www.cancer.org/97tabp6.html)
"Cancer Facts & Figures-1997" (Copyright 1997, Reprinted with permission from the American Cancer Society)

Estimated Death Rate by Female Breast Cancer in 1997

National Estimated Rate = 32.7 Deaths per 100,000 Female Population*

ALPHA ORDER

RANK	STATE	RATE
37	Alabama	30.3
48	Alaska	20.9
30	Arizona	31.4
11	Arkansas	36.6
46	California	26.6
44	Colorado	27.5
42	Connecticut	28.5
7	Delaware	38.0
3	Florida	39.7
47	Georgia	25.7
50	Hawaii	18.7
39	Idaho	29.2
13	Illinois	36.3
29	Indiana	32.2
2	Iowa	40.4
40	Kansas	29.1
23	Kentucky	32.7
20	Louisiana	33.7
9	Maine	37.7
26	Maryland	32.4
15	Massachusetts	34.9
34	Michigan	30.6
32	Minnesota	30.8
34	Mississippi	30.6
36	Missouri	30.5
17	Montana	34.3
28	Nebraska	32.3
16	Nevada	34.6
4	New Hampshire	39.4
5	New Jersey	39.0
43	New Mexico	28.1
14	New York	36.1
26	North Carolina	32.4
10	North Dakota	37.3
12	Ohio	36.4
41	Oklahoma	28.6
32	Oregon	30.8
1	Pennsylvania	43.1
6	Rhode Island	38.9
24	South Carolina	32.6
8	South Dakota	37.9
21	Tennessee	33.5
38	Texas	29.5
49	Utah	20.4
45	Vermont	26.9
25	Virginia	32.5
31	Washington	31.1
19	West Virginia	33.8
18	Wisconsin	34.1
21	Wyoming	33.5

RANK ORDER

RANK	STATE	RATE
1	Pennsylvania	43.1
2	Iowa	40.4
3	Florida	39.7
4	New Hampshire	39.4
5	New Jersey	39.0
6	Rhode Island	38.9
7	Delaware	38.0
8	South Dakota	37.9
9	Maine	37.7
10	North Dakota	37.3
11	Arkansas	36.6
12	Ohio	36.4
13	Illinois	36.3
14	New York	36.1
15	Massachusetts	34.9
16	Nevada	34.6
17	Montana	34.3
18	Wisconsin	34.1
19	West Virginia	33.8
20	Louisiana	33.7
21	Tennessee	33.5
21	Wyoming	33.5
23	Kentucky	32.7
24	South Carolina	32.6
25	Virginia	32.5
26	Maryland	32.4
26	North Carolina	32.4
28	Nebraska	32.3
29	Indiana	32.2
30	Arizona	31.4
31	Washington	31.1
32	Minnesota	30.8
32	Oregon	30.8
34	Michigan	30.6
34	Mississippi	30.6
36	Missouri	30.5
37	Alabama	30.3
38	Texas	29.5
39	Idaho	29.2
40	Kansas	29.1
41	Oklahoma	28.6
42	Connecticut	28.5
43	New Mexico	28.1
44	Colorado	27.5
45	Vermont	26.9
46	California	26.6
47	Georgia	25.7
48	Alaska	20.9
49	Utah	20.4
50	Hawaii	18.7

District of Columbia   44.1

Source: Morgan Quitno Press using data from American Cancer Society (http://www.cancer.org/97tabp6.html)
"Cancer Facts & Figures-1997" (Copyright 1997, Reprinted with permission from the American Cancer Society)
*Rates calculated using 1995 Census resident female population estimates. Not age adjusted.

Estimated Deaths by Colon and Rectum Cancer in 1997

National Estimated Total = 54,900 Deaths

ALPHA ORDER

RANK	STATE	DEATHS	% of USA
28	Alabama	660	1.20%
50	Alaska	50	0.09%
23	Arizona	810	1.48%
29	Arkansas	610	1.11%
1	California	4,700	8.56%
30	Colorado	590	1.07%
26	Connecticut	690	1.26%
47	Delaware	140	0.26%
3	Florida	3,700	6.74%
16	Georgia	1,100	2.00%
41	Hawaii	220	0.40%
43	Idaho	190	0.35%
6	Illinois	2,700	4.92%
12	Indiana	1,300	2.37%
25	Iowa	770	1.40%
32	Kansas	550	1.00%
19	Kentucky	940	1.71%
21	Louisiana	920	1.68%
36	Maine	310	0.56%
16	Maryland	1,100	2.00%
10	Massachusetts	1,600	2.91%
8	Michigan	2,100	3.83%
22	Minnesota	860	1.57%
33	Mississippi	510	0.93%
12	Missouri	1,300	2.37%
43	Montana	190	0.35%
35	Nebraska	380	0.69%
36	Nevada	310	0.56%
39	New Hampshire	240	0.44%
9	New Jersey	1,900	3.46%
41	New Mexico	220	0.40%
2	New York	3,900	7.10%
11	North Carolina	1,500	2.73%
46	North Dakota	150	0.27%
7	Ohio	2,600	4.74%
27	Oklahoma	680	1.24%
30	Oregon	590	1.07%
5	Pennsylvania	3,300	6.01%
38	Rhode Island	280	0.51%
24	South Carolina	800	1.46%
45	South Dakota	160	0.29%
15	Tennessee	1,200	2.19%
4	Texas	3,600	6.56%
40	Utah	230	0.42%
48	Vermont	100	0.18%
12	Virginia	1,300	2.37%
20	Washington	930	1.69%
34	West Virginia	490	0.89%
18	Wisconsin	1,000	1.82%
49	Wyoming	70	0.13%

RANK ORDER

RANK	STATE	DEATHS	% of USA
1	California	4,700	8.56%
2	New York	3,900	7.10%
3	Florida	3,700	6.74%
4	Texas	3,600	6.56%
5	Pennsylvania	3,300	6.01%
6	Illinois	2,700	4.92%
7	Ohio	2,600	4.74%
8	Michigan	2,100	3.83%
9	New Jersey	1,900	3.46%
10	Massachusetts	1,600	2.91%
11	North Carolina	1,500	2.73%
12	Indiana	1,300	2.37%
12	Missouri	1,300	2.37%
12	Virginia	1,300	2.37%
15	Tennessee	1,200	2.19%
16	Georgia	1,100	2.00%
16	Maryland	1,100	2.00%
18	Wisconsin	1,000	1.82%
19	Kentucky	940	1.71%
20	Washington	930	1.69%
21	Louisiana	920	1.68%
22	Minnesota	860	1.57%
23	Arizona	810	1.48%
24	South Carolina	800	1.46%
25	Iowa	770	1.40%
26	Connecticut	690	1.26%
27	Oklahoma	680	1.24%
28	Alabama	660	1.20%
29	Arkansas	610	1.11%
30	Colorado	590	1.07%
30	Oregon	590	1.07%
32	Kansas	550	1.00%
33	Mississippi	510	0.93%
34	West Virginia	490	0.89%
35	Nebraska	380	0.69%
36	Maine	310	0.56%
36	Nevada	310	0.56%
38	Rhode Island	280	0.51%
39	New Hampshire	240	0.44%
40	Utah	230	0.42%
41	Hawaii	220	0.40%
41	New Mexico	220	0.40%
43	Idaho	190	0.35%
43	Montana	190	0.35%
45	South Dakota	160	0.29%
46	North Dakota	150	0.27%
47	Delaware	140	0.26%
48	Vermont	100	0.18%
49	Wyoming	70	0.13%
50	Alaska	50	0.09%
	District of Columbia	130	0.24%

Source: American Cancer Society (http://www.cancer.org/97tabp6.html)
"Cancer Facts & Figures-1997" (Copyright 1997, Reprinted with permission from the American Cancer Society)

Estimated Death Rate by Colon and Rectum Cancer in 1997

National Estimated Rate = 20.7 Deaths per 100,000 Population*

RANK	STATE	RATE
43	Alabama	15.4
50	Alaska	8.2
39	Arizona	18.3
8	Arkansas	24.3
46	California	14.7
43	Colorado	15.4
25	Connecticut	21.1
32	Delaware	19.3
6	Florida	25.7
45	Georgia	15.0
36	Hawaii	18.6
42	Idaho	16.0
15	Illinois	22.8
17	Indiana	22.3
3	Iowa	27.0
23	Kansas	21.4
10	Kentucky	24.2
25	Louisiana	21.1
7	Maine	24.9
20	Maryland	21.7
5	Massachusetts	26.3
18	Michigan	21.9
37	Minnesota	18.5
34	Mississippi	18.8
8	Missouri	24.3
21	Montana	21.6
14	Nebraska	23.0
32	Nevada	19.3
27	New Hampshire	20.7
11	New Jersey	23.8
48	New Mexico	12.8
23	New York	21.4
29	North Carolina	20.5
12	North Dakota	23.3
12	Ohio	23.3
28	Oklahoma	20.6
38	Oregon	18.4
2	Pennsylvania	27.4
1	Rhode Island	28.3
21	South Carolina	21.6
18	South Dakota	21.9
16	Tennessee	22.6
34	Texas	18.8
49	Utah	11.5
40	Vermont	17.0
30	Virginia	19.5
41	Washington	16.8
4	West Virginia	26.8
31	Wisconsin	19.4
47	Wyoming	14.6

RANK	STATE	RATE
1	Rhode Island	28.3
2	Pennsylvania	27.4
3	Iowa	27.0
4	West Virginia	26.8
5	Massachusetts	26.3
6	Florida	25.7
7	Maine	24.9
8	Arkansas	24.3
8	Missouri	24.3
10	Kentucky	24.2
11	New Jersey	23.8
12	North Dakota	23.3
12	Ohio	23.3
14	Nebraska	23.0
15	Illinois	22.8
16	Tennessee	22.6
17	Indiana	22.3
18	Michigan	21.9
18	South Dakota	21.9
20	Maryland	21.7
21	Montana	21.6
21	South Carolina	21.6
23	Kansas	21.4
23	New York	21.4
25	Connecticut	21.1
25	Louisiana	21.1
27	New Hampshire	20.7
28	Oklahoma	20.6
29	North Carolina	20.5
30	Virginia	19.5
31	Wisconsin	19.4
32	Delaware	19.3
32	Nevada	19.3
34	Mississippi	18.8
34	Texas	18.8
36	Hawaii	18.6
37	Minnesota	18.5
38	Oregon	18.4
39	Arizona	18.3
40	Vermont	17.0
41	Washington	16.8
42	Idaho	16.0
43	Alabama	15.4
43	Colorado	15.4
45	Georgia	15.0
46	California	14.7
47	Wyoming	14.6
48	New Mexico	12.8
49	Utah	11.5
50	Alaska	8.2

| | District of Columbia | 23.9 |

Source: Morgan Quitno Press using data from American Cancer Society (http://www.cancer.org/97tabp6.html)
"Cancer Facts & Figures-1997" (Copyright 1997, Reprinted with permission from the American Cancer Society)
*Rates calculated using 1996 Census resident population estimates. Not age adjusted.

Estimated Deaths by Leukemia in 1996

National Estimated Total = 21,000 Deaths

ALPHA ORDER

RANK	STATE	DEATHS	% of USA
20	Alabama	380	1.81%
50	Alaska	10	0.05%
18	Arizona	420	2.00%
33	Arkansas	210	1.00%
1	California	2,100	10.00%
28	Colorado	250	1.19%
26	Connecticut	280	1.33%
46	Delaware	50	0.24%
2	Florida	1,400	6.67%
13	Georgia	480	2.29%
46	Hawaii	50	0.24%
40	Idaho	80	0.38%
6	Illinois	1,100	5.24%
13	Indiana	480	2.29%
25	Iowa	300	1.43%
30	Kansas	240	1.14%
23	Kentucky	340	1.62%
20	Louisiana	380	1.81%
35	Maine	120	0.57%
24	Maryland	330	1.57%
11	Massachusetts	520	2.48%
8	Michigan	800	3.81%
16	Minnesota	450	2.14%
32	Mississippi	220	1.05%
12	Missouri	500	2.38%
40	Montana	80	0.38%
38	Nebraska	100	0.48%
35	Nevada	120	0.57%
44	New Hampshire	60	0.29%
9	New Jersey	680	3.24%
35	New Mexico	120	0.57%
3	New York	1,300	6.19%
10	North Carolina	530	2.52%
44	North Dakota	60	0.29%
7	Ohio	920	4.38%
28	Oklahoma	250	1.19%
27	Oregon	270	1.29%
5	Pennsylvania	1,200	5.71%
39	Rhode Island	90	0.43%
31	South Carolina	230	1.10%
43	South Dakota	70	0.33%
20	Tennessee	380	1.81%
3	Texas	1,300	6.19%
40	Utah	80	0.38%
48	Vermont	40	0.19%
15	Virginia	460	2.19%
16	Washington	450	2.14%
34	West Virginia	170	0.81%
19	Wisconsin	400	1.90%
48	Wyoming	40	0.19%

RANK ORDER

RANK	STATE	DEATHS	% of USA
1	California	2,100	10.00%
2	Florida	1,400	6.67%
3	New York	1,300	6.19%
3	Texas	1,300	6.19%
5	Pennsylvania	1,200	5.71%
6	Illinois	1,100	5.24%
7	Ohio	920	4.38%
8	Michigan	800	3.81%
9	New Jersey	680	3.24%
10	North Carolina	530	2.52%
11	Massachusetts	520	2.48%
12	Missouri	500	2.38%
13	Georgia	480	2.29%
13	Indiana	480	2.29%
15	Virginia	460	2.19%
16	Minnesota	450	2.14%
16	Washington	450	2.14%
18	Arizona	420	2.00%
19	Wisconsin	400	1.90%
20	Alabama	380	1.81%
20	Louisiana	380	1.81%
20	Tennessee	380	1.81%
23	Kentucky	340	1.62%
24	Maryland	330	1.57%
25	Iowa	300	1.43%
26	Connecticut	280	1.33%
27	Oregon	270	1.29%
28	Colorado	250	1.19%
28	Oklahoma	250	1.19%
30	Kansas	240	1.14%
31	South Carolina	230	1.10%
32	Mississippi	220	1.05%
33	Arkansas	210	1.00%
34	West Virginia	170	0.81%
35	Maine	120	0.57%
35	Nevada	120	0.57%
35	New Mexico	120	0.57%
38	Nebraska	100	0.48%
39	Rhode Island	90	0.43%
40	Idaho	80	0.38%
40	Montana	80	0.38%
40	Utah	80	0.38%
43	South Dakota	70	0.33%
44	New Hampshire	60	0.29%
44	North Dakota	60	0.29%
46	Delaware	50	0.24%
46	Hawaii	50	0.24%
48	Vermont	40	0.19%
48	Wyoming	40	0.19%
50	Alaska	10	0.05%
	District of Columbia	60	0.29%

Source: American Cancer Society
"Cancer Facts & Figures-1996" (Copyright 1996, Reprinted with permission from the American Cancer Society)

Estimated Death Rate by Leukemia in 1996

National Estimated Rate = 8.0 Deaths per 100,000 Population*

RANK	STATE	RATE
15	Alabama	8.9
50	Alaska	1.7
2	Arizona	10.0
21	Arkansas	8.5
43	California	6.6
41	Colorado	6.7
21	Connecticut	8.5
36	Delaware	7.0
3	Florida	9.9
41	Georgia	6.7
48	Hawaii	4.2
38	Idaho	6.9
11	Illinois	9.3
24	Indiana	8.3
1	Iowa	10.6
8	Kansas	9.4
16	Kentucky	8.8
16	Louisiana	8.8
6	Maine	9.7
44	Maryland	6.5
18	Massachusetts	8.6
23	Michigan	8.4
5	Minnesota	9.8
28	Mississippi	8.2
8	Missouri	9.4
13	Montana	9.2
46	Nebraska	6.1
29	Nevada	7.8
47	New Hampshire	5.2
18	New Jersey	8.6
35	New Mexico	7.1
33	New York	7.2
32	North Carolina	7.4
8	North Dakota	9.4
24	Ohio	8.3
31	Oklahoma	7.6
18	Oregon	8.6
3	Pennsylvania	9.9
14	Rhode Island	9.1
45	South Carolina	6.3
7	South Dakota	9.6
33	Tennessee	7.2
38	Texas	6.9
49	Utah	4.1
40	Vermont	6.8
36	Virginia	7.0
24	Washington	8.3
11	West Virginia	9.3
29	Wisconsin	7.8
24	Wyoming	8.3

RANK	STATE	RATE
1	Iowa	10.6
2	Arizona	10.0
3	Florida	9.9
3	Pennsylvania	9.9
5	Minnesota	9.8
6	Maine	9.7
7	South Dakota	9.6
8	Kansas	9.4
8	Missouri	9.4
8	North Dakota	9.4
11	Illinois	9.3
11	West Virginia	9.3
13	Montana	9.2
14	Rhode Island	9.1
15	Alabama	8.9
16	Kentucky	8.8
16	Louisiana	8.8
18	Massachusetts	8.6
18	New Jersey	8.6
18	Oregon	8.6
21	Arkansas	8.5
21	Connecticut	8.5
23	Michigan	8.4
24	Indiana	8.3
24	Ohio	8.3
24	Washington	8.3
24	Wyoming	8.3
28	Mississippi	8.2
29	Nevada	7.8
29	Wisconsin	7.8
31	Oklahoma	7.6
32	North Carolina	7.4
33	New York	7.2
33	Tennessee	7.2
35	New Mexico	7.1
36	Delaware	7.0
36	Virginia	7.0
38	Idaho	6.9
38	Texas	6.9
40	Vermont	6.8
41	Colorado	6.7
41	Georgia	6.7
43	California	6.6
44	Maryland	6.5
45	South Carolina	6.3
46	Nebraska	6.1
47	New Hampshire	5.2
48	Hawaii	4.2
49	Utah	4.1
50	Alaska	1.7
	District of Columbia	10.8

Source: Morgan Quitno Press using data from American Cancer Society
"Cancer Facts & Figures-1996" (Copyright 1996, Reprinted with permission from the American Cancer Society)
Rates calculated using 1995 Census resident population estimates. Not age adjusted.

Estimated Deaths by Lung Cancer in 1997

National Estimated Total = 160,400 Deaths

<u>ALPHA ORDER</u>

RANK	STATE	DEATHS	% of USA
21	Alabama	2,800	1.75%
50	Alaska	190	0.12%
23	Arizona	2,600	1.62%
26	Arkansas	2,200	1.37%
1	California	13,800	8.60%
33	Colorado	1,500	0.94%
29	Connecticut	1,800	1.12%
41	Delaware	540	0.34%
2	Florida	12,100	7.54%
13	Georgia	3,900	2.43%
44	Hawaii	490	0.31%
42	Idaho	510	0.32%
7	Illinois	7,100	4.43%
12	Indiana	4,000	2.49%
29	Iowa	1,800	1.12%
33	Kansas	1,500	0.94%
17	Kentucky	3,300	2.06%
19	Louisiana	3,000	1.87%
36	Maine	1,000	0.62%
19	Maryland	3,000	1.87%
14	Massachusetts	3,800	2.37%
8	Michigan	6,100	3.80%
26	Minnesota	2,200	1.37%
31	Mississippi	1,700	1.06%
11	Missouri	4,100	2.56%
42	Montana	510	0.32%
37	Nebraska	890	0.55%
35	Nevada	1,100	0.69%
38	New Hampshire	720	0.45%
10	New Jersey	4,700	2.93%
40	New Mexico	660	0.41%
4	New York	10,200	6.36%
9	North Carolina	4,800	2.99%
48	North Dakota	310	0.19%
6	Ohio	7,700	4.80%
25	Oklahoma	2,300	1.43%
26	Oregon	2,200	1.37%
5	Pennsylvania	8,500	5.30%
39	Rhode Island	710	0.44%
24	South Carolina	2,400	1.50%
46	South Dakota	400	0.25%
14	Tennessee	3,800	2.37%
3	Texas	10,800	6.73%
45	Utah	460	0.29%
47	Vermont	360	0.22%
16	Virginia	3,700	2.31%
18	Washington	3,200	2.00%
32	West Virginia	1,600	1.00%
22	Wisconsin	2,700	1.68%
49	Wyoming	240	0.15%

<u>RANK ORDER</u>

RANK	STATE	DEATHS	% of USA
1	California	13,800	8.60%
2	Florida	12,100	7.54%
3	Texas	10,800	6.73%
4	New York	10,200	6.36%
5	Pennsylvania	8,500	5.30%
6	Ohio	7,700	4.80%
7	Illinois	7,100	4.43%
8	Michigan	6,100	3.80%
9	North Carolina	4,800	2.99%
10	New Jersey	4,700	2.93%
11	Missouri	4,100	2.56%
12	Indiana	4,000	2.49%
13	Georgia	3,900	2.43%
14	Massachusetts	3,800	2.37%
14	Tennessee	3,800	2.37%
16	Virginia	3,700	2.31%
17	Kentucky	3,300	2.06%
18	Washington	3,200	2.00%
19	Louisiana	3,000	1.87%
19	Maryland	3,000	1.87%
21	Alabama	2,800	1.75%
22	Wisconsin	2,700	1.68%
23	Arizona	2,600	1.62%
24	South Carolina	2,400	1.50%
25	Oklahoma	2,300	1.43%
26	Arkansas	2,200	1.37%
26	Minnesota	2,200	1.37%
26	Oregon	2,200	1.37%
29	Connecticut	1,800	1.12%
29	Iowa	1,800	1.12%
31	Mississippi	1,700	1.06%
32	West Virginia	1,600	1.00%
33	Colorado	1,500	0.94%
33	Kansas	1,500	0.94%
35	Nevada	1,100	0.69%
36	Maine	1,000	0.62%
37	Nebraska	890	0.55%
38	New Hampshire	720	0.45%
39	Rhode Island	710	0.44%
40	New Mexico	660	0.41%
41	Delaware	540	0.34%
42	Idaho	510	0.32%
42	Montana	510	0.32%
44	Hawaii	490	0.31%
45	Utah	460	0.29%
46	South Dakota	400	0.25%
47	Vermont	360	0.22%
48	North Dakota	310	0.19%
49	Wyoming	240	0.15%
50	Alaska	190	0.12%
	District of Columbia	330	0.21%

Source: American Cancer Society (http://www.cancer.org/97tabp6.html)
"Cancer Facts & Figures-1997" (Copyright 1997, Reprinted with permission from the American Cancer Society)

Estimated Death Rate by Lung Cancer in 1997

National Estimated Rate = 60.5 Deaths per 100,000 Population*

ALPHA ORDER

RANK	STATE	RATE
17	Alabama	65.5
49	Alaska	31.3
29	Arizona	58.7
1	Arkansas	87.6
44	California	43.3
47	Colorado	39.2
36	Connecticut	55.0
7	Delaware	74.5
4	Florida	84.0
39	Georgia	53.0
46	Hawaii	41.4
45	Idaho	42.9
26	Illinois	59.9
16	Indiana	68.5
21	Iowa	63.1
30	Kansas	58.3
3	Kentucky	85.0
12	Louisiana	68.9
5	Maine	80.5
27	Maryland	59.1
23	Massachusetts	62.4
20	Michigan	63.6
43	Minnesota	47.2
22	Mississippi	62.6
6	Missouri	76.5
31	Montana	58.0
38	Nebraska	53.9
15	Nevada	68.6
24	New Hampshire	62.0
28	New Jersey	58.8
48	New Mexico	38.5
34	New York	56.1
17	North Carolina	65.5
42	North Dakota	48.1
12	Ohio	68.9
11	Oklahoma	69.7
14	Oregon	68.7
10	Pennsylvania	70.5
8	Rhode Island	71.7
19	South Carolina	64.9
37	South Dakota	54.6
9	Tennessee	71.4
33	Texas	56.5
50	Utah	23.0
25	Vermont	61.1
35	Virginia	55.4
32	Washington	57.8
1	West Virginia	87.6
40	Wisconsin	52.3
41	Wyoming	49.9

RANK ORDER

RANK	STATE	RATE
1	Arkansas	87.6
1	West Virginia	87.6
3	Kentucky	85.0
4	Florida	84.0
5	Maine	80.5
6	Missouri	76.5
7	Delaware	74.5
8	Rhode Island	71.7
9	Tennessee	71.4
10	Pennsylvania	70.5
11	Oklahoma	69.7
12	Louisiana	68.9
12	Ohio	68.9
14	Oregon	68.7
15	Nevada	68.6
16	Indiana	68.5
17	Alabama	65.5
17	North Carolina	65.5
19	South Carolina	64.9
20	Michigan	63.6
21	Iowa	63.1
22	Mississippi	62.6
23	Massachusetts	62.4
24	New Hampshire	62.0
25	Vermont	61.1
26	Illinois	59.9
27	Maryland	59.1
28	New Jersey	58.8
29	Arizona	58.7
30	Kansas	58.3
31	Montana	58.0
32	Washington	57.8
33	Texas	56.5
34	New York	56.1
35	Virginia	55.4
36	Connecticut	55.0
37	South Dakota	54.6
38	Nebraska	53.9
39	Georgia	53.0
40	Wisconsin	52.3
41	Wyoming	49.9
42	North Dakota	48.1
43	Minnesota	47.2
44	California	43.3
45	Idaho	42.9
46	Hawaii	41.4
47	Colorado	39.2
48	New Mexico	38.5
49	Alaska	31.3
50	Utah	23.0

| | District of Columbia | 60.8 |

Source: Morgan Quitno Press using data from American Cancer Society (http://www.cancer.org/97tabp6.html)
"Cancer Facts & Figures-1997" (Copyright 1997, Reprinted with permission from the American Cancer Society)
*Rates calculated using 1996 Census resident population estimates. Not age adjusted.

Estimated Deaths by Non-Hodgkin's Lymphoma in 1997

National Estimated Total = 23,800 Deaths

ALPHA ORDER

RANK	STATE	DEATHS	% of USA
21	Alabama	380	1.60%
50	Alaska	10	0.04%
19	Arizona	390	1.64%
29	Arkansas	270	1.13%
1	California	2,200	9.24%
30	Colorado	260	1.09%
26	Connecticut	320	1.34%
46	Delaware	80	0.34%
3	Florida	1,700	7.14%
19	Georgia	390	1.64%
42	Hawaii	100	0.42%
43	Idaho	90	0.38%
6	Illinois	1,100	4.62%
16	Indiana	490	2.06%
24	Iowa	350	1.47%
32	Kansas	250	1.05%
24	Kentucky	350	1.47%
26	Louisiana	320	1.34%
36	Maine	150	0.63%
21	Maryland	380	1.60%
10	Massachusetts	650	2.73%
8	Michigan	860	3.61%
14	Minnesota	530	2.23%
33	Mississippi	200	0.84%
12	Missouri	550	2.31%
43	Montana	90	0.38%
34	Nebraska	170	0.71%
37	Nevada	140	0.59%
40	New Hampshire	120	0.50%
9	New Jersey	760	3.19%
40	New Mexico	120	0.50%
2	New York	1,800	7.56%
11	North Carolina	640	2.69%
43	North Dakota	90	0.38%
6	Ohio	1,100	4.62%
23	Oklahoma	360	1.51%
28	Oregon	310	1.30%
5	Pennsylvania	1,400	5.88%
39	Rhode Island	130	0.55%
30	South Carolina	260	1.09%
47	South Dakota	50	0.21%
17	Tennessee	480	2.02%
4	Texas	1,600	6.72%
37	Utah	140	0.59%
47	Vermont	50	0.21%
15	Virginia	520	2.18%
18	Washington	450	1.89%
34	West Virginia	170	0.71%
13	Wisconsin	540	2.27%
49	Wyoming	30	0.13%

RANK ORDER

RANK	STATE	DEATHS	% of USA
1	California	2,200	9.24%
2	New York	1,800	7.56%
3	Florida	1,700	7.14%
4	Texas	1,600	6.72%
5	Pennsylvania	1,400	5.88%
6	Illinois	1,100	4.62%
6	Ohio	1,100	4.62%
8	Michigan	860	3.61%
9	New Jersey	760	3.19%
10	Massachusetts	650	2.73%
11	North Carolina	640	2.69%
12	Missouri	550	2.31%
13	Wisconsin	540	2.27%
14	Minnesota	530	2.23%
15	Virginia	520	2.18%
16	Indiana	490	2.06%
17	Tennessee	480	2.02%
18	Washington	450	1.89%
19	Arizona	390	1.64%
19	Georgia	390	1.64%
21	Alabama	380	1.60%
21	Maryland	380	1.60%
23	Oklahoma	360	1.51%
24	Iowa	350	1.47%
24	Kentucky	350	1.47%
26	Connecticut	320	1.34%
26	Louisiana	320	1.34%
28	Oregon	310	1.30%
29	Arkansas	270	1.13%
30	Colorado	260	1.09%
30	South Carolina	260	1.09%
32	Kansas	250	1.05%
33	Mississippi	200	0.84%
34	Nebraska	170	0.71%
34	West Virginia	170	0.71%
36	Maine	150	0.63%
37	Nevada	140	0.59%
37	Utah	140	0.59%
39	Rhode Island	130	0.55%
40	New Hampshire	120	0.50%
40	New Mexico	120	0.50%
42	Hawaii	100	0.42%
43	Idaho	90	0.38%
43	Montana	90	0.38%
43	North Dakota	90	0.38%
46	Delaware	80	0.34%
47	South Dakota	50	0.21%
47	Vermont	50	0.21%
49	Wyoming	30	0.13%
50	Alaska	10	0.04%
	District of Columbia	50	0.21%

Source: American Cancer Society (http://www.cancer.org/97tabp6.html)
"Cancer Facts & Figures-1997" (Copyright 1997, Reprinted with permission from the American Cancer Society)

Estimated Death Rate by Non-Hodgkin's Lymphoma in 1997

National Estimated Rate = 9.0 Deaths per 100,000 Population*

ALPHA ORDER

RANK	STATE	RATE
28	Alabama	8.9
50	Alaska	1.6
29	Arizona	8.8
10	Arkansas	10.8
45	California	6.9
46	Colorado	6.8
18	Connecticut	9.8
8	Delaware	11.0
5	Florida	11.8
49	Georgia	5.3
33	Hawaii	8.4
38	Idaho	7.6
23	Illinois	9.3
33	Indiana	8.4
3	Iowa	12.3
20	Kansas	9.7
25	Kentucky	9.0
40	Louisiana	7.4
4	Maine	12.1
39	Maryland	7.5
11	Massachusetts	10.7
25	Michigan	9.0
7	Minnesota	11.4
40	Mississippi	7.4
13	Missouri	10.3
16	Montana	10.2
13	Nebraska	10.3
30	Nevada	8.7
13	New Hampshire	10.3
22	New Jersey	9.5
42	New Mexico	7.0
17	New York	9.9
30	North Carolina	8.7
1	North Dakota	14.0
18	Ohio	9.8
9	Oklahoma	10.9
20	Oregon	9.7
6	Pennsylvania	11.6
2	Rhode Island	13.1
42	South Carolina	7.0
46	South Dakota	6.8
25	Tennessee	9.0
33	Texas	8.4
42	Utah	7.0
32	Vermont	8.5
37	Virginia	7.8
36	Washington	8.1
23	West Virginia	9.3
12	Wisconsin	10.5
48	Wyoming	6.2

RANK ORDER

RANK	STATE	RATE
1	North Dakota	14.0
2	Rhode Island	13.1
3	Iowa	12.3
4	Maine	12.1
5	Florida	11.8
6	Pennsylvania	11.6
7	Minnesota	11.4
8	Delaware	11.0
9	Oklahoma	10.9
10	Arkansas	10.8
11	Massachusetts	10.7
12	Wisconsin	10.5
13	Missouri	10.3
13	Nebraska	10.3
13	New Hampshire	10.3
16	Montana	10.2
17	New York	9.9
18	Connecticut	9.8
18	Ohio	9.8
20	Kansas	9.7
20	Oregon	9.7
22	New Jersey	9.5
23	Illinois	9.3
23	West Virginia	9.3
25	Kentucky	9.0
25	Michigan	9.0
25	Tennessee	9.0
28	Alabama	8.9
29	Arizona	8.8
30	Nevada	8.7
30	North Carolina	8.7
32	Vermont	8.5
33	Hawaii	8.4
33	Indiana	8.4
33	Texas	8.4
36	Washington	8.1
37	Virginia	7.8
38	Idaho	7.6
39	Maryland	7.5
40	Louisiana	7.4
40	Mississippi	7.4
42	New Mexico	7.0
42	South Carolina	7.0
42	Utah	7.0
45	California	6.9
46	Colorado	6.8
46	South Dakota	6.8
48	Wyoming	6.2
49	Georgia	5.3
50	Alaska	1.6

District of Columbia   9.2

*Source: Morgan Quitno Press using data from American Cancer Society (http://www.cancer.org/97tabp6.html)
"Cancer Facts & Figures-1997" (Copyright 1997, Reprinted with permission from the American Cancer Society)
Rates calculated using 1996 Census resident population estimates. Not age adjusted.

Estimated Deaths by Pancreatic Cancer in 1997

National Estimated Total = 28,100 Deaths

ALPHA ORDER

RANK	STATE	DEATHS	% of USA
23	Alabama	420	1.49%
50	Alaska	20	0.07%
22	Arizona	450	1.60%
32	Arkansas	280	1.00%
1	California	2,600	9.25%
27	Colorado	360	1.28%
26	Connecticut	370	1.32%
45	Delaware	80	0.28%
2	Florida	2,100	7.47%
13	Georgia	690	2.46%
39	Hawaii	130	0.46%
46	Idaho	70	0.25%
6	Illinois	1,200	4.27%
13	Indiana	690	2.46%
32	Iowa	280	1.00%
31	Kansas	290	1.03%
21	Kentucky	460	1.64%
18	Louisiana	530	1.89%
36	Maine	160	0.57%
20	Maryland	480	1.71%
12	Massachusetts	700	2.49%
8	Michigan	1,000	3.56%
23	Minnesota	420	1.49%
30	Mississippi	300	1.07%
17	Missouri	570	2.03%
42	Montana	100	0.36%
35	Nebraska	170	0.60%
36	Nevada	160	0.57%
39	New Hampshire	130	0.46%
9	New Jersey	940	3.35%
38	New Mexico	140	0.50%
2	New York	2,100	7.47%
10	North Carolina	760	2.70%
46	North Dakota	70	0.25%
6	Ohio	1,200	4.27%
29	Oklahoma	340	1.21%
25	Oregon	380	1.35%
5	Pennsylvania	1,500	5.34%
43	Rhode Island	90	0.32%
27	South Carolina	360	1.28%
43	South Dakota	90	0.32%
16	Tennessee	580	2.06%
4	Texas	1,900	6.76%
41	Utah	110	0.39%
48	Vermont	50	0.18%
11	Virginia	720	2.56%
19	Washington	520	1.85%
34	West Virginia	200	0.71%
15	Wisconsin	590	2.10%
49	Wyoming	40	0.14%

RANK ORDER

RANK	STATE	DEATHS	% of USA
1	California	2,600	9.25%
2	Florida	2,100	7.47%
2	New York	2,100	7.47%
4	Texas	1,900	6.76%
5	Pennsylvania	1,500	5.34%
6	Illinois	1,200	4.27%
6	Ohio	1,200	4.27%
8	Michigan	1,000	3.56%
9	New Jersey	940	3.35%
10	North Carolina	760	2.70%
11	Virginia	720	2.56%
12	Massachusetts	700	2.49%
13	Georgia	690	2.46%
13	Indiana	690	2.46%
15	Wisconsin	590	2.10%
16	Tennessee	580	2.06%
17	Missouri	570	2.03%
18	Louisiana	530	1.89%
19	Washington	520	1.85%
20	Maryland	480	1.71%
21	Kentucky	460	1.64%
22	Arizona	450	1.60%
23	Alabama	420	1.49%
23	Minnesota	420	1.49%
25	Oregon	380	1.35%
26	Connecticut	370	1.32%
27	Colorado	360	1.28%
27	South Carolina	360	1.28%
29	Oklahoma	340	1.21%
30	Mississippi	300	1.07%
31	Kansas	290	1.03%
32	Arkansas	280	1.00%
32	Iowa	280	1.00%
34	West Virginia	200	0.71%
35	Nebraska	170	0.60%
36	Maine	160	0.57%
36	Nevada	160	0.57%
38	New Mexico	140	0.50%
39	Hawaii	130	0.46%
39	New Hampshire	130	0.46%
41	Utah	110	0.39%
42	Montana	100	0.36%
43	Rhode Island	90	0.32%
43	South Dakota	90	0.32%
45	Delaware	80	0.28%
46	Idaho	70	0.25%
46	North Dakota	70	0.25%
48	Vermont	50	0.18%
49	Wyoming	40	0.14%
50	Alaska	20	0.07%
	District of Columbia	100	0.36%

Source: American Cancer Society (http://www.cancer.org/97tabp6.html)
"Cancer Facts & Figures-1997" (Copyright 1997, Reprinted with permission from the American Cancer Society)

Estimated Death Rate by Pancreatic Cancer in 1997

National Estimated Rate = 10.6 Deaths per 100,000 Population*

ALPHA ORDER				RANK ORDER		
RANK	STATE	RATE		RANK	STATE	RATE
35	Alabama	9.8		1	Florida	14.6
50	Alaska	3.3		2	Maine	12.9
31	Arizona	10.2		3	Pennsylvania	12.4
16	Arkansas	11.2		4	South Dakota	12.3
46	California	8.2		5	Louisiana	12.2
39	Colorado	9.4		6	Oregon	11.9
14	Connecticut	11.3		7	Indiana	11.8
18	Delaware	11.0		7	Kentucky	11.8
1	Florida	14.6		7	New Jersey	11.8
39	Georgia	9.4		10	Massachusetts	11.5
18	Hawaii	11.0		10	New York	11.5
48	Idaho	5.9		12	Montana	11.4
32	Illinois	10.1		12	Wisconsin	11.4
7	Indiana	11.8		14	Connecticut	11.3
35	Iowa	9.8		14	Kansas	11.3
14	Kansas	11.3		16	Arkansas	11.2
7	Kentucky	11.8		16	New Hampshire	11.2
5	Louisiana	12.2		18	Delaware	11.0
2	Maine	12.9		18	Hawaii	11.0
38	Maryland	9.5		18	Mississippi	11.0
10	Massachusetts	11.5		18	West Virginia	11.0
27	Michigan	10.4		22	North Dakota	10.9
43	Minnesota	9.0		22	Tennessee	10.9
18	Mississippi	11.0		24	Virginia	10.8
26	Missouri	10.6		25	Ohio	10.7
12	Montana	11.4		26	Missouri	10.6
29	Nebraska	10.3		27	Michigan	10.4
33	Nevada	10.0		27	North Carolina	10.4
16	New Hampshire	11.2		29	Nebraska	10.3
7	New Jersey	11.8		29	Oklahoma	10.3
46	New Mexico	8.2		31	Arizona	10.2
10	New York	11.5		32	Illinois	10.1
27	North Carolina	10.4		33	Nevada	10.0
22	North Dakota	10.9		34	Texas	9.9
25	Ohio	10.7		35	Alabama	9.8
29	Oklahoma	10.3		35	Iowa	9.8
6	Oregon	11.9		37	South Carolina	9.7
3	Pennsylvania	12.4		38	Maryland	9.5
42	Rhode Island	9.1		39	Colorado	9.4
37	South Carolina	9.7		39	Georgia	9.4
4	South Dakota	12.3		39	Washington	9.4
22	Tennessee	10.9		42	Rhode Island	9.1
34	Texas	9.9		43	Minnesota	9.0
49	Utah	5.5		44	Vermont	8.5
44	Vermont	8.5		45	Wyoming	8.3
24	Virginia	10.8		46	California	8.2
39	Washington	9.4		46	New Mexico	8.2
18	West Virginia	11.0		48	Idaho	5.9
12	Wisconsin	11.4		49	Utah	5.5
45	Wyoming	8.3		50	Alaska	3.3
					District of Columbia	18.4

Source: Morgan Quitno Press using data from American Cancer Society (http://www.cancer.org/97tabp6.html)
"Cancer Facts & Figures-1997" (Copyright 1997, Reprinted with permission from the American Cancer Society)
*Rates calculated using 1996 Census resident population estimates. Not age adjusted.

Estimated Deaths by Prostate Cancer in 1997

National Estimated Total = 41,800 Deaths

RANK	STATE	DEATHS	% of USA
23	Alabama	670	1.60%
50	Alaska	40	0.10%
20	Arizona	710	1.70%
27	Arkansas	530	1.27%
1	California	3,900	9.33%
31	Colorado	500	1.20%
29	Connecticut	520	1.24%
47	Delaware	110	0.26%
2	Florida	3,200	7.66%
14	Georgia	960	2.30%
44	Hawaii	140	0.33%
40	Idaho	180	0.43%
6	Illinois	1,900	4.55%
16	Indiana	850	2.03%
32	Iowa	490	1.17%
33	Kansas	430	1.03%
25	Kentucky	560	1.34%
22	Louisiana	690	1.65%
37	Maine	220	0.53%
17	Maryland	810	1.94%
11	Massachusetts	1,000	2.39%
8	Michigan	1,600	3.83%
21	Minnesota	700	1.67%
30	Mississippi	510	1.22%
15	Missouri	890	2.13%
40	Montana	180	0.43%
35	Nebraska	260	0.62%
37	Nevada	220	0.53%
43	New Hampshire	150	0.36%
9	New Jersey	1,400	3.35%
37	New Mexico	220	0.53%
3	New York	2,600	6.22%
10	North Carolina	1,300	3.11%
42	North Dakota	170	0.41%
7	Ohio	1,800	4.31%
27	Oklahoma	530	1.27%
25	Oregon	560	1.34%
5	Pennsylvania	2,400	5.74%
46	Rhode Island	120	0.29%
24	South Carolina	630	1.51%
44	South Dakota	140	0.33%
19	Tennessee	780	1.87%
3	Texas	2,600	6.22%
36	Utah	240	0.57%
48	Vermont	90	0.22%
13	Virginia	980	2.34%
17	Washington	810	1.94%
34	West Virginia	320	0.77%
11	Wisconsin	1,000	2.39%
49	Wyoming	80	0.19%

RANK	STATE	DEATHS	% of USA
1	California	3,900	9.33%
2	Florida	3,200	7.66%
3	New York	2,600	6.22%
3	Texas	2,600	6.22%
5	Pennsylvania	2,400	5.74%
6	Illinois	1,900	4.55%
7	Ohio	1,800	4.31%
8	Michigan	1,600	3.83%
9	New Jersey	1,400	3.35%
10	North Carolina	1,300	3.11%
11	Massachusetts	1,000	2.39%
11	Wisconsin	1,000	2.39%
13	Virginia	980	2.34%
14	Georgia	960	2.30%
15	Missouri	890	2.13%
16	Indiana	850	2.03%
17	Maryland	810	1.94%
17	Washington	810	1.94%
19	Tennessee	780	1.87%
20	Arizona	710	1.70%
21	Minnesota	700	1.67%
22	Louisiana	690	1.65%
23	Alabama	670	1.60%
24	South Carolina	630	1.51%
25	Kentucky	560	1.34%
25	Oregon	560	1.34%
27	Arkansas	530	1.27%
27	Oklahoma	530	1.27%
29	Connecticut	520	1.24%
30	Mississippi	510	1.22%
31	Colorado	500	1.20%
32	Iowa	490	1.17%
33	Kansas	430	1.03%
34	West Virginia	320	0.77%
35	Nebraska	260	0.62%
36	Utah	240	0.57%
37	Maine	220	0.53%
37	Nevada	220	0.53%
37	New Mexico	220	0.53%
40	Idaho	180	0.43%
40	Montana	180	0.43%
42	North Dakota	170	0.41%
43	New Hampshire	150	0.36%
44	Hawaii	140	0.33%
44	South Dakota	140	0.33%
46	Rhode Island	120	0.29%
47	Delaware	110	0.26%
48	Vermont	90	0.22%
49	Wyoming	80	0.19%
50	Alaska	40	0.10%
	District of Columbia	110	0.26%

Source: American Cancer Society (http://www.cancer.org/97tabp6.html)
"Cancer Facts & Figures-1997" (Copyright 1997, Reprinted with permission from the American Cancer Society)

Estimated Death Rate by Prostate Cancer in 1997

National Rate = 32.6 Deaths per 100,000 Male Population*

ALPHA ORDER				RANK ORDER		
RANK	STATE	RATE		RANK	STATE	RATE
27	Alabama	32.8		1	North Dakota	53.2
50	Alaska	12.6		2	Florida	46.6
20	Arizona	34.0		3	Arkansas	44.2
3	Arkansas	44.2		4	Montana	41.6
47	California	24.7		5	Pennsylvania	41.4
43	Colorado	26.9		6	Wisconsin	39.8
28	Connecticut	32.7		7	Mississippi	39.4
30	Delaware	31.5		8	South Dakota	39.0
2	Florida	46.6		9	North Carolina	37.2
42	Georgia	27.4		10	Maine	36.4
49	Hawaii	23.3		10	New Jersey	36.4
32	Idaho	31.0		10	West Virginia	36.4
25	Illinois	33.0		13	Oregon	36.1
36	Indiana	30.1		14	South Carolina	35.6
15	Iowa	35.4		15	Iowa	35.4
19	Kansas	34.1		16	Missouri	34.6
38	Kentucky	29.9		17	Michigan	34.4
25	Louisiana	33.0		18	Massachusetts	34.2
10	Maine	36.4		19	Kansas	34.1
22	Maryland	33.1		20	Arizona	34.0
18	Massachusetts	34.2		21	Ohio	33.4
17	Michigan	34.4		22	Maryland	33.1
33	Minnesota	30.9		22	Oklahoma	33.1
7	Mississippi	39.4		22	Wyoming	33.1
16	Missouri	34.6		25	Illinois	33.0
4	Montana	41.6		25	Louisiana	33.0
29	Nebraska	32.5		27	Alabama	32.8
40	Nevada	28.2		28	Connecticut	32.7
44	New Hampshire	26.6		29	Nebraska	32.5
10	New Jersey	36.4		30	Delaware	31.5
45	New Mexico	26.5		31	Vermont	31.3
39	New York	29.8		32	Idaho	31.0
9	North Carolina	37.2		33	Minnesota	30.9
1	North Dakota	53.2		34	Tennessee	30.8
21	Ohio	33.4		35	Virginia	30.3
22	Oklahoma	33.1		36	Indiana	30.1
13	Oregon	36.1		37	Washington	30.0
5	Pennsylvania	41.4		38	Kentucky	29.9
46	Rhode Island	25.2		39	New York	29.8
14	South Carolina	35.6		40	Nevada	28.2
8	South Dakota	39.0		40	Texas	28.2
34	Tennessee	30.8		42	Georgia	27.4
40	Texas	28.2		43	Colorado	26.9
47	Utah	24.7		44	New Hampshire	26.6
31	Vermont	31.3		45	New Mexico	26.5
35	Virginia	30.3		46	Rhode Island	25.2
37	Washington	30.0		47	California	24.7
10	West Virginia	36.4		47	Utah	24.7
6	Wisconsin	39.8		49	Hawaii	23.3
22	Wyoming	33.1		50	Alaska	12.6
					District of Columbia	42.4

Source: Morgan Quitno Press using data from American Cancer Society (http://www.cancer.org/97tabp6.html)
"Cancer Facts & Figures-1997" (Copyright 1997, Reprinted with permission from the American Cancer Society)
Rates calculated using 1995 Census resident male population estimates. Not age adjusted.

Estimated Deaths by Skin Melanoma in 1997

National Estimated Total = 7,300 Deaths

ALPHA ORDER

RANK	STATE	DEATHS	% of USA
18	Alabama	140	1.92%
50	Alaska	5	0.07%
19	Arizona	130	1.78%
34	Arkansas	60	0.82%
1	California	780	10.68%
29	Colorado	90	1.23%
26	Connecticut	100	1.37%
44	Delaware	20	0.27%
2	Florida	510	6.99%
14	Georgia	190	2.60%
48	Hawaii	10	0.14%
39	Idaho	30	0.41%
6	Illinois	340	4.66%
15	Indiana	170	2.33%
29	Iowa	90	1.23%
23	Kansas	110	1.51%
19	Kentucky	130	1.78%
23	Louisiana	110	1.51%
38	Maine	40	0.55%
23	Maryland	110	1.51%
10	Massachusetts	220	3.01%
10	Michigan	220	3.01%
26	Minnesota	100	1.37%
37	Mississippi	50	0.68%
15	Missouri	170	2.33%
44	Montana	20	0.27%
39	Nebraska	30	0.41%
34	Nevada	60	0.82%
39	New Hampshire	30	0.41%
8	New Jersey	230	3.15%
34	New Mexico	60	0.82%
4	New York	410	5.62%
8	North Carolina	230	3.15%
44	North Dakota	20	0.27%
7	Ohio	260	3.56%
26	Oklahoma	100	1.37%
22	Oregon	120	1.64%
5	Pennsylvania	390	5.34%
39	Rhode Island	30	0.41%
29	South Carolina	90	1.23%
48	South Dakota	10	0.14%
12	Tennessee	200	2.74%
3	Texas	450	6.16%
32	Utah	70	0.96%
39	Vermont	30	0.41%
12	Virginia	200	2.74%
17	Washington	150	2.05%
32	West Virginia	70	0.96%
19	Wisconsin	130	1.78%
44	Wyoming	20	0.27%

RANK ORDER

RANK	STATE	DEATHS	% of USA
1	California	780	10.68%
2	Florida	510	6.99%
3	Texas	450	6.16%
4	New York	410	5.62%
5	Pennsylvania	390	5.34%
6	Illinois	340	4.66%
7	Ohio	260	3.56%
8	New Jersey	230	3.15%
8	North Carolina	230	3.15%
10	Massachusetts	220	3.01%
10	Michigan	220	3.01%
12	Tennessee	200	2.74%
12	Virginia	200	2.74%
14	Georgia	190	2.60%
15	Indiana	170	2.33%
15	Missouri	170	2.33%
17	Washington	150	2.05%
18	Alabama	140	1.92%
19	Arizona	130	1.78%
19	Kentucky	130	1.78%
19	Wisconsin	130	1.78%
22	Oregon	120	1.64%
23	Kansas	110	1.51%
23	Louisiana	110	1.51%
23	Maryland	110	1.51%
26	Connecticut	100	1.37%
26	Minnesota	100	1.37%
26	Oklahoma	100	1.37%
29	Colorado	90	1.23%
29	Iowa	90	1.23%
29	South Carolina	90	1.23%
32	Utah	70	0.96%
32	West Virginia	70	0.96%
34	Arkansas	60	0.82%
34	Nevada	60	0.82%
34	New Mexico	60	0.82%
37	Mississippi	50	0.68%
38	Maine	40	0.55%
39	Idaho	30	0.41%
39	Nebraska	30	0.41%
39	New Hampshire	30	0.41%
39	Rhode Island	30	0.41%
39	Vermont	30	0.41%
44	Delaware	20	0.27%
44	Montana	20	0.27%
44	North Dakota	20	0.27%
44	Wyoming	20	0.27%
48	Hawaii	10	0.14%
48	South Dakota	10	0.14%
50	Alaska	5	0.07%
	District of Columbia	5	0.07%

Source: American Cancer Society (http://www.cancer.org/97tabp6.html)
"Cancer Facts & Figures-1997" (Copyright 1997, Reprinted with permission from the American Cancer Society)

Estimated Death Rate by Skin Melanoma in 1997

National Estimated Rate = 2.8 Deaths per 100,000 Population*

ALPHA ORDER

RANK	STATE	RATE
12	Alabama	3.3
49	Alaska	0.8
24	Arizona	2.9
35	Arkansas	2.4
35	California	2.4
35	Colorado	2.4
18	Connecticut	3.1
28	Delaware	2.8
9	Florida	3.5
30	Georgia	2.6
49	Hawaii	0.8
32	Idaho	2.5
24	Illinois	2.9
24	Indiana	2.9
14	Iowa	3.2
2	Kansas	4.3
12	Kentucky	3.3
32	Louisiana	2.5
14	Maine	3.2
44	Maryland	2.2
8	Massachusetts	3.6
40	Michigan	2.3
45	Minnesota	2.1
46	Mississippi	1.8
14	Missouri	3.2
40	Montana	2.3
46	Nebraska	1.8
6	Nevada	3.7
30	New Hampshire	2.6
24	New Jersey	2.9
9	New Mexico	3.5
40	New York	2.3
18	North Carolina	3.1
18	North Dakota	3.1
40	Ohio	2.3
21	Oklahoma	3.0
6	Oregon	3.7
14	Pennsylvania	3.2
21	Rhode Island	3.0
35	South Carolina	2.4
48	South Dakota	1.4
4	Tennessee	3.8
35	Texas	2.4
9	Utah	3.5
1	Vermont	5.1
21	Virginia	3.0
29	Washington	2.7
4	West Virginia	3.8
32	Wisconsin	2.5
3	Wyoming	4.2

RANK ORDER

RANK	STATE	RATE
1	Vermont	5.1
2	Kansas	4.3
3	Wyoming	4.2
4	Tennessee	3.8
4	West Virginia	3.8
6	Nevada	3.7
6	Oregon	3.7
8	Massachusetts	3.6
9	Florida	3.5
9	New Mexico	3.5
9	Utah	3.5
12	Alabama	3.3
12	Kentucky	3.3
14	Iowa	3.2
14	Maine	3.2
14	Missouri	3.2
14	Pennsylvania	3.2
18	Connecticut	3.1
18	North Carolina	3.1
18	North Dakota	3.1
21	Oklahoma	3.0
21	Rhode Island	3.0
21	Virginia	3.0
24	Arizona	2.9
24	Illinois	2.9
24	Indiana	2.9
24	New Jersey	2.9
28	Delaware	2.8
29	Washington	2.7
30	Georgia	2.6
30	New Hampshire	2.6
32	Idaho	2.5
32	Louisiana	2.5
32	Wisconsin	2.5
35	Arkansas	2.4
35	California	2.4
35	Colorado	2.4
35	South Carolina	2.4
35	Texas	2.4
40	Michigan	2.3
40	Montana	2.3
40	New York	2.3
40	Ohio	2.3
44	Maryland	2.2
45	Minnesota	2.1
46	Mississippi	1.8
46	Nebraska	1.8
48	South Dakota	1.4
49	Alaska	0.8
49	Hawaii	0.8

District of Columbia 0.9

Source: Morgan Quitno Press using data from American Cancer Society (http://www.cancer.org/97tabp6.html)
"Cancer Facts & Figures-1997" (Copyright 1997, Reprinted with permission from the American Cancer Society)
*Rates calculated using 1996 Census resident population estimates. Not age adjusted.

Estimated Deaths by Uterus (Cervix) Cancer in 1997

National Estimated Total = 4,800 Deaths*

ALPHA ORDER					RANK ORDER			
RANK	STATE		DEATHS	% of USA	RANK	STATE	DEATHS	% of USA
20	Alabama		80	1.67%	1	California	510	10.63%
48	Alaska		5	0.10%	2	New York	400	8.33%
26	Arizona		50	1.04%	2	Texas	400	8.33%
24	Arkansas		60	1.25%	4	Florida	380	7.92%
1	California		510	10.63%	5	Pennsylvania	270	5.63%
26	Colorado		50	1.04%	6	Illinois	240	5.00%
36	Connecticut		20	0.42%	7	Ohio	220	4.58%
36	Delaware		20	0.42%	8	Michigan	160	3.33%
4	Florida		380	7.92%	9	New Jersey	130	2.71%
13	Georgia		100	2.08%	10	Indiana	120	2.50%
43	Hawaii		10	0.21%	10	Missouri	120	2.50%
48	Idaho		5	0.10%	12	North Carolina	110	2.29%
6	Illinois		240	5.00%	13	Georgia	100	2.08%
10	Indiana		120	2.50%	13	Kentucky	100	2.08%
26	Iowa		50	1.04%	13	Maryland	100	2.08%
26	Kansas		50	1.04%	13	Tennessee	100	2.08%
13	Kentucky		100	2.08%	13	Virginia	100	2.08%
26	Louisiana		50	1.04%	13	Wisconsin	100	2.08%
36	Maine		20	0.42%	19	Massachusetts	90	1.88%
13	Maryland		100	2.08%	20	Alabama	80	1.67%
19	Massachusetts		90	1.88%	20	South Carolina	80	1.67%
8	Michigan		160	3.33%	22	Mississippi	70	1.46%
31	Minnesota		40	0.83%	22	Oklahoma	70	1.46%
22	Mississippi		70	1.46%	24	Arkansas	60	1.25%
10	Missouri		120	2.50%	24	Washington	60	1.25%
36	Montana		20	0.42%	26	Arizona	50	1.04%
43	Nebraska		10	0.21%	26	Colorado	50	1.04%
34	Nevada		30	0.63%	26	Iowa	50	1.04%
34	New Hampshire		30	0.63%	26	Kansas	50	1.04%
9	New Jersey		130	2.71%	26	Louisiana	50	1.04%
36	New Mexico		20	0.42%	31	Minnesota	40	0.83%
2	New York		400	8.33%	31	Oregon	40	0.83%
12	North Carolina		110	2.29%	31	West Virginia	40	0.83%
48	North Dakota		5	0.10%	34	Nevada	30	0.63%
7	Ohio		220	4.58%	34	New Hampshire	30	0.63%
22	Oklahoma		70	1.46%	36	Connecticut	20	0.42%
31	Oregon		40	0.83%	36	Delaware	20	0.42%
5	Pennsylvania		270	5.63%	36	Maine	20	0.42%
36	Rhode Island		20	0.42%	36	Montana	20	0.42%
20	South Carolina		80	1.67%	36	New Mexico	20	0.42%
43	South Dakota		10	0.21%	36	Rhode Island	20	0.42%
13	Tennessee		100	2.08%	36	Utah	20	0.42%
2	Texas		400	8.33%	43	Hawaii	10	0.21%
36	Utah		20	0.42%	43	Nebraska	10	0.21%
43	Vermont		10	0.21%	43	South Dakota	10	0.21%
13	Virginia		100	2.08%	43	Vermont	10	0.21%
24	Washington		60	1.25%	43	Wyoming	10	0.21%
31	West Virginia		40	0.83%	48	Alaska	5	0.10%
13	Wisconsin		100	2.08%	48	Idaho	5	0.10%
43	Wyoming		10	0.21%	48	North Dakota	5	0.10%
						District of Columbia	10	0.21%

Source: American Cancer Society (http://www.cancer.org/97tabp6.html)
    "Cancer Facts & Figures-1997" (Copyright 1997, Reprinted with permission from the American Cancer Society)
*Does not include estimated deaths by uterus (endometrial) cancer.

Estimated Death Rate by Uterus (Cervix) Cancer in 1997

National Estimated Rate = 3.6 Deaths per 100,000 Female Population*

ALPHA ORDER

RANK	STATE	RATE
25	Alabama	3.6
44	Alaska	1.7
39	Arizona	2.3
6	Arkansas	4.7
29	California	3.2
37	Colorado	2.6
48	Connecticut	1.2
1	Delaware	5.4
2	Florida	5.2
35	Georgia	2.7
44	Hawaii	1.7
50	Idaho	0.9
16	Illinois	4.0
16	Indiana	4.0
26	Iowa	3.4
21	Kansas	3.8
4	Kentucky	5.0
41	Louisiana	2.2
31	Maine	3.1
19	Maryland	3.9
34	Massachusetts	2.9
28	Michigan	3.3
44	Minnesota	1.7
4	Mississippi	5.0
8	Missouri	4.4
7	Montana	4.6
48	Nebraska	1.2
16	Nevada	4.0
3	New Hampshire	5.1
29	New Jersey	3.2
39	New Mexico	2.3
10	New York	4.2
32	North Carolina	3.0
47	North Dakota	1.6
21	Ohio	3.8
10	Oklahoma	4.2
38	Oregon	2.5
9	Pennsylvania	4.3
19	Rhode Island	3.9
10	South Carolina	4.2
35	South Dakota	2.7
24	Tennessee	3.7
10	Texas	4.2
43	Utah	2.0
26	Vermont	3.4
32	Virginia	3.0
41	Washington	2.2
10	West Virginia	4.2
21	Wisconsin	3.8
10	Wyoming	4.2

RANK ORDER

RANK	STATE	RATE
1	Delaware	5.4
2	Florida	5.2
3	New Hampshire	5.1
4	Kentucky	5.0
4	Mississippi	5.0
6	Arkansas	4.7
7	Montana	4.6
8	Missouri	4.4
9	Pennsylvania	4.3
10	New York	4.2
10	Oklahoma	4.2
10	South Carolina	4.2
10	Texas	4.2
10	West Virginia	4.2
10	Wyoming	4.2
16	Illinois	4.0
16	Indiana	4.0
16	Nevada	4.0
19	Maryland	3.9
19	Rhode Island	3.9
21	Kansas	3.8
21	Ohio	3.8
21	Wisconsin	3.8
24	Tennessee	3.7
25	Alabama	3.6
26	Iowa	3.4
26	Vermont	3.4
28	Michigan	3.3
29	California	3.2
29	New Jersey	3.2
31	Maine	3.1
32	North Carolina	3.0
32	Virginia	3.0
34	Massachusetts	2.9
35	Georgia	2.7
35	South Dakota	2.7
37	Colorado	2.6
38	Oregon	2.5
39	Arizona	2.3
39	New Mexico	2.3
41	Louisiana	2.2
41	Washington	2.2
43	Utah	2.0
44	Alaska	1.7
44	Hawaii	1.7
44	Minnesota	1.7
47	North Dakota	1.6
48	Connecticut	1.2
48	Nebraska	1.2
50	Idaho	0.9

District of Columbia	3.4

Source: Morgan Quitno Press using data from American Cancer Society (http://www.cancer.org/97tabp6.html)
"Cancer Facts & Figures-1997" (Copyright 1997, Reprinted with permission from the American Cancer Society)
*Rates calculated using 1995 Census resident female population estimates. Not age adjusted.

Deaths by Atherosclerosis in 1994

National Total = 17,116 Deaths*

ALPHA ORDER					RANK ORDER			
RANK	STATE	DEATHS	% of USA		RANK	STATE	DEATHS	% of USA
27	Alabama	221	1.29%		1	California	1,994	11.65%
49	Alaska	18	0.11%		2	Florida	1,103	6.44%
25	Arizona	290	1.69%		3	Texas	1,024	5.98%
31	Arkansas	173	1.01%		4	New York	871	5.09%
1	California	1,994	11.65%		5	Michigan	802	4.69%
14	Colorado	398	2.33%		6	Pennsylvania	777	4.54%
30	Connecticut	200	1.17%		7	Ohio	717	4.19%
48	Delaware	19	0.11%		8	Illinois	640	3.74%
2	Florida	1,103	6.44%		9	Indiana	523	3.06%
10	Georgia	488	2.85%		10	Georgia	488	2.85%
50	Hawaii	17	0.10%		11	New Jersey	428	2.50%
44	Idaho	58	0.34%		12	North Carolina	409	2.39%
8	Illinois	640	3.74%		13	Virginia	408	2.38%
9	Indiana	523	3.06%		14	Colorado	398	2.33%
16	Iowa	380	2.22%		15	Tennessee	386	2.26%
23	Kansas	297	1.74%		16	Iowa	380	2.22%
29	Kentucky	208	1.22%		17	Massachusetts	359	2.10%
24	Louisiana	293	1.71%		17	Washington	359	2.10%
37	Maine	102	0.60%		19	Missouri	358	2.09%
33	Maryland	158	0.92%		20	Oklahoma	357	2.09%
17	Massachusetts	359	2.10%		21	Wisconsin	333	1.95%
5	Michigan	802	4.69%		22	Minnesota	303	1.77%
22	Minnesota	303	1.77%		23	Kansas	297	1.74%
34	Mississippi	142	0.83%		24	Louisiana	293	1.71%
19	Missouri	358	2.09%		25	Arizona	290	1.69%
40	Montana	75	0.44%		26	Oregon	281	1.64%
28	Nebraska	210	1.23%		27	Alabama	221	1.29%
41	Nevada	72	0.42%		28	Nebraska	210	1.23%
37	New Hampshire	102	0.60%		29	Kentucky	208	1.22%
11	New Jersey	428	2.50%		30	Connecticut	200	1.17%
35	New Mexico	125	0.73%		31	Arkansas	173	1.01%
4	New York	871	5.09%		32	West Virginia	172	1.00%
12	North Carolina	409	2.39%		33	Maryland	158	0.92%
42	North Dakota	63	0.37%		34	Mississippi	142	0.83%
7	Ohio	717	4.19%		35	New Mexico	125	0.73%
20	Oklahoma	357	2.09%		36	South Carolina	114	0.67%
26	Oregon	281	1.64%		37	Maine	102	0.60%
6	Pennsylvania	777	4.54%		37	New Hampshire	102	0.60%
43	Rhode Island	61	0.36%		39	Utah	79	0.46%
36	South Carolina	114	0.67%		40	Montana	75	0.44%
44	South Dakota	58	0.34%		41	Nevada	72	0.42%
15	Tennessee	386	2.26%		42	North Dakota	63	0.37%
3	Texas	1,024	5.98%		43	Rhode Island	61	0.36%
39	Utah	79	0.46%		44	Idaho	58	0.34%
47	Vermont	28	0.16%		44	South Dakota	58	0.34%
13	Virginia	408	2.38%		46	Wyoming	34	0.20%
17	Washington	359	2.10%		47	Vermont	28	0.16%
32	West Virginia	172	1.00%		48	Delaware	19	0.11%
21	Wisconsin	333	1.95%		49	Alaska	18	0.11%
46	Wyoming	34	0.20%		50	Hawaii	17	0.10%
						District of Columbia	29	0.17%

Source: U.S. Department of Health and Human Services, National Center for Health Statistics
     unpublished data
*By state of residence. Atherosclerosis is a form of hardening of the arteries.

Death Rate by Atherosclerosis in 1994

National Rate = 6.57 Deaths per 100,000 Population*

ALPHA ORDER

RANK	STATE	RATE
40	Alabama	5.23
48	Alaska	2.96
19	Arizona	7.10
20	Arkansas	7.04
29	California	6.34
5	Colorado	10.88
32	Connecticut	6.10
49	Delaware	2.68
15	Florida	7.90
21	Georgia	6.91
50	Hawaii	1.44
41	Idaho	5.11
36	Illinois	5.44
9	Indiana	9.08
1	Iowa	13.42
3	Kansas	11.62
37	Kentucky	5.43
22	Louisiana	6.78
13	Maine	8.22
46	Maryland	3.15
33	Massachusetts	5.94
12	Michigan	8.44
25	Minnesota	6.63
39	Mississippi	5.31
22	Missouri	6.78
11	Montana	8.76
2	Nebraska	12.93
42	Nevada	4.93
10	New Hampshire	8.97
38	New Jersey	5.41
16	New Mexico	7.55
44	New York	4.79
34	North Carolina	5.78
6	North Dakota	9.87
27	Ohio	6.45
4	Oklahoma	10.96
8	Oregon	9.10
28	Pennsylvania	6.44
31	Rhode Island	6.12
47	South Carolina	3.11
14	South Dakota	8.04
17	Tennessee	7.45
35	Texas	5.56
45	Utah	4.13
43	Vermont	4.82
30	Virginia	6.22
24	Washington	6.71
7	West Virginia	9.43
26	Wisconsin	6.55
18	Wyoming	7.14

RANK ORDER

RANK	STATE	RATE
1	Iowa	13.42
2	Nebraska	12.93
3	Kansas	11.62
4	Oklahoma	10.96
5	Colorado	10.88
6	North Dakota	9.87
7	West Virginia	9.43
8	Oregon	9.10
9	Indiana	9.08
10	New Hampshire	8.97
11	Montana	8.76
12	Michigan	8.44
13	Maine	8.22
14	South Dakota	8.04
15	Florida	7.90
16	New Mexico	7.55
17	Tennessee	7.45
18	Wyoming	7.14
19	Arizona	7.10
20	Arkansas	7.04
21	Georgia	6.91
22	Louisiana	6.78
22	Missouri	6.78
24	Washington	6.71
25	Minnesota	6.63
26	Wisconsin	6.55
27	Ohio	6.45
28	Pennsylvania	6.44
29	California	6.34
30	Virginia	6.22
31	Rhode Island	6.12
32	Connecticut	6.10
33	Massachusetts	5.94
34	North Carolina	5.78
35	Texas	5.56
36	Illinois	5.44
37	Kentucky	5.43
38	New Jersey	5.41
39	Mississippi	5.31
40	Alabama	5.23
41	Idaho	5.11
42	Nevada	4.93
43	Vermont	4.82
44	New York	4.79
45	Utah	4.13
46	Maryland	3.15
47	South Carolina	3.11
48	Alaska	2.96
49	Delaware	2.68
50	Hawaii	1.44
	District of Columbia	5.07

Source: U.S. Department of Health and Human Services, National Center for Health Statistics
   unpublished data
*By state of residence. Atherosclerosis is a form of hardening of the arteries. Not age adjusted.

Deaths by Cerebrovascular Diseases in 1994

National Total = 153,306 Deaths*

ALPHA ORDER

RANK	STATE	DEATHS	% of USA
20	Alabama	2,614	1.71%
50	Alaska	123	0.08%
28	Arizona	2,133	1.39%
26	Arkansas	2,181	1.42%
1	California	15,773	10.29%
33	Colorado	1,542	1.01%
30	Connecticut	1,832	1.19%
47	Delaware	348	0.23%
2	Florida	9,600	6.26%
13	Georgia	3,898	2.54%
43	Hawaii	584	0.38%
40	Idaho	641	0.42%
6	Illinois	7,287	4.75%
11	Indiana	4,019	2.62%
29	Iowa	2,108	1.38%
32	Kansas	1,761	1.15%
23	Kentucky	2,484	1.62%
25	Louisiana	2,378	1.55%
37	Maine	761	0.50%
22	Maryland	2,518	1.64%
17	Massachusetts	3,341	2.18%
8	Michigan	5,699	3.72%
19	Minnesota	2,901	1.89%
31	Mississippi	1,779	1.16%
14	Missouri	3,824	2.49%
44	Montana	574	0.37%
35	Nebraska	1,140	0.74%
39	Nevada	646	0.42%
42	New Hampshire	585	0.38%
10	New Jersey	4,103	2.68%
36	New Mexico	774	0.50%
5	New York	8,229	5.37%
9	North Carolina	5,180	3.38%
45	North Dakota	509	0.33%
7	Ohio	6,417	4.19%
27	Oklahoma	2,148	1.40%
24	Oregon	2,386	1.56%
4	Pennsylvania	8,451	5.51%
41	Rhode Island	594	0.39%
21	South Carolina	2,544	1.66%
46	South Dakota	496	0.32%
12	Tennessee	3,981	2.60%
3	Texas	9,251	6.03%
38	Utah	717	0.47%
47	Vermont	348	0.23%
15	Virginia	3,658	2.39%
18	Washington	3,110	2.03%
34	West Virginia	1,224	0.80%
16	Wisconsin	3,514	2.29%
49	Wyoming	219	0.14%

RANK ORDER

RANK	STATE	DEATHS	% of USA
1	California	15,773	10.29%
2	Florida	9,600	6.26%
3	Texas	9,251	6.03%
4	Pennsylvania	8,451	5.51%
5	New York	8,229	5.37%
6	Illinois	7,287	4.75%
7	Ohio	6,417	4.19%
8	Michigan	5,699	3.72%
9	North Carolina	5,180	3.38%
10	New Jersey	4,103	2.68%
11	Indiana	4,019	2.62%
12	Tennessee	3,981	2.60%
13	Georgia	3,898	2.54%
14	Missouri	3,824	2.49%
15	Virginia	3,658	2.39%
16	Wisconsin	3,514	2.29%
17	Massachusetts	3,341	2.18%
18	Washington	3,110	2.03%
19	Minnesota	2,901	1.89%
20	Alabama	2,614	1.71%
21	South Carolina	2,544	1.66%
22	Maryland	2,518	1.64%
23	Kentucky	2,484	1.62%
24	Oregon	2,386	1.56%
25	Louisiana	2,378	1.55%
26	Arkansas	2,181	1.42%
27	Oklahoma	2,148	1.40%
28	Arizona	2,133	1.39%
29	Iowa	2,108	1.38%
30	Connecticut	1,832	1.19%
31	Mississippi	1,779	1.16%
32	Kansas	1,761	1.15%
33	Colorado	1,542	1.01%
34	West Virginia	1,224	0.80%
35	Nebraska	1,140	0.74%
36	New Mexico	774	0.50%
37	Maine	761	0.50%
38	Utah	717	0.47%
39	Nevada	646	0.42%
40	Idaho	641	0.42%
41	Rhode Island	594	0.39%
42	New Hampshire	585	0.38%
43	Hawaii	584	0.38%
44	Montana	574	0.37%
45	North Dakota	509	0.33%
46	South Dakota	496	0.32%
47	Delaware	348	0.23%
47	Vermont	348	0.23%
49	Wyoming	219	0.14%
50	Alaska	123	0.08%
	District of Columbia	379	0.25%

Source: U.S. Department of Health and Human Services, National Center for Health Statistics
    "Monthly Vital Statistics Report" (Vol. 45, No. 3(S), September 30, 1996)
*Final data by state of residence. Cerebrovascular diseases include stroke and other disorders of the blood vessels of the brain.

Death Rate by Cerebrovascular Diseases in 1994

National Rate = 58.9 Deaths per 100,000 Population*

ALPHA ORDER

RANK ORDER

RANK	STATE	RATE
22	Alabama	62.0
50	Alaska	20.3
36	Arizona	52.3
1	Arkansas	88.9
41	California	50.2
48	Colorado	42.2
31	Connecticut	55.9
43	Delaware	49.3
14	Florida	68.8
34	Georgia	55.2
42	Hawaii	49.6
30	Idaho	56.6
22	Illinois	62.0
10	Indiana	69.9
5	Iowa	74.5
13	Kansas	68.9
20	Kentucky	64.9
35	Louisiana	55.1
24	Maine	61.4
39	Maryland	50.3
33	Massachusetts	55.3
25	Michigan	60.0
21	Minnesota	63.5
18	Mississippi	66.7
7	Missouri	72.5
17	Montana	67.1
8	Nebraska	70.2
47	Nevada	44.3
38	New Hampshire	51.5
37	New Jersey	51.9
44	New Mexico	46.8
46	New York	45.3
6	North Carolina	73.3
2	North Dakota	79.8
29	Ohio	57.8
19	Oklahoma	65.9
3	Oregon	77.3
9	Pennsylvania	70.1
27	Rhode Island	59.6
11	South Carolina	69.4
14	South Dakota	68.8
4	Tennessee	76.9
39	Texas	50.3
49	Utah	37.6
25	Vermont	60.0
32	Virginia	55.8
28	Washington	58.2
16	West Virginia	67.2
12	Wisconsin	69.2
45	Wyoming	46.0

RANK	STATE	RATE
1	Arkansas	88.9
2	North Dakota	79.8
3	Oregon	77.3
4	Tennessee	76.9
5	Iowa	74.5
6	North Carolina	73.3
7	Missouri	72.5
8	Nebraska	70.2
9	Pennsylvania	70.1
10	Indiana	69.9
11	South Carolina	69.4
12	Wisconsin	69.2
13	Kansas	68.9
14	Florida	68.8
14	South Dakota	68.8
16	West Virginia	67.2
17	Montana	67.1
18	Mississippi	66.7
19	Oklahoma	65.9
20	Kentucky	64.9
21	Minnesota	63.5
22	Alabama	62.0
22	Illinois	62.0
24	Maine	61.4
25	Michigan	60.0
25	Vermont	60.0
27	Rhode Island	59.6
28	Washington	58.2
29	Ohio	57.8
30	Idaho	56.6
31	Connecticut	55.9
32	Virginia	55.8
33	Massachusetts	55.3
34	Georgia	55.2
35	Louisiana	55.1
36	Arizona	52.3
37	New Jersey	51.9
38	New Hampshire	51.5
39	Maryland	50.3
39	Texas	50.3
41	California	50.2
42	Hawaii	49.6
43	Delaware	49.3
44	New Mexico	46.8
45	Wyoming	46.0
46	New York	45.3
47	Nevada	44.3
48	Colorado	42.2
49	Utah	37.6
50	Alaska	20.3

| | District of Columbia | 66.5 |

Source: U.S. Department of Health and Human Services, National Center for Health Statistics
   "Monthly Vital Statistics Report" (Vol. 45, No. 3(S), September 30, 1996)
*Final data by state of residence. Cerebrovascular diseases include stroke and other disorders of the blood vessels of the brain. Not age adjusted.

Deaths by Chronic Liver Disease and Cirrhosis in 1994

National Total = 25,406 Deaths*

ALPHA ORDER

RANK	STATE	DEATHS	% of USA
20	Alabama	405	1.59%
50	Alaska	41	0.16%
13	Arizona	558	2.20%
32	Arkansas	219	0.86%
1	California	3,648	14.36%
24	Colorado	330	1.30%
27	Connecticut	303	1.19%
46	Delaware	58	0.23%
2	Florida	1,897	7.47%
11	Georgia	610	2.40%
41	Hawaii	88	0.35%
44	Idaho	73	0.29%
5	Illinois	1,221	4.81%
17	Indiana	443	1.74%
36	Iowa	163	0.64%
34	Kansas	183	0.72%
25	Kentucky	314	1.24%
21	Louisiana	368	1.45%
37	Maine	120	0.47%
19	Maryland	415	1.63%
12	Massachusetts	593	2.33%
7	Michigan	1,038	4.09%
26	Minnesota	307	1.21%
30	Mississippi	235	0.92%
18	Missouri	437	1.72%
45	Montana	70	0.28%
39	Nebraska	97	0.38%
33	Nevada	209	0.82%
40	New Hampshire	91	0.36%
8	New Jersey	880	3.46%
31	New Mexico	232	0.91%
4	New York	1,835	7.22%
10	North Carolina	701	2.76%
48	North Dakota	49	0.19%
9	Ohio	844	3.32%
28	Oklahoma	287	1.13%
29	Oregon	260	1.02%
6	Pennsylvania	1,156	4.55%
38	Rhode Island	108	0.43%
22	South Carolina	352	1.39%
42	South Dakota	86	0.34%
14	Tennessee	496	1.95%
3	Texas	1,866	7.34%
43	Utah	82	0.32%
49	Vermont	47	0.18%
16	Virginia	444	1.75%
15	Washington	479	1.89%
35	West Virginia	175	0.69%
23	Wisconsin	338	1.33%
47	Wyoming	50	0.20%

RANK ORDER

RANK	STATE	DEATHS	% of USA
1	California	3,648	14.36%
2	Florida	1,897	7.47%
3	Texas	1,866	7.34%
4	New York	1,835	7.22%
5	Illinois	1,221	4.81%
6	Pennsylvania	1,156	4.55%
7	Michigan	1,038	4.09%
8	New Jersey	880	3.46%
9	Ohio	844	3.32%
10	North Carolina	701	2.76%
11	Georgia	610	2.40%
12	Massachusetts	593	2.33%
13	Arizona	558	2.20%
14	Tennessee	496	1.95%
15	Washington	479	1.89%
16	Virginia	444	1.75%
17	Indiana	443	1.74%
18	Missouri	437	1.72%
19	Maryland	415	1.63%
20	Alabama	405	1.59%
21	Louisiana	368	1.45%
22	South Carolina	352	1.39%
23	Wisconsin	338	1.33%
24	Colorado	330	1.30%
25	Kentucky	314	1.24%
26	Minnesota	307	1.21%
27	Connecticut	303	1.19%
28	Oklahoma	287	1.13%
29	Oregon	260	1.02%
30	Mississippi	235	0.92%
31	New Mexico	232	0.91%
32	Arkansas	219	0.86%
33	Nevada	209	0.82%
34	Kansas	183	0.72%
35	West Virginia	175	0.69%
36	Iowa	163	0.64%
37	Maine	120	0.47%
38	Rhode Island	108	0.43%
39	Nebraska	97	0.38%
40	New Hampshire	91	0.36%
41	Hawaii	88	0.35%
42	South Dakota	86	0.34%
43	Utah	82	0.32%
44	Idaho	73	0.29%
45	Montana	70	0.28%
46	Delaware	58	0.23%
47	Wyoming	50	0.20%
48	North Dakota	49	0.19%
49	Vermont	47	0.18%
50	Alaska	41	0.16%
	District of Columbia	105	0.41%

Source: U.S. Department of Health and Human Services, National Center for Health Statistics
"Monthly Vital Statistics Report" (Vol. 45, No. 3(S), September 30, 1996)
*By state of residence. Cirrhosis of the liver is characterized by the replacement of normal tissue with fibrous tissue and the loss of functional liver cells. It can result from alcohol abuse, nutritional deprivation, or infection especially by the hepatitis virus.

Death Rate by Chronic Liver Disease and Cirrhosis in 1994

National Rate = 9.8 Death per 100,000 Population*

ALPHA ORDER			RANK ORDER		
RANK	**STATE**	**RATE**	**RANK**	**STATE**	**RATE**
17	Alabama	9.6	1	Nevada	14.3
43	Alaska	6.8	2	New Mexico	14.0
3	Arizona	13.7	3	Arizona	13.7
25	Arkansas	8.9	4	Florida	13.6
6	California	11.6	5	South Dakota	11.9
23	Colorado	9.0	6	California	11.6
22	Connecticut	9.3	7	New Jersey	11.1
33	Delaware	8.2	8	Michigan	10.9
4	Florida	13.6	9	Rhode Island	10.8
28	Georgia	8.6	10	Wyoming	10.5
41	Hawaii	7.5	11	Illinois	10.4
47	Idaho	6.4	12	Texas	10.2
11	Illinois	10.4	13	New York	10.1
38	Indiana	7.7	14	North Carolina	9.9
49	Iowa	5.8	15	Massachusetts	9.8
42	Kansas	7.2	16	Maine	9.7
33	Kentucky	8.2	17	Alabama	9.6
29	Louisiana	8.5	17	Pennsylvania	9.6
16	Maine	9.7	17	South Carolina	9.6
31	Maryland	8.3	17	Tennessee	9.6
15	Massachusetts	9.8	17	West Virginia	9.6
8	Michigan	10.9	22	Connecticut	9.3
45	Minnesota	6.7	23	Colorado	9.0
26	Mississippi	8.8	23	Washington	9.0
31	Missouri	8.3	25	Arkansas	8.9
33	Montana	8.2	26	Mississippi	8.8
48	Nebraska	6.0	26	Oklahoma	8.8
1	Nevada	14.3	28	Georgia	8.6
37	New Hampshire	8.0	29	Louisiana	8.5
7	New Jersey	11.1	30	Oregon	8.4
2	New Mexico	14.0	31	Maryland	8.3
13	New York	10.1	31	Missouri	8.3
14	North Carolina	9.9	33	Delaware	8.2
38	North Dakota	7.7	33	Kentucky	8.2
40	Ohio	7.6	33	Montana	8.2
26	Oklahoma	8.8	36	Vermont	8.1
30	Oregon	8.4	37	New Hampshire	8.0
17	Pennsylvania	9.6	38	Indiana	7.7
9	Rhode Island	10.8	38	North Dakota	7.7
17	South Carolina	9.6	40	Ohio	7.6
5	South Dakota	11.9	41	Hawaii	7.5
17	Tennessee	9.6	42	Kansas	7.2
12	Texas	10.2	43	Alaska	6.8
50	Utah	4.3	43	Virginia	6.8
36	Vermont	8.1	45	Minnesota	6.7
43	Virginia	6.8	45	Wisconsin	6.7
23	Washington	9.0	47	Idaho	6.4
17	West Virginia	9.6	48	Nebraska	6.0
45	Wisconsin	6.7	49	Iowa	5.8
10	Wyoming	10.5	50	Utah	4.3
				District of Columbia	18.4

Source: U.S. Department of Health and Human Services, National Center for Health Statistics
  "Monthly Vital Statistics Report" (Vol. 45, No. 3(S), September 30, 1996)
By state of residence. Cirrhosis of the liver is characterized by the replacement of normal tissue with fibrous tissue and the loss of functional liver cells. It can result from alcohol abuse, nutritional deprivation, or infection especially by the hepatitis virus. Not age adjusted.

Deaths by Chronic Obstructive Pulmonary Diseases in 1994

National Total = 101,628 Deaths*

	ALPHA ORDER				RANK ORDER		
RANK	STATE	DEATHS	% of USA	RANK	STATE	DEATHS	% of USA
21	Alabama	1,802	1.77%	1	California	11,054	10.88%
50	Alaska	100	0.10%	2	Florida	7,167	7.05%
20	Arizona	1,874	1.84%	3	Texas	6,256	6.16%
31	Arkansas	1,176	1.16%	4	New York	6,115	6.02%
1	California	11,054	10.88%	5	Pennsylvania	5,248	5.16%
25	Colorado	1,516	1.49%	6	Ohio	4,820	4.74%
30	Connecticut	1,184	1.17%	7	Illinois	4,298	4.23%
46	Delaware	268	0.26%	8	Michigan	3,455	3.40%
2	Florida	7,167	7.05%	9	New Jersey	2,648	2.61%
12	Georgia	2,447	2.41%	10	North Carolina	2,567	2.53%
49	Hawaii	210	0.21%	11	Missouri	2,468	2.43%
39	Idaho	495	0.49%	12	Georgia	2,447	2.41%
7	Illinois	4,298	4.23%	13	Indiana	2,429	2.39%
13	Indiana	2,429	2.39%	14	Massachusetts	2,354	2.32%
28	Iowa	1,315	1.29%	15	Washington	2,221	2.19%
32	Kansas	1,107	1.09%	16	Virginia	2,179	2.14%
19	Kentucky	1,892	1.86%	17	Tennessee	2,176	2.14%
26	Louisiana	1,461	1.44%	18	Wisconsin	1,938	1.91%
38	Maine	631	0.62%	19	Kentucky	1,892	1.86%
22	Maryland	1,654	1.63%	20	Arizona	1,874	1.84%
14	Massachusetts	2,354	2.32%	21	Alabama	1,802	1.77%
8	Michigan	3,455	3.40%	22	Maryland	1,654	1.63%
23	Minnesota	1,567	1.54%	23	Minnesota	1,567	1.54%
34	Mississippi	949	0.93%	24	Oklahoma	1,556	1.53%
11	Missouri	2,468	2.43%	25	Colorado	1,516	1.49%
40	Montana	487	0.48%	26	Louisiana	1,461	1.44%
36	Nebraska	752	0.74%	27	Oregon	1,428	1.41%
35	Nevada	775	0.76%	28	Iowa	1,315	1.29%
41	New Hampshire	483	0.48%	29	South Carolina	1,312	1.29%
9	New Jersey	2,648	2.61%	30	Connecticut	1,184	1.17%
37	New Mexico	653	0.64%	31	Arkansas	1,176	1.16%
4	New York	6,115	6.02%	32	Kansas	1,107	1.09%
10	North Carolina	2,567	2.53%	33	West Virginia	1,067	1.05%
48	North Dakota	233	0.23%	34	Mississippi	949	0.93%
6	Ohio	4,820	4.74%	35	Nevada	775	0.76%
24	Oklahoma	1,556	1.53%	36	Nebraska	752	0.74%
27	Oregon	1,428	1.41%	37	New Mexico	653	0.64%
5	Pennsylvania	5,248	5.16%	38	Maine	631	0.62%
43	Rhode Island	380	0.37%	39	Idaho	495	0.49%
29	South Carolina	1,312	1.29%	40	Montana	487	0.48%
44	South Dakota	300	0.30%	41	New Hampshire	483	0.48%
17	Tennessee	2,176	2.14%	42	Utah	453	0.45%
3	Texas	6,256	6.16%	43	Rhode Island	380	0.37%
42	Utah	453	0.45%	44	South Dakota	300	0.30%
47	Vermont	267	0.26%	45	Wyoming	270	0.27%
16	Virginia	2,179	2.14%	46	Delaware	268	0.26%
15	Washington	2,221	2.19%	47	Vermont	267	0.26%
33	West Virginia	1,067	1.05%	48	North Dakota	233	0.23%
18	Wisconsin	1,938	1.91%	49	Hawaii	210	0.21%
45	Wyoming	270	0.27%	50	Alaska	100	0.10%
					District of Columbia	171	0.17%

Source: U.S. Department of Health and Human Services, National Center for Health Statistics
   "Monthly Vital Statistics Report" (Vol. 45, No. 3(S), September 30, 1996)
*Final data by state of residence. Includes allied conditions.

Death Rate by Chronic Obstructive Pulmonary Diseases in 1994

National Rate = 39.0 Deaths per 100,000 Population*

ALPHA ORDER

RANK	STATE	RATE
20	Alabama	42.7
50	Alaska	16.5
14	Arizona	46.0
8	Arkansas	47.9
39	California	35.2
26	Colorado	41.5
36	Connecticut	36.1
31	Delaware	37.9
5	Florida	51.4
40	Georgia	34.7
49	Hawaii	17.8
16	Idaho	43.7
32	Illinois	36.6
22	Indiana	42.2
11	Iowa	46.5
19	Kansas	43.3
7	Kentucky	49.4
43	Louisiana	33.9
6	Maine	50.9
47	Maryland	33.0
28	Massachusetts	39.0
34	Michigan	36.4
41	Minnesota	34.3
38	Mississippi	35.6
10	Missouri	46.8
2	Montana	56.9
12	Nebraska	46.3
4	Nevada	53.2
21	New Hampshire	42.5
45	New Jersey	33.5
27	New Mexico	39.5
44	New York	33.7
35	North Carolina	36.3
33	North Dakota	36.5
18	Ohio	43.4
9	Oklahoma	47.8
12	Oregon	46.3
17	Pennsylvania	43.5
29	Rhode Island	38.1
37	South Carolina	35.8
24	South Dakota	41.6
23	Tennessee	42.0
42	Texas	34.0
48	Utah	23.7
14	Vermont	46.0
46	Virginia	33.3
24	Washington	41.6
1	West Virginia	58.6
29	Wisconsin	38.1
3	Wyoming	56.7

RANK ORDER

RANK	STATE	RATE
1	West Virginia	58.6
2	Montana	56.9
3	Wyoming	56.7
4	Nevada	53.2
5	Florida	51.4
6	Maine	50.9
7	Kentucky	49.4
8	Arkansas	47.9
9	Oklahoma	47.8
10	Missouri	46.8
11	Iowa	46.5
12	Nebraska	46.3
12	Oregon	46.3
14	Arizona	46.0
14	Vermont	46.0
16	Idaho	43.7
17	Pennsylvania	43.5
18	Ohio	43.4
19	Kansas	43.3
20	Alabama	42.7
21	New Hampshire	42.5
22	Indiana	42.2
23	Tennessee	42.0
24	South Dakota	41.6
24	Washington	41.6
26	Colorado	41.5
27	New Mexico	39.5
28	Massachusetts	39.0
29	Rhode Island	38.1
29	Wisconsin	38.1
31	Delaware	37.9
32	Illinois	36.6
33	North Dakota	36.5
34	Michigan	36.4
35	North Carolina	36.3
36	Connecticut	36.1
37	South Carolina	35.8
38	Mississippi	35.6
39	California	35.2
40	Georgia	34.7
41	Minnesota	34.3
42	Texas	34.0
43	Louisiana	33.9
44	New York	33.7
45	New Jersey	33.5
46	Virginia	33.3
47	Maryland	33.0
48	Utah	23.7
49	Hawaii	17.8
50	Alaska	16.5
	District of Columbia	30.0

Source: U.S. Department of Health and Human Services, National Center for Health Statistics
   "Monthly Vital Statistics Report" (Vol. 45, No. 3(S), September 30, 1996)
*Final data by state of residence. Includes allied conditions. Not age adjusted.

Deaths by Diabetes Mellitus in 1994

National Total = 56,692 Deaths*

ALPHA ORDER

RANK	STATE	DEATHS	% of USA
19	Alabama	1,067	1.88%
50	Alaska	48	0.08%
25	Arizona	768	1.35%
31	Arkansas	538	0.95%
1	California	4,936	8.71%
34	Colorado	459	0.81%
28	Connecticut	626	1.10%
46	Delaware	166	0.29%
4	Florida	3,357	5.92%
17	Georgia	1,086	1.92%
47	Hawaii	156	0.28%
42	Idaho	202	0.36%
7	Illinois	2,590	4.57%
12	Indiana	1,397	2.46%
30	Iowa	620	1.09%
32	Kansas	509	0.90%
22	Kentucky	940	1.66%
11	Louisiana	1,445	2.55%
37	Maine	318	0.56%
14	Maryland	1,324	2.34%
13	Massachusetts	1,351	2.38%
8	Michigan	2,235	3.94%
24	Minnesota	853	1.50%
33	Mississippi	498	0.88%
15	Missouri	1,195	2.11%
41	Montana	215	0.38%
38	Nebraska	282	0.50%
43	Nevada	191	0.34%
39	New Hampshire	256	0.45%
9	New Jersey	2,178	3.84%
35	New Mexico	417	0.74%
3	New York	3,658	6.45%
10	North Carolina	1,599	2.82%
45	North Dakota	172	0.30%
6	Ohio	3,145	5.55%
27	Oklahoma	634	1.12%
26	Oregon	637	1.12%
5	Pennsylvania	3,292	5.81%
40	Rhode Island	242	0.43%
23	South Carolina	929	1.64%
44	South Dakota	173	0.31%
20	Tennessee	1,060	1.87%
2	Texas	4,373	7.71%
36	Utah	339	0.60%
48	Vermont	136	0.24%
16	Virginia	1,128	1.99%
21	Washington	976	1.72%
29	West Virginia	622	1.10%
18	Wisconsin	1,081	1.91%
49	Wyoming	78	0.14%

RANK ORDER

RANK	STATE	DEATHS	% of USA
1	California	4,936	8.71%
2	Texas	4,373	7.71%
3	New York	3,658	6.45%
4	Florida	3,357	5.92%
5	Pennsylvania	3,292	5.81%
6	Ohio	3,145	5.55%
7	Illinois	2,590	4.57%
8	Michigan	2,235	3.94%
9	New Jersey	2,178	3.84%
10	North Carolina	1,599	2.82%
11	Louisiana	1,445	2.55%
12	Indiana	1,397	2.46%
13	Massachusetts	1,351	2.38%
14	Maryland	1,324	2.34%
15	Missouri	1,195	2.11%
16	Virginia	1,128	1.99%
17	Georgia	1,086	1.92%
18	Wisconsin	1,081	1.91%
19	Alabama	1,067	1.88%
20	Tennessee	1,060	1.87%
21	Washington	976	1.72%
22	Kentucky	940	1.66%
23	South Carolina	929	1.64%
24	Minnesota	853	1.50%
25	Arizona	768	1.35%
26	Oregon	637	1.12%
27	Oklahoma	634	1.12%
28	Connecticut	626	1.10%
29	West Virginia	622	1.10%
30	Iowa	620	1.09%
31	Arkansas	538	0.95%
32	Kansas	509	0.90%
33	Mississippi	498	0.88%
34	Colorado	459	0.81%
35	New Mexico	417	0.74%
36	Utah	339	0.60%
37	Maine	318	0.56%
38	Nebraska	282	0.50%
39	New Hampshire	256	0.45%
40	Rhode Island	242	0.43%
41	Montana	215	0.38%
42	Idaho	202	0.36%
43	Nevada	191	0.34%
44	South Dakota	173	0.31%
45	North Dakota	172	0.30%
46	Delaware	166	0.29%
47	Hawaii	156	0.28%
48	Vermont	136	0.24%
49	Wyoming	78	0.14%
50	Alaska	48	0.08%
	District of Columbia	195	0.34%

Source: U.S. Department of Health and Human Services, National Center for Health Statistics
"Monthly Vital Statistics Report" (Vol. 45, No. 3(S), September 30, 1996)
*Final data by state of residence.

Death Rate by Diabetes Mellitus in 1994

National Rate = 21.8 Deaths per 100,000 Population*

ALPHA ORDER

RANK	STATE	RATE
10	Alabama	25.3
50	Alaska	7.9
36	Arizona	18.8
27	Arkansas	21.9
45	California	15.7
49	Colorado	12.6
35	Connecticut	19.1
19	Delaware	23.5
16	Florida	24.1
46	Georgia	15.4
47	Hawaii	13.2
40	Idaho	17.8
26	Illinois	22.0
14	Indiana	24.3
27	Iowa	21.9
33	Kansas	19.9
13	Kentucky	24.6
2	Louisiana	33.5
8	Maine	25.6
7	Maryland	26.4
25	Massachusetts	22.4
19	Michigan	23.5
37	Minnesota	18.7
37	Mississippi	18.7
22	Missouri	22.6
12	Montana	25.1
42	Nebraska	17.4
48	Nevada	13.1
24	New Hampshire	22.5
4	New Jersey	27.6
11	New Mexico	25.2
32	New York	20.1
22	North Carolina	22.6
6	North Dakota	27.0
3	Ohio	28.3
34	Oklahoma	19.5
30	Oregon	20.6
5	Pennsylvania	27.3
14	Rhode Island	24.3
9	South Carolina	25.4
17	South Dakota	24.0
31	Tennessee	20.5
18	Texas	23.8
40	Utah	17.8
21	Vermont	23.4
43	Virginia	17.2
39	Washington	18.3
1	West Virginia	34.1
29	Wisconsin	21.3
44	Wyoming	16.4

RANK ORDER

RANK	STATE	RATE
1	West Virginia	34.1
2	Louisiana	33.5
3	Ohio	28.3
4	New Jersey	27.6
5	Pennsylvania	27.3
6	North Dakota	27.0
7	Maryland	26.4
8	Maine	25.6
9	South Carolina	25.4
10	Alabama	25.3
11	New Mexico	25.2
12	Montana	25.1
13	Kentucky	24.6
14	Indiana	24.3
14	Rhode Island	24.3
16	Florida	24.1
17	South Dakota	24.0
18	Texas	23.8
19	Delaware	23.5
19	Michigan	23.5
21	Vermont	23.4
22	Missouri	22.6
22	North Carolina	22.6
24	New Hampshire	22.5
25	Massachusetts	22.4
26	Illinois	22.0
27	Arkansas	21.9
27	Iowa	21.9
29	Wisconsin	21.3
30	Oregon	20.6
31	Tennessee	20.5
32	New York	20.1
33	Kansas	19.9
34	Oklahoma	19.5
35	Connecticut	19.1
36	Arizona	18.8
37	Minnesota	18.7
37	Mississippi	18.7
39	Washington	18.3
40	Idaho	17.8
40	Utah	17.8
42	Nebraska	17.4
43	Virginia	17.2
44	Wyoming	16.4
45	California	15.7
46	Georgia	15.4
47	Hawaii	13.2
48	Nevada	13.1
49	Colorado	12.6
50	Alaska	7.9
	District of Columbia	34.2

Source: U.S. Department of Health and Human Services, National Center for Health Statistics
"Monthly Vital Statistics Report" (Vol. 45, No. 3(S), September 30, 1996)
*Final data by state of residence. Not age adjusted.

Deaths by Diseases of the Heart in 1994

National Total = 732,409 Deaths*

ALPHA ORDER

RANK	STATE	DEATHS	% of USA
18	Alabama	13,171	1.80%
50	Alaska	536	0.07%
25	Arizona	9,984	1.36%
30	Arkansas	8,354	1.14%
1	California	68,807	9.39%
34	Colorado	6,331	0.86%
27	Connecticut	9,742	1.33%
45	Delaware	1,990	0.27%
3	Florida	48,652	6.64%
13	Georgia	17,032	2.33%
44	Hawaii	2,274	0.31%
42	Idaho	2,425	0.33%
6	Illinois	35,386	4.83%
12	Indiana	17,381	2.37%
29	Iowa	9,246	1.26%
32	Kansas	7,431	1.01%
19	Kentucky	12,244	1.67%
21	Louisiana	11,968	1.63%
36	Maine	3,577	0.49%
20	Maryland	12,039	1.64%
14	Massachusetts	16,920	2.31%
8	Michigan	28,255	3.86%
24	Minnesota	10,308	1.41%
28	Mississippi	9,658	1.32%
11	Missouri	18,246	2.49%
47	Montana	1,922	0.26%
35	Nebraska	5,032	0.69%
37	Nevada	3,448	0.47%
40	New Hampshire	2,823	0.39%
9	New Jersey	23,668	3.23%
39	New Mexico	3,063	0.42%
2	New York	63,219	8.63%
10	North Carolina	19,270	2.63%
46	North Dakota	1,931	0.26%
7	Ohio	34,746	4.74%
23	Oklahoma	11,158	1.52%
31	Oregon	7,433	1.01%
4	Pennsylvania	44,092	6.02%
38	Rhode Island	3,180	0.43%
26	South Carolina	9,921	1.35%
43	South Dakota	2,285	0.31%
15	Tennessee	16,194	2.21%
5	Texas	41,618	5.68%
40	Utah	2,823	0.39%
48	Vermont	1,522	0.21%
16	Virginia	15,941	2.18%
22	Washington	11,203	1.53%
33	West Virginia	6,872	0.94%
17	Wisconsin	14,373	1.96%
49	Wyoming	965	0.13%

RANK ORDER

RANK	STATE	DEATHS	% of USA
1	California	68,807	9.39%
2	New York	63,219	8.63%
3	Florida	48,652	6.64%
4	Pennsylvania	44,092	6.02%
5	Texas	41,618	5.68%
6	Illinois	35,386	4.83%
7	Ohio	34,746	4.74%
8	Michigan	28,255	3.86%
9	New Jersey	23,668	3.23%
10	North Carolina	19,270	2.63%
11	Missouri	18,246	2.49%
12	Indiana	17,381	2.37%
13	Georgia	17,032	2.33%
14	Massachusetts	16,920	2.31%
15	Tennessee	16,194	2.21%
16	Virginia	15,941	2.18%
17	Wisconsin	14,373	1.96%
18	Alabama	13,171	1.80%
19	Kentucky	12,244	1.67%
20	Maryland	12,039	1.64%
21	Louisiana	11,968	1.63%
22	Washington	11,203	1.53%
23	Oklahoma	11,158	1.52%
24	Minnesota	10,308	1.41%
25	Arizona	9,984	1.36%
26	South Carolina	9,921	1.35%
27	Connecticut	9,742	1.33%
28	Mississippi	9,658	1.32%
29	Iowa	9,246	1.26%
30	Arkansas	8,354	1.14%
31	Oregon	7,433	1.01%
32	Kansas	7,431	1.01%
33	West Virginia	6,872	0.94%
34	Colorado	6,331	0.86%
35	Nebraska	5,032	0.69%
36	Maine	3,577	0.49%
37	Nevada	3,448	0.47%
38	Rhode Island	3,180	0.43%
39	New Mexico	3,063	0.42%
40	New Hampshire	2,823	0.39%
40	Utah	2,823	0.39%
42	Idaho	2,425	0.33%
43	South Dakota	2,285	0.31%
44	Hawaii	2,274	0.31%
45	Delaware	1,990	0.27%
46	North Dakota	1,931	0.26%
47	Montana	1,922	0.26%
48	Vermont	1,522	0.21%
49	Wyoming	965	0.13%
50	Alaska	536	0.07%
	District of Columbia	1,750	0.24%

Source: U.S. Department of Health and Human Services, National Center for Health Statistics
"Monthly Vital Statistics Report" (Vol. 45, No. 3(S), September 30, 1996)
*Final data by state of residence.

Death Rate by Diseases of the Heart in 1994

National Rate = 281.3 Deaths per 100,000 Population*

ALPHA ORDER

RANK	STATE	RATE
15	Alabama	312.2
50	Alaska	88.4
33	Arizona	245.0
8	Arkansas	340.6
42	California	218.9
48	Colorado	173.2
22	Connecticut	297.4
26	Delaware	281.7
4	Florida	348.7
35	Georgia	241.4
46	Hawaii	192.9
43	Idaho	214.0
19	Illinois	301.1
18	Indiana	302.2
9	Iowa	326.8
23	Kansas	291.0
10	Kentucky	320.0
28	Louisiana	277.4
24	Maine	288.4
37	Maryland	240.5
27	Massachusetts	280.1
21	Michigan	297.5
40	Minnesota	225.7
3	Mississippi	361.8
6	Missouri	345.7
41	Montana	224.5
16	Nebraska	310.1
38	Nevada	236.6
32	New Hampshire	248.3
20	New Jersey	299.4
47	New Mexico	185.2
5	New York	347.9
29	North Carolina	272.6
17	North Dakota	302.7
13	Ohio	313.0
7	Oklahoma	342.5
36	Oregon	240.8
2	Pennsylvania	365.8
11	Rhode Island	319.0
30	South Carolina	270.8
12	South Dakota	316.8
14	Tennessee	312.9
39	Texas	226.5
49	Utah	148.0
31	Vermont	262.3
34	Virginia	243.3
44	Washington	209.7
1	West Virginia	377.2
25	Wisconsin	282.8
45	Wyoming	202.7

RANK ORDER

RANK	STATE	RATE
1	West Virginia	377.2
2	Pennsylvania	365.8
3	Mississippi	361.8
4	Florida	348.7
5	New York	347.9
6	Missouri	345.7
7	Oklahoma	342.5
8	Arkansas	340.6
9	Iowa	326.8
10	Kentucky	320.0
11	Rhode Island	319.0
12	South Dakota	316.8
13	Ohio	313.0
14	Tennessee	312.9
15	Alabama	312.2
16	Nebraska	310.1
17	North Dakota	302.7
18	Indiana	302.2
19	Illinois	301.1
20	New Jersey	299.4
21	Michigan	297.5
22	Connecticut	297.4
23	Kansas	291.0
24	Maine	288.4
25	Wisconsin	282.8
26	Delaware	281.7
27	Massachusetts	280.1
28	Louisiana	277.4
29	North Carolina	272.6
30	South Carolina	270.8
31	Vermont	262.3
32	New Hampshire	248.3
33	Arizona	245.0
34	Virginia	243.3
35	Georgia	241.4
36	Oregon	240.8
37	Maryland	240.5
38	Nevada	236.6
39	Texas	226.5
40	Minnesota	225.7
41	Montana	224.5
42	California	218.9
43	Idaho	214.0
44	Washington	209.7
45	Wyoming	202.7
46	Hawaii	192.9
47	New Mexico	185.2
48	Colorado	173.2
49	Utah	148.0
50	Alaska	88.4

District of Columbia	306.9

Source: U.S. Department of Health and Human Services, National Center for Health Statistics
    "Monthly Vital Statistics Report" (Vol. 45, No. 3(S), September 30, 1996)
Final data by state of residence. Not age adjusted.

Deaths by Malignant Neoplasms in 1994

National Total = 534,310 Deaths*

ALPHA ORDER

RANK	STATE	DEATHS	% of USA
20	Alabama	9,406	1.76%
50	Alaska	568	0.11%
24	Arizona	7,966	1.49%
30	Arkansas	5,914	1.11%
1	California	51,453	9.63%
32	Colorado	5,427	1.02%
26	Connecticut	7,126	1.33%
45	Delaware	1,626	0.30%
3	Florida	36,739	6.88%
13	Georgia	12,350	2.31%
43	Hawaii	1,765	0.33%
42	Idaho	1,848	0.35%
6	Illinois	25,142	4.71%
14	Indiana	12,105	2.27%
28	Iowa	6,608	1.24%
33	Kansas	5,366	1.00%
22	Kentucky	8,899	1.67%
21	Louisiana	8,959	1.68%
36	Maine	2,977	0.56%
18	Maryland	10,075	1.89%
11	Massachusetts	13,892	2.60%
8	Michigan	19,470	3.64%
23	Minnesota	8,574	1.60%
31	Mississippi	5,618	1.05%
15	Missouri	11,989	2.24%
44	Montana	1,746	0.33%
35	Nebraska	3,278	0.61%
37	Nevada	2,967	0.56%
40	New Hampshire	2,269	0.42%
9	New Jersey	18,375	3.44%
38	New Mexico	2,600	0.49%
2	New York	39,174	7.33%
10	North Carolina	14,594	2.73%
47	North Dakota	1,358	0.25%
7	Ohio	24,947	4.67%
27	Oklahoma	7,067	1.32%
29	Oregon	6,539	1.22%
5	Pennsylvania	30,359	5.68%
39	Rhode Island	2,429	0.45%
25	South Carolina	7,414	1.39%
46	South Dakota	1,472	0.28%
16	Tennessee	11,375	2.13%
4	Texas	31,421	5.88%
41	Utah	2,092	0.39%
48	Vermont	1,157	0.22%
12	Virginia	12,622	2.36%
19	Washington	9,701	1.82%
34	West Virginia	4,734	0.89%
17	Wisconsin	10,419	1.95%
49	Wyoming	777	0.15%

RANK ORDER

RANK	STATE	DEATHS	% of USA
1	California	51,453	9.63%
2	New York	39,174	7.33%
3	Florida	36,739	6.88%
4	Texas	31,421	5.88%
5	Pennsylvania	30,359	5.68%
6	Illinois	25,142	4.71%
7	Ohio	24,947	4.67%
8	Michigan	19,470	3.64%
9	New Jersey	18,375	3.44%
10	North Carolina	14,594	2.73%
11	Massachusetts	13,892	2.60%
12	Virginia	12,622	2.36%
13	Georgia	12,350	2.31%
14	Indiana	12,105	2.27%
15	Missouri	11,989	2.24%
16	Tennessee	11,375	2.13%
17	Wisconsin	10,419	1.95%
18	Maryland	10,075	1.89%
19	Washington	9,701	1.82%
20	Alabama	9,406	1.76%
21	Louisiana	8,959	1.68%
22	Kentucky	8,899	1.67%
23	Minnesota	8,574	1.60%
24	Arizona	7,966	1.49%
25	South Carolina	7,414	1.39%
26	Connecticut	7,126	1.33%
27	Oklahoma	7,067	1.32%
28	Iowa	6,608	1.24%
29	Oregon	6,539	1.22%
30	Arkansas	5,914	1.11%
31	Mississippi	5,618	1.05%
32	Colorado	5,427	1.02%
33	Kansas	5,366	1.00%
34	West Virginia	4,734	0.89%
35	Nebraska	3,278	0.61%
36	Maine	2,977	0.56%
37	Nevada	2,967	0.56%
38	New Mexico	2,600	0.49%
39	Rhode Island	2,429	0.45%
40	New Hampshire	2,269	0.42%
41	Utah	2,092	0.39%
42	Idaho	1,848	0.35%
43	Hawaii	1,765	0.33%
44	Montana	1,746	0.33%
45	Delaware	1,626	0.30%
46	South Dakota	1,472	0.28%
47	North Dakota	1,358	0.25%
48	Vermont	1,157	0.22%
49	Wyoming	777	0.15%
50	Alaska	568	0.11%
	District of Columbia	1,562	0.29%

Source: U.S. Department of Health and Human Services, National Center for Health Statistics
   "Monthly Vital Statistics Report" (Vol. 45, No. 3(S), September 30, 1996)
*Final data by state of residence. Neoplasms are abnormal tissue, tumors. Includes many cancers.

Death Rate by Malignant Neoplasms in 1994

National Rate = 205.2 Deaths per 100,000 Population*

<table>
<tr><td colspan="3">ALPHA ORDER</td><td colspan="3">RANK ORDER</td></tr>
<tr><td>RANK</td><td>STATE</td><td>RATE</td><td>RANK</td><td>STATE</td><td>RATE</td></tr>
<tr><td>14</td><td>Alabama</td><td>223.0</td><td>1</td><td>Florida</td><td>263.3</td></tr>
<tr><td>50</td><td>Alaska</td><td>93.7</td><td>2</td><td>West Virginia</td><td>259.8</td></tr>
<tr><td>37</td><td>Arizona</td><td>195.5</td><td>3</td><td>Pennsylvania</td><td>251.9</td></tr>
<tr><td>5</td><td>Arkansas</td><td>241.1</td><td>4</td><td>Rhode Island</td><td>243.7</td></tr>
<tr><td>43</td><td>California</td><td>163.7</td><td>5</td><td>Arkansas</td><td>241.1</td></tr>
<tr><td>48</td><td>Colorado</td><td>148.5</td><td>6</td><td>Maine</td><td>240.0</td></tr>
<tr><td>16</td><td>Connecticut</td><td>217.6</td><td>7</td><td>Iowa</td><td>233.6</td></tr>
<tr><td>10</td><td>Delaware</td><td>230.2</td><td>8</td><td>Kentucky</td><td>232.5</td></tr>
<tr><td>1</td><td>Florida</td><td>263.3</td><td>8</td><td>New Jersey</td><td>232.5</td></tr>
<tr><td>41</td><td>Georgia</td><td>175.0</td><td>10</td><td>Delaware</td><td>230.2</td></tr>
<tr><td>47</td><td>Hawaii</td><td>149.8</td><td>11</td><td>Massachusetts</td><td>230.0</td></tr>
<tr><td>45</td><td>Idaho</td><td>163.1</td><td>12</td><td>Missouri</td><td>227.2</td></tr>
<tr><td>19</td><td>Illinois</td><td>213.9</td><td>13</td><td>Ohio</td><td>224.7</td></tr>
<tr><td>23</td><td>Indiana</td><td>210.4</td><td>14</td><td>Alabama</td><td>223.0</td></tr>
<tr><td>7</td><td>Iowa</td><td>233.6</td><td>15</td><td>Tennessee</td><td>219.8</td></tr>
<tr><td>24</td><td>Kansas</td><td>210.1</td><td>16</td><td>Connecticut</td><td>217.6</td></tr>
<tr><td>8</td><td>Kentucky</td><td>232.5</td><td>17</td><td>Oklahoma</td><td>216.9</td></tr>
<tr><td>25</td><td>Louisiana</td><td>207.6</td><td>18</td><td>New York</td><td>215.6</td></tr>
<tr><td>6</td><td>Maine</td><td>240.0</td><td>19</td><td>Illinois</td><td>213.9</td></tr>
<tr><td>34</td><td>Maryland</td><td>201.2</td><td>20</td><td>North Dakota</td><td>212.9</td></tr>
<tr><td>11</td><td>Massachusetts</td><td>230.0</td><td>21</td><td>Oregon</td><td>211.9</td></tr>
<tr><td>27</td><td>Michigan</td><td>205.0</td><td>22</td><td>Mississippi</td><td>210.5</td></tr>
<tr><td>39</td><td>Minnesota</td><td>187.7</td><td>23</td><td>Indiana</td><td>210.4</td></tr>
<tr><td>22</td><td>Mississippi</td><td>210.5</td><td>24</td><td>Kansas</td><td>210.1</td></tr>
<tr><td>12</td><td>Missouri</td><td>227.2</td><td>25</td><td>Louisiana</td><td>207.6</td></tr>
<tr><td>30</td><td>Montana</td><td>204.0</td><td>26</td><td>North Carolina</td><td>206.4</td></tr>
<tr><td>33</td><td>Nebraska</td><td>202.0</td><td>27</td><td>Michigan</td><td>205.0</td></tr>
<tr><td>31</td><td>Nevada</td><td>203.6</td><td>27</td><td>Wisconsin</td><td>205.0</td></tr>
<tr><td>35</td><td>New Hampshire</td><td>199.6</td><td>29</td><td>South Dakota</td><td>204.1</td></tr>
<tr><td>8</td><td>New Jersey</td><td>232.5</td><td>30</td><td>Montana</td><td>204.0</td></tr>
<tr><td>46</td><td>New Mexico</td><td>157.2</td><td>31</td><td>Nevada</td><td>203.6</td></tr>
<tr><td>18</td><td>New York</td><td>215.6</td><td>32</td><td>South Carolina</td><td>202.3</td></tr>
<tr><td>26</td><td>North Carolina</td><td>206.4</td><td>33</td><td>Nebraska</td><td>202.0</td></tr>
<tr><td>20</td><td>North Dakota</td><td>212.9</td><td>34</td><td>Maryland</td><td>201.2</td></tr>
<tr><td>13</td><td>Ohio</td><td>224.7</td><td>35</td><td>New Hampshire</td><td>199.6</td></tr>
<tr><td>17</td><td>Oklahoma</td><td>216.9</td><td>36</td><td>Vermont</td><td>199.4</td></tr>
<tr><td>21</td><td>Oregon</td><td>211.9</td><td>37</td><td>Arizona</td><td>195.5</td></tr>
<tr><td>3</td><td>Pennsylvania</td><td>251.9</td><td>38</td><td>Virginia</td><td>192.7</td></tr>
<tr><td>4</td><td>Rhode Island</td><td>243.7</td><td>39</td><td>Minnesota</td><td>187.7</td></tr>
<tr><td>32</td><td>South Carolina</td><td>202.3</td><td>40</td><td>Washington</td><td>181.6</td></tr>
<tr><td>29</td><td>South Dakota</td><td>204.1</td><td>41</td><td>Georgia</td><td>175.0</td></tr>
<tr><td>15</td><td>Tennessee</td><td>219.8</td><td>42</td><td>Texas</td><td>171.0</td></tr>
<tr><td>42</td><td>Texas</td><td>171.0</td><td>43</td><td>California</td><td>163.7</td></tr>
<tr><td>49</td><td>Utah</td><td>109.6</td><td>44</td><td>Wyoming</td><td>163.2</td></tr>
<tr><td>36</td><td>Vermont</td><td>199.4</td><td>45</td><td>Idaho</td><td>163.1</td></tr>
<tr><td>38</td><td>Virginia</td><td>192.7</td><td>46</td><td>New Mexico</td><td>157.2</td></tr>
<tr><td>40</td><td>Washington</td><td>181.6</td><td>47</td><td>Hawaii</td><td>149.8</td></tr>
<tr><td>2</td><td>West Virginia</td><td>259.8</td><td>48</td><td>Colorado</td><td>148.5</td></tr>
<tr><td>27</td><td>Wisconsin</td><td>205.0</td><td>49</td><td>Utah</td><td>109.6</td></tr>
<tr><td>44</td><td>Wyoming</td><td>163.2</td><td>50</td><td>Alaska</td><td>93.7</td></tr>
<tr><td></td><td></td><td></td><td></td><td>District of Columbia</td><td>274.0</td></tr>
</table>

Source: U.S. Department of Health and Human Services, National Center for Health Statistics
    "Monthly Vital Statistics Report" (Vol. 45, No. 3(S), September 30, 1996)
*Final data by state of residence. Neoplasms are abnormal tissue, tumors. Includes many cancers. Not age adjusted.

Deaths by Pneumonia and Influenza in 1994

National Total = 81,473 Deaths*

ALPHA ORDER					RANK ORDER			
RANK	STATE	DEATHS	% of USA		RANK	STATE	DEATHS	% of USA
21	Alabama	1,424	1.75%		1	California	10,253	12.58%
50	Alaska	50	0.06%		2	New York	6,266	7.69%
24	Arizona	1,205	1.48%		3	Pennsylvania	4,241	5.21%
28	Arkansas	1,011	1.24%		4	Texas	3,921	4.81%
1	California	10,253	12.58%		5	Illinois	3,890	4.77%
32	Colorado	880	1.08%		6	Florida	3,798	4.66%
26	Connecticut	1,170	1.44%		7	Ohio	3,305	4.06%
47	Delaware	200	0.25%		8	Michigan	2,878	3.53%
6	Florida	3,798	4.66%		9	Massachusetts	2,633	3.23%
13	Georgia	2,059	2.53%		10	New Jersey	2,290	2.81%
44	Hawaii	279	0.34%		11	Missouri	2,246	2.76%
39	Idaho	345	0.42%		12	North Carolina	2,210	2.71%
5	Illinois	3,890	4.77%		13	Georgia	2,059	2.53%
15	Indiana	1,776	2.18%		14	Tennessee	2,036	2.50%
23	Iowa	1,222	1.50%		15	Indiana	1,776	2.18%
29	Kansas	947	1.16%		16	Virginia	1,755	2.15%
18	Kentucky	1,505	1.85%		17	Wisconsin	1,749	2.15%
27	Louisiana	1,081	1.33%		18	Kentucky	1,505	1.85%
38	Maine	353	0.43%		19	Washington	1,457	1.79%
25	Maryland	1,188	1.46%		20	Minnesota	1,456	1.79%
9	Massachusetts	2,633	3.23%		21	Alabama	1,424	1.75%
8	Michigan	2,878	3.53%		22	Oklahoma	1,393	1.71%
20	Minnesota	1,456	1.79%		23	Iowa	1,222	1.50%
30	Mississippi	929	1.14%		24	Arizona	1,205	1.48%
11	Missouri	2,246	2.76%		25	Maryland	1,188	1.46%
42	Montana	293	0.36%		26	Connecticut	1,170	1.44%
35	Nebraska	617	0.76%		27	Louisiana	1,081	1.33%
40	Nevada	319	0.39%		28	Arkansas	1,011	1.24%
45	New Hampshire	258	0.32%		29	Kansas	947	1.16%
10	New Jersey	2,290	2.81%		30	Mississippi	929	1.14%
37	New Mexico	414	0.51%		31	Oregon	897	1.10%
2	New York	6,266	7.69%		32	Colorado	880	1.08%
12	North Carolina	2,210	2.71%		33	South Carolina	845	1.04%
46	North Dakota	203	0.25%		34	West Virginia	679	0.83%
7	Ohio	3,305	4.06%		35	Nebraska	617	0.76%
22	Oklahoma	1,393	1.71%		36	Utah	469	0.58%
31	Oregon	897	1.10%		37	New Mexico	414	0.51%
3	Pennsylvania	4,241	5.21%		38	Maine	353	0.43%
41	Rhode Island	299	0.37%		39	Idaho	345	0.42%
33	South Carolina	845	1.04%		40	Nevada	319	0.39%
43	South Dakota	284	0.35%		41	Rhode Island	299	0.37%
14	Tennessee	2,036	2.50%		42	Montana	293	0.36%
4	Texas	3,921	4.81%		43	South Dakota	284	0.35%
36	Utah	469	0.58%		44	Hawaii	279	0.34%
48	Vermont	178	0.22%		45	New Hampshire	258	0.32%
16	Virginia	1,755	2.15%		46	North Dakota	203	0.25%
19	Washington	1,457	1.79%		47	Delaware	200	0.25%
34	West Virginia	679	0.83%		48	Vermont	178	0.22%
17	Wisconsin	1,749	2.15%		49	Wyoming	121	0.15%
49	Wyoming	121	0.15%		50	Alaska	50	0.06%
						District of Columbia	196	0.24%

Source: U.S. Department of Health and Human Services, National Center for Health Statistics
"Monthly Vital Statistics Report" (Vol. 45, No. 3(S), September 30, 1996)
*Final data by state of residence.

Death Rate by Pneumonia and Influenza in 1994

National Rate = 31.3 Deaths per 100,000 Population*

ALPHA ORDER   RANK ORDER

RANK	STATE	RATE		RANK	STATE	RATE
18	Alabama	33.8		1	Massachusetts	43.6
50	Alaska	8.2		2	Iowa	43.2
30	Arizona	29.6		3	Oklahoma	42.8
5	Arkansas	41.2		4	Missouri	42.6
20	California	32.6		5	Arkansas	41.2
43	Colorado	24.1		6	South Dakota	39.4
12	Connecticut	35.7		7	Kentucky	39.3
35	Delaware	28.3		7	Tennessee	39.3
37	Florida	27.2		9	Nebraska	38.0
31	Georgia	29.2		10	West Virginia	37.3
44	Hawaii	23.7		11	Kansas	37.1
25	Idaho	30.4		12	Connecticut	35.7
19	Illinois	33.1		13	Pennsylvania	35.2
24	Indiana	30.9		14	Mississippi	34.8
2	Iowa	43.2		15	New York	34.5
11	Kansas	37.1		16	Wisconsin	34.4
7	Kentucky	39.3		17	Montana	34.2
39	Louisiana	25.1		18	Alabama	33.8
34	Maine	28.5		19	Illinois	33.1
44	Maryland	23.7		20	California	32.6
1	Massachusetts	43.6		21	Minnesota	31.9
26	Michigan	30.3		22	North Dakota	31.8
21	Minnesota	31.9		23	North Carolina	31.3
14	Mississippi	34.8		24	Indiana	30.9
4	Missouri	42.6		25	Idaho	30.4
17	Montana	34.2		26	Michigan	30.3
9	Nebraska	38.0		27	Rhode Island	30.0
48	Nevada	21.9		27	Vermont	30.0
47	New Hampshire	22.7		29	Ohio	29.8
33	New Jersey	29.0		30	Arizona	29.6
40	New Mexico	25.0		31	Georgia	29.2
15	New York	34.5		32	Oregon	29.1
23	North Carolina	31.3		33	New Jersey	29.0
22	North Dakota	31.8		34	Maine	28.5
29	Ohio	29.8		35	Delaware	28.3
3	Oklahoma	42.8		36	Washington	27.3
32	Oregon	29.1		37	Florida	27.2
13	Pennsylvania	35.2		38	Virginia	26.8
27	Rhode Island	30.0		39	Louisiana	25.1
46	South Carolina	23.1		40	New Mexico	25.0
6	South Dakota	39.4		40	Wyoming	25.0
7	Tennessee	39.3		42	Utah	24.6
49	Texas	21.3		43	Colorado	24.1
42	Utah	24.6		44	Hawaii	23.7
27	Vermont	30.0		44	Maryland	23.7
38	Virginia	26.8		46	South Carolina	23.1
36	Washington	27.3		47	New Hampshire	22.7
10	West Virginia	37.3		48	Nevada	21.9
16	Wisconsin	34.4		49	Texas	21.3
40	Wyoming	25.0		50	Alaska	8.2

	District of Columbia	34.4

Source: U.S. Department of Health and Human Services, National Center for Health Statistics
        "Monthly Vital Statistics Report" (Vol. 45, No. 3(S), September 30, 1996)
*Final data by state of residence. Not age adjusted.

Deaths by Complications of Pregnancy and Childbirth in 1994

National Total = 328 Deaths*

ALPHA ORDER

RANK	STATE	DEATHS	% of USA
10	Alabama	10	3.05%
32	Alaska	1	0.30%
23	Arizona	3	0.91%
40	Arkansas	0	0.00%
1	California	55	16.77%
32	Colorado	1	0.30%
17	Connecticut	6	1.83%
40	Delaware	0	0.00%
4	Florida	18	5.49%
6	Georgia	15	4.57%
27	Hawaii	2	0.61%
27	Idaho	2	0.61%
7	Illinois	13	3.96%
32	Indiana	1	0.30%
40	Iowa	0	0.00%
27	Kansas	2	0.61%
23	Kentucky	3	0.91%
15	Louisiana	7	2.13%
40	Maine	0	0.00%
8	Maryland	12	3.66%
40	Massachusetts	0	0.00%
13	Michigan	8	2.44%
23	Minnesota	3	0.91%
19	Mississippi	5	1.52%
17	Missouri	6	1.83%
40	Montana	0	0.00%
32	Nebraska	1	0.30%
32	Nevada	1	0.30%
40	New Hampshire	0	0.00%
9	New Jersey	11	3.35%
19	New Mexico	5	1.52%
2	New York	38	11.59%
5	North Carolina	16	4.88%
27	North Dakota	2	0.61%
10	Ohio	10	3.05%
22	Oklahoma	4	1.22%
27	Oregon	2	0.61%
13	Pennsylvania	8	2.44%
40	Rhode Island	0	0.00%
19	South Carolina	5	1.52%
40	South Dakota	0	0.00%
10	Tennessee	10	3.05%
3	Texas	27	8.23%
32	Utah	1	0.30%
32	Vermont	1	0.30%
15	Virginia	7	2.13%
23	Washington	3	0.91%
32	West Virginia	1	0.30%
40	Wisconsin	0	0.00%
40	Wyoming	0	0.00%

RANK ORDER

RANK	STATE	DEATHS	% of USA
1	California	55	16.77%
2	New York	38	11.59%
3	Texas	27	8.23%
4	Florida	18	5.49%
5	North Carolina	16	4.88%
6	Georgia	15	4.57%
7	Illinois	13	3.96%
8	Maryland	12	3.66%
9	New Jersey	11	3.35%
10	Alabama	10	3.05%
10	Ohio	10	3.05%
10	Tennessee	10	3.05%
13	Michigan	8	2.44%
13	Pennsylvania	8	2.44%
15	Louisiana	7	2.13%
15	Virginia	7	2.13%
17	Connecticut	6	1.83%
17	Missouri	6	1.83%
19	Mississippi	5	1.52%
19	New Mexico	5	1.52%
19	South Carolina	5	1.52%
22	Oklahoma	4	1.22%
23	Arizona	3	0.91%
23	Kentucky	3	0.91%
23	Minnesota	3	0.91%
23	Washington	3	0.91%
27	Hawaii	2	0.61%
27	Idaho	2	0.61%
27	Kansas	2	0.61%
27	North Dakota	2	0.61%
27	Oregon	2	0.61%
32	Alaska	1	0.30%
32	Colorado	1	0.30%
32	Indiana	1	0.30%
32	Nebraska	1	0.30%
32	Nevada	1	0.30%
32	Utah	1	0.30%
32	Vermont	1	0.30%
32	West Virginia	1	0.30%
40	Arkansas	0	0.00%
40	Delaware	0	0.00%
40	Iowa	0	0.00%
40	Maine	0	0.00%
40	Massachusetts	0	0.00%
40	Montana	0	0.00%
40	New Hampshire	0	0.00%
40	Rhode Island	0	0.00%
40	South Dakota	0	0.00%
40	Wisconsin	0	0.00%
40	Wyoming	0	0.00%
	District of Columbia	2	0.61%

Source: U.S. Department of Health and Human Services, National Center for Health Statistics
unpublished (http://wonder.cdc.gov/WONDER/)
*By state of residence.

Death Rate by Complications of Pregnancy and Childbirth in 1994

National Rate = 0.12 Deaths per 100,000 Population*

<table>
<thead>
<tr><th colspan="3">ALPHA ORDER</th><th colspan="3">RANK ORDER</th></tr>
<tr><th>RANK</th><th>STATE</th><th>RATE</th><th>RANK</th><th>STATE</th><th>RATE</th></tr>
</thead>
<tbody>
<tr><td>3</td><td>Alabama</td><td>0.23</td><td>1</td><td>North Dakota</td><td>0.31</td></tr>
<tr><td>14</td><td>Alaska</td><td>0.16</td><td>2</td><td>New Mexico</td><td>0.30</td></tr>
<tr><td>27</td><td>Arizona</td><td>0.07</td><td>3</td><td>Alabama</td><td>0.23</td></tr>
<tr><td>40</td><td>Arkansas</td><td>0.00</td><td>3</td><td>Maryland</td><td>0.23</td></tr>
<tr><td>11</td><td>California</td><td>0.17</td><td>5</td><td>North Carolina</td><td>0.22</td></tr>
<tr><td>38</td><td>Colorado</td><td>0.02</td><td>6</td><td>Georgia</td><td>0.21</td></tr>
<tr><td>9</td><td>Connecticut</td><td>0.18</td><td>7</td><td>New York</td><td>0.20</td></tr>
<tr><td>40</td><td>Delaware</td><td>0.00</td><td>8</td><td>Tennessee</td><td>0.19</td></tr>
<tr><td>20</td><td>Florida</td><td>0.12</td><td>9</td><td>Connecticut</td><td>0.18</td></tr>
<tr><td>6</td><td>Georgia</td><td>0.21</td><td>9</td><td>Mississippi</td><td>0.18</td></tr>
<tr><td>14</td><td>Hawaii</td><td>0.16</td><td>11</td><td>California</td><td>0.17</td></tr>
<tr><td>11</td><td>Idaho</td><td>0.17</td><td>11</td><td>Idaho</td><td>0.17</td></tr>
<tr><td>22</td><td>Illinois</td><td>0.11</td><td>11</td><td>Vermont</td><td>0.17</td></tr>
<tr><td>39</td><td>Indiana</td><td>0.01</td><td>14</td><td>Alaska</td><td>0.16</td></tr>
<tr><td>40</td><td>Iowa</td><td>0.00</td><td>14</td><td>Hawaii</td><td>0.16</td></tr>
<tr><td>27</td><td>Kansas</td><td>0.07</td><td>14</td><td>Louisiana</td><td>0.16</td></tr>
<tr><td>27</td><td>Kentucky</td><td>0.07</td><td>17</td><td>Texas</td><td>0.14</td></tr>
<tr><td>14</td><td>Louisiana</td><td>0.16</td><td>18</td><td>New Jersey</td><td>0.13</td></tr>
<tr><td>40</td><td>Maine</td><td>0.00</td><td>18</td><td>South Carolina</td><td>0.13</td></tr>
<tr><td>3</td><td>Maryland</td><td>0.23</td><td>20</td><td>Florida</td><td>0.12</td></tr>
<tr><td>40</td><td>Massachusetts</td><td>0.00</td><td>20</td><td>Oklahoma</td><td>0.12</td></tr>
<tr><td>26</td><td>Michigan</td><td>0.08</td><td>22</td><td>Illinois</td><td>0.11</td></tr>
<tr><td>30</td><td>Minnesota</td><td>0.06</td><td>22</td><td>Missouri</td><td>0.11</td></tr>
<tr><td>9</td><td>Mississippi</td><td>0.18</td><td>24</td><td>Virginia</td><td>0.10</td></tr>
<tr><td>22</td><td>Missouri</td><td>0.11</td><td>25</td><td>Ohio</td><td>0.09</td></tr>
<tr><td>40</td><td>Montana</td><td>0.00</td><td>26</td><td>Michigan</td><td>0.08</td></tr>
<tr><td>30</td><td>Nebraska</td><td>0.06</td><td>27</td><td>Arizona</td><td>0.07</td></tr>
<tr><td>30</td><td>Nevada</td><td>0.06</td><td>27</td><td>Kansas</td><td>0.07</td></tr>
<tr><td>40</td><td>New Hampshire</td><td>0.00</td><td>27</td><td>Kentucky</td><td>0.07</td></tr>
<tr><td>18</td><td>New Jersey</td><td>0.13</td><td>30</td><td>Minnesota</td><td>0.06</td></tr>
<tr><td>2</td><td>New Mexico</td><td>0.30</td><td>30</td><td>Nebraska</td><td>0.06</td></tr>
<tr><td>7</td><td>New York</td><td>0.20</td><td>30</td><td>Nevada</td><td>0.06</td></tr>
<tr><td>5</td><td>North Carolina</td><td>0.22</td><td>30</td><td>Oregon</td><td>0.06</td></tr>
<tr><td>1</td><td>North Dakota</td><td>0.31</td><td>30</td><td>Pennsylvania</td><td>0.06</td></tr>
<tr><td>25</td><td>Ohio</td><td>0.09</td><td>35</td><td>Utah</td><td>0.05</td></tr>
<tr><td>20</td><td>Oklahoma</td><td>0.12</td><td>35</td><td>Washington</td><td>0.05</td></tr>
<tr><td>30</td><td>Oregon</td><td>0.06</td><td>35</td><td>West Virginia</td><td>0.05</td></tr>
<tr><td>30</td><td>Pennsylvania</td><td>0.06</td><td>38</td><td>Colorado</td><td>0.02</td></tr>
<tr><td>40</td><td>Rhode Island</td><td>0.00</td><td>39</td><td>Indiana</td><td>0.01</td></tr>
<tr><td>18</td><td>South Carolina</td><td>0.13</td><td>40</td><td>Arkansas</td><td>0.00</td></tr>
<tr><td>40</td><td>South Dakota</td><td>0.00</td><td>40</td><td>Delaware</td><td>0.00</td></tr>
<tr><td>8</td><td>Tennessee</td><td>0.19</td><td>40</td><td>Iowa</td><td>0.00</td></tr>
<tr><td>17</td><td>Texas</td><td>0.14</td><td>40</td><td>Maine</td><td>0.00</td></tr>
<tr><td>35</td><td>Utah</td><td>0.05</td><td>40</td><td>Massachusetts</td><td>0.00</td></tr>
<tr><td>11</td><td>Vermont</td><td>0.17</td><td>40</td><td>Montana</td><td>0.00</td></tr>
<tr><td>24</td><td>Virginia</td><td>0.10</td><td>40</td><td>New Hampshire</td><td>0.00</td></tr>
<tr><td>35</td><td>Washington</td><td>0.05</td><td>40</td><td>Rhode Island</td><td>0.00</td></tr>
<tr><td>35</td><td>West Virginia</td><td>0.05</td><td>40</td><td>South Dakota</td><td>0.00</td></tr>
<tr><td>40</td><td>Wisconsin</td><td>0.00</td><td>40</td><td>Wisconsin</td><td>0.00</td></tr>
<tr><td>40</td><td>Wyoming</td><td>0.00</td><td>40</td><td>Wyoming</td><td>0.00</td></tr>
<tr><td></td><td></td><td></td><td></td><td>District of Columbia</td><td>0.35</td></tr>
</tbody>
</table>

Source: U.S. Department of Health and Human Services, National Center for Health Statistics
    unpublished (http://wonder.cdc.gov/WONDER/)
*By state of residence. Not age adjusted.

Deaths by Tuberculosis in 1994

National Total = 1,478 Deaths*

ALPHA ORDER

RANK	STATE	DEATHS	% of USA
14	Alabama	30	2.03%
48	Alaska	1	0.07%
16	Arizona	26	1.76%
24	Arkansas	16	1.08%
1	California	198	13.40%
24	Colorado	16	1.08%
32	Connecticut	9	0.61%
33	Delaware	6	0.41%
4	Florida	112	7.58%
9	Georgia	45	3.04%
37	Hawaii	5	0.34%
50	Idaho	0	0.00%
5	Illinois	83	5.62%
30	Indiana	12	0.81%
37	Iowa	5	0.34%
33	Kansas	6	0.41%
15	Kentucky	27	1.83%
10	Louisiana	44	2.98%
40	Maine	4	0.27%
16	Maryland	26	1.76%
24	Massachusetts	16	1.08%
10	Michigan	44	2.98%
28	Minnesota	15	1.01%
20	Mississippi	20	1.35%
21	Missouri	19	1.29%
33	Montana	6	0.41%
40	Nebraska	4	0.27%
46	Nevada	2	0.14%
43	New Hampshire	3	0.20%
6	New Jersey	60	4.06%
21	New Mexico	19	1.29%
2	New York	153	10.35%
8	North Carolina	46	3.11%
48	North Dakota	1	0.07%
13	Ohio	32	2.17%
21	Oklahoma	19	1.29%
31	Oregon	11	0.74%
7	Pennsylvania	53	3.59%
43	Rhode Island	3	0.20%
18	South Carolina	25	1.69%
37	South Dakota	5	0.34%
12	Tennessee	39	2.64%
3	Texas	135	9.13%
40	Utah	4	0.27%
46	Vermont	2	0.14%
19	Virginia	21	1.42%
24	Washington	16	1.08%
33	West Virginia	6	0.41%
29	Wisconsin	14	0.95%
43	Wyoming	3	0.20%

RANK ORDER

RANK	STATE	DEATHS	% of USA
1	California	198	13.40%
2	New York	153	10.35%
3	Texas	135	9.13%
4	Florida	112	7.58%
5	Illinois	83	5.62%
6	New Jersey	60	4.06%
7	Pennsylvania	53	3.59%
8	North Carolina	46	3.11%
9	Georgia	45	3.04%
10	Louisiana	44	2.98%
10	Michigan	44	2.98%
12	Tennessee	39	2.64%
13	Ohio	32	2.17%
14	Alabama	30	2.03%
15	Kentucky	27	1.83%
16	Arizona	26	1.76%
16	Maryland	26	1.76%
18	South Carolina	25	1.69%
19	Virginia	21	1.42%
20	Mississippi	20	1.35%
21	Missouri	19	1.29%
21	New Mexico	19	1.29%
21	Oklahoma	19	1.29%
24	Arkansas	16	1.08%
24	Colorado	16	1.08%
24	Massachusetts	16	1.08%
24	Washington	16	1.08%
28	Minnesota	15	1.01%
29	Wisconsin	14	0.95%
30	Indiana	12	0.81%
31	Oregon	11	0.74%
32	Connecticut	9	0.61%
33	Delaware	6	0.41%
33	Kansas	6	0.41%
33	Montana	6	0.41%
33	West Virginia	6	0.41%
37	Hawaii	5	0.34%
37	Iowa	5	0.34%
37	South Dakota	5	0.34%
40	Maine	4	0.27%
40	Nebraska	4	0.27%
40	Utah	4	0.27%
43	New Hampshire	3	0.20%
43	Rhode Island	3	0.20%
43	Wyoming	3	0.20%
46	Nevada	2	0.14%
46	Vermont	2	0.14%
48	Alaska	1	0.07%
48	North Dakota	1	0.07%
50	Idaho	0	0.00%
	District of Columbia	11	0.74%

Source: U.S. Department of Health and Human Services, National Center for Health Statistics
    unpublished data
*By state of residence.

Deaths Rate by Tuberculosis in 1994

National Rate = 0.56 Deaths per 100,000 Population*

ALPHA ORDER

RANK	STATE	RATE
10	Alabama	0.71
47	Alaska	0.16
18	Arizona	0.63
16	Arkansas	0.65
21	California	0.62
25	Colorado	0.43
38	Connecticut	0.27
3	Delaware	0.84
5	Florida	0.80
18	Georgia	0.63
27	Hawaii	0.42
50	Idaho	0.00
11	Illinois	0.70
44	Indiana	0.20
46	Iowa	0.17
43	Kansas	0.23
11	Kentucky	0.70
2	Louisiana	1.01
31	Maine	0.32
23	Maryland	0.51
40	Massachusetts	0.26
24	Michigan	0.46
31	Minnesota	0.32
8	Mississippi	0.74
28	Missouri	0.35
11	Montana	0.70
42	Nebraska	0.24
49	Nevada	0.13
40	New Hampshire	0.26
6	New Jersey	0.75
1	New Mexico	1.14
3	New York	0.84
16	North Carolina	0.65
48	North Dakota	0.15
37	Ohio	0.28
22	Oklahoma	0.58
28	Oregon	0.35
25	Pennsylvania	0.43
35	Rhode Island	0.30
15	South Carolina	0.68
14	South Dakota	0.69
6	Tennessee	0.75
9	Texas	0.73
44	Utah	0.20
30	Vermont	0.34
31	Virginia	0.32
36	Washington	0.29
31	West Virginia	0.32
38	Wisconsin	0.27
18	Wyoming	0.63

RANK ORDER

RANK	STATE	RATE
1	New Mexico	1.14
2	Louisiana	1.01
3	Delaware	0.84
3	New York	0.84
5	Florida	0.80
6	New Jersey	0.75
6	Tennessee	0.75
8	Mississippi	0.74
9	Texas	0.73
10	Alabama	0.71
11	Illinois	0.70
11	Kentucky	0.70
11	Montana	0.70
14	South Dakota	0.69
15	South Carolina	0.68
16	Arkansas	0.65
16	North Carolina	0.65
18	Arizona	0.63
18	Georgia	0.63
18	Wyoming	0.63
21	California	0.62
22	Oklahoma	0.58
23	Maryland	0.51
24	Michigan	0.46
25	Colorado	0.43
25	Pennsylvania	0.43
27	Hawaii	0.42
28	Missouri	0.35
28	Oregon	0.35
30	Vermont	0.34
31	Maine	0.32
31	Minnesota	0.32
31	Virginia	0.32
31	West Virginia	0.32
35	Rhode Island	0.30
36	Washington	0.29
37	Ohio	0.28
38	Connecticut	0.27
38	Wisconsin	0.27
40	Massachusetts	0.26
40	New Hampshire	0.26
42	Nebraska	0.24
43	Kansas	0.23
44	Indiana	0.20
44	Utah	0.20
46	Iowa	0.17
47	Alaska	0.16
48	North Dakota	0.15
49	Nevada	0.13
50	Idaho	0.00
	District of Columbia	1.92

Source: U.S. Department of Health and Human Services, National Center for Health Statistics
unpublished data
*By state of residence. Not age adjusted.

Deaths by Injury in 1994

National Total = 140,940 Deaths*

RANK	STATE	DEATHS	% of USA
14	Alabama	3,350	2.38%
43	Alaska	488	0.35%
17	Arizona	3,119	2.21%
29	Arkansas	1,883	1.34%
1	California	17,370	12.32%
26	Colorado	2,252	1.60%
30	Connecticut	1,560	1.11%
47	Delaware	398	0.28%
3	Florida	8,560	6.07%
9	Georgia	4,553	3.23%
42	Hawaii	545	0.39%
39	Idaho	777	0.55%
4	Illinois	6,672	4.73%
16	Indiana	3,190	2.26%
31	Iowa	1,532	1.09%
32	Kansas	1,461	1.04%
22	Kentucky	2,482	1.76%
15	Louisiana	3,343	2.37%
40	Maine	623	0.44%
18	Maryland	2,976	2.11%
23	Massachusetts	2,451	1.74%
6	Michigan	5,213	3.70%
25	Minnesota	2,297	1.63%
24	Mississippi	2,332	1.65%
10	Missouri	3,688	2.62%
41	Montana	604	0.43%
38	Nebraska	847	0.60%
35	Nevada	1,117	0.79%
44	New Hampshire	437	0.31%
13	New Jersey	3,404	2.42%
33	New Mexico	1,352	0.96%
2	New York	8,678	6.16%
8	North Carolina	4,676	3.32%
49	North Dakota	322	0.23%
7	Ohio	5,002	3.55%
27	Oklahoma	2,220	1.58%
28	Oregon	1,986	1.41%
5	Pennsylvania	6,581	4.67%
46	Rhode Island	415	0.29%
21	South Carolina	2,502	1.78%
45	South Dakota	428	0.30%
11	Tennessee	3,681	2.61%
37	Texas	1,002	0.71%
36	Utah	1,063	0.75%
50	Vermont	245	0.17%
12	Virginia	3,640	2.58%
19	Washington	2,954	2.10%
34	West Virginia	1,150	0.82%
20	Wisconsin	2,604	1.85%
48	Wyoming	362	0.26%

RANK	STATE	DEATHS	% of USA
1	California	17,370	12.32%
2	New York	8,678	6.16%
3	Florida	8,560	6.07%
4	Illinois	6,672	4.73%
5	Pennsylvania	6,581	4.67%
6	Michigan	5,213	3.70%
7	Ohio	5,002	3.55%
8	North Carolina	4,676	3.32%
9	Georgia	4,553	3.23%
10	Missouri	3,688	2.62%
11	Tennessee	3,681	2.61%
12	Virginia	3,640	2.58%
13	New Jersey	3,404	2.42%
14	Alabama	3,350	2.38%
15	Louisiana	3,343	2.37%
16	Indiana	3,190	2.26%
17	Arizona	3,119	2.21%
18	Maryland	2,976	2.11%
19	Washington	2,954	2.10%
20	Wisconsin	2,604	1.85%
21	South Carolina	2,502	1.78%
22	Kentucky	2,482	1.76%
23	Massachusetts	2,451	1.74%
24	Mississippi	2,332	1.65%
25	Minnesota	2,297	1.63%
26	Colorado	2,252	1.60%
27	Oklahoma	2,220	1.58%
28	Oregon	1,986	1.41%
29	Arkansas	1,883	1.34%
30	Connecticut	1,560	1.11%
31	Iowa	1,532	1.09%
32	Kansas	1,461	1.04%
33	New Mexico	1,352	0.96%
34	West Virginia	1,150	0.82%
35	Nevada	1,117	0.79%
36	Utah	1,063	0.75%
37	Texas	1,002	0.71%
38	Nebraska	847	0.60%
39	Idaho	777	0.55%
40	Maine	623	0.44%
41	Montana	604	0.43%
42	Hawaii	545	0.39%
43	Alaska	488	0.35%
44	New Hampshire	437	0.31%
45	South Dakota	428	0.30%
46	Rhode Island	415	0.29%
47	Delaware	398	0.28%
48	Wyoming	362	0.26%
49	North Dakota	322	0.23%
50	Vermont	245	0.17%
	District of Columbia	553	0.39%

Source: Morgan Quitno Press using data from U.S. Dept. of HHS, National Center for Health Statistics
    unpublished (http://wonder.cdc.gov/WONDER/)
*Final data by state of residence. Injury as used here includes Accidents (including motor vehicle), Suicides, Homicides and "Other" undetermined.

Death Rate by Injury in 1994

National Rate = 54.13 Deaths by Injury per 100,000 Population*

ALPHA ORDER

RANK	STATE	RATE
4	Alabama	79.38
3	Alaska	80.48
8	Arizona	76.46
6	Arkansas	76.72
33	California	55.25
21	Colorado	61.57
43	Connecticut	47.61
28	Delaware	56.29
22	Florida	61.33
18	Georgia	64.49
44	Hawaii	46.22
13	Idaho	68.54
27	Illinois	56.74
31	Indiana	55.43
36	Iowa	54.13
26	Kansas	57.17
17	Kentucky	64.82
5	Louisiana	77.45
41	Maine	50.23
24	Maryland	59.45
49	Massachusetts	40.55
34	Michigan	54.87
40	Minnesota	50.27
1	Mississippi	87.33
12	Missouri	69.86
11	Montana	70.56
37	Nebraska	52.16
7	Nevada	76.57
50	New Hampshire	38.45
46	New Jersey	43.03
2	New Mexico	81.74
42	New York	47.75
16	North Carolina	66.11
39	North Dakota	50.45
45	Ohio	45.04
15	Oklahoma	68.16
19	Oregon	64.31
35	Pennsylvania	54.58
48	Rhode Island	41.65
14	South Carolina	68.32
25	South Dakota	59.35
10	Tennessee	71.10
23	Texas	59.82
29	Utah	55.64
47	Vermont	42.21
30	Virginia	55.54
32	Washington	55.28
20	West Virginia	63.10
38	Wisconsin	51.23
9	Wyoming	76.03

RANK ORDER

RANK	STATE	RATE
1	Mississippi	87.33
2	New Mexico	81.74
3	Alaska	80.48
4	Alabama	79.38
5	Louisiana	77.45
6	Arkansas	76.72
7	Nevada	76.57
8	Arizona	76.46
9	Wyoming	76.03
10	Tennessee	71.10
11	Montana	70.56
12	Missouri	69.86
13	Idaho	68.54
14	South Carolina	68.32
15	Oklahoma	68.16
16	North Carolina	66.11
17	Kentucky	64.82
18	Georgia	64.49
19	Oregon	64.31
20	West Virginia	63.10
21	Colorado	61.57
22	Florida	61.33
23	Texas	59.82
24	Maryland	59.45
25	South Dakota	59.35
26	Kansas	57.17
27	Illinois	56.74
28	Delaware	56.29
29	Utah	55.64
30	Virginia	55.54
31	Indiana	55.43
32	Washington	55.28
33	California	55.25
34	Michigan	54.87
35	Pennsylvania	54.58
36	Iowa	54.13
37	Nebraska	52.16
38	Wisconsin	51.23
39	North Dakota	50.45
40	Minnesota	50.27
41	Maine	50.23
42	New York	47.75
43	Connecticut	47.61
44	Hawaii	46.22
45	Ohio	45.04
46	New Jersey	43.03
47	Vermont	42.21
48	Rhode Island	41.65
49	Massachusetts	40.55
50	New Hampshire	38.45
	District of Columbia	96.80

Source: Morgan Quitno Press using data from U.S. Dept. of HHS, National Center for Health Statistics unpublished (http://wonder.cdc.gov/WONDER/)

Final data by state of residence. Injury as used here includes Accidents (including motor vehicle), Suicides, Homicides and "Other" undetermined. Not age adjusted.

Deaths by Accidents in 1994

National Total = 91,437 Deaths*

ALPHA ORDER					RANK ORDER			
RANK	STATE		DEATHS	% of USA	RANK	STATE	DEATHS	% of USA
15	Alabama		2,165	2.37%	1	California	9,469	10.36%
43	Alaska		326	0.36%	2	Texas	6,339	6.93%
17	Arizona		1,831	2.00%	3	Florida	5,090	5.57%
30	Arkansas		1,140	1.25%	4	New York	4,987	5.45%
1	California		9,469	10.36%	5	Pennsylvania	4,351	4.76%
27	Colorado		1,361	1.49%	6	Illinois	4,043	4.42%
32	Connecticut		1,009	1.10%	7	Ohio	3,278	3.58%
45	Delaware		282	0.31%	8	Michigan	2,994	3.27%
3	Florida		5,090	5.57%	9	North Carolina	2,923	3.20%
10	Georgia		2,820	3.08%	10	Georgia	2,820	3.08%
42	Hawaii		336	0.37%	11	Tennessee	2,399	2.62%
39	Idaho		522	0.57%	12	Missouri	2,286	2.50%
6	Illinois		4,043	4.42%	13	New Jersey	2,280	2.49%
16	Indiana		1,959	2.14%	14	Virginia	2,194	2.40%
31	Iowa		1,128	1.23%	15	Alabama	2,165	2.37%
33	Kansas		961	1.05%	16	Indiana	1,959	2.14%
21	Kentucky		1,697	1.86%	17	Arizona	1,831	2.00%
18	Louisiana		1,809	1.98%	18	Louisiana	1,809	1.98%
40	Maine		416	0.45%	19	Washington	1,776	1.94%
26	Maryland		1,382	1.51%	20	Wisconsin	1,735	1.90%
28	Massachusetts		1,319	1.44%	21	Kentucky	1,697	1.86%
8	Michigan		2,994	3.27%	22	Minnesota	1,625	1.78%
22	Minnesota		1,625	1.78%	23	South Carolina	1,621	1.77%
24	Mississippi		1,528	1.67%	24	Mississippi	1,528	1.67%
12	Missouri		2,286	2.50%	25	Oklahoma	1,467	1.60%
41	Montana		395	0.43%	26	Maryland	1,382	1.51%
37	Nebraska		574	0.63%	27	Colorado	1,361	1.49%
38	Nevada		528	0.58%	28	Massachusetts	1,319	1.44%
46	New Hampshire		271	0.30%	29	Oregon	1,262	1.38%
13	New Jersey		2,280	2.49%	30	Arkansas	1,140	1.25%
34	New Mexico		846	0.93%	31	Iowa	1,128	1.23%
4	New York		4,987	5.45%	32	Connecticut	1,009	1.10%
9	North Carolina		2,923	3.20%	33	Kansas	961	1.05%
47	North Dakota		232	0.25%	34	New Mexico	846	0.93%
7	Ohio		3,278	3.58%	35	West Virginia	750	0.82%
25	Oklahoma		1,467	1.60%	36	Utah	646	0.71%
29	Oregon		1,262	1.38%	37	Nebraska	574	0.63%
5	Pennsylvania		4,351	4.76%	38	Nevada	528	0.58%
49	Rhode Island		221	0.24%	39	Idaho	522	0.57%
23	South Carolina		1,621	1.77%	40	Maine	416	0.45%
44	South Dakota		302	0.33%	41	Montana	395	0.43%
11	Tennessee		2,399	2.62%	42	Hawaii	336	0.37%
2	Texas		6,339	6.93%	43	Alaska	326	0.36%
36	Utah		646	0.71%	44	South Dakota	302	0.33%
50	Vermont		173	0.19%	45	Delaware	282	0.31%
14	Virginia		2,194	2.40%	46	New Hampshire	271	0.30%
19	Washington		1,776	1.94%	47	North Dakota	232	0.25%
35	West Virginia		750	0.82%	48	Wyoming	225	0.25%
20	Wisconsin		1,735	1.90%	49	Rhode Island	221	0.24%
48	Wyoming		225	0.25%	50	Vermont	173	0.19%
						District of Columbia	164	0.18%

Source: U.S. Department of Health and Human Services, National Center for Health Statistics
"Monthly Vital Statistics Report" (Vol. 45, No. 3(S), September 30, 1996)
*Final data by state of residence. Includes motor vehicle deaths, poisoning, falls, drowning and other accidents.

Death Rate by Accidents in 1994

National Rate = 35.1 Deaths per 100,000 Population*

ALPHA ORDER				RANK ORDER		
RANK	STATE	RATE		RANK	STATE	RATE
3	Alabama	51.3		1	Mississippi	57.2
2	Alaska	53.8		2	Alaska	53.8
11	Arizona	44.9		3	Alabama	51.3
6	Arkansas	46.5		4	New Mexico	51.2
41	California	30.1		5	Wyoming	47.3
24	Colorado	37.2		6	Arkansas	46.5
40	Connecticut	30.8		7	Tennessee	46.4
21	Delaware	39.9		8	Idaho	46.1
25	Florida	36.5		8	Montana	46.1
20	Georgia	40.0		10	Oklahoma	45.0
45	Hawaii	28.5		11	Arizona	44.9
8	Idaho	46.1		12	Kentucky	44.3
32	Illinois	34.4		13	South Carolina	44.2
33	Indiana	34.1		14	Missouri	43.3
21	Iowa	39.9		15	Louisiana	41.9
23	Kansas	37.6		15	South Dakota	41.9
12	Kentucky	44.3		17	North Carolina	41.3
15	Louisiana	41.9		18	West Virginia	41.2
36	Maine	33.5		19	Oregon	40.9
46	Maryland	27.6		20	Georgia	40.0
50	Massachusetts	21.8		21	Delaware	39.9
39	Michigan	31.5		21	Iowa	39.9
29	Minnesota	35.6		23	Kansas	37.6
1	Mississippi	57.2		24	Colorado	37.2
14	Missouri	43.3		25	Florida	36.5
8	Montana	46.1		26	North Dakota	36.4
30	Nebraska	35.4		27	Nevada	36.2
27	Nevada	36.2		28	Pennsylvania	36.1
48	New Hampshire	23.8		29	Minnesota	35.6
44	New Jersey	28.8		30	Nebraska	35.4
4	New Mexico	51.2		31	Texas	34.5
47	New York	27.4		32	Illinois	34.4
17	North Carolina	41.3		33	Indiana	34.1
26	North Dakota	36.4		33	Wisconsin	34.1
43	Ohio	29.5		35	Utah	33.9
10	Oklahoma	45.0		36	Maine	33.5
19	Oregon	40.9		36	Virginia	33.5
28	Pennsylvania	36.1		38	Washington	33.2
49	Rhode Island	22.2		39	Michigan	31.5
13	South Carolina	44.2		40	Connecticut	30.8
15	South Dakota	41.9		41	California	30.1
7	Tennessee	46.4		42	Vermont	29.8
31	Texas	34.5		43	Ohio	29.5
35	Utah	33.9		44	New Jersey	28.8
42	Vermont	29.8		45	Hawaii	28.5
36	Virginia	33.5		46	Maryland	27.6
38	Washington	33.2		47	New York	27.4
18	West Virginia	41.2		48	New Hampshire	23.8
33	Wisconsin	34.1		49	Rhode Island	22.2
5	Wyoming	47.3		50	Massachusetts	21.8
					District of Columbia	28.8

Source: U.S. Department of Health and Human Services, National Center for Health Statistics
    "Monthly Vital Statistics Report" (Vol. 45, No. 3(S), September 30, 1996)
*Final data by state of residence. Includes motor vehicle deaths, poisoning, falls, drowning and other accidents.
Not age adjusted.

Deaths by Motor Vehicle Accidents in 1994

National Total = 42,524 Deaths*

ALPHA ORDER

RANK	STATE	DEATHS	% of USA
12	Alabama	1,132	2.66%
48	Alaska	84	0.20%
16	Arizona	880	2.07%
27	Arkansas	656	1.54%
1	California	4,509	10.60%
28	Colorado	648	1.52%
36	Connecticut	329	0.77%
44	Delaware	122	0.29%
3	Florida	2,712	6.38%
7	Georgia	1,492	3.51%
43	Hawaii	127	0.30%
39	Idaho	255	0.60%
5	Illinois	1,757	4.13%
14	Indiana	988	2.32%
29	Iowa	524	1.23%
32	Kansas	478	1.12%
20	Kentucky	794	1.87%
17	Louisiana	873	2.05%
40	Maine	206	0.48%
26	Maryland	661	1.55%
31	Massachusetts	484	1.14%
8	Michigan	1,485	3.49%
24	Minnesota	722	1.70%
18	Mississippi	849	2.00%
13	Missouri	1,104	2.60%
41	Montana	194	0.46%
38	Nebraska	275	0.65%
37	Nevada	282	0.66%
46	New Hampshire	118	0.28%
21	New Jersey	773	1.82%
33	New Mexico	422	0.99%
4	New York	1,830	4.30%
9	North Carolina	1,465	3.45%
47	North Dakota	86	0.20%
10	Ohio	1,394	3.28%
23	Oklahoma	737	1.73%
30	Oregon	488	1.15%
6	Pennsylvania	1,556	3.66%
49	Rhode Island	75	0.18%
19	South Carolina	827	1.94%
42	South Dakota	159	0.37%
11	Tennessee	1,272	2.99%
2	Texas	3,327	7.82%
35	Utah	363	0.85%
50	Vermont	72	0.17%
15	Virginia	916	2.15%
25	Washington	715	1.68%
34	West Virginia	375	0.88%
22	Wisconsin	747	1.76%
45	Wyoming	119	0.28%

RANK ORDER

RANK	STATE	DEATHS	% of USA
1	California	4,509	10.60%
2	Texas	3,327	7.82%
3	Florida	2,712	6.38%
4	New York	1,830	4.30%
5	Illinois	1,757	4.13%
6	Pennsylvania	1,556	3.66%
7	Georgia	1,492	3.51%
8	Michigan	1,485	3.49%
9	North Carolina	1,465	3.45%
10	Ohio	1,394	3.28%
11	Tennessee	1,272	2.99%
12	Alabama	1,132	2.66%
13	Missouri	1,104	2.60%
14	Indiana	988	2.32%
15	Virginia	916	2.15%
16	Arizona	880	2.07%
17	Louisiana	873	2.05%
18	Mississippi	849	2.00%
19	South Carolina	827	1.94%
20	Kentucky	794	1.87%
21	New Jersey	773	1.82%
22	Wisconsin	747	1.76%
23	Oklahoma	737	1.73%
24	Minnesota	722	1.70%
25	Washington	715	1.68%
26	Maryland	661	1.55%
27	Arkansas	656	1.54%
28	Colorado	648	1.52%
29	Iowa	524	1.23%
30	Oregon	488	1.15%
31	Massachusetts	484	1.14%
32	Kansas	478	1.12%
33	New Mexico	422	0.99%
34	West Virginia	375	0.88%
35	Utah	363	0.85%
36	Connecticut	329	0.77%
37	Nevada	282	0.66%
38	Nebraska	275	0.65%
39	Idaho	255	0.60%
40	Maine	206	0.48%
41	Montana	194	0.46%
42	South Dakota	159	0.37%
43	Hawaii	127	0.30%
44	Delaware	122	0.29%
45	Wyoming	119	0.28%
46	New Hampshire	118	0.28%
47	North Dakota	86	0.20%
48	Alaska	84	0.20%
49	Rhode Island	75	0.18%
50	Vermont	72	0.17%
	District of Columbia	66	0.16%

Source: U.S. Department of Health and Human Services, National Center for Health Statistics
unpublished (http://wonder.cdc.gov/WONDER/)
*Final data by state of residence. These numbers are compiled from death certificates by the Centers for Disease Control and Prevention. They may differ from motor vehicle deaths collected by the U.S. Department of Transportation from other sources.

Death Rate by Motor Vehicle Accidents in 1994

National Rate = 16.32 Deaths per 100,000 Population*

ALPHA ORDER

RANK ORDER

RANK	STATE	RATE
2	Alabama	26.82
37	Alaska	13.85
12	Arizona	21.57
3	Arkansas	26.73
35	California	14.34
25	Colorado	17.72
47	Connecticut	10.04
26	Delaware	17.25
19	Florida	19.43
13	Georgia	21.13
44	Hawaii	10.77
10	Idaho	22.49
33	Illinois	14.94
27	Indiana	17.17
23	Iowa	18.52
22	Kansas	18.70
15	Kentucky	20.73
18	Louisiana	20.22
29	Maine	16.61
40	Maryland	13.20
49	Massachusetts	8.00
32	Michigan	15.63
30	Minnesota	15.80
1	Mississippi	31.79
14	Missouri	20.91
7	Montana	22.66
28	Nebraska	16.93
20	Nevada	19.33
45	New Hampshire	10.38
48	New Jersey	9.77
4	New Mexico	25.51
46	New York	10.07
16	North Carolina	20.71
38	North Dakota	13.47
42	Ohio	12.55
8	Oklahoma	22.62
30	Oregon	15.80
41	Pennsylvania	12.90
50	Rhode Island	7.52
9	South Carolina	22.58
11	South Dakota	22.04
6	Tennessee	24.56
24	Texas	18.09
21	Utah	19.00
43	Vermont	12.40
36	Virginia	13.97
39	Washington	13.38
17	West Virginia	20.57
34	Wisconsin	14.69
5	Wyoming	24.99

RANK	STATE	RATE
1	Mississippi	31.79
2	Alabama	26.82
3	Arkansas	26.73
4	New Mexico	25.51
5	Wyoming	24.99
6	Tennessee	24.56
7	Montana	22.66
8	Oklahoma	22.62
9	South Carolina	22.58
10	Idaho	22.49
11	South Dakota	22.04
12	Arizona	21.57
13	Georgia	21.13
14	Missouri	20.91
15	Kentucky	20.73
16	North Carolina	20.71
17	West Virginia	20.57
18	Louisiana	20.22
19	Florida	19.43
20	Nevada	19.33
21	Utah	19.00
22	Kansas	18.70
23	Iowa	18.52
24	Texas	18.09
25	Colorado	17.72
26	Delaware	17.25
27	Indiana	17.17
28	Nebraska	16.93
29	Maine	16.61
30	Minnesota	15.80
30	Oregon	15.80
32	Michigan	15.63
33	Illinois	14.94
34	Wisconsin	14.69
35	California	14.34
36	Virginia	13.97
37	Alaska	13.85
38	North Dakota	13.47
39	Washington	13.38
40	Maryland	13.20
41	Pennsylvania	12.90
42	Ohio	12.55
43	Vermont	12.40
44	Hawaii	10.77
45	New Hampshire	10.38
46	New York	10.07
47	Connecticut	10.04
48	New Jersey	9.77
49	Massachusetts	8.00
50	Rhode Island	7.52
	District of Columbia	11.55

Source: U.S. Department of Health and Human Services, National Center for Health Statistics
    unpublished (http://wonder.cdc.gov/WONDER/)
*Final data by state of residence. These numbers are compiled from death certificates by the Centers for Disease Control and Prevention. They may differ from motor vehicle deaths collected by the U.S. Department of Transportation from other sources.

Deaths by Homicide in 1994

National Total = 24,926 Homicides*

ALPHA ORDER

RANK ORDER

RANK	STATE	HOMICIDES	% of USA
13	Alabama	601	2.41%
42	Alaska	36	0.14%
18	Arizona	458	1.84%
22	Arkansas	322	1.29%
1	California	3,938	15.80%
29	Colorado	207	0.83%
28	Connecticut	209	0.84%
45	Delaware	30	0.12%
5	Florida	1,319	5.29%
8	Georgia	820	3.29%
40	Hawaii	45	0.18%
41	Idaho	39	0.16%
4	Illinois	1,462	5.87%
19	Indiana	457	1.83%
36	Iowa	65	0.26%
30	Kansas	187	0.75%
26	Kentucky	234	0.94%
7	Louisiana	912	3.66%
44	Maine	33	0.13%
11	Maryland	651	2.61%
25	Massachusetts	236	0.95%
6	Michigan	1,038	4.16%
34	Minnesota	150	0.60%
17	Mississippi	460	1.85%
12	Missouri	610	2.45%
43	Montana	35	0.14%
38	Nebraska	54	0.22%
33	Nevada	165	0.66%
48	New Hampshire	22	0.09%
20	New Jersey	426	1.71%
31	New Mexico	184	0.74%
3	New York	2,054	8.24%
9	North Carolina	819	3.29%
49	North Dakota	6	0.02%
15	Ohio	568	2.28%
24	Oklahoma	281	1.13%
32	Oregon	179	0.72%
10	Pennsylvania	756	3.03%
39	Rhode Island	49	0.20%
21	South Carolina	396	1.59%
47	South Dakota	24	0.10%
16	Tennessee	548	2.20%
2	Texas	2,153	8.64%
37	Utah	63	0.25%
50	Vermont	4	0.02%
14	Virginia	585	2.35%
23	Washington	321	1.29%
35	West Virginia	114	0.46%
27	Wisconsin	225	0.90%
46	Wyoming	26	0.10%

RANK	STATE	HOMICIDES	% of USA
1	California	3,938	15.80%
2	Texas	2,153	8.64%
3	New York	2,054	8.24%
4	Illinois	1,462	5.87%
5	Florida	1,319	5.29%
6	Michigan	1,038	4.16%
7	Louisiana	912	3.66%
8	Georgia	820	3.29%
9	North Carolina	819	3.29%
10	Pennsylvania	756	3.03%
11	Maryland	651	2.61%
12	Missouri	610	2.45%
13	Alabama	601	2.41%
14	Virginia	585	2.35%
15	Ohio	568	2.28%
16	Tennessee	548	2.20%
17	Mississippi	460	1.85%
18	Arizona	458	1.84%
19	Indiana	457	1.83%
20	New Jersey	426	1.71%
21	South Carolina	396	1.59%
22	Arkansas	322	1.29%
23	Washington	321	1.29%
24	Oklahoma	281	1.13%
25	Massachusetts	236	0.95%
26	Kentucky	234	0.94%
27	Wisconsin	225	0.90%
28	Connecticut	209	0.84%
29	Colorado	207	0.83%
30	Kansas	187	0.75%
31	New Mexico	184	0.74%
32	Oregon	179	0.72%
33	Nevada	165	0.66%
34	Minnesota	150	0.60%
35	West Virginia	114	0.46%
36	Iowa	65	0.26%
37	Utah	63	0.25%
38	Nebraska	54	0.22%
39	Rhode Island	49	0.20%
40	Hawaii	45	0.18%
41	Idaho	39	0.16%
42	Alaska	36	0.14%
43	Montana	35	0.14%
44	Maine	33	0.13%
45	Delaware	30	0.12%
46	Wyoming	26	0.10%
47	South Dakota	24	0.10%
48	New Hampshire	22	0.09%
49	North Dakota	6	0.02%
50	Vermont	4	0.02%
	District of Columbia	350	1.40%

Source: U.S. Department of Health and Human Services, National Center for Health Statistics unpublished (http://wonder.cdc.gov/WONDER/)
Final data by state of residence. Includes legal intervention. Homicide data shown here are collected by the Centers for Disease Control and Prevention based on death certificates and differ from murder data collected by the F.B.I. from other sources.

Death Rate by Homicide in 1994

National Rate = 9.57 Deaths by Homicides per 100,000 Population*

ALPHA ORDER

RANK	STATE	RATE
3	Alabama	14.24
29	Alaska	5.93
14	Arizona	11.22
4	Arkansas	13.12
6	California	12.52
31	Colorado	5.65
24	Connecticut	6.37
37	Delaware	4.24
19	Florida	9.45
9	Georgia	11.61
40	Hawaii	3.81
41	Idaho	3.44
7	Illinois	12.43
22	Indiana	7.94
47	Iowa	2.29
23	Kansas	7.31
27	Kentucky	6.11
1	Louisiana	21.13
46	Maine	2.66
5	Maryland	13.00
39	Massachusetts	3.90
16	Michigan	10.92
45	Minnesota	3.28
2	Mississippi	17.22
11	Missouri	11.55
38	Montana	4.08
42	Nebraska	3.32
12	Nevada	11.31
48	New Hampshire	1.93
33	New Jersey	5.38
15	New Mexico	11.12
13	New York	11.30
10	North Carolina	11.57
49	North Dakota	0.94
34	Ohio	5.11
21	Oklahoma	8.62
30	Oregon	5.79
25	Pennsylvania	6.27
35	Rhode Island	4.91
17	South Carolina	10.81
42	South Dakota	3.32
18	Tennessee	10.58
8	Texas	11.70
44	Utah	3.29
50	Vermont	0.68
20	Virginia	8.92
28	Washington	6.00
26	West Virginia	6.25
36	Wisconsin	4.42
32	Wyoming	5.46

RANK ORDER

RANK	STATE	RATE
1	Louisiana	21.13
2	Mississippi	17.22
3	Alabama	14.24
4	Arkansas	13.12
5	Maryland	13.00
6	California	12.52
7	Illinois	12.43
8	Texas	11.70
9	Georgia	11.61
10	North Carolina	11.57
11	Missouri	11.55
12	Nevada	11.31
13	New York	11.30
14	Arizona	11.22
15	New Mexico	11.12
16	Michigan	10.92
17	South Carolina	10.81
18	Tennessee	10.58
19	Florida	9.45
20	Virginia	8.92
21	Oklahoma	8.62
22	Indiana	7.94
23	Kansas	7.31
24	Connecticut	6.37
25	Pennsylvania	6.27
26	West Virginia	6.25
27	Kentucky	6.11
28	Washington	6.00
29	Alaska	5.93
30	Oregon	5.79
31	Colorado	5.65
32	Wyoming	5.46
33	New Jersey	5.38
34	Ohio	5.11
35	Rhode Island	4.91
36	Wisconsin	4.42
37	Delaware	4.24
38	Montana	4.08
39	Massachusetts	3.90
40	Hawaii	3.81
41	Idaho	3.44
42	Nebraska	3.32
42	South Dakota	3.32
44	Utah	3.29
45	Minnesota	3.28
46	Maine	2.66
47	Iowa	2.29
48	New Hampshire	1.93
49	North Dakota	0.94
50	Vermont	0.68
	District of Columbia	61.26

Source: U.S. Department of Health and Human Services, National Center for Health Statistics unpublished (http://wonder.cdc.gov/WONDER/)

*Final data by state of residence. Includes legal intervention. Homicide data shown here are collected by the Centers for Disease Control and Prevention based on death certificates and differ from murder data collected by the F.B.I. from other sources.

Deaths by Suicide in 1994

National Total = 31,142 Deaths*

ALPHA ORDER

RANK	STATE	SUICIDES	% of USA
21	Alabama	532	1.71%
44	Alaska	121	0.39%
12	Arizona	767	2.46%
29	Arkansas	364	1.17%
1	California	3,712	11.92%
17	Colorado	614	1.97%
31	Connecticut	324	1.04%
48	Delaware	80	0.26%
3	Florida	2,075	6.66%
10	Georgia	835	2.68%
42	Hawaii	138	0.44%
38	Idaho	201	0.65%
7	Illinois	1,068	3.43%
15	Indiana	718	2.31%
32	Iowa	322	1.03%
35	Kansas	292	0.94%
23	Kentucky	517	1.66%
20	Louisiana	552	1.77%
40	Maine	168	0.54%
22	Maryland	528	1.70%
24	Massachusetts	512	1.64%
8	Michigan	1,036	3.33%
26	Minnesota	494	1.59%
33	Mississippi	315	1.01%
14	Missouri	728	2.34%
41	Montana	158	0.51%
39	Nebraska	188	0.60%
30	Nevada	341	1.09%
43	New Hampshire	137	0.44%
19	New Jersey	578	1.86%
34	New Mexico	303	0.97%
4	New York	1,498	4.81%
9	North Carolina	897	2.88%
48	North Dakota	80	0.26%
6	Ohio	1,101	3.54%
28	Oklahoma	451	1.45%
24	Oregon	512	1.64%
5	Pennsylvania	1,326	4.26%
47	Rhode Island	82	0.26%
27	South Carolina	468	1.50%
46	South Dakota	97	0.31%
16	Tennessee	660	2.12%
2	Texas	2,337	7.50%
36	Utah	291	0.93%
50	Vermont	58	0.19%
11	Virginia	821	2.64%
13	Washington	759	2.44%
37	West Virginia	258	0.83%
18	Wisconsin	592	1.90%
45	Wyoming	107	0.34%

RANK ORDER

RANK	STATE	SUICIDES	% of USA
1	California	3,712	11.92%
2	Texas	2,337	7.50%
3	Florida	2,075	6.66%
4	New York	1,498	4.81%
5	Pennsylvania	1,326	4.26%
6	Ohio	1,101	3.54%
7	Illinois	1,068	3.43%
8	Michigan	1,036	3.33%
9	North Carolina	897	2.88%
10	Georgia	835	2.68%
11	Virginia	821	2.64%
12	Arizona	767	2.46%
13	Washington	759	2.44%
14	Missouri	728	2.34%
15	Indiana	718	2.31%
16	Tennessee	660	2.12%
17	Colorado	614	1.97%
18	Wisconsin	592	1.90%
19	New Jersey	578	1.86%
20	Louisiana	552	1.77%
21	Alabama	532	1.71%
22	Maryland	528	1.70%
23	Kentucky	517	1.66%
24	Massachusetts	512	1.64%
24	Oregon	512	1.64%
26	Minnesota	494	1.59%
27	South Carolina	468	1.50%
28	Oklahoma	451	1.45%
29	Arkansas	364	1.17%
30	Nevada	341	1.09%
31	Connecticut	324	1.04%
32	Iowa	322	1.03%
33	Mississippi	315	1.01%
34	New Mexico	303	0.97%
35	Kansas	292	0.94%
36	Utah	291	0.93%
37	West Virginia	258	0.83%
38	Idaho	201	0.65%
39	Nebraska	188	0.60%
40	Maine	168	0.54%
41	Montana	158	0.51%
42	Hawaii	138	0.44%
43	New Hampshire	137	0.44%
44	Alaska	121	0.39%
45	Wyoming	107	0.34%
46	South Dakota	97	0.31%
47	Rhode Island	82	0.26%
48	Delaware	80	0.26%
48	North Dakota	80	0.26%
50	Vermont	58	0.19%
	District of Columbia	29	0.09%

*Source: U.S. Department of Health and Human Services, National Center for Health Statistics
"Monthly Vital Statistics Report" (Vol. 45, No. 3(S), September 30, 1996)
Final data by state of residence.

Death Rate by Suicide in 1994

National Rate = 12.0 Suicides per 100,000 Population*

ALPHA ORDER

RANK	STATE	RATE
25	Alabama	12.6
3	Alaska	20.0
4	Arizona	18.8
12	Arkansas	14.8
30	California	11.8
8	Colorado	16.8
44	Connecticut	9.9
38	Delaware	11.3
11	Florida	14.9
30	Georgia	11.8
33	Hawaii	11.7
7	Idaho	17.7
46	Illinois	9.1
26	Indiana	12.5
36	Iowa	11.4
36	Kansas	11.4
17	Kentucky	13.5
20	Louisiana	12.8
17	Maine	13.5
42	Maryland	10.5
47	Massachusetts	8.5
40	Michigan	10.9
41	Minnesota	10.8
30	Mississippi	11.8
15	Missouri	13.8
5	Montana	18.5
34	Nebraska	11.6
1	Nevada	23.4
29	New Hampshire	12.1
50	New Jersey	7.3
6	New Mexico	18.3
48	New York	8.2
23	North Carolina	12.7
26	North Dakota	12.5
44	Ohio	9.9
15	Oklahoma	13.8
9	Oregon	16.6
39	Pennsylvania	11.0
48	Rhode Island	8.2
20	South Carolina	12.8
17	South Dakota	13.5
20	Tennessee	12.8
23	Texas	12.7
10	Utah	15.3
43	Vermont	10.0
26	Virginia	12.5
13	Washington	14.2
13	West Virginia	14.2
34	Wisconsin	11.6
2	Wyoming	22.5

RANK ORDER

RANK	STATE	RATE
1	Nevada	23.4
2	Wyoming	22.5
3	Alaska	20.0
4	Arizona	18.8
5	Montana	18.5
6	New Mexico	18.3
7	Idaho	17.7
8	Colorado	16.8
9	Oregon	16.6
10	Utah	15.3
11	Florida	14.9
12	Arkansas	14.8
13	Washington	14.2
13	West Virginia	14.2
15	Missouri	13.8
15	Oklahoma	13.8
17	Kentucky	13.5
17	Maine	13.5
17	South Dakota	13.5
20	Louisiana	12.8
20	South Carolina	12.8
20	Tennessee	12.8
23	North Carolina	12.7
23	Texas	12.7
25	Alabama	12.6
26	Indiana	12.5
26	North Dakota	12.5
26	Virginia	12.5
29	New Hampshire	12.1
30	California	11.8
30	Georgia	11.8
30	Mississippi	11.8
33	Hawaii	11.7
34	Nebraska	11.6
34	Wisconsin	11.6
36	Iowa	11.4
36	Kansas	11.4
38	Delaware	11.3
39	Pennsylvania	11.0
40	Michigan	10.9
41	Minnesota	10.8
42	Maryland	10.5
43	Vermont	10.0
44	Connecticut	9.9
44	Ohio	9.9
46	Illinois	9.1
47	Massachusetts	8.5
48	New York	8.2
48	Rhode Island	8.2
50	New Jersey	7.3
	District of Columbia	5.1

*Source: U.S. Department of Health and Human Services, National Center for Health Statistics
"Monthly Vital Statistics Report" (Vol. 45, No. 3(S), September 30, 1996)*
Final data by state of residence. Not age adjusted.

Years Lost by Premature Death in 1994

National Average = 5,390.7 Years Lost per 100,000 Population*

ALPHA ORDER				RANK ORDER		
RANK	**STATE**	**YEARS**		**RANK**	**STATE**	**YEARS**
3	Alabama	6,665.2		1	Mississippi	7,436.2
23	Alaska	5,196.6		2	Louisiana	7,053.4
11	Arizona	5,949.7		3	Alabama	6,665.2
4	Arkansas	6,417.7		4	Arkansas	6,417.7
24	California	5,127.4		5	South Carolina	6,307.7
36	Colorado	4,652.2		6	Georgia	6,165.8
32	Connecticut	4,859.0		7	Florida	6,065.2
20	Delaware	5,372.1		8	Tennessee	6,037.9
7	Florida	6,065.2		9	Nevada	6,001.8
6	Georgia	6,165.8		10	North Carolina	5,995.7
42	Hawaii	4,258.2		11	Arizona	5,949.7
37	Idaho	4,528.7		12	New York	5,888.2
16	Illinois	5,743.2		13	Oklahoma	5,841.3
25	Indiana	5,118.1		14	Maryland	5,825.7
41	Iowa	4,282.2		15	New Mexico	5,752.4
33	Kansas	4,766.7		16	Illinois	5,743.2
21	Kentucky	5,328.5		17	Missouri	5,675.6
2	Louisiana	7,053.4		18	Texas	5,409.9
47	Maine	4,132.3		19	Michigan	5,372.9
14	Maryland	5,825.7		20	Delaware	5,372.1
44	Massachusetts	4,178.0		21	Kentucky	5,328.5
19	Michigan	5,372.9		22	New Jersey	5,243.3
48	Minnesota	4,015.5		23	Alaska	5,196.6
1	Mississippi	7,436.2		24	California	5,127.4
17	Missouri	5,675.6		25	Indiana	5,118.1
35	Montana	4,726.4		26	Pennsylvania	5,067.0
38	Nebraska	4,479.0		27	West Virginia	5,057.8
9	Nevada	6,001.8		28	South Dakota	5,032.7
50	New Hampshire	3,718.0		29	Wyoming	4,995.7
22	New Jersey	5,243.3		30	Virginia	4,934.8
15	New Mexico	5,752.4		31	Ohio	4,864.0
12	New York	5,888.2		32	Connecticut	4,859.0
10	North Carolina	5,995.7		33	Kansas	4,766.7
45	North Dakota	4,174.7		34	Oregon	4,763.7
31	Ohio	4,864.0		35	Montana	4,726.4
13	Oklahoma	5,841.3		36	Colorado	4,652.2
34	Oregon	4,763.7		37	Idaho	4,528.7
26	Pennsylvania	5,067.0		38	Nebraska	4,479.0
46	Rhode Island	4,156.3		39	Washington	4,382.9
5	South Carolina	6,307.7		40	Utah	4,367.3
28	South Dakota	5,032.7		41	Iowa	4,282.2
8	Tennessee	6,037.9		42	Hawaii	4,258.2
18	Texas	5,409.9		43	Wisconsin	4,242.1
40	Utah	4,367.3		44	Massachusetts	4,178.0
49	Vermont	3,794.1		45	North Dakota	4,174.7
30	Virginia	4,934.8		46	Rhode Island	4,156.3
39	Washington	4,382.9		47	Maine	4,132.3
27	West Virginia	5,057.8		48	Minnesota	4,015.5
43	Wisconsin	4,242.1		49	Vermont	3,794.1
29	Wyoming	4,995.7		50	New Hampshire	3,718.0
					District of Columbia	14,095.1

Source: U.S. Department of Health and Human Services, National Center for Health Statistics
"State Health Profiles"
*Age-adjusted years of potential life lost due to death before age 65.

Years Lost by Premature Death from Cancer in 1994

National Average = 804.2 Years Lost per 100,000 Population*

ALPHA ORDER

RANK	STATE	YEARS
3	Alabama	936.4
49	Alaska	570.8
34	Arizona	744.8
2	Arkansas	943.1
36	California	739.2
44	Colorado	656.4
33	Connecticut	761.8
11	Delaware	883.4
12	Florida	878.9
22	Georgia	817.1
40	Hawaii	675.5
46	Idaho	617.8
24	Illinois	811.0
25	Indiana	802.2
30	Iowa	769.2
21	Kansas	818.4
5	Kentucky	916.1
4	Louisiana	922.7
6	Maine	907.8
23	Maryland	812.0
31	Massachusetts	767.9
18	Michigan	834.1
38	Minnesota	693.1
1	Mississippi	952.1
15	Missouri	851.4
50	Montana	564.1
31	Nebraska	767.9
26	Nevada	795.2
29	New Hampshire	773.4
14	New Jersey	853.3
45	New Mexico	625.6
17	New York	834.3
16	North Carolina	842.1
39	North Dakota	679.9
19	Ohio	833.4
13	Oklahoma	858.6
35	Oregon	742.4
20	Pennsylvania	820.6
9	Rhode Island	894.8
7	South Carolina	899.5
43	South Dakota	663.6
10	Tennessee	890.2
28	Texas	783.6
47	Utah	608.6
42	Vermont	668.9
27	Virginia	788.7
41	Washington	673.5
8	West Virginia	897.1
37	Wisconsin	714.3
48	Wyoming	608.3

RANK ORDER

RANK	STATE	YEARS
1	Mississippi	952.1
2	Arkansas	943.1
3	Alabama	936.4
4	Louisiana	922.7
5	Kentucky	916.1
6	Maine	907.8
7	South Carolina	899.5
8	West Virginia	897.1
9	Rhode Island	894.8
10	Tennessee	890.2
11	Delaware	883.4
12	Florida	878.9
13	Oklahoma	858.6
14	New Jersey	853.3
15	Missouri	851.4
16	North Carolina	842.1
17	New York	834.3
18	Michigan	834.1
19	Ohio	833.4
20	Pennsylvania	820.6
21	Kansas	818.4
22	Georgia	817.1
23	Maryland	812.0
24	Illinois	811.0
25	Indiana	802.2
26	Nevada	795.2
27	Virginia	788.7
28	Texas	783.6
29	New Hampshire	773.4
30	Iowa	769.2
31	Massachusetts	767.9
31	Nebraska	767.9
33	Connecticut	761.8
34	Arizona	744.8
35	Oregon	742.4
36	California	739.2
37	Wisconsin	714.3
38	Minnesota	693.1
39	North Dakota	679.9
40	Hawaii	675.5
41	Washington	673.5
42	Vermont	668.9
43	South Dakota	663.6
44	Colorado	656.4
45	New Mexico	625.6
46	Idaho	617.8
47	Utah	608.6
48	Wyoming	608.3
49	Alaska	570.8
50	Montana	564.1

	District of Columbia	1,268.1

Source: U.S. Department of Health and Human Services, National Center for Health Statistics
    "State Health Profiles"
*Age-adjusted years of potential life lost due to death before age 65.

Years Lost by Premature Death from Heart Disease in 1994

National Average = 610.7 Years Lost per 100,000 Population*

ALPHA ORDER				RANK ORDER		
RANK	**STATE**	**YEARS**		**RANK**	**STATE**	**YEARS**
2	Alabama	869.1		1	Mississippi	1,082.7
42	Alaska	459.2		2	Alabama	869.1
30	Arizona	543.6		3	Louisiana	862.1
8	Arkansas	768.0		4	South Carolina	812.9
39	California	477.4		5	Oklahoma	795.4
46	Colorado	416.6		6	Tennessee	785.9
29	Connecticut	556.1		7	West Virginia	776.1
11	Delaware	726.4		8	Arkansas	768.0
26	Florida	584.2		9	Kentucky	755.8
10	Georgia	750.9		10	Georgia	750.9
24	Hawaii	597.8		11	Delaware	726.4
41	Idaho	467.9		12	North Carolina	705.5
15	Illinois	665.4		13	Missouri	702.5
19	Indiana	639.3		14	Michigan	677.0
36	Iowa	489.0		15	Illinois	665.4
38	Kansas	480.2		16	Maryland	657.1
9	Kentucky	755.8		17	Nevada	646.8
3	Louisiana	862.1		18	Ohio	642.3
33	Maine	504.4		19	Indiana	639.3
16	Maryland	657.1		20	Pennsylvania	636.5
32	Massachusetts	504.7		21	Texas	631.7
14	Michigan	677.0		22	Virginia	618.6
43	Minnesota	445.2		23	New York	610.0
1	Mississippi	1,082.7		24	Hawaii	597.8
13	Missouri	702.5		25	South Dakota	589.9
47	Montana	406.8		26	Florida	584.2
34	Nebraska	501.6		27	Wyoming	576.5
17	Nevada	646.8		28	New Jersey	570.1
40	New Hampshire	473.4		29	Connecticut	556.1
28	New Jersey	570.1		30	Arizona	543.6
49	New Mexico	393.0		31	Rhode Island	539.0
23	New York	610.0		32	Massachusetts	504.7
12	North Carolina	705.5		33	Maine	504.4
37	North Dakota	488.0		34	Nebraska	501.6
18	Ohio	642.3		35	Wisconsin	494.0
5	Oklahoma	795.4		36	Iowa	489.0
48	Oregon	401.8		37	North Dakota	488.0
20	Pennsylvania	636.5		38	Kansas	480.2
31	Rhode Island	539.0		39	California	477.4
4	South Carolina	812.9		40	New Hampshire	473.4
25	South Dakota	589.9		41	Idaho	467.9
6	Tennessee	785.9		42	Alaska	459.2
21	Texas	631.7		43	Minnesota	445.2
50	Utah	391.5		44	Vermont	441.2
44	Vermont	441.2		45	Washington	426.1
22	Virginia	618.6		46	Colorado	416.6
45	Washington	426.1		47	Montana	406.8
7	West Virginia	776.1		48	Oregon	401.8
35	Wisconsin	494.0		49	New Mexico	393.0
27	Wyoming	576.5		50	Utah	391.5
					District of Columbia	1,009.8

Source: U.S. Department of Health and Human Services, National Center for Health Statistics
"State Health Profiles"
*Age-adjusted years of potential life lost due to death before age 65.

Years Lost by Premature Death from HIV Infection in 1994

National Average = 432.8 Years Lost per 100,000 Population*

ALPHA ORDER				RANK ORDER		
RANK	STATE	YEARS		RANK	STATE	YEARS
22	Alabama	280.3		1	New York	1,124.1
46	Alaska	82.2		2	Florida	861.4
17	Arizona	306.6		3	New Jersey	769.5
32	Arkansas	194.3		4	Maryland	611.5
6	California	527.6		5	Georgia	549.6
25	Colorado	264.4		6	California	527.6
8	Connecticut	448.0		7	Delaware	520.3
7	Delaware	520.3		8	Connecticut	448.0
2	Florida	861.4		9	Louisiana	441.9
5	Georgia	549.6		10	Texas	418.4
23	Hawaii	273.4		11	Massachusetts	405.3
47	Idaho	79.1		12	South Carolina	403.6
16	Illinois	325.6		13	North Carolina	380.0
36	Indiana	149.8		14	Nevada	376.8
45	Iowa	88.3		15	Mississippi	335.5
40	Kansas	125.7		16	Illinois	325.6
38	Kentucky	139.3		17	Arizona	306.6
9	Louisiana	441.9		18	Pennsylvania	306.4
33	Maine	156.6		19	Rhode Island	299.6
4	Maryland	611.5		20	Virginia	287.9
11	Massachusetts	405.3		21	Washington	284.1
30	Michigan	219.7		22	Alabama	280.3
34	Minnesota	154.5		23	Hawaii	273.4
15	Mississippi	335.5		24	Oregon	267.2
27	Missouri	248.6		25	Colorado	264.4
44	Montana	89.6		26	Tennessee	262.2
37	Nebraska	148.9		27	Missouri	248.6
14	Nevada	376.8		28	Oklahoma	244.8
43	New Hampshire	93.0		29	New Mexico	241.5
3	New Jersey	769.5		30	Michigan	219.7
29	New Mexico	241.5		31	Ohio	205.3
1	New York	1,124.1		32	Arkansas	194.3
13	North Carolina	380.0		33	Maine	156.6
NA	North Dakota**	NA		34	Minnesota	154.5
31	Ohio	205.3		34	Vermont	154.5
28	Oklahoma	244.8		36	Indiana	149.8
24	Oregon	267.2		37	Nebraska	148.9
18	Pennsylvania	306.4		38	Kentucky	139.3
19	Rhode Island	299.6		39	Utah	133.2
12	South Carolina	403.6		40	Kansas	125.7
NA	South Dakota**	NA		41	Wisconsin	113.1
26	Tennessee	262.2		42	West Virginia	99.1
10	Texas	418.4		43	New Hampshire	93.0
39	Utah	133.2		44	Montana	89.6
34	Vermont	154.5		45	Iowa	88.3
20	Virginia	287.9		46	Alaska	82.2
21	Washington	284.1		47	Idaho	79.1
42	West Virginia	99.1		NA	North Dakota**	NA
41	Wisconsin	113.1		NA	South Dakota**	NA
NA	Wyoming**	NA		NA	Wyoming**	NA
					District of Columbia	2,790.6

Source: U.S. Department of Health and Human Services, National Center for Health Statistics
   "State Health Profiles"
*Age-adjusted years of potential life lost due to death before age 65.
**Data for states with fewer than 20 deaths from HIV infection for persons under 65 years of age are considered
unreliable and are not shown.

Years Lost by Premature Death from Homicide and Suicide in 1994

National Average = 709.5 Years Lost per 100,000 Population*

ALPHA ORDER

RANK	STATE	YEARS
10	Alabama	864.4
9	Alaska	869.9
3	Arizona	1,009.1
6	Arkansas	903.5
13	California	808.8
23	Colorado	674.5
33	Connecticut	577.3
37	Delaware	508.9
16	Florida	765.4
20	Georgia	728.3
44	Hawaii	438.7
30	Idaho	622.8
12	Illinois	812.2
24	Indiana	667.9
46	Iowa	430.6
27	Kansas	653.6
34	Kentucky	566.3
1	Louisiana	1,213.8
45	Maine	437.3
11	Maryland	834.8
49	Massachusetts	383.4
17	Michigan	763.1
43	Minnesota	446.5
4	Mississippi	971.3
8	Missouri	876.6
26	Montana	661.7
41	Nebraska	463.3
2	Nevada	1,046.8
48	New Hampshire	391.7
47	New Jersey	419.6
5	New Mexico	952.2
22	New York	690.2
15	North Carolina	788.4
39	North Dakota	475.1
40	Ohio	468.3
18	Oklahoma	731.6
28	Oregon	648.5
35	Pennsylvania	562.5
42	Rhode Island	456.5
21	South Carolina	724.3
32	South Dakota	578.8
19	Tennessee	730.3
14	Texas	805.3
31	Utah	590.0
50	Vermont	287.4
25	Virginia	666.4
29	Washington	627.2
36	West Virginia	535.9
38	Wisconsin	503.2
7	Wyoming	890.5

RANK ORDER

RANK	STATE	YEARS
1	Louisiana	1,213.8
2	Nevada	1,046.8
3	Arizona	1,009.1
4	Mississippi	971.3
5	New Mexico	952.2
6	Arkansas	903.5
7	Wyoming	890.5
8	Missouri	876.6
9	Alaska	869.9
10	Alabama	864.4
11	Maryland	834.8
12	Illinois	812.2
13	California	808.8
14	Texas	805.3
15	North Carolina	788.4
16	Florida	765.4
17	Michigan	763.1
18	Oklahoma	731.6
19	Tennessee	730.3
20	Georgia	728.3
21	South Carolina	724.3
22	New York	690.2
23	Colorado	674.5
24	Indiana	667.9
25	Virginia	666.4
26	Montana	661.7
27	Kansas	653.6
28	Oregon	648.5
29	Washington	627.2
30	Idaho	622.8
31	Utah	590.0
32	South Dakota	578.8
33	Connecticut	577.3
34	Kentucky	566.3
35	Pennsylvania	562.5
36	West Virginia	535.9
37	Delaware	508.9
38	Wisconsin	503.2
39	North Dakota	475.1
40	Ohio	468.3
41	Nebraska	463.3
42	Rhode Island	456.5
43	Minnesota	446.5
44	Hawaii	438.7
45	Maine	437.3
46	Iowa	430.6
47	New Jersey	419.6
48	New Hampshire	391.7
49	Massachusetts	383.4
50	Vermont	287.4

| | District of Columbia | 3,062.7 |

Source: U.S. Department of Health and Human Services, National Center for Health Statistics
"State Health Profiles"
*Age-adjusted years of potential life lost due to death before age 65.

Years Lost by Premature Death from Unintentional Injuries in 1994

National Average = 928.2 Years Lost per 100,000 Population*

ALPHA ORDER

RANK ORDER

RANK	STATE	YEARS
7	Alabama	1,361.3
1	Alaska	1,645.5
9	Arizona	1,269.3
6	Arkansas	1,372.9
36	California	840.0
26	Colorado	973.1
41	Connecticut	731.3
30	Delaware	917.5
22	Florida	1,019.3
20	Georgia	1,043.5
42	Hawaii	713.4
14	Idaho	1,213.8
28	Illinois	945.3
31	Indiana	914.7
23	Iowa	1,012.3
24	Kansas	1,003.2
15	Kentucky	1,166.3
13	Louisiana	1,217.0
37	Maine	826.3
43	Maryland	704.5
50	Massachusetts	433.2
34	Michigan	855.9
40	Minnesota	797.4
2	Mississippi	1,599.5
16	Missouri	1,138.5
5	Montana	1,392.1
29	Nebraska	927.3
17	Nevada	1,131.0
48	New Hampshire	615.4
46	New Jersey	673.4
3	New Mexico	1,493.2
47	New York	673.2
18	North Carolina	1,104.4
32	North Dakota	879.3
44	Ohio	687.3
12	Oklahoma	1,236.9
19	Oregon	1,044.6
35	Pennsylvania	849.3
49	Rhode Island	468.1
8	South Carolina	1,282.3
11	South Dakota	1,253.7
10	Tennessee	1,268.4
25	Texas	974.7
27	Utah	947.2
45	Vermont	682.1
39	Virginia	818.1
33	Washington	861.0
21	West Virginia	1,028.5
38	Wisconsin	822.2
4	Wyoming	1,480.4

RANK	STATE	YEARS
1	Alaska	1,645.5
2	Mississippi	1,599.5
3	New Mexico	1,493.2
4	Wyoming	1,480.4
5	Montana	1,392.1
6	Arkansas	1,372.9
7	Alabama	1,361.3
8	South Carolina	1,282.3
9	Arizona	1,269.3
10	Tennessee	1,268.4
11	South Dakota	1,253.7
12	Oklahoma	1,236.9
13	Louisiana	1,217.0
14	Idaho	1,213.8
15	Kentucky	1,166.3
16	Missouri	1,138.5
17	Nevada	1,131.0
18	North Carolina	1,104.4
19	Oregon	1,044.6
20	Georgia	1,043.5
21	West Virginia	1,028.5
22	Florida	1,019.3
23	Iowa	1,012.3
24	Kansas	1,003.2
25	Texas	974.7
26	Colorado	973.1
27	Utah	947.2
28	Illinois	945.3
29	Nebraska	927.3
30	Delaware	917.5
31	Indiana	914.7
32	North Dakota	879.3
33	Washington	861.0
34	Michigan	855.9
35	Pennsylvania	849.3
36	California	840.0
37	Maine	826.3
38	Wisconsin	822.2
39	Virginia	818.1
40	Minnesota	797.4
41	Connecticut	731.3
42	Hawaii	713.4
43	Maryland	704.5
44	Ohio	687.3
45	Vermont	682.1
46	New Jersey	673.4
47	New York	673.2
48	New Hampshire	615.4
49	Rhode Island	468.1
50	Massachusetts	433.2
	District of Columbia	721.4

Source: U.S. Department of Health and Human Services, National Center for Health Statistics "State Health Profiles"

*Age-adjusted years of potential life lost due to death before age 65. Includes such subcategories as falls, drowning, fires/burns, poisonings and motor vehicle injuries.

Estimated Years of Potential Life Lost Attributable to Smoking in 1990

National Estimated Total = 5,062,814 Years of Potential Life Lost*

ALPHA ORDER

RANK ORDER

RANK	STATE	YEARS	% of USA		RANK	STATE	YEARS	% of USA
20	Alabama	90,360	1.78%		1	California	498,297	9.84%
50	Alaska	6,720	0.13%		2	New York	377,530	7.46%
26	Arizona	66,959	1.32%		3	Florida	328,191	6.48%
29	Arkansas	58,742	1.16%		4	Texas	317,631	6.27%
1	California	498,297	9.84%		5	Pennsylvania	271,839	5.37%
33	Colorado	49,000	0.97%		6	Illinois	235,933	4.66%
27	Connecticut	60,535	1.20%		7	Ohio	231,497	4.57%
41	Delaware	15,248	0.30%		8	Michigan	195,600	3.86%
3	Florida	328,191	6.48%		9	New Jersey	151,773	3.00%
11	Georgia	134,168	2.65%		10	North Carolina	147,810	2.92%
42	Hawaii	15,222	0.30%		11	Georgia	134,168	2.65%
43	Idaho	14,708	0.29%		12	Tennessee	132,635	2.62%
6	Illinois	235,933	4.66%		13	Indiana	123,584	2.44%
13	Indiana	123,584	2.44%		14	Missouri	122,136	2.41%
32	Iowa	50,521	1.00%		15	Virginia	119,716	2.36%
34	Kansas	42,540	0.84%		16	Massachusetts	117,640	2.32%
18	Kentucky	94,602	1.87%		17	Louisiana	94,886	1.87%
17	Louisiana	94,886	1.87%		18	Kentucky	94,602	1.87%
37	Maine	27,419	0.54%		19	Maryland	92,197	1.82%
19	Maryland	92,197	1.82%		20	Alabama	90,360	1.78%
16	Massachusetts	117,640	2.32%		21	Washington	89,222	1.76%
8	Michigan	195,600	3.86%		22	Wisconsin	86,345	1.71%
25	Minnesota	67,835	1.34%		23	South Carolina	79,069	1.56%
30	Mississippi	57,839	1.14%		24	Oklahoma	73,057	1.44%
14	Missouri	122,136	2.41%		25	Minnesota	67,835	1.34%
45	Montana	14,491	0.29%		26	Arizona	66,959	1.32%
36	Nebraska	29,075	0.57%		27	Connecticut	60,535	1.20%
35	Nevada	30,254	0.60%		28	Oregon	59,217	1.17%
40	New Hampshire	18,993	0.38%		29	Arkansas	58,742	1.16%
9	New Jersey	151,773	3.00%		30	Mississippi	57,839	1.14%
39	New Mexico	21,156	0.42%		31	West Virginia	51,007	1.01%
2	New York	377,530	7.46%		32	Iowa	50,521	1.00%
10	North Carolina	147,810	2.92%		33	Colorado	49,000	0.97%
47	North Dakota	11,717	0.23%		34	Kansas	42,540	0.84%
7	Ohio	231,497	4.57%		35	Nevada	30,254	0.60%
24	Oklahoma	73,057	1.44%		36	Nebraska	29,075	0.57%
28	Oregon	59,217	1.17%		37	Maine	27,419	0.54%
5	Pennsylvania	271,839	5.37%		38	Rhode Island	21,541	0.43%
38	Rhode Island	21,541	0.43%		39	New Mexico	21,156	0.42%
23	South Carolina	79,069	1.56%		40	New Hampshire	18,993	0.38%
46	South Dakota	12,684	0.25%		41	Delaware	15,248	0.30%
12	Tennessee	132,635	2.62%		42	Hawaii	15,222	0.30%
4	Texas	317,631	6.27%		43	Idaho	14,708	0.29%
44	Utah	14,572	0.29%		44	Utah	14,572	0.29%
48	Vermont	10,631	0.21%		45	Montana	14,491	0.29%
15	Virginia	119,716	2.36%		46	South Dakota	12,684	0.25%
21	Washington	89,222	1.76%		47	North Dakota	11,717	0.23%
31	West Virginia	51,007	1.01%		48	Vermont	10,631	0.21%
22	Wisconsin	86,345	1.71%		49	Wyoming	7,298	0.14%
49	Wyoming	7,298	0.14%		50	Alaska	6,720	0.13%
						District of Columbia	21,172	0.42%

Source: U.S. Department of Health and Human Services, Centers for Disease Control and Prevention
"Surveillance for Smoking-Attributable Mortality, 1990" (MMWR, Vol. 43, No. SS-1, June 10, 1994)
*Calculated by using life expectancy at age of death.

Estimated Deaths Attributable to Smoking in 1990

National Estimated Total = 415,226 Deaths

ALPHA ORDER

RANK	STATE	DEATHS	% of USA
22	Alabama	6,801	1.64%
50	Alaska	402	0.10%
25	Arizona	5,697	1.37%
30	Arkansas	4,706	1.13%
1	California	42,574	10.25%
33	Colorado	4,171	1.00%
27	Connecticut	5,362	1.29%
44	Delaware	1,178	0.28%
3	Florida	28,596	6.89%
15	Georgia	9,694	2.33%
46	Hawaii	1,174	0.28%
42	Idaho	1,304	0.31%
6	Illinois	19,269	4.64%
12	Indiana	10,250	2.47%
29	Iowa	4,816	1.16%
34	Kansas	3,828	0.92%
19	Kentucky	7,449	1.79%
21	Louisiana	6,887	1.66%
36	Maine	2,376	0.57%
20	Maryland	7,370	1.77%
11	Massachusetts	10,430	2.51%
8	Michigan	15,454	3.72%
24	Minnesota	6,127	1.48%
31	Mississippi	4,458	1.07%
14	Missouri	10,177	2.45%
41	Montana	1,313	0.32%
35	Nebraska	2,675	0.64%
37	Nevada	2,234	0.54%
40	New Hampshire	1,655	0.40%
9	New Jersey	12,605	3.04%
39	New Mexico	1,741	0.42%
2	New York	30,992	7.46%
10	North Carolina	11,032	2.66%
47	North Dakota	1,031	0.25%
7	Ohio	18,114	4.36%
23	Oklahoma	6,138	1.48%
28	Oregon	5,226	1.26%
5	Pennsylvania	22,624	5.45%
38	Rhode Island	1,881	0.45%
26	South Carolina	5,619	1.35%
45	South Dakota	1,175	0.28%
13	Tennessee	10,214	2.46%
4	Texas	25,452	6.13%
43	Utah	1,228	0.30%
48	Vermont	913	0.22%
16	Virginia	9,237	2.22%
17	Washington	7,790	1.88%
32	West Virginia	4,221	1.02%
18	Wisconsin	7,620	1.84%
49	Wyoming	659	0.16%

RANK ORDER

RANK	STATE	DEATHS	% of USA
1	California	42,574	10.25%
2	New York	30,992	7.46%
3	Florida	28,596	6.89%
4	Texas	25,452	6.13%
5	Pennsylvania	22,624	5.45%
6	Illinois	19,269	4.64%
7	Ohio	18,114	4.36%
8	Michigan	15,454	3.72%
9	New Jersey	12,605	3.04%
10	North Carolina	11,032	2.66%
11	Massachusetts	10,430	2.51%
12	Indiana	10,250	2.47%
13	Tennessee	10,214	2.46%
14	Missouri	10,177	2.45%
15	Georgia	9,694	2.33%
16	Virginia	9,237	2.22%
17	Washington	7,790	1.88%
18	Wisconsin	7,620	1.84%
19	Kentucky	7,449	1.79%
20	Maryland	7,370	1.77%
21	Louisiana	6,887	1.66%
22	Alabama	6,801	1.64%
23	Oklahoma	6,138	1.48%
24	Minnesota	6,127	1.48%
25	Arizona	5,697	1.37%
26	South Carolina	5,619	1.35%
27	Connecticut	5,362	1.29%
28	Oregon	5,226	1.26%
29	Iowa	4,816	1.16%
30	Arkansas	4,706	1.13%
31	Mississippi	4,458	1.07%
32	West Virginia	4,221	1.02%
33	Colorado	4,171	1.00%
34	Kansas	3,828	0.92%
35	Nebraska	2,675	0.64%
36	Maine	2,376	0.57%
37	Nevada	2,234	0.54%
38	Rhode Island	1,881	0.45%
39	New Mexico	1,741	0.42%
40	New Hampshire	1,655	0.40%
41	Montana	1,313	0.32%
42	Idaho	1,304	0.31%
43	Utah	1,228	0.30%
44	Delaware	1,178	0.28%
45	South Dakota	1,175	0.28%
46	Hawaii	1,174	0.28%
47	North Dakota	1,031	0.25%
48	Vermont	913	0.22%
49	Wyoming	659	0.16%
50	Alaska	402	0.10%
	District of Columbia	1,287	0.31%

Source: U.S. Department of Health and Human Services, Centers for Disease Control and Prevention "Surveillance for Smoking-Attributable Mortality, 1990" (MMWR, Vol. 43, No. SS-1, June 10, 1994)

Estimated Death Rate Attributable to Smoking in 1990

National Estimated Median Rate = 363.3 Deaths per 100,000 Population*

ALPHA ORDER

RANK ORDER

RANK	STATE	RATE	RANK	STATE	RATE
29	Alabama	350.4	1	Nevada	478.1
5	Alaska	398.2	2	Tennessee	442.1
35	Arizona	339.6	3	West Virginia	433.6
16	Arkansas	376.3	4	Kentucky	428.7
24	California	366.3	5	Alaska	398.2
38	Colorado	331.4	6	Indiana	394.3
39	Connecticut	325.7	7	Delaware	393.1
7	Delaware	393.1	8	Oklahoma	390.4
27	Florida	357.5	9	Maine	389.4
13	Georgia	383.5	10	Texas	389.1
49	Hawaii	257.2	11	Louisiana	388.2
47	Idaho	293.2	12	Missouri	383.8
26	Illinois	360.0	13	Georgia	383.5
6	Indiana	394.3	14	South Carolina	380.1
44	Iowa	304.2	15	Maryland	378.1
45	Kansas	300.8	16	Arkansas	376.3
4	Kentucky	428.7	17	Mississippi	375.1
11	Louisiana	388.2	18	Michigan	372.5
9	Maine	389.4	19	Wyoming	371.0
15	Maryland	378.1	20	Oregon	369.3
34	Massachusetts	345.3	21	North Carolina	367.6
18	Michigan	372.5	22	Washington	367.4
46	Minnesota	295.2	23	Virginia	366.6
17	Mississippi	375.1	24	California	366.3
12	Missouri	383.8	25	Vermont	363.3
36	Montana	334.2	26	Illinois	360.0
40	Nebraska	321.0	27	Florida	357.5
1	Nevada	478.1	28	New York	352.8
31	New Hampshire	349.3	29	Alabama	350.4
37	New Jersey	334.1	30	Rhode Island	350.3
48	New Mexico	287.7	31	New Hampshire	349.3
28	New York	352.8	32	Ohio	347.7
21	North Carolina	367.6	33	Pennsylvania	346.8
42	North Dakota	308.2	34	Massachusetts	345.3
32	Ohio	347.7	35	Arizona	339.6
8	Oklahoma	390.4	36	Montana	334.2
20	Oregon	369.3	37	New Jersey	334.1
33	Pennsylvania	346.8	38	Colorado	331.4
30	Rhode Island	350.3	39	Connecticut	325.7
14	South Carolina	380.1	40	Nebraska	321.0
43	South Dakota	307.9	41	Wisconsin	313.3
2	Tennessee	442.1	42	North Dakota	308.2
10	Texas	389.1	43	South Dakota	307.9
50	Utah	218.0	44	Iowa	304.2
25	Vermont	363.3	45	Kansas	300.8
23	Virginia	366.6	46	Minnesota	295.2
22	Washington	367.4	47	Idaho	293.2
3	West Virginia	433.6	48	New Mexico	287.7
41	Wisconsin	313.3	49	Hawaii	257.2
19	Wyoming	371.0	50	Utah	218.0
				District of Columbia	444.7

Source: U.S. Department of Health and Human Services, Centers for Disease Control and Prevention
    "Surveillance for Smoking-Attributable Mortality, 1990" (MMWR, Vol. 43, No. SS-1, June 10, 1994)
*Per 100,000 population of adults 35 years old or older in 1990. Deaths among infants and bum deaths among persons 1 to 34 years were excluded from rate calculations.

Alcohol-Induced Deaths in 1994

National Total = 20,163 Deaths*

ALPHA ORDER

RANK	STATE	DEATHS	% of USA
23	Alabama	287	1.42%
40	Alaska	86	0.43%
13	Arizona	429	2.13%
33	Arkansas	153	0.76%
1	California	3,509	17.40%
16	Colorado	389	1.93%
31	Connecticut	173	0.86%
48	Delaware	47	0.23%
3	Florida	1,251	6.20%
9	Georgia	581	2.88%
49	Hawaii	42	0.21%
45	Idaho	65	0.32%
5	Illinois	769	3.81%
25	Indiana	274	1.36%
35	Iowa	143	0.71%
34	Kansas	144	0.71%
27	Kentucky	250	1.24%
26	Louisiana	257	1.27%
38	Maine	99	0.49%
22	Maryland	292	1.45%
20	Massachusetts	331	1.64%
6	Michigan	720	3.57%
24	Minnesota	281	1.39%
32	Mississippi	164	0.81%
18	Missouri	366	1.82%
39	Montana	87	0.43%
43	Nebraska	80	0.40%
30	Nevada	197	0.98%
42	New Hampshire	82	0.41%
8	New Jersey	584	2.90%
28	New Mexico	233	1.16%
2	New York	1,739	8.62%
7	North Carolina	718	3.56%
47	North Dakota	48	0.24%
11	Ohio	513	2.54%
29	Oklahoma	209	1.04%
21	Oregon	300	1.49%
10	Pennsylvania	579	2.87%
46	Rhode Island	62	0.31%
14	South Carolina	415	2.06%
41	South Dakota	83	0.41%
15	Tennessee	400	1.98%
4	Texas	1,135	5.63%
37	Utah	117	0.58%
49	Vermont	42	0.21%
17	Virginia	378	1.87%
12	Washington	443	2.20%
36	West Virginia	128	0.63%
19	Wisconsin	341	1.69%
44	Wyoming	66	0.33%

RANK ORDER

RANK	STATE	DEATHS	% of USA
1	California	3,509	17.40%
2	New York	1,739	8.62%
3	Florida	1,251	6.20%
4	Texas	1,135	5.63%
5	Illinois	769	3.81%
6	Michigan	720	3.57%
7	North Carolina	718	3.56%
8	New Jersey	584	2.90%
9	Georgia	581	2.88%
10	Pennsylvania	579	2.87%
11	Ohio	513	2.54%
12	Washington	443	2.20%
13	Arizona	429	2.13%
14	South Carolina	415	2.06%
15	Tennessee	400	1.98%
16	Colorado	389	1.93%
17	Virginia	378	1.87%
18	Missouri	366	1.82%
19	Wisconsin	341	1.69%
20	Massachusetts	331	1.64%
21	Oregon	300	1.49%
22	Maryland	292	1.45%
23	Alabama	287	1.42%
24	Minnesota	281	1.39%
25	Indiana	274	1.36%
26	Louisiana	257	1.27%
27	Kentucky	250	1.24%
28	New Mexico	233	1.16%
29	Oklahoma	209	1.04%
30	Nevada	197	0.98%
31	Connecticut	173	0.86%
32	Mississippi	164	0.81%
33	Arkansas	153	0.76%
34	Kansas	144	0.71%
35	Iowa	143	0.71%
36	West Virginia	128	0.63%
37	Utah	117	0.58%
38	Maine	99	0.49%
39	Montana	87	0.43%
40	Alaska	86	0.43%
41	South Dakota	83	0.41%
42	New Hampshire	82	0.41%
43	Nebraska	80	0.40%
44	Wyoming	66	0.33%
45	Idaho	65	0.32%
46	Rhode Island	62	0.31%
47	North Dakota	48	0.24%
48	Delaware	47	0.23%
49	Hawaii	42	0.21%
49	Vermont	42	0.21%
	District of Columbia	82	0.41%

Source: U.S. Department of Health and Human Services, National Center for Health Statistics
   (http://wonder.cdc.gov/WONDER/)

By state of residence. Includes excessive blood level of alcohol, accidental poisoning by alcohol and the following alcohol-related causes: psychoses, dependence syndrome, polyneuropathy, cardiomyopathy, gastritis, chronic liver disease and cirrhosis. Excludes accidents, homicides and other causes indirectly related to alcohol use.

Death Rate from Alcohol-Induced Deaths in 1994

National Rate = 7.74 Deaths per 100,000 Population*

ALPHA ORDER

RANK	STATE	RATE
26	Alabama	6.80
1	Alaska	14.18
9	Arizona	10.51
32	Arkansas	6.23
7	California	11.16
8	Colorado	10.63
44	Connecticut	5.28
28	Delaware	6.64
14	Florida	8.96
16	Georgia	8.23
50	Hawaii	3.56
41	Idaho	5.73
29	Illinois	6.54
48	Indiana	4.76
45	Iowa	5.05
42	Kansas	5.63
30	Kentucky	6.52
38	Louisiana	5.95
17	Maine	7.98
39	Maryland	5.83
43	Massachusetts	5.47
19	Michigan	7.57
35	Minnesota	6.15
36	Mississippi	6.14
25	Missouri	6.93
10	Montana	10.16
46	Nebraska	4.92
4	Nevada	13.50
23	New Hampshire	7.21
21	New Jersey	7.38
2	New Mexico	14.08
13	New York	9.57
11	North Carolina	10.15
20	North Dakota	7.52
49	Ohio	4.61
31	Oklahoma	6.41
12	Oregon	9.71
47	Pennsylvania	4.80
33	Rhode Island	6.22
6	South Carolina	11.33
5	South Dakota	11.50
18	Tennessee	7.72
34	Texas	6.17
37	Utah	6.12
22	Vermont	7.23
40	Virginia	5.76
15	Washington	8.29
24	West Virginia	7.02
27	Wisconsin	6.70
3	Wyoming	13.86

RANK ORDER

RANK	STATE	RATE
1	Alaska	14.18
2	New Mexico	14.08
3	Wyoming	13.86
4	Nevada	13.50
5	South Dakota	11.50
6	South Carolina	11.33
7	California	11.16
8	Colorado	10.63
9	Arizona	10.51
10	Montana	10.16
11	North Carolina	10.15
12	Oregon	9.71
13	New York	9.57
14	Florida	8.96
15	Washington	8.29
16	Georgia	8.23
17	Maine	7.98
18	Tennessee	7.72
19	Michigan	7.57
20	North Dakota	7.52
21	New Jersey	7.38
22	Vermont	7.23
23	New Hampshire	7.21
24	West Virginia	7.02
25	Missouri	6.93
26	Alabama	6.80
27	Wisconsin	6.70
28	Delaware	6.64
29	Illinois	6.54
30	Kentucky	6.52
31	Oklahoma	6.41
32	Arkansas	6.23
33	Rhode Island	6.22
34	Texas	6.17
35	Minnesota	6.15
36	Mississippi	6.14
37	Utah	6.12
38	Louisiana	5.95
39	Maryland	5.83
40	Virginia	5.76
41	Idaho	5.73
42	Kansas	5.63
43	Massachusetts	5.47
44	Connecticut	5.28
45	Iowa	5.05
46	Nebraska	4.92
47	Pennsylvania	4.80
48	Indiana	4.76
49	Ohio	4.61
50	Hawaii	3.56
	District of Columbia	14.35

Source: U.S. Department of Health and Human Services, National Center for Health Statistics
   (http://wonder.cdc.gov/WONDER/)
*By state of residence. Includes excessive blood level of alcohol, accidental poisoning by alcohol and the following alcohol-related causes: psychoses, dependence syndrome, polyneuropathy, cardiomyopathy, gastritis, chronic liver disease and cirrhosis. Excludes accidents, homicides and other causes indirectly related to alcohol use. Not age-adjusted.

Drug-Induced Deaths in 1994

National Total = 13,923 Deaths*

RANK	STATE	DEATHS	% of USA
32	Alabama	89	0.64%
45	Alaska	26	0.19%
12	Arizona	338	2.43%
33	Arkansas	86	0.62%
1	California	2,590	18.60%
19	Colorado	217	1.56%
17	Connecticut	230	1.65%
39	Delaware	54	0.39%
7	Florida	598	4.30%
14	Georgia	262	1.88%
34	Hawaii	81	0.58%
41	Idaho	51	0.37%
6	Illinois	601	4.32%
28	Indiana	134	0.96%
36	Iowa	68	0.49%
38	Kansas	65	0.47%
27	Kentucky	135	0.97%
22	Louisiana	175	1.26%
44	Maine	27	0.19%
9	Maryland	468	3.36%
8	Massachusetts	480	3.45%
10	Michigan	421	3.02%
29	Minnesota	109	0.78%
37	Mississippi	67	0.48%
21	Missouri	185	1.33%
42	Montana	39	0.28%
43	Nebraska	30	0.22%
25	Nevada	142	1.02%
46	New Hampshire	23	0.17%
5	New Jersey	739	5.31%
24	New Mexico	164	1.18%
2	New York	1,275	9.16%
18	North Carolina	224	1.61%
50	North Dakota	7	0.05%
13	Ohio	332	2.38%
31	Oklahoma	94	0.68%
16	Oregon	236	1.70%
3	Pennsylvania	837	6.01%
35	Rhode Island	72	0.52%
26	South Carolina	140	1.01%
49	South Dakota	13	0.09%
20	Tennessee	204	1.47%
4	Texas	788	5.66%
30	Utah	108	0.78%
46	Vermont	23	0.17%
15	Virginia	249	1.79%
11	Washington	370	2.66%
39	West Virginia	54	0.39%
23	Wisconsin	167	1.20%
48	Wyoming	18	0.13%

RANK	STATE	DEATHS	% of USA
1	California	2,590	18.60%
2	New York	1,275	9.16%
3	Pennsylvania	837	6.01%
4	Texas	788	5.66%
5	New Jersey	739	5.31%
6	Illinois	601	4.32%
7	Florida	598	4.30%
8	Massachusetts	480	3.45%
9	Maryland	468	3.36%
10	Michigan	421	3.02%
11	Washington	370	2.66%
12	Arizona	338	2.43%
13	Ohio	332	2.38%
14	Georgia	262	1.88%
15	Virginia	249	1.79%
16	Oregon	236	1.70%
17	Connecticut	230	1.65%
18	North Carolina	224	1.61%
19	Colorado	217	1.56%
20	Tennessee	204	1.47%
21	Missouri	185	1.33%
22	Louisiana	175	1.26%
23	Wisconsin	167	1.20%
24	New Mexico	164	1.18%
25	Nevada	142	1.02%
26	South Carolina	140	1.01%
27	Kentucky	135	0.97%
28	Indiana	134	0.96%
29	Minnesota	109	0.78%
30	Utah	108	0.78%
31	Oklahoma	94	0.68%
32	Alabama	89	0.64%
33	Arkansas	86	0.62%
34	Hawaii	81	0.58%
35	Rhode Island	72	0.52%
36	Iowa	68	0.49%
37	Mississippi	67	0.48%
38	Kansas	65	0.47%
39	Delaware	54	0.39%
39	West Virginia	54	0.39%
41	Idaho	51	0.37%
42	Montana	39	0.28%
43	Nebraska	30	0.22%
44	Maine	27	0.19%
45	Alaska	26	0.19%
46	New Hampshire	23	0.17%
46	Vermont	23	0.17%
48	Wyoming	18	0.13%
49	South Dakota	13	0.09%
50	North Dakota	7	0.05%
	District of Columbia	18	0.13%

Source: U.S. Department of Health and Human Services, National Center for Health Statistics (http://wonder.cdc.gov/WONDER/)

By state of residence. Includes drug psychoses, drug dependence, nondependent use excluding alcohol and tobacco, accidental poisoning or suicide by drugs, medicaments and biologicals. Excludes accidents, homicides and other causes indirectly related to drug use.

Death Rate from Drug-Induced Deaths in 1994

National Rate = 5.35 Deaths per 100,000 Population*

RANK	STATE	RATE
46	Alabama	2.10
22	Alaska	4.28
5	Arizona	8.28
33	Arkansas	3.50
6	California	8.23
16	Colorado	5.93
11	Connecticut	7.02
9	Delaware	7.63
22	Florida	4.28
31	Georgia	3.71
15	Hawaii	6.87
20	Idaho	4.49
18	Illinois	5.11
44	Indiana	2.32
42	Iowa	2.40
40	Kansas	2.54
32	Kentucky	3.52
25	Louisiana	4.05
45	Maine	2.17
3	Maryland	9.34
7	Massachusetts	7.94
21	Michigan	4.43
43	Minnesota	2.38
41	Mississippi	2.50
33	Missouri	3.50
19	Montana	4.55
48	Nebraska	1.84
2	Nevada	9.73
47	New Hampshire	2.02
3	New Jersey	9.34
1	New Mexico	9.91
12	New York	7.01
36	North Carolina	3.16
50	North Dakota	1.09
37	Ohio	2.98
39	Oklahoma	2.88
8	Oregon	7.64
13	Pennsylvania	6.94
10	Rhode Island	7.22
28	South Carolina	3.82
49	South Dakota	1.80
27	Tennessee	3.94
22	Texas	4.28
17	Utah	5.65
26	Vermont	3.96
29	Virginia	3.79
14	Washington	6.92
38	West Virginia	2.96
35	Wisconsin	3.28
30	Wyoming	3.78

RANK	STATE	RATE
1	New Mexico	9.91
2	Nevada	9.73
3	Maryland	9.34
3	New Jersey	9.34
5	Arizona	8.28
6	California	8.23
7	Massachusetts	7.94
8	Oregon	7.64
9	Delaware	7.63
10	Rhode Island	7.22
11	Connecticut	7.02
12	New York	7.01
13	Pennsylvania	6.94
14	Washington	6.92
15	Hawaii	6.87
16	Colorado	5.93
17	Utah	5.65
18	Illinois	5.11
19	Montana	4.55
20	Idaho	4.49
21	Michigan	4.43
22	Alaska	4.28
22	Florida	4.28
22	Texas	4.28
25	Louisiana	4.05
26	Vermont	3.96
27	Tennessee	3.94
28	South Carolina	3.82
29	Virginia	3.79
30	Wyoming	3.78
31	Georgia	3.71
32	Kentucky	3.52
33	Arkansas	3.50
33	Missouri	3.50
35	Wisconsin	3.28
36	North Carolina	3.16
37	Ohio	2.98
38	West Virginia	2.96
39	Oklahoma	2.88
40	Kansas	2.54
41	Mississippi	2.50
42	Iowa	2.40
43	Minnesota	2.38
44	Indiana	2.32
45	Maine	2.17
46	Alabama	2.10
47	New Hampshire	2.02
48	Nebraska	1.84
49	South Dakota	1.80
50	North Dakota	1.09

	District of Columbia	3.15

Source: U.S. Department of Health and Human Services, National Center for Health Statistics
(http://wonder.cdc.gov/WONDER/)

*By state of residence. Includes drug psychoses, drug dependence, nondependent use excluding alcohol and tobacco, accidental poisoning or suicide by drugs, medicaments and biologicals. Excludes accidents, homicides and other causes indirectly related to drug use. Not age adjusted.

Occupational Fatalities per 100,000 Workers: 1993 to 1995

National Rate = 4.4 Deaths per 100,000 Workers*

ALPHA ORDER				RANK ORDER		
RANK	STATE	RATE		RANK	STATE	RATE
28	Alabama	5.2		1	Alaska	36.3
1	Alaska	36.3		2	North Dakota	32.6
27	Arizona	5.6		3	Wyoming	29.3
21	Arkansas	7.7		4	Vermont	27.5
50	California	0.7		5	Montana	27.4
29	Colorado	5.1		6	South Dakota	27.1
22	Connecticut	7.2		7	Delaware	21.7
7	Delaware	21.7		8	Rhode Island	18.5
48	Florida	1.7		9	Maine	17.6
40	Georgia	3.0		10	Idaho	16.7
16	Hawaii	12.5		11	New Hampshire	16.6
10	Idaho	16.7		12	Nevada	15.1
47	Illinois	2.1		13	Nebraska	14.6
36	Indiana	4.2		14	West Virginia	14.2
19	Iowa	8.1		15	New Mexico	13.8
20	Kansas	8.0		16	Hawaii	12.5
24	Kentucky	6.6		17	Utah	12.4
26	Louisiana	5.9		18	Mississippi	9.3
9	Maine	17.6		19	Iowa	8.1
32	Maryland	4.8		20	Kansas	8.0
36	Massachusetts	4.2		21	Arkansas	7.7
42	Michigan	2.8		22	Connecticut	7.2
32	Minnesota	4.8		23	Oregon	7.0
18	Mississippi	9.3		24	Kentucky	6.6
36	Missouri	4.2		25	South Carolina	6.5
5	Montana	27.4		26	Louisiana	5.9
13	Nebraska	14.6		27	Arizona	5.6
12	Nevada	15.1		28	Alabama	5.2
11	New Hampshire	16.6		29	Colorado	5.1
40	New Jersey	3.0		29	Tennessee	5.1
15	New Mexico	13.8		31	Oklahoma	5.0
42	New York	2.8		32	Maryland	4.8
42	North Carolina	2.8		32	Minnesota	4.8
2	North Dakota	32.6		34	Wisconsin	4.6
45	Ohio	2.3		35	Washington	4.4
31	Oklahoma	5.0		36	Indiana	4.2
23	Oregon	7.0		36	Massachusetts	4.2
46	Pennsylvania	2.2		36	Missouri	4.2
8	Rhode Island	18.5		39	Virginia	3.5
25	South Carolina	6.5		40	Georgia	3.0
6	South Dakota	27.1		40	New Jersey	3.0
29	Tennessee	5.1		42	Michigan	2.8
49	Texas	1.1		42	New York	2.8
17	Utah	12.4		42	North Carolina	2.8
4	Vermont	27.5		45	Ohio	2.3
39	Virginia	3.5		46	Pennsylvania	2.2
35	Washington	4.4		47	Illinois	2.1
14	West Virginia	14.2		48	Florida	1.7
34	Wisconsin	4.6		49	Texas	1.1
3	Wyoming	29.3		50	California	0.7
					District of Columbia**	NA

Source: U.S. Department of Labor, Bureau of Labor Statistics
 "Census of Fatal Occupational Injuries"
Fatalities are adjusted to reflect differences in industry mixes from state to state.
**Not available.*

III. FACILITIES

Hospitals in 1995

National Total = 6,291 Hospitals*

RANK	STATE	HOSPITALS	% of USA
20	Alabama	133	2.11%
46	Alaska	27	0.43%
29	Arizona	89	1.41%
28	Arkansas	96	1.53%
1	California	499	7.93%
30	Colorado	87	1.38%
38	Connecticut	55	0.87%
50	Delaware	13	0.21%
5	Florida	264	4.20%
8	Georgia	195	3.10%
47	Hawaii	26	0.41%
41	Idaho	48	0.76%
6	Illinois	242	3.85%
18	Indiana	136	2.16%
22	Iowa	127	2.02%
13	Kansas	151	2.40%
23	Kentucky	121	1.92%
10	Louisiana	161	2.56%
42	Maine	45	0.72%
32	Maryland	80	1.27%
17	Massachusetts	139	2.21%
9	Michigan	190	3.02%
11	Minnesota	155	2.46%
25	Mississippi	109	1.73%
13	Missouri	151	2.40%
36	Montana	61	0.97%
27	Nebraska	101	1.61%
45	Nevada	28	0.45%
43	New Hampshire	36	0.57%
24	New Jersey	113	1.80%
36	New Mexico	61	0.97%
3	New York	286	4.55%
12	North Carolina	152	2.42%
39	North Dakota	51	0.81%
7	Ohio	210	3.34%
18	Oklahoma	136	2.16%
33	Oregon	71	1.13%
4	Pennsylvania	282	4.48%
49	Rhode Island	16	0.25%
31	South Carolina	84	1.34%
35	South Dakota	62	0.99%
15	Tennessee	148	2.35%
2	Texas	498	7.92%
40	Utah	50	0.79%
48	Vermont	17	0.27%
21	Virginia	128	2.03%
26	Washington	104	1.65%
34	West Virginia	67	1.07%
16	Wisconsin	144	2.29%
44	Wyoming	29	0.46%

RANK	STATE	HOSPITALS	% of USA
1	California	499	7.93%
2	Texas	498	7.92%
3	New York	286	4.55%
4	Pennsylvania	282	4.48%
5	Florida	264	4.20%
6	Illinois	242	3.85%
7	Ohio	210	3.34%
8	Georgia	195	3.10%
9	Michigan	190	3.02%
10	Louisiana	161	2.56%
11	Minnesota	155	2.46%
12	North Carolina	152	2.42%
13	Kansas	151	2.40%
13	Missouri	151	2.40%
15	Tennessee	148	2.35%
16	Wisconsin	144	2.29%
17	Massachusetts	139	2.21%
18	Indiana	136	2.16%
18	Oklahoma	136	2.16%
20	Alabama	133	2.11%
21	Virginia	128	2.03%
22	Iowa	127	2.02%
23	Kentucky	121	1.92%
24	New Jersey	113	1.80%
25	Mississippi	109	1.73%
26	Washington	104	1.65%
27	Nebraska	101	1.61%
28	Arkansas	96	1.53%
29	Arizona	89	1.41%
30	Colorado	87	1.38%
31	South Carolina	84	1.34%
32	Maryland	80	1.27%
33	Oregon	71	1.13%
34	West Virginia	67	1.07%
35	South Dakota	62	0.99%
36	Montana	61	0.97%
36	New Mexico	61	0.97%
38	Connecticut	55	0.87%
39	North Dakota	51	0.81%
40	Utah	50	0.79%
41	Idaho	48	0.76%
42	Maine	45	0.72%
43	New Hampshire	36	0.57%
44	Wyoming	29	0.46%
45	Nevada	28	0.45%
46	Alaska	27	0.43%
47	Hawaii	26	0.41%
48	Vermont	17	0.27%
49	Rhode Island	16	0.25%
50	Delaware	13	0.21%
	District of Columbia	17	0.27%

Source: American Hospital Association (Chicago, IL)
"Hospital Statistics" (1996-97 edition)
Federal and nonfederal hospitals.

Federal Hospitals in 1995

National Total = 299 Hospitals*

ALPHA ORDER

RANK ORDER

RANK	STATE	HOSPITALS	% of USA
11	Alabama	8	2.68%
16	Alaska	7	2.34%
3	Arizona	15	5.02%
34	Arkansas	3	1.00%
1	California	18	6.02%
19	Colorado	6	2.01%
41	Connecticut	2	0.67%
41	Delaware	2	0.67%
5	Florida	12	4.01%
11	Georgia	8	2.68%
46	Hawaii	1	0.33%
41	Idaho	2	0.67%
11	Illinois	8	2.68%
34	Indiana	3	1.00%
34	Iowa	3	1.00%
21	Kansas	5	1.67%
30	Kentucky	4	1.34%
21	Louisiana	5	1.67%
46	Maine	1	0.33%
11	Maryland	8	2.68%
30	Massachusetts	4	1.34%
21	Michigan	5	1.67%
30	Minnesota	4	1.34%
21	Mississippi	5	1.67%
16	Missouri	7	2.34%
21	Montana	5	1.67%
21	Nebraska	5	1.67%
34	Nevada	3	1.00%
46	New Hampshire	1	0.33%
34	New Jersey	3	1.00%
5	New Mexico	12	4.01%
4	New York	13	4.35%
9	North Carolina	9	3.01%
21	North Dakota	5	1.67%
21	Ohio	5	1.67%
7	Oklahoma	11	3.68%
41	Oregon	2	0.67%
8	Pennsylvania	10	3.34%
46	Rhode Island	1	0.33%
19	South Carolina	6	2.01%
9	South Dakota	9	3.01%
21	Tennessee	5	1.67%
1	Texas	18	6.02%
41	Utah	2	0.67%
46	Vermont	1	0.33%
11	Virginia	8	2.68%
16	Washington	7	2.34%
30	West Virginia	4	1.34%
34	Wisconsin	3	1.00%
34	Wyoming	3	1.00%

RANK	STATE	HOSPITALS	% of USA
1	California	18	6.02%
1	Texas	18	6.02%
3	Arizona	15	5.02%
4	New York	13	4.35%
5	Florida	12	4.01%
5	New Mexico	12	4.01%
7	Oklahoma	11	3.68%
8	Pennsylvania	10	3.34%
9	North Carolina	9	3.01%
9	South Dakota	9	3.01%
11	Alabama	8	2.68%
11	Georgia	8	2.68%
11	Illinois	8	2.68%
11	Maryland	8	2.68%
11	Virginia	8	2.68%
16	Alaska	7	2.34%
16	Missouri	7	2.34%
16	Washington	7	2.34%
19	Colorado	6	2.01%
19	South Carolina	6	2.01%
21	Kansas	5	1.67%
21	Louisiana	5	1.67%
21	Michigan	5	1.67%
21	Mississippi	5	1.67%
21	Montana	5	1.67%
21	Nebraska	5	1.67%
21	North Dakota	5	1.67%
21	Ohio	5	1.67%
21	Tennessee	5	1.67%
30	Kentucky	4	1.34%
30	Massachusetts	4	1.34%
30	Minnesota	4	1.34%
30	West Virginia	4	1.34%
34	Arkansas	3	1.00%
34	Indiana	3	1.00%
34	Iowa	3	1.00%
34	Nevada	3	1.00%
34	New Jersey	3	1.00%
34	Wisconsin	3	1.00%
34	Wyoming	3	1.00%
41	Connecticut	2	0.67%
41	Delaware	2	0.67%
41	Idaho	2	0.67%
41	Oregon	2	0.67%
41	Utah	2	0.67%
46	Hawaii	1	0.33%
46	Maine	1	0.33%
46	New Hampshire	1	0.33%
46	Rhode Island	1	0.33%
46	Vermont	1	0.33%
	District of Columbia	2	0.67%

Source: American Hospital Association (Chicago, IL)
"Hospital Statistics" (1996-97 edition)
*Federal hospitals are controlled by an agency or department of the federal government.

Nonfederal Hospitals in 1995

National Total = 5,992 Hospitals

RANK	STATE	HOSPITALS	% of USA
19	Alabama	125	2.09%
47	Alaska	20	0.33%
31	Arizona	74	1.23%
28	Arkansas	93	1.55%
1	California	481	8.03%
29	Colorado	81	1.35%
36	Connecticut	53	0.88%
50	Delaware	11	0.18%
5	Florida	252	4.21%
8	Georgia	187	3.12%
45	Hawaii	25	0.42%
40	Idaho	46	0.77%
6	Illinois	234	3.91%
18	Indiana	133	2.22%
21	Iowa	124	2.07%
12	Kansas	146	2.44%
23	Kentucky	117	1.95%
10	Louisiana	156	2.60%
42	Maine	44	0.73%
32	Maryland	72	1.20%
17	Massachusetts	135	2.25%
9	Michigan	185	3.09%
11	Minnesota	151	2.52%
25	Mississippi	104	1.74%
13	Missouri	144	2.40%
35	Montana	56	0.93%
27	Nebraska	96	1.60%
45	Nevada	25	0.42%
43	New Hampshire	35	0.58%
24	New Jersey	110	1.84%
38	New Mexico	49	0.82%
3	New York	273	4.56%
14	North Carolina	143	2.39%
40	North Dakota	46	0.77%
7	Ohio	205	3.42%
19	Oklahoma	125	2.09%
33	Oregon	69	1.15%
4	Pennsylvania	272	4.54%
49	Rhode Island	15	0.25%
30	South Carolina	78	1.30%
36	South Dakota	53	0.88%
14	Tennessee	143	2.39%
2	Texas	480	8.01%
39	Utah	48	0.80%
48	Vermont	16	0.27%
22	Virginia	120	2.00%
26	Washington	97	1.62%
34	West Virginia	63	1.05%
16	Wisconsin	141	2.35%
44	Wyoming	26	0.43%

RANK	STATE	HOSPITALS	% of USA
1	California	481	8.03%
2	Texas	480	8.01%
3	New York	273	4.56%
4	Pennsylvania	272	4.54%
5	Florida	252	4.21%
6	Illinois	234	3.91%
7	Ohio	205	3.42%
8	Georgia	187	3.12%
9	Michigan	185	3.09%
10	Louisiana	156	2.60%
11	Minnesota	151	2.52%
12	Kansas	146	2.44%
13	Missouri	144	2.40%
14	North Carolina	143	2.39%
14	Tennessee	143	2.39%
16	Wisconsin	141	2.35%
17	Massachusetts	135	2.25%
18	Indiana	133	2.22%
19	Alabama	125	2.09%
19	Oklahoma	125	2.09%
21	Iowa	124	2.07%
22	Virginia	120	2.00%
23	Kentucky	117	1.95%
24	New Jersey	110	1.84%
25	Mississippi	104	1.74%
26	Washington	97	1.62%
27	Nebraska	96	1.60%
28	Arkansas	93	1.55%
29	Colorado	81	1.35%
30	South Carolina	78	1.30%
31	Arizona	74	1.23%
32	Maryland	72	1.20%
33	Oregon	69	1.15%
34	West Virginia	63	1.05%
35	Montana	56	0.93%
36	Connecticut	53	0.88%
36	South Dakota	53	0.88%
38	New Mexico	49	0.82%
39	Utah	48	0.80%
40	Idaho	46	0.77%
40	North Dakota	46	0.77%
42	Maine	44	0.73%
43	New Hampshire	35	0.58%
44	Wyoming	26	0.43%
45	Hawaii	25	0.42%
45	Nevada	25	0.42%
47	Alaska	20	0.33%
48	Vermont	16	0.27%
49	Rhode Island	15	0.25%
50	Delaware	11	0.18%
	District of Columbia	15	0.25%

Source: American Hospital Association (Chicago, IL)
"Hospital Statistics" (1996-97 edition)

Psychiatric Hospitals in 1995

National Total = 675 Hospitals*

ALPHA ORDER				RANK ORDER			
RANK	STATE	HOSPITALS	% of USA	RANK	STATE	HOSPITALS	% of USA
26	Alabama	11	1.63%	1	Texas	51	7.56%
42	Alaska	3	0.44%	2	California	47	6.96%
22	Arizona	12	1.78%	3	Pennsylvania	40	5.93%
29	Arkansas	8	1.19%	4	New York	39	5.78%
2	California	47	6.96%	5	Florida	34	5.04%
27	Colorado	10	1.48%	6	Ohio	24	3.56%
16	Connecticut	15	2.22%	7	Georgia	23	3.41%
42	Delaware	3	0.44%	7	Illinois	23	3.41%
5	Florida	34	5.04%	7	Massachusetts	23	3.41%
7	Georgia	23	3.41%	10	Louisiana	22	3.26%
47	Hawaii	1	0.15%	11	North Carolina	20	2.96%
35	Idaho	5	0.74%	11	Virginia	20	2.96%
7	Illinois	23	3.41%	13	Indiana	19	2.81%
13	Indiana	19	2.81%	14	Maryland	17	2.52%
31	Iowa	7	1.04%	14	Michigan	17	2.52%
21	Kansas	13	1.93%	16	Connecticut	15	2.22%
22	Kentucky	12	1.78%	16	Tennessee	15	2.22%
10	Louisiana	22	3.26%	18	Missouri	14	2.07%
35	Maine	5	0.74%	18	Oklahoma	14	2.07%
14	Maryland	17	2.52%	18	Wisconsin	14	2.07%
7	Massachusetts	23	3.41%	21	Kansas	13	1.93%
14	Michigan	17	2.52%	22	Arizona	12	1.78%
29	Minnesota	8	1.19%	22	Kentucky	12	1.78%
31	Mississippi	7	1.04%	22	New Jersey	12	1.78%
18	Missouri	14	2.07%	22	New Mexico	12	1.78%
47	Montana	1	0.15%	26	Alabama	11	1.63%
39	Nebraska	4	0.59%	27	Colorado	10	1.48%
35	Nevada	5	0.74%	28	South Carolina	9	1.33%
39	New Hampshire	4	0.59%	29	Arkansas	8	1.19%
22	New Jersey	12	1.78%	29	Minnesota	8	1.19%
22	New Mexico	12	1.78%	31	Iowa	7	1.04%
4	New York	39	5.78%	31	Mississippi	7	1.04%
11	North Carolina	20	2.96%	33	Utah	6	0.89%
47	North Dakota	1	0.15%	33	Washington	6	0.89%
6	Ohio	24	3.56%	35	Idaho	5	0.74%
18	Oklahoma	14	2.07%	35	Maine	5	0.74%
35	Oregon	5	0.74%	35	Nevada	5	0.74%
3	Pennsylvania	40	5.93%	35	Oregon	5	0.74%
42	Rhode Island	3	0.44%	39	Nebraska	4	0.59%
28	South Carolina	9	1.33%	39	New Hampshire	4	0.59%
47	South Dakota	1	0.15%	39	West Virginia	4	0.59%
16	Tennessee	15	2.22%	42	Alaska	3	0.44%
1	Texas	51	7.56%	42	Delaware	3	0.44%
33	Utah	6	0.89%	42	Rhode Island	3	0.44%
45	Vermont	2	0.30%	45	Vermont	2	0.30%
11	Virginia	20	2.96%	45	Wyoming	2	0.30%
33	Washington	6	0.89%	47	Hawaii	1	0.15%
39	West Virginia	4	0.59%	47	Montana	1	0.15%
18	Wisconsin	14	2.07%	47	North Dakota	1	0.15%
45	Wyoming	2	0.30%	47	South Dakota	1	0.15%
				District of Columbia		2	0.30%

Source: American Hospital Association (Chicago, IL)
"Hospital Statistics" (1996-97 edition)
*Federal and nonfederal psychiatric hospitals.

Community Hospitals in 1995

National Total = 5,194 Hospitals*

RANK	STATE	HOSPITALS	% of USA
18	Alabama	115	2.21%
47	Alaska	17	0.33%
32	Arizona	61	1.17%
28	Arkansas	85	1.64%
1	California	424	8.16%
29	Colorado	69	1.33%
42	Connecticut	34	0.65%
50	Delaware	8	0.15%
5	Florida	212	4.08%
9	Georgia	160	3.08%
45	Hawaii	21	0.40%
39	Idaho	41	0.79%
6	Illinois	207	3.99%
18	Indiana	115	2.21%
17	Iowa	116	2.23%
11	Kansas	132	2.54%
21	Kentucky	104	2.00%
12	Louisiana	130	2.50%
40	Maine	39	0.75%
35	Maryland	50	0.96%
23	Massachusetts	96	1.85%
8	Michigan	167	3.22%
10	Minnesota	142	2.73%
22	Mississippi	97	1.87%
14	Missouri	126	2.43%
34	Montana	55	1.06%
26	Nebraska	91	1.75%
46	Nevada	20	0.39%
43	New Hampshire	29	0.56%
25	New Jersey	92	1.77%
41	New Mexico	36	0.69%
3	New York	230	4.43%
16	North Carolina	119	2.29%
37	North Dakota	43	0.83%
7	Ohio	180	3.47%
20	Oklahoma	110	2.12%
31	Oregon	64	1.23%
4	Pennsylvania	225	4.33%
49	Rhode Island	11	0.21%
30	South Carolina	66	1.27%
35	South Dakota	50	0.96%
14	Tennessee	126	2.43%
2	Texas	416	8.01%
38	Utah	42	0.81%
48	Vermont	14	0.27%
23	Virginia	96	1.85%
27	Washington	88	1.69%
33	West Virginia	59	1.14%
13	Wisconsin	127	2.45%
44	Wyoming	25	0.48%

RANK	STATE	HOSPITALS	% of USA
1	California	424	8.16%
2	Texas	416	8.01%
3	New York	230	4.43%
4	Pennsylvania	225	4.33%
5	Florida	212	4.08%
6	Illinois	207	3.99%
7	Ohio	180	3.47%
8	Michigan	167	3.22%
9	Georgia	160	3.08%
10	Minnesota	142	2.73%
11	Kansas	132	2.54%
12	Louisiana	130	2.50%
13	Wisconsin	127	2.45%
14	Missouri	126	2.43%
14	Tennessee	126	2.43%
16	North Carolina	119	2.29%
17	Iowa	116	2.23%
18	Alabama	115	2.21%
18	Indiana	115	2.21%
20	Oklahoma	110	2.12%
21	Kentucky	104	2.00%
22	Mississippi	97	1.87%
23	Massachusetts	96	1.85%
23	Virginia	96	1.85%
25	New Jersey	92	1.77%
26	Nebraska	91	1.75%
27	Washington	88	1.69%
28	Arkansas	85	1.64%
29	Colorado	69	1.33%
30	South Carolina	66	1.27%
31	Oregon	64	1.23%
32	Arizona	61	1.17%
33	West Virginia	59	1.14%
34	Montana	55	1.06%
35	Maryland	50	0.96%
35	South Dakota	50	0.96%
37	North Dakota	43	0.83%
38	Utah	42	0.81%
39	Idaho	41	0.79%
40	Maine	39	0.75%
41	New Mexico	36	0.69%
42	Connecticut	34	0.65%
43	New Hampshire	29	0.56%
44	Wyoming	25	0.48%
45	Hawaii	21	0.40%
46	Nevada	20	0.39%
47	Alaska	17	0.33%
48	Vermont	14	0.27%
49	Rhode Island	11	0.21%
50	Delaware	8	0.15%
	District of Columbia	12	0.23%

Source: American Hospital Association (Chicago, IL)
 "Hospital Statistics" (1996-97 edition)
*All nonfederal short-term general and other special hospitals whose facilities and services are available to the public. Community hospitals are a subset of nonfederal hospitals.

Community Hospitals per 100,000 Population in 1995

National Rate = 1.98 Community Hospitals per 100,000 Population*

ALPHA ORDER

RANK	STATE	RATE		RANK	STATE	RATE
17	Alabama	2.71		1	South Dakota	6.85
16	Alaska	2.82		2	North Dakota	6.70
42	Arizona	1.42		3	Montana	6.32
10	Arkansas	3.42		4	Nebraska	5.55
43	California	1.34		5	Wyoming	5.22
31	Colorado	1.84		6	Kansas	5.15
49	Connecticut	1.04		7	Iowa	4.08
47	Delaware	1.12		8	Mississippi	3.60
40	Florida	1.49		9	Idaho	3.52
24	Georgia	2.22		10	Arkansas	3.42
33	Hawaii	1.78		11	Oklahoma	3.36
9	Idaho	3.52		12	West Virginia	3.23
34	Illinois	1.76		13	Maine	3.15
29	Indiana	1.98		14	Minnesota	3.08
7	Iowa	4.08		15	Louisiana	3.00
6	Kansas	5.15		16	Alaska	2.82
18	Kentucky	2.70		17	Alabama	2.71
15	Louisiana	3.00		18	Kentucky	2.70
13	Maine	3.15		19	New Hampshire	2.53
50	Maryland	0.99		20	Wisconsin	2.48
39	Massachusetts	1.58		21	Tennessee	2.40
35	Michigan	1.75		22	Vermont	2.39
14	Minnesota	3.08		23	Missouri	2.37
8	Mississippi	3.60		24	Georgia	2.22
23	Missouri	2.37		25	Texas	2.21
3	Montana	6.32		26	Utah	2.15
4	Nebraska	5.55		27	New Mexico	2.13
44	Nevada	1.30		28	Oregon	2.03
19	New Hampshire	2.53		29	Indiana	1.98
46	New Jersey	1.16		30	Pennsylvania	1.87
27	New Mexico	2.13		31	Colorado	1.84
45	New York	1.26		32	South Carolina	1.80
36	North Carolina	1.65		33	Hawaii	1.78
2	North Dakota	6.70		34	Illinois	1.76
37	Ohio	1.62		35	Michigan	1.75
11	Oklahoma	3.36		36	North Carolina	1.65
28	Oregon	2.03		37	Ohio	1.62
30	Pennsylvania	1.87		37	Washington	1.62
48	Rhode Island	1.11		39	Massachusetts	1.58
32	South Carolina	1.80		40	Florida	1.49
1	South Dakota	6.85		41	Virginia	1.45
21	Tennessee	2.40		42	Arizona	1.42
25	Texas	2.21		43	California	1.34
26	Utah	2.15		44	Nevada	1.30
22	Vermont	2.39		45	New York	1.26
41	Virginia	1.45		46	New Jersey	1.16
37	Washington	1.62		47	Delaware	1.12
12	West Virginia	3.23		48	Rhode Island	1.11
20	Wisconsin	2.48		49	Connecticut	1.04
5	Wyoming	5.22		50	Maryland	0.99
					District of Columbia	2.16

Source: Morgan Quitno Press using data from American Hospital Association (Chicago, IL)
"Hospital Statistics" (1996-97 edition)
*All nonfederal short-term general and other special hospitals whose facilities and services are available to the public. Community hospitals are a subset of nonfederal hospitals.

Community Hospitals per 1,000 Square Miles in 1995

National Rate = 1.40 Community Hospitals*

ALPHA ORDER

RANK	STATE	RATE
23	Alabama	2.20
50	Alaska	0.03
43	Arizona	0.54
31	Arkansas	1.60
17	California	2.67
39	Colorado	0.66
4	Connecticut	6.13
11	Delaware	3.34
10	Florida	3.54
16	Georgia	2.71
12	Hawaii	3.25
44	Idaho	0.49
9	Illinois	3.57
13	Indiana	3.16
25	Iowa	2.06
31	Kansas	1.60
19	Kentucky	2.57
18	Louisiana	2.62
38	Maine	1.16
7	Maryland	4.07
2	Massachusetts	10.39
29	Michigan	1.73
30	Minnesota	1.63
26	Mississippi	2.01
28	Missouri	1.81
46	Montana	0.37
37	Nebraska	1.18
49	Nevada	0.18
14	New Hampshire	3.12
1	New Jersey	11.20
47	New Mexico	0.30
6	New York	4.26
22	North Carolina	2.26
42	North Dakota	0.61
8	Ohio	4.02
33	Oklahoma	1.57
39	Oregon	0.66
5	Pennsylvania	4.89
3	Rhode Island	8.94
24	South Carolina	2.12
41	South Dakota	0.65
15	Tennessee	2.99
34	Texas	1.56
44	Utah	0.49
35	Vermont	1.46
21	Virginia	2.27
36	Washington	1.25
20	West Virginia	2.43
27	Wisconsin	1.94
48	Wyoming	0.26

RANK ORDER

RANK	STATE	RATE
1	New Jersey	11.20
2	Massachusetts	10.39
3	Rhode Island	8.94
4	Connecticut	6.13
5	Pennsylvania	4.89
6	New York	4.26
7	Maryland	4.07
8	Ohio	4.02
9	Illinois	3.57
10	Florida	3.54
11	Delaware	3.34
12	Hawaii	3.25
13	Indiana	3.16
14	New Hampshire	3.12
15	Tennessee	2.99
16	Georgia	2.71
17	California	2.67
18	Louisiana	2.62
19	Kentucky	2.57
20	West Virginia	2.43
21	Virginia	2.27
22	North Carolina	2.26
23	Alabama	2.20
24	South Carolina	2.12
25	Iowa	2.06
26	Mississippi	2.01
27	Wisconsin	1.94
28	Missouri	1.81
29	Michigan	1.73
30	Minnesota	1.63
31	Arkansas	1.60
31	Kansas	1.60
33	Oklahoma	1.57
34	Texas	1.56
35	Vermont	1.46
36	Washington	1.25
37	Nebraska	1.18
38	Maine	1.16
39	Colorado	0.66
39	Oregon	0.66
41	South Dakota	0.65
42	North Dakota	0.61
43	Arizona	0.54
44	Idaho	0.49
44	Utah	0.49
46	Montana	0.37
47	New Mexico	0.30
48	Wyoming	0.26
49	Nevada	0.18
50	Alaska	0.03

District of Columbia** NA

Source: Morgan Quitno Press using data from American Hospital Association (Chicago, IL)
      "Hospital Statistics" (1996-97 edition)
*Based on revised 1990 Census land and water area figures. Community hospitals are nonfederal short-term general and other special hospitals, whose facilities and services are available to the public. They are a subset of nonfederal hospitals.
**The District of Columbia has 12 community hospitals for its 68 square miles.

Nongovernment Not-For-Profit Hospitals in 1995

National Total = 3,092 Hospitals*

ALPHA ORDER

RANK	STATE	HOSPITALS	% of USA
32	Alabama	36	1.16%
48	Alaska	7	0.23%
25	Arizona	44	1.42%
23	Arkansas	46	1.49%
1	California	229	7.41%
33	Colorado	35	1.13%
36	Connecticut	33	1.07%
47	Delaware	8	0.26%
9	Florida	93	3.01%
21	Georgia	50	1.62%
44	Hawaii	12	0.39%
45	Idaho	11	0.36%
4	Illinois	158	5.11%
17	Indiana	59	1.91%
19	Iowa	53	1.71%
18	Kansas	57	1.84%
16	Kentucky	69	2.23%
38	Louisiana	29	0.94%
33	Maine	35	1.13%
22	Maryland	48	1.55%
11	Massachusetts	84	2.72%
6	Michigan	143	4.62%
12	Minnesota	83	2.68%
37	Mississippi	31	1.00%
13	Missouri	78	2.52%
28	Montana	43	1.39%
23	Nebraska	46	1.49%
50	Nevada	6	0.19%
39	New Hampshire	24	0.78%
10	New Jersey	87	2.81%
42	New Mexico	20	0.65%
3	New York	191	6.18%
15	North Carolina	70	2.26%
29	North Dakota	42	1.36%
5	Ohio	153	4.95%
31	Oklahoma	37	1.20%
25	Oregon	44	1.42%
2	Pennsylvania	216	6.99%
45	Rhode Island	11	0.36%
41	South Carolina	21	0.68%
25	South Dakota	44	1.42%
20	Tennessee	51	1.65%
7	Texas	130	4.20%
40	Utah	22	0.71%
43	Vermont	14	0.45%
14	Virginia	77	2.49%
29	Washington	42	1.36%
35	West Virginia	34	1.10%
8	Wisconsin	119	3.85%
48	Wyoming	7	0.23%

RANK ORDER

RANK	STATE	HOSPITALS	% of USA
1	California	229	7.41%
2	Pennsylvania	216	6.99%
3	New York	191	6.18%
4	Illinois	158	5.11%
5	Ohio	153	4.95%
6	Michigan	143	4.62%
7	Texas	130	4.20%
8	Wisconsin	119	3.85%
9	Florida	93	3.01%
10	New Jersey	87	2.81%
11	Massachusetts	84	2.72%
12	Minnesota	83	2.68%
13	Missouri	78	2.52%
14	Virginia	77	2.49%
15	North Carolina	70	2.26%
16	Kentucky	69	2.23%
17	Indiana	59	1.91%
18	Kansas	57	1.84%
19	Iowa	53	1.71%
20	Tennessee	51	1.65%
21	Georgia	50	1.62%
22	Maryland	48	1.55%
23	Arkansas	46	1.49%
23	Nebraska	46	1.49%
25	Arizona	44	1.42%
25	Oregon	44	1.42%
25	South Dakota	44	1.42%
28	Montana	43	1.39%
29	North Dakota	42	1.36%
29	Washington	42	1.36%
31	Oklahoma	37	1.20%
32	Alabama	36	1.16%
33	Colorado	35	1.13%
33	Maine	35	1.13%
35	West Virginia	34	1.10%
36	Connecticut	33	1.07%
37	Mississippi	31	1.00%
38	Louisiana	29	0.94%
39	New Hampshire	24	0.78%
40	Utah	22	0.71%
41	South Carolina	21	0.68%
42	New Mexico	20	0.65%
43	Vermont	14	0.45%
44	Hawaii	12	0.39%
45	Idaho	11	0.36%
45	Rhode Island	11	0.36%
47	Delaware	8	0.26%
48	Alaska	7	0.23%
48	Wyoming	7	0.23%
50	Nevada	6	0.19%
	District of Columbia	10	0.32%

Source: American Hospital Association (Chicago, IL)
"Hospital Statistics" (1996-97 edition)
*Nongovernment not-for-profit hospitals are a subset of community hospitals.

Investor-Owned (For-Profit) Hospitals in 1995

National Total = 752 Hospitals*

ALPHA ORDER

RANK	STATE	HOSPITALS	% of USA
7	Alabama	33	4.39%
36	Alaska	1	0.13%
17	Arizona	12	1.60%
9	Arkansas	19	2.53%
2	California	106	14.10%
24	Colorado	6	0.80%
44	Connecticut	0	0.00%
44	Delaware	0	0.00%
3	Florida	96	12.77%
6	Georgia	36	4.79%
36	Hawaii	1	0.13%
31	Idaho	3	0.40%
13	Illinois	13	1.73%
22	Indiana	7	0.93%
36	Iowa	1	0.13%
21	Kansas	8	1.06%
8	Kentucky	22	2.93%
5	Louisiana	41	5.45%
36	Maine	1	0.13%
33	Maryland	2	0.27%
28	Massachusetts	4	0.53%
36	Michigan	1	0.13%
44	Minnesota	0	0.00%
13	Mississippi	13	1.73%
19	Missouri	11	1.46%
44	Montana	0	0.00%
33	Nebraska	2	0.27%
25	Nevada	5	0.66%
25	New Hampshire	5	0.66%
36	New Jersey	1	0.13%
28	New Mexico	4	0.53%
17	New York	12	1.60%
13	North Carolina	13	1.73%
36	North Dakota	1	0.13%
31	Ohio	3	0.40%
11	Oklahoma	15	1.99%
28	Oregon	4	0.53%
22	Pennsylvania	7	0.93%
44	Rhode Island	0	0.00%
10	South Carolina	18	2.39%
44	South Dakota	0	0.00%
4	Tennessee	45	5.98%
1	Texas	132	17.55%
19	Utah	11	1.46%
44	Vermont	0	0.00%
13	Virginia	13	1.73%
25	Washington	5	0.66%
11	West Virginia	15	1.99%
36	Wisconsin	1	0.13%
33	Wyoming	2	0.27%

RANK ORDER

RANK	STATE	HOSPITALS	% of USA
1	Texas	132	17.55%
2	California	106	14.10%
3	Florida	96	12.77%
4	Tennessee	45	5.98%
5	Louisiana	41	5.45%
6	Georgia	36	4.79%
7	Alabama	33	4.39%
8	Kentucky	22	2.93%
9	Arkansas	19	2.53%
10	South Carolina	18	2.39%
11	Oklahoma	15	1.99%
11	West Virginia	15	1.99%
13	Illinois	13	1.73%
13	Mississippi	13	1.73%
13	North Carolina	13	1.73%
13	Virginia	13	1.73%
17	Arizona	12	1.60%
17	New York	12	1.60%
19	Missouri	11	1.46%
19	Utah	11	1.46%
21	Kansas	8	1.06%
22	Indiana	7	0.93%
22	Pennsylvania	7	0.93%
24	Colorado	6	0.80%
25	Nevada	5	0.66%
25	New Hampshire	5	0.66%
25	Washington	5	0.66%
28	Massachusetts	4	0.53%
28	New Mexico	4	0.53%
28	Oregon	4	0.53%
31	Idaho	3	0.40%
31	Ohio	3	0.40%
33	Maryland	2	0.27%
33	Nebraska	2	0.27%
33	Wyoming	2	0.27%
36	Alaska	1	0.13%
36	Hawaii	1	0.13%
36	Iowa	1	0.13%
36	Maine	1	0.13%
36	Michigan	1	0.13%
36	New Jersey	1	0.13%
36	North Dakota	1	0.13%
36	Wisconsin	1	0.13%
44	Connecticut	0	0.00%
44	Delaware	0	0.00%
44	Minnesota	0	0.00%
44	Montana	0	0.00%
44	Rhode Island	0	0.00%
44	South Dakota	0	0.00%
44	Vermont	0	0.00%
	District of Columbia	1	0.13%

Source: American Hospital Association (Chicago, IL)
    "Hospital Statistics" (1996-97 edition)
Investor-owned (for-profit) hospitals are a subset of community hospitals.

State and Local Government-Owned Hospitals in 1995

National Total = 1,350 Hospitals*

ALPHA ORDER

RANK	STATE	HOSPITALS	% of USA
11	Alabama	46	3.41%
32	Alaska	9	0.67%
40	Arizona	5	0.37%
25	Arkansas	20	1.48%
2	California	89	6.59%
18	Colorado	28	2.07%
44	Connecticut	1	0.07%
45	Delaware	0	0.00%
23	Florida	23	1.70%
3	Georgia	74	5.48%
35	Hawaii	8	0.59%
19	Idaho	27	2.00%
15	Illinois	36	2.67%
10	Indiana	49	3.63%
5	Iowa	62	4.59%
4	Kansas	67	4.96%
28	Kentucky	13	0.96%
6	Louisiana	60	4.44%
42	Maine	3	0.22%
45	Maryland	0	0.00%
35	Massachusetts	8	0.59%
23	Michigan	23	1.70%
7	Minnesota	59	4.37%
9	Mississippi	53	3.93%
14	Missouri	37	2.74%
29	Montana	12	0.89%
12	Nebraska	43	3.19%
32	Nevada	9	0.67%
45	New Hampshire	0	0.00%
41	New Jersey	4	0.30%
29	New Mexico	12	0.89%
19	New York	27	2.00%
15	North Carolina	36	2.67%
45	North Dakota	0	0.00%
22	Ohio	24	1.78%
8	Oklahoma	58	4.30%
26	Oregon	16	1.19%
43	Pennsylvania	2	0.15%
45	Rhode Island	0	0.00%
19	South Carolina	27	2.00%
38	South Dakota	6	0.44%
17	Tennessee	30	2.22%
1	Texas	154	11.41%
32	Utah	9	0.67%
45	Vermont	0	0.00%
38	Virginia	6	0.44%
13	Washington	41	3.04%
31	West Virginia	10	0.74%
37	Wisconsin	7	0.52%
26	Wyoming	16	1.19%

RANK ORDER

RANK	STATE	HOSPITALS	% of USA
1	Texas	154	11.41%
2	California	89	6.59%
3	Georgia	74	5.48%
4	Kansas	67	4.96%
5	Iowa	62	4.59%
6	Louisiana	60	4.44%
7	Minnesota	59	4.37%
8	Oklahoma	58	4.30%
9	Mississippi	53	3.93%
10	Indiana	49	3.63%
11	Alabama	46	3.41%
12	Nebraska	43	3.19%
13	Washington	41	3.04%
14	Missouri	37	2.74%
15	Illinois	36	2.67%
15	North Carolina	36	2.67%
17	Tennessee	30	2.22%
18	Colorado	28	2.07%
19	Idaho	27	2.00%
19	New York	27	2.00%
19	South Carolina	27	2.00%
22	Ohio	24	1.78%
23	Florida	23	1.70%
23	Michigan	23	1.70%
25	Arkansas	20	1.48%
26	Oregon	16	1.19%
26	Wyoming	16	1.19%
28	Kentucky	13	0.96%
29	Montana	12	0.89%
29	New Mexico	12	0.89%
31	West Virginia	10	0.74%
32	Alaska	9	0.67%
32	Nevada	9	0.67%
32	Utah	9	0.67%
35	Hawaii	8	0.59%
35	Massachusetts	8	0.59%
37	Wisconsin	7	0.52%
38	South Dakota	6	0.44%
38	Virginia	6	0.44%
40	Arizona	5	0.37%
41	New Jersey	4	0.30%
42	Maine	3	0.22%
43	Pennsylvania	2	0.15%
44	Connecticut	1	0.07%
45	Delaware	0	0.00%
45	Maryland	0	0.00%
45	New Hampshire	0	0.00%
45	North Dakota	0	0.00%
45	Rhode Island	0	0.00%
45	Vermont	0	0.00%
	District of Columbia	1	0.07%

Source: American Hospital Association (Chicago, IL)
"Hospital Statistics" (1996-97 edition)
*State and local government-owned hospitals are a subset of community hospitals.

Hospital Beds in 1995

National Total = 1,080,601 Beds*

ALPHA ORDER

RANK	STATE	BEDS	% of USA
18	Alabama	22,336	2.07%
50	Alaska	1,812	0.17%
29	Arizona	12,869	1.19%
31	Arkansas	11,829	1.09%
2	California	92,790	8.59%
30	Colorado	11,912	1.10%
32	Connecticut	10,983	1.02%
48	Delaware	2,552	0.24%
5	Florida	58,406	5.40%
10	Georgia	33,403	3.09%
46	Hawaii	3,695	0.34%
44	Idaho	3,895	0.36%
6	Illinois	51,007	4.72%
17	Indiana	23,031	2.13%
24	Iowa	14,884	1.38%
25	Kansas	14,054	1.30%
21	Kentucky	17,787	1.65%
16	Louisiana	23,174	2.14%
39	Maine	5,007	0.46%
22	Maryland	17,774	1.64%
12	Massachusetts	26,631	2.46%
9	Michigan	33,932	3.14%
19	Minnesota	20,753	1.92%
23	Mississippi	16,106	1.49%
13	Missouri	26,020	2.41%
41	Montana	4,542	0.42%
34	Nebraska	9,267	0.86%
43	Nevada	4,201	0.39%
42	New Hampshire	4,315	0.40%
8	New Jersey	35,828	3.32%
36	New Mexico	5,702	0.53%
1	New York	93,074	8.61%
11	North Carolina	29,534	2.73%
40	North Dakota	4,794	0.44%
7	Ohio	43,317	4.01%
26	Oklahoma	13,727	1.27%
35	Oregon	9,256	0.86%
4	Pennsylvania	60,981	5.64%
45	Rhode Island	3,894	0.36%
28	South Carolina	13,632	1.26%
37	South Dakota	5,618	0.52%
15	Tennessee	25,493	2.36%
3	Texas	70,881	6.56%
38	Utah	5,171	0.48%
49	Vermont	2,113	0.20%
14	Virginia	25,740	2.38%
27	Washington	13,673	1.27%
33	West Virginia	9,799	0.91%
20	Wisconsin	20,528	1.90%
47	Wyoming	2,610	0.24%

RANK ORDER

RANK	STATE	BEDS	% of USA
1	New York	93,074	8.61%
2	California	92,790	8.59%
3	Texas	70,881	6.56%
4	Pennsylvania	60,981	5.64%
5	Florida	58,406	5.40%
6	Illinois	51,007	4.72%
7	Ohio	43,317	4.01%
8	New Jersey	35,828	3.32%
9	Michigan	33,932	3.14%
10	Georgia	33,403	3.09%
11	North Carolina	29,534	2.73%
12	Massachusetts	26,631	2.46%
13	Missouri	26,020	2.41%
14	Virginia	25,740	2.38%
15	Tennessee	25,493	2.36%
16	Louisiana	23,174	2.14%
17	Indiana	23,031	2.13%
18	Alabama	22,336	2.07%
19	Minnesota	20,753	1.92%
20	Wisconsin	20,528	1.90%
21	Kentucky	17,787	1.65%
22	Maryland	17,774	1.64%
23	Mississippi	16,106	1.49%
24	Iowa	14,884	1.38%
25	Kansas	14,054	1.30%
26	Oklahoma	13,727	1.27%
27	Washington	13,673	1.27%
28	South Carolina	13,632	1.26%
29	Arizona	12,869	1.19%
30	Colorado	11,912	1.10%
31	Arkansas	11,829	1.09%
32	Connecticut	10,983	1.02%
33	West Virginia	9,799	0.91%
34	Nebraska	9,267	0.86%
35	Oregon	9,256	0.86%
36	New Mexico	5,702	0.53%
37	South Dakota	5,618	0.52%
38	Utah	5,171	0.48%
39	Maine	5,007	0.46%
40	North Dakota	4,794	0.44%
41	Montana	4,542	0.42%
42	New Hampshire	4,315	0.40%
43	Nevada	4,201	0.39%
44	Idaho	3,895	0.36%
45	Rhode Island	3,894	0.36%
46	Hawaii	3,695	0.34%
47	Wyoming	2,610	0.24%
48	Delaware	2,552	0.24%
49	Vermont	2,113	0.20%
50	Alaska	1,812	0.17%
	District of Columbia	6,269	0.58%

Source: American Hospital Association (Chicago, IL)
"Hospital Statistics" (1996-97 edition)
In federal and nonfederal hospitals.

Hospital Beds per 100,000 Population in 1995

National Rate = 411 Beds per 100,000 Population*

ALPHA ORDER				RANK ORDER		
RANK	**STATE**	**RATE**		**RANK**	**STATE**	**RATE**
9	Alabama	526		1	South Dakota	770
44	Alaska	300		2	North Dakota	747
45	Arizona	299		3	Mississippi	597
16	Arkansas	476		4	Nebraska	565
46	California	294		5	Kansas	548
42	Colorado	318		6	Wyoming	545
40	Connecticut	336		7	West Virginia	537
36	Delaware	356		8	Louisiana	534
24	Florida	412		9	Alabama	526
17	Georgia	463		10	Iowa	524
43	Hawaii	313		11	Montana	522
41	Idaho	334		12	New York	512
22	Illinois	433		13	Pennsylvania	506
28	Indiana	397		14	Missouri	489
10	Iowa	524		15	Tennessee	486
5	Kansas	548		16	Arkansas	476
18	Kentucky	461		17	Georgia	463
8	Louisiana	534		18	Kentucky	461
26	Maine	404		19	New Jersey	451
38	Maryland	353		20	Minnesota	450
21	Massachusetts	439		21	Massachusetts	439
36	Michigan	356		22	Illinois	433
20	Minnesota	450		23	Oklahoma	419
3	Mississippi	597		24	Florida	412
14	Missouri	489		25	North Carolina	410
11	Montana	522		26	Maine	404
4	Nebraska	565		27	Wisconsin	401
48	Nevada	274		28	Indiana	397
33	New Hampshire	376		29	Rhode Island	393
19	New Jersey	451		30	Ohio	389
39	New Mexico	337		30	Virginia	389
12	New York	512		32	Texas	377
25	North Carolina	410		33	New Hampshire	376
2	North Dakota	747		34	South Carolina	372
30	Ohio	389		35	Vermont	361
23	Oklahoma	419		36	Delaware	356
46	Oregon	294		36	Michigan	356
13	Pennsylvania	506		38	Maryland	353
29	Rhode Island	393		39	New Mexico	337
34	South Carolina	372		40	Connecticut	336
1	South Dakota	770		41	Idaho	334
15	Tennessee	486		42	Colorado	318
32	Texas	377		43	Hawaii	313
49	Utah	264		44	Alaska	300
35	Vermont	361		45	Arizona	299
30	Virginia	389		46	California	294
50	Washington	251		46	Oregon	294
7	West Virginia	537		48	Nevada	274
27	Wisconsin	401		49	Utah	264
6	Wyoming	545		50	Washington	251
					District of Columbia	1,130

*Source: Morgan Quitno Press using data from American Hospital Association (Chicago, IL)
    "Hospital Statistics" (1996-97 edition)*
In federal and nonfederal hospitals.

Average Number of Beds per Hospital in 1995

National Average = 172 Beds per Hospital*

ALPHA ORDER

RANK	STATE	BEDS
20	Alabama	168
50	Alaska	67
26	Arizona	145
36	Arkansas	123
14	California	186
31	Colorado	137
10	Connecticut	200
11	Delaware	196
5	Florida	221
18	Georgia	171
29	Hawaii	142
48	Idaho	81
7	Illinois	211
19	Indiana	169
38	Iowa	117
43	Kansas	93
24	Kentucky	147
27	Louisiana	144
39	Maine	111
4	Maryland	222
13	Massachusetts	192
15	Michigan	179
32	Minnesota	134
23	Mississippi	148
16	Missouri	172
49	Montana	74
45	Nebraska	92
22	Nevada	150
37	New Hampshire	120
2	New Jersey	317
43	New Mexico	93
1	New York	325
12	North Carolina	194
42	North Dakota	94
8	Ohio	206
41	Oklahoma	101
34	Oregon	130
6	Pennsylvania	216
3	Rhode Island	243
21	South Carolina	162
46	South Dakota	91
16	Tennessee	172
29	Texas	142
40	Utah	103
35	Vermont	124
9	Virginia	201
33	Washington	131
25	West Virginia	146
28	Wisconsin	143
47	Wyoming	90

RANK ORDER

RANK	STATE	BEDS
1	New York	325
2	New Jersey	317
3	Rhode Island	243
4	Maryland	222
5	Florida	221
6	Pennsylvania	216
7	Illinois	211
8	Ohio	206
9	Virginia	201
10	Connecticut	200
11	Delaware	196
12	North Carolina	194
13	Massachusetts	192
14	California	186
15	Michigan	179
16	Missouri	172
16	Tennessee	172
18	Georgia	171
19	Indiana	169
20	Alabama	168
21	South Carolina	162
22	Nevada	150
23	Mississippi	148
24	Kentucky	147
25	West Virginia	146
26	Arizona	145
27	Louisiana	144
28	Wisconsin	143
29	Hawaii	142
29	Texas	142
31	Colorado	137
32	Minnesota	134
33	Washington	131
34	Oregon	130
35	Vermont	124
36	Arkansas	123
37	New Hampshire	120
38	Iowa	117
39	Maine	111
40	Utah	103
41	Oklahoma	101
42	North Dakota	94
43	Kansas	93
43	New Mexico	93
45	Nebraska	92
46	South Dakota	91
47	Wyoming	90
48	Idaho	81
49	Montana	74
50	Alaska	67

District of Columbia	369

Source: Morgan Quitno Press using data from American Hospital Association (Chicago, IL)
     "Hospital Statistics" (1996-97 edition)
*In federal and nonfederal hospitals.

Beds in Federal Hospitals in 1995

National Total = 77,079 Beds*

ALPHA ORDER

RANK ORDER

RANK	STATE	BEDS	% of USA
15	Alabama	1,886	2.45%
40	Alaska	349	0.45%
17	Arizona	1,636	2.12%
27	Arkansas	977	1.27%
3	California	5,418	7.03%
24	Colorado	1,123	1.46%
37	Connecticut	566	0.73%
45	Delaware	231	0.30%
5	Florida	3,943	5.12%
11	Georgia	2,037	2.64%
39	Hawaii	355	0.46%
48	Idaho	203	0.26%
6	Illinois	3,466	4.50%
30	Indiana	882	1.14%
28	Iowa	924	1.20%
29	Kansas	915	1.19%
23	Kentucky	1,149	1.49%
26	Louisiana	1,045	1.36%
41	Maine	326	0.42%
14	Maryland	1,917	2.49%
8	Massachusetts	2,277	2.95%
16	Michigan	1,749	2.27%
25	Minnesota	1,121	1.45%
22	Mississippi	1,215	1.58%
12	Missouri	1,999	2.59%
44	Montana	251	0.33%
36	Nebraska	567	0.74%
47	Nevada	216	0.28%
46	New Hampshire	228	0.30%
18	New Jersey	1,594	2.07%
35	New Mexico	664	0.86%
2	New York	6,184	8.02%
10	North Carolina	2,096	2.72%
43	North Dakota	275	0.36%
7	Ohio	2,729	3.54%
32	Oklahoma	837	1.09%
31	Oregon	840	1.09%
4	Pennsylvania	4,308	5.59%
50	Rhode Island	137	0.18%
34	South Carolina	759	0.98%
33	South Dakota	804	1.04%
9	Tennessee	2,136	2.77%
1	Texas	6,824	8.85%
42	Utah	292	0.38%
49	Vermont	150	0.19%
13	Virginia	1,938	2.51%
20	Washington	1,305	1.69%
21	West Virginia	1,243	1.61%
19	Wisconsin	1,335	1.73%
38	Wyoming	432	0.56%

RANK	STATE	BEDS	% of USA
1	Texas	6,824	8.85%
2	New York	6,184	8.02%
3	California	5,418	7.03%
4	Pennsylvania	4,308	5.59%
5	Florida	3,943	5.12%
6	Illinois	3,466	4.50%
7	Ohio	2,729	3.54%
8	Massachusetts	2,277	2.95%
9	Tennessee	2,136	2.77%
10	North Carolina	2,096	2.72%
11	Georgia	2,037	2.64%
12	Missouri	1,999	2.59%
13	Virginia	1,938	2.51%
14	Maryland	1,917	2.49%
15	Alabama	1,886	2.45%
16	Michigan	1,749	2.27%
17	Arizona	1,636	2.12%
18	New Jersey	1,594	2.07%
19	Wisconsin	1,335	1.73%
20	Washington	1,305	1.69%
21	West Virginia	1,243	1.61%
22	Mississippi	1,215	1.58%
23	Kentucky	1,149	1.49%
24	Colorado	1,123	1.46%
25	Minnesota	1,121	1.45%
26	Louisiana	1,045	1.36%
27	Arkansas	977	1.27%
28	Iowa	924	1.20%
29	Kansas	915	1.19%
30	Indiana	882	1.14%
31	Oregon	840	1.09%
32	Oklahoma	837	1.09%
33	South Dakota	804	1.04%
34	South Carolina	759	0.98%
35	New Mexico	664	0.86%
36	Nebraska	567	0.74%
37	Connecticut	566	0.73%
38	Wyoming	432	0.56%
39	Hawaii	355	0.46%
40	Alaska	349	0.45%
41	Maine	326	0.42%
42	Utah	292	0.38%
43	North Dakota	275	0.36%
44	Montana	251	0.33%
45	Delaware	231	0.30%
46	New Hampshire	228	0.30%
47	Nevada	216	0.28%
48	Idaho	203	0.26%
49	Vermont	150	0.19%
50	Rhode Island	137	0.18%
	District of Columbia	1,226	1.59%

Source: American Hospital Association (Chicago, IL)
"Hospital Statistics" (1996-97 edition)
*Federal hospitals are controlled by an agency or department of the federal government.

Beds in Nonfederal Hospitals in 1995

National Total = 1,003,522 Beds

ALPHA ORDER

RANK ORDER

RANK	STATE	BEDS	% of USA	RANK	STATE	BEDS	% of USA
18	Alabama	20,450	2.04%	1	California	87,372	8.71%
50	Alaska	1,463	0.15%	2	New York	86,890	8.66%
29	Arizona	11,233	1.12%	3	Texas	64,057	6.38%
30	Arkansas	10,852	1.08%	4	Pennsylvania	56,673	5.65%
1	California	87,372	8.71%	5	Florida	54,463	5.43%
31	Colorado	10,789	1.08%	6	Illinois	47,541	4.74%
32	Connecticut	10,417	1.04%	7	Ohio	40,588	4.04%
47	Delaware	2,321	0.23%	8	New Jersey	34,234	3.41%
5	Florida	54,463	5.43%	9	Michigan	32,183	3.21%
10	Georgia	31,366	3.13%	10	Georgia	31,366	3.13%
46	Hawaii	3,340	0.33%	11	North Carolina	27,438	2.73%
45	Idaho	3,692	0.37%	12	Massachusetts	24,354	2.43%
6	Illinois	47,541	4.74%	13	Missouri	24,021	2.39%
16	Indiana	22,149	2.21%	14	Virginia	23,802	2.37%
24	Iowa	13,960	1.39%	15	Tennessee	23,357	2.33%
25	Kansas	13,139	1.31%	16	Indiana	22,149	2.21%
21	Kentucky	16,638	1.66%	17	Louisiana	22,129	2.21%
17	Louisiana	22,129	2.21%	18	Alabama	20,450	2.04%
39	Maine	4,681	0.47%	19	Minnesota	19,632	1.96%
22	Maryland	15,857	1.58%	20	Wisconsin	19,193	1.91%
12	Massachusetts	24,354	2.43%	21	Kentucky	16,638	1.66%
9	Michigan	32,183	3.21%	22	Maryland	15,857	1.58%
19	Minnesota	19,632	1.96%	23	Mississippi	14,891	1.48%
23	Mississippi	14,891	1.48%	24	Iowa	13,960	1.39%
13	Missouri	24,021	2.39%	25	Kansas	13,139	1.31%
41	Montana	4,291	0.43%	26	Oklahoma	12,890	1.28%
33	Nebraska	8,700	0.87%	27	South Carolina	12,873	1.28%
43	Nevada	3,985	0.40%	28	Washington	12,368	1.23%
42	New Hampshire	4,087	0.41%	29	Arizona	11,233	1.12%
8	New Jersey	34,234	3.41%	30	Arkansas	10,852	1.08%
36	New Mexico	5,038	0.50%	31	Colorado	10,789	1.08%
2	New York	86,890	8.66%	32	Connecticut	10,417	1.04%
11	North Carolina	27,438	2.73%	33	Nebraska	8,700	0.87%
40	North Dakota	4,519	0.45%	34	West Virginia	8,556	0.85%
7	Ohio	40,588	4.04%	35	Oregon	8,416	0.84%
26	Oklahoma	12,890	1.28%	36	New Mexico	5,038	0.50%
35	Oregon	8,416	0.84%	37	Utah	4,879	0.49%
4	Pennsylvania	56,673	5.65%	38	South Dakota	4,814	0.48%
44	Rhode Island	3,757	0.37%	39	Maine	4,681	0.47%
27	South Carolina	12,873	1.28%	40	North Dakota	4,519	0.45%
38	South Dakota	4,814	0.48%	41	Montana	4,291	0.43%
15	Tennessee	23,357	2.33%	42	New Hampshire	4,087	0.41%
3	Texas	64,057	6.38%	43	Nevada	3,985	0.40%
37	Utah	4,879	0.49%	44	Rhode Island	3,757	0.37%
49	Vermont	1,963	0.20%	45	Idaho	3,692	0.37%
14	Virginia	23,802	2.37%	46	Hawaii	3,340	0.33%
28	Washington	12,368	1.23%	47	Delaware	2,321	0.23%
34	West Virginia	8,556	0.85%	48	Wyoming	2,178	0.22%
20	Wisconsin	19,193	1.91%	49	Vermont	1,963	0.20%
48	Wyoming	2,178	0.22%	50	Alaska	1,463	0.15%
					District of Columbia	5,043	0.50%

Source: American Hospital Association (Chicago, IL)
"Hospital Statistics" (1996-97 edition)

Beds in Psychiatric Hospitals in 1995

National Total = 120,363 Beds*

ALPHA ORDER				RANK ORDER			
RANK	STATE	BEDS	% of USA	RANK	STATE	BEDS	% of USA
16	Alabama	2,802	2.33%	1	New York	11,403	9.47%
46	Alaska	193	0.16%	2	California	10,424	8.66%
31	Arizona	1,323	1.10%	3	Pennsylvania	8,936	7.42%
34	Arkansas	708	0.59%	4	Texas	6,176	5.13%
2	California	10,424	8.66%	5	North Carolina	5,040	4.19%
25	Colorado	1,717	1.43%	6	Illinois	4,663	3.87%
22	Connecticut	2,041	1.70%	7	Virginia	4,588	3.81%
39	Delaware	456	0.38%	8	New Jersey	4,500	3.74%
9	Florida	4,318	3.59%	9	Florida	4,318	3.59%
13	Georgia	3,081	2.56%	10	Massachusetts	3,350	2.78%
47	Hawaii	187	0.16%	11	Ohio	3,338	2.77%
43	Idaho	309	0.26%	12	Indiana	3,267	2.71%
6	Illinois	4,663	3.87%	13	Georgia	3,081	2.56%
12	Indiana	3,267	2.71%	14	Michigan	3,021	2.51%
26	Iowa	1,627	1.35%	15	Maryland	2,803	2.33%
21	Kansas	2,294	1.91%	16	Alabama	2,802	2.33%
27	Kentucky	1,481	1.23%	17	Wisconsin	2,719	2.26%
19	Louisiana	2,451	2.04%	18	Minnesota	2,632	2.19%
36	Maine	670	0.56%	19	Louisiana	2,451	2.04%
15	Maryland	2,803	2.33%	20	Mississippi	2,301	1.91%
10	Massachusetts	3,350	2.78%	21	Kansas	2,294	1.91%
14	Michigan	3,021	2.51%	22	Connecticut	2,041	1.70%
18	Minnesota	2,632	2.19%	23	Tennessee	1,864	1.55%
20	Mississippi	2,301	1.91%	24	Missouri	1,818	1.51%
24	Missouri	1,818	1.51%	25	Colorado	1,717	1.43%
49	Montana	66	0.05%	26	Iowa	1,627	1.35%
37	Nebraska	617	0.51%	27	Kentucky	1,481	1.23%
42	Nevada	385	0.32%	28	South Carolina	1,439	1.20%
38	New Hampshire	559	0.46%	29	Washington	1,428	1.19%
8	New Jersey	4,500	3.74%	30	Oklahoma	1,392	1.16%
32	New Mexico	1,302	1.08%	31	Arizona	1,323	1.10%
1	New York	11,403	9.47%	32	New Mexico	1,302	1.08%
5	North Carolina	5,040	4.19%	33	Oregon	1,255	1.04%
44	North Dakota	283	0.24%	34	Arkansas	708	0.59%
11	Ohio	3,338	2.77%	35	Utah	695	0.58%
30	Oklahoma	1,392	1.16%	36	Maine	670	0.56%
33	Oregon	1,255	1.04%	37	Nebraska	617	0.51%
3	Pennsylvania	8,936	7.42%	38	New Hampshire	559	0.46%
45	Rhode Island	239	0.20%	39	Delaware	456	0.38%
28	South Carolina	1,439	1.20%	40	West Virginia	435	0.36%
50	South Dakota	60	0.05%	41	Wyoming	432	0.36%
23	Tennessee	1,864	1.55%	42	Nevada	385	0.32%
4	Texas	6,176	5.13%	43	Idaho	309	0.26%
35	Utah	695	0.58%	44	North Dakota	283	0.24%
48	Vermont	152	0.13%	45	Rhode Island	239	0.20%
7	Virginia	4,588	3.81%	46	Alaska	193	0.16%
29	Washington	1,428	1.19%	47	Hawaii	187	0.16%
40	West Virginia	435	0.36%	48	Vermont	152	0.13%
17	Wisconsin	2,719	2.26%	49	Montana	66	0.05%
41	Wyoming	432	0.36%	50	South Dakota	60	0.05%
					District of Columbia	1,123	0.93%

Source: American Hospital Association (Chicago, IL)
   "Hospital Statistics" (1996-97 edition)
*In federal and nonfederal psychiatric hospitals.

Beds in Community Hospitals in 1995

National Total = 872,736 Beds*

ALPHA ORDER

RANK	STATE	BEDS	% of USA
18	Alabama	18,252	2.09%
50	Alaska	1,270	0.15%
30	Arizona	9,852	1.13%
29	Arkansas	10,144	1.16%
1	California	75,016	8.60%
31	Colorado	9,258	1.06%
34	Connecticut	7,518	0.86%
48	Delaware	1,865	0.21%
4	Florida	49,690	5.69%
10	Georgia	26,124	2.99%
45	Hawaii	3,030	0.35%
43	Idaho	3,383	0.39%
6	Illinois	41,964	4.81%
14	Indiana	19,362	2.22%
22	Iowa	12,615	1.45%
28	Kansas	10,761	1.23%
21	Kentucky	15,131	1.73%
15	Louisiana	19,146	2.19%
40	Maine	4,011	0.46%
23	Maryland	12,607	1.44%
16	Massachusetts	18,860	2.16%
9	Michigan	29,636	3.40%
19	Minnesota	17,367	1.99%
24	Mississippi	12,590	1.44%
12	Missouri	21,851	2.50%
37	Montana	4,225	0.48%
33	Nebraska	7,851	0.90%
42	Nevada	3,600	0.41%
44	New Hampshire	3,375	0.39%
8	New Jersey	29,863	3.42%
41	New Mexico	3,675	0.42%
2	New York	73,908	8.47%
11	North Carolina	22,729	2.60%
39	North Dakota	4,168	0.48%
7	Ohio	37,766	4.33%
25	Oklahoma	11,462	1.31%
35	Oregon	7,161	0.82%
5	Pennsylvania	48,534	5.56%
46	Rhode Island	2,718	0.31%
26	South Carolina	11,307	1.30%
36	South Dakota	4,636	0.53%
13	Tennessee	20,909	2.40%
3	Texas	57,178	6.55%
38	Utah	4,184	0.48%
49	Vermont	1,811	0.21%
17	Virginia	18,579	2.13%
27	Washington	10,820	1.24%
32	West Virginia	8,121	0.93%
20	Wisconsin	17,009	1.95%
47	Wyoming	2,038	0.23%

RANK ORDER

RANK	STATE	BEDS	% of USA
1	California	75,016	8.60%
2	New York	73,908	8.47%
3	Texas	57,178	6.55%
4	Florida	49,690	5.69%
5	Pennsylvania	48,534	5.56%
6	Illinois	41,964	4.81%
7	Ohio	37,766	4.33%
8	New Jersey	29,863	3.42%
9	Michigan	29,636	3.40%
10	Georgia	26,124	2.99%
11	North Carolina	22,729	2.60%
12	Missouri	21,851	2.50%
13	Tennessee	20,909	2.40%
14	Indiana	19,362	2.22%
15	Louisiana	19,146	2.19%
16	Massachusetts	18,860	2.16%
17	Virginia	18,579	2.13%
18	Alabama	18,252	2.09%
19	Minnesota	17,367	1.99%
20	Wisconsin	17,009	1.95%
21	Kentucky	15,131	1.73%
22	Iowa	12,615	1.45%
23	Maryland	12,607	1.44%
24	Mississippi	12,590	1.44%
25	Oklahoma	11,462	1.31%
26	South Carolina	11,307	1.30%
27	Washington	10,820	1.24%
28	Kansas	10,761	1.23%
29	Arkansas	10,144	1.16%
30	Arizona	9,852	1.13%
31	Colorado	9,258	1.06%
32	West Virginia	8,121	0.93%
33	Nebraska	7,851	0.90%
34	Connecticut	7,518	0.86%
35	Oregon	7,161	0.82%
36	South Dakota	4,636	0.53%
37	Montana	4,225	0.48%
38	Utah	4,184	0.48%
39	North Dakota	4,168	0.48%
40	Maine	4,011	0.46%
41	New Mexico	3,675	0.42%
42	Nevada	3,600	0.41%
43	Idaho	3,383	0.39%
44	New Hampshire	3,375	0.39%
45	Hawaii	3,030	0.35%
46	Rhode Island	2,718	0.31%
47	Wyoming	2,038	0.23%
48	Delaware	1,865	0.21%
49	Vermont	1,811	0.21%
50	Alaska	1,270	0.15%
	District of Columbia	3,806	0.44%

Source: American Hospital Association (Chicago, IL)
       "Hospital Statistics" (1996-97 edition)
*All nonfederal short-term general and other special hospitals, whose facilities and services are available to the public. Community hospitals are a subset of nonfederal hospitals.

Rate of Beds in Community Hospitals in 1995

National Rate = 332 Beds per 100,000 Population*

ALPHA ORDER				RANK ORDER		
RANK	STATE	RATE		RANK	STATE	RATE
9	Alabama	430		1	North Dakota	649
49	Alaska	211		2	South Dakota	635
45	Arizona	229		3	Montana	486
13	Arkansas	408		4	Nebraska	479
42	California	238		5	Mississippi	467
41	Colorado	247		6	West Virginia	445
44	Connecticut	230		7	Iowa	444
38	Delaware	260		8	Louisiana	441
22	Florida	350		9	Alabama	430
20	Georgia	362		10	Wyoming	425
39	Hawaii	257		11	Kansas	420
35	Idaho	290		12	Missouri	411
21	Illinois	356		13	Arkansas	408
25	Indiana	334		14	New York	406
7	Iowa	444		15	Pennsylvania	402
11	Kansas	420		16	Tennessee	398
17	Kentucky	392		17	Kentucky	392
8	Louisiana	441		18	Minnesota	376
27	Maine	324		18	New Jersey	376
40	Maryland	250		20	Georgia	362
29	Massachusetts	311		21	Illinois	356
29	Michigan	311		22	Florida	350
18	Minnesota	376		22	Oklahoma	350
5	Mississippi	467		24	Ohio	339
12	Missouri	411		25	Indiana	334
3	Montana	486		26	Wisconsin	332
4	Nebraska	479		27	Maine	324
43	Nevada	235		28	North Carolina	316
34	New Hampshire	294		29	Massachusetts	311
18	New Jersey	376		29	Michigan	311
47	New Mexico	217		31	Vermont	310
14	New York	406		32	South Carolina	308
28	North Carolina	316		33	Texas	304
1	North Dakota	649		34	New Hampshire	294
24	Ohio	339		35	Idaho	290
22	Oklahoma	350		36	Virginia	281
46	Oregon	227		37	Rhode Island	274
15	Pennsylvania	402		38	Delaware	260
37	Rhode Island	274		39	Hawaii	257
32	South Carolina	308		40	Maryland	250
2	South Dakota	635		41	Colorado	247
16	Tennessee	398		42	California	238
33	Texas	304		43	Nevada	235
48	Utah	214		44	Connecticut	230
31	Vermont	310		45	Arizona	229
36	Virginia	281		46	Oregon	227
50	Washington	199		47	New Mexico	217
6	West Virginia	445		48	Utah	214
26	Wisconsin	332		49	Alaska	211
10	Wyoming	425		50	Washington	199
					District of Columbia	686

Source: Morgan Quitno Press using data from American Hospital Association (Chicago, IL)
   "Hospital Statistics" (1996-97 edition)

All nonfederal short-term general and other special hospitals, whose facilities and services are available to the public. Community hospitals are a subset of nonfederal hospitals.

Average Number of Beds per Community Hospital in 1995

National Average = 168 Beds per Community Hospital*

ALPHA ORDER				RANK ORDER		
RANK	STATE	BEDS		RANK	STATE	BEDS
22	Alabama	159		1	New Jersey	325
50	Alaska	75		2	New York	321
21	Arizona	162		3	Maryland	252
35	Arkansas	119		4	Rhode Island	247
14	California	177		5	Florida	234
29	Colorado	134		6	Connecticut	221
6	Connecticut	221		7	Pennsylvania	216
23	Delaware	155		8	Ohio	210
5	Florida	234		9	Illinois	203
20	Georgia	163		10	Massachusetts	196
26	Hawaii	144		11	Virginia	194
46	Idaho	83		12	North Carolina	191
9	Illinois	203		13	Nevada	180
18	Indiana	168		14	California	177
38	Iowa	109		14	Michigan	177
47	Kansas	82		16	Missouri	173
25	Kentucky	145		17	South Carolina	171
24	Louisiana	147		18	Indiana	168
40	Maine	103		19	Tennessee	166
3	Maryland	252		20	Georgia	163
10	Massachusetts	196		21	Arizona	162
14	Michigan	177		22	Alabama	159
34	Minnesota	122		23	Delaware	155
31	Mississippi	130		24	Louisiana	147
16	Missouri	173		25	Kentucky	145
49	Montana	77		26	Hawaii	144
45	Nebraska	86		27	West Virginia	138
13	Nevada	180		28	Texas	137
36	New Hampshire	116		29	Colorado	134
1	New Jersey	325		29	Wisconsin	134
41	New Mexico	102		31	Mississippi	130
2	New York	321		32	Vermont	129
12	North Carolina	191		33	Washington	123
43	North Dakota	97		34	Minnesota	122
8	Ohio	210		35	Arkansas	119
39	Oklahoma	104		36	New Hampshire	116
37	Oregon	112		37	Oregon	112
7	Pennsylvania	216		38	Iowa	109
4	Rhode Island	247		39	Oklahoma	104
17	South Carolina	171		40	Maine	103
44	South Dakota	93		41	New Mexico	102
19	Tennessee	166		42	Utah	100
28	Texas	137		43	North Dakota	97
42	Utah	100		44	South Dakota	93
32	Vermont	129		45	Nebraska	86
11	Virginia	194		46	Idaho	83
33	Washington	123		47	Kansas	82
27	West Virginia	138		47	Wyoming	82
29	Wisconsin	134		49	Montana	77
47	Wyoming	82		50	Alaska	75
					District of Columbia	476

Source: Morgan Quitno Press using data from American Hospital Association (Chicago, IL)
    "Hospital Statistics" (1996-97 edition)
All nonfederal short-term general and other special hospitals, whose facilities and services are available to the public. Community hospitals are a subset of nonfederal hospitals.

Beds in Nongovernment Not-For-Profit Hospitals in 1995

National Total = 609,729 Beds*

ALPHA ORDER

RANK	STATE	BEDS	% of USA
24	Alabama	7,409	1.22%
49	Alaska	790	0.13%
22	Arizona	7,648	1.25%
26	Arkansas	6,761	1.11%
3	California	47,621	7.81%
27	Colorado	6,431	1.05%
25	Connecticut	7,286	1.19%
45	Delaware	1,865	0.31%
9	Florida	24,039	3.94%
18	Georgia	11,407	1.87%
44	Hawaii	1,972	0.32%
47	Idaho	1,308	0.21%
4	Illinois	35,986	5.90%
14	Indiana	13,143	2.16%
21	Iowa	8,249	1.35%
30	Kansas	6,070	1.00%
20	Kentucky	10,175	1.67%
28	Louisiana	6,192	1.02%
38	Maine	3,788	0.62%
16	Maryland	12,318	2.02%
11	Massachusetts	16,626	2.73%
7	Michigan	27,021	4.43%
17	Minnesota	12,088	1.98%
33	Mississippi	5,228	0.86%
10	Missouri	16,999	2.79%
39	Montana	3,727	0.61%
34	Nebraska	5,147	0.84%
48	Nevada	1,069	0.18%
40	New Hampshire	2,944	0.48%
6	New Jersey	27,222	4.46%
43	New Mexico	2,052	0.34%
1	New York	59,740	9.80%
15	North Carolina	13,019	2.14%
37	North Dakota	3,907	0.64%
5	Ohio	33,333	5.47%
31	Oklahoma	5,749	0.94%
32	Oregon	5,691	0.93%
2	Pennsylvania	47,893	7.85%
41	Rhode Island	2,718	0.45%
35	South Carolina	4,678	0.77%
36	South Dakota	4,304	0.71%
19	Tennessee	11,172	1.83%
8	Texas	25,812	4.23%
42	Utah	2,333	0.38%
46	Vermont	1,811	0.30%
13	Virginia	13,450	2.21%
23	Washington	7,633	1.25%
29	West Virginia	6,143	1.01%
12	Wisconsin	15,778	2.59%
50	Wyoming	546	0.09%

RANK ORDER

RANK	STATE	BEDS	% of USA
1	New York	59,740	9.80%
2	Pennsylvania	47,893	7.85%
3	California	47,621	7.81%
4	Illinois	35,986	5.90%
5	Ohio	33,333	5.47%
6	New Jersey	27,222	4.46%
7	Michigan	27,021	4.43%
8	Texas	25,812	4.23%
9	Florida	24,039	3.94%
10	Missouri	16,999	2.79%
11	Massachusetts	16,626	2.73%
12	Wisconsin	15,778	2.59%
13	Virginia	13,450	2.21%
14	Indiana	13,143	2.16%
15	North Carolina	13,019	2.14%
16	Maryland	12,318	2.02%
17	Minnesota	12,088	1.98%
18	Georgia	11,407	1.87%
19	Tennessee	11,172	1.83%
20	Kentucky	10,175	1.67%
21	Iowa	8,249	1.35%
22	Arizona	7,648	1.25%
23	Washington	7,633	1.25%
24	Alabama	7,409	1.22%
25	Connecticut	7,286	1.19%
26	Arkansas	6,761	1.11%
27	Colorado	6,431	1.05%
28	Louisiana	6,192	1.02%
29	West Virginia	6,143	1.01%
30	Kansas	6,070	1.00%
31	Oklahoma	5,749	0.94%
32	Oregon	5,691	0.93%
33	Mississippi	5,228	0.86%
34	Nebraska	5,147	0.84%
35	South Carolina	4,678	0.77%
36	South Dakota	4,304	0.71%
37	North Dakota	3,907	0.64%
38	Maine	3,788	0.62%
39	Montana	3,727	0.61%
40	New Hampshire	2,944	0.48%
41	Rhode Island	2,718	0.45%
42	Utah	2,333	0.38%
43	New Mexico	2,052	0.34%
44	Hawaii	1,972	0.32%
45	Delaware	1,865	0.31%
46	Vermont	1,811	0.30%
47	Idaho	1,308	0.21%
48	Nevada	1,069	0.18%
49	Alaska	790	0.13%
50	Wyoming	546	0.09%
	District of Columbia	3,438	0.56%

Source: American Hospital Association (Chicago, IL)
   "Hospital Statistics" (1996-97 edition)
*Nongovernment not-for-profit hospitals are a subset of community hospitals.

Beds in Investor-Owned (For-Profit) Hospitals in 1995

National Total = 105,737 Beds*

ALPHA ORDER

RANK ORDER

RANK	STATE	BEDS	% of USA
7	Alabama	4,058	3.84%
36	Alaska	238	0.23%
18	Arizona	1,493	1.41%
14	Arkansas	1,952	1.85%
3	California	13,725	12.98%
24	Colorado	805	0.76%
44	Connecticut	0	0.00%
44	Delaware	0	0.00%
2	Florida	17,900	16.93%
6	Georgia	4,269	4.04%
40	Hawaii	143	0.14%
29	Idaho	448	0.42%
12	Illinois	2,177	2.06%
23	Indiana	815	0.77%
39	Iowa	150	0.14%
20	Kansas	1,226	1.16%
8	Kentucky	3,235	3.06%
4	Louisiana	5,714	5.40%
41	Maine	76	0.07%
34	Maryland	289	0.27%
26	Massachusetts	617	0.58%
42	Michigan	65	0.06%
44	Minnesota	0	0.00%
19	Mississippi	1,406	1.33%
15	Missouri	1,735	1.64%
44	Montana	0	0.00%
30	Nebraska	441	0.42%
17	Nevada	1,549	1.46%
31	New Hampshire	431	0.41%
38	New Jersey	155	0.15%
25	New Mexico	630	0.60%
11	New York	2,539	2.40%
16	North Carolina	1,601	1.51%
35	North Dakota	261	0.25%
28	Ohio	449	0.42%
13	Oklahoma	1,984	1.88%
33	Oregon	366	0.35%
27	Pennsylvania	562	0.53%
44	Rhode Island	0	0.00%
10	South Carolina	2,617	2.48%
44	South Dakota	0	0.00%
5	Tennessee	5,309	5.02%
1	Texas	18,306	17.31%
22	Utah	1,144	1.08%
44	Vermont	0	0.00%
9	Virginia	2,928	2.77%
32	Washington	409	0.39%
21	West Virginia	1,189	1.12%
43	Wisconsin	49	0.05%
37	Wyoming	172	0.16%

RANK	STATE	BEDS	% of USA
1	Texas	18,306	17.31%
2	Florida	17,900	16.93%
3	California	13,725	12.98%
4	Louisiana	5,714	5.40%
5	Tennessee	5,309	5.02%
6	Georgia	4,269	4.04%
7	Alabama	4,058	3.84%
8	Kentucky	3,235	3.06%
9	Virginia	2,928	2.77%
10	South Carolina	2,617	2.48%
11	New York	2,539	2.40%
12	Illinois	2,177	2.06%
13	Oklahoma	1,984	1.88%
14	Arkansas	1,952	1.85%
15	Missouri	1,735	1.64%
16	North Carolina	1,601	1.51%
17	Nevada	1,549	1.46%
18	Arizona	1,493	1.41%
19	Mississippi	1,406	1.33%
20	Kansas	1,226	1.16%
21	West Virginia	1,189	1.12%
22	Utah	1,144	1.08%
23	Indiana	815	0.77%
24	Colorado	805	0.76%
25	New Mexico	630	0.60%
26	Massachusetts	617	0.58%
27	Pennsylvania	562	0.53%
28	Ohio	449	0.42%
29	Idaho	448	0.42%
30	Nebraska	441	0.42%
31	New Hampshire	431	0.41%
32	Washington	409	0.39%
33	Oregon	366	0.35%
34	Maryland	289	0.27%
35	North Dakota	261	0.25%
36	Alaska	238	0.23%
37	Wyoming	172	0.16%
38	New Jersey	155	0.15%
39	Iowa	150	0.14%
40	Hawaii	143	0.14%
41	Maine	76	0.07%
42	Michigan	65	0.06%
43	Wisconsin	49	0.05%
44	Connecticut	0	0.00%
44	Delaware	0	0.00%
44	Minnesota	0	0.00%
44	Montana	0	0.00%
44	Rhode Island	0	0.00%
44	South Dakota	0	0.00%
44	Vermont	0	0.00%
	District of Columbia	110	0.10%

Source: American Hospital Association (Chicago, IL)
"Hospital Statistics" (1996-97 edition)
*Investor-owned (for-profit) hospitals are a subset of community hospitals.

Beds in State and Local Government-Owned Hospitals in 1995

National Total = 157,270 Beds*

ALPHA ORDER

RANK	STATE	BEDS	% of USA
8	Alabama	6,785	4.31%
41	Alaska	242	0.15%
37	Arizona	711	0.45%
29	Arkansas	1,431	0.91%
1	California	13,670	8.69%
25	Colorado	2,022	1.29%
42	Connecticut	232	0.15%
45	Delaware	0	0.00%
6	Florida	7,751	4.93%
4	Georgia	10,448	6.64%
35	Hawaii	915	0.58%
27	Idaho	1,627	1.03%
16	Illinois	3,801	2.42%
10	Indiana	5,404	3.44%
13	Iowa	4,216	2.68%
18	Kansas	3,465	2.20%
26	Kentucky	1,721	1.09%
7	Louisiana	7,240	4.60%
43	Maine	147	0.09%
45	Maryland	0	0.00%
28	Massachusetts	1,617	1.03%
21	Michigan	2,550	1.62%
11	Minnesota	5,279	3.36%
9	Mississippi	5,956	3.79%
19	Missouri	3,117	1.98%
39	Montana	498	0.32%
23	Nebraska	2,263	1.44%
34	Nevada	982	0.62%
45	New Hampshire	0	0.00%
22	New Jersey	2,486	1.58%
33	New Mexico	993	0.63%
3	New York	11,629	7.39%
5	North Carolina	8,109	5.16%
45	North Dakota	0	0.00%
15	Ohio	3,984	2.53%
17	Oklahoma	3,729	2.37%
32	Oregon	1,104	0.70%
44	Pennsylvania	79	0.05%
45	Rhode Island	0	0.00%
14	South Carolina	4,012	2.55%
40	South Dakota	332	0.21%
12	Tennessee	4,428	2.82%
2	Texas	13,060	8.30%
38	Utah	707	0.45%
45	Vermont	0	0.00%
24	Virginia	2,201	1.40%
20	Washington	2,778	1.77%
36	West Virginia	789	0.50%
31	Wisconsin	1,182	0.75%
30	Wyoming	1,320	0.84%

RANK ORDER

RANK	STATE	BEDS	% of USA
1	California	13,670	8.69%
2	Texas	13,060	8.30%
3	New York	11,629	7.39%
4	Georgia	10,448	6.64%
5	North Carolina	8,109	5.16%
6	Florida	7,751	4.93%
7	Louisiana	7,240	4.60%
8	Alabama	6,785	4.31%
9	Mississippi	5,956	3.79%
10	Indiana	5,404	3.44%
11	Minnesota	5,279	3.36%
12	Tennessee	4,428	2.82%
13	Iowa	4,216	2.68%
14	South Carolina	4,012	2.55%
15	Ohio	3,984	2.53%
16	Illinois	3,801	2.42%
17	Oklahoma	3,729	2.37%
18	Kansas	3,465	2.20%
19	Missouri	3,117	1.98%
20	Washington	2,778	1.77%
21	Michigan	2,550	1.62%
22	New Jersey	2,486	1.58%
23	Nebraska	2,263	1.44%
24	Virginia	2,201	1.40%
25	Colorado	2,022	1.29%
26	Kentucky	1,721	1.09%
27	Idaho	1,627	1.03%
28	Massachusetts	1,617	1.03%
29	Arkansas	1,431	0.91%
30	Wyoming	1,320	0.84%
31	Wisconsin	1,182	0.75%
32	Oregon	1,104	0.70%
33	New Mexico	993	0.63%
34	Nevada	982	0.62%
35	Hawaii	915	0.58%
36	West Virginia	789	0.50%
37	Arizona	711	0.45%
38	Utah	707	0.45%
39	Montana	498	0.32%
40	South Dakota	332	0.21%
41	Alaska	242	0.15%
42	Connecticut	232	0.15%
43	Maine	147	0.09%
44	Pennsylvania	79	0.05%
45	Delaware	0	0.00%
45	Maryland	0	0.00%
45	New Hampshire	0	0.00%
45	North Dakota	0	0.00%
45	Rhode Island	0	0.00%
45	Vermont	0	0.00%
	District of Columbia	258	0.16%

Source: American Hospital Association (Chicago, IL)
    "Hospital Statistics" (1996-97 edition)
*State and local government-owned hospitals are a subset of community hospitals.

Hospital Admissions in 1995

National Total = 33,282,124 Admissions*

ALPHA ORDER

RANK	STATE	ADMISSIONS	% of USA
17	Alabama	680,169	2.04%
48	Alaska	63,196	0.19%
24	Arizona	485,628	1.46%
30	Arkansas	369,046	1.11%
1	California	3,203,317	9.62%
28	Colorado	380,786	1.14%
31	Connecticut	363,163	1.09%
47	Delaware	88,748	0.27%
4	Florida	1,910,738	5.74%
10	Georgia	961,029	2.89%
42	Hawaii	115,361	0.35%
43	Idaho	111,620	0.34%
6	Illinois	1,539,098	4.62%
16	Indiana	728,315	2.19%
29	Iowa	378,184	1.14%
32	Kansas	321,962	0.97%
21	Kentucky	577,312	1.73%
18	Louisiana	671,855	2.02%
39	Maine	151,467	0.46%
19	Maryland	635,705	1.91%
12	Massachusetts	805,938	2.42%
8	Michigan	1,162,369	3.49%
22	Minnesota	521,558	1.57%
26	Mississippi	424,166	1.27%
14	Missouri	788,168	2.37%
45	Montana	104,736	0.31%
35	Nebraska	203,705	0.61%
38	Nevada	162,190	0.49%
41	New Hampshire	117,945	0.35%
9	New Jersey	1,096,326	3.29%
36	New Mexico	194,278	0.58%
2	New York	2,506,198	7.53%
11	North Carolina	922,302	2.77%
46	North Dakota	100,632	0.30%
7	Ohio	1,435,042	4.31%
27	Oklahoma	413,747	1.24%
33	Oregon	315,158	0.95%
5	Pennsylvania	1,892,489	5.69%
40	Rhode Island	126,176	0.38%
25	South Carolina	452,367	1.36%
44	South Dakota	109,215	0.33%
13	Tennessee	790,252	2.37%
3	Texas	2,240,243	6.73%
37	Utah	184,810	0.56%
49	Vermont	60,042	0.18%
15	Virginia	782,259	2.35%
23	Washington	520,309	1.56%
34	West Virginia	291,828	0.88%
20	Wisconsin	582,792	1.75%
50	Wyoming	48,686	0.15%

RANK ORDER

RANK	STATE	ADMISSIONS	% of USA
1	California	3,203,317	9.62%
2	New York	2,506,198	7.53%
3	Texas	2,240,243	6.73%
4	Florida	1,910,738	5.74%
5	Pennsylvania	1,892,489	5.69%
6	Illinois	1,539,098	4.62%
7	Ohio	1,435,042	4.31%
8	Michigan	1,162,369	3.49%
9	New Jersey	1,096,326	3.29%
10	Georgia	961,029	2.89%
11	North Carolina	922,302	2.77%
12	Massachusetts	805,938	2.42%
13	Tennessee	790,252	2.37%
14	Missouri	788,168	2.37%
15	Virginia	782,259	2.35%
16	Indiana	728,315	2.19%
17	Alabama	680,169	2.04%
18	Louisiana	671,855	2.02%
19	Maryland	635,705	1.91%
20	Wisconsin	582,792	1.75%
21	Kentucky	577,312	1.73%
22	Minnesota	521,558	1.57%
23	Washington	520,309	1.56%
24	Arizona	485,628	1.46%
25	South Carolina	452,367	1.36%
26	Mississippi	424,166	1.27%
27	Oklahoma	413,747	1.24%
28	Colorado	380,786	1.14%
29	Iowa	378,184	1.14%
30	Arkansas	369,046	1.11%
31	Connecticut	363,163	1.09%
32	Kansas	321,962	0.97%
33	Oregon	315,158	0.95%
34	West Virginia	291,828	0.88%
35	Nebraska	203,705	0.61%
36	New Mexico	194,278	0.58%
37	Utah	184,810	0.56%
38	Nevada	162,190	0.49%
39	Maine	151,467	0.46%
40	Rhode Island	126,176	0.38%
41	New Hampshire	117,945	0.35%
42	Hawaii	115,361	0.35%
43	Idaho	111,620	0.34%
44	South Dakota	109,215	0.33%
45	Montana	104,736	0.31%
46	North Dakota	100,632	0.30%
47	Delaware	88,748	0.27%
48	Alaska	63,196	0.19%
49	Vermont	60,042	0.18%
50	Wyoming	48,686	0.15%
	District of Columbia	189,499	0.57%

*Source: American Hospital Association (Chicago, IL)
"Hospital Statistics" (1996-97 edition)*
*Admissions in federal and nonfederal hospitals.

Admissions to Federal Hospitals in 1995

National Total = 1,559,089 Admissions*

ALPHA ORDER

RANK	STATE	ADMISSIONS	% of USA
21	Alabama	26,954	1.73%
26	Alaska	20,401	1.31%
10	Arizona	47,533	3.05%
28	Arkansas	19,003	1.22%
2	California	112,930	7.24%
18	Colorado	30,064	1.93%
39	Connecticut	11,386	0.73%
48	Delaware	3,859	0.25%
3	Florida	98,883	6.34%
8	Georgia	55,596	3.57%
30	Hawaii	17,714	1.14%
44	Idaho	5,398	0.35%
7	Illinois	55,866	3.58%
32	Indiana	15,154	0.97%
37	Iowa	13,154	0.84%
27	Kansas	19,364	1.24%
19	Kentucky	29,574	1.90%
23	Louisiana	26,241	1.68%
46	Maine	4,253	0.27%
12	Maryland	45,060	2.89%
24	Massachusetts	23,876	1.53%
25	Michigan	23,666	1.52%
29	Minnesota	18,652	1.20%
22	Mississippi	26,507	1.70%
6	Missouri	57,564	3.69%
42	Montana	8,402	0.54%
33	Nebraska	15,093	0.97%
43	Nevada	7,753	0.50%
50	New Hampshire	2,715	0.17%
38	New Jersey	13,135	0.84%
20	New Mexico	29,408	1.89%
4	New York	67,783	4.35%
9	North Carolina	54,313	3.48%
40	North Dakota	9,996	0.64%
14	Ohio	36,514	2.34%
15	Oklahoma	31,717	2.03%
34	Oregon	14,958	0.96%
13	Pennsylvania	38,257	2.45%
47	Rhode Island	4,018	0.26%
16	South Carolina	31,386	2.01%
36	South Dakota	14,376	0.92%
17	Tennessee	31,127	2.00%
1	Texas	152,065	9.75%
41	Utah	9,698	0.62%
49	Vermont	3,595	0.23%
5	Virginia	61,097	3.92%
11	Washington	45,633	2.93%
31	West Virginia	15,762	1.01%
35	Wisconsin	14,871	0.95%
45	Wyoming	4,906	0.31%

RANK ORDER

RANK	STATE	ADMISSIONS	% of USA
1	Texas	152,065	9.75%
2	California	112,930	7.24%
3	Florida	98,883	6.34%
4	New York	67,783	4.35%
5	Virginia	61,097	3.92%
6	Missouri	57,564	3.69%
7	Illinois	55,866	3.58%
8	Georgia	55,596	3.57%
9	North Carolina	54,313	3.48%
10	Arizona	47,533	3.05%
11	Washington	45,633	2.93%
12	Maryland	45,060	2.89%
13	Pennsylvania	38,257	2.45%
14	Ohio	36,514	2.34%
15	Oklahoma	31,717	2.03%
16	South Carolina	31,386	2.01%
17	Tennessee	31,127	2.00%
18	Colorado	30,064	1.93%
19	Kentucky	29,574	1.90%
20	New Mexico	29,408	1.89%
21	Alabama	26,954	1.73%
22	Mississippi	26,507	1.70%
23	Louisiana	26,241	1.68%
24	Massachusetts	23,876	1.53%
25	Michigan	23,666	1.52%
26	Alaska	20,401	1.31%
27	Kansas	19,364	1.24%
28	Arkansas	19,003	1.22%
29	Minnesota	18,652	1.20%
30	Hawaii	17,714	1.14%
31	West Virginia	15,762	1.01%
32	Indiana	15,154	0.97%
33	Nebraska	15,093	0.97%
34	Oregon	14,958	0.96%
35	Wisconsin	14,871	0.95%
36	South Dakota	14,376	0.92%
37	Iowa	13,154	0.84%
38	New Jersey	13,135	0.84%
39	Connecticut	11,386	0.73%
40	North Dakota	9,996	0.64%
41	Utah	9,698	0.62%
42	Montana	8,402	0.54%
43	Nevada	7,753	0.50%
44	Idaho	5,398	0.35%
45	Wyoming	4,906	0.31%
46	Maine	4,253	0.27%
47	Rhode Island	4,018	0.26%
48	Delaware	3,859	0.25%
49	Vermont	3,595	0.23%
50	New Hampshire	2,715	0.17%
	District of Columbia	31,859	2.04%

Source: American Hospital Association (Chicago, IL)
"Hospital Statistics" (1996-97 edition)
*Federal hospitals are controlled by an agency or department of the federal government.

Admissions to Nonfederal Hospitals in 1995

National Total = 31,723,035 Admissions

RANK	STATE	ADMISSIONS	% of USA
17	Alabama	653,215	2.06%
50	Alaska	42,795	0.13%
24	Arizona	438,095	1.38%
31	Arkansas	350,043	1.10%
1	California	3,090,387	9.74%
30	Colorado	350,722	1.11%
29	Connecticut	351,777	1.11%
47	Delaware	87,889	0.28%
5	Florida	1,811,855	5.71%
10	Georgia	905,433	2.85%
43	Hawaii	97,647	0.31%
42	Idaho	106,222	0.33%
6	Illinois	1,483,232	4.68%
16	Indiana	713,161	2.25%
28	Iowa	365,030	1.15%
32	Kansas	302,598	0.95%
21	Kentucky	547,738	1.73%
18	Louisiana	645,614	2.03%
39	Maine	147,214	0.46%
19	Maryland	590,645	1.86%
12	Massachusetts	782,062	2.47%
8	Michigan	1,138,703	3.59%
22	Minnesota	502,906	1.59%
26	Mississippi	397,659	1.25%
14	Missouri	730,604	2.30%
44	Montana	96,334	0.30%
35	Nebraska	188,612	0.59%
38	Nevada	154,437	0.49%
41	New Hampshire	115,230	0.36%
9	New Jersey	1,083,191	3.41%
37	New Mexico	164,870	0.52%
2	New York	2,438,415	7.69%
11	North Carolina	867,989	2.74%
46	North Dakota	90,636	0.29%
7	Ohio	1,398,528	4.41%
27	Oklahoma	382,030	1.20%
33	Oregon	300,200	0.95%
4	Pennsylvania	1,854,232	5.84%
40	Rhode Island	122,158	0.39%
25	South Carolina	420,981	1.33%
45	South Dakota	94,839	0.30%
13	Tennessee	759,125	2.39%
3	Texas	2,088,178	6.58%
36	Utah	175,112	0.55%
48	Vermont	56,447	0.18%
15	Virginia	721,162	2.27%
23	Washington	474,676	1.50%
34	West Virginia	276,066	0.87%
20	Wisconsin	567,921	1.79%
49	Wyoming	43,780	0.14%

RANK	STATE	ADMISSIONS	% of USA
1	California	3,090,387	9.74%
2	New York	2,438,415	7.69%
3	Texas	2,088,178	6.58%
4	Pennsylvania	1,854,232	5.84%
5	Florida	1,811,855	5.71%
6	Illinois	1,483,232	4.68%
7	Ohio	1,398,528	4.41%
8	Michigan	1,138,703	3.59%
9	New Jersey	1,083,191	3.41%
10	Georgia	905,433	2.85%
11	North Carolina	867,989	2.74%
12	Massachusetts	782,062	2.47%
13	Tennessee	759,125	2.39%
14	Missouri	730,604	2.30%
15	Virginia	721,162	2.27%
16	Indiana	713,161	2.25%
17	Alabama	653,215	2.06%
18	Louisiana	645,614	2.03%
19	Maryland	590,645	1.86%
20	Wisconsin	567,921	1.79%
21	Kentucky	547,738	1.73%
22	Minnesota	502,906	1.59%
23	Washington	474,676	1.50%
24	Arizona	438,095	1.38%
25	South Carolina	420,981	1.33%
26	Mississippi	397,659	1.25%
27	Oklahoma	382,030	1.20%
28	Iowa	365,030	1.15%
29	Connecticut	351,777	1.11%
30	Colorado	350,722	1.11%
31	Arkansas	350,043	1.10%
32	Kansas	302,598	0.95%
33	Oregon	300,200	0.95%
34	West Virginia	276,066	0.87%
35	Nebraska	188,612	0.59%
36	Utah	175,112	0.55%
37	New Mexico	164,870	0.52%
38	Nevada	154,437	0.49%
39	Maine	147,214	0.46%
40	Rhode Island	122,158	0.39%
41	New Hampshire	115,230	0.36%
42	Idaho	106,222	0.33%
43	Hawaii	97,647	0.31%
44	Montana	96,334	0.30%
45	South Dakota	94,839	0.30%
46	North Dakota	90,636	0.29%
47	Delaware	87,889	0.28%
48	Vermont	56,447	0.18%
49	Wyoming	43,780	0.14%
50	Alaska	42,795	0.13%
	District of Columbia	157,640	0.50%

Source: American Hospital Association (Chicago, IL)
"Hospital Statistics" (1996-97 edition)

Admissions to Psychiatric Hospitals in 1995

National Total = 765,729 Admissions*

ALPHA ORDER

RANK	STATE	ADMISSIONS	% of USA
20	Alabama	14,581	1.90%
42	Alaska	2,705	0.35%
25	Arizona	11,085	1.45%
30	Arkansas	8,363	1.09%
2	California	52,670	6.88%
26	Colorado	10,288	1.34%
23	Connecticut	12,612	1.65%
40	Delaware	3,991	0.52%
6	Florida	36,522	4.77%
4	Georgia	42,098	5.50%
50	Hawaii	117	0.02%
43	Idaho	2,677	0.35%
10	Illinois	27,695	3.62%
12	Indiana	21,239	2.77%
33	Iowa	6,573	0.86%
24	Kansas	11,486	1.50%
22	Kentucky	14,122	1.84%
11	Louisiana	22,223	2.90%
38	Maine	4,942	0.65%
17	Maryland	17,071	2.23%
9	Massachusetts	28,350	3.70%
13	Michigan	21,135	2.76%
31	Minnesota	7,776	1.02%
27	Mississippi	9,262	1.21%
19	Missouri	15,158	1.98%
49	Montana	180	0.02%
34	Nebraska	5,558	0.73%
36	Nevada	5,128	0.67%
37	New Hampshire	5,116	0.67%
18	New Jersey	15,211	1.99%
28	New Mexico	8,912	1.16%
5	New York	41,407	5.41%
7	North Carolina	35,115	4.59%
47	North Dakota	1,620	0.21%
8	Ohio	28,647	3.74%
21	Oklahoma	14,344	1.87%
41	Oregon	3,921	0.51%
3	Pennsylvania	45,590	5.95%
44	Rhode Island	2,304	0.30%
29	South Carolina	8,896	1.16%
48	South Dakota	738	0.10%
16	Tennessee	18,841	2.46%
1	Texas	55,195	7.21%
39	Utah	4,367	0.57%
46	Vermont	1,639	0.21%
14	Virginia	20,575	2.69%
32	Washington	6,919	0.90%
35	West Virginia	5,176	0.68%
15	Wisconsin	19,876	2.60%
45	Wyoming	2,263	0.30%

RANK ORDER

RANK	STATE	ADMISSIONS	% of USA
1	Texas	55,195	7.21%
2	California	52,670	6.88%
3	Pennsylvania	45,590	5.95%
4	Georgia	42,098	5.50%
5	New York	41,407	5.41%
6	Florida	36,522	4.77%
7	North Carolina	35,115	4.59%
8	Ohio	28,647	3.74%
9	Massachusetts	28,350	3.70%
10	Illinois	27,695	3.62%
11	Louisiana	22,223	2.90%
12	Indiana	21,239	2.77%
13	Michigan	21,135	2.76%
14	Virginia	20,575	2.69%
15	Wisconsin	19,876	2.60%
16	Tennessee	18,841	2.46%
17	Maryland	17,071	2.23%
18	New Jersey	15,211	1.99%
19	Missouri	15,158	1.98%
20	Alabama	14,581	1.90%
21	Oklahoma	14,344	1.87%
22	Kentucky	14,122	1.84%
23	Connecticut	12,612	1.65%
24	Kansas	11,486	1.50%
25	Arizona	11,085	1.45%
26	Colorado	10,288	1.34%
27	Mississippi	9,262	1.21%
28	New Mexico	8,912	1.16%
29	South Carolina	8,896	1.16%
30	Arkansas	8,363	1.09%
31	Minnesota	7,776	1.02%
32	Washington	6,919	0.90%
33	Iowa	6,573	0.86%
34	Nebraska	5,558	0.73%
35	West Virginia	5,176	0.68%
36	Nevada	5,128	0.67%
37	New Hampshire	5,116	0.67%
38	Maine	4,942	0.65%
39	Utah	4,367	0.57%
40	Delaware	3,991	0.52%
41	Oregon	3,921	0.51%
42	Alaska	2,705	0.35%
43	Idaho	2,677	0.35%
44	Rhode Island	2,304	0.30%
45	Wyoming	2,263	0.30%
46	Vermont	1,639	0.21%
47	North Dakota	1,620	0.21%
48	South Dakota	738	0.10%
49	Montana	180	0.02%
50	Hawaii	117	0.02%
	District of Columbia	3,450	0.45%

Source: American Hospital Association (Chicago, IL)
   "Hospital Statistics" (1996-97 edition)
Admissions to federal and nonfederal psychiatric hospitals.

Admissions to Community Hospitals in 1995

National Total = 30,945,357 Admissions*

ALPHA ORDER				RANK ORDER			
RANK	STATE	ADMISSIONS	% of USA	RANK	STATE	ADMISSIONS	% of USA
17	Alabama	642,023	2.07%	1	California	3,028,686	9.79%
50	Alaska	40,090	0.13%	2	New York	2,397,920	7.75%
24	Arizona	426,627	1.38%	3	Texas	2,029,050	6.56%
29	Arkansas	341,680	1.10%	4	Pennsylvania	1,810,118	5.85%
1	California	3,028,686	9.79%	5	Florida	1,771,689	5.73%
30	Colorado	340,349	1.10%	6	Illinois	1,451,929	4.69%
31	Connecticut	337,503	1.09%	7	Ohio	1,375,335	4.44%
47	Delaware	80,898	0.26%	8	Michigan	1,120,065	3.62%
5	Florida	1,771,689	5.73%	9	New Jersey	1,068,336	3.45%
10	Georgia	858,702	2.77%	10	Georgia	858,702	2.77%
43	Hawaii	97,268	0.31%	11	North Carolina	832,848	2.69%
42	Idaho	103,545	0.33%	12	Massachusetts	750,807	2.43%
6	Illinois	1,451,929	4.69%	13	Tennessee	739,502	2.39%
16	Indiana	699,101	2.26%	14	Missouri	714,037	2.31%
28	Iowa	360,949	1.17%	15	Virginia	699,223	2.26%
33	Kansas	290,750	0.94%	16	Indiana	699,101	2.26%
21	Kentucky	533,564	1.72%	17	Alabama	642,023	2.07%
18	Louisiana	622,168	2.01%	18	Louisiana	622,168	2.01%
39	Maine	142,272	0.46%	19	Maryland	574,075	1.86%
19	Maryland	574,075	1.86%	20	Wisconsin	550,438	1.78%
12	Massachusetts	750,807	2.43%	21	Kentucky	533,564	1.72%
8	Michigan	1,120,065	3.62%	22	Minnesota	496,085	1.60%
22	Minnesota	496,085	1.60%	23	Washington	466,694	1.51%
26	Mississippi	388,397	1.26%	24	Arizona	426,627	1.38%
14	Missouri	714,037	2.31%	25	South Carolina	410,159	1.33%
44	Montana	96,154	0.31%	26	Mississippi	388,397	1.26%
35	Nebraska	182,686	0.59%	27	Oklahoma	367,580	1.19%
38	Nevada	149,309	0.48%	28	Iowa	360,949	1.17%
41	New Hampshire	109,708	0.35%	29	Arkansas	341,680	1.10%
9	New Jersey	1,068,336	3.45%	30	Colorado	340,349	1.10%
37	New Mexico	155,695	0.50%	31	Connecticut	337,503	1.09%
2	New York	2,397,920	7.75%	32	Oregon	296,279	0.96%
11	North Carolina	832,848	2.69%	33	Kansas	290,750	0.94%
46	North Dakota	88,792	0.29%	34	West Virginia	270,890	0.88%
7	Ohio	1,375,335	4.44%	35	Nebraska	182,686	0.59%
27	Oklahoma	367,580	1.19%	36	Utah	170,745	0.55%
32	Oregon	296,279	0.96%	37	New Mexico	155,695	0.50%
4	Pennsylvania	1,810,118	5.85%	38	Nevada	149,309	0.48%
40	Rhode Island	118,585	0.38%	39	Maine	142,272	0.46%
25	South Carolina	410,159	1.33%	40	Rhode Island	118,585	0.38%
45	South Dakota	93,950	0.30%	41	New Hampshire	109,708	0.35%
13	Tennessee	739,502	2.39%	42	Idaho	103,545	0.33%
3	Texas	2,029,050	6.56%	43	Hawaii	97,268	0.31%
36	Utah	170,745	0.55%	44	Montana	96,154	0.31%
48	Vermont	54,808	0.18%	45	South Dakota	93,950	0.30%
15	Virginia	699,223	2.26%	46	North Dakota	88,792	0.29%
23	Washington	466,694	1.51%	47	Delaware	80,898	0.26%
34	West Virginia	270,890	0.88%	48	Vermont	54,808	0.18%
20	Wisconsin	550,438	1.78%	49	Wyoming	43,364	0.14%
49	Wyoming	43,364	0.14%	50	Alaska	40,090	0.13%
					District of Columbia	153,930	0.50%

Source: American Hospital Association (Chicago, IL)
"Hospital Statistics" (1996-97 edition)
*Admissions to all nonfederal short-term general and other special hospitals, whose facilities and services are available to the public. Community hospitals are a subset of nonfederal hospitals.

Admissions to Nongovernment Not-For-Profit Hospitals in 1995

National Total = 22,556,693 Admissions*

ALPHA ORDER

RANK	STATE	ADMISSIONS	% of USA
24	Alabama	270,270	1.20%
49	Alaska	27,617	0.12%
21	Arizona	348,540	1.55%
27	Arkansas	242,589	1.08%
1	California	1,994,898	8.84%
28	Colorado	239,622	1.06%
23	Connecticut	330,255	1.46%
43	Delaware	80,898	0.36%
9	Florida	904,812	4.01%
18	Georgia	416,733	1.85%
45	Hawaii	69,083	0.31%
47	Idaho	50,286	0.22%
4	Illinois	1,272,162	5.64%
15	Indiana	501,529	2.22%
25	Iowa	251,772	1.12%
32	Kansas	179,506	0.80%
20	Kentucky	376,806	1.67%
29	Louisiana	220,455	0.98%
35	Maine	136,255	0.60%
12	Maryland	561,014	2.49%
10	Massachusetts	685,965	3.04%
6	Michigan	1,059,548	4.70%
19	Minnesota	395,321	1.75%
34	Mississippi	166,058	0.74%
11	Missouri	579,242	2.57%
40	Montana	90,916	0.40%
36	Nebraska	128,673	0.57%
48	Nevada	40,100	0.18%
39	New Hampshire	97,700	0.43%
7	New Jersey	1,033,688	4.58%
42	New Mexico	89,387	0.40%
2	New York	1,986,144	8.81%
16	North Carolina	475,267	2.11%
44	North Dakota	78,825	0.35%
5	Ohio	1,231,765	5.46%
31	Oklahoma	193,035	0.86%
26	Oregon	250,569	1.11%
3	Pennsylvania	1,797,198	7.97%
37	Rhode Island	118,585	0.53%
33	South Carolina	178,791	0.79%
41	South Dakota	89,809	0.40%
17	Tennessee	432,950	1.92%
8	Texas	985,325	4.37%
38	Utah	107,240	0.48%
46	Vermont	54,808	0.24%
13	Virginia	516,894	2.29%
22	Washington	347,675	1.54%
30	West Virginia	205,621	0.91%
14	Wisconsin	511,479	2.27%
50	Wyoming	12,868	0.06%

RANK ORDER

RANK	STATE	ADMISSIONS	% of USA
1	California	1,994,898	8.84%
2	New York	1,986,144	8.81%
3	Pennsylvania	1,797,198	7.97%
4	Illinois	1,272,162	5.64%
5	Ohio	1,231,765	5.46%
6	Michigan	1,059,548	4.70%
7	New Jersey	1,033,688	4.58%
8	Texas	985,325	4.37%
9	Florida	904,812	4.01%
10	Massachusetts	685,965	3.04%
11	Missouri	579,242	2.57%
12	Maryland	561,014	2.49%
13	Virginia	516,894	2.29%
14	Wisconsin	511,479	2.27%
15	Indiana	501,529	2.22%
16	North Carolina	475,267	2.11%
17	Tennessee	432,950	1.92%
18	Georgia	416,733	1.85%
19	Minnesota	395,321	1.75%
20	Kentucky	376,806	1.67%
21	Arizona	348,540	1.55%
22	Washington	347,675	1.54%
23	Connecticut	330,255	1.46%
24	Alabama	270,270	1.20%
25	Iowa	251,772	1.12%
26	Oregon	250,569	1.11%
27	Arkansas	242,589	1.08%
28	Colorado	239,622	1.06%
29	Louisiana	220,455	0.98%
30	West Virginia	205,621	0.91%
31	Oklahoma	193,035	0.86%
32	Kansas	179,506	0.80%
33	South Carolina	178,791	0.79%
34	Mississippi	166,058	0.74%
35	Maine	136,255	0.60%
36	Nebraska	128,673	0.57%
37	Rhode Island	118,585	0.53%
38	Utah	107,240	0.48%
39	New Hampshire	97,700	0.43%
40	Montana	90,916	0.40%
41	South Dakota	89,809	0.40%
42	New Mexico	89,387	0.40%
43	Delaware	80,898	0.36%
44	North Dakota	78,825	0.35%
45	Hawaii	69,083	0.31%
46	Vermont	54,808	0.24%
47	Idaho	50,286	0.22%
48	Nevada	40,100	0.18%
49	Alaska	27,617	0.12%
50	Wyoming	12,868	0.06%
	District of Columbia	140,145	0.62%

Source: American Hospital Association (Chicago, IL)
     "Hospital Statistics" (1996-97 edition)
*Nongovernment not-for-profit hospitals are a subset of community hospitals.

Admissions to Investor-Owned (For-Profit) Hospitals in 1995

National Total = 3,427,850 Admissions*

RANK	STATE	ADMISSIONS	% of USA
6	Alabama	133,416	3.89%
36	Alaska	6,434	0.19%
16	Arizona	51,801	1.51%
15	Arkansas	56,170	1.64%
3	California	474,490	13.84%
23	Colorado	35,611	1.04%
44	Connecticut	0	0.00%
44	Delaware	0	0.00%
2	Florida	598,981	17.47%
7	Georgia	131,704	3.84%
37	Hawaii	6,124	0.18%
27	Idaho	15,519	0.45%
13	Illinois	74,596	2.18%
24	Indiana	21,780	0.64%
40	Iowa	1,728	0.05%
21	Kansas	41,893	1.22%
8	Kentucky	105,832	3.09%
5	Louisiana	145,113	4.23%
41	Maine	877	0.03%
29	Maryland	13,061	0.38%
35	Massachusetts	9,388	0.27%
42	Michigan	773	0.02%
44	Minnesota	0	0.00%
19	Mississippi	43,683	1.27%
18	Missouri	47,257	1.38%
44	Montana	0	0.00%
30	Nebraska	13,002	0.38%
12	Nevada	75,290	2.20%
31	New Hampshire	12,008	0.35%
39	New Jersey	1,976	0.06%
25	New Mexico	20,150	0.59%
11	New York	78,934	2.30%
17	North Carolina	50,589	1.48%
33	North Dakota	9,967	0.29%
26	Ohio	16,731	0.49%
14	Oklahoma	57,807	1.69%
32	Oregon	10,237	0.30%
34	Pennsylvania	9,941	0.29%
44	Rhode Island	0	0.00%
10	South Carolina	93,987	2.74%
44	South Dakota	0	0.00%
4	Tennessee	164,172	4.79%
1	Texas	599,587	17.49%
20	Utah	42,545	1.24%
44	Vermont	0	0.00%
9	Virginia	95,186	2.78%
28	Washington	14,212	0.41%
22	West Virginia	38,483	1.12%
43	Wisconsin	663	0.02%
38	Wyoming	3,876	0.11%

RANK	STATE	ADMISSIONS	% of USA
1	Texas	599,587	17.49%
2	Florida	598,981	17.47%
3	California	474,490	13.84%
4	Tennessee	164,172	4.79%
5	Louisiana	145,113	4.23%
6	Alabama	133,416	3.89%
7	Georgia	131,704	3.84%
8	Kentucky	105,832	3.09%
9	Virginia	95,186	2.78%
10	South Carolina	93,987	2.74%
11	New York	78,934	2.30%
12	Nevada	75,290	2.20%
13	Illinois	74,596	2.18%
14	Oklahoma	57,807	1.69%
15	Arkansas	56,170	1.64%
16	Arizona	51,801	1.51%
17	North Carolina	50,589	1.48%
18	Missouri	47,257	1.38%
19	Mississippi	43,683	1.27%
20	Utah	42,545	1.24%
21	Kansas	41,893	1.22%
22	West Virginia	38,483	1.12%
23	Colorado	35,611	1.04%
24	Indiana	21,780	0.64%
25	New Mexico	20,150	0.59%
26	Ohio	16,731	0.49%
27	Idaho	15,519	0.45%
28	Washington	14,212	0.41%
29	Maryland	13,061	0.38%
30	Nebraska	13,002	0.38%
31	New Hampshire	12,008	0.35%
32	Oregon	10,237	0.30%
33	North Dakota	9,967	0.29%
34	Pennsylvania	9,941	0.29%
35	Massachusetts	9,388	0.27%
36	Alaska	6,434	0.19%
37	Hawaii	6,124	0.18%
38	Wyoming	3,876	0.11%
39	New Jersey	1,976	0.06%
40	Iowa	1,728	0.05%
41	Maine	877	0.03%
42	Michigan	773	0.02%
43	Wisconsin	663	0.02%
44	Connecticut	0	0.00%
44	Delaware	0	0.00%
44	Minnesota	0	0.00%
44	Montana	0	0.00%
44	Rhode Island	0	0.00%
44	South Dakota	0	0.00%
44	Vermont	0	0.00%
	District of Columbia	2,276	0.07%

Source: American Hospital Association (Chicago, IL)
"Hospital Statistics" (1996-97 edition)
Investor-owned (for-profit) hospitals are a subset of community hospitals.

Admissions to State and Local Government-Owned Hospitals in 1995

National Total = 4,960,814 Admissions*

ALPHA ORDER

RANK	STATE	ADMISSIONS	% of USA
8	Alabama	238,337	4.80%
40	Alaska	6,039	0.12%
36	Arizona	26,286	0.53%
27	Arkansas	42,921	0.87%
1	California	559,298	11.27%
22	Colorado	65,116	1.31%
39	Connecticut	7,248	0.15%
45	Delaware	0	0.00%
6	Florida	267,896	5.40%
4	Georgia	310,265	6.25%
37	Hawaii	22,061	0.44%
30	Idaho	37,740	0.76%
16	Illinois	105,171	2.12%
10	Indiana	175,792	3.54%
15	Iowa	107,449	2.17%
21	Kansas	69,351	1.40%
25	Kentucky	50,926	1.03%
7	Louisiana	256,600	5.17%
42	Maine	5,140	0.10%
45	Maryland	0	0.00%
24	Massachusetts	55,454	1.12%
23	Michigan	59,744	1.20%
18	Minnesota	100,764	2.03%
9	Mississippi	178,656	3.60%
19	Missouri	87,538	1.76%
41	Montana	5,238	0.11%
28	Nebraska	41,011	0.83%
32	Nevada	33,919	0.68%
45	New Hampshire	0	0.00%
33	New Jersey	32,672	0.66%
26	New Mexico	46,158	0.93%
3	New York	332,842	6.71%
5	North Carolina	306,992	6.19%
45	North Dakota	0	0.00%
13	Ohio	126,839	2.56%
14	Oklahoma	116,738	2.35%
31	Oregon	35,473	0.72%
44	Pennsylvania	2,979	0.06%
45	Rhode Island	0	0.00%
12	South Carolina	137,381	2.77%
43	South Dakota	4,141	0.08%
11	Tennessee	142,380	2.87%
2	Texas	444,138	8.95%
38	Utah	20,960	0.42%
45	Vermont	0	0.00%
20	Virginia	87,143	1.76%
17	Washington	104,807	2.11%
34	West Virginia	26,786	0.54%
29	Wisconsin	38,296	0.77%
35	Wyoming	26,620	0.54%

RANK ORDER

RANK	STATE	ADMISSIONS	% of USA
1	California	559,298	11.27%
2	Texas	444,138	8.95%
3	New York	332,842	6.71%
4	Georgia	310,265	6.25%
5	North Carolina	306,992	6.19%
6	Florida	267,896	5.40%
7	Louisiana	256,600	5.17%
8	Alabama	238,337	4.80%
9	Mississippi	178,656	3.60%
10	Indiana	175,792	3.54%
11	Tennessee	142,380	2.87%
12	South Carolina	137,381	2.77%
13	Ohio	126,839	2.56%
14	Oklahoma	116,738	2.35%
15	Iowa	107,449	2.17%
16	Illinois	105,171	2.12%
17	Washington	104,807	2.11%
18	Minnesota	100,764	2.03%
19	Missouri	87,538	1.76%
20	Virginia	87,143	1.76%
21	Kansas	69,351	1.40%
22	Colorado	65,116	1.31%
23	Michigan	59,744	1.20%
24	Massachusetts	55,454	1.12%
25	Kentucky	50,926	1.03%
26	New Mexico	46,158	0.93%
27	Arkansas	42,921	0.87%
28	Nebraska	41,011	0.83%
29	Wisconsin	38,296	0.77%
30	Idaho	37,740	0.76%
31	Oregon	35,473	0.72%
32	Nevada	33,919	0.68%
33	New Jersey	32,672	0.66%
34	West Virginia	26,786	0.54%
35	Wyoming	26,620	0.54%
36	Arizona	26,286	0.53%
37	Hawaii	22,061	0.44%
38	Utah	20,960	0.42%
39	Connecticut	7,248	0.15%
40	Alaska	6,039	0.12%
41	Montana	5,238	0.11%
42	Maine	5,140	0.10%
43	South Dakota	4,141	0.08%
44	Pennsylvania	2,979	0.06%
45	Delaware	0	0.00%
45	Maryland	0	0.00%
45	New Hampshire	0	0.00%
45	North Dakota	0	0.00%
45	Rhode Island	0	0.00%
45	Vermont	0	0.00%
	District of Columbia	11,509	0.23%

Source: American Hospital Association (Chicago, IL)
"Hospital Statistics" (1996-97 edition)
State and local government-owned hospitals are a subset of community hospitals.

Inpatient Days in Community Hospitals in 1995

National Total = 199,876,367 Inpatient Days*

ALPHA ORDER

ALPHA ORDER

RANK	STATE	DAYS	% of USA
18	Alabama	3,923,611	1.96%
50	Alaska	243,452	0.12%
30	Arizona	2,028,168	1.01%
28	Arkansas	2,185,843	1.09%
2	California	16,417,556	8.21%
32	Colorado	1,980,497	0.99%
31	Connecticut	1,993,466	1.00%
47	Delaware	551,484	0.28%
5	Florida	10,725,645	5.37%
10	Georgia	5,762,413	2.88%
40	Hawaii	881,248	0.44%
46	Idaho	664,507	0.33%
6	Illinois	9,137,222	4.57%
17	Indiana	4,111,951	2.06%
25	Iowa	2,582,644	1.29%
29	Kansas	2,106,950	1.05%
21	Kentucky	3,273,564	1.64%
19	Louisiana	3,880,875	1.94%
39	Maine	945,419	0.47%
22	Maryland	3,209,692	1.61%
12	Massachusetts	4,754,666	2.38%
9	Michigan	7,043,976	3.52%
16	Minnesota	4,138,607	2.07%
23	Mississippi	2,790,942	1.40%
13	Missouri	4,603,760	2.30%
38	Montana	997,759	0.50%
34	Nebraska	1,635,017	0.82%
41	Nevada	816,749	0.41%
44	New Hampshire	753,739	0.38%
8	New Jersey	7,813,768	3.91%
43	New Mexico	776,782	0.39%
1	New York	21,563,886	10.79%
11	North Carolina	5,651,064	2.83%
37	North Dakota	1,002,029	0.50%
7	Ohio	8,096,794	4.05%
26	Oklahoma	2,214,996	1.11%
35	Oregon	1,380,844	0.69%
3	Pennsylvania	12,346,057	6.18%
45	Rhode Island	673,092	0.34%
24	South Carolina	2,645,554	1.32%
36	South Dakota	1,081,335	0.54%
14	Tennessee	4,561,488	2.28%
4	Texas	11,366,956	5.69%
42	Utah	800,052	0.40%
48	Vermont	461,004	0.23%
15	Virginia	4,205,374	2.10%
27	Washington	2,208,038	1.10%
33	West Virginia	1,781,452	0.89%
20	Wisconsin	3,725,049	1.86%
49	Wyoming	386,460	0.19%

RANK ORDER

RANK	STATE	DAYS	% of USA
1	New York	21,563,886	10.79%
2	California	16,417,556	8.21%
3	Pennsylvania	12,346,057	6.18%
4	Texas	11,366,956	5.69%
5	Florida	10,725,645	5.37%
6	Illinois	9,137,222	4.57%
7	Ohio	8,096,794	4.05%
8	New Jersey	7,813,768	3.91%
9	Michigan	7,043,976	3.52%
10	Georgia	5,762,413	2.88%
11	North Carolina	5,651,064	2.83%
12	Massachusetts	4,754,666	2.38%
13	Missouri	4,603,760	2.30%
14	Tennessee	4,561,488	2.28%
15	Virginia	4,205,374	2.10%
16	Minnesota	4,138,607	2.07%
17	Indiana	4,111,951	2.06%
18	Alabama	3,923,611	1.96%
19	Louisiana	3,880,875	1.94%
20	Wisconsin	3,725,049	1.86%
21	Kentucky	3,273,564	1.64%
22	Maryland	3,209,692	1.61%
23	Mississippi	2,790,942	1.40%
24	South Carolina	2,645,554	1.32%
25	Iowa	2,582,644	1.29%
26	Oklahoma	2,214,996	1.11%
27	Washington	2,208,038	1.10%
28	Arkansas	2,185,843	1.09%
29	Kansas	2,106,950	1.05%
30	Arizona	2,028,168	1.01%
31	Connecticut	1,993,466	1.00%
32	Colorado	1,980,497	0.99%
33	West Virginia	1,781,452	0.89%
34	Nebraska	1,635,017	0.82%
35	Oregon	1,380,844	0.69%
36	South Dakota	1,081,335	0.54%
37	North Dakota	1,002,029	0.50%
38	Montana	997,759	0.50%
39	Maine	945,419	0.47%
40	Hawaii	881,248	0.44%
41	Nevada	816,749	0.41%
42	Utah	800,052	0.40%
43	New Mexico	776,782	0.39%
44	New Hampshire	753,739	0.38%
45	Rhode Island	673,092	0.34%
46	Idaho	664,507	0.33%
47	Delaware	551,484	0.28%
48	Vermont	461,004	0.23%
49	Wyoming	386,460	0.19%
50	Alaska	243,452	0.12%
	District of Columbia	992,871	0.50%

Source: American Hospital Association (Chicago, IL)
    "Hospital Statistics" (1996-97 edition)
*Inpatient days in all nonfederal short-term general and other special hospitals, whose facilities and services are available to the public. Community hospitals are a subset of nonfederal hospitals.

Average Daily Census in Community Hospitals in 1995

National Average = 548,303 Inpatients*

RANK	STATE	INPATIENTS	% of USA
18	Alabama	10,753	1.96%
50	Alaska	667	0.12%
30	Arizona	5,558	1.01%
28	Arkansas	6,017	1.10%
2	California	45,060	8.22%
32	Colorado	5,426	0.99%
31	Connecticut	5,461	1.00%
47	Delaware	1,511	0.28%
5	Florida	29,416	5.36%
10	Georgia	15,785	2.88%
40	Hawaii	2,414	0.44%
44	Idaho	2,095	0.38%
6	Illinois	25,056	4.57%
17	Indiana	11,265	2.05%
25	Iowa	7,075	1.29%
29	Kansas	5,733	1.05%
21	Kentucky	8,968	1.64%
19	Louisiana	10,698	1.95%
39	Maine	2,590	0.47%
22	Maryland	8,794	1.60%
12	Massachusetts	13,027	2.38%
9	Michigan	19,300	3.52%
16	Minnesota	11,338	2.07%
23	Mississippi	7,673	1.40%
13	Missouri	12,612	2.30%
38	Montana	2,734	0.50%
34	Nebraska	4,478	0.82%
41	Nevada	2,237	0.41%
45	New Hampshire	2,065	0.38%
8	New Jersey	21,407	3.90%
43	New Mexico	2,128	0.39%
1	New York	59,078	10.77%
11	North Carolina	15,483	2.82%
37	North Dakota	2,744	0.50%
7	Ohio	22,188	4.05%
26	Oklahoma	6,068	1.11%
35	Oregon	3,783	0.69%
3	Pennsylvania	33,825	6.17%
46	Rhode Island	1,844	0.34%
24	South Carolina	7,250	1.32%
36	South Dakota	2,963	0.54%
14	Tennessee	12,513	2.28%
4	Texas	31,191	5.69%
42	Utah	2,192	0.40%
48	Vermont	1,263	0.23%
15	Virginia	11,540	2.10%
27	Washington	6,052	1.10%
33	West Virginia	4,883	0.89%
20	Wisconsin	10,323	1.88%
49	Wyoming	1,059	0.19%

RANK	STATE	INPATIENTS	% of USA
1	New York	59,078	10.77%
2	California	45,060	8.22%
3	Pennsylvania	33,825	6.17%
4	Texas	31,191	5.69%
5	Florida	29,416	5.36%
6	Illinois	25,056	4.57%
7	Ohio	22,188	4.05%
8	New Jersey	21,407	3.90%
9	Michigan	19,300	3.52%
10	Georgia	15,785	2.88%
11	North Carolina	15,483	2.82%
12	Massachusetts	13,027	2.38%
13	Missouri	12,612	2.30%
14	Tennessee	12,513	2.28%
15	Virginia	11,540	2.10%
16	Minnesota	11,338	2.07%
17	Indiana	11,265	2.05%
18	Alabama	10,753	1.96%
19	Louisiana	10,698	1.95%
20	Wisconsin	10,323	1.88%
21	Kentucky	8,968	1.64%
22	Maryland	8,794	1.60%
23	Mississippi	7,673	1.40%
24	South Carolina	7,250	1.32%
25	Iowa	7,075	1.29%
26	Oklahoma	6,068	1.11%
27	Washington	6,052	1.10%
28	Arkansas	6,017	1.10%
29	Kansas	5,733	1.05%
30	Arizona	5,558	1.01%
31	Connecticut	5,461	1.00%
32	Colorado	5,426	0.99%
33	West Virginia	4,883	0.89%
34	Nebraska	4,478	0.82%
35	Oregon	3,783	0.69%
36	South Dakota	2,963	0.54%
37	North Dakota	2,744	0.50%
38	Montana	2,734	0.50%
39	Maine	2,590	0.47%
40	Hawaii	2,414	0.44%
41	Nevada	2,237	0.41%
42	Utah	2,192	0.40%
43	New Mexico	2,128	0.39%
44	Idaho	2,095	0.38%
45	New Hampshire	2,065	0.38%
46	Rhode Island	1,844	0.34%
47	Delaware	1,511	0.28%
48	Vermont	1,263	0.23%
49	Wyoming	1,059	0.19%
50	Alaska	667	0.12%
	District of Columbia	2,720	0.50%

Source: American Hospital Association (Chicago, IL)
    "Hospital Statistics" (1996-97 edition)
*Average total of inpatients receiving care in all nonfederal short-term general and other special hospitals, whose facilities and services are available to the public. Excludes newborns. Community hospitals are a subset of nonfederal hospitals.

Average Stay in Community Hospitals in 1995

National Average = 6.5 Days*

ALPHA ORDER				RANK ORDER		
RANK	STATE	DAYS		RANK	STATE	DAYS
31	Alabama	6.1		1	South Dakota	11.5
31	Alaska	6.1		2	North Dakota	11.3
47	Arizona	4.8		3	Montana	10.4
23	Arkansas	6.4		4	Hawaii	9.1
45	California	5.4		5	New York	9.0
40	Colorado	5.8		6	Nebraska	8.9
37	Connecticut	5.9		6	Wyoming	8.9
15	Delaware	6.8		8	Vermont	8.4
31	Florida	6.1		9	Minnesota	8.3
19	Georgia	6.7		10	New Jersey	7.3
4	Hawaii	9.1		11	Iowa	7.2
23	Idaho	6.4		11	Kansas	7.2
26	Illinois	6.3		11	Mississippi	7.2
37	Indiana	5.9		14	New Hampshire	6.9
11	Iowa	7.2		15	Delaware	6.8
11	Kansas	7.2		15	North Carolina	6.8
31	Kentucky	6.1		15	Pennsylvania	6.8
29	Louisiana	6.2		15	Wisconsin	6.8
20	Maine	6.6		19	Georgia	6.7
42	Maryland	5.6		20	Maine	6.6
26	Massachusetts	6.3		20	West Virginia	6.6
26	Michigan	6.3		22	South Carolina	6.5
9	Minnesota	8.3		23	Arkansas	6.4
11	Mississippi	7.2		23	Idaho	6.4
23	Missouri	6.4		23	Missouri	6.4
3	Montana	10.4		26	Illinois	6.3
6	Nebraska	8.9		26	Massachusetts	6.3
44	Nevada	5.5		26	Michigan	6.3
14	New Hampshire	6.9		29	Louisiana	6.2
10	New Jersey	7.3		29	Tennessee	6.2
46	New Mexico	5.0		31	Alabama	6.1
5	New York	9.0		31	Alaska	6.1
15	North Carolina	6.8		31	Florida	6.1
2	North Dakota	11.3		31	Kentucky	6.1
37	Ohio	5.9		35	Oklahoma	6.0
35	Oklahoma	6.0		35	Virginia	6.0
48	Oregon	4.7		37	Connecticut	5.9
15	Pennsylvania	6.8		37	Indiana	5.9
41	Rhode Island	5.7		37	Ohio	5.9
22	South Carolina	6.5		40	Colorado	5.8
1	South Dakota	11.5		41	Rhode Island	5.7
29	Tennessee	6.2		42	Maryland	5.6
42	Texas	5.6		42	Texas	5.6
48	Utah	4.7		44	Nevada	5.5
8	Vermont	8.4		45	California	5.4
35	Virginia	6.0		46	New Mexico	5.0
48	Washington	4.7		47	Arizona	4.8
20	West Virginia	6.6		48	Oregon	4.7
15	Wisconsin	6.8		48	Utah	4.7
6	Wyoming	8.9		48	Washington	4.7
					District of Columbia	6.5

Source: American Hospital Association (Chicago, IL)
"Hospital Statistics" (1996-97 edition)

*All nonfederal short-term general and other special hospitals, whose facilities and services are available to the public. Community hospitals are a subset of nonfederal hospitals.

Occupancy Rate in Community Hospitals in 1995

National Rate = 62.8% of Community Hospital Beds Occupied*

ALPHA ORDER				RANK ORDER		
RANK	STATE	PERCENT		RANK	STATE	PERCENT
33	Alabama	58.9		1	Delaware	81.0
48	Alaska	52.5		2	New York	79.9
40	Arizona	56.4		3	Hawaii	79.7
30	Arkansas	59.3		4	Connecticut	72.6
26	California	60.1		5	New Jersey	71.7
35	Colorado	58.6		6	Maryland	69.8
4	Connecticut	72.6		7	Pennsylvania	69.7
1	Delaware	81.0		7	Vermont	69.7
32	Florida	59.2		9	Massachusetts	69.1
25	Georgia	60.4		10	North Carolina	68.1
3	Hawaii	79.7		11	Rhode Island	67.8
21	Idaho	61.9		12	North Dakota	65.8
29	Illinois	59.7		13	Minnesota	65.3
36	Indiana	58.2		14	Michigan	65.1
41	Iowa	56.1		15	Montana	64.7
45	Kansas	53.3		16	Maine	64.6
30	Kentucky	59.3		17	South Carolina	64.1
42	Louisiana	55.9		18	South Dakota	63.9
16	Maine	64.6		19	Nevada	62.1
6	Maryland	69.8		19	Virginia	62.1
9	Massachusetts	69.1		21	Idaho	61.9
14	Michigan	65.1		22	New Hampshire	61.2
13	Minnesota	65.3		23	Mississippi	60.9
23	Mississippi	60.9		24	Wisconsin	60.7
38	Missouri	57.7		25	Georgia	60.4
15	Montana	64.7		26	California	60.1
39	Nebraska	57.0		26	West Virginia	60.1
19	Nevada	62.1		28	Tennessee	59.8
22	New Hampshire	61.2		29	Illinois	59.7
5	New Jersey	71.7		30	Arkansas	59.3
37	New Mexico	57.9		30	Kentucky	59.3
2	New York	79.9		32	Florida	59.2
10	North Carolina	68.1		33	Alabama	58.9
12	North Dakota	65.8		34	Ohio	58.8
34	Ohio	58.8		35	Colorado	58.6
46	Oklahoma	52.9		36	Indiana	58.2
47	Oregon	52.8		37	New Mexico	57.9
7	Pennsylvania	69.7		38	Missouri	57.7
11	Rhode Island	67.8		39	Nebraska	57.0
17	South Carolina	64.1		40	Arizona	56.4
18	South Dakota	63.9		41	Iowa	56.1
28	Tennessee	59.8		42	Louisiana	55.9
44	Texas	54.6		42	Washington	55.9
49	Utah	52.4		44	Texas	54.6
7	Vermont	69.7		45	Kansas	53.3
19	Virginia	62.1		46	Oklahoma	52.9
42	Washington	55.9		47	Oregon	52.8
26	West Virginia	60.1		48	Alaska	52.5
24	Wisconsin	60.7		49	Utah	52.4
50	Wyoming	52.0		50	Wyoming	52.0
				District of Columbia		71.5

Source: Morgan Quitno Press using data from American Hospital Association (Chicago, IL)
    "Hospital Statistics" (1996-97 edition)
*Average daily census compared to number of community hospital beds.

Outpatient Visits to Hospitals in 1995

National Total = 483,194,920 Visits*

ALPHA ORDER

RANK	STATE	VISITS	% of USA
21	Alabama	7,588,958	1.57%
42	Alaska	1,948,115	0.40%
24	Arizona	6,562,743	1.36%
33	Arkansas	4,224,830	0.87%
1	California	45,423,380	9.40%
22	Colorado	7,230,558	1.50%
23	Connecticut	6,593,282	1.36%
48	Delaware	1,623,224	0.34%
7	Florida	20,812,375	4.31%
12	Georgia	12,256,961	2.54%
38	Hawaii	2,964,982	0.61%
43	Idaho	1,928,711	0.40%
6	Illinois	22,742,668	4.71%
11	Indiana	12,269,459	2.54%
25	Iowa	6,527,609	1.35%
31	Kansas	4,906,624	1.02%
20	Kentucky	7,628,250	1.58%
17	Louisiana	9,172,873	1.90%
39	Maine	2,698,324	0.56%
26	Maryland	6,422,874	1.33%
9	Massachusetts	14,963,967	3.10%
8	Michigan	20,205,151	4.18%
27	Minnesota	6,355,927	1.32%
34	Mississippi	4,140,052	0.86%
13	Missouri	11,796,215	2.44%
46	Montana	1,720,715	0.36%
37	Nebraska	3,148,016	0.65%
40	Nevada	1,979,744	0.41%
41	New Hampshire	1,962,721	0.41%
10	New Jersey	13,576,833	2.81%
35	New Mexico	4,116,237	0.85%
2	New York	42,220,199	8.74%
14	North Carolina	11,300,184	2.34%
45	North Dakota	1,878,550	0.39%
5	Ohio	23,309,547	4.82%
29	Oklahoma	5,634,688	1.17%
28	Oregon	6,194,151	1.28%
4	Pennsylvania	28,504,979	5.90%
44	Rhode Island	1,903,861	0.39%
30	South Carolina	5,410,137	1.12%
47	South Dakota	1,646,704	0.34%
19	Tennessee	8,547,980	1.77%
3	Texas	28,595,321	5.92%
36	Utah	3,576,080	0.74%
49	Vermont	1,152,471	0.24%
15	Virginia	10,820,185	2.24%
16	Washington	10,584,440	2.19%
32	West Virginia	4,454,629	0.92%
18	Wisconsin	8,879,457	1.84%
50	Wyoming	926,232	0.19%

RANK ORDER

RANK	STATE	VISITS	% of USA
1	California	45,423,380	9.40%
2	New York	42,220,199	8.74%
3	Texas	28,595,321	5.92%
4	Pennsylvania	28,504,979	5.90%
5	Ohio	23,309,547	4.82%
6	Illinois	22,742,668	4.71%
7	Florida	20,812,375	4.31%
8	Michigan	20,205,151	4.18%
9	Massachusetts	14,963,967	3.10%
10	New Jersey	13,576,833	2.81%
11	Indiana	12,269,459	2.54%
12	Georgia	12,256,961	2.54%
13	Missouri	11,796,215	2.44%
14	North Carolina	11,300,184	2.34%
15	Virginia	10,820,185	2.24%
16	Washington	10,584,440	2.19%
17	Louisiana	9,172,873	1.90%
18	Wisconsin	8,879,457	1.84%
19	Tennessee	8,547,980	1.77%
20	Kentucky	7,628,250	1.58%
21	Alabama	7,588,958	1.57%
22	Colorado	7,230,558	1.50%
23	Connecticut	6,593,282	1.36%
24	Arizona	6,562,743	1.36%
25	Iowa	6,527,609	1.35%
26	Maryland	6,422,874	1.33%
27	Minnesota	6,355,927	1.32%
28	Oregon	6,194,151	1.28%
29	Oklahoma	5,634,688	1.17%
30	South Carolina	5,410,137	1.12%
31	Kansas	4,906,624	1.02%
32	West Virginia	4,454,629	0.92%
33	Arkansas	4,224,830	0.87%
34	Mississippi	4,140,052	0.86%
35	New Mexico	4,116,237	0.85%
36	Utah	3,576,080	0.74%
37	Nebraska	3,148,016	0.65%
38	Hawaii	2,964,982	0.61%
39	Maine	2,698,324	0.56%
40	Nevada	1,979,744	0.41%
41	New Hampshire	1,962,721	0.41%
42	Alaska	1,948,115	0.40%
43	Idaho	1,928,711	0.40%
44	Rhode Island	1,903,861	0.39%
45	North Dakota	1,878,550	0.39%
46	Montana	1,720,715	0.36%
47	South Dakota	1,646,704	0.34%
48	Delaware	1,623,224	0.34%
49	Vermont	1,152,471	0.24%
50	Wyoming	926,232	0.19%
	District of Columbia	2,162,747	0.45%

Source: American Hospital Association (Chicago, IL)
"Hospital Statistics" (1996-97 edition)
*To federal and nonfederal hospitals. Includes emergency and other visits.

Emergency Outpatient Visits to Hospitals in 1995

National Total = 99,911,108 Visits*

ALPHA ORDER

RANK	STATE	VISITS	% of USA
18	Alabama	2,097,114	2.10%
43	Alaska	331,144	0.33%
23	Arizona	1,539,755	1.54%
30	Arkansas	1,076,174	1.08%
1	California	9,167,532	9.18%
29	Colorado	1,143,839	1.14%
25	Connecticut	1,389,502	1.39%
45	Delaware	295,500	0.30%
4	Florida	5,190,266	5.19%
9	Georgia	3,197,005	3.20%
47	Hawaii	272,489	0.27%
42	Idaho	381,034	0.38%
7	Illinois	4,528,365	4.53%
16	Indiana	2,270,149	2.27%
32	Iowa	1,018,731	1.02%
34	Kansas	828,731	0.83%
20	Kentucky	1,788,188	1.79%
14	Louisiana	2,349,511	2.35%
35	Maine	636,823	0.64%
21	Maryland	1,662,508	1.66%
11	Massachusetts	2,753,741	2.76%
8	Michigan	3,574,357	3.58%
28	Minnesota	1,205,460	1.21%
26	Mississippi	1,388,553	1.39%
17	Missouri	2,264,320	2.27%
44	Montana	318,022	0.32%
40	Nebraska	453,473	0.45%
38	Nevada	499,453	0.50%
39	New Hampshire	453,545	0.45%
13	New Jersey	2,600,562	2.60%
36	New Mexico	626,519	0.63%
2	New York	7,144,918	7.15%
10	North Carolina	3,165,617	3.17%
46	North Dakota	294,566	0.29%
6	Ohio	4,993,227	5.00%
27	Oklahoma	1,236,554	1.24%
33	Oregon	999,182	1.00%
5	Pennsylvania	5,033,505	5.04%
41	Rhode Island	447,014	0.45%
24	South Carolina	1,442,505	1.44%
48	South Dakota	251,422	0.25%
15	Tennessee	2,346,802	2.35%
3	Texas	6,544,457	6.55%
37	Utah	605,158	0.61%
49	Vermont	215,947	0.22%
12	Virginia	2,601,509	2.60%
19	Washington	1,953,410	1.96%
31	West Virginia	1,057,635	1.06%
22	Wisconsin	1,642,066	1.64%
50	Wyoming	200,105	0.20%

RANK ORDER

RANK	STATE	VISITS	% of USA
1	California	9,167,532	9.18%
2	New York	7,144,918	7.15%
3	Texas	6,544,457	6.55%
4	Florida	5,190,266	5.19%
5	Pennsylvania	5,033,505	5.04%
6	Ohio	4,993,227	5.00%
7	Illinois	4,528,365	4.53%
8	Michigan	3,574,357	3.58%
9	Georgia	3,197,005	3.20%
10	North Carolina	3,165,617	3.17%
11	Massachusetts	2,753,741	2.76%
12	Virginia	2,601,509	2.60%
13	New Jersey	2,600,562	2.60%
14	Louisiana	2,349,511	2.35%
15	Tennessee	2,346,802	2.35%
16	Indiana	2,270,149	2.27%
17	Missouri	2,264,320	2.27%
18	Alabama	2,097,114	2.10%
19	Washington	1,953,410	1.96%
20	Kentucky	1,788,188	1.79%
21	Maryland	1,662,508	1.66%
22	Wisconsin	1,642,066	1.64%
23	Arizona	1,539,755	1.54%
24	South Carolina	1,442,505	1.44%
25	Connecticut	1,389,502	1.39%
26	Mississippi	1,388,553	1.39%
27	Oklahoma	1,236,554	1.24%
28	Minnesota	1,205,460	1.21%
29	Colorado	1,143,839	1.14%
30	Arkansas	1,076,174	1.08%
31	West Virginia	1,057,635	1.06%
32	Iowa	1,018,731	1.02%
33	Oregon	999,182	1.00%
34	Kansas	828,731	0.83%
35	Maine	636,823	0.64%
36	New Mexico	626,519	0.63%
37	Utah	605,158	0.61%
38	Nevada	499,453	0.50%
39	New Hampshire	453,545	0.45%
40	Nebraska	453,473	0.45%
41	Rhode Island	447,014	0.45%
42	Idaho	381,034	0.38%
43	Alaska	331,144	0.33%
44	Montana	318,022	0.32%
45	Delaware	295,500	0.30%
46	North Dakota	294,566	0.29%
47	Hawaii	272,489	0.27%
48	South Dakota	251,422	0.25%
49	Vermont	215,947	0.22%
50	Wyoming	200,105	0.20%
	District of Columbia	433,144	0.43%

Source: American Hospital Association (Chicago, IL)
"Hospital Statistics" (1996-97 edition)
*To federal and nonfederal hospitals.

Surgical Operations in Hospitals in 1995

National Total = 24,044,287 Surgical Operations*

RANK	STATE	OPERATIONS	% of USA
18	Alabama	476,988	1.98%
48	Alaska	50,226	0.21%
25	Arizona	327,472	1.36%
32	Arkansas	249,300	1.04%
1	California	2,051,572	8.53%
28	Colorado	296,916	1.23%
30	Connecticut	266,248	1.11%
45	Delaware	76,300	0.32%
5	Florida	1,269,379	5.28%
9	Georgia	700,915	2.92%
44	Hawaii	80,135	0.33%
41	Idaho	87,245	0.36%
7	Illinois	1,045,025	4.35%
14	Indiana	592,226	2.46%
24	Iowa	332,769	1.38%
34	Kansas	235,934	0.98%
23	Kentucky	399,935	1.66%
21	Louisiana	411,813	1.71%
38	Maine	123,094	0.51%
17	Maryland	520,806	2.17%
12	Massachusetts	646,360	2.69%
8	Michigan	948,602	3.95%
22	Minnesota	409,796	1.70%
31	Mississippi	256,827	1.07%
16	Missouri	556,157	2.31%
46	Montana	75,486	0.31%
35	Nebraska	189,603	0.79%
39	Nevada	113,947	0.47%
42	New Hampshire	83,874	0.35%
10	New Jersey	662,702	2.76%
37	New Mexico	140,215	0.58%
2	New York	1,674,516	6.96%
11	North Carolina	658,528	2.74%
43	North Dakota	80,850	0.34%
6	Ohio	1,216,806	5.06%
27	Oklahoma	299,989	1.25%
29	Oregon	266,630	1.11%
4	Pennsylvania	1,463,335	6.09%
40	Rhode Island	105,011	0.44%
26	South Carolina	317,647	1.32%
47	South Dakota	74,662	0.31%
15	Tennessee	556,432	2.31%
3	Texas	1,559,624	6.49%
36	Utah	151,613	0.63%
49	Vermont	45,171	0.19%
13	Virginia	612,237	2.55%
20	Washington	421,990	1.76%
33	West Virginia	241,839	1.01%
19	Wisconsin	461,364	1.92%
50	Wyoming	35,823	0.15%

RANK	STATE	OPERATIONS	% of USA
1	California	2,051,572	8.53%
2	New York	1,674,516	6.96%
3	Texas	1,559,624	6.49%
4	Pennsylvania	1,463,335	6.09%
5	Florida	1,269,379	5.28%
6	Ohio	1,216,806	5.06%
7	Illinois	1,045,025	4.35%
8	Michigan	948,602	3.95%
9	Georgia	700,915	2.92%
10	New Jersey	662,702	2.76%
11	North Carolina	658,528	2.74%
12	Massachusetts	646,360	2.69%
13	Virginia	612,237	2.55%
14	Indiana	592,226	2.46%
15	Tennessee	556,432	2.31%
16	Missouri	556,157	2.31%
17	Maryland	520,806	2.17%
18	Alabama	476,988	1.98%
19	Wisconsin	461,364	1.92%
20	Washington	421,990	1.76%
21	Louisiana	411,813	1.71%
22	Minnesota	409,796	1.70%
23	Kentucky	399,935	1.66%
24	Iowa	332,769	1.38%
25	Arizona	327,472	1.36%
26	South Carolina	317,647	1.32%
27	Oklahoma	299,989	1.25%
28	Colorado	296,916	1.23%
29	Oregon	266,630	1.11%
30	Connecticut	266,248	1.11%
31	Mississippi	256,827	1.07%
32	Arkansas	249,300	1.04%
33	West Virginia	241,839	1.01%
34	Kansas	235,934	0.98%
35	Nebraska	189,603	0.79%
36	Utah	151,613	0.63%
37	New Mexico	140,215	0.58%
38	Maine	123,094	0.51%
39	Nevada	113,947	0.47%
40	Rhode Island	105,011	0.44%
41	Idaho	87,245	0.36%
42	New Hampshire	83,874	0.35%
43	North Dakota	80,850	0.34%
44	Hawaii	80,135	0.33%
45	Delaware	76,300	0.32%
46	Montana	75,486	0.31%
47	South Dakota	74,662	0.31%
48	Alaska	50,226	0.21%
49	Vermont	45,171	0.19%
50	Wyoming	35,823	0.15%
	District of Columbia	122,353	0.51%

Source: American Hospital Association (Chicago, IL)
"Hospital Statistics" (1996-97 edition)
*In federal and nonfederal hospital operating rooms.

Medicare and Medicaid Certified Hospitals in 1997

National Total = 6,225 Hospitals*

ALPHA ORDER

RANK	STATE	HOSPITALS	% of USA
20	Alabama	129	2.07%
47	Alaska	25	0.40%
29	Arizona	87	1.40%
28	Arkansas	93	1.49%
1	California	516	8.29%
30	Colorado	82	1.32%
41	Connecticut	47	0.76%
50	Delaware	11	0.18%
3	Florida	271	4.35%
8	Georgia	199	3.20%
46	Hawaii	27	0.43%
40	Idaho	48	0.77%
6	Illinois	226	3.63%
11	Indiana	157	2.52%
22	Iowa	121	1.94%
18	Kansas	144	2.31%
21	Kentucky	122	1.96%
9	Louisiana	185	2.97%
42	Maine	44	0.71%
32	Maryland	72	1.16%
19	Massachusetts	134	2.15%
9	Michigan	185	2.97%
12	Minnesota	152	2.44%
25	Mississippi	108	1.73%
15	Missouri	146	2.35%
35	Montana	61	0.98%
26	Nebraska	99	1.59%
43	Nevada	36	0.58%
44	New Hampshire	31	0.50%
24	New Jersey	112	1.80%
37	New Mexico	56	0.90%
3	New York	271	4.35%
15	North Carolina	146	2.35%
39	North Dakota	49	0.79%
7	Ohio	211	3.39%
14	Oklahoma	150	2.41%
33	Oregon	67	1.08%
5	Pennsylvania	259	4.16%
48	Rhode Island	17	0.27%
31	South Carolina	76	1.22%
35	South Dakota	61	0.98%
13	Tennessee	151	2.43%
2	Texas	499	8.02%
38	Utah	51	0.82%
49	Vermont	16	0.26%
22	Virginia	121	1.94%
26	Washington	99	1.59%
34	West Virginia	65	1.04%
17	Wisconsin	145	2.33%
45	Wyoming	29	0.47%

RANK ORDER

RANK	STATE	HOSPITALS	% of USA
1	California	516	8.29%
2	Texas	499	8.02%
3	Florida	271	4.35%
3	New York	271	4.35%
5	Pennsylvania	259	4.16%
6	Illinois	226	3.63%
7	Ohio	211	3.39%
8	Georgia	199	3.20%
9	Louisiana	185	2.97%
9	Michigan	185	2.97%
11	Indiana	157	2.52%
12	Minnesota	152	2.44%
13	Tennessee	151	2.43%
14	Oklahoma	150	2.41%
15	Missouri	146	2.35%
15	North Carolina	146	2.35%
17	Wisconsin	145	2.33%
18	Kansas	144	2.31%
19	Massachusetts	134	2.15%
20	Alabama	129	2.07%
21	Kentucky	122	1.96%
22	Iowa	121	1.94%
22	Virginia	121	1.94%
24	New Jersey	112	1.80%
25	Mississippi	108	1.73%
26	Nebraska	99	1.59%
26	Washington	99	1.59%
28	Arkansas	93	1.49%
29	Arizona	87	1.40%
30	Colorado	82	1.32%
31	South Carolina	76	1.22%
32	Maryland	72	1.16%
33	Oregon	67	1.08%
34	West Virginia	65	1.04%
35	Montana	61	0.98%
35	South Dakota	61	0.98%
37	New Mexico	56	0.90%
38	Utah	51	0.82%
39	North Dakota	49	0.79%
40	Idaho	48	0.77%
41	Connecticut	47	0.76%
42	Maine	44	0.71%
43	Nevada	36	0.58%
44	New Hampshire	31	0.50%
45	Wyoming	29	0.47%
46	Hawaii	27	0.43%
47	Alaska	25	0.40%
48	Rhode Island	17	0.27%
49	Vermont	16	0.26%
50	Delaware	11	0.18%
	District of Columbia	16	0.26%

Source: U.S. Department of Health and Human Services, Health Care Financing Administration unpublished data (February 26, 1997)
*Certified by HCFA to participate in the Medicare/Medicaid programs. National total does not include 62 certified hospitals in U.S. territories.

Medicare and Medicaid Certified Hospices in 1997

National Total = 2,125 Hospices*

ALPHA ORDER					RANK ORDER			
RANK	STATE	HOSPICES	% of USA		RANK	STATE	HOSPICES	% of USA
16	Alabama	50	2.35%		1	California	183	8.61%
50	Alaska	3	0.14%		2	Texas	138	6.49%
24	Arizona	38	1.79%		3	Pennsylvania	113	5.32%
10	Arkansas	58	2.73%		4	Ohio	90	4.24%
1	California	183	8.61%		5	Illinois	83	3.91%
27	Colorado	34	1.60%		6	Missouri	76	3.58%
31	Connecticut	28	1.32%		7	Michigan	72	3.39%
49	Delaware	5	0.24%		8	North Carolina	71	3.34%
22	Florida	39	1.84%		9	Tennessee	63	2.96%
14	Georgia	52	2.45%		10	Arkansas	58	2.73%
47	Hawaii	7	0.33%		11	Indiana	54	2.54%
34	Idaho	27	1.27%		11	Minnesota	54	2.54%
5	Illinois	83	3.91%		11	New York	54	2.54%
11	Indiana	54	2.54%		14	Georgia	52	2.45%
16	Iowa	50	2.35%		15	Wisconsin	51	2.40%
28	Kansas	32	1.51%		16	Alabama	50	2.35%
31	Kentucky	28	1.32%		16	Iowa	50	2.35%
22	Louisiana	39	1.84%		18	Oklahoma	45	2.12%
40	Maine	14	0.66%		19	Massachusetts	44	2.07%
26	Maryland	36	1.69%		19	New Jersey	44	2.07%
19	Massachusetts	44	2.07%		21	Virginia	41	1.93%
7	Michigan	72	3.39%		22	Florida	39	1.84%
11	Minnesota	54	2.54%		22	Louisiana	39	1.84%
30	Mississippi	29	1.36%		24	Arizona	38	1.79%
6	Missouri	76	3.58%		24	Oregon	38	1.79%
39	Montana	15	0.71%		26	Maryland	36	1.69%
36	Nebraska	25	1.18%		27	Colorado	34	1.60%
48	Nevada	6	0.28%		28	Kansas	32	1.51%
38	New Hampshire	18	0.85%		28	South Carolina	32	1.51%
19	New Jersey	44	2.07%		30	Mississippi	29	1.36%
34	New Mexico	27	1.27%		31	Connecticut	28	1.32%
11	New York	54	2.54%		31	Kentucky	28	1.32%
8	North Carolina	71	3.34%		31	Washington	28	1.32%
42	North Dakota	13	0.61%		34	Idaho	27	1.27%
4	Ohio	90	4.24%		34	New Mexico	27	1.27%
18	Oklahoma	45	2.12%		36	Nebraska	25	1.18%
24	Oregon	38	1.79%		37	West Virginia	21	0.99%
3	Pennsylvania	113	5.32%		38	New Hampshire	18	0.85%
45	Rhode Island	9	0.42%		39	Montana	15	0.71%
28	South Carolina	32	1.51%		40	Maine	14	0.66%
43	South Dakota	12	0.56%		40	Utah	14	0.66%
9	Tennessee	63	2.96%		42	North Dakota	13	0.61%
2	Texas	138	6.49%		43	South Dakota	12	0.56%
40	Utah	14	0.66%		44	Wyoming	11	0.52%
46	Vermont	8	0.38%		45	Rhode Island	9	0.42%
21	Virginia	41	1.93%		46	Vermont	8	0.38%
31	Washington	28	1.32%		47	Hawaii	7	0.33%
37	West Virginia	21	0.99%		48	Nevada	6	0.28%
15	Wisconsin	51	2.40%		49	Delaware	5	0.24%
44	Wyoming	11	0.52%		50	Alaska	3	0.14%
						District of Columbia	3	0.14%

Source: U.S. Department of Health and Human Services, Health Care Financing Administration unpublished data (February 26, 1997)
Certified by HCFA to participate in the Medicare/Medicaid programs. National total does not include 36 certified hospices in U.S. territories. An hospice provides specialized services for terminally ill people and their families.

Medicare and Medicaid Certified Rural Health Clinics in 1997

National Total = 3,283 Rural Health Clinics*

<u>ALPHA ORDER</u>

RANK	STATE	CLINICS	% of USA
16	Alabama	75	2.28%
39	Alaska	12	0.37%
40	Arizona	10	0.30%
12	Arkansas	101	3.08%
2	California	191	5.82%
29	Colorado	37	1.13%
46	Connecticut	0	0.00%
46	Delaware	0	0.00%
8	Florida	125	3.81%
7	Georgia	129	3.93%
43	Hawaii	1	0.03%
31	Idaho	25	0.76%
6	Illinois	152	4.63%
30	Indiana	26	0.79%
10	Iowa	122	3.72%
4	Kansas	168	5.12%
20	Kentucky	59	1.80%
18	Louisiana	73	2.22%
28	Maine	40	1.22%
46	Maryland	0	0.00%
46	Massachusetts	0	0.00%
11	Michigan	106	3.23%
23	Minnesota	52	1.58%
3	Mississippi	170	5.18%
5	Missouri	165	5.03%
33	Montana	22	0.67%
19	Nebraska	72	2.19%
43	Nevada	1	0.03%
34	New Hampshire	21	0.64%
46	New Jersey	0	0.00%
37	New Mexico	15	0.46%
40	New York	10	0.30%
8	North Carolina	125	3.81%
15	North Dakota	78	2.38%
42	Ohio	8	0.24%
13	Oklahoma	90	2.74%
32	Oregon	23	0.70%
26	Pennsylvania	47	1.43%
43	Rhode Island	1	0.03%
14	South Carolina	83	2.53%
22	South Dakota	57	1.74%
17	Tennessee	74	2.25%
1	Texas	463	14.10%
36	Utah	16	0.49%
34	Vermont	21	0.64%
24	Virginia	51	1.55%
25	Washington	48	1.46%
21	West Virginia	58	1.77%
27	Wisconsin	46	1.40%
38	Wyoming	14	0.43%

<u>RANK ORDER</u>

RANK	STATE	CLINICS	% of USA
1	Texas	463	14.10%
2	California	191	5.82%
3	Mississippi	170	5.18%
4	Kansas	168	5.12%
5	Missouri	165	5.03%
6	Illinois	152	4.63%
7	Georgia	129	3.93%
8	Florida	125	3.81%
8	North Carolina	125	3.81%
10	Iowa	122	3.72%
11	Michigan	106	3.23%
12	Arkansas	101	3.08%
13	Oklahoma	90	2.74%
14	South Carolina	83	2.53%
15	North Dakota	78	2.38%
16	Alabama	75	2.28%
17	Tennessee	74	2.25%
18	Louisiana	73	2.22%
19	Nebraska	72	2.19%
20	Kentucky	59	1.80%
21	West Virginia	58	1.77%
22	South Dakota	57	1.74%
23	Minnesota	52	1.58%
24	Virginia	51	1.55%
25	Washington	48	1.46%
26	Pennsylvania	47	1.43%
27	Wisconsin	46	1.40%
28	Maine	40	1.22%
29	Colorado	37	1.13%
30	Indiana	26	0.79%
31	Idaho	25	0.76%
32	Oregon	23	0.70%
33	Montana	22	0.67%
34	New Hampshire	21	0.64%
34	Vermont	21	0.64%
36	Utah	16	0.49%
37	New Mexico	15	0.46%
38	Wyoming	14	0.43%
39	Alaska	12	0.37%
40	Arizona	10	0.30%
40	New York	10	0.30%
42	Ohio	8	0.24%
43	Hawaii	1	0.03%
43	Nevada	1	0.03%
43	Rhode Island	1	0.03%
46	Connecticut	0	0.00%
46	Delaware	0	0.00%
46	Maryland	0	0.00%
46	Massachusetts	0	0.00%
46	New Jersey	0	0.00%
	District of Columbia	0	0.00%

Source: U.S. Department of Health and Human Services, Health Care Financing Administration unpublished data (February 26, 1997)

Certified by HCFA to participate in the Medicare/Medicaid programs. There are no certified rural health clinics in U.S. territories.

Medicare and Medicaid Certified Home Health Agencies in 1997

National Total = 10,007 Home Health Agencies*

ALPHA ORDER					RANK ORDER			
RANK	**STATE**		**AGENCIES**	**% of USA**	**RANK**	**STATE**	**AGENCIES**	**% of USA**
21	Alabama		181	1.81%	1	Texas	1,664	16.63%
48	Alaska		25	0.25%	2	California	839	8.38%
24	Arizona		129	1.29%	3	Louisiana	528	5.28%
18	Arkansas		204	2.04%	4	Ohio	438	4.38%
2	California		839	8.38%	5	Florida	374	3.74%
19	Colorado		201	2.01%	5	Pennsylvania	374	3.74%
25	Connecticut		110	1.10%	7	Illinois	366	3.66%
49	Delaware		20	0.20%	8	Oklahoma	348	3.48%
5	Florida		374	3.74%	9	Indiana	283	2.83%
28	Georgia		98	0.98%	10	Missouri	271	2.71%
46	Hawaii		28	0.28%	11	Minnesota	258	2.58%
35	Idaho		78	0.78%	12	Tennessee	241	2.41%
7	Illinois		366	3.66%	13	New York	226	2.26%
9	Indiana		283	2.83%	14	Kansas	221	2.21%
17	Iowa		205	2.05%	14	Virginia	221	2.21%
14	Kansas		221	2.21%	16	Michigan	206	2.06%
27	Kentucky		106	1.06%	17	Iowa	205	2.05%
3	Louisiana		528	5.28%	18	Arkansas	204	2.04%
43	Maine		48	0.48%	19	Colorado	201	2.01%
34	Maryland		79	0.79%	20	Massachusetts	199	1.99%
20	Massachusetts		199	1.99%	21	Alabama	181	1.81%
16	Michigan		206	2.06%	22	Wisconsin	172	1.72%
11	Minnesota		258	2.58%	23	North Carolina	160	1.60%
36	Mississippi		70	0.70%	24	Arizona	129	1.29%
10	Missouri		271	2.71%	25	Connecticut	110	1.10%
39	Montana		60	0.60%	26	New Mexico	109	1.09%
31	Nebraska		86	0.86%	27	Kentucky	106	1.06%
42	Nevada		54	0.54%	28	Georgia	98	0.98%
44	New Hampshire		45	0.45%	29	Oregon	89	0.89%
41	New Jersey		55	0.55%	29	West Virginia	89	0.89%
26	New Mexico		109	1.09%	31	Nebraska	86	0.86%
13	New York		226	2.26%	31	Utah	86	0.86%
23	North Carolina		160	1.60%	33	South Carolina	80	0.80%
45	North Dakota		37	0.37%	34	Maryland	79	0.79%
4	Ohio		438	4.38%	35	Idaho	78	0.78%
8	Oklahoma		348	3.48%	36	Mississippi	70	0.70%
29	Oregon		89	0.89%	37	Washington	67	0.67%
5	Pennsylvania		374	3.74%	38	Wyoming	61	0.61%
46	Rhode Island		28	0.28%	39	Montana	60	0.60%
33	South Carolina		80	0.80%	40	South Dakota	56	0.56%
40	South Dakota		56	0.56%	41	New Jersey	55	0.55%
12	Tennessee		241	2.41%	42	Nevada	54	0.54%
1	Texas		1,664	16.63%	43	Maine	48	0.48%
31	Utah		86	0.86%	44	New Hampshire	45	0.45%
50	Vermont		13	0.13%	45	North Dakota	37	0.37%
14	Virginia		221	2.21%	46	Hawaii	28	0.28%
37	Washington		67	0.67%	46	Rhode Island	28	0.28%
29	West Virginia		89	0.89%	48	Alaska	25	0.25%
22	Wisconsin		172	1.72%	49	Delaware	20	0.20%
38	Wyoming		61	0.61%	50	Vermont	13	0.13%
						District of Columbia	21	0.21%

Source: U.S. Department of Health and Human Services, Health Care Financing Administration
unpublished data (February 26, 1997)

*Certified by HCFA to participate in the Medicare/Medicaid programs. National total does not include 48 certified home health agencies in U.S. territories. A home health agency provides health services to individuals in their homes for the purpose of promoting, maintaining or restoring health or maximizing the level of independence, while minimizing the effects of disability and illness.

Medicare and Medicaid Certified Community Mental Health Centers in 1997

National Total = 1,237 Centers*

ALPHA ORDER

RANK	STATE	CENTERS	% of USA
3	Alabama	113	9.14%
43	Alaska	1	0.08%
4	Arizona	74	5.98%
27	Arkansas	11	0.89%
6	California	60	4.85%
18	Colorado	18	1.46%
32	Connecticut	7	0.57%
47	Delaware	0	0.00%
1	Florida	239	19.32%
27	Georgia	11	0.89%
47	Hawaii	0	0.00%
42	Idaho	2	0.16%
12	Illinois	32	2.59%
25	Indiana	13	1.05%
30	Iowa	10	0.81%
14	Kansas	20	1.62%
23	Kentucky	14	1.13%
9	Louisiana	38	3.07%
37	Maine	4	0.32%
27	Maryland	11	0.89%
21	Massachusetts	15	1.21%
15	Michigan	19	1.54%
20	Minnesota	16	1.29%
30	Mississippi	10	0.81%
13	Missouri	25	2.02%
35	Montana	5	0.40%
43	Nebraska	1	0.08%
37	Nevada	4	0.32%
35	New Hampshire	5	0.40%
9	New Jersey	38	3.07%
18	New Mexico	18	1.46%
26	New York	12	0.97%
8	North Carolina	39	3.15%
47	North Dakota	0	0.00%
11	Ohio	33	2.67%
21	Oklahoma	15	1.21%
15	Oregon	19	1.54%
5	Pennsylvania	65	5.25%
43	Rhode Island	1	0.08%
23	South Carolina	14	1.13%
40	South Dakota	3	0.24%
15	Tennessee	19	1.54%
2	Texas	115	9.30%
34	Utah	6	0.49%
47	Vermont	0	0.00%
32	Virginia	7	0.57%
7	Washington	47	3.80%
40	West Virginia	3	0.24%
43	Wisconsin	1	0.08%
37	Wyoming	4	0.32%

RANK ORDER

RANK	STATE	CENTERS	% of USA
1	Florida	239	19.32%
2	Texas	115	9.30%
3	Alabama	113	9.14%
4	Arizona	74	5.98%
5	Pennsylvania	65	5.25%
6	California	60	4.85%
7	Washington	47	3.80%
8	North Carolina	39	3.15%
9	Louisiana	38	3.07%
9	New Jersey	38	3.07%
11	Ohio	33	2.67%
12	Illinois	32	2.59%
13	Missouri	25	2.02%
14	Kansas	20	1.62%
15	Michigan	19	1.54%
15	Oregon	19	1.54%
15	Tennessee	19	1.54%
18	Colorado	18	1.46%
18	New Mexico	18	1.46%
20	Minnesota	16	1.29%
21	Massachusetts	15	1.21%
21	Oklahoma	15	1.21%
23	Kentucky	14	1.13%
23	South Carolina	14	1.13%
25	Indiana	13	1.05%
26	New York	12	0.97%
27	Arkansas	11	0.89%
27	Georgia	11	0.89%
27	Maryland	11	0.89%
30	Iowa	10	0.81%
30	Mississippi	10	0.81%
32	Connecticut	7	0.57%
32	Virginia	7	0.57%
34	Utah	6	0.49%
35	Montana	5	0.40%
35	New Hampshire	5	0.40%
37	Maine	4	0.32%
37	Nevada	4	0.32%
37	Wyoming	4	0.32%
40	South Dakota	3	0.24%
40	West Virginia	3	0.24%
42	Idaho	2	0.16%
43	Alaska	1	0.08%
43	Nebraska	1	0.08%
43	Rhode Island	1	0.08%
43	Wisconsin	1	0.08%
47	Delaware	0	0.00%
47	Hawaii	0	0.00%
47	North Dakota	0	0.00%
47	Vermont	0	0.00%
	District of Columbia	0	0.00%

Source: U.S. Department of Health and Human Services, Health Care Financing Administration unpublished data (February 26, 1997)

*Certified by HCFA to participate in the Medicare/Medicaid programs. National total does not include 9 certified mental health centers in U.S. territories.

Medicare and Medicaid Certified Nursing Care Facilities in 1997

National Total = 17,307 Nursing Care Facilities*

ALPHA ORDER

RANK	STATE	FACILITIES	% of USA
29	Alabama	223	1.29%
50	Alaska	16	0.09%
34	Arizona	161	0.93%
24	Arkansas	285	1.65%
1	California	1,416	8.18%
29	Colorado	223	1.29%
26	Connecticut	263	1.52%
46	Delaware	44	0.25%
6	Florida	702	4.06%
18	Georgia	355	2.05%
47	Hawaii	43	0.25%
43	Idaho	82	0.47%
4	Illinois	862	4.98%
9	Indiana	575	3.32%
11	Iowa	472	2.73%
15	Kansas	431	2.49%
22	Kentucky	314	1.81%
19	Louisiana	345	1.99%
36	Maine	136	0.79%
27	Maryland	254	1.47%
10	Massachusetts	567	3.28%
14	Michigan	448	2.59%
13	Minnesota	456	2.63%
31	Mississippi	203	1.17%
8	Missouri	591	3.41%
38	Montana	103	0.60%
28	Nebraska	237	1.37%
47	Nevada	43	0.25%
44	New Hampshire	81	0.47%
21	New Jersey	332	1.92%
42	New Mexico	86	0.50%
7	New York	661	3.82%
17	North Carolina	400	2.31%
41	North Dakota	88	0.51%
3	Ohio	1,026	5.93%
12	Oklahoma	458	2.65%
33	Oregon	164	0.95%
5	Pennsylvania	774	4.47%
39	Rhode Island	99	0.57%
32	South Carolina	173	1.00%
37	South Dakota	114	0.66%
20	Tennessee	343	1.98%
2	Texas	1,336	7.72%
40	Utah	95	0.55%
45	Vermont	45	0.26%
25	Virginia	278	1.61%
23	Washington	286	1.65%
35	West Virginia	139	0.80%
16	Wisconsin	420	2.43%
49	Wyoming	38	0.22%

RANK ORDER

RANK	STATE	FACILITIES	% of USA
1	California	1,416	8.18%
2	Texas	1,336	7.72%
3	Ohio	1,026	5.93%
4	Illinois	862	4.98%
5	Pennsylvania	774	4.47%
6	Florida	702	4.06%
7	New York	661	3.82%
8	Missouri	591	3.41%
9	Indiana	575	3.32%
10	Massachusetts	567	3.28%
11	Iowa	472	2.73%
12	Oklahoma	458	2.65%
13	Minnesota	456	2.63%
14	Michigan	448	2.59%
15	Kansas	431	2.49%
16	Wisconsin	420	2.43%
17	North Carolina	400	2.31%
18	Georgia	355	2.05%
19	Louisiana	345	1.99%
20	Tennessee	343	1.98%
21	New Jersey	332	1.92%
22	Kentucky	314	1.81%
23	Washington	286	1.65%
24	Arkansas	285	1.65%
25	Virginia	278	1.61%
26	Connecticut	263	1.52%
27	Maryland	254	1.47%
28	Nebraska	237	1.37%
29	Alabama	223	1.29%
29	Colorado	223	1.29%
31	Mississippi	203	1.17%
32	South Carolina	173	1.00%
33	Oregon	164	0.95%
34	Arizona	161	0.93%
35	West Virginia	139	0.80%
36	Maine	136	0.79%
37	South Dakota	114	0.66%
38	Montana	103	0.60%
39	Rhode Island	99	0.57%
40	Utah	95	0.55%
41	North Dakota	88	0.51%
42	New Mexico	86	0.50%
43	Idaho	82	0.47%
44	New Hampshire	81	0.47%
45	Vermont	45	0.26%
46	Delaware	44	0.25%
47	Hawaii	43	0.25%
47	Nevada	43	0.25%
49	Wyoming	38	0.22%
50	Alaska	16	0.09%
	District of Columbia	21	0.12%

Source: U.S. Department of Health and Human Services, Health Care Financing Administration
unpublished data (February 26, 1997)
*Certified by HCFA to participate in the Medicare/Medicaid programs. National total does not include eight certified nursing care facilities in U.S. territories.

Nursing Home Beds in 1991

National Total = 1,559,394 Nursing Home Beds

ALPHA ORDER					RANK ORDER			
RANK	STATE	BEDS	% of USA		RANK	STATE	BEDS	% of USA
28	Alabama	21,323	1.37%		1	Texas	108,285	6.94%
50	Alaska	780	0.05%		2	California	105,781	6.78%
33	Arizona	13,265	0.85%		3	Illinois	95,465	6.12%
27	Arkansas	21,706	1.39%		4	New York	94,884	6.08%
2	California	105,781	6.78%		5	Pennsylvania	85,387	5.48%
30	Colorado	17,609	1.13%		6	Ohio	82,516	5.29%
21	Connecticut	27,983	1.79%		7	Florida	63,752	4.09%
45	Delaware	4,101	0.26%		8	Indiana	55,701	3.57%
7	Florida	63,752	4.09%		9	Missouri	51,652	3.31%
16	Georgia	35,011	2.25%		10	Massachusetts	50,133	3.21%
49	Hawaii	1,958	0.13%		11	Michigan	48,886	3.13%
44	Idaho	4,887	0.31%		12	Wisconsin	48,710	3.12%
3	Illinois	95,465	6.12%		13	Minnesota	42,001	2.69%
8	Indiana	55,701	3.57%		14	New Jersey	39,970	2.56%
17	Iowa	34,521	2.21%		15	Louisiana	36,644	2.35%
23	Kansas	27,115	1.74%		16	Georgia	35,011	2.25%
26	Kentucky	25,685	1.65%		17	Iowa	34,521	2.21%
15	Louisiana	36,644	2.35%		18	Tennessee	32,493	2.08%
37	Maine	9,192	0.59%		19	Oklahoma	32,421	2.08%
22	Maryland	27,163	1.74%		20	North Carolina	28,259	1.81%
10	Massachusetts	50,133	3.21%		21	Connecticut	27,983	1.79%
11	Michigan	48,886	3.13%		22	Maryland	27,163	1.74%
13	Minnesota	42,001	2.69%		23	Kansas	27,115	1.74%
31	Mississippi	14,431	0.93%		24	Washington	26,506	1.70%
9	Missouri	51,652	3.31%		25	Virginia	26,324	1.69%
43	Montana	5,713	0.37%		26	Kentucky	25,685	1.65%
29	Nebraska	17,846	1.14%		27	Arkansas	21,706	1.39%
47	Nevada	3,171	0.20%		28	Alabama	21,323	1.37%
39	New Hampshire	7,493	0.48%		29	Nebraska	17,846	1.14%
14	New Jersey	39,970	2.56%		30	Colorado	17,609	1.13%
42	New Mexico	5,933	0.38%		31	Mississippi	14,431	0.93%
4	New York	94,884	6.08%		32	Oregon	14,382	0.92%
20	North Carolina	28,259	1.81%		33	Arizona	13,265	0.85%
41	North Dakota	6,056	0.39%		34	South Carolina	13,122	0.84%
6	Ohio	82,516	5.29%		35	Rhode Island	9,915	0.64%
19	Oklahoma	32,421	2.08%		36	West Virginia	9,792	0.63%
32	Oregon	14,382	0.92%		37	Maine	9,192	0.59%
5	Pennsylvania	85,387	5.48%		38	South Dakota	8,448	0.54%
35	Rhode Island	9,915	0.64%		39	New Hampshire	7,493	0.48%
34	South Carolina	13,122	0.84%		40	Utah	6,292	0.40%
38	South Dakota	8,448	0.54%		41	North Dakota	6,056	0.39%
18	Tennessee	32,493	2.08%		42	New Mexico	5,933	0.38%
1	Texas	108,285	6.94%		43	Montana	5,713	0.37%
40	Utah	6,292	0.40%		44	Idaho	4,887	0.31%
46	Vermont	3,478	0.22%		45	Delaware	4,101	0.26%
25	Virginia	26,324	1.69%		46	Vermont	3,478	0.22%
24	Washington	26,506	1.70%		47	Nevada	3,171	0.20%
36	West Virginia	9,792	0.63%		48	Wyoming	2,243	0.14%
12	Wisconsin	48,710	3.12%		49	Hawaii	1,958	0.13%
48	Wyoming	2,243	0.14%		50	Alaska	780	0.05%
						District of Columbia	3,010	0.19%

Source: U.S. Department of Health and Human Services, National Center for Health Statistics
    unpublished data

Rate of Nursing Home Beds in 1991

National Rate = 49.1 Nursing Home Beds per 1,000 Population Age 65 and Older

ALPHA ORDER

RANK	STATE	RATE
35	Alabama	40.2
45	Alaska	32.5
47	Arizona	26.7
16	Arkansas	61.3
44	California	33.2
24	Colorado	51.8
14	Connecticut	61.9
28	Delaware	50.0
48	Florida	26.2
23	Georgia	52.3
50	Hawaii	15.1
37	Idaho	39.1
11	Illinois	65.8
4	Indiana	78.7
2	Iowa	80.1
5	Kansas	78.4
21	Kentucky	54.4
6	Louisiana	77.3
20	Maine	55.7
26	Maryland	51.3
17	Massachusetts	60.7
33	Michigan	43.3
7	Minnesota	75.5
32	Mississippi	44.8
10	Missouri	71.2
22	Montana	52.9
3	Nebraska	79.0
49	Nevada	23.1
18	New Hampshire	58.1
39	New Jersey	38.3
42	New Mexico	35.3
35	New York	40.2
43	North Carolina	34.2
13	North Dakota	65.1
19	Ohio	57.5
8	Oklahoma	75.4
41	Oregon	35.9
29	Pennsylvania	46.0
12	Rhode Island	65.7
46	South Carolina	32.3
1	South Dakota	82.0
25	Tennessee	51.6
15	Texas	61.6
34	Utah	40.6
27	Vermont	51.1
38	Virginia	38.6
31	Washington	45.0
40	West Virginia	36.0
9	Wisconsin	73.7
30	Wyoming	45.8

RANK ORDER

RANK	STATE	RATE
1	South Dakota	82.0
2	Iowa	80.1
3	Nebraska	79.0
4	Indiana	78.7
5	Kansas	78.4
6	Louisiana	77.3
7	Minnesota	75.5
8	Oklahoma	75.4
9	Wisconsin	73.7
10	Missouri	71.2
11	Illinois	65.8
12	Rhode Island	65.7
13	North Dakota	65.1
14	Connecticut	61.9
15	Texas	61.6
16	Arkansas	61.3
17	Massachusetts	60.7
18	New Hampshire	58.1
19	Ohio	57.5
20	Maine	55.7
21	Kentucky	54.4
22	Montana	52.9
23	Georgia	52.3
24	Colorado	51.8
25	Tennessee	51.6
26	Maryland	51.3
27	Vermont	51.1
28	Delaware	50.0
29	Pennsylvania	46.0
30	Wyoming	45.8
31	Washington	45.0
32	Mississippi	44.8
33	Michigan	43.3
34	Utah	40.6
35	Alabama	40.2
35	New York	40.2
37	Idaho	39.1
38	Virginia	38.6
39	New Jersey	38.3
40	West Virginia	36.0
41	Oregon	35.9
42	New Mexico	35.3
43	North Carolina	34.2
44	California	33.2
45	Alaska	32.5
46	South Carolina	32.3
47	Arizona	26.7
48	Florida	26.2
49	Nevada	23.1
50	Hawaii	15.1
	District of Columbia	38.6

Source: U.S. Department of Health and Human Services, National Center for Health Statistics unpublished data

Nursing Home Population in 1991

National Total = 1,478,903 Persons in Nursing Homes*

<u>ALPHA ORDER</u>

RANK	STATE	POPULATION	% of USA
27	Alabama	21,675	1.47%
50	Alaska	808	0.05%
34	Arizona	12,103	0.82%
28	Arkansas	20,298	1.37%
2	California	98,885	6.69%
30	Colorado	15,871	1.07%
20	Connecticut	27,921	1.89%
45	Delaware	4,308	0.29%
7	Florida	59,878	4.05%
15	Georgia	34,728	2.35%
48	Hawaii	2,840	0.19%
44	Idaho	4,871	0.33%
4	Illinois	87,540	5.92%
10	Indiana	46,231	3.13%
16	Iowa	33,214	2.25%
24	Kansas	25,304	1.71%
25	Kentucky	24,966	1.69%
17	Louisiana	32,367	2.19%
37	Maine	9,241	0.62%
22	Maryland	25,977	1.76%
8	Massachusetts	48,276	3.26%
11	Michigan	46,198	3.12%
13	Minnesota	43,298	2.93%
31	Mississippi	14,819	1.00%
12	Missouri	45,745	3.09%
41	Montana	6,297	0.43%
29	Nebraska	17,779	1.20%
47	Nevada	3,043	0.21%
39	New Hampshire	7,523	0.51%
14	New Jersey	40,068	2.71%
42	New Mexico	5,834	0.39%
1	New York	99,372	6.72%
19	North Carolina	28,546	1.93%
40	North Dakota	6,784	0.46%
6	Ohio	77,676	5.25%
21	Oklahoma	27,456	1.86%
32	Oregon	13,392	0.91%
5	Pennsylvania	83,107	5.62%
36	Rhode Island	9,440	0.64%
33	South Carolina	13,089	0.89%
38	South Dakota	8,192	0.55%
18	Tennessee	32,304	2.18%
3	Texas	90,405	6.11%
43	Utah	5,544	0.37%
46	Vermont	3,591	0.24%
23	Virginia	25,775	1.74%
26	Washington	24,525	1.66%
35	West Virginia	9,809	0.66%
9	Wisconsin	46,898	3.17%
49	Wyoming	2,211	0.15%

<u>RANK ORDER</u>

RANK	STATE	POPULATION	% of USA
1	New York	99,372	6.72%
2	California	98,885	6.69%
3	Texas	90,405	6.11%
4	Illinois	87,540	5.92%
5	Pennsylvania	83,107	5.62%
6	Ohio	77,676	5.25%
7	Florida	59,878	4.05%
8	Massachusetts	48,276	3.26%
9	Wisconsin	46,898	3.17%
10	Indiana	46,231	3.13%
11	Michigan	46,198	3.12%
12	Missouri	45,745	3.09%
13	Minnesota	43,298	2.93%
14	New Jersey	40,068	2.71%
15	Georgia	34,728	2.35%
16	Iowa	33,214	2.25%
17	Louisiana	32,367	2.19%
18	Tennessee	32,304	2.18%
19	North Carolina	28,546	1.93%
20	Connecticut	27,921	1.89%
21	Oklahoma	27,456	1.86%
22	Maryland	25,977	1.76%
23	Virginia	25,775	1.74%
24	Kansas	25,304	1.71%
25	Kentucky	24,966	1.69%
26	Washington	24,525	1.66%
27	Alabama	21,675	1.47%
28	Arkansas	20,298	1.37%
29	Nebraska	17,779	1.20%
30	Colorado	15,871	1.07%
31	Mississippi	14,819	1.00%
32	Oregon	13,392	0.91%
33	South Carolina	13,089	0.89%
34	Arizona	12,103	0.82%
35	West Virginia	9,809	0.66%
36	Rhode Island	9,440	0.64%
37	Maine	9,241	0.62%
38	South Dakota	8,192	0.55%
39	New Hampshire	7,523	0.51%
40	North Dakota	6,784	0.46%
41	Montana	6,297	0.43%
42	New Mexico	5,834	0.39%
43	Utah	5,544	0.37%
44	Idaho	4,871	0.33%
45	Delaware	4,308	0.29%
46	Vermont	3,591	0.24%
47	Nevada	3,043	0.21%
48	Hawaii	2,840	0.19%
49	Wyoming	2,211	0.15%
50	Alaska	808	0.05%
	District of Columbia	2,881	0.19%

Source: U.S. Department of Health and Human Services, National Center for Health Statistics
   "National Health Provider Inventory" (Advance Data, No. 266, September 19, 1995)
A nursing home is facility with three or more beds that is either licensed as a nursing home, certified as a nursing facility under Medicare or Medicaid, identified as a nursing care unit of a retirement center or determined to provide nursing or medical care.

Percent of Nursing Home Population 65 Years Old or Older in 1991

National Percent = 92.3% of Nursing Home Population*

<table>
<tr><td colspan="3">ALPHA ORDER</td><td colspan="3">RANK ORDER</td></tr>
<tr><td>RANK</td><td>STATE</td><td>PERCENT</td><td>RANK</td><td>STATE</td><td>PERCENT</td></tr>
<tr><td>25</td><td>Alabama</td><td>92.5</td><td>1</td><td>Rhode Island</td><td>96.5</td></tr>
<tr><td>50</td><td>Alaska</td><td>78.7</td><td>2</td><td>South Dakota</td><td>95.7</td></tr>
<tr><td>36</td><td>Arizona</td><td>91.9</td><td>3</td><td>Maine</td><td>95.6</td></tr>
<tr><td>44</td><td>Arkansas</td><td>90.5</td><td>4</td><td>North Dakota</td><td>95.4</td></tr>
<tr><td>47</td><td>California</td><td>88.8</td><td>5</td><td>Iowa</td><td>95.2</td></tr>
<tr><td>41</td><td>Colorado</td><td>90.9</td><td>6</td><td>New Hampshire</td><td>95.1</td></tr>
<tr><td>28</td><td>Connecticut</td><td>92.3</td><td>7</td><td>Florida</td><td>94.9</td></tr>
<tr><td>28</td><td>Delaware</td><td>92.3</td><td>8</td><td>Vermont</td><td>94.5</td></tr>
<tr><td>7</td><td>Florida</td><td>94.9</td><td>9</td><td>Minnesota</td><td>94.3</td></tr>
<tr><td>42</td><td>Georgia</td><td>90.7</td><td>10</td><td>West Virginia</td><td>94.2</td></tr>
<tr><td>33</td><td>Hawaii</td><td>92.0</td><td>11</td><td>New York</td><td>94.1</td></tr>
<tr><td>42</td><td>Idaho</td><td>90.7</td><td>12</td><td>Pennsylvania</td><td>94.0</td></tr>
<tr><td>46</td><td>Illinois</td><td>89.0</td><td>13</td><td>Nebraska</td><td>93.9</td></tr>
<tr><td>40</td><td>Indiana</td><td>91.1</td><td>14</td><td>Wyoming</td><td>93.6</td></tr>
<tr><td>5</td><td>Iowa</td><td>95.2</td><td>15</td><td>Massachusetts</td><td>93.5</td></tr>
<tr><td>22</td><td>Kansas</td><td>92.7</td><td>16</td><td>New Jersey</td><td>93.4</td></tr>
<tr><td>31</td><td>Kentucky</td><td>92.1</td><td>17</td><td>Missouri</td><td>93.1</td></tr>
<tr><td>45</td><td>Louisiana</td><td>89.1</td><td>18</td><td>Oregon</td><td>93.0</td></tr>
<tr><td>3</td><td>Maine</td><td>95.6</td><td>18</td><td>Texas</td><td>93.0</td></tr>
<tr><td>33</td><td>Maryland</td><td>92.0</td><td>20</td><td>Mississippi</td><td>92.9</td></tr>
<tr><td>15</td><td>Massachusetts</td><td>93.5</td><td>21</td><td>Oklahoma</td><td>92.8</td></tr>
<tr><td>39</td><td>Michigan</td><td>91.5</td><td>22</td><td>Kansas</td><td>92.7</td></tr>
<tr><td>9</td><td>Minnesota</td><td>94.3</td><td>22</td><td>Tennessee</td><td>92.7</td></tr>
<tr><td>20</td><td>Mississippi</td><td>92.9</td><td>24</td><td>South Carolina</td><td>92.6</td></tr>
<tr><td>17</td><td>Missouri</td><td>93.1</td><td>25</td><td>Alabama</td><td>92.5</td></tr>
<tr><td>25</td><td>Montana</td><td>92.5</td><td>25</td><td>Montana</td><td>92.5</td></tr>
<tr><td>13</td><td>Nebraska</td><td>93.9</td><td>27</td><td>Virginia</td><td>92.4</td></tr>
<tr><td>48</td><td>Nevada</td><td>88.0</td><td>28</td><td>Connecticut</td><td>92.3</td></tr>
<tr><td>6</td><td>New Hampshire</td><td>95.1</td><td>28</td><td>Delaware</td><td>92.3</td></tr>
<tr><td>16</td><td>New Jersey</td><td>93.4</td><td>28</td><td>North Carolina</td><td>92.3</td></tr>
<tr><td>33</td><td>New Mexico</td><td>92.0</td><td>31</td><td>Kentucky</td><td>92.1</td></tr>
<tr><td>11</td><td>New York</td><td>94.1</td><td>31</td><td>Washington</td><td>92.1</td></tr>
<tr><td>28</td><td>North Carolina</td><td>92.3</td><td>33</td><td>Hawaii</td><td>92.0</td></tr>
<tr><td>4</td><td>North Dakota</td><td>95.4</td><td>33</td><td>Maryland</td><td>92.0</td></tr>
<tr><td>37</td><td>Ohio</td><td>91.7</td><td>33</td><td>New Mexico</td><td>92.0</td></tr>
<tr><td>21</td><td>Oklahoma</td><td>92.8</td><td>36</td><td>Arizona</td><td>91.9</td></tr>
<tr><td>18</td><td>Oregon</td><td>93.0</td><td>37</td><td>Ohio</td><td>91.7</td></tr>
<tr><td>12</td><td>Pennsylvania</td><td>94.0</td><td>38</td><td>Wisconsin</td><td>91.6</td></tr>
<tr><td>1</td><td>Rhode Island</td><td>96.5</td><td>39</td><td>Michigan</td><td>91.5</td></tr>
<tr><td>24</td><td>South Carolina</td><td>92.6</td><td>40</td><td>Indiana</td><td>91.1</td></tr>
<tr><td>2</td><td>South Dakota</td><td>95.7</td><td>41</td><td>Colorado</td><td>90.9</td></tr>
<tr><td>22</td><td>Tennessee</td><td>92.7</td><td>42</td><td>Georgia</td><td>90.7</td></tr>
<tr><td>18</td><td>Texas</td><td>93.0</td><td>42</td><td>Idaho</td><td>90.7</td></tr>
<tr><td>49</td><td>Utah</td><td>86.5</td><td>44</td><td>Arkansas</td><td>90.5</td></tr>
<tr><td>8</td><td>Vermont</td><td>94.5</td><td>45</td><td>Louisiana</td><td>89.1</td></tr>
<tr><td>27</td><td>Virginia</td><td>92.4</td><td>46</td><td>Illinois</td><td>89.0</td></tr>
<tr><td>31</td><td>Washington</td><td>92.1</td><td>47</td><td>California</td><td>88.8</td></tr>
<tr><td>10</td><td>West Virginia</td><td>94.2</td><td>48</td><td>Nevada</td><td>88.0</td></tr>
<tr><td>38</td><td>Wisconsin</td><td>91.6</td><td>49</td><td>Utah</td><td>86.5</td></tr>
<tr><td>14</td><td>Wyoming</td><td>93.6</td><td>50</td><td>Alaska</td><td>78.7</td></tr>
<tr><td></td><td></td><td></td><td></td><td>District of Columbia</td><td>93.3</td></tr>
</table>

Source: U.S. Department of Health and Human Services, National Center for Health Statistics
"National Health Provider Inventory" (Advance Data, No. 266, September 19, 1995)
*A nursing home is facility with three or more beds that is either licensed as a nursing home, certified as a nursing facility under Medicare or Medicaid, identified as a nursing care unit of a retirement center or determined to provide nursing or medical care.

Percent of Nursing Home Population 85 Years Old or Older in 1991

National Percent = 33.7% of Nursing Home Population*

ALPHA ORDER

RANK	STATE	PERCENT
43	Alabama	28.6
48	Alaska	24.9
20	Arizona	34.8
44	Arkansas	28.5
34	California	31.3
15	Colorado	37.3
37	Connecticut	31.1
15	Delaware	37.3
22	Florida	34.6
37	Georgia	31.1
2	Hawaii	46.8
29	Idaho	32.6
32	Illinois	31.8
31	Indiana	32.1
5	Iowa	42.8
8	Kansas	40.0
39	Kentucky	30.8
50	Louisiana	23.8
6	Maine	41.4
46	Maryland	27.8
11	Massachusetts	38.5
26	Michigan	33.4
12	Minnesota	38.4
47	Mississippi	27.5
23	Missouri	33.9
17	Montana	37.1
4	Nebraska	43.8
49	Nevada	24.2
1	New Hampshire	49.0
18	New Jersey	35.6
20	New Mexico	34.8
13	New York	38.3
45	North Carolina	28.4
7	North Dakota	41.3
32	Ohio	31.8
27	Oklahoma	33.2
29	Oregon	32.6
28	Pennsylvania	33.0
10	Rhode Island	39.9
23	South Carolina	33.9
3	South Dakota	45.5
36	Tennessee	31.2
34	Texas	31.3
42	Utah	29.3
8	Vermont	40.0
23	Virginia	33.9
41	Washington	30.4
40	West Virginia	30.5
14	Wisconsin	37.7
19	Wyoming	35.2

RANK ORDER

RANK	STATE	PERCENT
1	New Hampshire	49.0
2	Hawaii	46.8
3	South Dakota	45.5
4	Nebraska	43.8
5	Iowa	42.8
6	Maine	41.4
7	North Dakota	41.3
8	Kansas	40.0
8	Vermont	40.0
10	Rhode Island	39.9
11	Massachusetts	38.5
12	Minnesota	38.4
13	New York	38.3
14	Wisconsin	37.7
15	Colorado	37.3
15	Delaware	37.3
17	Montana	37.1
18	New Jersey	35.6
19	Wyoming	35.2
20	Arizona	34.8
20	New Mexico	34.8
22	Florida	34.6
23	Missouri	33.9
23	South Carolina	33.9
23	Virginia	33.9
26	Michigan	33.4
27	Oklahoma	33.2
28	Pennsylvania	33.0
29	Idaho	32.6
29	Oregon	32.6
31	Indiana	32.1
32	Illinois	31.8
32	Ohio	31.8
34	California	31.3
34	Texas	31.3
36	Tennessee	31.2
37	Connecticut	31.1
37	Georgia	31.1
39	Kentucky	30.8
40	West Virginia	30.5
41	Washington	30.4
42	Utah	29.3
43	Alabama	28.6
44	Arkansas	28.5
45	North Carolina	28.4
46	Maryland	27.8
47	Mississippi	27.5
48	Alaska	24.9
49	Nevada	24.2
50	Louisiana	23.8

District of Columbia 26.5

Source: Morgan Quitno Press using data from U.S. Dept of Health & Human Serv's, Nat'l Center for Health Statistics "National Health Provider Inventory" (unpublished data)

*A nursing home is facility with three or more beds that is either licensed as a nursing home, certified as a nursing facility under Medicare or Medicaid, identified as a nursing care unit of a retirement center or determined to provide nursing or medical care.

Percent of Population in Nursing Homes in 1991

National Percent = 0.59% of Population*

ALPHA ORDER

RANK	STATE	PERCENT
29	Alabama	0.53
50	Alaska	0.14
46	Arizona	0.32
11	Arkansas	0.86
45	California	0.33
37	Colorado	0.47
12	Connecticut	0.85
24	Delaware	0.63
40	Florida	0.45
31	Georgia	0.52
48	Hawaii	0.25
37	Idaho	0.47
16	Illinois	0.76
13	Indiana	0.82
1	Iowa	1.19
5	Kansas	1.02
22	Kentucky	0.67
16	Louisiana	0.76
18	Maine	0.75
29	Maryland	0.53
14	Massachusetts	0.80
34	Michigan	0.49
6	Minnesota	0.98
26	Mississippi	0.57
9	Missouri	0.89
15	Montana	0.78
3	Nebraska	1.12
49	Nevada	0.24
21	New Hampshire	0.68
31	New Jersey	0.52
43	New Mexico	0.38
27	New York	0.55
41	North Carolina	0.42
4	North Dakota	1.07
19	Ohio	0.71
10	Oklahoma	0.87
39	Oregon	0.46
20	Pennsylvania	0.70
8	Rhode Island	0.94
44	South Carolina	0.37
2	South Dakota	1.17
23	Tennessee	0.65
31	Texas	0.52
47	Utah	0.31
24	Vermont	0.63
42	Virginia	0.41
34	Washington	0.49
27	West Virginia	0.55
7	Wisconsin	0.95
36	Wyoming	0.48

RANK ORDER

RANK	STATE	PERCENT
1	Iowa	1.19
2	South Dakota	1.17
3	Nebraska	1.12
4	North Dakota	1.07
5	Kansas	1.02
6	Minnesota	0.98
7	Wisconsin	0.95
8	Rhode Island	0.94
9	Missouri	0.89
10	Oklahoma	0.87
11	Arkansas	0.86
12	Connecticut	0.85
13	Indiana	0.82
14	Massachusetts	0.80
15	Montana	0.78
16	Illinois	0.76
16	Louisiana	0.76
18	Maine	0.75
19	Ohio	0.71
20	Pennsylvania	0.70
21	New Hampshire	0.68
22	Kentucky	0.67
23	Tennessee	0.65
24	Delaware	0.63
24	Vermont	0.63
26	Mississippi	0.57
27	New York	0.55
27	West Virginia	0.55
29	Alabama	0.53
29	Maryland	0.53
31	Georgia	0.52
31	New Jersey	0.52
31	Texas	0.52
34	Michigan	0.49
34	Washington	0.49
36	Wyoming	0.48
37	Colorado	0.47
37	Idaho	0.47
39	Oregon	0.46
40	Florida	0.45
41	North Carolina	0.42
42	Virginia	0.41
43	New Mexico	0.38
44	South Carolina	0.37
45	California	0.33
46	Arizona	0.32
47	Utah	0.31
48	Hawaii	0.25
49	Nevada	0.24
50	Alaska	0.14
	District of Columbia	0.49

Source: Morgan Quitno Press using data from U.S. Dept of Health & Human Serv's, Nat'l Center for Health Statistics "National Health Provider Inventory" (Advance Data, No. 266, September 19, 1995)
*A nursing home is facility with three or more beds that is either licensed as a nursing home, certified as a nursing facility under Medicare or Medicaid, identified as a nursing care unit of a retirement center or determined to provide nursing or medical care.

Nursing Home Population in 1980

National Total = 1,426,371 Persons in Nursing Homes

ALPHA ORDER

RANK	STATE	POPULATION	% of USA
27	Alabama	18,702	1.31%
50	Alaska	854	0.06%
35	Arizona	8,424	0.59%
28	Arkansas	18,631	1.31%
1	California	134,756	9.45%
30	Colorado	16,109	1.13%
19	Connecticut	27,873	1.95%
46	Delaware	2,771	0.19%
13	Florida	36,306	2.55%
17	Georgia	29,376	2.06%
45	Hawaii	3,159	0.22%
42	Idaho	5,084	0.36%
4	Illinois	80,410	5.64%
11	Indiana	40,112	2.81%
14	Iowa	36,217	2.54%
21	Kansas	24,545	1.72%
23	Kentucky	23,591	1.65%
24	Louisiana	22,776	1.60%
34	Maine	9,570	0.67%
26	Maryland	19,821	1.39%
8	Massachusetts	49,728	3.49%
7	Michigan	55,805	3.91%
10	Minnesota	44,553	3.12%
32	Mississippi	12,753	0.89%
12	Missouri	37,942	2.66%
41	Montana	5,479	0.38%
29	Nebraska	17,650	1.24%
48	Nevada	2,339	0.16%
39	New Hampshire	6,673	0.47%
15	New Jersey	34,414	2.41%
47	New Mexico	2,585	0.18%
2	New York	114,276	8.01%
16	North Carolina	29,596	2.07%
38	North Dakota	7,486	0.52%
6	Ohio	71,479	5.01%
20	Oklahoma	25,732	1.80%
31	Oregon	16,052	1.13%
5	Pennsylvania	72,285	5.07%
36	Rhode Island	8,146	0.57%
33	South Carolina	11,666	0.82%
37	South Dakota	8,087	0.57%
25	Tennessee	22,014	1.54%
3	Texas	89,275	6.26%
43	Utah	4,921	0.35%
44	Vermont	4,354	0.31%
22	Virginia	24,323	1.71%
18	Washington	27,970	1.96%
40	West Virginia	6,355	0.45%
9	Wisconsin	48,282	3.38%
49	Wyoming	2,198	0.15%

RANK ORDER

RANK	STATE	POPULATION	% of USA
1	California	134,756	9.45%
2	New York	114,276	8.01%
3	Texas	89,275	6.26%
4	Illinois	80,410	5.64%
5	Pennsylvania	72,285	5.07%
6	Ohio	71,479	5.01%
7	Michigan	55,805	3.91%
8	Massachusetts	49,728	3.49%
9	Wisconsin	48,282	3.38%
10	Minnesota	44,553	3.12%
11	Indiana	40,112	2.81%
12	Missouri	37,942	2.66%
13	Florida	36,306	2.55%
14	Iowa	36,217	2.54%
15	New Jersey	34,414	2.41%
16	North Carolina	29,596	2.07%
17	Georgia	29,376	2.06%
18	Washington	27,970	1.96%
19	Connecticut	27,873	1.95%
20	Oklahoma	25,732	1.80%
21	Kansas	24,545	1.72%
22	Virginia	24,323	1.71%
23	Kentucky	23,591	1.65%
24	Louisiana	22,776	1.60%
25	Tennessee	22,014	1.54%
26	Maryland	19,821	1.39%
27	Alabama	18,702	1.31%
28	Arkansas	18,631	1.31%
29	Nebraska	17,650	1.24%
30	Colorado	16,109	1.13%
31	Oregon	16,052	1.13%
32	Mississippi	12,753	0.89%
33	South Carolina	11,666	0.82%
34	Maine	9,570	0.67%
35	Arizona	8,424	0.59%
36	Rhode Island	8,146	0.57%
37	South Dakota	8,087	0.57%
38	North Dakota	7,486	0.52%
39	New Hampshire	6,673	0.47%
40	West Virginia	6,355	0.45%
41	Montana	5,479	0.38%
42	Idaho	5,084	0.36%
43	Utah	4,921	0.35%
44	Vermont	4,354	0.31%
45	Hawaii	3,159	0.22%
46	Delaware	2,771	0.19%
47	New Mexico	2,585	0.18%
48	Nevada	2,339	0.16%
49	Wyoming	2,198	0.15%
50	Alaska	854	0.06%
	District of Columbia	2,866	0.20%

Source: U.S. Bureau of the Census
"Nursing Homes Persons in Institutions and Other Group Quarters" (PC80-2-4D)

Percent of Population in Nursing Homes in 1980

National Percent = 0.63% of Population in Nursing Homes

ALPHA ORDER

RANK ORDER

RANK	STATE	PERCENT	RANK	STATE	PERCENT
35	Alabama	0.48	1	Iowa	1.24
49	Alaska	0.21	2	South Dakota	1.17
47	Arizona	0.31	3	North Dakota	1.15
14	Arkansas	0.81	4	Nebraska	1.12
28	California	0.57	5	Minnesota	1.09
29	Colorado	0.56	6	Kansas	1.04
8	Connecticut	0.90	7	Wisconsin	1.03
37	Delaware	0.47	8	Connecticut	0.90
42	Florida	0.37	9	Massachusetts	0.87
30	Georgia	0.54	10	Rhode Island	0.86
45	Hawaii	0.33	11	Maine	0.85
30	Idaho	0.54	11	Oklahoma	0.85
18	Illinois	0.70	11	Vermont	0.85
16	Indiana	0.73	14	Arkansas	0.81
1	Iowa	1.24	15	Missouri	0.77
6	Kansas	1.04	16	Indiana	0.73
23	Kentucky	0.64	17	New Hampshire	0.72
30	Louisiana	0.54	18	Illinois	0.70
11	Maine	0.85	18	Montana	0.70
37	Maryland	0.47	20	Washington	0.68
9	Massachusetts	0.87	21	Ohio	0.66
27	Michigan	0.60	22	New York	0.65
5	Minnesota	1.09	23	Kentucky	0.64
33	Mississippi	0.51	24	Texas	0.63
15	Missouri	0.77	25	Oregon	0.61
18	Montana	0.70	25	Pennsylvania	0.61
4	Nebraska	1.12	27	Michigan	0.60
48	Nevada	0.29	28	California	0.57
17	New Hampshire	0.72	29	Colorado	0.56
37	New Jersey	0.47	30	Georgia	0.54
50	New Mexico	0.20	30	Idaho	0.54
22	New York	0.65	30	Louisiana	0.54
34	North Carolina	0.50	33	Mississippi	0.51
3	North Dakota	1.15	34	North Carolina	0.50
21	Ohio	0.66	35	Alabama	0.48
11	Oklahoma	0.85	35	Tennessee	0.48
25	Oregon	0.61	37	Delaware	0.47
25	Pennsylvania	0.61	37	Maryland	0.47
10	Rhode Island	0.86	37	New Jersey	0.47
42	South Carolina	0.37	37	Wyoming	0.47
2	South Dakota	1.17	41	Virginia	0.45
35	Tennessee	0.48	42	Florida	0.37
24	Texas	0.63	42	South Carolina	0.37
44	Utah	0.34	44	Utah	0.34
11	Vermont	0.85	45	Hawaii	0.33
41	Virginia	0.45	45	West Virginia	0.33
20	Washington	0.68	47	Arizona	0.31
45	West Virginia	0.33	48	Nevada	0.29
7	Wisconsin	1.03	49	Alaska	0.21
37	Wyoming	0.47	50	New Mexico	0.20
				District of Columbia	0.45

Source: Morgan Quitno Press using data from U.S. Bureau of the Census
"Nursing Homes Persons in Institutions and Other Group Quarters" (PC80-2-4D)

Change in Nursing Home Population: 1980 to 1990

National Change = 345,661 Increase in Nursing Home Population

ALPHA ORDER

RANK	STATE	INCREASE	% of USA
21	Alabama	5,329	1.54%
47	Alaska	348	0.10%
19	Arizona	6,048	1.75%
26	Arkansas	3,178	0.92%
6	California	13,606	3.94%
30	Colorado	2,397	0.69%
27	Connecticut	3,089	0.89%
35	Delaware	1,825	0.53%
1	Florida	43,992	12.73%
15	Georgia	7,173	2.08%
50	Hawaii	66	0.02%
43	Idaho	1,234	0.36%
8	Illinois	13,252	3.83%
13	Indiana	10,733	3.11%
49	Iowa	238	0.07%
37	Kansas	1,610	0.47%
23	Kentucky	4,283	1.24%
14	Louisiana	9,296	2.69%
48	Maine	285	0.08%
16	Maryland	7,063	2.04%
20	Massachusetts	5,934	1.72%
36	Michigan	1,817	0.53%
29	Minnesota	2,498	0.72%
28	Mississippi	3,050	0.88%
5	Missouri	14,118	4.08%
31	Montana	2,285	0.66%
39	Nebraska	1,521	0.44%
42	Nevada	1,266	0.37%
38	New Hampshire	1,529	0.44%
10	New Jersey	12,640	3.66%
25	New Mexico	3,691	1.07%
11	New York	11,899	3.44%
4	North Carolina	17,418	5.04%
44	North Dakota	673	0.19%
3	Ohio	22,290	6.45%
24	Oklahoma	3,934	1.14%
32	Oregon	2,148	0.62%
2	Pennsylvania	34,169	9.89%
34	Rhode Island	2,010	0.58%
17	South Carolina	6,562	1.90%
41	South Dakota	1,269	0.37%
9	Tennessee	13,178	3.81%
12	Texas	11,730	3.39%
40	Utah	1,301	0.38%
46	Vermont	455	0.13%
7	Virginia	13,439	3.89%
22	Washington	4,870	1.41%
18	West Virginia	6,236	1.80%
33	Wisconsin	2,063	0.60%
45	Wyoming	481	0.14%

RANK ORDER

RANK	STATE	INCREASE	% of USA
1	Florida	43,992	12.73%
2	Pennsylvania	34,169	9.89%
3	Ohio	22,290	6.45%
4	North Carolina	17,418	5.04%
5	Missouri	14,118	4.08%
6	California	13,606	3.94%
7	Virginia	13,439	3.89%
8	Illinois	13,252	3.83%
9	Tennessee	13,178	3.81%
10	New Jersey	12,640	3.66%
11	New York	11,899	3.44%
12	Texas	11,730	3.39%
13	Indiana	10,733	3.11%
14	Louisiana	9,296	2.69%
15	Georgia	7,173	2.08%
16	Maryland	7,063	2.04%
17	South Carolina	6,562	1.90%
18	West Virginia	6,236	1.80%
19	Arizona	6,048	1.75%
20	Massachusetts	5,934	1.72%
21	Alabama	5,329	1.54%
22	Washington	4,870	1.41%
23	Kentucky	4,283	1.24%
24	Oklahoma	3,934	1.14%
25	New Mexico	3,691	1.07%
26	Arkansas	3,178	0.92%
27	Connecticut	3,089	0.89%
28	Mississippi	3,050	0.88%
29	Minnesota	2,498	0.72%
30	Colorado	2,397	0.69%
31	Montana	2,285	0.66%
32	Oregon	2,148	0.62%
33	Wisconsin	2,063	0.60%
34	Rhode Island	2,010	0.58%
35	Delaware	1,825	0.53%
36	Michigan	1,817	0.53%
37	Kansas	1,610	0.47%
38	New Hampshire	1,529	0.44%
39	Nebraska	1,521	0.44%
40	Utah	1,301	0.38%
41	South Dakota	1,269	0.37%
42	Nevada	1,266	0.37%
43	Idaho	1,234	0.36%
44	North Dakota	673	0.19%
45	Wyoming	481	0.14%
46	Vermont	455	0.13%
47	Alaska	348	0.10%
48	Maine	285	0.08%
49	Iowa	238	0.07%
50	Hawaii	66	0.02%
	District of Columbia	4,142	1.20%

Source: Morgan Quitno Press using data from U.S. Bureau of the Census
"Nursing Homes Persons in Institutions and Other Group Quarters" (PC80-2-4D) and
"Nursing Home Population 1990" (CPH-L-137)

Percent Change in Nursing Home Population: 1980 to 1990

National Percent Change = 24.2% Increase

ALPHA ORDER				RANK ORDER		
RANK	STATE	PERCENT		RANK	STATE	PERCENT
19	Alabama	28.5		1	New Mexico	142.8
14	Alaska	40.7		2	Florida	121.2
4	Arizona	71.8		3	West Virginia	98.1
30	Arkansas	17.1		4	Arizona	71.8
41	California	10.1		5	Delaware	65.9
34	Colorado	14.9		6	Tennessee	59.9
38	Connecticut	11.1		7	North Carolina	58.9
5	Delaware	65.9		8	South Carolina	56.2
2	Florida	121.2		9	Virginia	55.3
23	Georgia	24.4		10	Nevada	54.1
49	Hawaii	2.1		11	Pennsylvania	47.3
24	Idaho	24.3		12	Montana	41.7
31	Illinois	16.5		13	Louisiana	40.8
20	Indiana	26.8		14	Alaska	40.7
50	Iowa	0.7		15	Missouri	37.2
44	Kansas	6.6		16	New Jersey	36.7
28	Kentucky	18.2		17	Maryland	35.6
13	Louisiana	40.8		18	Ohio	31.2
48	Maine	3.0		19	Alabama	28.5
17	Maryland	35.6		20	Indiana	26.8
37	Massachusetts	11.9		21	Utah	26.4
47	Michigan	3.3		22	Rhode Island	24.7
45	Minnesota	5.6		23	Georgia	24.4
25	Mississippi	23.9		24	Idaho	24.3
15	Missouri	37.2		25	Mississippi	23.9
12	Montana	41.7		26	New Hampshire	22.9
43	Nebraska	8.6		27	Wyoming	21.9
10	Nevada	54.1		28	Kentucky	18.2
26	New Hampshire	22.9		29	Washington	17.4
16	New Jersey	36.7		30	Arkansas	17.1
1	New Mexico	142.8		31	Illinois	16.5
40	New York	10.4		32	South Dakota	15.7
7	North Carolina	58.9		33	Oklahoma	15.3
42	North Dakota	9.0		34	Colorado	14.9
18	Ohio	31.2		35	Oregon	13.4
33	Oklahoma	15.3		36	Texas	13.1
35	Oregon	13.4		37	Massachusetts	11.9
11	Pennsylvania	47.3		38	Connecticut	11.1
22	Rhode Island	24.7		39	Vermont	10.5
8	South Carolina	56.2		40	New York	10.4
32	South Dakota	15.7		41	California	10.1
6	Tennessee	59.9		42	North Dakota	9.0
36	Texas	13.1		43	Nebraska	8.6
21	Utah	26.4		44	Kansas	6.6
39	Vermont	10.5		45	Minnesota	5.6
9	Virginia	55.3		46	Wisconsin	4.3
29	Washington	17.4		47	Michigan	3.3
3	West Virginia	98.1		48	Maine	3.0
46	Wisconsin	4.3		49	Hawaii	2.1
27	Wyoming	21.9		50	Iowa	0.7
					District of Columbia	144.5

Source: Morgan Quitno Press using data from U.S. Bureau of the Census
"Nursing Homes Persons in Institutions and Other Group Quarters" (PC80-2-4D) and
"Nursing Home Population 1990" (CPH-L-137)

Health Service Establishments in 1994

National Total = 476,204 Establishments*

ALPHA ORDER

RANK	STATE	ESTABLISH'S	% of USA
26	Alabama	6,135	1.29%
48	Alaska	987	0.21%
20	Arizona	7,812	1.64%
32	Arkansas	3,976	0.83%
1	California	63,112	13.25%
21	Colorado	7,684	1.61%
23	Connecticut	7,074	1.49%
45	Delaware	1,299	0.27%
4	Florida	32,082	6.74%
10	Georgia	12,072	2.54%
39	Hawaii	2,411	0.51%
43	Idaho	1,937	0.41%
6	Illinois	20,117	4.22%
16	Indiana	9,497	1.99%
30	Iowa	4,632	0.97%
31	Kansas	4,356	0.91%
25	Kentucky	6,147	1.29%
22	Louisiana	7,463	1.57%
40	Maine	2,377	0.50%
15	Maryland	9,816	2.06%
11	Massachusetts	11,355	2.38%
9	Michigan	16,881	3.54%
24	Minnesota	6,814	1.43%
33	Mississippi	3,370	0.71%
17	Missouri	9,029	1.90%
44	Montana	1,723	0.36%
37	Nebraska	2,633	0.55%
38	Nevada	2,604	0.55%
42	New Hampshire	2,002	0.42%
8	New Jersey	17,585	3.69%
36	New Mexico	2,679	0.56%
2	New York	34,910	7.33%
14	North Carolina	9,879	2.07%
49	North Dakota	943	0.20%
7	Ohio	19,973	4.19%
28	Oklahoma	5,774	1.21%
27	Oregon	5,908	1.24%
5	Pennsylvania	23,737	4.98%
41	Rhode Island	2,031	0.43%
29	South Carolina	5,185	1.09%
46	South Dakota	1,178	0.25%
18	Tennessee	8,945	1.88%
3	Texas	32,275	6.78%
34	Utah	3,255	0.68%
47	Vermont	1,082	0.23%
12	Virginia	10,378	2.18%
13	Washington	9,916	2.08%
35	West Virginia	3,013	0.63%
19	Wisconsin	7,901	1.66%
50	Wyoming	846	0.18%

RANK ORDER

RANK	STATE	ESTABLISH'S	% of USA
1	California	63,112	13.25%
2	New York	34,910	7.33%
3	Texas	32,275	6.78%
4	Florida	32,082	6.74%
5	Pennsylvania	23,737	4.98%
6	Illinois	20,117	4.22%
7	Ohio	19,973	4.19%
8	New Jersey	17,585	3.69%
9	Michigan	16,881	3.54%
10	Georgia	12,072	2.54%
11	Massachusetts	11,355	2.38%
12	Virginia	10,378	2.18%
13	Washington	9,916	2.08%
14	North Carolina	9,879	2.07%
15	Maryland	9,816	2.06%
16	Indiana	9,497	1.99%
17	Missouri	9,029	1.90%
18	Tennessee	8,945	1.88%
19	Wisconsin	7,901	1.66%
20	Arizona	7,812	1.64%
21	Colorado	7,684	1.61%
22	Louisiana	7,463	1.57%
23	Connecticut	7,074	1.49%
24	Minnesota	6,814	1.43%
25	Kentucky	6,147	1.29%
26	Alabama	6,135	1.29%
27	Oregon	5,908	1.24%
28	Oklahoma	5,774	1.21%
29	South Carolina	5,185	1.09%
30	Iowa	4,632	0.97%
31	Kansas	4,356	0.91%
32	Arkansas	3,976	0.83%
33	Mississippi	3,370	0.71%
34	Utah	3,255	0.68%
35	West Virginia	3,013	0.63%
36	New Mexico	2,679	0.56%
37	Nebraska	2,633	0.55%
38	Nevada	2,604	0.55%
39	Hawaii	2,411	0.51%
40	Maine	2,377	0.50%
41	Rhode Island	2,031	0.43%
42	New Hampshire	2,002	0.42%
43	Idaho	1,937	0.41%
44	Montana	1,723	0.36%
45	Delaware	1,299	0.27%
46	South Dakota	1,178	0.25%
47	Vermont	1,082	0.23%
48	Alaska	987	0.21%
49	North Dakota	943	0.20%
50	Wyoming	846	0.18%
	District of Columbia	1,414	0.30%

Source: U.S. Bureau of the Census
"1994 County Business Patterns"
*Includes establishments exempt from, as well as subject to, the federal income tax. Includes those establishments within the Standard Industry Classification (SIC) 8000. These include those primarily engaged in furnishing medical, surgical and other health services to persons.

Offices and Clinics of Doctors of Medicine in 1992

National Total = 197,701 Establishments*

ALPHA ORDER

ALPHA ORDER

RANK	STATE	ESTABLISH'S	% of USA
23	Alabama	2,611	1.32%
47	Alaska	349	0.18%
20	Arizona	3,150	1.59%
29	Arkansas	1,664	0.84%
1	California	28,494	14.41%
22	Colorado	2,698	1.36%
21	Connecticut	3,039	1.54%
45	Delaware	587	0.30%
3	Florida	14,487	7.33%
10	Georgia	5,214	2.64%
37	Hawaii	1,066	0.54%
43	Idaho	728	0.37%
6	Illinois	8,424	4.26%
16	Indiana	3,744	1.89%
33	Iowa	1,349	0.68%
32	Kansas	1,382	0.70%
24	Kentucky	2,565	1.30%
18	Louisiana	3,293	1.67%
39	Maine	914	0.46%
11	Maryland	4,760	2.41%
13	Massachusetts	4,524	2.29%
9	Michigan	5,935	3.00%
30	Minnesota	1,480	0.75%
31	Mississippi	1,458	0.74%
19	Missouri	3,280	1.66%
44	Montana	599	0.30%
41	Nebraska	886	0.45%
36	Nevada	1,096	0.55%
42	New Hampshire	754	0.38%
8	New Jersey	7,718	3.90%
38	New Mexico	1,033	0.52%
2	New York	16,226	8.21%
15	North Carolina	3,826	1.94%
50	North Dakota	243	0.12%
7	Ohio	8,004	4.05%
28	Oklahoma	2,052	1.04%
26	Oregon	2,263	1.14%
5	Pennsylvania	9,347	4.73%
40	Rhode Island	889	0.45%
27	South Carolina	2,219	1.12%
47	South Dakota	349	0.18%
14	Tennessee	3,840	1.94%
4	Texas	14,367	7.27%
35	Utah	1,261	0.64%
46	Vermont	393	0.20%
12	Virginia	4,724	2.39%
17	Washington	3,464	1.75%
34	West Virginia	1,340	0.68%
25	Wisconsin	2,546	1.29%
49	Wyoming	294	0.15%

RANK ORDER

RANK	STATE	ESTABLISH'S	% of USA
1	California	28,494	14.41%
2	New York	16,226	8.21%
3	Florida	14,487	7.33%
4	Texas	14,367	7.27%
5	Pennsylvania	9,347	4.73%
6	Illinois	8,424	4.26%
7	Ohio	8,004	4.05%
8	New Jersey	7,718	3.90%
9	Michigan	5,935	3.00%
10	Georgia	5,214	2.64%
11	Maryland	4,760	2.41%
12	Virginia	4,724	2.39%
13	Massachusetts	4,524	2.29%
14	Tennessee	3,840	1.94%
15	North Carolina	3,826	1.94%
16	Indiana	3,744	1.89%
17	Washington	3,464	1.75%
18	Louisiana	3,293	1.67%
19	Missouri	3,280	1.66%
20	Arizona	3,150	1.59%
21	Connecticut	3,039	1.54%
22	Colorado	2,698	1.36%
23	Alabama	2,611	1.32%
24	Kentucky	2,565	1.30%
25	Wisconsin	2,546	1.29%
26	Oregon	2,263	1.14%
27	South Carolina	2,219	1.12%
28	Oklahoma	2,052	1.04%
29	Arkansas	1,664	0.84%
30	Minnesota	1,480	0.75%
31	Mississippi	1,458	0.74%
32	Kansas	1,382	0.70%
33	Iowa	1,349	0.68%
34	West Virginia	1,340	0.68%
35	Utah	1,261	0.64%
36	Nevada	1,096	0.55%
37	Hawaii	1,066	0.54%
38	New Mexico	1,033	0.52%
39	Maine	914	0.46%
40	Rhode Island	889	0.45%
41	Nebraska	886	0.45%
42	New Hampshire	754	0.38%
43	Idaho	728	0.37%
44	Montana	599	0.30%
45	Delaware	587	0.30%
46	Vermont	393	0.20%
47	Alaska	349	0.18%
47	South Dakota	349	0.18%
49	Wyoming	294	0.15%
50	North Dakota	243	0.12%
	District of Columbia	773	0.39%

Source: U.S. Bureau of the Census
   "1992 Census of Service Industries, Geographic Area Series, United States" (SC92-A-52)
*Includes only establishments subject to the federal income tax.

Offices and Clinics of Dentists in 1992

National Total = 108,804 Establishments*

ALPHA ORDER

RANK	STATE	ESTABLISH'S	% of USA
27	Alabama	1,331	1.22%
45	Alaska	262	0.24%
25	Arizona	1,522	1.40%
33	Arkansas	822	0.76%
1	California	14,806	13.61%
21	Colorado	1,911	1.76%
22	Connecticut	1,740	1.60%
49	Delaware	215	0.20%
4	Florida	5,374	4.94%
13	Georgia	2,346	2.16%
36	Hawaii	640	0.59%
42	Idaho	455	0.42%
6	Illinois	5,156	4.74%
16	Indiana	2,177	2.00%
30	Iowa	1,149	1.06%
31	Kansas	1,003	0.92%
26	Kentucky	1,462	1.34%
24	Louisiana	1,548	1.42%
41	Maine	458	0.42%
15	Maryland	2,195	2.02%
10	Massachusetts	2,941	2.70%
8	Michigan	4,348	4.00%
19	Minnesota	2,010	1.85%
34	Mississippi	784	0.72%
18	Missouri	2,047	1.88%
44	Montana	397	0.36%
35	Nebraska	747	0.69%
40	Nevada	478	0.44%
39	New Hampshire	514	0.47%
9	New Jersey	4,033	3.71%
38	New Mexico	532	0.49%
2	New York	8,560	7.87%
17	North Carolina	2,162	1.99%
47	North Dakota	250	0.23%
7	Ohio	4,497	4.13%
28	Oklahoma	1,229	1.13%
23	Oregon	1,587	1.46%
5	Pennsylvania	5,316	4.89%
43	Rhode Island	406	0.37%
29	South Carolina	1,153	1.06%
46	South Dakota	260	0.24%
20	Tennessee	1,984	1.82%
3	Texas	6,233	5.73%
32	Utah	974	0.90%
48	Vermont	245	0.23%
12	Virginia	2,524	2.32%
11	Washington	2,674	2.46%
37	West Virginia	563	0.52%
14	Wisconsin	2,235	2.05%
50	Wyoming	202	0.19%

RANK ORDER

RANK	STATE	ESTABLISH'S	% of USA
1	California	14,806	13.61%
2	New York	8,560	7.87%
3	Texas	6,233	5.73%
4	Florida	5,374	4.94%
5	Pennsylvania	5,316	4.89%
6	Illinois	5,156	4.74%
7	Ohio	4,497	4.13%
8	Michigan	4,348	4.00%
9	New Jersey	4,033	3.71%
10	Massachusetts	2,941	2.70%
11	Washington	2,674	2.46%
12	Virginia	2,524	2.32%
13	Georgia	2,346	2.16%
14	Wisconsin	2,235	2.05%
15	Maryland	2,195	2.02%
16	Indiana	2,177	2.00%
17	North Carolina	2,162	1.99%
18	Missouri	2,047	1.88%
19	Minnesota	2,010	1.85%
20	Tennessee	1,984	1.82%
21	Colorado	1,911	1.76%
22	Connecticut	1,740	1.60%
23	Oregon	1,587	1.46%
24	Louisiana	1,548	1.42%
25	Arizona	1,522	1.40%
26	Kentucky	1,462	1.34%
27	Alabama	1,331	1.22%
28	Oklahoma	1,229	1.13%
29	South Carolina	1,153	1.06%
30	Iowa	1,149	1.06%
31	Kansas	1,003	0.92%
32	Utah	974	0.90%
33	Arkansas	822	0.76%
34	Mississippi	784	0.72%
35	Nebraska	747	0.69%
36	Hawaii	640	0.59%
37	West Virginia	563	0.52%
38	New Mexico	532	0.49%
39	New Hampshire	514	0.47%
40	Nevada	478	0.44%
41	Maine	458	0.42%
42	Idaho	455	0.42%
43	Rhode Island	406	0.37%
44	Montana	397	0.36%
45	Alaska	262	0.24%
46	South Dakota	260	0.24%
47	North Dakota	250	0.23%
48	Vermont	245	0.23%
49	Delaware	215	0.20%
50	Wyoming	202	0.19%
	District of Columbia	347	0.32%

Source: U.S. Bureau of the Census
"1992 Census of Service Industries, Geographic Area Series, United States" (SC92-A-52)
*Includes only establishments subject to the federal income tax.

Offices and Clinics of Doctors of Osteopathy in 1992

National Total = 8,708 Establishments*

ALPHA ORDER

RANK	STATE	ESTABLISH'S	% of USA
31	Alabama	32	0.37%
41	Alaska	11	0.13%
10	Arizona	317	3.64%
32	Arkansas	26	0.30%
9	California	322	3.70%
11	Colorado	207	2.38%
38	Connecticut	14	0.16%
26	Delaware	50	0.57%
4	Florida	762	8.75%
17	Georgia	124	1.42%
41	Hawaii	11	0.13%
39	Idaho	13	0.15%
14	Illinois	173	1.99%
16	Indiana	142	1.63%
13	Iowa	193	2.22%
20	Kansas	97	1.11%
30	Kentucky	38	0.44%
47	Louisiana	6	0.07%
18	Maine	120	1.38%
36	Maryland	16	0.18%
28	Massachusetts	40	0.46%
1	Michigan	1,201	13.79%
36	Minnesota	16	0.18%
34	Mississippi	20	0.23%
6	Missouri	446	5.12%
40	Montana	12	0.14%
49	Nebraska	2	0.02%
27	Nevada	41	0.47%
45	New Hampshire	9	0.10%
7	New Jersey	399	4.58%
23	New Mexico	57	0.65%
12	New York	201	2.31%
35	North Carolina	19	0.22%
49	North Dakota	2	0.02%
3	Ohio	821	9.43%
8	Oklahoma	328	3.77%
19	Oregon	112	1.29%
2	Pennsylvania	1,062	12.20%
24	Rhode Island	55	0.63%
33	South Carolina	21	0.24%
45	South Dakota	9	0.10%
25	Tennessee	52	0.60%
5	Texas	707	8.12%
43	Utah	10	0.11%
47	Vermont	6	0.07%
29	Virginia	39	0.45%
15	Washington	149	1.71%
22	West Virginia	90	1.03%
21	Wisconsin	96	1.10%
43	Wyoming	10	0.11%

RANK ORDER

RANK	STATE	ESTABLISH'S	% of USA
1	Michigan	1,201	13.79%
2	Pennsylvania	1,062	12.20%
3	Ohio	821	9.43%
4	Florida	762	8.75%
5	Texas	707	8.12%
6	Missouri	446	5.12%
7	New Jersey	399	4.58%
8	Oklahoma	328	3.77%
9	California	322	3.70%
10	Arizona	317	3.64%
11	Colorado	207	2.38%
12	New York	201	2.31%
13	Iowa	193	2.22%
14	Illinois	173	1.99%
15	Washington	149	1.71%
16	Indiana	142	1.63%
17	Georgia	124	1.42%
18	Maine	120	1.38%
19	Oregon	112	1.29%
20	Kansas	97	1.11%
21	Wisconsin	96	1.10%
22	West Virginia	90	1.03%
23	New Mexico	57	0.65%
24	Rhode Island	55	0.63%
25	Tennessee	52	0.60%
26	Delaware	50	0.57%
27	Nevada	41	0.47%
28	Massachusetts	40	0.46%
29	Virginia	39	0.45%
30	Kentucky	38	0.44%
31	Alabama	32	0.37%
32	Arkansas	26	0.30%
33	South Carolina	21	0.24%
34	Mississippi	20	0.23%
35	North Carolina	19	0.22%
36	Maryland	16	0.18%
36	Minnesota	16	0.18%
38	Connecticut	14	0.16%
39	Idaho	13	0.15%
40	Montana	12	0.14%
41	Alaska	11	0.13%
41	Hawaii	11	0.13%
43	Utah	10	0.11%
43	Wyoming	10	0.11%
45	New Hampshire	9	0.10%
45	South Dakota	9	0.10%
47	Louisiana	6	0.07%
47	Vermont	6	0.07%
49	Nebraska	2	0.02%
49	North Dakota	2	0.02%
	District of Columbia	2	0.02%

Source: U.S. Bureau of the Census
"1992 Census of Service Industries, Geographic Area Series, United States" (SC92-A-52)
*Includes only establishments subject to the federal income tax.

Offices and Clinics of Chiropractors in 1992

National Total = 27,329 Establishments*

ALPHA ORDER

RANK	STATE	ESTABLISH'S	% of USA
29	Alabama	282	1.03%
47	Alaska	71	0.26%
14	Arizona	622	2.28%
31	Arkansas	237	0.87%
1	California	4,364	15.97%
16	Colorado	589	2.16%
24	Connecticut	347	1.27%
49	Delaware	50	0.18%
2	Florida	1,847	6.76%
12	Georgia	760	2.78%
39	Hawaii	119	0.44%
37	Idaho	134	0.49%
7	Illinois	1,068	3.91%
20	Indiana	436	1.60%
18	Iowa	446	1.63%
25	Kansas	321	1.17%
30	Kentucky	269	0.98%
28	Louisiana	284	1.04%
38	Maine	126	0.46%
32	Maryland	231	0.85%
17	Massachusetts	575	2.10%
8	Michigan	938	3.43%
10	Minnesota	824	3.02%
42	Mississippi	113	0.41%
15	Missouri	598	2.19%
41	Montana	117	0.43%
35	Nebraska	163	0.60%
34	Nevada	166	0.61%
43	New Hampshire	108	0.40%
6	New Jersey	1,245	4.56%
33	New Mexico	185	0.68%
3	New York	1,741	6.37%
19	North Carolina	439	1.61%
45	North Dakota	90	0.33%
9	Ohio	871	3.19%
27	Oklahoma	316	1.16%
21	Oregon	428	1.57%
5	Pennsylvania	1,310	4.79%
46	Rhode Island	79	0.29%
26	South Carolina	319	1.17%
40	South Dakota	118	0.43%
22	Tennessee	356	1.30%
4	Texas	1,426	5.22%
36	Utah	153	0.56%
48	Vermont	65	0.24%
23	Virginia	355	1.30%
11	Washington	804	2.94%
44	West Virginia	105	0.38%
13	Wisconsin	665	2.43%
50	Wyoming	41	0.15%

RANK ORDER

RANK	STATE	ESTABLISH'S	% of USA
1	California	4,364	15.97%
2	Florida	1,847	6.76%
3	New York	1,741	6.37%
4	Texas	1,426	5.22%
5	Pennsylvania	1,310	4.79%
6	New Jersey	1,245	4.56%
7	Illinois	1,068	3.91%
8	Michigan	938	3.43%
9	Ohio	871	3.19%
10	Minnesota	824	3.02%
11	Washington	804	2.94%
12	Georgia	760	2.78%
13	Wisconsin	665	2.43%
14	Arizona	622	2.28%
15	Missouri	598	2.19%
16	Colorado	589	2.16%
17	Massachusetts	575	2.10%
18	Iowa	446	1.63%
19	North Carolina	439	1.61%
20	Indiana	436	1.60%
21	Oregon	428	1.57%
22	Tennessee	356	1.30%
23	Virginia	355	1.30%
24	Connecticut	347	1.27%
25	Kansas	321	1.17%
26	South Carolina	319	1.17%
27	Oklahoma	316	1.16%
28	Louisiana	284	1.04%
29	Alabama	282	1.03%
30	Kentucky	269	0.98%
31	Arkansas	237	0.87%
32	Maryland	231	0.85%
33	New Mexico	185	0.68%
34	Nevada	166	0.61%
35	Nebraska	163	0.60%
36	Utah	153	0.56%
37	Idaho	134	0.49%
38	Maine	126	0.46%
39	Hawaii	119	0.44%
40	South Dakota	118	0.43%
41	Montana	117	0.43%
42	Mississippi	113	0.41%
43	New Hampshire	108	0.40%
44	West Virginia	105	0.38%
45	North Dakota	90	0.33%
46	Rhode Island	79	0.29%
47	Alaska	71	0.26%
48	Vermont	65	0.24%
49	Delaware	50	0.18%
50	Wyoming	41	0.15%
	District of Columbia	13	0.05%

Source: U.S. Bureau of the Census
"1992 Census of Service Industries, Geographic Area Series, United States" (SC92-A-52)
Includes only establishments subject to the federal income tax.

Offices and Clinics of Optometrists in 1992

National Total = 17,135 Establishments*

ALPHA ORDER					RANK ORDER				
RANK	STATE		ESTABLISH'S	% of USA	RANK	STATE		ESTABLISH'S	% of USA
26	Alabama		229	1.34%	1	California		2,382	13.90%
49	Alaska		44	0.26%	2	Texas		1,100	6.42%
32	Arizona		189	1.10%	3	Pennsylvania		869	5.07%
29	Arkansas		202	1.18%	4	Florida		854	4.98%
1	California		2,382	13.90%	5	Ohio		836	4.88%
22	Colorado		257	1.50%	6	New York		791	4.62%
27	Connecticut		228	1.33%	7	Illinois		698	4.07%
50	Delaware		40	0.23%	8	Michigan		607	3.54%
4	Florida		854	4.98%	9	New Jersey		550	3.21%
13	Georgia		373	2.18%	10	North Carolina		498	2.91%
40	Hawaii		99	0.58%	11	Indiana		463	2.70%
41	Idaho		94	0.55%	12	Virginia		436	2.54%
7	Illinois		698	4.07%	13	Georgia		373	2.18%
11	Indiana		463	2.70%	14	Massachusetts		370	2.16%
21	Iowa		270	1.58%	15	Tennessee		364	2.12%
24	Kansas		247	1.44%	16	Wisconsin		347	2.03%
23	Kentucky		248	1.45%	17	Washington		341	1.99%
31	Louisiana		196	1.14%	18	Oklahoma		317	1.85%
35	Maine		123	0.72%	19	Missouri		301	1.76%
25	Maryland		235	1.37%	20	Minnesota		281	1.64%
14	Massachusetts		370	2.16%	21	Iowa		270	1.58%
8	Michigan		607	3.54%	22	Colorado		257	1.50%
20	Minnesota		281	1.64%	23	Kentucky		248	1.45%
34	Mississippi		148	0.86%	24	Kansas		247	1.44%
19	Missouri		301	1.76%	25	Maryland		235	1.37%
39	Montana		103	0.60%	26	Alabama		229	1.34%
36	Nebraska		121	0.71%	27	Connecticut		228	1.33%
37	Nevada		110	0.64%	28	Oregon		222	1.30%
44	New Hampshire		74	0.43%	29	Arkansas		202	1.18%
9	New Jersey		550	3.21%	30	South Carolina		198	1.16%
38	New Mexico		104	0.61%	31	Louisiana		196	1.14%
6	New York		791	4.62%	32	Arizona		189	1.10%
10	North Carolina		498	2.91%	33	West Virginia		151	0.88%
46	North Dakota		64	0.37%	34	Mississippi		148	0.86%
5	Ohio		836	4.88%	35	Maine		123	0.72%
18	Oklahoma		317	1.85%	36	Nebraska		121	0.71%
28	Oregon		222	1.30%	37	Nevada		110	0.64%
3	Pennsylvania		869	5.07%	38	New Mexico		104	0.61%
45	Rhode Island		72	0.42%	39	Montana		103	0.60%
30	South Carolina		198	1.16%	40	Hawaii		99	0.58%
43	South Dakota		80	0.47%	41	Idaho		94	0.55%
15	Tennessee		364	2.12%	42	Utah		81	0.47%
2	Texas		1,100	6.42%	43	South Dakota		80	0.47%
42	Utah		81	0.47%	44	New Hampshire		74	0.43%
48	Vermont		50	0.29%	45	Rhode Island		72	0.42%
12	Virginia		436	2.54%	46	North Dakota		64	0.37%
17	Washington		341	1.99%	47	Wyoming		54	0.32%
33	West Virginia		151	0.88%	48	Vermont		50	0.29%
16	Wisconsin		347	2.03%	49	Alaska		44	0.26%
47	Wyoming		54	0.32%	50	Delaware		40	0.23%
						District of Columbia		24	0.14%

Source: U.S. Bureau of the Census
  "1992 Census of Service Industries, Geographic Area Series, United States" (SC92-A-52)
*Includes only establishments subject to the federal income tax.

Offices and Clinics of Podiatrists in 1992

National Total = 7,948 Establishments*

ALPHA ORDER

RANK	STATE	ESTABLISH'S	% of USA
29	Alabama	49	0.62%
49	Alaska	5	0.06%
18	Arizona	121	1.52%
41	Arkansas	20	0.25%
2	California	930	11.70%
22	Colorado	88	1.11%
14	Connecticut	152	1.91%
39	Delaware	25	0.31%
4	Florida	564	7.10%
17	Georgia	139	1.75%
44	Hawaii	16	0.20%
43	Idaho	17	0.21%
7	Illinois	419	5.27%
12	Indiana	166	2.09%
23	Iowa	75	0.94%
26	Kansas	55	0.69%
31	Kentucky	46	0.58%
30	Louisiana	48	0.60%
34	Maine	36	0.45%
10	Maryland	211	2.65%
11	Massachusetts	208	2.62%
8	Michigan	400	5.03%
25	Minnesota	60	0.75%
42	Mississippi	18	0.23%
20	Missouri	98	1.23%
44	Montana	16	0.20%
35	Nebraska	34	0.43%
37	Nevada	28	0.35%
40	New Hampshire	24	0.30%
6	New Jersey	449	5.65%
36	New Mexico	33	0.42%
1	New York	938	11.80%
16	North Carolina	140	1.76%
48	North Dakota	7	0.09%
5	Ohio	490	6.17%
27	Oklahoma	52	0.65%
24	Oregon	61	0.77%
3	Pennsylvania	589	7.41%
28	Rhode Island	50	0.63%
33	South Carolina	40	0.50%
46	South Dakota	14	0.18%
21	Tennessee	90	1.13%
9	Texas	382	4.81%
32	Utah	44	0.55%
47	Vermont	9	0.11%
13	Virginia	164	2.06%
15	Washington	146	1.84%
38	West Virginia	26	0.33%
19	Wisconsin	119	1.50%
49	Wyoming	5	0.06%

RANK ORDER

RANK	STATE	ESTABLISH'S	% of USA
1	New York	938	11.80%
2	California	930	11.70%
3	Pennsylvania	589	7.41%
4	Florida	564	7.10%
5	Ohio	490	6.17%
6	New Jersey	449	5.65%
7	Illinois	419	5.27%
8	Michigan	400	5.03%
9	Texas	382	4.81%
10	Maryland	211	2.65%
11	Massachusetts	208	2.62%
12	Indiana	166	2.09%
13	Virginia	164	2.06%
14	Connecticut	152	1.91%
15	Washington	146	1.84%
16	North Carolina	140	1.76%
17	Georgia	139	1.75%
18	Arizona	121	1.52%
19	Wisconsin	119	1.50%
20	Missouri	98	1.23%
21	Tennessee	90	1.13%
22	Colorado	88	1.11%
23	Iowa	75	0.94%
24	Oregon	61	0.77%
25	Minnesota	60	0.75%
26	Kansas	55	0.69%
27	Oklahoma	52	0.65%
28	Rhode Island	50	0.63%
29	Alabama	49	0.62%
30	Louisiana	48	0.60%
31	Kentucky	46	0.58%
32	Utah	44	0.55%
33	South Carolina	40	0.50%
34	Maine	36	0.45%
35	Nebraska	34	0.43%
36	New Mexico	33	0.42%
37	Nevada	28	0.35%
38	West Virginia	26	0.33%
39	Delaware	25	0.31%
40	New Hampshire	24	0.30%
41	Arkansas	20	0.25%
42	Mississippi	18	0.23%
43	Idaho	17	0.21%
44	Hawaii	16	0.20%
44	Montana	16	0.20%
46	South Dakota	14	0.18%
47	Vermont	9	0.11%
48	North Dakota	7	0.09%
49	Alaska	5	0.06%
49	Wyoming	5	0.06%
	District of Columbia	32	0.40%

Source: U.S. Bureau of the Census
"1992 Census of Service Industries, Geographic Area Series, United States" (SC92-A-52)
*Includes only establishments subject to the federal income tax.

Offices and Clinics of Other Health Practitioners in 1992

National Total = 22,260 Establishments*

ALPHA ORDER					RANK ORDER			
RANK	STATE	ESTABLISH'S	% of USA		RANK	STATE	ESTABLISH'S	% of USA
28	Alabama	174	0.78%		1	California	3,954	17.76%
47	Alaska	60	0.27%		2	Florida	1,644	7.39%
17	Arizona	447	2.01%		3	Texas	1,636	7.35%
33	Arkansas	156	0.70%		4	New York	1,344	6.04%
1	California	3,954	17.76%		5	Pennsylvania	899	4.04%
14	Colorado	515	2.31%		6	Ohio	860	3.86%
24	Connecticut	312	1.40%		7	Illinois	722	3.24%
43	Delaware	76	0.34%		8	Michigan	669	3.01%
2	Florida	1,644	7.39%		9	New Jersey	666	2.99%
12	Georgia	544	2.44%		10	Washington	620	2.79%
37	Hawaii	120	0.54%		11	Maryland	592	2.66%
42	Idaho	79	0.35%		12	Georgia	544	2.44%
7	Illinois	722	3.24%		13	Massachusetts	526	2.36%
25	Indiana	275	1.24%		14	Colorado	515	2.31%
33	Iowa	156	0.70%		15	North Carolina	497	2.23%
32	Kansas	158	0.71%		16	Virginia	485	2.18%
27	Kentucky	212	0.95%		17	Arizona	447	2.01%
23	Louisiana	324	1.46%		18	Missouri	374	1.68%
38	Maine	112	0.50%		19	Minnesota	361	1.62%
11	Maryland	592	2.66%		19	Oregon	361	1.62%
13	Massachusetts	526	2.36%		21	Wisconsin	340	1.53%
8	Michigan	669	3.01%		22	Tennessee	330	1.48%
19	Minnesota	361	1.62%		23	Louisiana	324	1.46%
40	Mississippi	102	0.46%		24	Connecticut	312	1.40%
18	Missouri	374	1.68%		25	Indiana	275	1.24%
41	Montana	86	0.39%		26	Oklahoma	228	1.02%
39	Nebraska	107	0.48%		27	Kentucky	212	0.95%
35	Nevada	130	0.58%		28	Alabama	174	0.78%
36	New Hampshire	128	0.58%		29	South Carolina	169	0.76%
9	New Jersey	666	2.99%		30	New Mexico	167	0.75%
30	New Mexico	167	0.75%		31	Utah	166	0.75%
4	New York	1,344	6.04%		32	Kansas	158	0.71%
15	North Carolina	497	2.23%		33	Arkansas	156	0.70%
50	North Dakota	31	0.14%		33	Iowa	156	0.70%
6	Ohio	860	3.86%		35	Nevada	130	0.58%
26	Oklahoma	228	1.02%		36	New Hampshire	128	0.58%
19	Oregon	361	1.62%		37	Hawaii	120	0.54%
5	Pennsylvania	899	4.04%		38	Maine	112	0.50%
46	Rhode Island	66	0.30%		39	Nebraska	107	0.48%
29	South Carolina	169	0.76%		40	Mississippi	102	0.46%
48	South Dakota	37	0.17%		41	Montana	86	0.39%
22	Tennessee	330	1.48%		42	Idaho	79	0.35%
3	Texas	1,636	7.35%		43	Delaware	76	0.34%
31	Utah	166	0.75%		44	Vermont	69	0.31%
44	Vermont	69	0.31%		44	West Virginia	69	0.31%
16	Virginia	485	2.18%		46	Rhode Island	66	0.30%
10	Washington	620	2.79%		47	Alaska	60	0.27%
44	West Virginia	69	0.31%		48	South Dakota	37	0.17%
21	Wisconsin	340	1.53%		48	Wyoming	37	0.17%
48	Wyoming	37	0.17%		50	North Dakota	31	0.14%
						District of Columbia	68	0.31%

Source: U.S. Bureau of the Census
   "1992 Census of Service Industries, Geographic Area Series, United States" (SC92-A-52)
*Includes only establishments subject to the federal income tax. Includes health practitioners not otherwise classified such as acupuncturists, midwives, nutritionists, physical and occupational therapists and psychologists.

IV. FINANCE

IV. FINANCE (Continued)

Persons Not Covered by Health Insurance in 1995

National Total = 40,485,060 Uninsured*

ALPHA ORDER

RANK	STATE	UNINSURED	% of USA
22	Alabama	573,210	1.42%
48	Alaska	75,375	0.19%
14	Arizona	878,220	2.17%
27	Arkansas	444,815	1.10%
1	California	6,502,390	16.06%
24	Colorado	554,704	1.37%
34	Connecticut	287,848	0.71%
43	Delaware	112,569	0.28%
4	Florida	2,595,672	6.41%
7	Georgia	1,290,411	3.19%
45	Hawaii	104,931	0.26%
39	Idaho	163,240	0.40%
6	Illinois	1,296,900	3.20%
18	Indiana	730,422	1.80%
32	Iowa	321,259	0.79%
33	Kansas	317,936	0.79%
23	Kentucky	563,122	1.39%
13	Louisiana	889,290	2.20%
38	Maine	167,265	0.41%
17	Maryland	770,967	1.90%
20	Massachusetts	673,881	1.66%
11	Michigan	925,186	2.29%
31	Minnesota	369,200	0.91%
26	Mississippi	531,112	1.31%
15	Missouri	776,574	1.92%
44	Montana	110,490	0.27%
40	Nebraska	147,510	0.36%
35	Nevada	286,671	0.71%
42	New Hampshire	114,800	0.28%
9	New Jersey	1,128,900	2.79%
28	New Mexico	432,640	1.07%
3	New York	2,765,032	6.83%
10	North Carolina	1,029,886	2.54%
50	North Dakota	53,286	0.13%
5	Ohio	1,324,946	3.27%
21	Oklahoma	628,800	1.55%
29	Oregon	393,625	0.97%
8	Pennsylvania	1,193,940	2.95%
41	Rhode Island	127,968	0.32%
25	South Carolina	535,382	1.32%
49	South Dakota	68,620	0.17%
16	Tennessee	776,556	1.92%
2	Texas	4,606,245	11.38%
37	Utah	229,086	0.57%
46	Vermont	77,220	0.19%
12	Virginia	893,025	2.21%
19	Washington	675,552	1.67%
36	West Virginia	279,225	0.69%
30	Wisconsin	373,906	0.92%
47	Wyoming	76,161	0.19%

RANK ORDER

RANK	STATE	UNINSURED	% of USA
1	California	6,502,390	16.06%
2	Texas	4,606,245	11.38%
3	New York	2,765,032	6.83%
4	Florida	2,595,672	6.41%
5	Ohio	1,324,946	3.27%
6	Illinois	1,296,900	3.20%
7	Georgia	1,290,411	3.19%
8	Pennsylvania	1,193,940	2.95%
9	New Jersey	1,128,900	2.79%
10	North Carolina	1,029,886	2.54%
11	Michigan	925,186	2.29%
12	Virginia	893,025	2.21%
13	Louisiana	889,290	2.20%
14	Arizona	878,220	2.17%
15	Missouri	776,574	1.92%
16	Tennessee	776,556	1.92%
17	Maryland	770,967	1.90%
18	Indiana	730,422	1.80%
19	Washington	675,552	1.67%
20	Massachusetts	673,881	1.66%
21	Oklahoma	628,800	1.55%
22	Alabama	573,210	1.42%
23	Kentucky	563,122	1.39%
24	Colorado	554,704	1.37%
25	South Carolina	535,382	1.32%
26	Mississippi	531,112	1.31%
27	Arkansas	444,815	1.10%
28	New Mexico	432,640	1.07%
29	Oregon	393,625	0.97%
30	Wisconsin	373,906	0.92%
31	Minnesota	369,200	0.91%
32	Iowa	321,259	0.79%
33	Kansas	317,936	0.79%
34	Connecticut	287,848	0.71%
35	Nevada	286,671	0.71%
36	West Virginia	279,225	0.69%
37	Utah	229,086	0.57%
38	Maine	167,265	0.41%
39	Idaho	163,240	0.40%
40	Nebraska	147,510	0.36%
41	Rhode Island	127,968	0.32%
42	New Hampshire	114,800	0.28%
43	Delaware	112,569	0.28%
44	Montana	110,490	0.27%
45	Hawaii	104,931	0.26%
46	Vermont	77,220	0.19%
47	Wyoming	76,161	0.19%
48	Alaska	75,375	0.19%
49	South Dakota	68,620	0.17%
50	North Dakota	53,286	0.13%
	District of Columbia	96,015	0.24%

Source: Morgan Quitno Press using data from U.S. Bureau of the Census
   "Health Insurance Coverage: 1995" (Current Population Reports, Series P60-195)
*Calculated by multiplying latest 1995 population estimates by percent of population uninsured.

Percent of Population Not Covered by Health Insurance in 1995

National Percent = 15.4% Not Covered by Health Insurance*

ALPHA ORDER

RANK	STATE	PERCENT
25	Alabama	13.5
32	Alaska	12.5
5	Arizona	20.4
10	Arkansas	17.9
3	California	20.6
17	Colorado	14.8
47	Connecticut	8.8
13	Delaware	15.7
9	Florida	18.3
10	Georgia	17.9
46	Hawaii	8.9
24	Idaho	14.0
40	Illinois	11.0
31	Indiana	12.6
38	Iowa	11.3
34	Kansas	12.4
19	Kentucky	14.6
4	Louisiana	20.5
25	Maine	13.5
14	Maryland	15.3
39	Massachusetts	11.1
43	Michigan	9.7
49	Minnesota	8.0
6	Mississippi	19.7
19	Missouri	14.6
30	Montana	12.7
45	Nebraska	9.0
8	Nevada	18.7
41	New Hampshire	10.0
23	New Jersey	14.2
1	New Mexico	25.6
16	New York	15.2
22	North Carolina	14.3
48	North Dakota	8.3
36	Ohio	11.9
7	Oklahoma	19.2
32	Oregon	12.5
42	Pennsylvania	9.9
29	Rhode Island	12.9
19	South Carolina	14.6
44	South Dakota	9.4
17	Tennessee	14.8
2	Texas	24.5
37	Utah	11.7
28	Vermont	13.2
25	Virginia	13.5
34	Washington	12.4
14	West Virginia	15.3
50	Wisconsin	7.3
12	Wyoming	15.9

RANK ORDER

RANK	STATE	PERCENT
1	New Mexico	25.6
2	Texas	24.5
3	California	20.6
4	Louisiana	20.5
5	Arizona	20.4
6	Mississippi	19.7
7	Oklahoma	19.2
8	Nevada	18.7
9	Florida	18.3
10	Arkansas	17.9
10	Georgia	17.9
12	Wyoming	15.9
13	Delaware	15.7
14	Maryland	15.3
14	West Virginia	15.3
16	New York	15.2
17	Colorado	14.8
17	Tennessee	14.8
19	Kentucky	14.6
19	Missouri	14.6
19	South Carolina	14.6
22	North Carolina	14.3
23	New Jersey	14.2
24	Idaho	14.0
25	Alabama	13.5
25	Maine	13.5
25	Virginia	13.5
28	Vermont	13.2
29	Rhode Island	12.9
30	Montana	12.7
31	Indiana	12.6
32	Alaska	12.5
32	Oregon	12.5
34	Kansas	12.4
34	Washington	12.4
36	Ohio	11.9
37	Utah	11.7
38	Iowa	11.3
39	Massachusetts	11.1
40	Illinois	11.0
41	New Hampshire	10.0
42	Pennsylvania	9.9
43	Michigan	9.7
44	South Dakota	9.4
45	Nebraska	9.0
46	Hawaii	8.9
47	Connecticut	8.8
48	North Dakota	8.3
49	Minnesota	8.0
50	Wisconsin	7.3
	District of Columbia	17.3

Source: U.S. Bureau of the Census
  "Health Insurance Coverage: 1995" (Current Population Reports, Series P60-195)
*Of those insured, 70.3% were covered by private insurance, 12.1% by Medicaid, 13.1% by Medicare and 3.5% by military health care coverage.

Persons Covered by Health Insurance in 1995

National Total = 222,404,940 Insured*

ALPHA ORDER

RANK	STATE	INSURED	% of USA
21	Alabama	3,672,790	1.65%
48	Alaska	527,625	0.24%
23	Arizona	3,426,780	1.54%
33	Arkansas	2,040,185	0.92%
1	California	25,062,610	11.27%
25	Colorado	3,193,296	1.44%
27	Connecticut	2,983,152	1.34%
46	Delaware	604,431	0.27%
4	Florida	11,588,328	5.21%
11	Georgia	5,918,589	2.66%
39	Hawaii	1,074,069	0.48%
42	Idaho	1,002,760	0.45%
6	Illinois	10,493,100	4.72%
14	Indiana	5,066,578	2.28%
30	Iowa	2,521,741	1.13%
31	Kansas	2,246,064	1.01%
24	Kentucky	3,293,878	1.48%
22	Louisiana	3,448,710	1.55%
40	Maine	1,071,735	0.48%
19	Maryland	4,268,033	1.92%
13	Massachusetts	5,397,119	2.43%
8	Michigan	8,612,814	3.87%
20	Minnesota	4,245,800	1.91%
32	Mississippi	2,164,888	0.97%
17	Missouri	4,542,426	2.04%
44	Montana	759,510	0.34%
36	Nebraska	1,491,490	0.67%
38	Nevada	1,246,329	0.56%
41	New Hampshire	1,033,200	0.46%
9	New Jersey	6,821,100	3.07%
37	New Mexico	1,257,360	0.57%
2	New York	15,425,968	6.94%
10	North Carolina	6,172,114	2.78%
47	North Dakota	588,714	0.26%
7	Ohio	9,809,054	4.41%
29	Oklahoma	2,646,200	1.19%
28	Oregon	2,755,375	1.24%
5	Pennsylvania	10,866,060	4.89%
43	Rhode Island	864,032	0.39%
26	South Carolina	3,131,618	1.41%
45	South Dakota	661,380	0.30%
18	Tennessee	4,470,444	2.01%
3	Texas	14,194,755	6.38%
34	Utah	1,728,914	0.78%
49	Vermont	507,780	0.23%
12	Virginia	5,721,975	2.57%
15	Washington	4,772,448	2.15%
35	West Virginia	1,545,775	0.70%
16	Wisconsin	4,748,094	2.13%
50	Wyoming	402,839	0.18%

RANK ORDER

RANK	STATE	INSURED	% of USA
1	California	25,062,610	11.27%
2	New York	15,425,968	6.94%
3	Texas	14,194,755	6.38%
4	Florida	11,588,328	5.21%
5	Pennsylvania	10,866,060	4.89%
6	Illinois	10,493,100	4.72%
7	Ohio	9,809,054	4.41%
8	Michigan	8,612,814	3.87%
9	New Jersey	6,821,100	3.07%
10	North Carolina	6,172,114	2.78%
11	Georgia	5,918,589	2.66%
12	Virginia	5,721,975	2.57%
13	Massachusetts	5,397,119	2.43%
14	Indiana	5,066,578	2.28%
15	Washington	4,772,448	2.15%
16	Wisconsin	4,748,094	2.13%
17	Missouri	4,542,426	2.04%
18	Tennessee	4,470,444	2.01%
19	Maryland	4,268,033	1.92%
20	Minnesota	4,245,800	1.91%
21	Alabama	3,672,790	1.65%
22	Louisiana	3,448,710	1.55%
23	Arizona	3,426,780	1.54%
24	Kentucky	3,293,878	1.48%
25	Colorado	3,193,296	1.44%
26	South Carolina	3,131,618	1.41%
27	Connecticut	2,983,152	1.34%
28	Oregon	2,755,375	1.24%
29	Oklahoma	2,646,200	1.19%
30	Iowa	2,521,741	1.13%
31	Kansas	2,246,064	1.01%
32	Mississippi	2,164,888	0.97%
33	Arkansas	2,040,185	0.92%
34	Utah	1,728,914	0.78%
35	West Virginia	1,545,775	0.70%
36	Nebraska	1,491,490	0.67%
37	New Mexico	1,257,360	0.57%
38	Nevada	1,246,329	0.56%
39	Hawaii	1,074,069	0.48%
40	Maine	1,071,735	0.48%
41	New Hampshire	1,033,200	0.46%
42	Idaho	1,002,760	0.45%
43	Rhode Island	864,032	0.39%
44	Montana	759,510	0.34%
45	South Dakota	661,380	0.30%
46	Delaware	604,431	0.27%
47	North Dakota	588,714	0.26%
48	Alaska	527,625	0.24%
49	Vermont	507,780	0.23%
50	Wyoming	402,839	0.18%
	District of Columbia	458,985	0.21%

Source: Morgan Quitno Press using data from U.S. Bureau of the Census
"Health Insurance Coverage: 1995" (Current Population Reports, Series P60-195)
Calculated by the editors by subtracting number of uninsured reported by Census from latest 1995 Census population estimates.

Percent of Population Covered by Health Insurance in 1995

National Percent = 84.6% of Population Covered by Health Insurance*

ALPHA ORDER

RANK ORDER

RANK	STATE	PERCENT		RANK	STATE	PERCENT
24	Alabama	86.5		1	Wisconsin	92.7
18	Alaska	87.5		2	Minnesota	92.0
46	Arizona	79.6		3	North Dakota	91.7
40	Arkansas	82.1		4	Connecticut	91.2
48	California	79.4		5	Hawaii	91.1
33	Colorado	85.2		6	Nebraska	91.0
4	Connecticut	91.2		7	South Dakota	90.6
38	Delaware	84.3		8	Michigan	90.3
42	Florida	81.7		9	Pennsylvania	90.1
40	Georgia	82.1		10	New Hampshire	90.0
5	Hawaii	91.1		11	Illinois	89.0
27	Idaho	86.0		12	Massachusetts	88.9
11	Illinois	89.0		13	Iowa	88.7
20	Indiana	87.4		14	Utah	88.3
13	Iowa	88.7		15	Ohio	88.1
16	Kansas	87.6		16	Kansas	87.6
30	Kentucky	85.4		16	Washington	87.6
47	Louisiana	79.5		18	Alaska	87.5
24	Maine	86.5		18	Oregon	87.5
36	Maryland	84.7		20	Indiana	87.4
12	Massachusetts	88.9		21	Montana	87.3
8	Michigan	90.3		22	Rhode Island	87.1
2	Minnesota	92.0		23	Vermont	86.8
45	Mississippi	80.3		24	Alabama	86.5
30	Missouri	85.4		24	Maine	86.5
21	Montana	87.3		24	Virginia	86.5
6	Nebraska	91.0		27	Idaho	86.0
43	Nevada	81.3		28	New Jersey	85.8
10	New Hampshire	90.0		29	North Carolina	85.7
28	New Jersey	85.8		30	Kentucky	85.4
50	New Mexico	74.4		30	Missouri	85.4
35	New York	84.8		30	South Carolina	85.4
29	North Carolina	85.7		33	Colorado	85.2
3	North Dakota	91.7		33	Tennessee	85.2
15	Ohio	88.1		35	New York	84.8
44	Oklahoma	80.8		36	Maryland	84.7
18	Oregon	87.5		36	West Virginia	84.7
9	Pennsylvania	90.1		38	Delaware	84.3
22	Rhode Island	87.1		39	Wyoming	84.1
30	South Carolina	85.4		40	Arkansas	82.1
7	South Dakota	90.6		40	Georgia	82.1
33	Tennessee	85.2		42	Florida	81.7
49	Texas	75.5		43	Nevada	81.3
14	Utah	88.3		44	Oklahoma	80.8
23	Vermont	86.8		45	Mississippi	80.3
24	Virginia	86.5		46	Arizona	79.6
16	Washington	87.6		47	Louisiana	79.5
36	West Virginia	84.7		48	California	79.4
1	Wisconsin	92.7		49	Texas	75.5
39	Wyoming	84.1		50	New Mexico	74.4
					District of Columbia	82.7

Source: Morgan Quitno Press using data from U.S. Bureau of the Census
"Health Insurance Coverage: 1995" (Current Population Reports, Series P60-195)
*This is the reverse of percent of population not covered in each state issued by Census.

Persons Not Covered by Health Insurance in 1991

National Total = 36,306,864 Uninsured*

RANK	STATE	UNINSURED	% of USA
14	Alabama	739,747	2.04%
46	Alaska	77,953	0.21%
18	Arizona	659,472	1.82%
29	Arkansas	374,618	1.03%
1	California	5,900,704	16.25%
30	Colorado	347,110	0.96%
35	Connecticut	250,116	0.69%
44	Delaware	92,480	0.25%
3	Florida	2,511,432	6.92%
10	Georgia	940,608	2.59%
45	Hawaii	80,514	0.22%
38	Idaho	187,020	0.52%
5	Illinois	1,359,950	3.75%
15	Indiana	733,993	2.02%
34	Iowa	251,280	0.69%
32	Kansas	286,580	0.79%
24	Kentucky	486,665	1.34%
11	Louisiana	886,369	2.44%
39	Maine	137,307	0.38%
19	Maryland	641,388	1.77%
16	Massachusetts	666,222	1.83%
13	Michigan	852,670	2.35%
27	Minnesota	411,897	1.13%
23	Mississippi	495,454	1.36%
20	Missouri	634,434	1.75%
42	Montana	103,424	0.28%
40	Nebraska	132,136	0.36%
37	Nevada	242,865	0.67%
41	New Hampshire	111,908	0.31%
12	New Jersey	854,370	2.35%
31	New Mexico	341,887	0.94%
4	New York	2,291,207	6.31%
8	North Carolina	1,012,800	2.79%
50	North Dakota	47,550	0.13%
6	Ohio	1,125,996	3.10%
21	Oklahoma	586,080	1.61%
26	Oregon	426,320	1.17%
9	Pennsylvania	955,760	2.63%
43	Rhode Island	103,412	0.28%
25	South Carolina	473,081	1.30%
48	South Dakota	70,200	0.19%
17	Tennessee	663,300	1.83%
2	Texas	3,954,432	10.89%
36	Utah	247,380	0.68%
47	Vermont	72,704	0.20%
7	Virginia	1,031,068	2.84%
22	Washington	531,908	1.47%
33	West Virginia	282,443	0.78%
28	Wisconsin	400,869	1.10%
49	Wyoming	51,296	0.14%

RANK	STATE	UNINSURED	% of USA
1	California	5,900,704	16.25%
2	Texas	3,954,432	10.89%
3	Florida	2,511,432	6.92%
4	New York	2,291,207	6.31%
5	Illinois	1,359,950	3.75%
6	Ohio	1,125,996	3.10%
7	Virginia	1,031,068	2.84%
8	North Carolina	1,012,800	2.79%
9	Pennsylvania	955,760	2.63%
10	Georgia	940,608	2.59%
11	Louisiana	886,369	2.44%
12	New Jersey	854,370	2.35%
13	Michigan	852,670	2.35%
14	Alabama	739,747	2.04%
15	Indiana	733,993	2.02%
16	Massachusetts	666,222	1.83%
17	Tennessee	663,300	1.83%
18	Arizona	659,472	1.82%
19	Maryland	641,388	1.77%
20	Missouri	634,434	1.75%
21	Oklahoma	586,080	1.61%
22	Washington	531,908	1.47%
23	Mississippi	495,454	1.36%
24	Kentucky	486,665	1.34%
25	South Carolina	473,081	1.30%
26	Oregon	426,320	1.17%
27	Minnesota	411,897	1.13%
28	Wisconsin	400,869	1.10%
29	Arkansas	374,618	1.03%
30	Colorado	347,110	0.96%
31	New Mexico	341,887	0.94%
32	Kansas	286,580	0.79%
33	West Virginia	282,443	0.78%
34	Iowa	251,280	0.69%
35	Connecticut	250,116	0.69%
36	Utah	247,380	0.68%
37	Nevada	242,865	0.67%
38	Idaho	187,020	0.52%
39	Maine	137,307	0.38%
40	Nebraska	132,136	0.36%
41	New Hampshire	111,908	0.31%
42	Montana	103,424	0.28%
43	Rhode Island	103,412	0.28%
44	Delaware	92,480	0.25%
45	Hawaii	80,514	0.22%
46	Alaska	77,953	0.21%
47	Vermont	72,704	0.20%
48	South Dakota	70,200	0.19%
49	Wyoming	51,296	0.14%
50	North Dakota	47,550	0.13%
	District of Columbia	155,628	0.43%

Source: Morgan Quitno Press using data from U.S. Bureau of the Census
"Health Insurance Coverage - 1993" (Statistical Brief, SB/94-28, October 1994)
*Based on percent of uninsured in each state issued by Census and 1991 state population estimates. National total calculated using 1991 national population estimate multiplied by Census national uninsured figure of 14.4%.

Percent of Persons Not Covered by Health Insurance in 1991

National Percent = 14.4% Uninsured

ALPHA ORDER

RANK	STATE	PERCENT
9	Alabama	18.1
19	Alaska	13.7
11	Arizona	17.6
13	Arkansas	15.8
4	California	19.4
37	Colorado	10.3
48	Connecticut	7.6
20	Delaware	13.6
6	Florida	18.9
17	Georgia	14.2
50	Hawaii	7.1
10	Idaho	18.0
30	Illinois	11.8
24	Indiana	13.1
44	Iowa	9.0
31	Kansas	11.5
24	Kentucky	13.1
3	Louisiana	20.9
33	Maine	11.1
23	Maryland	13.2
33	Massachusetts	11.1
43	Michigan	9.1
42	Minnesota	9.3
5	Mississippi	19.1
29	Missouri	12.3
26	Montana	12.8
45	Nebraska	8.3
6	Nevada	18.9
40	New Hampshire	10.1
35	New Jersey	11.0
2	New Mexico	22.1
28	New York	12.7
15	North Carolina	15.0
49	North Dakota	7.5
37	Ohio	10.3
8	Oklahoma	18.5
16	Oregon	14.6
47	Pennsylvania	8.0
37	Rhode Island	10.3
22	South Carolina	13.3
41	South Dakota	10.0
21	Tennessee	13.4
1	Texas	22.8
18	Utah	14.0
26	Vermont	12.8
12	Virginia	16.4
36	Washington	10.6
14	West Virginia	15.7
46	Wisconsin	8.1
32	Wyoming	11.2

RANK ORDER

RANK	STATE	PERCENT
1	Texas	22.8
2	New Mexico	22.1
3	Louisiana	20.9
4	California	19.4
5	Mississippi	19.1
6	Florida	18.9
6	Nevada	18.9
8	Oklahoma	18.5
9	Alabama	18.1
10	Idaho	18.0
11	Arizona	17.6
12	Virginia	16.4
13	Arkansas	15.8
14	West Virginia	15.7
15	North Carolina	15.0
16	Oregon	14.6
17	Georgia	14.2
18	Utah	14.0
19	Alaska	13.7
20	Delaware	13.6
21	Tennessee	13.4
22	South Carolina	13.3
23	Maryland	13.2
24	Indiana	13.1
24	Kentucky	13.1
26	Montana	12.8
26	Vermont	12.8
28	New York	12.7
29	Missouri	12.3
30	Illinois	11.8
31	Kansas	11.5
32	Wyoming	11.2
33	Maine	11.1
33	Massachusetts	11.1
35	New Jersey	11.0
36	Washington	10.6
37	Colorado	10.3
37	Ohio	10.3
37	Rhode Island	10.3
40	New Hampshire	10.1
41	South Dakota	10.0
42	Minnesota	9.3
43	Michigan	9.1
44	Iowa	9.0
45	Nebraska	8.3
46	Wisconsin	8.1
47	Pennsylvania	8.0
48	Connecticut	7.6
49	North Dakota	7.5
50	Hawaii	7.1
	District of Columbia	26.2

Source: U.S. Bureau of the Census
"Health Insurance Coverage - 1993" (Statistical Brief, SB/94-28, October 1994)

Change in Number of Uninsured Persons: 1991 to 1995

National Change = 4,178,196 Increase

RANK	STATE	CHANGE
50	Alabama	(166,537)
40	Alaska	(2,578)
7	Arizona	218,748
18	Arkansas	70,197
2	California	601,686
8	Colorado	207,594
23	Connecticut	37,732
30	Delaware	20,089
15	Florida	84,240
4	Georgia	349,803
29	Hawaii	24,417
44	Idaho	(23,780)
48	Illinois	(63,050)
42	Indiana	(3,571)
19	Iowa	69,979
25	Kansas	31,356
16	Kentucky	76,457
37	Louisiana	2,921
26	Maine	29,958
12	Maryland	129,579
33	Massachusetts	7,659
17	Michigan	72,516
47	Minnesota	(42,697)
24	Mississippi	35,658
11	Missouri	142,140
34	Montana	7,066
32	Nebraska	15,374
21	Nevada	43,806
38	New Hampshire	2,892
5	New Jersey	274,530
14	New Mexico	90,753
3	New York	473,825
31	North Carolina	17,086
35	North Dakota	5,736
9	Ohio	198,950
22	Oklahoma	42,720
46	Oregon	(32,695)
6	Pennsylvania	238,180
28	Rhode Island	24,556
20	South Carolina	62,301
39	South Dakota	(1,580)
13	Tennessee	113,256
1	Texas	651,813
43	Utah	(18,294)
36	Vermont	4,516
49	Virginia	(138,043)
10	Washington	143,644
41	West Virginia	(3,218)
45	Wisconsin	(26,963)
27	Wyoming	24,865

RANK ORDER

RANK	STATE	CHANGE
1	Texas	651,813
2	California	601,686
3	New York	473,825
4	Georgia	349,803
5	New Jersey	274,530
6	Pennsylvania	238,180
7	Arizona	218,748
8	Colorado	207,594
9	Ohio	198,950
10	Washington	143,644
11	Missouri	142,140
12	Maryland	129,579
13	Tennessee	113,256
14	New Mexico	90,753
15	Florida	84,240
16	Kentucky	76,457
17	Michigan	72,516
18	Arkansas	70,197
19	Iowa	69,979
20	South Carolina	62,301
21	Nevada	43,806
22	Oklahoma	42,720
23	Connecticut	37,732
24	Mississippi	35,658
25	Kansas	31,356
26	Maine	29,958
27	Wyoming	24,865
28	Rhode Island	24,556
29	Hawaii	24,417
30	Delaware	20,089
31	North Carolina	17,086
32	Nebraska	15,374
33	Massachusetts	7,659
34	Montana	7,066
35	North Dakota	5,736
36	Vermont	4,516
37	Louisiana	2,921
38	New Hampshire	2,892
39	South Dakota	(1,580)
40	Alaska	(2,578)
41	West Virginia	(3,218)
42	Indiana	(3,571)
43	Utah	(18,294)
44	Idaho	(23,780)
45	Wisconsin	(26,963)
46	Oregon	(32,695)
47	Minnesota	(42,697)
48	Illinois	(63,050)
49	Virginia	(138,043)
50	Alabama	(166,537)
	District of Columbia	(59,613)

Source: Morgan Quitno Press using data from U.S. Bureau of the Census
"Health Insurance Coverage: 1995" (Current Population Reports, Series P60-195) and
"Health Insurance Coverage: 1993" (Statistical Brief, SB/94-28, October 1994)

Percent Change in Number of Uninsured: 1991 to 1995

National Percent Change = 11.51% Increase

RANK	STATE	PERCENT CHANGE
50	Alabama	(22.51)
42	Alaska	(3.31)
4	Arizona	33.17
17	Arkansas	18.74
28	California	10.20
1	Colorado	59.81
23	Connecticut	15.09
14	Delaware	21.72
34	Florida	3.35
3	Georgia	37.19
6	Hawaii	30.33
48	Idaho	(12.72)
43	Illinois	(4.64)
39	Indiana	(0.49)
7	Iowa	27.85
27	Kansas	10.94
22	Kentucky	15.71
38	Louisiana	0.33
13	Maine	21.82
16	Maryland	20.20
37	Massachusetts	1.15
29	Michigan	8.50
47	Minnesota	(10.37)
31	Mississippi	7.20
12	Missouri	22.40
32	Montana	6.83
26	Nebraska	11.63
18	Nevada	18.04
35	New Hampshire	2.58
5	New Jersey	32.13
9	New Mexico	26.54
15	New York	20.68
36	North Carolina	1.69
25	North Dakota	12.06
19	Ohio	17.67
30	Oklahoma	7.29
46	Oregon	(7.67)
10	Pennsylvania	24.92
11	Rhode Island	23.75
24	South Carolina	13.17
41	South Dakota	(2.25)
20	Tennessee	17.07
21	Texas	16.48
45	Utah	(7.40)
33	Vermont	6.21
49	Virginia	(13.39)
8	Washington	27.01
40	West Virginia	(1.14)
44	Wisconsin	(6.73)
2	Wyoming	48.47

RANK	STATE	PERCENT CHANGE
1	Colorado	59.81
2	Wyoming	48.47
3	Georgia	37.19
4	Arizona	33.17
5	New Jersey	32.13
6	Hawaii	30.33
7	Iowa	27.85
8	Washington	27.01
9	New Mexico	26.54
10	Pennsylvania	24.92
11	Rhode Island	23.75
12	Missouri	22.40
13	Maine	21.82
14	Delaware	21.72
15	New York	20.68
16	Maryland	20.20
17	Arkansas	18.74
18	Nevada	18.04
19	Ohio	17.67
20	Tennessee	17.07
21	Texas	16.48
22	Kentucky	15.71
23	Connecticut	15.09
24	South Carolina	13.17
25	North Dakota	12.06
26	Nebraska	11.63
27	Kansas	10.94
28	California	10.20
29	Michigan	8.50
30	Oklahoma	7.29
31	Mississippi	7.20
32	Montana	6.83
33	Vermont	6.21
34	Florida	3.35
35	New Hampshire	2.58
36	North Carolina	1.69
37	Massachusetts	1.15
38	Louisiana	0.33
39	Indiana	(0.49)
40	West Virginia	(1.14)
41	South Dakota	(2.25)
42	Alaska	(3.31)
43	Illinois	(4.64)
44	Wisconsin	(6.73)
45	Utah	(7.40)
46	Oregon	(7.67)
47	Minnesota	(10.37)
48	Idaho	(12.72)
49	Virginia	(13.39)
50	Alabama	(22.51)
	District of Columbia	(38.30)

Source: Morgan Quitno Press using data from U.S. Bureau of the Census
"Health Insurance Coverage: 1995" (Current Population Reports, Series P60-195) and
"Health Insurance Coverage: 1993" (Statistical Brief, SB/94-28, October 1994)

Change in Percent of Population Uninsured: 1991 to 1995

National Percent Change = 6.94% Increase

ALPHA ORDER

RANK	STATE	PERCENT CHANGE
50	Alabama	(25.41)
43	Alaska	(8.76)
13	Arizona	15.91
19	Arkansas	13.29
28	California	6.19
1	Colorado	43.69
16	Connecticut	15.79
18	Delaware	15.44
38	Florida	(3.17)
4	Georgia	26.06
6	Hawaii	25.35
49	Idaho	(22.22)
42	Illinois	(6.78)
39	Indiana	(3.82)
5	Iowa	25.56
25	Kansas	7.83
20	Kentucky	11.45
36	Louisiana	(1.91)
9	Maine	21.62
13	Maryland	15.91
32	Massachusetts	0.00
27	Michigan	6.59
45	Minnesota	(13.98)
30	Mississippi	3.14
11	Missouri	18.70
33	Montana	(0.78)
24	Nebraska	8.43
35	Nevada	(1.06)
34	New Hampshire	(0.99)
3	New Jersey	29.09
15	New Mexico	15.84
10	New York	19.69
40	North Carolina	(4.67)
21	North Dakota	10.67
17	Ohio	15.53
29	Oklahoma	3.78
46	Oregon	(14.38)
8	Pennsylvania	23.75
7	Rhode Island	25.24
23	South Carolina	9.77
41	South Dakota	(6.00)
22	Tennessee	10.45
26	Texas	7.46
47	Utah	(16.43)
31	Vermont	3.13
48	Virginia	(17.68)
12	Washington	16.98
37	West Virginia	(2.55)
44	Wisconsin	(9.88)
2	Wyoming	41.96

RANK ORDER

RANK	STATE	PERCENT CHANGE
1	Colorado	43.69
2	Wyoming	41.96
3	New Jersey	29.09
4	Georgia	26.06
5	Iowa	25.56
6	Hawaii	25.35
7	Rhode Island	25.24
8	Pennsylvania	23.75
9	Maine	21.62
10	New York	19.69
11	Missouri	18.70
12	Washington	16.98
13	Arizona	15.91
13	Maryland	15.91
15	New Mexico	15.84
16	Connecticut	15.79
17	Ohio	15.53
18	Delaware	15.44
19	Arkansas	13.29
20	Kentucky	11.45
21	North Dakota	10.67
22	Tennessee	10.45
23	South Carolina	9.77
24	Nebraska	8.43
25	Kansas	7.83
26	Texas	7.46
27	Michigan	6.59
28	California	6.19
29	Oklahoma	3.78
30	Mississippi	3.14
31	Vermont	3.13
32	Massachusetts	0.00
33	Montana	(0.78)
34	New Hampshire	(0.99)
35	Nevada	(1.06)
36	Louisiana	(1.91)
37	West Virginia	(2.55)
38	Florida	(3.17)
39	Indiana	(3.82)
40	North Carolina	(4.67)
41	South Dakota	(6.00)
42	Illinois	(6.78)
43	Alaska	(8.76)
44	Wisconsin	(9.88)
45	Minnesota	(13.98)
46	Oregon	(14.38)
47	Utah	(16.43)
48	Virginia	(17.68)
49	Idaho	(22.22)
50	Alabama	(25.41)
	District of Columbia	(33.97)

Source: Morgan Quitno Press using data from U.S. Bureau of the Census
"Health Insurance Coverage: 1995" (Current Population Reports, Series P60-195) and
"Health Insurance Coverage: 1993" (Statistical Brief, SB/94-28, October 1994)

Managed Care Organizations (MCOs) in 1995

National Total = 1,691 MCOs*

ALPHA ORDER

RANK	STATE	MCOs	% of USA
21	Alabama	35	2.07%
46	Alaska	3	0.18%
12	Arizona	47	2.78%
36	Arkansas	15	0.89%
2	California	114	6.74%
15	Colorado	40	2.37%
26	Connecticut	27	1.60%
38	Delaware	12	0.71%
1	Florida	118	6.98%
10	Georgia	52	3.08%
37	Hawaii	13	0.77%
46	Idaho	3	0.18%
6	Illinois	72	4.26%
14	Indiana	45	2.66%
33	Iowa	18	1.06%
28	Kansas	26	1.54%
30	Kentucky	22	1.30%
15	Louisiana	40	2.37%
39	Maine	11	0.65%
18	Maryland	37	2.19%
19	Massachusetts	36	2.13%
13	Michigan	46	2.72%
25	Minnesota	28	1.66%
40	Mississippi	8	0.47%
11	Missouri	48	2.84%
49	Montana	2	0.12%
34	Nebraska	17	1.01%
23	Nevada	33	1.95%
40	New Hampshire	8	0.47%
24	New Jersey	32	1.89%
35	New Mexico	16	0.95%
7	New York	57	3.37%
17	North Carolina	39	2.31%
45	North Dakota	4	0.24%
4	Ohio	82	4.85%
26	Oklahoma	27	1.60%
32	Oregon	19	1.12%
5	Pennsylvania	76	4.49%
43	Rhode Island	6	0.35%
29	South Carolina	23	1.36%
44	South Dakota	5	0.30%
7	Tennessee	57	3.37%
3	Texas	105	6.21%
31	Utah	21	1.24%
46	Vermont	3	0.18%
19	Virginia	36	2.13%
22	Washington	34	2.01%
40	West Virginia	8	0.47%
9	Wisconsin	53	3.13%
50	Wyoming	0	0.00%

RANK ORDER

RANK	STATE	MCOs	% of USA
1	Florida	118	6.98%
2	California	114	6.74%
3	Texas	105	6.21%
4	Ohio	82	4.85%
5	Pennsylvania	76	4.49%
6	Illinois	72	4.26%
7	New York	57	3.37%
7	Tennessee	57	3.37%
9	Wisconsin	53	3.13%
10	Georgia	52	3.08%
11	Missouri	48	2.84%
12	Arizona	47	2.78%
13	Michigan	46	2.72%
14	Indiana	45	2.66%
15	Colorado	40	2.37%
15	Louisiana	40	2.37%
17	North Carolina	39	2.31%
18	Maryland	37	2.19%
19	Massachusetts	36	2.13%
19	Virginia	36	2.13%
21	Alabama	35	2.07%
22	Washington	34	2.01%
23	Nevada	33	1.95%
24	New Jersey	32	1.89%
25	Minnesota	28	1.66%
26	Connecticut	27	1.60%
26	Oklahoma	27	1.60%
28	Kansas	26	1.54%
29	South Carolina	23	1.36%
30	Kentucky	22	1.30%
31	Utah	21	1.24%
32	Oregon	19	1.12%
33	Iowa	18	1.06%
34	Nebraska	17	1.01%
35	New Mexico	16	0.95%
36	Arkansas	15	0.89%
37	Hawaii	13	0.77%
38	Delaware	12	0.71%
39	Maine	11	0.65%
40	Mississippi	8	0.47%
40	New Hampshire	8	0.47%
40	West Virginia	8	0.47%
43	Rhode Island	6	0.35%
44	South Dakota	5	0.30%
45	North Dakota	4	0.24%
46	Alaska	3	0.18%
46	Idaho	3	0.18%
46	Vermont	3	0.18%
49	Montana	2	0.12%
50	Wyoming	0	0.00%
	District of Columbia	9	0.53%

Source: Morgan Quitno Press using data from American Association of Health Plans
"1995-1996 Managed Health Care Overview"
*As of October 1995. Managed Care Organizations (MCOs) are a combination of Health Maintenance
Organizations (HMOs) and Preferred Provider Organizations (PPOs). Total does not include MCOs in Guam or
Puerto Rico. Health plans are allocated to states based upon their primary service areas. This means each plan is
counted once. However, many plans serve more than one state.

Enrollment in Managed Care Organizations (MCOs) in 1994

National Total = 136,092,671 Enrollees*

RANK	STATE	ENROLLEES	% of USA
28	Alabama	1,201,925	0.88%
49	Alaska	135,764	0.10%
20	Arizona	2,419,360	1.78%
36	Arkansas	662,168	0.49%
1	California	19,776,089	14.53%
25	Colorado	2,035,070	1.50%
24	Connecticut	2,043,761	1.50%
43	Delaware	260,781	0.19%
5	Florida	7,276,214	5.35%
15	Georgia	3,199,759	2.35%
35	Hawaii*	753,942	0.55%
44	Idaho	238,108	0.17%
6	Illinois	6,840,835	5.03%
19	Indiana	2,551,244	1.87%
27	Iowa	1,399,578	1.03%
31	Kansas	988,869	0.73%
26	Kentucky	1,417,466	1.04%
21	Louisiana	2,336,434	1.72%
42	Maine	327,029	0.24%
9	Maryland	3,975,222	2.92%
11	Massachusetts	3,795,701	2.79%
8	Michigan	4,876,209	3.58%
10	Minnesota	3,833,657	2.82%
38	Mississippi	603,075	0.44%
16	Missouri	2,939,247	2.16%
46	Montana	182,542	0.13%
37	Nebraska	621,263	0.46%
33	Nevada	843,816	0.62%
40	New Hampshire	432,635	0.32%
12	New Jersey	3,769,843	2.77%
34	New Mexico	779,386	0.57%
3	New York	8,398,596	6.17%
14	North Carolina	3,240,256	2.38%
45	North Dakota	185,217	0.14%
7	Ohio	6,057,577	4.45%
29	Oklahoma	1,144,255	0.84%
23	Oregon	2,077,673	1.53%
4	Pennsylvania	7,299,494	5.36%
41	Rhode Island	412,425	0.30%
30	South Carolina	1,027,572	0.76%
47	South Dakota	179,752	0.13%
13	Tennessee	3,500,036	2.57%
2	Texas	10,296,211	7.57%
32	Utah	966,574	0.71%
48	Vermont	164,127	0.12%
22	Virginia	2,226,008	1.64%
18	Washington	2,710,393	1.99%
39	West Virginia	442,034	0.32%
17	Wisconsin	2,773,074	2.04%
50	Wyoming	92,969	0.07%

RANK ORDER

RANK	STATE	ENROLLEES	% of USA
1	California	19,776,089	14.53%
2	Texas	10,296,211	7.57%
3	New York	8,398,596	6.17%
4	Pennsylvania	7,299,494	5.36%
5	Florida	7,276,214	5.35%
6	Illinois	6,840,835	5.03%
7	Ohio	6,057,577	4.45%
8	Michigan	4,876,209	3.58%
9	Maryland	3,975,222	2.92%
10	Minnesota	3,833,657	2.82%
11	Massachusetts	3,795,701	2.79%
12	New Jersey	3,769,843	2.77%
13	Tennessee	3,500,036	2.57%
14	North Carolina	3,240,256	2.38%
15	Georgia	3,199,759	2.35%
16	Missouri	2,939,247	2.16%
17	Wisconsin	2,773,074	2.04%
18	Washington	2,710,393	1.99%
19	Indiana	2,551,244	1.87%
20	Arizona	2,419,360	1.78%
21	Louisiana	2,336,434	1.72%
22	Virginia	2,226,008	1.64%
23	Oregon	2,077,673	1.53%
24	Connecticut	2,043,761	1.50%
25	Colorado	2,035,070	1.50%
26	Kentucky	1,417,466	1.04%
27	Iowa	1,399,578	1.03%
28	Alabama	1,201,925	0.88%
29	Oklahoma	1,144,255	0.84%
30	South Carolina	1,027,572	0.76%
31	Kansas	988,869	0.73%
32	Utah	966,574	0.71%
33	Nevada	843,816	0.62%
34	New Mexico	779,386	0.57%
35	Hawaii*	753,942	0.55%
36	Arkansas	662,168	0.49%
37	Nebraska	621,263	0.46%
38	Mississippi	603,075	0.44%
39	West Virginia	442,034	0.32%
40	New Hampshire	432,635	0.32%
41	Rhode Island	412,425	0.30%
42	Maine	327,029	0.24%
43	Delaware	260,781	0.19%
44	Idaho	238,108	0.17%
45	North Dakota	185,217	0.14%
46	Montana	182,542	0.13%
47	South Dakota	179,752	0.13%
48	Vermont	164,127	0.12%
49	Alaska	135,764	0.10%
50	Wyoming	92,969	0.07%
	District of Columbia	381,436	0.28%

Source: American Association of Health Plans (formerly American Managed Care and Review Association)
   "Managed Care Covered Lives, Year-end 1994"
*As of December 31, 1994 except Hawaii is December 31, 1993. Managed Care Organizations (MCOs) are a combination of Health Maintenance Organizations (HMOs) and Preferred Provider Organizations (PPOs). Total excludes 234,768 enrollees in Puerto Rico and 81,087 enrollees in Guam.

Percent of Population Enrolled in a
Managed Care Organization (MCO) in 1994
National Percent = 52.2% of Population*

ALPHA ORDER				RANK ORDER		
RANK	STATE	PERCENT		RANK	STATE	PERCENT
39	Alabama	28.5		1	Minnesota	83.9
47	Alaska	22.4		2	Maryland	79.4
10	Arizona	59.4		3	Tennessee	67.6
42	Arkansas	27.0		4	Oregon	67.3
6	California	62.9		5	Hawaii*	63.9
14	Colorado	55.7		6	California	62.9
8	Connecticut	62.4		7	Massachusetts	62.8
35	Delaware	36.9		8	Connecticut	62.4
19	Florida	52.1		9	Pennsylvania	60.6
28	Georgia	45.4		10	Arizona	59.4
5	Hawaii*	63.9		11	Illinois	58.2
49	Idaho	21.0		12	Nevada	57.9
11	Illinois	58.2		13	Texas	56.0
29	Indiana	44.4		14	Colorado	55.7
23	Iowa	49.5		14	Missouri	55.7
31	Kansas	38.7		16	Ohio	54.6
34	Kentucky	37.0		16	Wisconsin	54.6
18	Louisiana	54.1		18	Louisiana	54.1
43	Maine	26.4		19	Florida	52.1
2	Maryland	79.4		20	Michigan	51.4
7	Massachusetts	62.8		21	Utah	50.7
20	Michigan	51.4		21	Washington	50.7
1	Minnesota	83.9		23	Iowa	49.5
46	Mississippi	22.6		24	New Jersey	47.7
14	Missouri	55.7		25	New Mexico	47.1
48	Montana	21.3		26	New York	46.2
32	Nebraska	38.3		27	North Carolina	45.8
12	Nevada	57.9		28	Georgia	45.4
33	New Hampshire	38.1		29	Indiana	44.4
24	New Jersey	47.7		30	Rhode Island	41.4
25	New Mexico	47.1		31	Kansas	38.7
26	New York	46.2		32	Nebraska	38.3
27	North Carolina	45.8		33	New Hampshire	38.1
38	North Dakota	29.0		34	Kentucky	37.0
16	Ohio	54.6		35	Delaware	36.9
36	Oklahoma	35.1		36	Oklahoma	35.1
4	Oregon	67.3		37	Virginia	34.0
9	Pennsylvania	60.6		38	North Dakota	29.0
30	Rhode Island	41.4		39	Alabama	28.5
41	South Carolina	28.0		40	Vermont	28.3
44	South Dakota	24.9		41	South Carolina	28.0
3	Tennessee	67.6		42	Arkansas	27.0
13	Texas	56.0		43	Maine	26.4
21	Utah	50.7		44	South Dakota	24.9
40	Vermont	28.3		45	West Virginia	24.3
37	Virginia	34.0		46	Mississippi	22.6
21	Washington	50.7		47	Alaska	22.4
45	West Virginia	24.3		48	Montana	21.3
16	Wisconsin	54.6		49	Idaho	21.0
50	Wyoming	19.5		50	Wyoming	19.5
				District of Columbia		66.9

Source: American Association of Health Plans (formerly American Managed Care and Review Association)
"Managed Care Covered Lives, Year-end 1994"
*As of December 31, 1994 except Hawaii is December 31, 1993. Managed Care Organizations (MCOs) are a combination of Health Maintenance Organizations (HMOs) and Preferred Provider Organizations (PPOs).

Health Maintenance Organizations (HMOs) in 1995

National Total = 668 HMOs*

ALPHA ORDER					RANK ORDER			
RANK	STATE		HMOs	% of USA	RANK	STATE	HMOs	% of USA
26	Alabama		10	1.50%	1	Florida	46	6.89%
49	Alaska		0	0.00%	2	California	42	6.29%
10	Arizona		20	2.99%	3	Ohio	38	5.69%
32	Arkansas		7	1.05%	4	New York	35	5.24%
2	California		42	6.29%	5	Texas	34	5.09%
23	Colorado		12	1.80%	6	Wisconsin	27	4.04%
16	Connecticut		16	2.40%	7	Illinois	26	3.89%
32	Delaware		7	1.05%	8	Missouri	23	3.44%
1	Florida		46	6.89%	9	Pennsylvania	22	3.29%
18	Georgia		15	2.25%	10	Arizona	20	2.99%
31	Hawaii		8	1.20%	10	Tennessee	20	2.99%
42	Idaho		2	0.30%	12	Maryland	19	2.84%
7	Illinois		26	3.89%	12	Michigan	19	2.84%
18	Indiana		15	2.25%	14	Virginia	18	2.69%
38	Iowa		5	0.75%	15	Massachusetts	17	2.54%
27	Kansas		9	1.35%	16	Connecticut	16	2.40%
35	Kentucky		6	0.90%	16	North Carolina	16	2.40%
20	Louisiana		14	2.10%	18	Georgia	15	2.25%
39	Maine		4	0.60%	18	Indiana	15	2.25%
12	Maryland		19	2.84%	20	Louisiana	14	2.10%
15	Massachusetts		17	2.54%	21	New Jersey	13	1.95%
12	Michigan		19	2.84%	21	Washington	13	1.95%
23	Minnesota		12	1.80%	23	Colorado	12	1.80%
46	Mississippi		1	0.15%	23	Minnesota	12	1.80%
8	Missouri		23	3.44%	23	Utah	12	1.80%
42	Montana		2	0.30%	26	Alabama	10	1.50%
35	Nebraska		6	0.90%	27	Kansas	9	1.35%
27	Nevada		9	1.35%	27	Nevada	9	1.35%
39	New Hampshire		4	0.60%	27	Oklahoma	9	1.35%
21	New Jersey		13	1.95%	27	Oregon	9	1.35%
32	New Mexico		7	1.05%	31	Hawaii	8	1.20%
4	New York		35	5.24%	32	Arkansas	7	1.05%
16	North Carolina		16	2.40%	32	Delaware	7	1.05%
41	North Dakota		3	0.45%	32	New Mexico	7	1.05%
3	Ohio		38	5.69%	35	Kentucky	6	0.90%
27	Oklahoma		9	1.35%	35	Nebraska	6	0.90%
27	Oregon		9	1.35%	35	South Carolina	6	0.90%
9	Pennsylvania		22	3.29%	38	Iowa	5	0.75%
42	Rhode Island		2	0.30%	39	Maine	4	0.60%
35	South Carolina		6	0.90%	39	New Hampshire	4	0.60%
46	South Dakota		1	0.15%	41	North Dakota	3	0.45%
10	Tennessee		20	2.99%	42	Idaho	2	0.30%
5	Texas		34	5.09%	42	Montana	2	0.30%
23	Utah		12	1.80%	42	Rhode Island	2	0.30%
46	Vermont		1	0.15%	42	West Virginia	2	0.30%
14	Virginia		18	2.69%	46	Mississippi	1	0.15%
21	Washington		13	1.95%	46	South Dakota	1	0.15%
42	West Virginia		2	0.30%	46	Vermont	1	0.15%
6	Wisconsin		27	4.04%	49	Alaska	0	0.00%
49	Wyoming		0	0.00%	49	Wyoming	0	0.00%
						District of Columbia	3	0.45%

Source: American Association of Health Plans (formerly Group Health Association of America)
   "1995-1996 Managed Health Care Overview"
*As of October 1995. Total does not include two HMOs in Guam or two in Puerto Rico. Health plans are allocated
to states based upon their primary service areas. This means each plan is counted once. However, many plans
serve more than one state.

Enrollees in Health Maintenance Organizations (HMOs) in 1996

National Total = 59,090,989 Enrollees*

ALPHA ORDER

RANK	STATE	ENROLLEES	% of USA
29	Alabama	340,284	0.58%
NA	Alaska**	NA	0.00%
17	Arizona	1,208,289	2.04%
28	Arkansas	381,140	0.65%
1	California	12,994,240	21.99%
18	Colorado	980,201	1.66%
19	Connecticut	979,280	1.66%
37	Delaware	212,504	0.36%
4	Florida	3,285,403	5.56%
22	Georgia	692,161	1.17%
33	Hawaii	262,580	0.44%
44	Idaho	44,466	0.08%
7	Illinois	2,342,163	3.96%
26	Indiana	571,489	0.97%
40	Iowa	137,938	0.23%
39	Kansas	161,556	0.27%
24	Kentucky	595,604	1.01%
27	Louisiana	477,561	0.81%
42	Maine	119,241	0.20%
11	Maryland	1,576,981	2.67%
5	Massachusetts	2,368,886	4.01%
8	Michigan	2,128,378	3.60%
14	Minnesota	1,328,530	2.25%
45	Mississippi	31,785	0.05%
16	Missouri	1,279,165	2.16%
46	Montana	26,102	0.04%
38	Nebraska	174,919	0.30%
32	Nevada	287,049	0.49%
35	New Hampshire	253,882	0.43%
10	New Jersey	1,829,144	3.10%
34	New Mexico	260,150	0.44%
2	New York	5,341,695	9.04%
20	North Carolina	809,145	1.37%
48	North Dakota	7,886	0.01%
9	Ohio	2,053,285	3.47%
30	Oklahoma	339,627	0.57%
12	Oregon	1,435,294	2.43%
3	Pennsylvania	3,309,632	5.60%
36	Rhode Island	235,499	0.40%
31	South Carolina	336,762	0.57%
47	South Dakota	20,408	0.03%
21	Tennessee	733,316	1.24%
6	Texas	2,347,386	3.97%
23	Utah	602,548	1.02%
43	Vermont	78,471	0.13%
25	Virginia	586,657	0.99%
15	Washington	1,305,125	2.21%
41	West Virginia	127,376	0.22%
13	Wisconsin	1,417,928	2.40%
NA	Wyoming**	NA	0.00%

RANK ORDER

RANK	STATE	ENROLLEES	% of USA
1	California	12,994,240	21.99%
2	New York	5,341,695	9.04%
3	Pennsylvania	3,309,632	5.60%
4	Florida	3,285,403	5.56%
5	Massachusetts	2,368,886	4.01%
6	Texas	2,347,386	3.97%
7	Illinois	2,342,163	3.96%
8	Michigan	2,128,378	3.60%
9	Ohio	2,053,285	3.47%
10	New Jersey	1,829,144	3.10%
11	Maryland	1,576,981	2.67%
12	Oregon	1,435,294	2.43%
13	Wisconsin	1,417,928	2.40%
14	Minnesota	1,328,530	2.25%
15	Washington	1,305,125	2.21%
16	Missouri	1,279,165	2.16%
17	Arizona	1,208,289	2.04%
18	Colorado	980,201	1.66%
19	Connecticut	979,280	1.66%
20	North Carolina	809,145	1.37%
21	Tennessee	733,316	1.24%
22	Georgia	692,161	1.17%
23	Utah	602,548	1.02%
24	Kentucky	595,604	1.01%
25	Virginia	586,657	0.99%
26	Indiana	571,489	0.97%
27	Louisiana	477,561	0.81%
28	Arkansas	381,140	0.65%
29	Alabama	340,284	0.58%
30	Oklahoma	339,627	0.57%
31	South Carolina	336,762	0.57%
32	Nevada	287,049	0.49%
33	Hawaii	262,580	0.44%
34	New Mexico	260,150	0.44%
35	New Hampshire	253,882	0.43%
36	Rhode Island	235,499	0.40%
37	Delaware	212,504	0.36%
38	Nebraska	174,919	0.30%
39	Kansas	161,556	0.27%
40	Iowa	137,938	0.23%
41	West Virginia	127,376	0.22%
42	Maine	119,241	0.20%
43	Vermont	78,471	0.13%
44	Idaho	44,466	0.08%
45	Mississippi	31,785	0.05%
46	Montana	26,102	0.04%
47	South Dakota	20,408	0.03%
48	North Dakota	7,886	0.01%
NA	Alaska**	NA	0.00%
NA	Wyoming**	NA	0.00%
	District of Columbia	585,077	0.99%

Source: InterStudy Publications (Minneapolis, MN)
  "The Competitive Edge Industry Report 6.2" (October 1996)
As of January 1, 1996. National total does not include 86,801 enrollees in Guam.
**Not available.*

Percent Change in Enrollees in Health Maintenance Organizations (HMOs): 1995 to 1996
National Percent Change = 16.7% Increase*

ALPHA ORDER

ALPHA ORDER

RANK	STATE	PERCENT CHANGE
36	Alabama	9.4
NA	Alaska**	NA
26	Arizona	15.1
1	Arkansas	307.8
34	California	11.4
32	Colorado	13.6
8	Connecticut	40.9
5	Delaware	60.7
20	Florida	23.1
14	Georgia	28.6
45	Hawaii	2.6
2	Idaho	165.7
26	Illinois	15.1
25	Indiana	17.7
40	Iowa	6.3
12	Kansas	31.7
48	Kentucky	(3.7)
7	Louisiana	52.7
9	Maine	38.4
42	Maryland	5.4
46	Massachusetts	1.5
37	Michigan	8.6
39	Minnesota	8.4
4	Mississippi	63.3
13	Missouri	30.8
17	Montana	26.3
19	Nebraska	23.2
21	Nevada	22.2
22	New Hampshire	21.4
6	New Jersey	56.5
44	New Mexico	2.8
35	New York	10.6
11	North Carolina	37.0
41	North Dakota	5.8
33	Ohio	12.6
10	Oklahoma	37.5
31	Oregon	14.1
16	Pennsylvania	26.8
24	Rhode Island	20.0
3	South Carolina	64.2
47	South Dakota	(2.1)
29	Tennessee	14.6
42	Texas	5.4
18	Utah	23.7
38	Vermont	8.5
28	Virginia	15.0
15	Washington	27.1
23	West Virginia	20.1
30	Wisconsin	14.3
NA	Wyoming**	NA

RANK ORDER

RANK	STATE	PERCENT CHANGE
1	Arkansas	307.8
2	Idaho	165.7
3	South Carolina	64.2
4	Mississippi	63.3
5	Delaware	60.7
6	New Jersey	56.5
7	Louisiana	52.7
8	Connecticut	40.9
9	Maine	38.4
10	Oklahoma	37.5
11	North Carolina	37.0
12	Kansas	31.7
13	Missouri	30.8
14	Georgia	28.6
15	Washington	27.1
16	Pennsylvania	26.8
17	Montana	26.3
18	Utah	23.7
19	Nebraska	23.2
20	Florida	23.1
21	Nevada	22.2
22	New Hampshire	21.4
23	West Virginia	20.1
24	Rhode Island	20.0
25	Indiana	17.7
26	Arizona	15.1
26	Illinois	15.1
28	Virginia	15.0
29	Tennessee	14.6
30	Wisconsin	14.3
31	Oregon	14.1
32	Colorado	13.6
33	Ohio	12.6
34	California	11.4
35	New York	10.6
36	Alabama	9.4
37	Michigan	8.6
38	Vermont	8.5
39	Minnesota	8.4
40	Iowa	6.3
41	North Dakota	5.8
42	Maryland	5.4
42	Texas	5.4
44	New Mexico	2.8
45	Hawaii	2.6
46	Massachusetts	1.5
47	South Dakota	(2.1)
48	Kentucky	(3.7)
NA	Alaska**	NA
NA	Wyoming**	NA
	District of Columbia**	NA

Source: InterStudy Publications (Minneapolis, MN)
"The Competitive Edge Industry Report 6.2" (October 1996)
*As of January 1, 1996.
**Not available.

Percent of Population Enrolled in Health Maintenance Organizations (HMOs) in 1996
National Percent = 22.3% Enrolled in HMOs*

ALPHA ORDER

RANK	STATE	PERCENT
40	Alabama	7.9
NA	Alaska**	NA
9	Arizona	29.0
27	Arkansas	15.2
2	California	40.3
13	Colorado	25.8
6	Connecticut	29.8
7	Delaware	29.3
17	Florida	23.0
37	Georgia	9.4
21	Hawaii	21.6
44	Idaho	3.7
22	Illinois	20.0
35	Indiana	9.9
43	Iowa	4.9
42	Kansas	6.3
26	Kentucky	15.3
32	Louisiana	11.0
36	Maine	9.5
4	Maryland	30.9
3	Massachusetts	39.0
19	Michigan	22.2
10	Minnesota	28.6
47	Mississippi	1.2
14	Missouri	24.0
45	Montana	2.9
33	Nebraska	10.8
23	Nevada	18.7
20	New Hampshire	21.9
17	New Jersey	23.0
25	New Mexico	15.5
8	New York	29.2
31	North Carolina	11.1
47	North Dakota	1.2
24	Ohio	18.5
34	Oklahoma	10.3
1	Oregon	44.8
12	Pennsylvania	27.4
15	Rhode Island	23.7
38	South Carolina	9.0
46	South Dakota	2.8
28	Tennessee	13.9
30	Texas	12.3
5	Utah	30.1
29	Vermont	13.4
39	Virginia	8.7
16	Washington	23.2
41	West Virginia	7.0
11	Wisconsin	27.6
NA	Wyoming**	NA

RANK ORDER

RANK	STATE	PERCENT
1	Oregon	44.8
2	California	40.3
3	Massachusetts	39.0
4	Maryland	30.9
5	Utah	30.1
6	Connecticut	29.8
7	Delaware	29.3
8	New York	29.2
9	Arizona	29.0
10	Minnesota	28.6
11	Wisconsin	27.6
12	Pennsylvania	27.4
13	Colorado	25.8
14	Missouri	24.0
15	Rhode Island	23.7
16	Washington	23.2
17	Florida	23.0
17	New Jersey	23.0
19	Michigan	22.2
20	New Hampshire	21.9
21	Hawaii	21.6
22	Illinois	20.0
23	Nevada	18.7
24	Ohio	18.5
25	New Mexico	15.5
26	Kentucky	15.3
27	Arkansas	15.2
28	Tennessee	13.9
29	Vermont	13.4
30	Texas	12.3
31	North Carolina	11.1
32	Louisiana	11.0
33	Nebraska	10.8
34	Oklahoma	10.3
35	Indiana	9.9
36	Maine	9.5
37	Georgia	9.4
38	South Carolina	9.0
39	Virginia	8.7
40	Alabama	7.9
41	West Virginia	7.0
42	Kansas	6.3
43	Iowa	4.9
44	Idaho	3.7
45	Montana	2.9
46	South Dakota	2.8
47	Mississippi	1.2
47	North Dakota	1.2
NA	Alaska**	NA
NA	Wyoming**	NA
	District of Columbia**	NA

Source: InterStudy Publications (Minneapolis, MN)
"The Competitive Edge Industry Report 6.2" (October 1996)
*As of January 1, 1996.
**Not available.

Percent of Insured Population
Enrolled in Health Maintenance Organizations (HMOs) in 1996
National Percent = 26.5% of Insured are Enrolled in HMOs*

<table>
<tr><th colspan="3">ALPHA ORDER</th><th colspan="3">RANK ORDER</th></tr>
<tr><th>RANK</th><th>STATE</th><th>PERCENT</th><th>RANK</th><th>STATE</th><th>PERCENT</th></tr>
<tr><td>40</td><td>Alabama</td><td>9.3</td><td>1</td><td>Oregon</td><td>52.1</td></tr>
<tr><td>49</td><td>Alaska</td><td>0.0</td><td>2</td><td>California</td><td>51.8</td></tr>
<tr><td>5</td><td>Arizona</td><td>35.3</td><td>3</td><td>Massachusetts</td><td>43.9</td></tr>
<tr><td>26</td><td>Arkansas</td><td>18.7</td><td>4</td><td>Maryland</td><td>36.9</td></tr>
<tr><td>2</td><td>California</td><td>51.8</td><td>5</td><td>Arizona</td><td>35.3</td></tr>
<tr><td>11</td><td>Colorado</td><td>30.7</td><td>6</td><td>Delaware</td><td>35.2</td></tr>
<tr><td>9</td><td>Connecticut</td><td>32.8</td><td>7</td><td>Utah</td><td>34.9</td></tr>
<tr><td>6</td><td>Delaware</td><td>35.2</td><td>8</td><td>New York</td><td>34.6</td></tr>
<tr><td>14</td><td>Florida</td><td>28.4</td><td>9</td><td>Connecticut</td><td>32.8</td></tr>
<tr><td>34</td><td>Georgia</td><td>11.7</td><td>10</td><td>Minnesota</td><td>31.3</td></tr>
<tr><td>21</td><td>Hawaii</td><td>24.4</td><td>11</td><td>Colorado</td><td>30.7</td></tr>
<tr><td>44</td><td>Idaho</td><td>4.4</td><td>12</td><td>Pennsylvania</td><td>30.5</td></tr>
<tr><td>23</td><td>Illinois</td><td>22.3</td><td>13</td><td>Wisconsin</td><td>29.9</td></tr>
<tr><td>36</td><td>Indiana</td><td>11.3</td><td>14</td><td>Florida</td><td>28.4</td></tr>
<tr><td>43</td><td>Iowa</td><td>5.5</td><td>15</td><td>Missouri</td><td>28.2</td></tr>
<tr><td>42</td><td>Kansas</td><td>7.2</td><td>16</td><td>Rhode Island</td><td>27.3</td></tr>
<tr><td>27</td><td>Kentucky</td><td>18.1</td><td>16</td><td>Washington</td><td>27.3</td></tr>
<tr><td>31</td><td>Louisiana</td><td>13.8</td><td>18</td><td>New Jersey</td><td>26.8</td></tr>
<tr><td>37</td><td>Maine</td><td>11.1</td><td>19</td><td>Michigan</td><td>24.7</td></tr>
<tr><td>4</td><td>Maryland</td><td>36.9</td><td>20</td><td>New Hampshire</td><td>24.6</td></tr>
<tr><td>3</td><td>Massachusetts</td><td>43.9</td><td>21</td><td>Hawaii</td><td>24.4</td></tr>
<tr><td>19</td><td>Michigan</td><td>24.7</td><td>22</td><td>Nevada</td><td>23.0</td></tr>
<tr><td>10</td><td>Minnesota</td><td>31.3</td><td>23</td><td>Illinois</td><td>22.3</td></tr>
<tr><td>47</td><td>Mississippi</td><td>1.5</td><td>24</td><td>Ohio</td><td>20.9</td></tr>
<tr><td>15</td><td>Missouri</td><td>28.2</td><td>25</td><td>New Mexico</td><td>20.7</td></tr>
<tr><td>45</td><td>Montana</td><td>3.4</td><td>26</td><td>Arkansas</td><td>18.7</td></tr>
<tr><td>34</td><td>Nebraska</td><td>11.7</td><td>27</td><td>Kentucky</td><td>18.1</td></tr>
<tr><td>22</td><td>Nevada</td><td>23.0</td><td>28</td><td>Texas</td><td>16.5</td></tr>
<tr><td>20</td><td>New Hampshire</td><td>24.6</td><td>29</td><td>Tennessee</td><td>16.4</td></tr>
<tr><td>18</td><td>New Jersey</td><td>26.8</td><td>30</td><td>Vermont</td><td>15.5</td></tr>
<tr><td>25</td><td>New Mexico</td><td>20.7</td><td>31</td><td>Louisiana</td><td>13.8</td></tr>
<tr><td>8</td><td>New York</td><td>34.6</td><td>32</td><td>North Carolina</td><td>13.1</td></tr>
<tr><td>32</td><td>North Carolina</td><td>13.1</td><td>33</td><td>Oklahoma</td><td>12.8</td></tr>
<tr><td>48</td><td>North Dakota</td><td>1.3</td><td>34</td><td>Georgia</td><td>11.7</td></tr>
<tr><td>24</td><td>Ohio</td><td>20.9</td><td>34</td><td>Nebraska</td><td>11.7</td></tr>
<tr><td>33</td><td>Oklahoma</td><td>12.8</td><td>36</td><td>Indiana</td><td>11.3</td></tr>
<tr><td>1</td><td>Oregon</td><td>52.1</td><td>37</td><td>Maine</td><td>11.1</td></tr>
<tr><td>12</td><td>Pennsylvania</td><td>30.5</td><td>38</td><td>South Carolina</td><td>10.8</td></tr>
<tr><td>16</td><td>Rhode Island</td><td>27.3</td><td>39</td><td>Virginia</td><td>10.3</td></tr>
<tr><td>38</td><td>South Carolina</td><td>10.8</td><td>40</td><td>Alabama</td><td>9.3</td></tr>
<tr><td>46</td><td>South Dakota</td><td>3.1</td><td>41</td><td>West Virginia</td><td>8.2</td></tr>
<tr><td>29</td><td>Tennessee</td><td>16.4</td><td>42</td><td>Kansas</td><td>7.2</td></tr>
<tr><td>28</td><td>Texas</td><td>16.5</td><td>43</td><td>Iowa</td><td>5.5</td></tr>
<tr><td>7</td><td>Utah</td><td>34.9</td><td>44</td><td>Idaho</td><td>4.4</td></tr>
<tr><td>30</td><td>Vermont</td><td>15.5</td><td>45</td><td>Montana</td><td>3.4</td></tr>
<tr><td>39</td><td>Virginia</td><td>10.3</td><td>46</td><td>South Dakota</td><td>3.1</td></tr>
<tr><td>16</td><td>Washington</td><td>27.3</td><td>47</td><td>Mississippi</td><td>1.5</td></tr>
<tr><td>41</td><td>West Virginia</td><td>8.2</td><td>48</td><td>North Dakota</td><td>1.3</td></tr>
<tr><td>13</td><td>Wisconsin</td><td>29.9</td><td>49</td><td>Alaska</td><td>0.0</td></tr>
<tr><td>49</td><td>Wyoming</td><td>0.0</td><td>49</td><td>Wyoming</td><td>0.0</td></tr>
<tr><td></td><td></td><td></td><td></td><td>District of Columbia**</td><td>NA</td></tr>
</table>

Source: Morgan Quitno Press using data from InterStudy Publications (Minneapolis, MN)
   "The Competitive Edge Industry Report 6.2" (October 1996)
*As of January 1, 1996. Calculated using estimated number of insured as of 1995.
**Not available.

Preferred Provider Organizations (PPOs) in 1995

National Total = 1,023 PPOs*

ALPHA ORDER

RANK	STATE	PPOs	% of USA
15	Alabama	25	2.44%
45	Alaska	3	0.29%
11	Arizona	27	2.64%
36	Arkansas	8	0.78%
1	California	72	7.04%
10	Colorado	28	2.74%
31	Connecticut	11	1.08%
40	Delaware	5	0.49%
1	Florida	72	7.04%
7	Georgia	37	3.62%
40	Hawaii	5	0.49%
47	Idaho	1	0.10%
5	Illinois	46	4.50%
9	Indiana	30	2.93%
30	Iowa	13	1.27%
26	Kansas	17	1.66%
28	Kentucky	16	1.56%
13	Louisiana	26	2.54%
37	Maine	7	0.68%
23	Maryland	18	1.76%
21	Massachusetts	19	1.86%
11	Michigan	27	2.64%
28	Minnesota	16	1.56%
37	Mississippi	7	0.68%
15	Missouri	25	2.44%
49	Montana	0	0.00%
31	Nebraska	11	1.08%
17	Nevada	24	2.35%
42	New Hampshire	4	0.39%
21	New Jersey	19	1.86%
34	New Mexico	9	0.88%
19	New York	22	2.15%
18	North Carolina	23	2.25%
47	North Dakota	1	0.10%
6	Ohio	44	4.30%
23	Oklahoma	18	1.76%
33	Oregon	10	0.98%
4	Pennsylvania	54	5.28%
42	Rhode Island	4	0.39%
26	South Carolina	17	1.66%
42	South Dakota	4	0.39%
7	Tennessee	37	3.62%
3	Texas	71	6.94%
34	Utah	9	0.88%
46	Vermont	2	0.20%
23	Virginia	18	1.76%
20	Washington	21	2.05%
39	West Virginia	6	0.59%
13	Wisconsin	26	2.54%
49	Wyoming	0	0.00%

RANK ORDER

RANK	STATE	PPOs	% of USA
1	California	72	7.04%
1	Florida	72	7.04%
3	Texas	71	6.94%
4	Pennsylvania	54	5.28%
5	Illinois	46	4.50%
6	Ohio	44	4.30%
7	Georgia	37	3.62%
7	Tennessee	37	3.62%
9	Indiana	30	2.93%
10	Colorado	28	2.74%
11	Arizona	27	2.64%
11	Michigan	27	2.64%
13	Louisiana	26	2.54%
13	Wisconsin	26	2.54%
15	Alabama	25	2.44%
15	Missouri	25	2.44%
17	Nevada	24	2.35%
18	North Carolina	23	2.25%
19	New York	22	2.15%
20	Washington	21	2.05%
21	Massachusetts	19	1.86%
21	New Jersey	19	1.86%
23	Maryland	18	1.76%
23	Oklahoma	18	1.76%
23	Virginia	18	1.76%
26	Kansas	17	1.66%
26	South Carolina	17	1.66%
28	Kentucky	16	1.56%
28	Minnesota	16	1.56%
30	Iowa	13	1.27%
31	Connecticut	11	1.08%
31	Nebraska	11	1.08%
33	Oregon	10	0.98%
34	New Mexico	9	0.88%
34	Utah	9	0.88%
36	Arkansas	8	0.78%
37	Maine	7	0.68%
37	Mississippi	7	0.68%
39	West Virginia	6	0.59%
40	Delaware	5	0.49%
40	Hawaii	5	0.49%
42	New Hampshire	4	0.39%
42	Rhode Island	4	0.39%
42	South Dakota	4	0.39%
45	Alaska	3	0.29%
46	Vermont	2	0.20%
47	Idaho	1	0.10%
47	North Dakota	1	0.10%
49	Montana	0	0.00%
49	Wyoming	0	0.00%
	District of Columbia	6	0.59%

Source: American Association of Health Plans (formerly American Managed Care and Review Association)
    "1995-1996 Managed Health Care Overview"
*As of October 1995. Total does not include two PPOs in Puerto Rico. Health plans are allocated to states based upon their primary service areas. This means each plan is counted once. However, many plans serve more than one state.

Enrollment in Preferred Provider Organizations (PPOs) in 1994

National Total = 82,718,223 Enrollees*

ALPHA ORDER

RANK	STATE	ENROLLEES	% of USA
28	Alabama	894,189	1.08%
48	Alaska	135,764	0.16%
24	Arizona	1,139,211	1.38%
34	Arkansas	543,067	0.66%
1	California	8,158,166	9.86%
25	Colorado	1,047,306	1.27%
22	Connecticut	1,216,321	1.47%
47	Delaware	142,408	0.17%
5	Florida	4,441,239	5.37%
12	Georgia	2,548,488	3.08%
36	Hawaii*	476,921	0.58%
42	Idaho	223,436	0.27%
3	Illinois	4,492,062	5.43%
15	Indiana	2,019,924	2.44%
21	Iowa	1,273,853	1.54%
30	Kansas	828,451	1.00%
26	Kentucky	997,952	1.21%
16	Louisiana	1,905,941	2.30%
41	Maine	237,285	0.29%
14	Maryland	2,030,314	2.45%
23	Massachusetts	1,212,304	1.47%
8	Michigan	2,993,934	3.62%
11	Minnesota	2,551,797	3.08%
33	Mississippi	595,775	0.72%
17	Missouri	1,765,073	2.13%
45	Montana	164,302	0.20%
39	Nebraska	429,040	0.52%
32	Nevada	758,716	0.92%
40	New Hampshire	247,763	0.30%
13	New Jersey	2,473,101	2.99%
35	New Mexico	502,898	0.61%
7	New York	3,736,986	4.52%
10	North Carolina	2,653,587	3.21%
44	North Dakota	175,524	0.21%
6	Ohio	3,834,255	4.64%
31	Oklahoma	797,987	0.96%
27	Oregon	944,388	1.14%
4	Pennsylvania	4,477,910	5.41%
43	Rhode Island	206,880	0.25%
29	South Carolina	846,363	1.02%
46	South Dakota	158,904	0.19%
9	Tennessee	2,758,071	3.33%
2	Texas	7,695,401	9.30%
37	Utah	471,422	0.57%
49	Vermont	116,900	0.14%
19	Virginia	1,640,166	1.98%
18	Washington	1,674,736	2.02%
38	West Virginia	442,034	0.53%
20	Wisconsin	1,402,472	1.70%
50	Wyoming	92,969	0.11%

RANK ORDER

RANK	STATE	ENROLLEES	% of USA
1	California	8,158,166	9.86%
2	Texas	7,695,401	9.30%
3	Illinois	4,492,062	5.43%
4	Pennsylvania	4,477,910	5.41%
5	Florida	4,441,239	5.37%
6	Ohio	3,834,255	4.64%
7	New York	3,736,986	4.52%
8	Michigan	2,993,934	3.62%
9	Tennessee	2,758,071	3.33%
10	North Carolina	2,653,587	3.21%
11	Minnesota	2,551,797	3.08%
12	Georgia	2,548,488	3.08%
13	New Jersey	2,473,101	2.99%
14	Maryland	2,030,314	2.45%
15	Indiana	2,019,924	2.44%
16	Louisiana	1,905,941	2.30%
17	Missouri	1,765,073	2.13%
18	Washington	1,674,736	2.02%
19	Virginia	1,640,166	1.98%
20	Wisconsin	1,402,472	1.70%
21	Iowa	1,273,853	1.54%
22	Connecticut	1,216,321	1.47%
23	Massachusetts	1,212,304	1.47%
24	Arizona	1,139,211	1.38%
25	Colorado	1,047,306	1.27%
26	Kentucky	997,952	1.21%
27	Oregon	944,388	1.14%
28	Alabama	894,189	1.08%
29	South Carolina	846,363	1.02%
30	Kansas	828,451	1.00%
31	Oklahoma	797,987	0.96%
32	Nevada	758,716	0.92%
33	Mississippi	595,775	0.72%
34	Arkansas	543,067	0.66%
35	New Mexico	502,898	0.61%
36	Hawaii*	476,921	0.58%
37	Utah	471,422	0.57%
38	West Virginia	442,034	0.53%
39	Nebraska	429,040	0.52%
40	New Hampshire	247,763	0.30%
41	Maine	237,285	0.29%
42	Idaho	223,436	0.27%
43	Rhode Island	206,880	0.25%
44	North Dakota	175,524	0.21%
45	Montana	164,302	0.20%
46	South Dakota	158,904	0.19%
47	Delaware	142,408	0.17%
48	Alaska	135,764	0.16%
49	Vermont	116,900	0.14%
50	Wyoming	92,969	0.11%
	District of Columbia	144,267	0.17%

Source: American Association of Health Plans (formerly American Managed Care and Review Association)
"Managed Care Covered Lives, Year-end 1994"
*As of December 31, 1994 except Hawaii is December 31, 1993. Total excludes 234,768 enrollees in Puerto Rico.

Percent of Population Enrolled in a
Preferred Provider Organization (PPO) in 1994
National Percent = 31.7% of Population*

ALPHA ORDER

RANK	STATE	PERCENT
41	Alabama	21.2
36	Alaska	22.4
25	Arizona	28.0
38	Arkansas	22.1
30	California	26.0
24	Colorado	28.6
12	Connecticut	37.1
44	Delaware	20.2
18	Florida	31.8
13	Georgia	36.1
8	Hawaii*	40.5
47	Idaho	19.7
9	Illinois	38.2
14	Indiana	35.1
4	Iowa	45.0
17	Kansas	32.4
29	Kentucky	26.1
5	Louisiana	44.2
50	Maine	19.1
7	Maryland	40.6
46	Massachusetts	20.1
19	Michigan	31.5
1	Minnesota	55.9
37	Mississippi	22.3
16	Missouri	33.4
49	Montana	19.2
28	Nebraska	26.4
3	Nevada	52.1
40	New Hampshire	21.8
20	New Jersey	31.3
23	New Mexico	30.4
43	New York	20.6
10	North Carolina	37.5
27	North Dakota	27.5
15	Ohio	34.5
33	Oklahoma	24.5
22	Oregon	30.6
11	Pennsylvania	37.2
42	Rhode Island	20.8
35	South Carolina	23.1
39	South Dakota	22.0
2	Tennessee	53.3
6	Texas	41.9
32	Utah	24.7
44	Vermont	20.2
31	Virginia	25.0
20	Washington	31.3
34	West Virginia	24.3
26	Wisconsin	27.6
48	Wyoming	19.5

RANK ORDER

RANK	STATE	PERCENT
1	Minnesota	55.9
2	Tennessee	53.3
3	Nevada	52.1
4	Iowa	45.0
5	Louisiana	44.2
6	Texas	41.9
7	Maryland	40.6
8	Hawaii*	40.5
9	Illinois	38.2
10	North Carolina	37.5
11	Pennsylvania	37.2
12	Connecticut	37.1
13	Georgia	36.1
14	Indiana	35.1
15	Ohio	34.5
16	Missouri	33.4
17	Kansas	32.4
18	Florida	31.8
19	Michigan	31.5
20	New Jersey	31.3
20	Washington	31.3
22	Oregon	30.6
23	New Mexico	30.4
24	Colorado	28.6
25	Arizona	28.0
26	Wisconsin	27.6
27	North Dakota	27.5
28	Nebraska	26.4
29	Kentucky	26.1
30	California	26.0
31	Virginia	25.0
32	Utah	24.7
33	Oklahoma	24.5
34	West Virginia	24.3
35	South Carolina	23.1
36	Alaska	22.4
37	Mississippi	22.3
38	Arkansas	22.1
39	South Dakota	22.0
40	New Hampshire	21.8
41	Alabama	21.2
42	Rhode Island	20.8
43	New York	20.6
44	Delaware	20.2
44	Vermont	20.2
46	Massachusetts	20.1
47	Idaho	19.7
48	Wyoming	19.5
49	Montana	19.2
50	Maine	19.1
	District of Columbia	25.3

Source: American Association of Health Plans (formerly American Managed Care and Review Association)
   "Managed Care Covered Lives, Year-end 1994"
*As of December 31, 1994 except Hawaii is December 31, 1993. National rate excludes enrollees in Puerto Rico.

Percent of Insured Population in a Preferred Provider Organization (PPO) in 1994
National Percent = 37.20% of Insured Population*

ALPHA ORDER

RANK	STATE	PERCENT
39	Alabama	25.70
38	Alaska	26.46
24	Arizona	33.71
36	Arkansas	27.22
25	California	32.61
26	Colorado	31.93
11	Connecticut	42.51
42	Delaware	24.18
19	Florida	37.59
12	Georgia	42.01
7	Hawaii	47.45
46	Idaho	22.80
10	Illinois	42.82
17	Indiana	37.72
6	Iowa	50.05
18	Kansas	37.64
28	Kentucky	30.54
4	Louisiana	54.07
47	Maine	22.71
8	Maryland	46.00
45	Massachusetts	23.05
22	Michigan	35.24
1	Minnesota	62.74
34	Mississippi	27.97
14	Missouri	39.33
49	Montana	22.51
32	Nebraska	29.15
2	Nevada	59.09
40	New Hampshire	24.85
21	New Jersey	35.87
15	New Mexico	38.74
41	New York	24.38
9	North Carolina	44.32
29	North Dakota	30.47
16	Ohio	38.61
30	Oklahoma	30.03
23	Oregon	34.34
13	Pennsylvania	41.74
43	Rhode Island	24.14
37	South Carolina	26.98
44	South Dakota	23.86
3	Tennessee	57.40
5	Texas	53.62
35	Utah	27.62
50	Vermont	21.57
33	Virginia	28.12
20	Washington	36.45
31	West Virginia	29.24
27	Wisconsin	30.75
48	Wyoming	22.62

RANK ORDER

RANK	STATE	PERCENT
1	Minnesota	62.74
2	Nevada	59.09
3	Tennessee	57.40
4	Louisiana	54.07
5	Texas	53.62
6	Iowa	50.05
7	Hawaii	47.45
8	Maryland	46.00
9	North Carolina	44.32
10	Illinois	42.82
11	Connecticut	42.51
12	Georgia	42.01
13	Pennsylvania	41.74
14	Missouri	39.33
15	New Mexico	38.74
16	Ohio	38.61
17	Indiana	37.72
18	Kansas	37.64
19	Florida	37.59
20	Washington	36.45
21	New Jersey	35.87
22	Michigan	35.24
23	Oregon	34.34
24	Arizona	33.71
25	California	32.61
26	Colorado	31.93
27	Wisconsin	30.75
28	Kentucky	30.54
29	North Dakota	30.47
30	Oklahoma	30.03
31	West Virginia	29.24
32	Nebraska	29.15
33	Virginia	28.12
34	Mississippi	27.97
35	Utah	27.62
36	Arkansas	27.22
37	South Carolina	26.98
38	Alaska	26.46
39	Alabama	25.70
40	New Hampshire	24.85
41	New York	24.38
42	Delaware	24.18
43	Rhode Island	24.14
44	South Dakota	23.86
45	Massachusetts	23.05
46	Idaho	22.80
47	Maine	22.71
48	Wyoming	22.62
49	Montana	22.51
50	Vermont	21.57
	District of Columbia	28.23

Source: MQ Press using data from American Assn. of Health Plans (formerly American Managed Care & Review Assn.) "Managed Care Covered Lives, Year-end 1994"

As of December 31, 1994. National rate includes enrollees for whom state of resident is not known but excludes enrollees in Puerto Rico.

Persons Eligible for the Civilian Health and Medical Program Of the Uniformed Services (CHAMPUS) in 1997
National Total = 5,080,746 Eligible to Enroll*

ALPHA ORDER

RANK ORDER

RANK	STATE	ELIGIBLE	% of USA
11	Alabama	124,856	2.46%
30	Alaska	47,188	0.93%
12	Arizona	110,954	2.18%
27	Arkansas	51,689	1.02%
1	California	580,641	11.43%
10	Colorado	128,597	2.53%
36	Connecticut	29,114	0.57%
43	Delaware	18,285	0.36%
4	Florida	417,120	8.21%
6	Georgia	250,425	4.93%
16	Hawaii	91,916	1.81%
39	Idaho	24,771	0.49%
18	Illinois	82,861	1.63%
31	Indiana	41,494	0.82%
45	Iowa	17,392	0.34%
23	Kansas	66,494	1.31%
22	Kentucky	74,896	1.47%
17	Louisiana	84,030	1.65%
37	Maine	27,719	0.55%
9	Maryland	141,456	2.78%
33	Massachusetts	35,830	0.71%
29	Michigan	48,078	0.95%
40	Minnesota	23,749	0.47%
24	Mississippi	65,927	1.30%
21	Missouri	76,994	1.52%
42	Montana	18,552	0.37%
32	Nebraska	39,702	0.78%
26	Nevada	54,289	1.07%
47	New Hampshire	15,479	0.30%
28	New Jersey	50,171	0.99%
25	New Mexico	61,471	1.21%
19	New York	82,277	1.62%
5	North Carolina	252,607	4.97%
41	North Dakota	22,248	0.44%
15	Ohio	92,243	1.82%
14	Oklahoma	102,508	2.02%
34	Oregon	34,189	0.67%
20	Pennsylvania	77,591	1.53%
48	Rhode Island	13,967	0.27%
8	South Carolina	143,141	2.82%
46	South Dakota	16,996	0.33%
13	Tennessee	102,676	2.02%
2	Texas	468,335	9.22%
35	Utah	30,822	0.61%
50	Vermont	4,677	0.09%
3	Virginia	452,690	8.91%
7	Washington	219,610	4.32%
44	West Virginia	17,639	0.35%
38	Wisconsin	26,551	0.52%
49	Wyoming	12,809	0.25%

RANK	STATE	ELIGIBLE	% of USA
1	California	580,641	11.43%
2	Texas	468,335	9.22%
3	Virginia	452,690	8.91%
4	Florida	417,120	8.21%
5	North Carolina	252,607	4.97%
6	Georgia	250,425	4.93%
7	Washington	219,610	4.32%
8	South Carolina	143,141	2.82%
9	Maryland	141,456	2.78%
10	Colorado	128,597	2.53%
11	Alabama	124,856	2.46%
12	Arizona	110,954	2.18%
13	Tennessee	102,676	2.02%
14	Oklahoma	102,508	2.02%
15	Ohio	92,243	1.82%
16	Hawaii	91,916	1.81%
17	Louisiana	84,030	1.65%
18	Illinois	82,861	1.63%
19	New York	82,277	1.62%
20	Pennsylvania	77,591	1.53%
21	Missouri	76,994	1.52%
22	Kentucky	74,896	1.47%
23	Kansas	66,494	1.31%
24	Mississippi	65,927	1.30%
25	New Mexico	61,471	1.21%
26	Nevada	54,289	1.07%
27	Arkansas	51,689	1.02%
28	New Jersey	50,171	0.99%
29	Michigan	48,078	0.95%
30	Alaska	47,188	0.93%
31	Indiana	41,494	0.82%
32	Nebraska	39,702	0.78%
33	Massachusetts	35,830	0.71%
34	Oregon	34,189	0.67%
35	Utah	30,822	0.61%
36	Connecticut	29,114	0.57%
37	Maine	27,719	0.55%
38	Wisconsin	26,551	0.52%
39	Idaho	24,771	0.49%
40	Minnesota	23,749	0.47%
41	North Dakota	22,248	0.44%
42	Montana	18,552	0.37%
43	Delaware	18,285	0.36%
44	West Virginia	17,639	0.35%
45	Iowa	17,392	0.34%
46	South Dakota	16,996	0.33%
47	New Hampshire	15,479	0.30%
48	Rhode Island	13,967	0.27%
49	Wyoming	12,809	0.25%
50	Vermont	4,677	0.09%
	District of Columbia	5,030	0.10%

Source: U.S. Department of Defense, Office of CHAMPUS
"Defense Enrollment Eligibility Reporting System (DEERS) Report" (January 2, 1997)
As of January 2, 1997. National total does not include 28,898 eligible in U.S. territories and possessions.
CHAMPUS provides health care coverage for current or former U.S. military personnel and their dependents.

Percent of Population Eligible for CHAMPUS in 1997

National Percent = 1.92% of Population Eligible*

ALPHA ORDER				RANK ORDER		
RANK	STATE	PERCENT		RANK	STATE	PERCENT
13	Alabama	2.92		1	Alaska	7.77
1	Alaska	7.77		2	Hawaii	7.76
19	Arizona	2.51		3	Virginia	6.78
27	Arkansas	2.06		4	Washington	3.97
31	California	1.82		5	South Carolina	3.87
11	Colorado	3.36		6	New Mexico	3.59
38	Connecticut	0.89		7	North Carolina	3.45
18	Delaware	2.52		7	North Dakota	3.45
14	Florida	2.90		9	Georgia	3.41
9	Georgia	3.41		10	Nevada	3.39
2	Hawaii	7.76		11	Colorado	3.36
26	Idaho	2.08		12	Oklahoma	3.11
42	Illinois	0.70		13	Alabama	2.92
41	Indiana	0.71		14	Florida	2.90
45	Iowa	0.61		15	Maryland	2.79
17	Kansas	2.59		16	Wyoming	2.66
28	Kentucky	1.93		17	Kansas	2.59
28	Louisiana	1.93		18	Delaware	2.52
24	Maine	2.23		19	Arizona	2.51
15	Maryland	2.79		20	Texas	2.45
46	Massachusetts	0.59		21	Mississippi	2.43
49	Michigan	0.50		22	Nebraska	2.40
47	Minnesota	0.51		23	South Dakota	2.32
21	Mississippi	2.43		24	Maine	2.23
33	Missouri	1.44		25	Montana	2.11
25	Montana	2.11		26	Idaho	2.08
22	Nebraska	2.40		27	Arkansas	2.06
10	Nevada	3.39		28	Kentucky	1.93
35	New Hampshire	1.33		28	Louisiana	1.93
44	New Jersey	0.63		28	Tennessee	1.93
6	New Mexico	3.59		31	California	1.82
50	New York	0.45		32	Utah	1.54
7	North Carolina	3.45		33	Missouri	1.44
7	North Dakota	3.45		34	Rhode Island	1.41
39	Ohio	0.83		35	New Hampshire	1.33
12	Oklahoma	3.11		36	Oregon	1.07
36	Oregon	1.07		37	West Virginia	0.97
43	Pennsylvania	0.64		38	Connecticut	0.89
34	Rhode Island	1.41		39	Ohio	0.83
5	South Carolina	3.87		40	Vermont	0.79
23	South Dakota	2.32		41	Indiana	0.71
28	Tennessee	1.93		42	Illinois	0.70
20	Texas	2.45		43	Pennsylvania	0.64
32	Utah	1.54		44	New Jersey	0.63
40	Vermont	0.79		45	Iowa	0.61
3	Virginia	6.78		46	Massachusetts	0.59
4	Washington	3.97		47	Minnesota	0.51
37	West Virginia	0.97		47	Wisconsin	0.51
47	Wisconsin	0.51		49	Michigan	0.50
16	Wyoming	2.66		50	New York	0.45
					District of Columbia	0.93

Source: Morgan Quitno Press using data from U.S. Department of Defense, Office of CHAMPUS
"Defense Enrollment Eligibility Reporting System (DEERS) Report" (January 2, 1997)
*As of January 2, 1997. National rate does not include those eligible in U.S. territories and possessions.
CHAMPUS provides health care coverage for current or former U.S. military personnel and their dependents.
Percentages calculated using Census estimates as of July 1, 1996.

Personal Health Care Expenditures in 1993

National Total = $778,510,000,000*

ALPHA ORDER

RANK	STATE	EXPENDITURES	% of USA
23	Alabama	$12,060,000,000	1.55%
48	Alaska	1,573,000,000	0.20%
24	Arizona	10,635,000,000	1.37%
33	Arkansas	6,111,000,000	0.78%
1	California	94,178,000,000	12.10%
26	Colorado	10,066,000,000	1.29%
22	Connecticut	12,216,000,000	1.57%
44	Delaware	2,260,000,000	0.29%
4	Florida	44,811,000,000	5.76%
11	Georgia	20,104,000,000	2.58%
39	Hawaii	3,485,000,000	0.45%
43	Idaho	2,277,000,000	0.29%
6	Illinois	34,747,000,000	4.46%
14	Indiana	16,401,000,000	2.11%
30	Iowa	7,341,000,000	0.94%
31	Kansas	6,903,000,000	0.89%
25	Kentucky	10,384,000,000	1.33%
21	Louisiana	13,014,000,000	1.67%
41	Maine	3,433,000,000	0.44%
17	Maryland	15,154,000,000	1.95%
10	Massachusetts	23,421,000,000	3.01%
8	Michigan	27,136,000,000	3.49%
20	Minnesota	14,194,000,000	1.82%
32	Mississippi	6,187,000,000	0.79%
16	Missouri	15,949,000,000	2.05%
45	Montana	2,103,000,000	0.27%
35	Nebraska	4,400,000,000	0.57%
38	Nevada	3,747,000,000	0.48%
40	New Hampshire	3,452,000,000	0.44%
9	New Jersey	25,741,000,000	3.31%
37	New Mexico	3,878,000,000	0.50%
2	New York	67,033,000,000	8.61%
12	North Carolina	18,241,000,000	2.34%
46	North Dakota	2,021,000,000	0.26%
7	Ohio	33,456,000,000	4.30%
28	Oklahoma	8,041,000,000	1.03%
29	Oregon	7,999,000,000	1.03%
5	Pennsylvania	41,521,000,000	5.33%
42	Rhode Island	3,428,000,000	0.44%
27	South Carolina	9,029,000,000	1.16%
47	South Dakota	1,953,000,000	0.25%
15	Tennessee	16,203,000,000	2.08%
3	Texas	49,816,000,000	6.40%
36	Utah	4,118,000,000	0.53%
49	Vermont	1,499,000,000	0.19%
13	Virginia	16,682,000,000	2.14%
18	Washington	15,129,000,000	1.94%
34	West Virginia	5,197,000,000	0.67%
19	Wisconsin	14,502,000,000	1.86%
50	Wyoming	998,000,000	0.13%

RANK ORDER

RANK	STATE	EXPENDITURES	% of USA
1	California	$94,178,000,000	12.10%
2	New York	67,033,000,000	8.61%
3	Texas	49,816,000,000	6.40%
4	Florida	44,811,000,000	5.76%
5	Pennsylvania	41,521,000,000	5.33%
6	Illinois	34,747,000,000	4.46%
7	Ohio	33,456,000,000	4.30%
8	Michigan	27,136,000,000	3.49%
9	New Jersey	25,741,000,000	3.31%
10	Massachusetts	23,421,000,000	3.01%
11	Georgia	20,104,000,000	2.58%
12	North Carolina	18,241,000,000	2.34%
13	Virginia	16,682,000,000	2.14%
14	Indiana	16,401,000,000	2.11%
15	Tennessee	16,203,000,000	2.08%
16	Missouri	15,949,000,000	2.05%
17	Maryland	15,154,000,000	1.95%
18	Washington	15,129,000,000	1.94%
19	Wisconsin	14,502,000,000	1.86%
20	Minnesota	14,194,000,000	1.82%
21	Louisiana	13,014,000,000	1.67%
22	Connecticut	12,216,000,000	1.57%
23	Alabama	12,060,000,000	1.55%
24	Arizona	10,635,000,000	1.37%
25	Kentucky	10,384,000,000	1.33%
26	Colorado	10,066,000,000	1.29%
27	South Carolina	9,029,000,000	1.16%
28	Oklahoma	8,041,000,000	1.03%
29	Oregon	7,999,000,000	1.03%
30	Iowa	7,341,000,000	0.94%
31	Kansas	6,903,000,000	0.89%
32	Mississippi	6,187,000,000	0.79%
33	Arkansas	6,111,000,000	0.78%
34	West Virginia	5,197,000,000	0.67%
35	Nebraska	4,400,000,000	0.57%
36	Utah	4,118,000,000	0.53%
37	New Mexico	3,878,000,000	0.50%
38	Nevada	3,747,000,000	0.48%
39	Hawaii	3,485,000,000	0.45%
40	New Hampshire	3,452,000,000	0.44%
41	Maine	3,433,000,000	0.44%
42	Rhode Island	3,428,000,000	0.44%
43	Idaho	2,277,000,000	0.29%
44	Delaware	2,260,000,000	0.29%
45	Montana	2,103,000,000	0.27%
46	North Dakota	2,021,000,000	0.26%
47	South Dakota	1,953,000,000	0.25%
48	Alaska	1,573,000,000	0.20%
49	Vermont	1,499,000,000	0.19%
50	Wyoming	998,000,000	0.13%
	District of Columbia	4,285,000,000	0.55%

Source: U.S. Department of Health and Human Services, Health Care Financing Administration
"State Health Expenditure Accounts" (Health Care Financing Review, Fall 1995, Volume 17, Number 1)
*By state of provider. Includes hospital care, physician services, dental services, home health care, drugs, vision products and other personal health care services and products.

Health Care Expenditures as a Percent of Gross State Product in 1992

National Percent = 12.1% of Total Gross State Product*

ALPHA ORDER				RANK ORDER		
RANK	STATE	PERCENT		RANK	STATE	PERCENT
6	Alabama	14.4		1	West Virginia	15.7
50	Alaska	5.7		2	Florida	15.6
9	Arizona	13.4		3	North Dakota	14.7
12	Arkansas	13.1		3	Rhode Island	14.7
35	California	11.2		5	Pennsylvania	14.5
34	Colorado	11.3		6	Alabama	14.4
30	Connecticut	11.7		7	Tennessee	13.9
48	Delaware	8.8		8	Massachusetts	13.6
2	Florida	15.6		9	Arizona	13.4
25	Georgia	12.1		10	Maine	13.3
46	Hawaii	9.8		10	Missouri	13.3
45	Idaho	10.0		12	Arkansas	13.1
35	Illinois	11.2		13	Ohio	13.0
18	Indiana	12.5		14	Kentucky	12.9
30	Iowa	11.7		15	Mississippi	12.8
30	Kansas	11.7		16	Montana	12.7
14	Kentucky	12.9		17	New York	12.6
18	Louisiana	12.5		18	Indiana	12.5
10	Maine	13.3		18	Louisiana	12.5
23	Maryland	12.2		18	Michigan	12.5
8	Massachusetts	13.6		18	Oklahoma	12.5
18	Michigan	12.5		22	Wisconsin	12.4
25	Minnesota	12.1		23	Maryland	12.2
15	Mississippi	12.8		23	New Hampshire	12.2
10	Missouri	13.3		25	Georgia	12.1
16	Montana	12.7		25	Minnesota	12.1
38	Nebraska	11.1		27	South Carolina	12.0
47	Nevada	9.4		27	South Dakota	12.0
23	New Hampshire	12.2		29	Vermont	11.8
42	New Jersey	10.7		30	Connecticut	11.7
35	New Mexico	11.2		30	Iowa	11.7
17	New York	12.6		30	Kansas	11.7
43	North Carolina	10.6		30	Oregon	11.7
3	North Dakota	14.7		34	Colorado	11.3
13	Ohio	13.0		35	California	11.2
18	Oklahoma	12.5		35	Illinois	11.2
30	Oregon	11.7		35	New Mexico	11.2
5	Pennsylvania	14.5		38	Nebraska	11.1
3	Rhode Island	14.7		38	Texas	11.1
27	South Carolina	12.0		40	Washington	11.0
27	South Dakota	12.0		41	Utah	10.8
7	Tennessee	13.9		42	New Jersey	10.7
38	Texas	11.1		43	North Carolina	10.6
41	Utah	10.8		44	Virginia	10.2
29	Vermont	11.8		45	Idaho	10.0
44	Virginia	10.2		46	Hawaii	9.8
40	Washington	11.0		47	Nevada	9.4
1	West Virginia	15.7		48	Delaware	8.8
22	Wisconsin	12.4		49	Wyoming	7.0
49	Wyoming	7.0		50	Alaska	5.7
					District of Columbia	9.9

Source: U.S. Department of Health and Human Services, Health Care Financing Administration
   "State Health Expenditure Accounts" (Health Care Financing Review, Fall 1995, Volume 17, Number 1)
*By state of provider. Includes hospital care, physician services, dental services, home health care, drugs, vision products and other personal health care services and products.

Per Capita Personal Health Care Expenditures in 1993

National Per Capita = $3,020*

ALPHA ORDER			RANK ORDER		
RANK	STATE	PER CAPITA	RANK	STATE	PER CAPITA
21	Alabama	$2,884	1	Massachusetts	$3,892
37	Alaska	2,630	2	Connecticut	3,727
35	Arizona	2,697	3	New York	3,693
42	Arkansas	2,520	4	Pennsylvania	3,451
17	California	3,017	5	Rhode Island	3,431
27	Colorado	2,821	6	New Jersey	3,275
2	Connecticut	3,727	7	Florida	3,266
8	Delaware	3,233	8	Delaware	3,233
7	Florida	3,266	9	Tennessee	3,181
20	Georgia	2,913	10	North Dakota	3,173
18	Hawaii	2,989	11	Minnesota	3,137
50	Idaho	2,068	12	New Hampshire	3,074
19	Illinois	2,972	13	Maryland	3,060
24	Indiana	2,874	14	Missouri	3,047
40	Iowa	2,601	15	Louisiana	3,034
31	Kansas	2,726	16	Ohio	3,025
30	Kentucky	2,738	17	California	3,017
15	Louisiana	3,034	18	Hawaii	2,989
28	Maine	2,771	19	Illinois	2,972
13	Maryland	3,060	20	Georgia	2,913
1	Massachusetts	3,892	21	Alabama	2,884
25	Michigan	2,869	22	Washington	2,879
11	Minnesota	3,137	23	Wisconsin	2,875
47	Mississippi	2,344	24	Indiana	2,874
14	Missouri	3,047	25	Michigan	2,869
43	Montana	2,501	26	West Virginia	2,859
31	Nebraska	2,726	27	Colorado	2,821
34	Nevada	2,705	28	Maine	2,771
12	New Hampshire	3,074	29	Texas	2,760
6	New Jersey	3,275	30	Kentucky	2,738
46	New Mexico	2,400	31	Kansas	2,726
3	New York	3,693	31	Nebraska	2,726
38	North Carolina	2,623	33	South Dakota	2,724
10	North Dakota	3,173	34	Nevada	2,705
16	Ohio	3,025	35	Arizona	2,697
45	Oklahoma	2,488	36	Oregon	2,636
36	Oregon	2,636	37	Alaska	2,630
4	Pennsylvania	3,451	38	North Carolina	2,623
5	Rhode Island	3,431	39	Vermont	2,602
44	South Carolina	2,489	40	Iowa	2,601
33	South Dakota	2,724	41	Virginia	2,576
9	Tennessee	3,181	42	Arkansas	2,520
29	Texas	2,760	43	Montana	2,501
48	Utah	2,214	44	South Carolina	2,489
39	Vermont	2,602	45	Oklahoma	2,488
41	Virginia	2,576	46	New Mexico	2,400
22	Washington	2,879	47	Mississippi	2,344
26	West Virginia	2,859	48	Utah	2,214
23	Wisconsin	2,875	49	Wyoming	2,123
49	Wyoming	2,123	50	Idaho	2,068
				District of Columbia	7,413

Source: Morgan Quitno Press using data from U.S. Dept of Health & Human Services, Health Care Financing Admin. "State Health Expenditure Accounts" (Health Care Financing Review, Fall 1995, Volume 17, Number 1)
By state of provider. Includes hospital care, physician services, dental services, home health care, drugs, vision products and other personal health care services and products.

Percent Change in Personal Health Care Expenditures: 1990 to 1993

National Percent Change = 28.0% Increase*

ALPHA ORDER

RANK	STATE	PERCENT CHANGE
13	Alabama	31.7
32	Alaska	27.0
41	Arizona	25.4
37	Arkansas	26.1
30	California	27.1
20	Colorado	30.3
48	Connecticut	22.5
12	Delaware	32.2
28	Florida	27.6
15	Georgia	31.5
29	Hawaii	27.5
1	Idaho	37.4
34	Illinois	26.7
19	Indiana	30.7
50	Iowa	21.9
43	Kansas	25.3
11	Kentucky	32.7
14	Louisiana	31.6
30	Maine	27.1
27	Maryland	28.0
49	Massachusetts	22.2
46	Michigan	23.5
47	Minnesota	23.3
16	Mississippi	31.2
34	Missouri	26.7
17	Montana	30.9
36	Nebraska	26.5
3	Nevada	35.4
2	New Hampshire	36.9
23	New Jersey	29.0
6	New Mexico	34.0
44	New York	24.8
8	North Carolina	33.1
44	North Dakota	24.8
41	Ohio	25.4
24	Oklahoma	28.1
20	Oregon	30.3
24	Pennsylvania	28.1
40	Rhode Island	25.5
5	South Carolina	34.8
18	South Dakota	30.8
8	Tennessee	33.1
7	Texas	33.7
22	Utah	29.9
33	Vermont	26.8
38	Virginia	25.9
3	Washington	35.4
8	West Virginia	33.1
24	Wisconsin	28.1
39	Wyoming	25.7

RANK ORDER

RANK	STATE	PERCENT CHANGE
1	Idaho	37.4
2	New Hampshire	36.9
3	Nevada	35.4
3	Washington	35.4
5	South Carolina	34.8
6	New Mexico	34.0
7	Texas	33.7
8	North Carolina	33.1
8	Tennessee	33.1
8	West Virginia	33.1
11	Kentucky	32.7
12	Delaware	32.2
13	Alabama	31.7
14	Louisiana	31.6
15	Georgia	31.5
16	Mississippi	31.2
17	Montana	30.9
18	South Dakota	30.8
19	Indiana	30.7
20	Colorado	30.3
20	Oregon	30.3
22	Utah	29.9
23	New Jersey	29.0
24	Oklahoma	28.1
24	Pennsylvania	28.1
24	Wisconsin	28.1
27	Maryland	28.0
28	Florida	27.6
29	Hawaii	27.5
30	California	27.1
30	Maine	27.1
32	Alaska	27.0
33	Vermont	26.8
34	Illinois	26.7
34	Missouri	26.7
36	Nebraska	26.5
37	Arkansas	26.1
38	Virginia	25.9
39	Wyoming	25.7
40	Rhode Island	25.5
41	Arizona	25.4
41	Ohio	25.4
43	Kansas	25.3
44	New York	24.8
44	North Dakota	24.8
46	Michigan	23.5
47	Minnesota	23.3
48	Connecticut	22.5
49	Massachusetts	22.2
50	Iowa	21.9
	District of Columbia	21.2

Source: Morgan Quitno Press using data from U.S. Dept of Health & Human Services, Health Care Financing Admin. "State Health Expenditure Accounts" (Health Care Financing Review, Fall 1995, Volume 17, Number 1)
By state of provider. Includes hospital care, physician services, dental services, home health care, drugs, vision products and other personal health care services and products.

Percent Change in Per Capita Expenditures for
Personal Health Care: 1990 to 1993
National Percent Change = 23.5% Increase*

RANK	STATE	PERCENT CHANGE
8	Alabama	27.2
49	Alaska	16.7
50	Arizona	16.6
35	Arkansas	22.2
41	California	21.1
42	Colorado	20.3
33	Connecticut	22.8
16	Delaware	25.9
42	Florida	20.3
31	Georgia	23.4
40	Hawaii	21.2
18	Idaho	25.7
26	Illinois	23.9
11	Indiana	26.9
46	Iowa	20.0
34	Kansas	22.6
5	Kentucky	29.0
3	Louisiana	29.5
14	Maine	26.0
30	Maryland	23.6
36	Massachusetts	22.1
38	Michigan	21.4
47	Minnesota	19.3
6	Mississippi	28.0
27	Missouri	23.8
23	Montana	24.4
28	Nebraska	23.7
48	Nevada	17.5
1	New Hampshire	35.2
11	New Jersey	26.9
19	New Mexico	25.6
28	New York	23.7
9	North Carolina	27.0
21	North Dakota	25.2
32	Ohio	23.0
22	Oklahoma	24.6
36	Oregon	22.1
13	Pennsylvania	26.5
14	Rhode Island	26.0
3	South Carolina	29.5
9	South Dakota	27.0
7	Tennessee	27.4
17	Texas	25.8
42	Utah	20.3
25	Vermont	24.0
42	Virginia	20.3
20	Washington	25.4
2	West Virginia	31.3
24	Wisconsin	24.2
38	Wyoming	21.4

RANK	STATE	PERCENT CHANGE
1	New Hampshire	35.2
2	West Virginia	31.3
3	Louisiana	29.5
3	South Carolina	29.5
5	Kentucky	29.0
6	Mississippi	28.0
7	Tennessee	27.4
8	Alabama	27.2
9	North Carolina	27.0
9	South Dakota	27.0
11	Indiana	26.9
11	New Jersey	26.9
13	Pennsylvania	26.5
14	Maine	26.0
14	Rhode Island	26.0
16	Delaware	25.9
17	Texas	25.8
18	Idaho	25.7
19	New Mexico	25.6
20	Washington	25.4
21	North Dakota	25.2
22	Oklahoma	24.6
23	Montana	24.4
24	Wisconsin	24.2
25	Vermont	24.0
26	Illinois	23.9
27	Missouri	23.8
28	Nebraska	23.7
28	New York	23.7
30	Maryland	23.6
31	Georgia	23.4
32	Ohio	23.0
33	Connecticut	22.8
34	Kansas	22.6
35	Arkansas	22.2
36	Massachusetts	22.1
36	Oregon	22.1
38	Michigan	21.4
38	Wyoming	21.4
40	Hawaii	21.2
41	California	21.1
42	Colorado	20.3
42	Florida	20.3
42	Utah	20.3
42	Virginia	20.3
46	Iowa	20.0
47	Minnesota	19.3
48	Nevada	17.5
49	Alaska	16.7
50	Arizona	16.6
	District of Columbia	27.3

*Source: Morgan Quitno Press using data from U.S. Dept of Health & Human Services, Health Care Financing Admin.
"State Health Expenditure Accounts" (Health Care Financing Review, Fall 1995, Volume 17, Number 1)*
By state of provider. Includes hospital care, physician services, dental services, home health care, drugs, vision products and other personal health care services and products.

Average Annual Change in Expenditures for Personal Health Care: 1980 to 1993
National Percent = 10.3% Average Annual Growth*

ALPHA ORDER

RANK	STATE	PERCENT
16	Alabama	10.9
27	Alaska	10.2
5	Arizona	11.9
32	Arkansas	10.1
27	California	10.2
23	Colorado	10.5
15	Connecticut	11.0
9	Delaware	11.3
2	Florida	12.4
4	Georgia	12.1
19	Hawaii	10.8
24	Idaho	10.4
47	Illinois	8.7
26	Indiana	10.3
50	Iowa	8.3
45	Kansas	9.0
16	Kentucky	10.9
24	Louisiana	10.4
21	Maine	10.6
21	Maryland	10.6
27	Massachusetts	10.2
49	Michigan	8.5
37	Minnesota	9.7
32	Mississippi	10.1
39	Missouri	9.6
35	Montana	9.8
46	Nebraska	8.9
3	Nevada	12.2
1	New Hampshire	13.0
10	New Jersey	11.2
8	New Mexico	11.7
37	New York	9.7
5	North Carolina	11.9
43	North Dakota	9.4
39	Ohio	9.6
44	Oklahoma	9.1
34	Oregon	9.9
27	Pennsylvania	10.2
27	Rhode Island	10.2
5	South Carolina	11.9
35	South Dakota	9.8
10	Tennessee	11.2
12	Texas	11.1
12	Utah	11.1
19	Vermont	10.8
16	Virginia	10.9
12	Washington	11.1
39	West Virginia	9.6
42	Wisconsin	9.5
47	Wyoming	8.7

RANK ORDER

RANK	STATE	PERCENT
1	New Hampshire	13.0
2	Florida	12.4
3	Nevada	12.2
4	Georgia	12.1
5	Arizona	11.9
5	North Carolina	11.9
5	South Carolina	11.9
8	New Mexico	11.7
9	Delaware	11.3
10	New Jersey	11.2
10	Tennessee	11.2
12	Texas	11.1
12	Utah	11.1
12	Washington	11.1
15	Connecticut	11.0
16	Alabama	10.9
16	Kentucky	10.9
16	Virginia	10.9
19	Hawaii	10.8
19	Vermont	10.8
21	Maine	10.6
21	Maryland	10.6
23	Colorado	10.5
24	Idaho	10.4
24	Louisiana	10.4
26	Indiana	10.3
27	Alaska	10.2
27	California	10.2
27	Massachusetts	10.2
27	Pennsylvania	10.2
27	Rhode Island	10.2
32	Arkansas	10.1
32	Mississippi	10.1
34	Oregon	9.9
35	Montana	9.8
35	South Dakota	9.8
37	Minnesota	9.7
37	New York	9.7
39	Missouri	9.6
39	Ohio	9.6
39	West Virginia	9.6
42	Wisconsin	9.5
43	North Dakota	9.4
44	Oklahoma	9.1
45	Kansas	9.0
46	Nebraska	8.9
47	Illinois	8.7
47	Wyoming	8.7
49	Michigan	8.5
50	Iowa	8.3
	District of Columbia	9.1

Source: U.S. Department of Health and Human Services, Health Care Financing Administration
"State Health Expenditure Accounts" (Health Care Financing Review, Fall 1995, Volume 17, Number 1)
*By state of provider. Includes hospital care, physician services, dental services, home health care, drugs, vision products and other personal health care services and products.

Average Annual Change in Per Capita Expenditures
For Personal Health Care: 1980 to 1993
National Percent = 9.3% Average Annual Increase*

<table>
<tr><td colspan="3">ALPHA ORDER</td><td colspan="3">RANK ORDER</td></tr>
<tr><td>RANK</td><td>STATE</td><td>PERCENT</td><td>RANK</td><td>STATE</td><td>PERCENT</td></tr>
<tr><td>7</td><td>Alabama</td><td>10.3</td><td>1</td><td>New Hampshire</td><td>11.3</td></tr>
<tr><td>50</td><td>Alaska</td><td>6.8</td><td>2</td><td>New Jersey</td><td>10.7</td></tr>
<tr><td>38</td><td>Arizona</td><td>8.8</td><td>3</td><td>Kentucky</td><td>10.6</td></tr>
<tr><td>21</td><td>Arkansas</td><td>9.6</td><td>3</td><td>South Carolina</td><td>10.6</td></tr>
<tr><td>48</td><td>California</td><td>7.9</td><td>5</td><td>Connecticut</td><td>10.5</td></tr>
<tr><td>38</td><td>Colorado</td><td>8.8</td><td>5</td><td>North Carolina</td><td>10.5</td></tr>
<tr><td>5</td><td>Connecticut</td><td>10.5</td><td>7</td><td>Alabama</td><td>10.3</td></tr>
<tr><td>13</td><td>Delaware</td><td>10.0</td><td>7</td><td>Louisiana</td><td>10.3</td></tr>
<tr><td>23</td><td>Florida</td><td>9.5</td><td>7</td><td>Tennessee</td><td>10.3</td></tr>
<tr><td>11</td><td>Georgia</td><td>10.1</td><td>10</td><td>West Virginia</td><td>10.2</td></tr>
<tr><td>30</td><td>Hawaii</td><td>9.2</td><td>11</td><td>Georgia</td><td>10.1</td></tr>
<tr><td>31</td><td>Idaho</td><td>9.1</td><td>11</td><td>Pennsylvania</td><td>10.1</td></tr>
<tr><td>45</td><td>Illinois</td><td>8.5</td><td>13</td><td>Delaware</td><td>10.0</td></tr>
<tr><td>13</td><td>Indiana</td><td>10.0</td><td>13</td><td>Indiana</td><td>10.0</td></tr>
<tr><td>42</td><td>Iowa</td><td>8.6</td><td>15</td><td>New Mexico</td><td>9.9</td></tr>
<tr><td>46</td><td>Kansas</td><td>8.4</td><td>16</td><td>Maine</td><td>9.8</td></tr>
<tr><td>3</td><td>Kentucky</td><td>10.6</td><td>16</td><td>Massachusetts</td><td>9.8</td></tr>
<tr><td>7</td><td>Louisiana</td><td>10.3</td><td>16</td><td>Vermont</td><td>9.8</td></tr>
<tr><td>16</td><td>Maine</td><td>9.8</td><td>19</td><td>Mississippi</td><td>9.7</td></tr>
<tr><td>27</td><td>Maryland</td><td>9.3</td><td>19</td><td>Rhode Island</td><td>9.7</td></tr>
<tr><td>16</td><td>Massachusetts</td><td>9.8</td><td>21</td><td>Arkansas</td><td>9.6</td></tr>
<tr><td>46</td><td>Michigan</td><td>8.4</td><td>21</td><td>North Dakota</td><td>9.6</td></tr>
<tr><td>37</td><td>Minnesota</td><td>8.9</td><td>23</td><td>Florida</td><td>9.5</td></tr>
<tr><td>19</td><td>Mississippi</td><td>9.7</td><td>23</td><td>South Dakota</td><td>9.5</td></tr>
<tr><td>31</td><td>Missouri</td><td>9.1</td><td>25</td><td>New York</td><td>9.4</td></tr>
<tr><td>27</td><td>Montana</td><td>9.3</td><td>25</td><td>Ohio</td><td>9.4</td></tr>
<tr><td>42</td><td>Nebraska</td><td>8.6</td><td>27</td><td>Maryland</td><td>9.3</td></tr>
<tr><td>49</td><td>Nevada</td><td>7.6</td><td>27</td><td>Montana</td><td>9.3</td></tr>
<tr><td>1</td><td>New Hampshire</td><td>11.3</td><td>27</td><td>Virginia</td><td>9.3</td></tr>
<tr><td>2</td><td>New Jersey</td><td>10.7</td><td>30</td><td>Hawaii</td><td>9.2</td></tr>
<tr><td>15</td><td>New Mexico</td><td>9.9</td><td>31</td><td>Idaho</td><td>9.1</td></tr>
<tr><td>25</td><td>New York</td><td>9.4</td><td>31</td><td>Missouri</td><td>9.1</td></tr>
<tr><td>5</td><td>North Carolina</td><td>10.5</td><td>31</td><td>Texas</td><td>9.1</td></tr>
<tr><td>21</td><td>North Dakota</td><td>9.6</td><td>31</td><td>Washington</td><td>9.1</td></tr>
<tr><td>25</td><td>Ohio</td><td>9.4</td><td>35</td><td>Utah</td><td>9.0</td></tr>
<tr><td>42</td><td>Oklahoma</td><td>8.6</td><td>35</td><td>Wisconsin</td><td>9.0</td></tr>
<tr><td>40</td><td>Oregon</td><td>8.7</td><td>37</td><td>Minnesota</td><td>8.9</td></tr>
<tr><td>11</td><td>Pennsylvania</td><td>10.1</td><td>38</td><td>Arizona</td><td>8.8</td></tr>
<tr><td>19</td><td>Rhode Island</td><td>9.7</td><td>38</td><td>Colorado</td><td>8.8</td></tr>
<tr><td>3</td><td>South Carolina</td><td>10.6</td><td>40</td><td>Oregon</td><td>8.7</td></tr>
<tr><td>23</td><td>South Dakota</td><td>9.5</td><td>40</td><td>Wyoming</td><td>8.7</td></tr>
<tr><td>7</td><td>Tennessee</td><td>10.3</td><td>42</td><td>Iowa</td><td>8.6</td></tr>
<tr><td>31</td><td>Texas</td><td>9.1</td><td>42</td><td>Nebraska</td><td>8.6</td></tr>
<tr><td>35</td><td>Utah</td><td>9.0</td><td>42</td><td>Oklahoma</td><td>8.6</td></tr>
<tr><td>16</td><td>Vermont</td><td>9.8</td><td>45</td><td>Illinois</td><td>8.5</td></tr>
<tr><td>27</td><td>Virginia</td><td>9.3</td><td>46</td><td>Kansas</td><td>8.4</td></tr>
<tr><td>31</td><td>Washington</td><td>9.1</td><td>46</td><td>Michigan</td><td>8.4</td></tr>
<tr><td>10</td><td>West Virginia</td><td>10.2</td><td>48</td><td>California</td><td>7.9</td></tr>
<tr><td>35</td><td>Wisconsin</td><td>9.0</td><td>49</td><td>Nevada</td><td>7.6</td></tr>
<tr><td>40</td><td>Wyoming</td><td>8.7</td><td>50</td><td>Alaska</td><td>6.8</td></tr>
<tr><td></td><td></td><td></td><td></td><td>District of Columbia</td><td>9.9</td></tr>
</table>

Source: Morgan Quitno Press using data from U.S. Dept of Health & Human Services, Health Care Financing Admin.
"State Health Expenditure Accounts" (Health Care Financing Review, Fall 1995, Volume 17, Number 1)
*By state of provider. Includes hospital care, physician services, dental services, home health care, drugs, vision products and other personal health care services and products.

Expenditures for Hospital Care in 1993

National Total = $323,919,000,000*

ALPHA ORDER					RANK ORDER			
RANK	STATE	EXPENDITURES	% of USA		RANK	STATE	EXPENDITURES	% of USA
21	Alabama	$5,301,000,000	1.64%		1	California	$34,827,000,000	10.77%
48	Alaska	701,000,000	0.22%		2	New York	28,001,000,000	8.66%
26	Arizona	3,999,000,000	1.24%		3	Texas	21,592,000,000	6.68%
33	Arkansas	2,723,000,000	0.84%		4	Pennsylvania	19,540,000,000	6.04%
1	California	34,827,000,000	10.77%		5	Florida	17,131,000,000	5.30%
27	Colorado	3,932,000,000	1.22%		6	Illinois	15,621,000,000	4.83%
24	Connecticut	4,380,000,000	1.35%		7	Ohio	14,305,000,000	4.42%
43	Delaware	937,000,000	0.29%		8	Michigan	11,711,000,000	3.62%
5	Florida	17,131,000,000	5.30%		9	New Jersey	10,312,000,000	3.19%
11	Georgia	8,704,000,000	2.69%		10	Massachusetts	10,034,000,000	3.10%
38	Hawaii	1,460,000,000	0.45%		11	Georgia	8,704,000,000	2.69%
46	Idaho	900,000,000	0.28%		12	North Carolina	7,801,000,000	2.41%
6	Illinois	15,621,000,000	4.83%		13	Missouri	7,652,000,000	2.37%
16	Indiana	6,998,000,000	2.16%		14	Tennessee	7,208,000,000	2.23%
29	Iowa	3,111,000,000	0.96%		15	Virginia	7,031,000,000	2.17%
32	Kansas	2,868,000,000	0.89%		16	Indiana	6,998,000,000	2.16%
23	Kentucky	4,515,000,000	1.40%		17	Louisiana	5,956,000,000	1.84%
17	Louisiana	5,956,000,000	1.84%		18	Maryland	5,926,000,000	1.83%
40	Maine	1,376,000,000	0.43%		19	Wisconsin	5,537,000,000	1.71%
18	Maryland	5,926,000,000	1.83%		20	Washington	5,305,000,000	1.64%
10	Massachusetts	10,034,000,000	3.10%		21	Alabama	5,301,000,000	1.64%
8	Michigan	11,711,000,000	3.62%		22	Minnesota	4,796,000,000	1.48%
22	Minnesota	4,796,000,000	1.48%		23	Kentucky	4,515,000,000	1.40%
31	Mississippi	2,897,000,000	0.90%		24	Connecticut	4,380,000,000	1.35%
13	Missouri	7,652,000,000	2.37%		25	South Carolina	4,221,000,000	1.30%
47	Montana	894,000,000	0.28%		26	Arizona	3,999,000,000	1.24%
35	Nebraska	2,003,000,000	0.62%		27	Colorado	3,932,000,000	1.22%
41	Nevada	1,362,000,000	0.42%		28	Oklahoma	3,329,000,000	1.03%
39	New Hampshire	1,388,000,000	0.43%		29	Iowa	3,111,000,000	0.96%
9	New Jersey	10,312,000,000	3.19%		30	Oregon	2,966,000,000	0.92%
36	New Mexico	1,848,000,000	0.57%		31	Mississippi	2,897,000,000	0.90%
2	New York	28,001,000,000	8.66%		32	Kansas	2,868,000,000	0.89%
12	North Carolina	7,801,000,000	2.41%		33	Arkansas	2,723,000,000	0.84%
45	North Dakota	903,000,000	0.28%		34	West Virginia	2,346,000,000	0.73%
7	Ohio	14,305,000,000	4.42%		35	Nebraska	2,003,000,000	0.62%
28	Oklahoma	3,329,000,000	1.03%		36	New Mexico	1,848,000,000	0.57%
30	Oregon	2,966,000,000	0.92%		37	Utah	1,743,000,000	0.54%
4	Pennsylvania	19,540,000,000	6.04%		38	Hawaii	1,460,000,000	0.45%
42	Rhode Island	1,314,000,000	0.41%		39	New Hampshire	1,388,000,000	0.43%
25	South Carolina	4,221,000,000	1.30%		40	Maine	1,376,000,000	0.43%
44	South Dakota	920,000,000	0.28%		41	Nevada	1,362,000,000	0.42%
14	Tennessee	7,208,000,000	2.23%		42	Rhode Island	1,314,000,000	0.41%
3	Texas	21,592,000,000	6.68%		43	Delaware	937,000,000	0.29%
37	Utah	1,743,000,000	0.54%		44	South Dakota	920,000,000	0.28%
49	Vermont	562,000,000	0.17%		45	North Dakota	903,000,000	0.28%
15	Virginia	7,031,000,000	2.17%		46	Idaho	900,000,000	0.28%
20	Washington	5,305,000,000	1.64%		47	Montana	894,000,000	0.28%
34	West Virginia	2,346,000,000	0.73%		48	Alaska	701,000,000	0.22%
19	Wisconsin	5,537,000,000	1.71%		49	Vermont	562,000,000	0.17%
50	Wyoming	417,000,000	0.13%		50	Wyoming	417,000,000	0.13%
						District of Columbia	2,612,000,000	0.81%

Source: U.S. Department of Health and Human Services, Health Care Financing Administration
"State Health Expenditure Accounts" (Health Care Financing Review, Fall 1995, Volume 17, Number 1)
By state of provider.

Percent of Total Personal Health Care Expenditures
Spent on Hospital Care in 1993
National Percent = 41.6%*

ALPHA ORDER

RANK	STATE	PERCENT
15	Alabama	44.0
12	Alaska	44.6
43	Arizona	37.6
12	Arkansas	44.6
46	California	37.0
38	Colorado	39.1
48	Connecticut	35.9
31	Delaware	41.5
41	Florida	38.2
17	Georgia	43.3
28	Hawaii	41.9
37	Idaho	39.5
10	Illinois	45.0
23	Indiana	42.7
25	Iowa	42.4
31	Kansas	41.5
16	Kentucky	43.5
7	Louisiana	45.8
35	Maine	40.1
38	Maryland	39.1
20	Massachusetts	42.8
19	Michigan	43.2
50	Minnesota	33.8
5	Mississippi	46.8
1	Missouri	48.0
24	Montana	42.5
8	Nebraska	45.5
47	Nevada	36.3
34	New Hampshire	40.2
35	New Jersey	40.1
2	New Mexico	47.7
29	New York	41.8
20	North Carolina	42.8
11	North Dakota	44.7
20	Ohio	42.8
33	Oklahoma	41.4
45	Oregon	37.1
3	Pennsylvania	47.1
40	Rhode Island	38.3
6	South Carolina	46.7
3	South Dakota	47.1
14	Tennessee	44.5
17	Texas	43.3
26	Utah	42.3
44	Vermont	37.5
27	Virginia	42.1
49	Washington	35.1
9	West Virginia	45.1
41	Wisconsin	38.2
29	Wyoming	41.8

RANK ORDER

RANK	STATE	PERCENT
1	Missouri	48.0
2	New Mexico	47.7
3	Pennsylvania	47.1
3	South Dakota	47.1
5	Mississippi	46.8
6	South Carolina	46.7
7	Louisiana	45.8
8	Nebraska	45.5
9	West Virginia	45.1
10	Illinois	45.0
11	North Dakota	44.7
12	Alaska	44.6
12	Arkansas	44.6
14	Tennessee	44.5
15	Alabama	44.0
16	Kentucky	43.5
17	Georgia	43.3
17	Texas	43.3
19	Michigan	43.2
20	Massachusetts	42.8
20	North Carolina	42.8
20	Ohio	42.8
23	Indiana	42.7
24	Montana	42.5
25	Iowa	42.4
26	Utah	42.3
27	Virginia	42.1
28	Hawaii	41.9
29	New York	41.8
29	Wyoming	41.8
31	Delaware	41.5
31	Kansas	41.5
33	Oklahoma	41.4
34	New Hampshire	40.2
35	Maine	40.1
35	New Jersey	40.1
37	Idaho	39.5
38	Colorado	39.1
38	Maryland	39.1
40	Rhode Island	38.3
41	Florida	38.2
41	Wisconsin	38.2
43	Arizona	37.6
44	Vermont	37.5
45	Oregon	37.1
46	California	37.0
47	Nevada	36.3
48	Connecticut	35.9
49	Washington	35.1
50	Minnesota	33.8

	District of Columbia	61.0

Source: Morgan Quitno Press using data from U.S. Dept of Health & Human Services, Health Care Financing Admin.
"State Health Expenditure Accounts" (Health Care Financing Review, Fall 1995, Volume 17, Number 1)
*By state of provider.

Per Capita Expenditures for Hospital Care in 1993

National Per Capita = $1,256*

ALPHA ORDER

RANK	STATE	PER CAPITA
16	Alabama	$1,268
27	Alaska	1,172
43	Arizona	1,014
31	Arkansas	1,123
33	California	1,116
35	Colorado	1,102
9	Connecticut	1,336
8	Delaware	1,340
19	Florida	1,248
17	Georgia	1,261
18	Hawaii	1,252
50	Idaho	817
9	Illinois	1,336
23	Indiana	1,226
35	Iowa	1,102
30	Kansas	1,133
26	Kentucky	1,190
7	Louisiana	1,389
34	Maine	1,111
24	Maryland	1,197
1	Massachusetts	1,667
21	Michigan	1,238
41	Minnesota	1,060
37	Mississippi	1,098
4	Missouri	1,462
40	Montana	1,063
20	Nebraska	1,241
45	Nevada	983
22	New Hampshire	1,236
12	New Jersey	1,312
29	New Mexico	1,144
3	New York	1,542
32	North Carolina	1,122
5	North Dakota	1,418
13	Ohio	1,293
42	Oklahoma	1,030
46	Oregon	977
2	Pennsylvania	1,624
11	Rhode Island	1,315
28	South Carolina	1,164
15	South Dakota	1,283
6	Tennessee	1,415
25	Texas	1,196
48	Utah	937
47	Vermont	976
39	Virginia	1,086
44	Washington	1,010
14	West Virginia	1,290
37	Wisconsin	1,098
49	Wyoming	887

RANK ORDER

RANK	STATE	PER CAPITA
1	Massachusetts	$1,667
2	Pennsylvania	1,624
3	New York	1,542
4	Missouri	1,462
5	North Dakota	1,418
6	Tennessee	1,415
7	Louisiana	1,389
8	Delaware	1,340
9	Connecticut	1,336
9	Illinois	1,336
11	Rhode Island	1,315
12	New Jersey	1,312
13	Ohio	1,293
14	West Virginia	1,290
15	South Dakota	1,283
16	Alabama	1,268
17	Georgia	1,261
18	Hawaii	1,252
19	Florida	1,248
20	Nebraska	1,241
21	Michigan	1,238
22	New Hampshire	1,236
23	Indiana	1,226
24	Maryland	1,197
25	Texas	1,196
26	Kentucky	1,190
27	Alaska	1,172
28	South Carolina	1,164
29	New Mexico	1,144
30	Kansas	1,133
31	Arkansas	1,123
32	North Carolina	1,122
33	California	1,116
34	Maine	1,111
35	Colorado	1,102
35	Iowa	1,102
37	Mississippi	1,098
37	Wisconsin	1,098
39	Virginia	1,086
40	Montana	1,063
41	Minnesota	1,060
42	Oklahoma	1,030
43	Arizona	1,014
44	Washington	1,010
45	Nevada	983
46	Oregon	977
47	Vermont	976
48	Utah	937
49	Wyoming	887
50	Idaho	817
	District of Columbia**	4,519

Source: Morgan Quitno Press using data from U.S. Dept of Health & Human Services, Health Care Financing Admin. "State Health Expenditure Accounts" (Health Care Financing Review, Fall 1995, Volume 17, Number 1)

*By state of provider.

**The District of Columbia's per capita is greatly affected by residents of Maryland and Virginia receiving services.

Percent Change in Expenditures for Hospital Care: 1990 to 1993

National Percent Change = 27.4% Increase*

ALPHA ORDER

RANK	STATE	PERCENT
12	Alabama	32.0
33	Alaska	25.9
40	Arizona	24.3
22	Arkansas	29.1
38	California	24.6
29	Colorado	26.8
47	Connecticut	19.5
10	Delaware	32.2
26	Florida	27.3
21	Georgia	30.2
28	Hawaii	27.2
4	Idaho	35.3
32	Illinois	26.0
9	Indiana	32.3
48	Iowa	18.1
37	Kansas	24.7
15	Kentucky	31.4
24	Louisiana	28.7
44	Maine	23.0
26	Maryland	27.3
44	Massachusetts	23.0
42	Michigan	23.3
50	Minnesota	17.1
8	Mississippi	32.5
25	Missouri	27.8
13	Montana	31.7
31	Nebraska	26.2
20	Nevada	30.6
15	New Hampshire	31.4
18	New Jersey	31.2
2	New Mexico	35.5
43	New York	23.1
10	North Carolina	32.2
33	North Dakota	25.9
36	Ohio	25.3
39	Oklahoma	24.5
22	Oregon	29.1
15	Pennsylvania	31.4
46	Rhode Island	20.0
1	South Carolina	35.8
7	South Dakota	32.6
19	Tennessee	30.8
2	Texas	35.5
14	Utah	31.5
35	Vermont	25.7
41	Virginia	24.2
5	Washington	33.9
6	West Virginia	33.1
30	Wisconsin	26.5
48	Wyoming	18.1

RANK ORDER

RANK	STATE	PERCENT
1	South Carolina	35.8
2	New Mexico	35.5
2	Texas	35.5
4	Idaho	35.3
5	Washington	33.9
6	West Virginia	33.1
7	South Dakota	32.6
8	Mississippi	32.5
9	Indiana	32.3
10	Delaware	32.2
10	North Carolina	32.2
12	Alabama	32.0
13	Montana	31.7
14	Utah	31.5
15	Kentucky	31.4
15	New Hampshire	31.4
15	Pennsylvania	31.4
18	New Jersey	31.2
19	Tennessee	30.8
20	Nevada	30.6
21	Georgia	30.2
22	Arkansas	29.1
22	Oregon	29.1
24	Louisiana	28.7
25	Missouri	27.8
26	Florida	27.3
26	Maryland	27.3
28	Hawaii	27.2
29	Colorado	26.8
30	Wisconsin	26.5
31	Nebraska	26.2
32	Illinois	26.0
33	Alaska	25.9
33	North Dakota	25.9
35	Vermont	25.7
36	Ohio	25.3
37	Kansas	24.7
38	California	24.6
39	Oklahoma	24.5
40	Arizona	24.3
41	Virginia	24.2
42	Michigan	23.3
43	New York	23.1
44	Maine	23.0
44	Massachusetts	23.0
46	Rhode Island	20.0
47	Connecticut	19.5
48	Iowa	18.1
48	Wyoming	18.1
50	Minnesota	17.1

| | District of Columbia | 22.5 |

Source: Morgan Quitno Press using data from U.S. Dept of Health & Human Services, Health Care Financing Admin.
"State Health Expenditure Accounts" (Health Care Financing Review, Fall 1995, Volume 17, Number 1)
*By state of provider.

Percent Change in Per Capita Expenditures for Hospital Care: 1990 to 1993

National Percent Change = 22.9% Increase*

ALPHA ORDER

RANK	STATE	PERCENT CHANGE
10	Alabama	27.6
46	Alaska	15.7
47	Arizona	15.5
17	Arkansas	25.2
42	California	18.8
44	Colorado	17.1
41	Connecticut	19.8
16	Delaware	25.8
40	Florida	19.9
30	Georgia	22.2
38	Hawaii	20.8
22	Idaho	23.8
24	Illinois	23.1
8	Indiana	28.5
45	Iowa	16.1
31	Kansas	22.1
9	Kentucky	27.7
13	Louisiana	26.7
32	Maine	22.0
25	Maryland	22.9
25	Massachusetts	22.9
36	Michigan	21.1
49	Minnesota	13.2
5	Mississippi	29.3
20	Missouri	25.0
19	Montana	25.1
23	Nebraska	23.4
49	Nevada	13.2
3	New Hampshire	29.8
6	New Jersey	29.1
12	New Mexico	27.1
32	New York	22.0
15	North Carolina	26.1
14	North Dakota	26.4
28	Ohio	22.8
35	Oklahoma	21.2
37	Oregon	20.9
4	Pennsylvania	29.7
39	Rhode Island	20.4
2	South Carolina	30.5
7	South Dakota	28.7
17	Tennessee	25.2
11	Texas	27.5
34	Utah	21.8
25	Vermont	22.9
43	Virginia	18.7
21	Washington	24.1
1	West Virginia	31.2
29	Wisconsin	22.7
48	Wyoming	14.0

RANK ORDER

RANK	STATE	PERCENT CHANGE
1	West Virginia	31.2
2	South Carolina	30.5
3	New Hampshire	29.8
4	Pennsylvania	29.7
5	Mississippi	29.3
6	New Jersey	29.1
7	South Dakota	28.7
8	Indiana	28.5
9	Kentucky	27.7
10	Alabama	27.6
11	Texas	27.5
12	New Mexico	27.1
13	Louisiana	26.7
14	North Dakota	26.4
15	North Carolina	26.1
16	Delaware	25.8
17	Arkansas	25.2
17	Tennessee	25.2
19	Montana	25.1
20	Missouri	25.0
21	Washington	24.1
22	Idaho	23.8
23	Nebraska	23.4
24	Illinois	23.1
25	Maryland	22.9
25	Massachusetts	22.9
25	Vermont	22.9
28	Ohio	22.8
29	Wisconsin	22.7
30	Georgia	22.2
31	Kansas	22.1
32	Maine	22.0
32	New York	22.0
34	Utah	21.8
35	Oklahoma	21.2
36	Michigan	21.1
37	Oregon	20.9
38	Hawaii	20.8
39	Rhode Island	20.4
40	Florida	19.9
41	Connecticut	19.8
42	California	18.8
43	Virginia	18.7
44	Colorado	17.1
45	Iowa	16.1
46	Alaska	15.7
47	Arizona	15.5
48	Wyoming	14.0
49	Minnesota	13.2
49	Nevada	13.2

District of Columbia   28.6

Source: Morgan Quitno Press using data from U.S. Dept of Health & Human Services, Health Care Financing Admin. "State Health Expenditure Accounts" (Health Care Financing Review, Fall 1995, Volume 17, Number 1)
*By state of provider.

Average Annual Change in Expenditures for Hospital Care: 1980 to 1993

National Percent = 9.4% Average Annual Growth*

ALPHA ORDER				RANK ORDER		
RANK	STATE	PERCENT		RANK	STATE	PERCENT
23	Alabama	9.8		1	New Hampshire	12.2
19	Alaska	10.2		2	South Carolina	12.0
15	Arizona	10.5		3	Hawaii	11.5
13	Arkansas	10.6		3	New Mexico	11.5
33	California	8.8		5	Georgia	11.4
27	Colorado	9.5		6	North Carolina	11.3
31	Connecticut	9.2		7	Florida	11.1
16	Delaware	10.4		7	Texas	11.1
7	Florida	11.1		9	Utah	11.0
5	Georgia	11.4		10	Washington	10.9
3	Hawaii	11.5		11	Idaho	10.7
11	Idaho	10.7		11	New Jersey	10.7
50	Illinois	7.4		13	Arkansas	10.6
26	Indiana	9.7		13	Kentucky	10.6
47	Iowa	7.8		15	Arizona	10.5
47	Kansas	7.8		16	Delaware	10.4
13	Kentucky	10.6		17	Nevada	10.3
20	Louisiana	10.0		17	Tennessee	10.3
33	Maine	8.8		19	Alaska	10.2
37	Maryland	8.6		20	Louisiana	10.0
45	Massachusetts	8.1		21	Montana	9.9
49	Michigan	7.7		21	Virginia	9.9
44	Minnesota	8.2		23	Alabama	9.8
23	Mississippi	9.8		23	Mississippi	9.8
32	Missouri	8.9		23	South Dakota	9.8
21	Montana	9.9		26	Indiana	9.7
33	Nebraska	8.8		27	Colorado	9.5
17	Nevada	10.3		27	Pennsylvania	9.5
1	New Hampshire	12.2		27	Vermont	9.5
11	New Jersey	10.7		30	Oregon	9.4
3	New Mexico	11.5		31	Connecticut	9.2
37	New York	8.6		32	Missouri	8.9
6	North Carolina	11.3		33	California	8.8
39	North Dakota	8.5		33	Maine	8.8
33	Ohio	8.8		33	Nebraska	8.8
39	Oklahoma	8.5		33	Ohio	8.8
30	Oregon	9.4		37	Maryland	8.6
27	Pennsylvania	9.5		37	New York	8.6
45	Rhode Island	8.1		39	North Dakota	8.5
2	South Carolina	12.0		39	Oklahoma	8.5
23	South Dakota	9.8		39	Wyoming	8.5
17	Tennessee	10.3		42	West Virginia	8.4
7	Texas	11.1		42	Wisconsin	8.4
9	Utah	11.0		44	Minnesota	8.2
27	Vermont	9.5		45	Massachusetts	8.1
21	Virginia	9.9		45	Rhode Island	8.1
10	Washington	10.9		47	Iowa	7.8
42	West Virginia	8.4		47	Kansas	7.8
42	Wisconsin	8.4		49	Michigan	7.7
39	Wyoming	8.5		50	Illinois	7.4
				District of Columbia		8.4

Source: U.S. Department of Health and Human Services, Health Care Financing Administration
"State Health Expenditure Accounts" (Health Care Financing Review, Fall 1995, Volume 17, Number 1)
*By state of provider.

271

Average Annual Change in Per Capita Expenditures
For Hospital Care: 1980 to 1993
National Percent = 8.3% Average Annual Increase*

ALPHA ORDER

RANK	STATE	PERCENT
18	Alabama	9.1
48	Alaska	6.9
43	Arizona	7.4
5	Arkansas	10.0
49	California	6.5
39	Colorado	7.7
24	Connecticut	8.7
19	Delaware	9.0
32	Florida	8.2
10	Georgia	9.4
6	Hawaii	9.8
14	Idaho	9.3
44	Illinois	7.2
14	Indiana	9.3
35	Iowa	8.0
44	Kansas	7.2
3	Kentucky	10.2
8	Louisiana	9.7
35	Maine	8.0
44	Maryland	7.2
39	Massachusetts	7.7
42	Michigan	7.5
44	Minnesota	7.2
14	Mississippi	9.3
27	Missouri	8.4
14	Montana	9.3
27	Nebraska	8.4
50	Nevada	5.6
2	New Hampshire	10.4
4	New Jersey	10.1
9	New Mexico	9.6
31	New York	8.3
6	North Carolina	9.8
24	North Dakota	8.7
26	Ohio	8.6
37	Oklahoma	7.8
32	Oregon	8.2
10	Pennsylvania	9.4
41	Rhode Island	7.6
1	South Carolina	10.6
10	South Dakota	9.4
10	Tennessee	9.4
19	Texas	9.0
21	Utah	8.9
27	Vermont	8.4
32	Virginia	8.2
23	Washington	8.8
21	West Virginia	8.9
37	Wisconsin	7.8
27	Wyoming	8.4

RANK ORDER

RANK	STATE	PERCENT
1	South Carolina	10.6
2	New Hampshire	10.4
3	Kentucky	10.2
4	New Jersey	10.1
5	Arkansas	10.0
6	Hawaii	9.8
6	North Carolina	9.8
8	Louisiana	9.7
9	New Mexico	9.6
10	Georgia	9.4
10	Pennsylvania	9.4
10	South Dakota	9.4
10	Tennessee	9.4
14	Idaho	9.3
14	Indiana	9.3
14	Mississippi	9.3
14	Montana	9.3
18	Alabama	9.1
19	Delaware	9.0
19	Texas	9.0
21	Utah	8.9
21	West Virginia	8.9
23	Washington	8.8
24	Connecticut	8.7
24	North Dakota	8.7
26	Ohio	8.6
27	Missouri	8.4
27	Nebraska	8.4
27	Vermont	8.4
27	Wyoming	8.4
31	New York	8.3
32	Florida	8.2
32	Oregon	8.2
32	Virginia	8.2
35	Iowa	8.0
35	Maine	8.0
37	Oklahoma	7.8
37	Wisconsin	7.8
39	Colorado	7.7
39	Massachusetts	7.7
41	Rhode Island	7.6
42	Michigan	7.5
43	Arizona	7.4
44	Illinois	7.2
44	Kansas	7.2
44	Maryland	7.2
44	Minnesota	7.2
48	Alaska	6.9
49	California	6.5
50	Nevada	5.6

District of Columbia 9.3

Source: Morgan Quitno Press using data from U.S. Dept of Health & Human Services, Health Care Financing Admin.
"State Health Expenditure Accounts" (Health Care Financing Review, Fall 1995, Volume 17, Number 1)
*By state of provider.

Expenditures for Physician Services in 1993

National Total = $171,226,000,000*

<table>
<tr><td colspan="4">ALPHA ORDER</td><td colspan="4">RANK ORDER</td></tr>
<tr><td>RANK</td><td>STATE</td><td>EXPENDITURES</td><td>% of USA</td><td>RANK</td><td>STATE</td><td>EXPENDITURES</td><td>% of USA</td></tr>
<tr><td>22</td><td>Alabama</td><td>$2,631,000,000</td><td>1.54%</td><td>1</td><td>California</td><td>$28,981,000,000</td><td>16.93%</td></tr>
<tr><td>48</td><td>Alaska</td><td>301,000,000</td><td>0.18%</td><td>2</td><td>New York</td><td>12,003,000,000</td><td>7.01%</td></tr>
<tr><td>21</td><td>Arizona</td><td>2,799,000,000</td><td>1.63%</td><td>3</td><td>Texas</td><td>10,526,000,000</td><td>6.15%</td></tr>
<tr><td>32</td><td>Arkansas</td><td>1,244,000,000</td><td>0.73%</td><td>4</td><td>Florida</td><td>10,498,000,000</td><td>6.13%</td></tr>
<tr><td>1</td><td>California</td><td>28,981,000,000</td><td>16.93%</td><td>5</td><td>Pennsylvania</td><td>7,460,000,000</td><td>4.36%</td></tr>
<tr><td>25</td><td>Colorado</td><td>2,452,000,000</td><td>1.43%</td><td>6</td><td>Ohio</td><td>7,118,000,000</td><td>4.16%</td></tr>
<tr><td>23</td><td>Connecticut</td><td>2,587,000,000</td><td>1.51%</td><td>7</td><td>Illinois</td><td>6,970,000,000</td><td>4.07%</td></tr>
<tr><td>44</td><td>Delaware</td><td>466,000,000</td><td>0.27%</td><td>8</td><td>New Jersey</td><td>5,776,000,000</td><td>3.37%</td></tr>
<tr><td>4</td><td>Florida</td><td>10,498,000,000</td><td>6.13%</td><td>9</td><td>Michigan</td><td>5,562,000,000</td><td>3.25%</td></tr>
<tr><td>10</td><td>Georgia</td><td>4,543,000,000</td><td>2.65%</td><td>10</td><td>Georgia</td><td>4,543,000,000</td><td>2.65%</td></tr>
<tr><td>39</td><td>Hawaii</td><td>771,000,000</td><td>0.45%</td><td>11</td><td>Massachusetts</td><td>4,442,000,000</td><td>2.59%</td></tr>
<tr><td>43</td><td>Idaho</td><td>486,000,000</td><td>0.28%</td><td>12</td><td>Virginia</td><td>3,769,000,000</td><td>2.20%</td></tr>
<tr><td>7</td><td>Illinois</td><td>6,970,000,000</td><td>4.07%</td><td>13</td><td>Washington</td><td>3,720,000,000</td><td>2.17%</td></tr>
<tr><td>18</td><td>Indiana</td><td>3,263,000,000</td><td>1.91%</td><td>14</td><td>North Carolina</td><td>3,717,000,000</td><td>2.17%</td></tr>
<tr><td>31</td><td>Iowa</td><td>1,376,000,000</td><td>0.80%</td><td>15</td><td>Maryland</td><td>3,704,000,000</td><td>2.16%</td></tr>
<tr><td>30</td><td>Kansas</td><td>1,425,000,000</td><td>0.83%</td><td>16</td><td>Minnesota</td><td>3,617,000,000</td><td>2.11%</td></tr>
<tr><td>26</td><td>Kentucky</td><td>2,038,000,000</td><td>1.19%</td><td>17</td><td>Wisconsin</td><td>3,362,000,000</td><td>1.96%</td></tr>
<tr><td>24</td><td>Louisiana</td><td>2,537,000,000</td><td>1.48%</td><td>18</td><td>Indiana</td><td>3,263,000,000</td><td>1.91%</td></tr>
<tr><td>41</td><td>Maine</td><td>601,000,000</td><td>0.35%</td><td>19</td><td>Tennessee</td><td>3,137,000,000</td><td>1.83%</td></tr>
<tr><td>15</td><td>Maryland</td><td>3,704,000,000</td><td>2.16%</td><td>20</td><td>Missouri</td><td>2,958,000,000</td><td>1.73%</td></tr>
<tr><td>11</td><td>Massachusetts</td><td>4,442,000,000</td><td>2.59%</td><td>21</td><td>Arizona</td><td>2,799,000,000</td><td>1.63%</td></tr>
<tr><td>9</td><td>Michigan</td><td>5,562,000,000</td><td>3.25%</td><td>22</td><td>Alabama</td><td>2,631,000,000</td><td>1.54%</td></tr>
<tr><td>16</td><td>Minnesota</td><td>3,617,000,000</td><td>2.11%</td><td>23</td><td>Connecticut</td><td>2,587,000,000</td><td>1.51%</td></tr>
<tr><td>33</td><td>Mississippi</td><td>1,107,000,000</td><td>0.65%</td><td>24</td><td>Louisiana</td><td>2,537,000,000</td><td>1.48%</td></tr>
<tr><td>20</td><td>Missouri</td><td>2,958,000,000</td><td>1.73%</td><td>25</td><td>Colorado</td><td>2,452,000,000</td><td>1.43%</td></tr>
<tr><td>46</td><td>Montana</td><td>392,000,000</td><td>0.23%</td><td>26</td><td>Kentucky</td><td>2,038,000,000</td><td>1.19%</td></tr>
<tr><td>37</td><td>Nebraska</td><td>825,000,000</td><td>0.48%</td><td>27</td><td>Oregon</td><td>1,904,000,000</td><td>1.11%</td></tr>
<tr><td>34</td><td>Nevada</td><td>1,029,000,000</td><td>0.60%</td><td>28</td><td>South Carolina</td><td>1,685,000,000</td><td>0.98%</td></tr>
<tr><td>38</td><td>New Hampshire</td><td>780,000,000</td><td>0.46%</td><td>29</td><td>Oklahoma</td><td>1,640,000,000</td><td>0.96%</td></tr>
<tr><td>8</td><td>New Jersey</td><td>5,776,000,000</td><td>3.37%</td><td>30</td><td>Kansas</td><td>1,425,000,000</td><td>0.83%</td></tr>
<tr><td>40</td><td>New Mexico</td><td>716,000,000</td><td>0.42%</td><td>31</td><td>Iowa</td><td>1,376,000,000</td><td>0.80%</td></tr>
<tr><td>2</td><td>New York</td><td>12,003,000,000</td><td>7.01%</td><td>32</td><td>Arkansas</td><td>1,244,000,000</td><td>0.73%</td></tr>
<tr><td>14</td><td>North Carolina</td><td>3,717,000,000</td><td>2.17%</td><td>33</td><td>Mississippi</td><td>1,107,000,000</td><td>0.65%</td></tr>
<tr><td>45</td><td>North Dakota</td><td>445,000,000</td><td>0.26%</td><td>34</td><td>Nevada</td><td>1,029,000,000</td><td>0.60%</td></tr>
<tr><td>6</td><td>Ohio</td><td>7,118,000,000</td><td>4.16%</td><td>35</td><td>West Virginia</td><td>988,000,000</td><td>0.58%</td></tr>
<tr><td>29</td><td>Oklahoma</td><td>1,640,000,000</td><td>0.96%</td><td>36</td><td>Utah</td><td>864,000,000</td><td>0.50%</td></tr>
<tr><td>27</td><td>Oregon</td><td>1,904,000,000</td><td>1.11%</td><td>37</td><td>Nebraska</td><td>825,000,000</td><td>0.48%</td></tr>
<tr><td>5</td><td>Pennsylvania</td><td>7,460,000,000</td><td>4.36%</td><td>38</td><td>New Hampshire</td><td>780,000,000</td><td>0.46%</td></tr>
<tr><td>42</td><td>Rhode Island</td><td>575,000,000</td><td>0.34%</td><td>39</td><td>Hawaii</td><td>771,000,000</td><td>0.45%</td></tr>
<tr><td>28</td><td>South Carolina</td><td>1,685,000,000</td><td>0.98%</td><td>40</td><td>New Mexico</td><td>716,000,000</td><td>0.42%</td></tr>
<tr><td>47</td><td>South Dakota</td><td>342,000,000</td><td>0.20%</td><td>41</td><td>Maine</td><td>601,000,000</td><td>0.35%</td></tr>
<tr><td>19</td><td>Tennessee</td><td>3,137,000,000</td><td>1.83%</td><td>42</td><td>Rhode Island</td><td>575,000,000</td><td>0.34%</td></tr>
<tr><td>3</td><td>Texas</td><td>10,526,000,000</td><td>6.15%</td><td>43</td><td>Idaho</td><td>486,000,000</td><td>0.28%</td></tr>
<tr><td>36</td><td>Utah</td><td>864,000,000</td><td>0.50%</td><td>44</td><td>Delaware</td><td>466,000,000</td><td>0.27%</td></tr>
<tr><td>49</td><td>Vermont</td><td>265,000,000</td><td>0.15%</td><td>45</td><td>North Dakota</td><td>445,000,000</td><td>0.26%</td></tr>
<tr><td>12</td><td>Virginia</td><td>3,769,000,000</td><td>2.20%</td><td>46</td><td>Montana</td><td>392,000,000</td><td>0.23%</td></tr>
<tr><td>13</td><td>Washington</td><td>3,720,000,000</td><td>2.17%</td><td>47</td><td>South Dakota</td><td>342,000,000</td><td>0.20%</td></tr>
<tr><td>35</td><td>West Virginia</td><td>988,000,000</td><td>0.58%</td><td>48</td><td>Alaska</td><td>301,000,000</td><td>0.18%</td></tr>
<tr><td>17</td><td>Wisconsin</td><td>3,362,000,000</td><td>1.96%</td><td>49</td><td>Vermont</td><td>265,000,000</td><td>0.15%</td></tr>
<tr><td>50</td><td>Wyoming</td><td>160,000,000</td><td>0.09%</td><td>50</td><td>Wyoming</td><td>160,000,000</td><td>0.09%</td></tr>
<tr><td></td><td></td><td></td><td></td><td></td><td>District of Columbia</td><td>672,000,000</td><td>0.39%</td></tr>
</table>

Source: U.S. Department of Health and Human Services, Health Care Financing Administration
"State Health Expenditure Accounts" (Health Care Financing Review, Fall 1995, Volume 17, Number 1)
*By state of provider.

Percent of Total Personal Health Care Expenditures
Spent on Physician Services in 1993
National Percent = 22.0%*

ALPHA ORDER

RANK	STATE	PERCENT
17	Alabama	21.8
34	Alaska	19.1
3	Arizona	26.3
26	Arkansas	20.4
1	California	30.8
6	Colorado	24.4
20	Connecticut	21.2
23	Delaware	20.6
9	Florida	23.4
11	Georgia	22.6
15	Hawaii	22.1
18	Idaho	21.3
29	Illinois	20.1
30	Indiana	19.9
38	Iowa	18.7
23	Kansas	20.6
31	Kentucky	19.6
32	Louisiana	19.5
47	Maine	17.5
6	Maryland	24.4
35	Massachusetts	19.0
25	Michigan	20.5
4	Minnesota	25.5
44	Mississippi	17.9
41	Missouri	18.5
40	Montana	18.6
37	Nebraska	18.8
2	Nevada	27.5
11	New Hampshire	22.6
14	New Jersey	22.4
41	New Mexico	18.5
44	New York	17.9
26	North Carolina	20.4
16	North Dakota	22.0
18	Ohio	21.3
26	Oklahoma	20.4
8	Oregon	23.8
43	Pennsylvania	18.0
49	Rhode Island	16.8
38	South Carolina	18.7
47	South Dakota	17.5
33	Tennessee	19.4
21	Texas	21.1
22	Utah	21.0
46	Vermont	17.7
11	Virginia	22.6
5	Washington	24.6
35	West Virginia	19.0
10	Wisconsin	23.2
50	Wyoming	16.0

RANK ORDER

RANK	STATE	PERCENT
1	California	30.8
2	Nevada	27.5
3	Arizona	26.3
4	Minnesota	25.5
5	Washington	24.6
6	Colorado	24.4
6	Maryland	24.4
8	Oregon	23.8
9	Florida	23.4
10	Wisconsin	23.2
11	Georgia	22.6
11	New Hampshire	22.6
11	Virginia	22.6
14	New Jersey	22.4
15	Hawaii	22.1
16	North Dakota	22.0
17	Alabama	21.8
18	Idaho	21.3
18	Ohio	21.3
20	Connecticut	21.2
21	Texas	21.1
22	Utah	21.0
23	Delaware	20.6
23	Kansas	20.6
25	Michigan	20.5
26	Arkansas	20.4
26	North Carolina	20.4
26	Oklahoma	20.4
29	Illinois	20.1
30	Indiana	19.9
31	Kentucky	19.6
32	Louisiana	19.5
33	Tennessee	19.4
34	Alaska	19.1
35	Massachusetts	19.0
35	West Virginia	19.0
37	Nebraska	18.8
38	Iowa	18.7
38	South Carolina	18.7
40	Montana	18.6
41	Missouri	18.5
41	New Mexico	18.5
43	Pennsylvania	18.0
44	Mississippi	17.9
44	New York	17.9
46	Vermont	17.7
47	Maine	17.5
47	South Dakota	17.5
49	Rhode Island	16.8
50	Wyoming	16.0

| | District of Columbia | 15.7 |

Source: Morgan Quitno Press using data from U.S. Dept of Health & Human Services, Health Care Financing Admin.
"State Health Expenditure Accounts" (Health Care Financing Review, Fall 1995, Volume 17, Number 1)
*By state of provider.

Per Capita Expenditures for Physician Services in 1993

National Per Capita = $664*

ALPHA ORDER

RANK	STATE	PER CAPITA
20	Alabama	$629
39	Alaska	503
9	Arizona	710
36	Arkansas	513
1	California	928
13	Colorado	687
3	Connecticut	789
14	Delaware	667
4	Florida	765
18	Georgia	658
16	Hawaii	661
48	Idaho	441
24	Illinois	596
30	Indiana	572
40	Iowa	488
32	Kansas	563
34	Kentucky	537
25	Louisiana	592
41	Maine	485
5	Maryland	748
7	Massachusetts	738
26	Michigan	588
2	Minnesota	800
49	Mississippi	419
31	Missouri	565
43	Montana	466
37	Nebraska	511
6	Nevada	743
12	New Hampshire	695
8	New Jersey	735
47	New Mexico	443
16	New York	661
35	North Carolina	535
11	North Dakota	699
19	Ohio	644
38	Oklahoma	507
21	Oregon	627
22	Pennsylvania	620
29	Rhode Island	576
44	South Carolina	465
42	South Dakota	477
23	Tennessee	616
27	Texas	583
44	Utah	465
46	Vermont	460
28	Virginia	582
10	Washington	708
33	West Virginia	543
14	Wisconsin	667
50	Wyoming	340

RANK ORDER

RANK	STATE	PER CAPITA
1	California	$928
2	Minnesota	800
3	Connecticut	789
4	Florida	765
5	Maryland	748
6	Nevada	743
7	Massachusetts	738
8	New Jersey	735
9	Arizona	710
10	Washington	708
11	North Dakota	699
12	New Hampshire	695
13	Colorado	687
14	Delaware	667
14	Wisconsin	667
16	Hawaii	661
16	New York	661
18	Georgia	658
19	Ohio	644
20	Alabama	629
21	Oregon	627
22	Pennsylvania	620
23	Tennessee	616
24	Illinois	596
25	Louisiana	592
26	Michigan	588
27	Texas	583
28	Virginia	582
29	Rhode Island	576
30	Indiana	572
31	Missouri	565
32	Kansas	563
33	West Virginia	543
34	Kentucky	537
35	North Carolina	535
36	Arkansas	513
37	Nebraska	511
38	Oklahoma	507
39	Alaska	503
40	Iowa	488
41	Maine	485
42	South Dakota	477
43	Montana	466
44	South Carolina	465
44	Utah	465
46	Vermont	460
47	New Mexico	443
48	Idaho	441
49	Mississippi	419
50	Wyoming	340

District of Columbia**   1,163

Source: Morgan Quitno Press using data from U.S. Dept of Health & Human Services, Health Care Financing Admin.
"State Health Expenditure Accounts" (Health Care Financing Review, Fall 1995, Volume 17, Number 1)
*By state of provider.
**The District of Columbia's per capita is greatly affected by residents of Maryland and Virginia receiving services.

Percent Change in Expenditures for Physician Services: 1990 to 1993

National Percent Change = 21.9% Increase*

ALPHA ORDER

RANK	STATE	PERCENT CHANGE
42	Alabama	17.1
44	Alaska	16.7
46	Arizona	12.0
49	Arkansas	9.7
6	California	29.6
5	Colorado	29.7
37	Connecticut	18.4
19	Delaware	23.6
48	Florida	11.2
15	Georgia	24.6
20	Hawaii	22.6
4	Idaho	29.9
34	Illinois	18.9
23	Indiana	21.8
25	Iowa	20.5
40	Kansas	17.7
16	Kentucky	24.3
30	Louisiana	19.2
11	Maine	25.2
12	Maryland	24.8
38	Massachusetts	18.0
30	Michigan	19.2
21	Minnesota	22.3
28	Mississippi	19.7
33	Missouri	19.0
10	Montana	26.0
26	Nebraska	19.9
9	Nevada	26.7
1	New Hampshire	58.9
7	New Jersey	27.8
14	New Mexico	24.7
17	New York	23.8
18	North Carolina	23.7
24	North Dakota	20.9
40	Ohio	17.7
36	Oklahoma	18.7
30	Oregon	19.2
29	Pennsylvania	19.3
47	Rhode Island	11.9
8	South Carolina	27.2
12	South Dakota	24.8
22	Tennessee	22.1
38	Texas	18.0
43	Utah	16.9
26	Vermont	19.9
35	Virginia	18.8
2	Washington	31.3
45	West Virginia	15.4
3	Wisconsin	31.1
50	Wyoming	9.6

RANK ORDER

RANK	STATE	PERCENT CHANGE
1	New Hampshire	58.9
2	Washington	31.3
3	Wisconsin	31.1
4	Idaho	29.9
5	Colorado	29.7
6	California	29.6
7	New Jersey	27.8
8	South Carolina	27.2
9	Nevada	26.7
10	Montana	26.0
11	Maine	25.2
12	Maryland	24.8
12	South Dakota	24.8
14	New Mexico	24.7
15	Georgia	24.6
16	Kentucky	24.3
17	New York	23.8
18	North Carolina	23.7
19	Delaware	23.6
20	Hawaii	22.6
21	Minnesota	22.3
22	Tennessee	22.1
23	Indiana	21.8
24	North Dakota	20.9
25	Iowa	20.5
26	Nebraska	19.9
26	Vermont	19.9
28	Mississippi	19.7
29	Pennsylvania	19.3
30	Louisiana	19.2
30	Michigan	19.2
30	Oregon	19.2
33	Missouri	19.0
34	Illinois	18.9
35	Virginia	18.8
36	Oklahoma	18.7
37	Connecticut	18.4
38	Massachusetts	18.0
38	Texas	18.0
40	Kansas	17.7
40	Ohio	17.7
42	Alabama	17.1
43	Utah	16.9
44	Alaska	16.7
45	West Virginia	15.4
46	Arizona	12.0
47	Rhode Island	11.9
48	Florida	11.2
49	Arkansas	9.7
50	Wyoming	9.6
	District of Columbia	2.3

Source: Morgan Quitno Press using data from U.S. Dept of Health & Human Services, Health Care Financing Admin.
"State Health Expenditure Accounts" (Health Care Financing Review, Fall 1995, Volume 17, Number 1)
*By state of provider.

Percent Change in Per Capita Expenditures for Physician Services: 1990 to 1993

National Percent Change = 17.5% Increase*

<table>
<tr><td colspan="3">ALPHA ORDER</td><td colspan="3">RANK ORDER</td></tr>
<tr><td>RANK</td><td>STATE</td><td>PERCENT CHANGE</td><td>RANK</td><td>STATE</td><td>PERCENT CHANGE</td></tr>
<tr><td>40</td><td>Alabama</td><td>13.1</td><td>1</td><td>New Hampshire</td><td>56.9</td></tr>
<tr><td>46</td><td>Alaska</td><td>7.2</td><td>2</td><td>Wisconsin</td><td>27.3</td></tr>
<tr><td>50</td><td>Arizona</td><td>4.1</td><td>3</td><td>New Jersey</td><td>25.6</td></tr>
<tr><td>47</td><td>Arkansas</td><td>6.4</td><td>4</td><td>Maine</td><td>24.0</td></tr>
<tr><td>5</td><td>California</td><td>23.4</td><td>5</td><td>California</td><td>23.4</td></tr>
<tr><td>14</td><td>Colorado</td><td>19.7</td><td>6</td><td>New York</td><td>22.6</td></tr>
<tr><td>17</td><td>Connecticut</td><td>18.6</td><td>7</td><td>South Carolina</td><td>22.4</td></tr>
<tr><td>23</td><td>Delaware</td><td>17.8</td><td>8</td><td>Washington</td><td>21.6</td></tr>
<tr><td>49</td><td>Florida</td><td>4.8</td><td>9</td><td>North Dakota</td><td>21.4</td></tr>
<tr><td>28</td><td>Georgia</td><td>16.9</td><td>10</td><td>South Dakota</td><td>21.1</td></tr>
<tr><td>32</td><td>Hawaii</td><td>16.4</td><td>11</td><td>Kentucky</td><td>20.7</td></tr>
<tr><td>15</td><td>Idaho</td><td>18.9</td><td>12</td><td>Maryland</td><td>20.5</td></tr>
<tr><td>34</td><td>Illinois</td><td>16.2</td><td>13</td><td>Montana</td><td>19.8</td></tr>
<tr><td>18</td><td>Indiana</td><td>18.4</td><td>14</td><td>Colorado</td><td>19.7</td></tr>
<tr><td>16</td><td>Iowa</td><td>18.7</td><td>15</td><td>Idaho</td><td>18.9</td></tr>
<tr><td>37</td><td>Kansas</td><td>15.1</td><td>16</td><td>Iowa</td><td>18.7</td></tr>
<tr><td>11</td><td>Kentucky</td><td>20.7</td><td>17</td><td>Connecticut</td><td>18.6</td></tr>
<tr><td>24</td><td>Louisiana</td><td>17.2</td><td>18</td><td>Indiana</td><td>18.4</td></tr>
<tr><td>4</td><td>Maine</td><td>24.0</td><td>19</td><td>Minnesota</td><td>18.3</td></tr>
<tr><td>12</td><td>Maryland</td><td>20.5</td><td>20</td><td>North Carolina</td><td>18.1</td></tr>
<tr><td>21</td><td>Massachusetts</td><td>17.9</td><td>21</td><td>Massachusetts</td><td>17.9</td></tr>
<tr><td>26</td><td>Michigan</td><td>17.1</td><td>21</td><td>Pennsylvania</td><td>17.9</td></tr>
<tr><td>19</td><td>Minnesota</td><td>18.3</td><td>23</td><td>Delaware</td><td>17.8</td></tr>
<tr><td>31</td><td>Mississippi</td><td>16.7</td><td>24</td><td>Louisiana</td><td>17.2</td></tr>
<tr><td>33</td><td>Missouri</td><td>16.3</td><td>24</td><td>Nebraska</td><td>17.2</td></tr>
<tr><td>13</td><td>Montana</td><td>19.8</td><td>26</td><td>Michigan</td><td>17.1</td></tr>
<tr><td>24</td><td>Nebraska</td><td>17.2</td><td>27</td><td>Vermont</td><td>17.0</td></tr>
<tr><td>44</td><td>Nevada</td><td>9.9</td><td>28</td><td>Georgia</td><td>16.9</td></tr>
<tr><td>1</td><td>New Hampshire</td><td>56.9</td><td>28</td><td>New Mexico</td><td>16.9</td></tr>
<tr><td>3</td><td>New Jersey</td><td>25.6</td><td>28</td><td>Tennessee</td><td>16.9</td></tr>
<tr><td>28</td><td>New Mexico</td><td>16.9</td><td>31</td><td>Mississippi</td><td>16.7</td></tr>
<tr><td>6</td><td>New York</td><td>22.6</td><td>32</td><td>Hawaii</td><td>16.4</td></tr>
<tr><td>20</td><td>North Carolina</td><td>18.1</td><td>33</td><td>Missouri</td><td>16.3</td></tr>
<tr><td>9</td><td>North Dakota</td><td>21.4</td><td>34</td><td>Illinois</td><td>16.2</td></tr>
<tr><td>36</td><td>Ohio</td><td>15.4</td><td>35</td><td>Oklahoma</td><td>15.5</td></tr>
<tr><td>35</td><td>Oklahoma</td><td>15.5</td><td>36</td><td>Ohio</td><td>15.4</td></tr>
<tr><td>42</td><td>Oregon</td><td>11.6</td><td>37</td><td>Kansas</td><td>15.1</td></tr>
<tr><td>21</td><td>Pennsylvania</td><td>17.9</td><td>38</td><td>West Virginia</td><td>13.8</td></tr>
<tr><td>41</td><td>Rhode Island</td><td>12.5</td><td>39</td><td>Virginia</td><td>13.5</td></tr>
<tr><td>7</td><td>South Carolina</td><td>22.4</td><td>40</td><td>Alabama</td><td>13.1</td></tr>
<tr><td>10</td><td>South Dakota</td><td>21.1</td><td>41</td><td>Rhode Island</td><td>12.5</td></tr>
<tr><td>28</td><td>Tennessee</td><td>16.9</td><td>42</td><td>Oregon</td><td>11.6</td></tr>
<tr><td>43</td><td>Texas</td><td>11.0</td><td>43</td><td>Texas</td><td>11.0</td></tr>
<tr><td>45</td><td>Utah</td><td>8.4</td><td>44</td><td>Nevada</td><td>9.9</td></tr>
<tr><td>27</td><td>Vermont</td><td>17.0</td><td>45</td><td>Utah</td><td>8.4</td></tr>
<tr><td>39</td><td>Virginia</td><td>13.5</td><td>46</td><td>Alaska</td><td>7.2</td></tr>
<tr><td>8</td><td>Washington</td><td>21.6</td><td>47</td><td>Arkansas</td><td>6.4</td></tr>
<tr><td>38</td><td>West Virginia</td><td>13.8</td><td>48</td><td>Wyoming</td><td>5.6</td></tr>
<tr><td>2</td><td>Wisconsin</td><td>27.3</td><td>49</td><td>Florida</td><td>4.8</td></tr>
<tr><td>48</td><td>Wyoming</td><td>5.6</td><td>50</td><td>Arizona</td><td>4.1</td></tr>
<tr><td></td><td></td><td></td><td></td><td>District of Columbia</td><td>7.5</td></tr>
</table>

Source: Morgan Quitno Press using data from U.S. Dept of Health & Human Services, Health Care Financing Admin.
"State Health Expenditure Accounts" (Health Care Financing Review, Fall 1995, Volume 17, Number 1)
*By state of provider.

Average Annual Change in Expenditures for Physician Services: 1980 to 1993

National Percent = 10.8% Average Annual Increase*

ALPHA ORDER

RANK	STATE	PERCENT CHANGE
14	Alabama	11.6
41	Alaska	9.1
5	Arizona	12.1
36	Arkansas	9.7
14	California	11.6
16	Colorado	11.4
5	Connecticut	12.1
20	Delaware	11.0
11	Florida	11.7
3	Georgia	12.5
41	Hawaii	9.1
29	Idaho	10.1
38	Illinois	9.6
24	Indiana	10.5
48	Iowa	8.3
41	Kansas	9.1
25	Kentucky	10.4
32	Louisiana	9.9
11	Maine	11.7
5	Maryland	12.1
4	Massachusetts	12.3
49	Michigan	8.2
21	Minnesota	10.9
33	Mississippi	9.8
33	Missouri	9.8
47	Montana	8.4
45	Nebraska	8.8
2	Nevada	13.1
1	New Hampshire	14.8
9	New Jersey	11.8
18	New Mexico	11.1
25	New York	10.4
8	North Carolina	11.9
39	North Dakota	9.4
36	Ohio	9.7
44	Oklahoma	9.0
40	Oregon	9.3
21	Pennsylvania	10.9
31	Rhode Island	10.0
11	South Carolina	11.7
33	South Dakota	9.8
23	Tennessee	10.7
29	Texas	10.1
28	Utah	10.2
18	Vermont	11.1
9	Virginia	11.8
16	Washington	11.4
45	West Virginia	8.8
27	Wisconsin	10.3
50	Wyoming	7.3

RANK ORDER

RANK	STATE	PERCENT CHANGE
1	New Hampshire	14.8
2	Nevada	13.1
3	Georgia	12.5
4	Massachusetts	12.3
5	Arizona	12.1
5	Connecticut	12.1
5	Maryland	12.1
8	North Carolina	11.9
9	New Jersey	11.8
9	Virginia	11.8
11	Florida	11.7
11	Maine	11.7
11	South Carolina	11.7
14	Alabama	11.6
14	California	11.6
16	Colorado	11.4
16	Washington	11.4
18	New Mexico	11.1
18	Vermont	11.1
20	Delaware	11.0
21	Minnesota	10.9
21	Pennsylvania	10.9
23	Tennessee	10.7
24	Indiana	10.5
25	Kentucky	10.4
25	New York	10.4
27	Wisconsin	10.3
28	Utah	10.2
29	Idaho	10.1
29	Texas	10.1
31	Rhode Island	10.0
32	Louisiana	9.9
33	Mississippi	9.8
33	Missouri	9.8
33	South Dakota	9.8
36	Arkansas	9.7
36	Ohio	9.7
38	Illinois	9.6
39	North Dakota	9.4
40	Oregon	9.3
41	Alaska	9.1
41	Hawaii	9.1
41	Kansas	9.1
44	Oklahoma	9.0
45	Nebraska	8.8
45	West Virginia	8.8
47	Montana	8.4
48	Iowa	8.3
49	Michigan	8.2
50	Wyoming	7.3

District of Columbia	8.4

Source: U.S. Department of Health and Human Services, Health Care Financing Administration
   "State Health Expenditure Accounts" (Health Care Financing Review, Fall 1995, Volume 17, Number 1)
*By state of provider.

Average Annual Change in Per Capita Expenditures
For Physician Services: 1980 to 1993
National Percent = 9.7% Average Annual Increase*

ALPHA ORDER

RANK	STATE	PERCENT
5	Alabama	11.0
50	Alaska	5.8
35	Arizona	8.9
33	Arkansas	9.2
33	California	9.2
21	Colorado	9.6
3	Connecticut	11.6
21	Delaware	9.6
36	Florida	8.8
9	Georgia	10.4
48	Hawaii	7.5
36	Idaho	8.8
26	Illinois	9.4
12	Indiana	10.2
38	Iowa	8.6
39	Kansas	8.5
13	Kentucky	10.1
20	Louisiana	9.7
6	Maine	10.9
7	Maryland	10.8
2	Massachusetts	12.0
46	Michigan	8.0
16	Minnesota	10.0
26	Mississippi	9.4
31	Missouri	9.3
47	Montana	7.8
39	Nebraska	8.5
41	Nevada	8.4
1	New Hampshire	13.1
4	New Jersey	11.2
31	New Mexico	9.3
13	New York	10.1
9	North Carolina	10.4
21	North Dakota	9.6
25	Ohio	9.5
41	Oklahoma	8.4
43	Oregon	8.2
7	Pennsylvania	10.8
21	Rhode Island	9.6
9	South Carolina	10.4
26	South Dakota	9.4
18	Tennessee	9.8
45	Texas	8.1
43	Utah	8.2
16	Vermont	10.0
13	Virginia	10.1
26	Washington	9.4
26	West Virginia	9.4
18	Wisconsin	9.8
49	Wyoming	7.3

RANK ORDER

RANK	STATE	PERCENT
1	New Hampshire	13.1
2	Massachusetts	12.0
3	Connecticut	11.6
4	New Jersey	11.2
5	Alabama	11.0
6	Maine	10.9
7	Maryland	10.8
7	Pennsylvania	10.8
9	Georgia	10.4
9	North Carolina	10.4
9	South Carolina	10.4
12	Indiana	10.2
13	Kentucky	10.1
13	New York	10.1
13	Virginia	10.1
16	Minnesota	10.0
16	Vermont	10.0
18	Tennessee	9.8
18	Wisconsin	9.8
20	Louisiana	9.7
21	Colorado	9.6
21	Delaware	9.6
21	North Dakota	9.6
21	Rhode Island	9.6
25	Ohio	9.5
26	Illinois	9.4
26	Mississippi	9.4
26	South Dakota	9.4
26	Washington	9.4
26	West Virginia	9.4
31	Missouri	9.3
31	New Mexico	9.3
33	Arkansas	9.2
33	California	9.2
35	Arizona	8.9
36	Florida	8.8
36	Idaho	8.8
38	Iowa	8.6
39	Kansas	8.5
39	Nebraska	8.5
41	Nevada	8.4
41	Oklahoma	8.4
43	Oregon	8.2
43	Utah	8.2
45	Texas	8.1
46	Michigan	8.0
47	Montana	7.8
48	Hawaii	7.5
49	Wyoming	7.3
50	Alaska	5.8

District of Columbia   9.2

Source: Morgan Quitno Press using data from U.S. Dept of Health & Human Services, Health Care Financing Admin.
"State Health Expenditure Accounts" (Health Care Financing Review, Fall 1995, Volume 17, Number 1)
*By state of provider.

Expenditures for Dental Service in 1993

National Total = $37,383,000,000*

ALPHA ORDER					RANK ORDER			
RANK	STATE	EXPENDITURES	% of USA		RANK	STATE	EXPENDITURES	% of USA
25	Alabama	$456,000,000	1.22%		1	California	$5,664,000,000	15.15%
44	Alaska	124,000,000	0.33%		2	New York	2,837,000,000	7.59%
24	Arizona	551,000,000	1.47%		3	Texas	2,081,000,000	5.57%
33	Arkansas	242,000,000	0.65%		4	Florida	2,029,000,000	5.43%
1	California	5,664,000,000	15.15%		5	Pennsylvania	1,634,000,000	4.37%
21	Colorado	605,000,000	1.62%		6	Illinois	1,588,000,000	4.25%
19	Connecticut	685,000,000	1.83%		7	Michigan	1,531,000,000	4.10%
45	Delaware	104,000,000	0.28%		8	New Jersey	1,460,000,000	3.91%
4	Florida	2,029,000,000	5.43%		9	Ohio	1,398,000,000	3.74%
12	Georgia	898,000,000	2.40%		10	Washington	1,189,000,000	3.18%
34	Hawaii	235,000,000	0.63%		11	Massachusetts	1,022,000,000	2.73%
41	Idaho	163,000,000	0.44%		12	Georgia	898,000,000	2.40%
6	Illinois	1,588,000,000	4.25%		13	Virginia	863,000,000	2.31%
18	Indiana	692,000,000	1.85%		14	North Carolina	810,000,000	2.17%
30	Iowa	341,000,000	0.91%		15	Wisconsin	765,000,000	2.05%
31	Kansas	325,000,000	0.87%		16	Maryland	749,000,000	2.00%
28	Kentucky	369,000,000	0.99%		17	Minnesota	741,000,000	1.98%
26	Louisiana	432,000,000	1.16%		18	Indiana	692,000,000	1.85%
42	Maine	157,000,000	0.42%		19	Connecticut	685,000,000	1.83%
16	Maryland	749,000,000	2.00%		20	Tennessee	609,000,000	1.63%
11	Massachusetts	1,022,000,000	2.73%		21	Colorado	605,000,000	1.62%
7	Michigan	1,531,000,000	4.10%		22	Missouri	602,000,000	1.61%
17	Minnesota	741,000,000	1.98%		23	Oregon	578,000,000	1.55%
36	Mississippi	214,000,000	0.57%		24	Arizona	551,000,000	1.47%
22	Missouri	602,000,000	1.61%		25	Alabama	456,000,000	1.22%
46	Montana	103,000,000	0.28%		26	Louisiana	432,000,000	1.16%
37	Nebraska	191,000,000	0.51%		27	South Carolina	387,000,000	1.04%
35	Nevada	215,000,000	0.58%		28	Kentucky	369,000,000	0.99%
39	New Hampshire	177,000,000	0.47%		29	Oklahoma	356,000,000	0.95%
8	New Jersey	1,460,000,000	3.91%		30	Iowa	341,000,000	0.91%
40	New Mexico	175,000,000	0.47%		31	Kansas	325,000,000	0.87%
2	New York	2,837,000,000	7.59%		32	Utah	276,000,000	0.74%
14	North Carolina	810,000,000	2.17%		33	Arkansas	242,000,000	0.65%
49	North Dakota	78,000,000	0.21%		34	Hawaii	235,000,000	0.63%
9	Ohio	1,398,000,000	3.74%		35	Nevada	215,000,000	0.58%
29	Oklahoma	356,000,000	0.95%		36	Mississippi	214,000,000	0.57%
23	Oregon	578,000,000	1.55%		37	Nebraska	191,000,000	0.51%
5	Pennsylvania	1,634,000,000	4.37%		38	West Virginia	182,000,000	0.49%
43	Rhode Island	150,000,000	0.40%		39	New Hampshire	177,000,000	0.47%
27	South Carolina	387,000,000	1.04%		40	New Mexico	175,000,000	0.47%
47	South Dakota	87,000,000	0.23%		41	Idaho	163,000,000	0.44%
20	Tennessee	609,000,000	1.63%		42	Maine	157,000,000	0.42%
3	Texas	2,081,000,000	5.57%		43	Rhode Island	150,000,000	0.40%
32	Utah	276,000,000	0.74%		44	Alaska	124,000,000	0.33%
48	Vermont	84,000,000	0.22%		45	Delaware	104,000,000	0.28%
13	Virginia	863,000,000	2.31%		46	Montana	103,000,000	0.28%
10	Washington	1,189,000,000	3.18%		47	South Dakota	87,000,000	0.23%
38	West Virginia	182,000,000	0.49%		48	Vermont	84,000,000	0.22%
15	Wisconsin	765,000,000	2.05%		49	North Dakota	78,000,000	0.21%
50	Wyoming	57,000,000	0.15%		50	Wyoming	57,000,000	0.15%
						District of Columbia	119,000,000	0.32%

Source: U.S. Department of Health and Human Services, Health Care Financing Administration
"State Health Expenditure Accounts" (Health Care Financing Review, Fall 1995, Volume 17, Number 1)
*By state of provider.

Percent of Total Personal Health Care Expenditures
Spent on Dental Service in 1993
National Percent = 4.8%*

ALPHA ORDER

RANK	STATE	PERCENT
44	Alabama	3.8
1	Alaska	7.9
16	Arizona	5.2
41	Arkansas	4.0
7	California	6.0
7	Colorado	6.0
12	Connecticut	5.6
23	Delaware	4.6
27	Florida	4.5
27	Georgia	4.5
5	Hawaii	6.7
3	Idaho	7.2
23	Illinois	4.6
37	Indiana	4.2
23	Iowa	4.6
22	Kansas	4.7
47	Kentucky	3.6
50	Louisiana	3.3
23	Maine	4.6
20	Maryland	4.9
31	Massachusetts	4.4
12	Michigan	5.6
16	Minnesota	5.2
48	Mississippi	3.5
44	Missouri	3.8
20	Montana	4.9
35	Nebraska	4.3
9	Nevada	5.7
19	New Hampshire	5.1
9	New Jersey	5.7
27	New Mexico	4.5
37	New York	4.2
31	North Carolina	4.4
42	North Dakota	3.9
37	Ohio	4.2
31	Oklahoma	4.4
3	Oregon	7.2
42	Pennsylvania	3.9
31	Rhode Island	4.4
35	South Carolina	4.3
27	South Dakota	4.5
44	Tennessee	3.8
37	Texas	4.2
5	Utah	6.7
12	Vermont	5.6
16	Virginia	5.2
1	Washington	7.9
48	West Virginia	3.5
15	Wisconsin	5.3
9	Wyoming	5.7

RANK ORDER

RANK	STATE	PERCENT
1	Alaska	7.9
1	Washington	7.9
3	Idaho	7.2
3	Oregon	7.2
5	Hawaii	6.7
5	Utah	6.7
7	California	6.0
7	Colorado	6.0
9	Nevada	5.7
9	New Jersey	5.7
9	Wyoming	5.7
12	Connecticut	5.6
12	Michigan	5.6
12	Vermont	5.6
15	Wisconsin	5.3
16	Arizona	5.2
16	Minnesota	5.2
16	Virginia	5.2
19	New Hampshire	5.1
20	Maryland	4.9
20	Montana	4.9
22	Kansas	4.7
23	Delaware	4.6
23	Illinois	4.6
23	Iowa	4.6
23	Maine	4.6
27	Florida	4.5
27	Georgia	4.5
27	New Mexico	4.5
27	South Dakota	4.5
31	Massachusetts	4.4
31	North Carolina	4.4
31	Oklahoma	4.4
31	Rhode Island	4.4
35	Nebraska	4.3
35	South Carolina	4.3
37	Indiana	4.2
37	New York	4.2
37	Ohio	4.2
37	Texas	4.2
41	Arkansas	4.0
42	North Dakota	3.9
42	Pennsylvania	3.9
44	Alabama	3.8
44	Missouri	3.8
44	Tennessee	3.8
47	Kentucky	3.6
48	Mississippi	3.5
48	West Virginia	3.5
50	Louisiana	3.3

| | District of Columbia | 2.8 |

Source: Morgan Quitno Press using data from U.S. Dept of Health & Human Services, Health Care Financing Admin.
"State Health Expenditure Accounts" (Health Care Financing Review, Fall 1995, Volume 17, Number 1)
*By state of provider.

Per Capita Expenditures for Dental Service in 1993

National Per Capita = $145*

ALPHA ORDER

RANK	STATE	PER CAPITA
43	Alabama	$109
3	Alaska	207
23	Arizona	140
47	Arkansas	100
7	California	181
8	Colorado	170
2	Connecticut	209
18	Delaware	149
19	Florida	148
27	Georgia	130
4	Hawaii	202
19	Idaho	148
24	Illinois	136
33	Indiana	121
33	Iowa	121
28	Kansas	128
49	Kentucky	97
46	Louisiana	101
29	Maine	127
16	Maryland	151
8	Massachusetts	170
11	Michigan	162
10	Minnesota	164
50	Mississippi	81
40	Missouri	115
31	Montana	122
38	Nebraska	118
14	Nevada	155
12	New Hampshire	158
6	New Jersey	186
44	New Mexico	108
13	New York	156
39	North Carolina	116
31	North Dakota	122
30	Ohio	126
42	Oklahoma	110
5	Oregon	190
24	Pennsylvania	136
17	Rhode Island	150
45	South Carolina	107
33	South Dakota	121
37	Tennessee	120
40	Texas	115
19	Utah	148
22	Vermont	146
26	Virginia	133
1	Washington	226
47	West Virginia	100
15	Wisconsin	152
33	Wyoming	121

RANK ORDER

RANK	STATE	PER CAPITA
1	Washington	$226
2	Connecticut	209
3	Alaska	207
4	Hawaii	202
5	Oregon	190
6	New Jersey	186
7	California	181
8	Colorado	170
8	Massachusetts	170
10	Minnesota	164
11	Michigan	162
12	New Hampshire	158
13	New York	156
14	Nevada	155
15	Wisconsin	152
16	Maryland	151
17	Rhode Island	150
18	Delaware	149
19	Florida	148
19	Idaho	148
19	Utah	148
22	Vermont	146
23	Arizona	140
24	Illinois	136
24	Pennsylvania	136
26	Virginia	133
27	Georgia	130
28	Kansas	128
29	Maine	127
30	Ohio	126
31	Montana	122
31	North Dakota	122
33	Indiana	121
33	Iowa	121
33	South Dakota	121
33	Wyoming	121
37	Tennessee	120
38	Nebraska	118
39	North Carolina	116
40	Missouri	115
40	Texas	115
42	Oklahoma	110
43	Alabama	109
44	New Mexico	108
45	South Carolina	107
46	Louisiana	101
47	Arkansas	100
47	West Virginia	100
49	Kentucky	97
50	Mississippi	81

| | District of Columbia | 206 |

Source: Morgan Quitno Press using data from U.S. Dept of Health & Human Services, Health Care Financing Admin.
"State Health Expenditure Accounts" (Health Care Financing Review, Fall 1995, Volume 17, Number 1)
*By state of provider.

Average Annual Change in Expenditures for Dental Service: 1980 to 1993

National Percent = 8.3% Average Annual Growth*

ALPHA ORDER			RANK ORDER		
RANK	STATE	PERCENT	RANK	STATE	PERCENT
29	Alabama	8.3	1	Alaska	10.6
1	Alaska	10.6	2	New Hampshire	10.4
8	Arizona	9.7	3	Maine	10.1
26	Arkansas	8.5	3	Utah	10.1
31	California	8.1	5	Florida	10.0
14	Colorado	9.2	5	Nevada	10.0
19	Connecticut	8.8	7	South Carolina	9.8
19	Delaware	8.8	8	Arizona	9.7
5	Florida	10.0	8	Georgia	9.7
8	Georgia	9.7	10	Vermont	9.5
24	Hawaii	8.6	11	Virginia	9.4
14	Idaho	9.2	12	Rhode Island	9.3
44	Illinois	7.0	12	Washington	9.3
32	Indiana	7.9	14	Colorado	9.2
49	Iowa	6.5	14	Idaho	9.2
37	Kansas	7.7	16	Maryland	9.1
26	Kentucky	8.5	16	North Carolina	9.1
44	Louisiana	7.0	16	South Dakota	9.1
3	Maine	10.1	19	Connecticut	8.8
16	Maryland	9.1	19	Delaware	8.8
29	Massachusetts	8.3	19	Texas	8.8
50	Michigan	6.4	22	New Jersey	8.7
32	Minnesota	7.9	22	New Mexico	8.7
32	Mississippi	7.9	24	Hawaii	8.6
37	Missouri	7.7	24	Tennessee	8.6
48	Montana	6.8	26	Arkansas	8.5
44	Nebraska	7.0	26	Kentucky	8.5
5	Nevada	10.0	26	Oregon	8.5
2	New Hampshire	10.4	29	Alabama	8.3
22	New Jersey	8.7	29	Massachusetts	8.3
22	New Mexico	8.7	31	California	8.1
37	New York	7.7	32	Indiana	7.9
16	North Carolina	9.1	32	Minnesota	7.9
40	North Dakota	7.4	32	Mississippi	7.9
43	Ohio	7.2	32	Pennsylvania	7.9
41	Oklahoma	7.3	32	West Virginia	7.9
26	Oregon	8.5	37	Kansas	7.7
32	Pennsylvania	7.9	37	Missouri	7.7
12	Rhode Island	9.3	37	New York	7.7
7	South Carolina	9.8	40	North Dakota	7.4
16	South Dakota	9.1	41	Oklahoma	7.3
24	Tennessee	8.6	41	Wisconsin	7.3
19	Texas	8.8	43	Ohio	7.2
3	Utah	10.1	44	Illinois	7.0
10	Vermont	9.5	44	Louisiana	7.0
11	Virginia	9.4	44	Nebraska	7.0
12	Washington	9.3	44	Wyoming	7.0
32	West Virginia	7.9	48	Montana	6.8
41	Wisconsin	7.3	49	Iowa	6.5
44	Wyoming	7.0	50	Michigan	6.4
				District of Columbia	8.4

Source: U.S. Department of Health and Human Services, Health Care Financing Administration
   "State Health Expenditure Accounts" (Health Care Financing Review, Fall 1995, Volume 17, Number 1)
*By state of provider.

Expenditures for Other Professional Health Care Services in 1993

National Total = $51,200,000,000*

ALPHA ORDER

RANK	STATE	EXPENDITURES	% of USA
26	Alabama	$641,000,000	1.25%
45	Alaska	127,000,000	0.25%
21	Arizona	821,000,000	1.60%
32	Arkansas	332,000,000	0.65%
1	California	6,859,000,000	13.39%
23	Colorado	751,000,000	1.47%
22	Connecticut	769,000,000	1.50%
44	Delaware	156,000,000	0.30%
4	Florida	3,505,000,000	6.84%
11	Georgia	1,226,000,000	2.39%
40	Hawaii	222,000,000	0.43%
46	Idaho	126,000,000	0.25%
6	Illinois	2,063,000,000	4.03%
16	Indiana	993,000,000	1.94%
31	Iowa	431,000,000	0.84%
30	Kansas	470,000,000	0.92%
25	Kentucky	691,000,000	1.35%
24	Louisiana	736,000,000	1.44%
42	Maine	210,000,000	0.41%
18	Maryland	942,000,000	1.84%
10	Massachusetts	1,524,000,000	2.98%
9	Michigan	1,844,000,000	3.60%
19	Minnesota	933,000,000	1.82%
35	Mississippi	288,000,000	0.56%
15	Missouri	1,013,000,000	1.98%
43	Montana	166,000,000	0.32%
39	Nebraska	225,000,000	0.44%
34	Nevada	307,000,000	0.60%
36	New Hampshire	269,000,000	0.53%
8	New Jersey	1,870,000,000	3.65%
37	New Mexico	254,000,000	0.50%
2	New York	3,717,000,000	7.26%
13	North Carolina	1,102,000,000	2.15%
49	North Dakota	93,000,000	0.18%
7	Ohio	1,969,000,000	3.84%
28	Oklahoma	504,000,000	0.98%
27	Oregon	530,000,000	1.03%
5	Pennsylvania	3,005,000,000	5.87%
38	Rhode Island	239,000,000	0.47%
29	South Carolina	472,000,000	0.92%
48	South Dakota	117,000,000	0.23%
12	Tennessee	1,166,000,000	2.28%
3	Texas	3,591,000,000	7.01%
41	Utah	220,000,000	0.43%
47	Vermont	122,000,000	0.24%
17	Virginia	970,000,000	1.89%
13	Washington	1,102,000,000	2.15%
33	West Virginia	326,000,000	0.64%
20	Wisconsin	875,000,000	1.71%
50	Wyoming	68,000,000	0.13%

RANK ORDER

RANK	STATE	EXPENDITURES	% of USA
1	California	$6,859,000,000	13.39%
2	New York	3,717,000,000	7.26%
3	Texas	3,591,000,000	7.01%
4	Florida	3,505,000,000	6.84%
5	Pennsylvania	3,005,000,000	5.87%
6	Illinois	2,063,000,000	4.03%
7	Ohio	1,969,000,000	3.84%
8	New Jersey	1,870,000,000	3.65%
9	Michigan	1,844,000,000	3.60%
10	Massachusetts	1,524,000,000	2.98%
11	Georgia	1,226,000,000	2.39%
12	Tennessee	1,166,000,000	2.28%
13	North Carolina	1,102,000,000	2.15%
13	Washington	1,102,000,000	2.15%
15	Missouri	1,013,000,000	1.98%
16	Indiana	993,000,000	1.94%
17	Virginia	970,000,000	1.89%
18	Maryland	942,000,000	1.84%
19	Minnesota	933,000,000	1.82%
20	Wisconsin	875,000,000	1.71%
21	Arizona	821,000,000	1.60%
22	Connecticut	769,000,000	1.50%
23	Colorado	751,000,000	1.47%
24	Louisiana	736,000,000	1.44%
25	Kentucky	691,000,000	1.35%
26	Alabama	641,000,000	1.25%
27	Oregon	530,000,000	1.03%
28	Oklahoma	504,000,000	0.98%
29	South Carolina	472,000,000	0.92%
30	Kansas	470,000,000	0.92%
31	Iowa	431,000,000	0.84%
32	Arkansas	332,000,000	0.65%
33	West Virginia	326,000,000	0.64%
34	Nevada	307,000,000	0.60%
35	Mississippi	288,000,000	0.56%
36	New Hampshire	269,000,000	0.53%
37	New Mexico	254,000,000	0.50%
38	Rhode Island	239,000,000	0.47%
39	Nebraska	225,000,000	0.44%
40	Hawaii	222,000,000	0.43%
41	Utah	220,000,000	0.43%
42	Maine	210,000,000	0.41%
43	Montana	166,000,000	0.32%
44	Delaware	156,000,000	0.30%
45	Alaska	127,000,000	0.25%
46	Idaho	126,000,000	0.25%
47	Vermont	122,000,000	0.24%
48	South Dakota	117,000,000	0.23%
49	North Dakota	93,000,000	0.18%
50	Wyoming	68,000,000	0.13%
	District of Columbia	267,000,000	0.52%

Source: U.S. Department of Health and Human Services, Health Care Financing Administration
"State Health Expenditure Accounts" (Health Care Financing Review, Fall 1995, Volume 17, Number 1)
By state of provider. Includes services by chiropractors, optometrists and podiatrists. Also includes spending in kidney dialysis clinics, alcohol treatment centers, rehabilitation clinics and other health care establishments not elsewhere classified. Medicare ambulance expenditures are also included.

Percent of Total Personal Health Care Expenditures
Spent on Other Professional Services in 1993
National Percent = 6.6%*

ALPHA ORDER

RANK ORDER

RANK	STATE	PERCENT		RANK	STATE	PERCENT
45	Alabama	5.3		1	Nevada	8.2
2	Alaska	8.1		2	Alaska	8.1
7	Arizona	7.7		2	Vermont	8.1
44	Arkansas	5.4		4	Montana	7.9
9	California	7.3		5	Florida	7.8
8	Colorado	7.5		5	New Hampshire	7.8
27	Connecticut	6.3		7	Arizona	7.7
16	Delaware	6.9		8	Colorado	7.5
5	Florida	7.8		9	California	7.3
31	Georgia	6.1		9	New Jersey	7.3
25	Hawaii	6.4		9	Washington	7.3
42	Idaho	5.5		12	Pennsylvania	7.2
37	Illinois	5.9		12	Tennessee	7.2
31	Indiana	6.1		12	Texas	7.2
37	Iowa	5.9		15	Rhode Island	7.0
17	Kansas	6.8		16	Delaware	6.9
20	Kentucky	6.7		17	Kansas	6.8
41	Louisiana	5.7		17	Michigan	6.8
31	Maine	6.1		17	Wyoming	6.8
30	Maryland	6.2		20	Kentucky	6.7
23	Massachusetts	6.5		21	Minnesota	6.6
17	Michigan	6.8		21	Oregon	6.6
21	Minnesota	6.6		23	Massachusetts	6.5
49	Mississippi	4.7		23	New Mexico	6.5
25	Missouri	6.4		25	Hawaii	6.4
4	Montana	7.9		25	Missouri	6.4
48	Nebraska	5.1		27	Connecticut	6.3
1	Nevada	8.2		27	Oklahoma	6.3
5	New Hampshire	7.8		27	West Virginia	6.3
9	New Jersey	7.3		30	Maryland	6.2
23	New Mexico	6.5		31	Georgia	6.1
42	New York	5.5		31	Indiana	6.1
34	North Carolina	6.0		31	Maine	6.1
50	North Dakota	4.6		34	North Carolina	6.0
37	Ohio	5.9		34	South Dakota	6.0
27	Oklahoma	6.3		34	Wisconsin	6.0
21	Oregon	6.6		37	Illinois	5.9
12	Pennsylvania	7.2		37	Iowa	5.9
15	Rhode Island	7.0		37	Ohio	5.9
47	South Carolina	5.2		40	Virginia	5.8
34	South Dakota	6.0		41	Louisiana	5.7
12	Tennessee	7.2		42	Idaho	5.5
12	Texas	7.2		42	New York	5.5
45	Utah	5.3		44	Arkansas	5.4
2	Vermont	8.1		45	Alabama	5.3
40	Virginia	5.8		45	Utah	5.3
9	Washington	7.3		47	South Carolina	5.2
27	West Virginia	6.3		48	Nebraska	5.1
34	Wisconsin	6.0		49	Mississippi	4.7
17	Wyoming	6.8		50	North Dakota	4.6

District of Columbia 6.2

Source: Morgan Quitno Press using data from U.S. Dept of Health & Human Services, Health Care Financing Admin.
"State Health Expenditure Accounts" (Health Care Financing Review, Fall 1995, Volume 17, Number 1)
*By state of provider. Includes services by chiropractors, optometrists and podiatrists. Also includes spending in kidney dialysis clinics, alcohol treatment centers, rehabilitation clinics and other health care establishments not elsewhere classified. Medicare ambulance expenditures are also included.

Per Capita Expenditures for Other Professional Health Care Services in 1993

National Per Capita = $199*

ALPHA ORDER				RANK ORDER		
RANK	STATE	PER CAPITA		RANK	STATE	PER CAPITA
40	Alabama	$153		1	Florida	$255
12	Alaska	212		2	Massachusetts	253
16	Arizona	208		3	Pennsylvania	250
46	Arkansas	137		4	New Hampshire	240
11	California	220		5	Rhode Island	239
14	Colorado	210		6	New Jersey	238
7	Connecticut	235		7	Connecticut	235
9	Delaware	223		8	Tennessee	229
1	Florida	255		9	Delaware	223
28	Georgia	178		10	Nevada	222
23	Hawaii	190		11	California	220
49	Idaho	114		12	Alaska	212
30	Illinois	176		12	Vermont	212
32	Indiana	174		14	Colorado	210
40	Iowa	153		14	Washington	210
25	Kansas	186		16	Arizona	208
26	Kentucky	182		17	Minnesota	206
34	Louisiana	172		18	New York	205
35	Maine	169		19	Texas	199
23	Maryland	190		20	Montana	197
2	Massachusetts	253		21	Michigan	195
21	Michigan	195		22	Missouri	194
17	Minnesota	206		23	Hawaii	190
50	Mississippi	109		23	Maryland	190
22	Missouri	194		25	Kansas	186
20	Montana	197		26	Kentucky	182
45	Nebraska	139		27	West Virginia	179
10	Nevada	222		28	Georgia	178
4	New Hampshire	240		28	Ohio	178
6	New Jersey	238		30	Illinois	176
38	New Mexico	157		31	Oregon	175
18	New York	205		32	Indiana	174
37	North Carolina	158		33	Wisconsin	173
43	North Dakota	146		34	Louisiana	172
28	Ohio	178		35	Maine	169
39	Oklahoma	156		36	South Dakota	163
31	Oregon	175		37	North Carolina	158
3	Pennsylvania	250		38	New Mexico	157
5	Rhode Island	239		39	Oklahoma	156
47	South Carolina	130		40	Alabama	153
36	South Dakota	163		40	Iowa	153
8	Tennessee	229		42	Virginia	150
19	Texas	199		43	North Dakota	146
48	Utah	118		44	Wyoming	145
12	Vermont	212		45	Nebraska	139
42	Virginia	150		46	Arkansas	137
14	Washington	210		47	South Carolina	130
27	West Virginia	179		48	Utah	118
33	Wisconsin	173		49	Idaho	114
44	Wyoming	145		50	Mississippi	109
					District of Columbia	462

Source: Morgan Quitno Press using data from U.S. Dept of Health & Human Services, Health Care Financing Admin. "State Health Expenditure Accounts" (Health Care Financing Review, Fall 1995, Volume 17, Number 1)
By state of provider. Includes services by chiropractors, optometrists and podiatrists. Also includes spending in kidney dialysis clinics, alcohol treatment centers, rehabilitation clinics and other health care establishments not elsewhere classified. Medicare ambulance expenditures are also included.

Average Annual Change in Expenditures for Other Professional Health Care Services: 1980 to 1993
National Percent = 17.4% Average Annual Increase*

ALPHA ORDER

ALPHA ORDER

RANK ORDER

RANK	STATE	PERCENT		RANK	STATE	PERCENT
17	Alabama	18.6		1	Nevada	21.3
30	Alaska	16.3		2	Delaware	20.6
12	Arizona	19.1		3	Georgia	20.3
44	Arkansas	15.3		4	Maryland	19.8
34	California	16.2		4	North Carolina	19.8
14	Colorado	18.7		6	Texas	19.7
14	Connecticut	18.7		7	Florida	19.6
2	Delaware	20.6		7	Tennessee	19.6
7	Florida	19.6		9	Hawaii	19.4
3	Georgia	20.3		9	New Jersey	19.4
9	Hawaii	19.4		11	Virginia	19.2
49	Idaho	13.1		12	Arizona	19.1
45	Illinois	15.2		13	New Hampshire	18.9
36	Indiana	15.7		14	Colorado	18.7
50	Iowa	13.0		14	Connecticut	18.7
41	Kansas	15.5		14	Massachusetts	18.7
22	Kentucky	17.5		17	Alabama	18.6
18	Louisiana	18.4		18	Louisiana	18.4
29	Maine	16.4		19	Pennsylvania	18.2
4	Maryland	19.8		20	Utah	18.1
14	Massachusetts	18.7		21	South Carolina	17.8
43	Michigan	15.4		22	Kentucky	17.5
46	Minnesota	15.0		23	Missouri	17.4
35	Mississippi	16.0		24	Rhode Island	17.3
23	Missouri	17.4		25	New York	17.2
37	Montana	15.6		25	Vermont	17.2
41	Nebraska	15.5		27	Wisconsin	17.0
1	Nevada	21.3		28	Oregon	16.9
13	New Hampshire	18.9		29	Maine	16.4
9	New Jersey	19.4		30	Alaska	16.3
30	New Mexico	16.3		30	New Mexico	16.3
25	New York	17.2		30	Washington	16.3
4	North Carolina	19.8		30	West Virginia	16.3
47	North Dakota	14.9		34	California	16.2
37	Ohio	15.6		35	Mississippi	16.0
37	Oklahoma	15.6		36	Indiana	15.7
28	Oregon	16.9		37	Montana	15.6
19	Pennsylvania	18.2		37	Ohio	15.6
24	Rhode Island	17.3		37	Oklahoma	15.6
21	South Carolina	17.8		37	South Dakota	15.6
37	South Dakota	15.6		41	Kansas	15.5
7	Tennessee	19.6		41	Nebraska	15.5
6	Texas	19.7		43	Michigan	15.4
20	Utah	18.1		44	Arkansas	15.3
25	Vermont	17.2		45	Illinois	15.2
11	Virginia	19.2		46	Minnesota	15.0
30	Washington	16.3		47	North Dakota	14.9
30	West Virginia	16.3		48	Wyoming	13.2
27	Wisconsin	17.0		49	Idaho	13.1
48	Wyoming	13.2		50	Iowa	13.0

District of Columbia — 15.9

Source: U.S. Department of Health and Human Services, Health Care Financing Administration "State Health Expenditure Accounts" (Health Care Financing Review, Fall 1995, Volume 17, Number 1)
By state of provider. Includes services by chiropractors, optometrists and podiatrists. Also includes spending in kidney dialysis clinics, alcohol treatment centers, rehabilitation clinics and other health care establishments not elsewhere classified. Medicare ambulance expenditures are also included.

Expenditures for Home Health Care in 1993

National Total = $22,982,000,000*

ALPHA ORDER				
RANK	STATE	EXPENDITURES	% of USA	
13	Alabama	$602,000,000	2.62%	
50	Alaska	5,000,000	0.02%	
22	Arizona	317,000,000	1.38%	
32	Arkansas	145,000,000	0.63%	
3	California	1,640,000,000	7.14%	
29	Colorado	195,000,000	0.85%	
17	Connecticut	391,000,000	1.70%	
43	Delaware	51,000,000	0.22%	
2	Florida	2,323,000,000	10.11%	
9	Georgia	729,000,000	3.17%	
46	Hawaii	32,000,000	0.14%	
45	Idaho	49,000,000	0.21%	
6	Illinois	853,000,000	3.71%	
24	Indiana	308,000,000	1.34%	
33	Iowa	137,000,000	0.60%	
30	Kansas	152,000,000	0.66%	
20	Kentucky	357,000,000	1.55%	
16	Louisiana	410,000,000	1.78%	
36	Maine	104,000,000	0.45%	
23	Maryland	314,000,000	1.37%	
7	Massachusetts	835,000,000	3.63%	
11	Michigan	714,000,000	3.11%	
15	Minnesota	414,000,000	1.80%	
25	Mississippi	300,000,000	1.31%	
21	Missouri	347,000,000	1.51%	
44	Montana	50,000,000	0.22%	
39	Nebraska	74,000,000	0.32%	
35	Nevada	120,000,000	0.52%	
40	New Hampshire	71,000,000	0.31%	
10	New Jersey	718,000,000	3.12%	
41	New Mexico	62,000,000	0.27%	
1	New York	3,562,000,000	15.50%	
14	North Carolina	541,000,000	2.35%	
48	North Dakota	16,000,000	0.07%	
12	Ohio	649,000,000	2.82%	
26	Oklahoma	273,000,000	1.19%	
34	Oregon	122,000,000	0.53%	
8	Pennsylvania	796,000,000	3.46%	
37	Rhode Island	103,000,000	0.45%	
28	South Carolina	216,000,000	0.94%	
48	South Dakota	16,000,000	0.07%	
5	Tennessee	899,000,000	3.91%	
4	Texas	1,583,000,000	6.89%	
38	Utah	100,000,000	0.44%	
42	Vermont	52,000,000	0.23%	
19	Virginia	368,000,000	1.60%	
18	Washington	380,000,000	1.65%	
31	West Virginia	150,000,000	0.65%	
27	Wisconsin	265,000,000	1.15%	
47	Wyoming	29,000,000	0.13%	

RANK ORDER			
RANK	STATE	EXPENDITURES	% of USA
1	New York	$3,562,000,000	15.50%
2	Florida	2,323,000,000	10.11%
3	California	1,640,000,000	7.14%
4	Texas	1,583,000,000	6.89%
5	Tennessee	899,000,000	3.91%
6	Illinois	853,000,000	3.71%
7	Massachusetts	835,000,000	3.63%
8	Pennsylvania	796,000,000	3.46%
9	Georgia	729,000,000	3.17%
10	New Jersey	718,000,000	3.12%
11	Michigan	714,000,000	3.11%
12	Ohio	649,000,000	2.82%
13	Alabama	602,000,000	2.62%
14	North Carolina	541,000,000	2.35%
15	Minnesota	414,000,000	1.80%
16	Louisiana	410,000,000	1.78%
17	Connecticut	391,000,000	1.70%
18	Washington	380,000,000	1.65%
19	Virginia	368,000,000	1.60%
20	Kentucky	357,000,000	1.55%
21	Missouri	347,000,000	1.51%
22	Arizona	317,000,000	1.38%
23	Maryland	314,000,000	1.37%
24	Indiana	308,000,000	1.34%
25	Mississippi	300,000,000	1.31%
26	Oklahoma	273,000,000	1.19%
27	Wisconsin	265,000,000	1.15%
28	South Carolina	216,000,000	0.94%
29	Colorado	195,000,000	0.85%
30	Kansas	152,000,000	0.66%
31	West Virginia	150,000,000	0.65%
32	Arkansas	145,000,000	0.63%
33	Iowa	137,000,000	0.60%
34	Oregon	122,000,000	0.53%
35	Nevada	120,000,000	0.52%
36	Maine	104,000,000	0.45%
37	Rhode Island	103,000,000	0.45%
38	Utah	100,000,000	0.44%
39	Nebraska	74,000,000	0.32%
40	New Hampshire	71,000,000	0.31%
41	New Mexico	62,000,000	0.27%
42	Vermont	52,000,000	0.23%
43	Delaware	51,000,000	0.22%
44	Montana	50,000,000	0.22%
45	Idaho	49,000,000	0.21%
46	Hawaii	32,000,000	0.14%
47	Wyoming	29,000,000	0.13%
48	North Dakota	16,000,000	0.07%
48	South Dakota	16,000,000	0.07%
50	Alaska	5,000,000	0.02%
	District of Columbia	45,000,000	0.20%

Source: U.S. Department of Health and Human Services, Health Care Financing Administration
    "State Health Expenditure Accounts" (Health Care Financing Review, Fall 1995, Volume 17, Number 1)
By state of provider. Includes spending for services and products by public and private freestanding home health agencies. Excludes home health care services provided by hospital-based agencies which are included in hospital expenditures.

Percent of Total Personal Health Care Expenditures
Spent on Home Health Care in 1993
National Percent = 3.0%*

ALPHA ORDER

RANK	STATE	PERCENT
4	Alabama	5.0
50	Alaska	0.3
15	Arizona	3.0
26	Arkansas	2.4
43	California	1.7
37	Colorado	1.9
11	Connecticut	3.2
30	Delaware	2.3
3	Florida	5.2
6	Georgia	3.6
47	Hawaii	0.9
31	Idaho	2.2
24	Illinois	2.5
37	Indiana	1.9
37	Iowa	1.9
31	Kansas	2.2
9	Kentucky	3.4
11	Louisiana	3.2
15	Maine	3.0
35	Maryland	2.1
6	Massachusetts	3.6
23	Michigan	2.6
19	Minnesota	2.9
5	Mississippi	4.8
31	Missouri	2.2
26	Montana	2.4
43	Nebraska	1.7
11	Nevada	3.2
35	New Hampshire	2.1
22	New Jersey	2.8
45	New Mexico	1.6
2	New York	5.3
15	North Carolina	3.0
48	North Dakota	0.8
37	Ohio	1.9
9	Oklahoma	3.4
46	Oregon	1.5
37	Pennsylvania	1.9
15	Rhode Island	3.0
26	South Carolina	2.4
48	South Dakota	0.8
1	Tennessee	5.5
11	Texas	3.2
26	Utah	2.4
8	Vermont	3.5
31	Virginia	2.2
24	Washington	2.5
19	West Virginia	2.9
42	Wisconsin	1.8
19	Wyoming	2.9

RANK ORDER

RANK	STATE	PERCENT
1	Tennessee	5.5
2	New York	5.3
3	Florida	5.2
4	Alabama	5.0
5	Mississippi	4.8
6	Georgia	3.6
6	Massachusetts	3.6
8	Vermont	3.5
9	Kentucky	3.4
9	Oklahoma	3.4
11	Connecticut	3.2
11	Louisiana	3.2
11	Nevada	3.2
11	Texas	3.2
15	Arizona	3.0
15	Maine	3.0
15	North Carolina	3.0
15	Rhode Island	3.0
19	Minnesota	2.9
19	West Virginia	2.9
19	Wyoming	2.9
22	New Jersey	2.8
23	Michigan	2.6
24	Illinois	2.5
24	Washington	2.5
26	Arkansas	2.4
26	Montana	2.4
26	South Carolina	2.4
26	Utah	2.4
30	Delaware	2.3
31	Idaho	2.2
31	Kansas	2.2
31	Missouri	2.2
31	Virginia	2.2
35	Maryland	2.1
35	New Hampshire	2.1
37	Colorado	1.9
37	Indiana	1.9
37	Iowa	1.9
37	Ohio	1.9
37	Pennsylvania	1.9
42	Wisconsin	1.8
43	California	1.7
43	Nebraska	1.7
45	New Mexico	1.6
46	Oregon	1.5
47	Hawaii	0.9
48	North Dakota	0.8
48	South Dakota	0.8
50	Alaska	0.3
	District of Columbia	1.1

Source: Morgan Quitno Press using data from U.S. Dept of Health & Human Services, Health Care Financing Admin. "State Health Expenditure Accounts" (Health Care Financing Review, Fall 1995, Volume 17, Number 1)
By state of provider. Includes spending for services and products by public and private freestanding home health agencies. Excludes home health care services provided by hospital-based agencies which are included in hospital expenditures.

Per Capita Expenditures for Home Health Care in 1993

National Per Capita = $89*

ALPHA ORDER

RANK	STATE	PER CAPITA
4	Alabama	$144
50	Alaska	8
20	Arizona	80
31	Arkansas	60
40	California	53
37	Colorado	55
6	Connecticut	119
23	Delaware	73
3	Florida	169
8	Georgia	106
47	Hawaii	27
44	Idaho	45
23	Illinois	73
38	Indiana	54
42	Iowa	49
31	Kansas	60
11	Kentucky	94
10	Louisiana	96
17	Maine	84
28	Maryland	63
5	Massachusetts	139
22	Michigan	75
12	Minnesota	92
7	Mississippi	114
26	Missouri	66
34	Montana	59
43	Nebraska	46
16	Nevada	87
28	New Hampshire	63
13	New Jersey	91
46	New Mexico	38
1	New York	196
21	North Carolina	78
48	North Dakota	25
34	Ohio	59
17	Oklahoma	84
45	Oregon	40
26	Pennsylvania	66
9	Rhode Island	103
31	South Carolina	60
49	South Dakota	22
2	Tennessee	177
15	Texas	88
38	Utah	54
14	Vermont	90
36	Virginia	57
25	Washington	72
19	West Virginia	83
40	Wisconsin	53
30	Wyoming	62

RANK ORDER

RANK	STATE	PER CAPITA
1	New York	$196
2	Tennessee	177
3	Florida	169
4	Alabama	144
5	Massachusetts	139
6	Connecticut	119
7	Mississippi	114
8	Georgia	106
9	Rhode Island	103
10	Louisiana	96
11	Kentucky	94
12	Minnesota	92
13	New Jersey	91
14	Vermont	90
15	Texas	88
16	Nevada	87
17	Maine	84
17	Oklahoma	84
19	West Virginia	83
20	Arizona	80
21	North Carolina	78
22	Michigan	75
23	Delaware	73
23	Illinois	73
25	Washington	72
26	Missouri	66
26	Pennsylvania	66
28	Maryland	63
28	New Hampshire	63
30	Wyoming	62
31	Arkansas	60
31	Kansas	60
31	South Carolina	60
34	Montana	59
34	Ohio	59
36	Virginia	57
37	Colorado	55
38	Indiana	54
38	Utah	54
40	California	53
40	Wisconsin	53
42	Iowa	49
43	Nebraska	46
44	Idaho	45
45	Oregon	40
46	New Mexico	38
47	Hawaii	27
48	North Dakota	25
49	South Dakota	22
50	Alaska	8
	District of Columbia	78

Source: Morgan Quitno Press using data from U.S. Dept of Health & Human Services, Health Care Financing Admin. "State Health Expenditure Accounts" (Health Care Financing Review, Fall 1995, Volume 17, Number 1)
By state of provider. Includes spending for services and products by public and private freestanding home health agencies. Excludes home health care services provided by hospital-based agencies which are included in hospital expenditures.

Annual Average Growth in Expenditures for Home Health Care: 1980 to 1993

National Percent = 19.1% Average Annual Increase*

ALPHA ORDER

RANK	STATE	PERCENT
9	Alabama	26.0
3	Alaska	31.8
5	Arizona	30.5
25	Arkansas	20.4
33	California	17.6
37	Colorado	17.0
30	Connecticut	18.7
24	Delaware	20.7
18	Florida	22.3
11	Georgia	25.2
39	Hawaii	16.7
42	Idaho	16.0
38	Illinois	16.9
19	Indiana	21.5
30	Iowa	18.7
15	Kansas	23.3
8	Kentucky	26.8
7	Louisiana	27.7
36	Maine	17.3
34	Maryland	17.5
28	Massachusetts	19.2
28	Michigan	19.2
14	Minnesota	23.5
16	Mississippi	22.8
48	Missouri	15.2
23	Montana	20.9
16	Nebraska	22.8
1	Nevada	35.2
44	New Hampshire	15.7
50	New Jersey	11.1
26	New Mexico	20.2
44	New York	15.7
6	North Carolina	29.1
19	North Dakota	21.5
34	Ohio	17.5
30	Oklahoma	18.7
47	Oregon	15.3
46	Pennsylvania	15.4
48	Rhode Island	15.2
21	South Carolina	21.2
26	South Dakota	20.2
4	Tennessee	31.2
13	Texas	24.3
2	Utah	33.9
42	Vermont	16.0
21	Virginia	21.2
40	Washington	16.6
12	West Virginia	24.4
41	Wisconsin	16.3
10	Wyoming	25.7

RANK ORDER

RANK	STATE	PERCENT
1	Nevada	35.2
2	Utah	33.9
3	Alaska	31.8
4	Tennessee	31.2
5	Arizona	30.5
6	North Carolina	29.1
7	Louisiana	27.7
8	Kentucky	26.8
9	Alabama	26.0
10	Wyoming	25.7
11	Georgia	25.2
12	West Virginia	24.4
13	Texas	24.3
14	Minnesota	23.5
15	Kansas	23.3
16	Mississippi	22.8
16	Nebraska	22.8
18	Florida	22.3
19	Indiana	21.5
19	North Dakota	21.5
21	South Carolina	21.2
21	Virginia	21.2
23	Montana	20.9
24	Delaware	20.7
25	Arkansas	20.4
26	New Mexico	20.2
26	South Dakota	20.2
28	Massachusetts	19.2
28	Michigan	19.2
30	Connecticut	18.7
30	Iowa	18.7
30	Oklahoma	18.7
33	California	17.6
34	Maryland	17.5
34	Ohio	17.5
36	Maine	17.3
37	Colorado	17.0
38	Illinois	16.9
39	Hawaii	16.7
40	Washington	16.6
41	Wisconsin	16.3
42	Idaho	16.0
42	Vermont	16.0
44	New Hampshire	15.7
44	New York	15.7
46	Pennsylvania	15.4
47	Oregon	15.3
48	Missouri	15.2
48	Rhode Island	15.2
50	New Jersey	11.1
	District of Columbia	11.7

Source: U.S. Department of Health and Human Services, Health Care Financing Administration
   "State Health Expenditure Accounts" (Health Care Financing Review, Fall 1995, Volume 17, Number 1)
*By state of provider. Includes spending for services and products by public and private freestanding home health agencies. Excludes home health care services provided by hospital-based agencies which are included in hospital expenditures.

Expenditures for Drug and Other Medical Non-Durables in 1993

National Total = $74,956,000,000*

ALPHA ORDER

RANK	STATE	EXPENDITURES	% of USA
21	Alabama	$1,247,000,000	1.66%
46	Alaska	165,000,000	0.22%
24	Arizona	1,124,000,000	1.50%
33	Arkansas	684,000,000	0.91%
1	California	9,017,000,000	12.03%
27	Colorado	919,000,000	1.23%
25	Connecticut	996,000,000	1.33%
44	Delaware	214,000,000	0.29%
4	Florida	4,450,000,000	5.94%
10	Georgia	2,117,000,000	2.82%
37	Hawaii	416,000,000	0.55%
43	Idaho	265,000,000	0.35%
6	Illinois	3,263,000,000	4.35%
16	Indiana	1,594,000,000	2.13%
30	Iowa	743,000,000	0.99%
32	Kansas	695,000,000	0.93%
22	Kentucky	1,196,000,000	1.60%
20	Louisiana	1,269,000,000	1.69%
40	Maine	333,000,000	0.44%
14	Maryland	1,749,000,000	2.33%
13	Massachusetts	1,961,000,000	2.62%
8	Michigan	2,937,000,000	3.92%
23	Minnesota	1,146,000,000	1.53%
31	Mississippi	720,000,000	0.96%
18	Missouri	1,420,000,000	1.89%
45	Montana	209,000,000	0.28%
36	Nebraska	421,000,000	0.56%
39	Nevada	408,000,000	0.54%
41	New Hampshire	319,000,000	0.43%
9	New Jersey	2,452,000,000	3.27%
38	New Mexico	409,000,000	0.55%
3	New York	5,081,000,000	6.78%
11	North Carolina	2,027,000,000	2.70%
49	North Dakota	160,000,000	0.21%
7	Ohio	3,218,000,000	4.29%
28	Oklahoma	874,000,000	1.17%
29	Oregon	762,000,000	1.02%
5	Pennsylvania	3,519,000,000	4.69%
42	Rhode Island	310,000,000	0.41%
26	South Carolina	978,000,000	1.30%
47	South Dakota	163,000,000	0.22%
15	Tennessee	1,635,000,000	2.18%
2	Texas	5,131,000,000	6.85%
35	Utah	439,000,000	0.59%
48	Vermont	161,000,000	0.21%
12	Virginia	2,015,000,000	2.69%
17	Washington	1,474,000,000	1.97%
34	West Virginia	574,000,000	0.77%
19	Wisconsin	1,290,000,000	1.72%
50	Wyoming	113,000,000	0.15%

RANK ORDER

RANK	STATE	EXPENDITURES	% of USA
1	California	$9,017,000,000	12.03%
2	Texas	5,131,000,000	6.85%
3	New York	5,081,000,000	6.78%
4	Florida	4,450,000,000	5.94%
5	Pennsylvania	3,519,000,000	4.69%
6	Illinois	3,263,000,000	4.35%
7	Ohio	3,218,000,000	4.29%
8	Michigan	2,937,000,000	3.92%
9	New Jersey	2,452,000,000	3.27%
10	Georgia	2,117,000,000	2.82%
11	North Carolina	2,027,000,000	2.70%
12	Virginia	2,015,000,000	2.69%
13	Massachusetts	1,961,000,000	2.62%
14	Maryland	1,749,000,000	2.33%
15	Tennessee	1,635,000,000	2.18%
16	Indiana	1,594,000,000	2.13%
17	Washington	1,474,000,000	1.97%
18	Missouri	1,420,000,000	1.89%
19	Wisconsin	1,290,000,000	1.72%
20	Louisiana	1,269,000,000	1.69%
21	Alabama	1,247,000,000	1.66%
22	Kentucky	1,196,000,000	1.60%
23	Minnesota	1,146,000,000	1.53%
24	Arizona	1,124,000,000	1.50%
25	Connecticut	996,000,000	1.33%
26	South Carolina	978,000,000	1.30%
27	Colorado	919,000,000	1.23%
28	Oklahoma	874,000,000	1.17%
29	Oregon	762,000,000	1.02%
30	Iowa	743,000,000	0.99%
31	Mississippi	720,000,000	0.96%
32	Kansas	695,000,000	0.93%
33	Arkansas	684,000,000	0.91%
34	West Virginia	574,000,000	0.77%
35	Utah	439,000,000	0.59%
36	Nebraska	421,000,000	0.56%
37	Hawaii	416,000,000	0.55%
38	New Mexico	409,000,000	0.55%
39	Nevada	408,000,000	0.54%
40	Maine	333,000,000	0.44%
41	New Hampshire	319,000,000	0.43%
42	Rhode Island	310,000,000	0.41%
43	Idaho	265,000,000	0.35%
44	Delaware	214,000,000	0.29%
45	Montana	209,000,000	0.28%
46	Alaska	165,000,000	0.22%
47	South Dakota	163,000,000	0.22%
48	Vermont	161,000,000	0.21%
49	North Dakota	160,000,000	0.21%
50	Wyoming	113,000,000	0.15%
	District of Columbia	175,000,000	0.23%

Source: U.S. Department of Health and Human Services, Health Care Financing Administration
   "State Health Expenditure Accounts" (Health Care Financing Review, Fall 1995, Volume 17, Number 1)
*By state of provider. Includes prescription and over-the-counter drugs and sundries. Limited to spending that occurs in retail outlets such as food stores, drug stores, HMO pharmacies or through mail-order pharmacies.

Percent of Total Personal Health Care Expenditures
Spent on Drugs and Other Medical Non-Durables in 1993
National Percent = 9.6%*

ALPHA ORDER

RANK	STATE	PERCENT
21	Alabama	10.3
18	Alaska	10.5
17	Arizona	10.6
8	Arkansas	11.2
32	California	9.6
40	Colorado	9.1
47	Connecticut	8.2
35	Delaware	9.5
26	Florida	9.9
18	Georgia	10.5
2	Hawaii	11.9
3	Idaho	11.6
38	Illinois	9.4
29	Indiana	9.7
23	Iowa	10.1
23	Kansas	10.1
5	Kentucky	11.5
28	Louisiana	9.8
29	Maine	9.7
5	Maryland	11.5
45	Massachusetts	8.4
13	Michigan	10.8
48	Minnesota	8.1
3	Mississippi	11.6
42	Missouri	8.9
26	Montana	9.9
32	Nebraska	9.6
11	Nevada	10.9
39	New Hampshire	9.2
35	New Jersey	9.5
18	New Mexico	10.5
50	New York	7.6
9	North Carolina	11.1
49	North Dakota	7.9
32	Ohio	9.6
11	Oklahoma	10.9
35	Oregon	9.5
44	Pennsylvania	8.5
41	Rhode Island	9.0
13	South Carolina	10.8
46	South Dakota	8.3
23	Tennessee	10.1
21	Texas	10.3
15	Utah	10.7
15	Vermont	10.7
1	Virginia	12.1
29	Washington	9.7
10	West Virginia	11.0
42	Wisconsin	8.9
7	Wyoming	11.3

RANK ORDER

RANK	STATE	PERCENT
1	Virginia	12.1
2	Hawaii	11.9
3	Idaho	11.6
3	Mississippi	11.6
5	Kentucky	11.5
5	Maryland	11.5
7	Wyoming	11.3
8	Arkansas	11.2
9	North Carolina	11.1
10	West Virginia	11.0
11	Nevada	10.9
11	Oklahoma	10.9
13	Michigan	10.8
13	South Carolina	10.8
15	Utah	10.7
15	Vermont	10.7
17	Arizona	10.6
18	Alaska	10.5
18	Georgia	10.5
18	New Mexico	10.5
21	Alabama	10.3
21	Texas	10.3
23	Iowa	10.1
23	Kansas	10.1
23	Tennessee	10.1
26	Florida	9.9
26	Montana	9.9
28	Louisiana	9.8
29	Indiana	9.7
29	Maine	9.7
29	Washington	9.7
32	California	9.6
32	Nebraska	9.6
32	Ohio	9.6
35	Delaware	9.5
35	New Jersey	9.5
35	Oregon	9.5
38	Illinois	9.4
39	New Hampshire	9.2
40	Colorado	9.1
41	Rhode Island	9.0
42	Missouri	8.9
42	Wisconsin	8.9
44	Pennsylvania	8.5
45	Massachusetts	8.4
46	South Dakota	8.3
47	Connecticut	8.2
48	Minnesota	8.1
49	North Dakota	7.9
50	New York	7.6

District of Columbia — 4.1

Source: Morgan Quitno Press using data from U.S. Dept of Health & Human Services, Health Care Financing Admin.
"State Health Expenditure Accounts" (Health Care Financing Review, Fall 1995, Volume 17, Number 1)
*By state of provider. Includes prescription and over-the-counter drugs and sundries. Limited to spending that occurs in retail outlets such as food stores, drug stores, HMO pharmacies or through mail-order pharmacies.

Per Capita Expenditures for Drugs and Other Medical Non-Durables in 1993

National Per Capita = $291*

ALPHA ORDER

RANK	STATE	PER CAPITA
15	Alabama	$298
31	Alaska	276
22	Arizona	285
25	Arkansas	282
21	California	289
40	Colorado	258
14	Connecticut	304
13	Delaware	306
4	Florida	324
12	Georgia	307
1	Hawaii	357
47	Idaho	241
29	Illinois	279
29	Indiana	279
38	Iowa	263
32	Kansas	274
7	Kentucky	315
16	Louisiana	296
37	Maine	269
2	Maryland	353
3	Massachusetts	326
9	Michigan	311
42	Minnesota	253
33	Mississippi	273
34	Missouri	271
46	Montana	249
39	Nebraska	261
17	Nevada	295
23	New Hampshire	284
8	New Jersey	312
42	New Mexico	253
26	New York	280
18	North Carolina	292
44	North Dakota	251
20	Ohio	291
35	Oklahoma	270
44	Oregon	251
18	Pennsylvania	292
11	Rhode Island	310
35	South Carolina	270
50	South Dakota	227
5	Tennessee	321
23	Texas	284
49	Utah	236
26	Vermont	280
9	Virginia	311
26	Washington	280
6	West Virginia	316
41	Wisconsin	256
48	Wyoming	240

RANK ORDER

RANK	STATE	PER CAPITA
1	Hawaii	$357
2	Maryland	353
3	Massachusetts	326
4	Florida	324
5	Tennessee	321
6	West Virginia	316
7	Kentucky	315
8	New Jersey	312
9	Michigan	311
9	Virginia	311
11	Rhode Island	310
12	Georgia	307
13	Delaware	306
14	Connecticut	304
15	Alabama	298
16	Louisiana	296
17	Nevada	295
18	North Carolina	292
18	Pennsylvania	292
20	Ohio	291
21	California	289
22	Arizona	285
23	New Hampshire	284
23	Texas	284
25	Arkansas	282
26	New York	280
26	Vermont	280
26	Washington	280
29	Illinois	279
29	Indiana	279
31	Alaska	276
32	Kansas	274
33	Mississippi	273
34	Missouri	271
35	Oklahoma	270
35	South Carolina	270
37	Maine	269
38	Iowa	263
39	Nebraska	261
40	Colorado	258
41	Wisconsin	256
42	Minnesota	253
42	New Mexico	253
44	North Dakota	251
44	Oregon	251
46	Montana	249
47	Idaho	241
48	Wyoming	240
49	Utah	236
50	South Dakota	227
	District of Columbia	303

Source: Morgan Quitno Press using data from U.S. Dept of Health & Human Services, Health Care Financing Admin. "State Health Expenditure Accounts" (Health Care Financing Review, Fall 1995, Volume 17, Number 1)
By state of provider. Includes prescription and over-the-counter drugs and sundries. Limited to spending that occurs in retail outlets such as food stores, drug stores, HMO pharmacies or through mail-order pharmacies.

Average Annual Change in Expenditures for Drugs and Other Medical Non-Durables: 1980 to 1993
National Percent = 10.0% Average Annual Growth*

ALPHA ORDER				RANK ORDER		
RANK	**STATE**	**PERCENT**		**RANK**	**STATE**	**PERCENT**
25	Alabama	9.9		1	Nevada	12.6
14	Alaska	10.8		2	Florida	12.1
3	Arizona	11.9		3	Arizona	11.9
45	Arkansas	8.7		4	Maryland	11.7
19	California	10.3		4	New Hampshire	11.7
17	Colorado	10.4		6	Vermont	11.6
26	Connecticut	9.8		7	Georgia	11.4
11	Delaware	10.9		8	Maine	11.3
2	Florida	12.1		8	Virginia	11.3
7	Georgia	11.4		10	New Mexico	11.2
11	Hawaii	10.9		11	Delaware	10.9
34	Idaho	9.3		11	Hawaii	10.9
37	Illinois	9.2		11	Rhode Island	10.9
42	Indiana	9.0		14	Alaska	10.8
45	Iowa	8.7		15	Massachusetts	10.7
37	Kansas	9.2		15	Utah	10.7
30	Kentucky	9.7		17	Colorado	10.4
47	Louisiana	8.6		17	Washington	10.4
8	Maine	11.3		19	California	10.3
4	Maryland	11.7		19	North Carolina	10.3
15	Massachusetts	10.7		19	South Carolina	10.3
31	Michigan	9.5		22	New Jersey	10.2
26	Minnesota	9.8		22	Tennessee	10.2
34	Mississippi	9.3		24	Wisconsin	10.1
44	Missouri	8.8		25	Alabama	9.9
31	Montana	9.5		26	Connecticut	9.8
42	Nebraska	9.0		26	Minnesota	9.8
1	Nevada	12.6		26	New York	9.8
4	New Hampshire	11.7		26	Texas	9.8
22	New Jersey	10.2		30	Kentucky	9.7
10	New Mexico	11.2		31	Michigan	9.5
26	New York	9.8		31	Montana	9.5
19	North Carolina	10.3		31	Pennsylvania	9.5
37	North Dakota	9.2		34	Idaho	9.3
40	Ohio	9.1		34	Mississippi	9.3
49	Oklahoma	8.4		34	South Dakota	9.3
48	Oregon	8.5		37	Illinois	9.2
31	Pennsylvania	9.5		37	Kansas	9.2
11	Rhode Island	10.9		37	North Dakota	9.2
19	South Carolina	10.3		40	Ohio	9.1
34	South Dakota	9.3		40	West Virginia	9.1
22	Tennessee	10.2		42	Indiana	9.0
26	Texas	9.8		42	Nebraska	9.0
15	Utah	10.7		44	Missouri	8.8
6	Vermont	11.6		45	Arkansas	8.7
8	Virginia	11.3		45	Iowa	8.7
17	Washington	10.4		47	Louisiana	8.6
40	West Virginia	9.1		48	Oregon	8.5
24	Wisconsin	10.1		49	Oklahoma	8.4
50	Wyoming	7.8		50	Wyoming	7.8
					District of Columbia	8.6

Source: U.S. Department of Health and Human Services, Health Care Financing Administration
"State Health Expenditure Accounts" (Health Care Financing Review, Fall 1995, Volume 17, Number 1)
*By state of provider. Includes prescription and over-the-counter drugs and sundries. Limited to spending that occurs in retail outlets such as food stores, drug stores, HMO pharmacies or through mail-order pharmacies.

Expenditures for Prescription Drugs in 1993

National Total = $48,840,000,000*

ALPHA ORDER					RANK ORDER			

RANK	STATE	EXPENDITURES	% of USA		RANK	STATE	EXPENDITURES	% of USA
18	Alabama	$904,000,000	1.85%		1	California	$5,501,000,000	11.26%
49	Alaska	85,000,000	0.17%		2	New York	3,232,000,000	6.62%
24	Arizona	728,000,000	1.49%		3	Texas	3,153,000,000	6.46%
31	Arkansas	484,000,000	0.99%		4	Florida	2,832,000,000	5.80%
1	California	5,501,000,000	11.26%		5	Pennsylvania	2,386,000,000	4.89%
28	Colorado	534,000,000	1.09%		6	Illinois	2,206,000,000	4.52%
26	Connecticut	650,000,000	1.33%		7	Ohio	2,095,000,000	4.29%
44	Delaware	129,000,000	0.26%		8	Michigan	2,054,000,000	4.21%
4	Florida	2,832,000,000	5.80%		9	New Jersey	1,601,000,000	3.28%
10	Georgia	1,397,000,000	2.86%		10	Georgia	1,397,000,000	2.86%
41	Hawaii	197,000,000	0.40%		11	North Carolina	1,392,000,000	2.85%
43	Idaho	182,000,000	0.37%		12	Virginia	1,343,000,000	2.75%
6	Illinois	2,206,000,000	4.52%		13	Massachusetts	1,337,000,000	2.74%
16	Indiana	1,106,000,000	2.26%		14	Tennessee	1,153,000,000	2.36%
29	Iowa	516,000,000	1.06%		15	Maryland	1,140,000,000	2.33%
32	Kansas	465,000,000	0.95%		16	Indiana	1,106,000,000	2.26%
21	Kentucky	846,000,000	1.73%		17	Missouri	975,000,000	2.00%
22	Louisiana	832,000,000	1.70%		18	Alabama	904,000,000	1.85%
39	Maine	213,000,000	0.44%		19	Wisconsin	899,000,000	1.84%
15	Maryland	1,140,000,000	2.33%		20	Washington	853,000,000	1.75%
13	Massachusetts	1,337,000,000	2.74%		21	Kentucky	846,000,000	1.73%
8	Michigan	2,054,000,000	4.21%		22	Louisiana	832,000,000	1.70%
23	Minnesota	739,000,000	1.51%		23	Minnesota	739,000,000	1.51%
30	Mississippi	499,000,000	1.02%		24	Arizona	728,000,000	1.49%
17	Missouri	975,000,000	2.00%		25	South Carolina	665,000,000	1.36%
45	Montana	120,000,000	0.25%		26	Connecticut	650,000,000	1.33%
36	Nebraska	293,000,000	0.60%		27	Oklahoma	569,000,000	1.17%
38	Nevada	246,000,000	0.50%		28	Colorado	534,000,000	1.09%
41	New Hampshire	197,000,000	0.40%		29	Iowa	516,000,000	1.06%
9	New Jersey	1,601,000,000	3.28%		30	Mississippi	499,000,000	1.02%
37	New Mexico	259,000,000	0.53%		31	Arkansas	484,000,000	0.99%
2	New York	3,232,000,000	6.62%		32	Kansas	465,000,000	0.95%
11	North Carolina	1,392,000,000	2.85%		33	Oregon	431,000,000	0.88%
48	North Dakota	103,000,000	0.21%		34	West Virginia	412,000,000	0.84%
7	Ohio	2,095,000,000	4.29%		35	Utah	302,000,000	0.62%
27	Oklahoma	569,000,000	1.17%		36	Nebraska	293,000,000	0.60%
33	Oregon	431,000,000	0.88%		37	New Mexico	259,000,000	0.53%
5	Pennsylvania	2,386,000,000	4.89%		38	Nevada	246,000,000	0.50%
40	Rhode Island	206,000,000	0.42%		39	Maine	213,000,000	0.44%
25	South Carolina	665,000,000	1.36%		40	Rhode Island	206,000,000	0.42%
47	South Dakota	104,000,000	0.21%		41	Hawaii	197,000,000	0.40%
14	Tennessee	1,153,000,000	2.36%		41	New Hampshire	197,000,000	0.40%
3	Texas	3,153,000,000	6.46%		43	Idaho	182,000,000	0.37%
35	Utah	302,000,000	0.62%		44	Delaware	129,000,000	0.26%
46	Vermont	108,000,000	0.22%		45	Montana	120,000,000	0.25%
12	Virginia	1,343,000,000	2.75%		46	Vermont	108,000,000	0.22%
20	Washington	853,000,000	1.75%		47	South Dakota	104,000,000	0.21%
34	West Virginia	412,000,000	0.84%		48	North Dakota	103,000,000	0.21%
19	Wisconsin	899,000,000	1.84%		49	Alaska	85,000,000	0.17%
50	Wyoming	64,000,000	0.13%		50	Wyoming	64,000,000	0.13%
						District of Columbia	103,000,000	0.21%

Source: U.S. Department of Health and Human Services, Health Care Financing Administration
"State Health Expenditure Accounts" (Health Care Financing Review, Fall 1995, Volume 17, Number 1)
*Purchases in retail outlets. By state of outlet. This is a subset of overall "Drug and Other Medical Non-Durable Expenditures" shown elsewhere in this book.

Percent of Total Personal Health Care Expenditures
Spent on Prescription Drugs in 1993
National Percent = 6.3%*

ALPHA ORDER

RANK	STATE	PERCENT
9	Alabama	7.5
43	Alaska	5.4
18	Arizona	6.8
5	Arkansas	7.9
35	California	5.8
45	Colorado	5.3
45	Connecticut	5.3
36	Delaware	5.7
26	Florida	6.3
17	Georgia	6.9
36	Hawaii	5.7
4	Idaho	8.0
26	Illinois	6.3
19	Indiana	6.7
16	Iowa	7.0
19	Kansas	6.7
1	Kentucky	8.1
24	Louisiana	6.4
30	Maine	6.2
9	Maryland	7.5
36	Massachusetts	5.7
7	Michigan	7.6
48	Minnesota	5.2
1	Mississippi	8.1
33	Missouri	6.1
36	Montana	5.7
19	Nebraska	6.7
23	Nevada	6.6
36	New Hampshire	5.7
30	New Jersey	6.2
19	New Mexico	6.7
50	New York	4.8
7	North Carolina	7.6
49	North Dakota	5.1
26	Ohio	6.3
14	Oklahoma	7.1
43	Oregon	5.4
36	Pennsylvania	5.7
34	Rhode Island	6.0
11	South Carolina	7.4
45	South Dakota	5.3
14	Tennessee	7.1
26	Texas	6.3
12	Utah	7.3
13	Vermont	7.2
1	Virginia	8.1
42	Washington	5.6
5	West Virginia	7.9
30	Wisconsin	6.2
24	Wyoming	6.4

RANK ORDER

RANK	STATE	PERCENT
1	Kentucky	8.1
1	Mississippi	8.1
1	Virginia	8.1
4	Idaho	8.0
5	Arkansas	7.9
5	West Virginia	7.9
7	Michigan	7.6
7	North Carolina	7.6
9	Alabama	7.5
9	Maryland	7.5
11	South Carolina	7.4
12	Utah	7.3
13	Vermont	7.2
14	Oklahoma	7.1
14	Tennessee	7.1
16	Iowa	7.0
17	Georgia	6.9
18	Arizona	6.8
19	Indiana	6.7
19	Kansas	6.7
19	Nebraska	6.7
19	New Mexico	6.7
23	Nevada	6.6
24	Louisiana	6.4
24	Wyoming	6.4
26	Florida	6.3
26	Illinois	6.3
26	Ohio	6.3
26	Texas	6.3
30	Maine	6.2
30	New Jersey	6.2
30	Wisconsin	6.2
33	Missouri	6.1
34	Rhode Island	6.0
35	California	5.8
36	Delaware	5.7
36	Hawaii	5.7
36	Massachusetts	5.7
36	Montana	5.7
36	New Hampshire	5.7
36	Pennsylvania	5.7
42	Washington	5.6
43	Alaska	5.4
43	Oregon	5.4
45	Colorado	5.3
45	Connecticut	5.3
45	South Dakota	5.3
48	Minnesota	5.2
49	North Dakota	5.1
50	New York	4.8

District of Columbia 2.4

Source: Morgan Quitno Press using data from U.S. Dept of Health & Human Services, Health Care Financing Admin.
"State Health Expenditure Accounts" (Health Care Financing Review, Fall 1995, Volume 17, Number 1)
Purchases in retail outlets. By state of outlet. This is a subset of overall "Drug and Other Medical Non-Durable Expenditures" shown elsewhere in this book.

Per Capita Expenditures for Prescription Drugs in 1993

National Per Capita = $189*

ALPHA ORDER				RANK ORDER		
RANK	STATE	PER CAPITA		RANK	STATE	PER CAPITA
7	Alabama	$216		1	Maryland	$230
48	Alaska	142		2	West Virginia	227
24	Arizona	185		3	Tennessee	226
13	Arkansas	200		4	Kentucky	223
33	California	176		5	Massachusetts	222
45	Colorado	150		6	Michigan	217
15	Connecticut	198		7	Alabama	216
24	Delaware	185		8	Virginia	207
9	Florida	206		9	Florida	206
12	Georgia	202		9	Rhode Island	206
38	Hawaii	169		11	New Jersey	204
39	Idaho	165		12	Georgia	202
19	Illinois	189		13	Arkansas	200
17	Indiana	194		13	North Carolina	200
27	Iowa	183		15	Connecticut	198
26	Kansas	184		15	Pennsylvania	198
4	Kentucky	223		17	Indiana	194
17	Louisiana	194		17	Louisiana	194
37	Maine	172		19	Illinois	189
1	Maryland	230		19	Mississippi	189
5	Massachusetts	222		19	Ohio	189
6	Michigan	217		22	Vermont	188
40	Minnesota	163		23	Missouri	186
19	Mississippi	189		24	Arizona	185
23	Missouri	186		24	Delaware	185
47	Montana	143		26	Kansas	184
29	Nebraska	182		27	Iowa	183
30	Nevada	178		27	South Carolina	183
35	New Hampshire	175		29	Nebraska	182
11	New Jersey	204		30	Nevada	178
44	New Mexico	160		30	New York	178
30	New York	178		30	Wisconsin	178
13	North Carolina	200		33	California	176
41	North Dakota	162		33	Oklahoma	176
19	Ohio	189		35	New Hampshire	175
33	Oklahoma	176		35	Texas	175
48	Oregon	142		37	Maine	172
15	Pennsylvania	198		38	Hawaii	169
9	Rhode Island	206		39	Idaho	165
27	South Carolina	183		40	Minnesota	163
46	South Dakota	145		41	North Dakota	162
3	Tennessee	226		41	Utah	162
35	Texas	175		41	Washington	162
41	Utah	162		44	New Mexico	160
22	Vermont	188		45	Colorado	150
8	Virginia	207		46	South Dakota	145
41	Washington	162		47	Montana	143
2	West Virginia	227		48	Alaska	142
30	Wisconsin	178		48	Oregon	142
50	Wyoming	136		50	Wyoming	136
					District of Columbia	178

Source: Morgan Quitno Press using data from U.S. Dept of Health & Human Services, Health Care Financing Admin. "State Health Expenditure Accounts" (Health Care Financing Review, Fall 1995, Volume 17, Number 1)
*Purchases in retail outlets. By state of outlet. This is a subset of overall "Drug and Other Medical Non-Durable Expenditures" shown elsewhere in this book.

Percent Change in Expenditures for Prescription Drugs: 1990 to 1993

National Percent Change = 27.9% Increase*

ALPHA ORDER

RANK ORDER

RANK	STATE	PERCENT CHANGE	RANK	STATE	PERCENT CHANGE
23	Alabama	27.9	1	Nevada	55.7
2	Alaska	46.6	2	Alaska	46.6
6	Arizona	38.4	3	Idaho	41.1
28	Arkansas	26.7	4	Colorado	40.9
19	California	30.3	5	Utah	38.5
4	Colorado	40.9	6	Arizona	38.4
49	Connecticut	19.5	7	Washington	38.0
15	Delaware	31.6	8	New Mexico	36.3
14	Florida	32.6	9	Oregon	35.5
10	Georgia	35.0	10	Georgia	35.0
13	Hawaii	33.1	11	Texas	34.4
3	Idaho	41.1	12	Montana	33.3
35	Illinois	24.6	13	Hawaii	33.1
29	Indiana	26.5	14	Florida	32.6
42	Iowa	23.2	15	Delaware	31.6
33	Kansas	24.7	16	North Carolina	31.2
26	Kentucky	26.8	17	Virginia	30.9
35	Louisiana	24.6	18	Wyoming	30.6
45	Maine	22.4	19	California	30.3
22	Maryland	28.4	20	South Carolina	30.1
47	Massachusetts	20.1	20	Tennessee	30.1
39	Michigan	24.2	22	Maryland	28.4
24	Minnesota	27.4	23	Alabama	27.9
32	Mississippi	25.1	24	Minnesota	27.4
37	Missouri	24.5	25	Wisconsin	27.0
12	Montana	33.3	26	Kentucky	26.8
33	Nebraska	24.7	26	South Dakota	26.8
1	Nevada	55.7	28	Arkansas	26.7
43	New Hampshire	23.1	29	Indiana	26.5
41	New Jersey	23.3	30	Oklahoma	26.4
8	New Mexico	36.3	31	Vermont	25.6
46	New York	21.3	32	Mississippi	25.1
16	North Carolina	31.2	33	Kansas	24.7
48	North Dakota	19.8	33	Nebraska	24.7
38	Ohio	24.4	35	Illinois	24.6
30	Oklahoma	26.4	35	Louisiana	24.6
9	Oregon	35.5	37	Missouri	24.5
44	Pennsylvania	22.5	38	Ohio	24.4
50	Rhode Island	18.4	39	Michigan	24.2
20	South Carolina	30.1	40	West Virginia	23.7
26	South Dakota	26.8	41	New Jersey	23.3
20	Tennessee	30.1	42	Iowa	23.2
11	Texas	34.4	43	New Hampshire	23.1
5	Utah	38.5	44	Pennsylvania	22.5
31	Vermont	25.6	45	Maine	22.4
17	Virginia	30.9	46	New York	21.3
7	Washington	38.0	47	Massachusetts	20.1
40	West Virginia	23.7	48	North Dakota	19.8
25	Wisconsin	27.0	49	Connecticut	19.5
18	Wyoming	30.6	50	Rhode Island	18.4
				District of Columbia	10.8

Source: Morgan Quitno Press using data from U.S. Dept of Health & Human Services, Health Care Financing Admin.
"State Health Expenditure Accounts" (Health Care Financing Review, Fall 1995, Volume 17, Number 1)
*Purchases in retail outlets. By state of outlet. This is a subset of overall "Drug and Other Medical Non-Durable
Expenditures" shown elsewhere in this book.

Percent Change in Per Capita Expenditures for Prescription Drugs: 1990 to 1993

National Percent Change = 22.7% Increase*

RANK	STATE	PERCENT CHANGE	RANK	STATE	PERCENT CHANGE
24	Alabama	23.4	1	Nevada	35.9
2	Alaska	35.2	2	Alaska	35.2
5	Arizona	28.5	3	Colorado	30.4
23	Arkansas	23.5	4	Idaho	28.9
21	California	23.9	5	Arizona	28.5
3	Colorado	30.4	6	New Mexico	28.0
49	Connecticut	19.3	7	Utah	27.6
14	Delaware	25.9	7	Washington	27.6
17	Florida	24.8	9	Oregon	26.8
12	Georgia	26.3	9	Texas	26.8
13	Hawaii	26.1	11	Montana	26.5
4	Idaho	28.9	12	Georgia	26.3
35	Illinois	21.9	13	Hawaii	26.1
29	Indiana	22.8	14	Delaware	25.9
43	Iowa	21.2	14	Wyoming	25.9
35	Kansas	21.9	16	North Carolina	25.0
25	Kentucky	23.2	17	Florida	24.8
29	Louisiana	22.8	18	Virginia	24.7
44	Maine	21.1	19	South Carolina	24.5
22	Maryland	23.7	20	Tennessee	24.2
47	Massachusetts	20.0	21	California	23.9
35	Michigan	21.9	22	Maryland	23.7
32	Minnesota	22.6	23	Arkansas	23.5
35	Mississippi	21.9	24	Alabama	23.4
40	Missouri	21.6	25	Kentucky	23.2
11	Montana	26.5	26	Oklahoma	23.1
33	Nebraska	22.1	27	South Dakota	22.9
1	Nevada	35.9	27	Vermont	22.9
41	New Hampshire	21.5	29	Indiana	22.8
42	New Jersey	21.4	29	Louisiana	22.8
6	New Mexico	28.0	29	Wisconsin	22.8
46	New York	20.3	32	Minnesota	22.6
16	North Carolina	25.0	33	Nebraska	22.1
47	North Dakota	20.0	34	West Virginia	22.0
35	Ohio	21.9	35	Illinois	21.9
26	Oklahoma	23.1	35	Kansas	21.9
9	Oregon	26.8	35	Michigan	21.9
45	Pennsylvania	20.7	35	Mississippi	21.9
50	Rhode Island	19.1	35	Ohio	21.9
19	South Carolina	24.5	40	Missouri	21.6
27	South Dakota	22.9	41	New Hampshire	21.5
20	Tennessee	24.2	42	New Jersey	21.4
9	Texas	26.8	43	Iowa	21.2
7	Utah	27.6	44	Maine	21.1
27	Vermont	22.9	45	Pennsylvania	20.7
18	Virginia	24.7	46	New York	20.3
7	Washington	27.6	47	Massachusetts	20.0
34	West Virginia	22.0	47	North Dakota	20.0
29	Wisconsin	22.8	49	Connecticut	19.3
14	Wyoming	25.9	50	Rhode Island	19.1
				District of Columbia	16.3

Source: Morgan Quitno Press using data from U.S. Dept of Health & Human Services, Health Care Financing Admin. "State Health Expenditure Accounts" (Health Care Financing Review, Fall 1995, Volume 17, Number 1)
Purchases in retail outlets. By state of outlet. This is a subset of overall "Drug and Other Medical Non-Durable Expenditures" shown elsewhere in this book.

Average Annual Change in Expenditures for Prescription Drugs: 1980 to 1993

National Percent = 11.4% Average Annual Increase*

<table>
<tr><td colspan="3">ALPHA ORDER</td><td colspan="3">RANK ORDER</td></tr>
<tr><td>RANK</td><td>STATE</td><td>PERCENT</td><td>RANK</td><td>STATE</td><td>PERCENT</td></tr>
<tr><td>32</td><td>Alabama</td><td>10.9</td><td>1</td><td>Nevada</td><td>15.8</td></tr>
<tr><td>4</td><td>Alaska</td><td>13.7</td><td>2</td><td>Arizona</td><td>14.7</td></tr>
<tr><td>2</td><td>Arizona</td><td>14.7</td><td>3</td><td>Utah</td><td>14.2</td></tr>
<tr><td>49</td><td>Arkansas</td><td>9.3</td><td>4</td><td>Alaska</td><td>13.7</td></tr>
<tr><td>16</td><td>California</td><td>11.8</td><td>4</td><td>Florida</td><td>13.7</td></tr>
<tr><td>18</td><td>Colorado</td><td>11.7</td><td>6</td><td>Delaware</td><td>13.3</td></tr>
<tr><td>33</td><td>Connecticut</td><td>10.7</td><td>6</td><td>Maryland</td><td>13.3</td></tr>
<tr><td>6</td><td>Delaware</td><td>13.3</td><td>6</td><td>New Hampshire</td><td>13.3</td></tr>
<tr><td>4</td><td>Florida</td><td>13.7</td><td>9</td><td>New Mexico</td><td>13.2</td></tr>
<tr><td>12</td><td>Georgia</td><td>12.7</td><td>10</td><td>Vermont</td><td>13.0</td></tr>
<tr><td>14</td><td>Hawaii</td><td>12.2</td><td>10</td><td>Virginia</td><td>13.0</td></tr>
<tr><td>20</td><td>Idaho</td><td>11.6</td><td>12</td><td>Georgia</td><td>12.7</td></tr>
<tr><td>26</td><td>Illinois</td><td>11.1</td><td>13</td><td>Massachusetts</td><td>12.5</td></tr>
<tr><td>39</td><td>Indiana</td><td>10.4</td><td>14</td><td>Hawaii</td><td>12.2</td></tr>
<tr><td>46</td><td>Iowa</td><td>9.6</td><td>15</td><td>South Carolina</td><td>11.9</td></tr>
<tr><td>37</td><td>Kansas</td><td>10.5</td><td>16</td><td>California</td><td>11.8</td></tr>
<tr><td>33</td><td>Kentucky</td><td>10.7</td><td>16</td><td>Rhode Island</td><td>11.8</td></tr>
<tr><td>47</td><td>Louisiana</td><td>9.5</td><td>18</td><td>Colorado</td><td>11.7</td></tr>
<tr><td>20</td><td>Maine</td><td>11.6</td><td>18</td><td>New Jersey</td><td>11.7</td></tr>
<tr><td>6</td><td>Maryland</td><td>13.3</td><td>20</td><td>Idaho</td><td>11.6</td></tr>
<tr><td>13</td><td>Massachusetts</td><td>12.5</td><td>20</td><td>Maine</td><td>11.6</td></tr>
<tr><td>28</td><td>Michigan</td><td>11.0</td><td>22</td><td>North Carolina</td><td>11.5</td></tr>
<tr><td>28</td><td>Minnesota</td><td>11.0</td><td>22</td><td>Wisconsin</td><td>11.5</td></tr>
<tr><td>42</td><td>Mississippi</td><td>10.1</td><td>24</td><td>Washington</td><td>11.3</td></tr>
<tr><td>41</td><td>Missouri</td><td>10.2</td><td>25</td><td>Tennessee</td><td>11.2</td></tr>
<tr><td>28</td><td>Montana</td><td>11.0</td><td>26</td><td>Illinois</td><td>11.1</td></tr>
<tr><td>37</td><td>Nebraska</td><td>10.5</td><td>26</td><td>New York</td><td>11.1</td></tr>
<tr><td>1</td><td>Nevada</td><td>15.8</td><td>28</td><td>Michigan</td><td>11.0</td></tr>
<tr><td>6</td><td>New Hampshire</td><td>13.3</td><td>28</td><td>Minnesota</td><td>11.0</td></tr>
<tr><td>18</td><td>New Jersey</td><td>11.7</td><td>28</td><td>Montana</td><td>11.0</td></tr>
<tr><td>9</td><td>New Mexico</td><td>13.2</td><td>28</td><td>Pennsylvania</td><td>11.0</td></tr>
<tr><td>26</td><td>New York</td><td>11.1</td><td>32</td><td>Alabama</td><td>10.9</td></tr>
<tr><td>22</td><td>North Carolina</td><td>11.5</td><td>33</td><td>Connecticut</td><td>10.7</td></tr>
<tr><td>35</td><td>North Dakota</td><td>10.6</td><td>33</td><td>Kentucky</td><td>10.7</td></tr>
<tr><td>43</td><td>Ohio</td><td>10.0</td><td>35</td><td>North Dakota</td><td>10.6</td></tr>
<tr><td>47</td><td>Oklahoma</td><td>9.5</td><td>35</td><td>Texas</td><td>10.6</td></tr>
<tr><td>43</td><td>Oregon</td><td>10.0</td><td>37</td><td>Kansas</td><td>10.5</td></tr>
<tr><td>28</td><td>Pennsylvania</td><td>11.0</td><td>37</td><td>Nebraska</td><td>10.5</td></tr>
<tr><td>16</td><td>Rhode Island</td><td>11.8</td><td>39</td><td>Indiana</td><td>10.4</td></tr>
<tr><td>15</td><td>South Carolina</td><td>11.9</td><td>40</td><td>West Virginia</td><td>10.3</td></tr>
<tr><td>43</td><td>South Dakota</td><td>10.0</td><td>41</td><td>Missouri</td><td>10.2</td></tr>
<tr><td>25</td><td>Tennessee</td><td>11.2</td><td>42</td><td>Mississippi</td><td>10.1</td></tr>
<tr><td>35</td><td>Texas</td><td>10.6</td><td>43</td><td>Ohio</td><td>10.0</td></tr>
<tr><td>3</td><td>Utah</td><td>14.2</td><td>43</td><td>Oregon</td><td>10.0</td></tr>
<tr><td>10</td><td>Vermont</td><td>13.0</td><td>43</td><td>South Dakota</td><td>10.0</td></tr>
<tr><td>10</td><td>Virginia</td><td>13.0</td><td>46</td><td>Iowa</td><td>9.6</td></tr>
<tr><td>24</td><td>Washington</td><td>11.3</td><td>47</td><td>Louisiana</td><td>9.5</td></tr>
<tr><td>40</td><td>West Virginia</td><td>10.3</td><td>47</td><td>Oklahoma</td><td>9.5</td></tr>
<tr><td>22</td><td>Wisconsin</td><td>11.5</td><td>49</td><td>Arkansas</td><td>9.3</td></tr>
<tr><td>50</td><td>Wyoming</td><td>8.2</td><td>50</td><td>Wyoming</td><td>8.2</td></tr>
<tr><td></td><td></td><td></td><td></td><td>District of Columbia</td><td>9.5</td></tr>
</table>

Source: U.S. Department of Health and Human Services, Health Care Financing Administration
   "State Health Expenditure Accounts" (Health Care Financing Review, Fall 1995, Volume 17, Number 1)
*Purchases in retail outlets. By state of outlet. This is a subset of overall "Drug and Other Medical Non-Durable Expenditures" shown elsewhere in this book.

Average Annual Change in Per Capita Expenditures
For Prescription Drugs: 1980 to 1993
National Percent = 10.3% Average Annual Increase*

ALPHA ORDER

RANK	STATE	PERCENT
27	Alabama	10.4
30	Alaska	10.2
7	Arizona	11.5
48	Arkansas	8.8
43	California	9.4
36	Colorado	9.9
30	Connecticut	10.2
1	Delaware	12.1
20	Florida	10.7
20	Georgia	10.7
24	Hawaii	10.5
32	Idaho	10.1
14	Illinois	10.9
33	Indiana	10.0
38	Iowa	9.8
36	Kansas	9.9
24	Kentucky	10.5
43	Louisiana	9.4
14	Maine	10.9
5	Maryland	11.8
2	Massachusetts	12.0
17	Michigan	10.8
33	Minnesota	10.0
38	Mississippi	9.8
42	Missouri	9.7
24	Montana	10.5
28	Nebraska	10.3
11	Nevada	11.2
6	New Hampshire	11.6
12	New Jersey	11.1
9	New Mexico	11.3
17	New York	10.8
33	North Carolina	10.0
20	North Dakota	10.7
38	Ohio	9.8
46	Oklahoma	8.9
46	Oregon	8.9
17	Pennsylvania	10.8
9	Rhode Island	11.3
20	South Carolina	10.7
38	South Dakota	9.8
28	Tennessee	10.3
49	Texas	8.6
2	Utah	12.0
2	Vermont	12.0
8	Virginia	11.4
45	Washington	9.3
14	West Virginia	10.9
13	Wisconsin	11.0
50	Wyoming	8.2

RANK ORDER

RANK	STATE	PERCENT
1	Delaware	12.1
2	Massachusetts	12.0
2	Utah	12.0
2	Vermont	12.0
5	Maryland	11.8
6	New Hampshire	11.6
7	Arizona	11.5
8	Virginia	11.4
9	New Mexico	11.3
9	Rhode Island	11.3
11	Nevada	11.2
12	New Jersey	11.1
13	Wisconsin	11.0
14	Illinois	10.9
14	Maine	10.9
14	West Virginia	10.9
17	Michigan	10.8
17	New York	10.8
17	Pennsylvania	10.8
20	Florida	10.7
20	Georgia	10.7
20	North Dakota	10.7
20	South Carolina	10.7
24	Hawaii	10.5
24	Kentucky	10.5
24	Montana	10.5
27	Alabama	10.4
28	Nebraska	10.3
28	Tennessee	10.3
30	Alaska	10.2
30	Connecticut	10.2
32	Idaho	10.1
33	Indiana	10.0
33	Minnesota	10.0
33	North Carolina	10.0
36	Colorado	9.9
36	Kansas	9.9
38	Iowa	9.8
38	Mississippi	9.8
38	Ohio	9.8
38	South Dakota	9.8
42	Missouri	9.7
43	California	9.4
43	Louisiana	9.4
45	Washington	9.3
46	Oklahoma	8.9
46	Oregon	8.9
48	Arkansas	8.8
49	Texas	8.6
50	Wyoming	8.2

District of Columbia	10.3

Source: Morgan Quitno Press using data from U.S. Dept of Health & Human Services, Health Care Financing Admin.
"State Health Expenditure Accounts" (Health Care Financing Review, Fall 1995, Volume 17, Number 1)
*Purchases in retail outlets. By state of outlet. This is a subset of overall "Drug and Other Medical Non-Durable Expenditures" shown elsewhere in this book.

Expenditures for Vision Products and Other Medical Durables in 1993

National Total = $12,636,000,000*

RANK	STATE	EXPENDITURES	% of USA
25	Alabama	$155,000,000	1.23%
48	Alaska	26,000,000	0.21%
21	Arizona	227,000,000	1.80%
39	Arkansas	56,000,000	0.44%
1	California	1,522,000,000	12.04%
22	Colorado	226,000,000	1.79%
23	Connecticut	192,000,000	1.52%
43	Delaware	35,000,000	0.28%
4	Florida	872,000,000	6.90%
10	Georgia	331,000,000	2.62%
37	Hawaii	64,000,000	0.51%
43	Idaho	35,000,000	0.28%
6	Illinois	604,000,000	4.78%
14	Indiana	270,000,000	2.14%
26	Iowa	148,000,000	1.17%
31	Kansas	107,000,000	0.85%
27	Kentucky	141,000,000	1.12%
24	Louisiana	160,000,000	1.27%
40	Maine	46,000,000	0.36%
13	Maryland	272,000,000	2.15%
15	Massachusetts	269,000,000	2.13%
8	Michigan	457,000,000	3.62%
12	Minnesota	277,000,000	2.19%
38	Mississippi	60,000,000	0.47%
17	Missouri	244,000,000	1.93%
42	Montana	36,000,000	0.28%
33	Nebraska	80,000,000	0.63%
34	Nevada	76,000,000	0.60%
41	New Hampshire	43,000,000	0.34%
8	New Jersey	457,000,000	3.62%
36	New Mexico	69,000,000	0.55%
2	New York	1,090,000,000	8.63%
16	North Carolina	268,000,000	2.12%
47	North Dakota	28,000,000	0.22%
7	Ohio	531,000,000	4.20%
28	Oklahoma	121,000,000	0.96%
32	Oregon	91,000,000	0.72%
5	Pennsylvania	617,000,000	4.88%
45	Rhode Island	33,000,000	0.26%
30	South Carolina	115,000,000	0.91%
46	South Dakota	30,000,000	0.24%
20	Tennessee	228,000,000	1.80%
3	Texas	883,000,000	6.99%
29	Utah	117,000,000	0.93%
49	Vermont	24,000,000	0.19%
11	Virginia	295,000,000	2.33%
18	Washington	242,000,000	1.92%
35	West Virginia	74,000,000	0.59%
19	Wisconsin	240,000,000	1.90%
50	Wyoming	17,000,000	0.13%

RANK	STATE	EXPENDITURES	% of USA
1	California	$1,522,000,000	12.04%
2	New York	1,090,000,000	8.63%
3	Texas	883,000,000	6.99%
4	Florida	872,000,000	6.90%
5	Pennsylvania	617,000,000	4.88%
6	Illinois	604,000,000	4.78%
7	Ohio	531,000,000	4.20%
8	Michigan	457,000,000	3.62%
8	New Jersey	457,000,000	3.62%
10	Georgia	331,000,000	2.62%
11	Virginia	295,000,000	2.33%
12	Minnesota	277,000,000	2.19%
13	Maryland	272,000,000	2.15%
14	Indiana	270,000,000	2.14%
15	Massachusetts	269,000,000	2.13%
16	North Carolina	268,000,000	2.12%
17	Missouri	244,000,000	1.93%
18	Washington	242,000,000	1.92%
19	Wisconsin	240,000,000	1.90%
20	Tennessee	228,000,000	1.80%
21	Arizona	227,000,000	1.80%
22	Colorado	226,000,000	1.79%
23	Connecticut	192,000,000	1.52%
24	Louisiana	160,000,000	1.27%
25	Alabama	155,000,000	1.23%
26	Iowa	148,000,000	1.17%
27	Kentucky	141,000,000	1.12%
28	Oklahoma	121,000,000	0.96%
29	Utah	117,000,000	0.93%
30	South Carolina	115,000,000	0.91%
31	Kansas	107,000,000	0.85%
32	Oregon	91,000,000	0.72%
33	Nebraska	80,000,000	0.63%
34	Nevada	76,000,000	0.60%
35	West Virginia	74,000,000	0.59%
36	New Mexico	69,000,000	0.55%
37	Hawaii	64,000,000	0.51%
38	Mississippi	60,000,000	0.47%
39	Arkansas	56,000,000	0.44%
40	Maine	46,000,000	0.36%
41	New Hampshire	43,000,000	0.34%
42	Montana	36,000,000	0.28%
43	Delaware	35,000,000	0.28%
43	Idaho	35,000,000	0.28%
45	Rhode Island	33,000,000	0.26%
46	South Dakota	30,000,000	0.24%
47	North Dakota	28,000,000	0.22%
48	Alaska	26,000,000	0.21%
49	Vermont	24,000,000	0.19%
50	Wyoming	17,000,000	0.13%
	District of Columbia	34,000,000	0.27%

Source: U.S. Department of Health and Human Services, Health Care Financing Administration
    "State Health Expenditure Accounts" (Health Care Financing Review, Fall 1995, Volume 17, Number 1)
*By state of provider. Includes eyeglasses, hearing aids, surgical appliances and supplies, bulk and cylinder oxygen and medical equipment rentals.

Percent of Total Personal Health Care Expenditures
Spent on Vision Products and Other Medical Durables in 1993
National Percent = 1.6%*

ALPHA ORDER

RANK	STATE	PERCENT
41	Alabama	1.3
15	Alaska	1.7
3	Arizona	2.1
50	Arkansas	0.9
21	California	1.6
2	Colorado	2.2
21	Connecticut	1.6
30	Delaware	1.5
7	Florida	1.9
21	Georgia	1.6
8	Hawaii	1.8
30	Idaho	1.5
15	Illinois	1.7
21	Indiana	1.6
4	Iowa	2.0
21	Kansas	1.6
37	Kentucky	1.4
44	Louisiana	1.2
41	Maine	1.3
8	Maryland	1.8
46	Massachusetts	1.1
15	Michigan	1.7
4	Minnesota	2.0
48	Mississippi	1.0
30	Missouri	1.5
15	Montana	1.7
8	Nebraska	1.8
4	Nevada	2.0
44	New Hampshire	1.2
8	New Jersey	1.8
8	New Mexico	1.8
21	New York	1.6
30	North Carolina	1.5
37	North Dakota	1.4
21	Ohio	1.6
30	Oklahoma	1.5
46	Oregon	1.1
30	Pennsylvania	1.5
48	Rhode Island	1.0
41	South Carolina	1.3
30	South Dakota	1.5
37	Tennessee	1.4
8	Texas	1.8
1	Utah	2.8
21	Vermont	1.6
8	Virginia	1.8
21	Washington	1.6
37	West Virginia	1.4
15	Wisconsin	1.7
15	Wyoming	1.7

RANK ORDER

RANK	STATE	PERCENT
1	Utah	2.8
2	Colorado	2.2
3	Arizona	2.1
4	Iowa	2.0
4	Minnesota	2.0
4	Nevada	2.0
7	Florida	1.9
8	Hawaii	1.8
8	Maryland	1.8
8	Nebraska	1.8
8	New Jersey	1.8
8	New Mexico	1.8
8	Texas	1.8
8	Virginia	1.8
15	Alaska	1.7
15	Illinois	1.7
15	Michigan	1.7
15	Montana	1.7
15	Wisconsin	1.7
15	Wyoming	1.7
21	California	1.6
21	Connecticut	1.6
21	Georgia	1.6
21	Indiana	1.6
21	Kansas	1.6
21	New York	1.6
21	Ohio	1.6
21	Vermont	1.6
21	Washington	1.6
30	Delaware	1.5
30	Idaho	1.5
30	Missouri	1.5
30	North Carolina	1.5
30	Oklahoma	1.5
30	Pennsylvania	1.5
30	South Dakota	1.5
37	Kentucky	1.4
37	North Dakota	1.4
37	Tennessee	1.4
37	West Virginia	1.4
41	Alabama	1.3
41	Maine	1.3
41	South Carolina	1.3
44	Louisiana	1.2
44	New Hampshire	1.2
46	Massachusetts	1.1
46	Oregon	1.1
48	Mississippi	1.0
48	Rhode Island	1.0
50	Arkansas	0.9

District of Columbia 0.8

Source: Morgan Quitno Press using data from U.S. Dept of Health & Human Services, Health Care Financing Admin.
"State Health Expenditure Accounts" (Health Care Financing Review, Fall 1995, Volume 17, Number 1)
*By state of provider. Includes eyeglasses, hearing aids, surgical appliances and supplies, bulk and cylinder oxygen and medical equipment rentals.

Per Capita Expenditures for Vision Products and Other Medical Durables in 1993

National Per Capita = $49*

ALPHA ORDER				RANK ORDER		
RANK	STATE	PER CAPITA		RANK	STATE	PER CAPITA
39	Alabama	$37		1	Florida	$64
30	Alaska	43		2	Colorado	63
7	Arizona	58		2	Utah	63
49	Arkansas	23		4	Minnesota	61
17	California	49		5	New York	60
2	Colorado	63		6	Connecticut	59
6	Connecticut	59		7	Arizona	58
15	Delaware	50		7	New Jersey	58
1	Florida	64		9	Hawaii	55
19	Georgia	48		9	Maryland	55
9	Hawaii	55		9	Nevada	55
46	Idaho	32		12	Illinois	52
12	Illinois	52		12	Iowa	52
23	Indiana	47		14	Pennsylvania	51
12	Iowa	52		15	Delaware	50
33	Kansas	42		15	Nebraska	50
39	Kentucky	37		17	California	49
39	Louisiana	37		17	Texas	49
39	Maine	37		19	Georgia	48
9	Maryland	55		19	Michigan	48
27	Massachusetts	45		19	Ohio	48
19	Michigan	48		19	Wisconsin	48
4	Minnesota	61		23	Indiana	47
49	Mississippi	23		23	Missouri	47
23	Missouri	47		25	Virginia	46
30	Montana	43		25	Washington	46
15	Nebraska	50		27	Massachusetts	45
9	Nevada	55		27	Tennessee	45
38	New Hampshire	38		29	North Dakota	44
7	New Jersey	58		30	Alaska	43
30	New Mexico	43		30	Montana	43
5	New York	60		30	New Mexico	43
37	North Carolina	39		33	Kansas	42
29	North Dakota	44		33	South Dakota	42
19	Ohio	48		33	Vermont	42
39	Oklahoma	37		36	West Virginia	41
48	Oregon	30		37	North Carolina	39
14	Pennsylvania	51		38	New Hampshire	38
45	Rhode Island	33		39	Alabama	37
46	South Carolina	32		39	Kentucky	37
33	South Dakota	42		39	Louisiana	37
27	Tennessee	45		39	Maine	37
17	Texas	49		39	Oklahoma	37
2	Utah	63		44	Wyoming	36
33	Vermont	42		45	Rhode Island	33
25	Virginia	46		46	Idaho	32
25	Washington	46		46	South Carolina	32
36	West Virginia	41		48	Oregon	30
19	Wisconsin	48		49	Arkansas	23
44	Wyoming	36		49	Mississippi	23
					District of Columbia	59

Source: Morgan Quitno Press using data from U.S. Dept of Health & Human Services, Health Care Financing Admin.
"State Health Expenditure Accounts" (Health Care Financing Review, Fall 1995, Volume 17, Number 1)
*By state of provider. Includes eyeglasses, hearing aids, surgical appliances and supplies, bulk and cylinder oxygen and medical equipment rentals.

Average Annual Change in Expenditures for
Vision Products and Other Medical Durables: 1980 to 1993
National Percent = 8.3% Average Annual Growth*

ALPHA ORDER

RANK	STATE	PERCENT
15	Alabama	8.7
49	Alaska	5.3
1	Arizona	10.5
26	Arkansas	8.0
8	California	9.4
12	Colorado	8.9
18	Connecticut	8.5
33	Delaware	7.4
6	Florida	9.9
8	Georgia	9.4
23	Hawaii	8.1
36	Idaho	7.1
30	Illinois	7.8
29	Indiana	7.9
39	Iowa	7.0
39	Kansas	7.0
21	Kentucky	8.3
46	Louisiana	6.7
19	Maine	8.4
19	Maryland	8.4
15	Massachusetts	8.7
33	Michigan	7.4
30	Minnesota	7.8
44	Mississippi	6.8
36	Missouri	7.1
44	Montana	6.8
48	Nebraska	5.7
3	Nevada	10.2
2	New Hampshire	10.3
15	New Jersey	8.7
11	New Mexico	9.3
23	New York	8.1
5	North Carolina	10.1
36	North Dakota	7.1
43	Ohio	6.9
39	Oklahoma	7.0
47	Oregon	6.4
32	Pennsylvania	7.7
22	Rhode Island	8.2
3	South Carolina	10.2
39	South Dakota	7.0
7	Tennessee	9.6
35	Texas	7.2
8	Utah	9.4
12	Vermont	8.9
14	Virginia	8.8
26	Washington	8.0
23	West Virginia	8.1
26	Wisconsin	8.0
50	Wyoming	5.1

RANK ORDER

RANK	STATE	PERCENT
1	Arizona	10.5
2	New Hampshire	10.3
3	Nevada	10.2
3	South Carolina	10.2
5	North Carolina	10.1
6	Florida	9.9
7	Tennessee	9.6
8	California	9.4
8	Georgia	9.4
8	Utah	9.4
11	New Mexico	9.3
12	Colorado	8.9
12	Vermont	8.9
14	Virginia	8.8
15	Alabama	8.7
15	Massachusetts	8.7
15	New Jersey	8.7
18	Connecticut	8.5
19	Maine	8.4
19	Maryland	8.4
21	Kentucky	8.3
22	Rhode Island	8.2
23	Hawaii	8.1
23	New York	8.1
23	West Virginia	8.1
26	Arkansas	8.0
26	Washington	8.0
26	Wisconsin	8.0
29	Indiana	7.9
30	Illinois	7.8
30	Minnesota	7.8
32	Pennsylvania	7.7
33	Delaware	7.4
33	Michigan	7.4
35	Texas	7.2
36	Idaho	7.1
36	Missouri	7.1
36	North Dakota	7.1
39	Iowa	7.0
39	Kansas	7.0
39	Oklahoma	7.0
39	South Dakota	7.0
43	Ohio	6.9
44	Mississippi	6.8
44	Montana	6.8
46	Louisiana	6.7
47	Oregon	6.4
48	Nebraska	5.7
49	Alaska	5.3
50	Wyoming	5.1
	District of Columbia	4.6

Source: U.S. Department of Health and Human Services, Health Care Financing Administration
   "State Health Expenditure Accounts" (Health Care Financing Review, Fall 1995, Volume 17, Number 1)
*By state of provider. Includes eyeglasses, hearing aids, surgical appliances and supplies, bulk and cylinder oxygen and medical equipment rentals.

Expenditures for Nursing Home Care in 1993

National Total = $66,201,000,000*

ALPHA ORDER

RANK ORDER

RANK	STATE	EXPENDITURES	% of USA
27	Alabama	$703,000,000	1.06%
50	Alaska	56,000,000	0.08%
31	Arizona	567,000,000	0.86%
32	Arkansas	558,000,000	0.84%
3	California	4,103,000,000	6.20%
28	Colorado	661,000,000	1.00%
14	Connecticut	1,749,000,000	2.64%
41	Delaware	217,000,000	0.33%
7	Florida	3,089,000,000	4.67%
21	Georgia	1,038,000,000	1.57%
45	Hawaii	181,000,000	0.27%
44	Idaho	197,000,000	0.30%
5	Illinois	3,148,000,000	4.76%
10	Indiana	2,018,000,000	3.05%
23	Iowa	927,000,000	1.40%
26	Kansas	721,000,000	1.09%
24	Kentucky	850,000,000	1.28%
18	Louisiana	1,186,000,000	1.79%
36	Maine	453,000,000	0.68%
19	Maryland	1,185,000,000	1.79%
8	Massachusetts	2,737,000,000	4.13%
12	Michigan	1,849,000,000	2.79%
11	Minnesota	1,884,000,000	2.85%
35	Mississippi	460,000,000	0.69%
16	Missouri	1,368,000,000	2.07%
46	Montana	178,000,000	0.27%
34	Nebraska	482,000,000	0.73%
47	Nevada	164,000,000	0.25%
38	New Hampshire	268,000,000	0.40%
9	New Jersey	2,128,000,000	3.21%
43	New Mexico	215,000,000	0.32%
1	New York	9,106,000,000	13.76%
15	North Carolina	1,562,000,000	2.36%
40	North Dakota	246,000,000	0.37%
4	Ohio	3,758,000,000	5.68%
25	Oklahoma	748,000,000	1.13%
29	Oregon	656,000,000	0.99%
2	Pennsylvania	4,153,000,000	6.27%
33	Rhode Island	485,000,000	0.73%
30	South Carolina	638,000,000	0.96%
42	South Dakota	216,000,000	0.33%
20	Tennessee	1,085,000,000	1.64%
6	Texas	3,104,000,000	4.69%
39	Utah	260,000,000	0.39%
48	Vermont	148,000,000	0.22%
22	Virginia	976,000,000	1.47%
17	Washington	1,291,000,000	1.95%
37	West Virginia	365,000,000	0.55%
13	Wisconsin	1,752,000,000	2.65%
49	Wyoming	83,000,000	0.13%

RANK	STATE	EXPENDITURES	% of USA
1	New York	$9,106,000,000	13.76%
2	Pennsylvania	4,153,000,000	6.27%
3	California	4,103,000,000	6.20%
4	Ohio	3,758,000,000	5.68%
5	Illinois	3,148,000,000	4.76%
6	Texas	3,104,000,000	4.69%
7	Florida	3,089,000,000	4.67%
8	Massachusetts	2,737,000,000	4.13%
9	New Jersey	2,128,000,000	3.21%
10	Indiana	2,018,000,000	3.05%
11	Minnesota	1,884,000,000	2.85%
12	Michigan	1,849,000,000	2.79%
13	Wisconsin	1,752,000,000	2.65%
14	Connecticut	1,749,000,000	2.64%
15	North Carolina	1,562,000,000	2.36%
16	Missouri	1,368,000,000	2.07%
17	Washington	1,291,000,000	1.95%
18	Louisiana	1,186,000,000	1.79%
19	Maryland	1,185,000,000	1.79%
20	Tennessee	1,085,000,000	1.64%
21	Georgia	1,038,000,000	1.57%
22	Virginia	976,000,000	1.47%
23	Iowa	927,000,000	1.40%
24	Kentucky	850,000,000	1.28%
25	Oklahoma	748,000,000	1.13%
26	Kansas	721,000,000	1.09%
27	Alabama	703,000,000	1.06%
28	Colorado	661,000,000	1.00%
29	Oregon	656,000,000	0.99%
30	South Carolina	638,000,000	0.96%
31	Arizona	567,000,000	0.86%
32	Arkansas	558,000,000	0.84%
33	Rhode Island	485,000,000	0.73%
34	Nebraska	482,000,000	0.73%
35	Mississippi	460,000,000	0.69%
36	Maine	453,000,000	0.68%
37	West Virginia	365,000,000	0.55%
38	New Hampshire	268,000,000	0.40%
39	Utah	260,000,000	0.39%
40	North Dakota	246,000,000	0.37%
41	Delaware	217,000,000	0.33%
42	South Dakota	216,000,000	0.33%
43	New Mexico	215,000,000	0.32%
44	Idaho	197,000,000	0.30%
45	Hawaii	181,000,000	0.27%
46	Montana	178,000,000	0.27%
47	Nevada	164,000,000	0.25%
48	Vermont	148,000,000	0.22%
49	Wyoming	83,000,000	0.13%
50	Alaska	56,000,000	0.08%
	District of Columbia	231,000,000	0.35%

Source: U.S. Department of Health and Human Services, Health Care Financing Administration
    "State Health Expenditure Accounts" (Health Care Financing Review, Fall 1995, Volume 17, Number 1)
*By state of provider. Includes freestanding nursing and personal-care facilities. Includes Medicare- and Medicaid-certified skilled nursing and intermediate care facilities as well as facilities that are not certified. Excludes hospital-based facilities as they are counted in hospital care expenditures.

Percent of Total Personal Health Care Expenditures
Spent on Nursing Home Care in 1993
National Percent = 8.5%*

ALPHA ORDER

RANK	STATE	PERCENT
43	Alabama	5.8
50	Alaska	3.6
45	Arizona	5.3
19	Arkansas	9.1
48	California	4.4
39	Colorado	6.6
1	Connecticut	14.3
17	Delaware	9.6
36	Florida	6.9
46	Georgia	5.2
46	Hawaii	5.2
22	Idaho	8.7
19	Illinois	9.1
7	Indiana	12.3
6	Iowa	12.6
14	Kansas	10.4
29	Kentucky	8.2
19	Louisiana	9.1
5	Maine	13.2
31	Maryland	7.8
10	Massachusetts	11.7
37	Michigan	6.8
4	Minnesota	13.3
33	Mississippi	7.4
23	Missouri	8.6
25	Montana	8.5
13	Nebraska	11.0
48	Nevada	4.4
31	New Hampshire	7.8
27	New Jersey	8.3
44	New Mexico	5.5
3	New York	13.6
23	North Carolina	8.6
8	North Dakota	12.2
11	Ohio	11.2
18	Oklahoma	9.3
29	Oregon	8.2
15	Pennsylvania	10.0
2	Rhode Island	14.1
34	South Carolina	7.1
12	South Dakota	11.1
38	Tennessee	6.7
41	Texas	6.2
40	Utah	6.3
16	Vermont	9.9
42	Virginia	5.9
25	Washington	8.5
35	West Virginia	7.0
9	Wisconsin	12.1
27	Wyoming	8.3

RANK ORDER

RANK	STATE	PERCENT
1	Connecticut	14.3
2	Rhode Island	14.1
3	New York	13.6
4	Minnesota	13.3
5	Maine	13.2
6	Iowa	12.6
7	Indiana	12.3
8	North Dakota	12.2
9	Wisconsin	12.1
10	Massachusetts	11.7
11	Ohio	11.2
12	South Dakota	11.1
13	Nebraska	11.0
14	Kansas	10.4
15	Pennsylvania	10.0
16	Vermont	9.9
17	Delaware	9.6
18	Oklahoma	9.3
19	Arkansas	9.1
19	Illinois	9.1
19	Louisiana	9.1
22	Idaho	8.7
23	Missouri	8.6
23	North Carolina	8.6
25	Montana	8.5
25	Washington	8.5
27	New Jersey	8.3
27	Wyoming	8.3
29	Kentucky	8.2
29	Oregon	8.2
31	Maryland	7.8
31	New Hampshire	7.8
33	Mississippi	7.4
34	South Carolina	7.1
35	West Virginia	7.0
36	Florida	6.9
37	Michigan	6.8
38	Tennessee	6.7
39	Colorado	6.6
40	Utah	6.3
41	Texas	6.2
42	Virginia	5.9
43	Alabama	5.8
44	New Mexico	5.5
45	Arizona	5.3
46	Georgia	5.2
46	Hawaii	5.2
48	California	4.4
48	Nevada	4.4
50	Alaska	3.6
	District of Columbia	5.4

Source: Morgan Quitno Press using data from U.S. Dept of Health & Human Services, Health Care Financing Admin.
"State Health Expenditure Accounts" (Health Care Financing Review, Fall 1995, Volume 17, Number 1)
*By state of provider. Includes freestanding nursing and personal-care facilities. Includes Medicare- and
Medicaid-certified skilled nursing and intermediate care facilities as well as facilities that are not certified.
Excludes hospital-based facilities as they are counted in hospital care expenditures.

Per Capita Expenditures for Nursing Home Care in 1993

National Per Capita = $257*

ALPHA ORDER

RANK	STATE	PER CAPITA
41	Alabama	$168
50	Alaska	94
45	Arizona	144
26	Arkansas	230
48	California	131
35	Colorado	185
1	Connecticut	534
13	Delaware	310
27	Florida	225
44	Georgia	150
42	Hawaii	155
36	Idaho	179
19	Illinois	269
8	Indiana	354
12	Iowa	328
16	Kansas	285
29	Kentucky	224
17	Louisiana	277
7	Maine	366
23	Maryland	239
4	Massachusetts	455
34	Michigan	196
5	Minnesota	416
39	Mississippi	174
20	Missouri	261
32	Montana	212
15	Nebraska	299
49	Nevada	118
23	New Hampshire	239
18	New Jersey	271
47	New Mexico	133
2	New York	502
27	North Carolina	225
6	North Dakota	386
11	Ohio	340
25	Oklahoma	231
30	Oregon	216
10	Pennsylvania	345
3	Rhode Island	485
38	South Carolina	176
14	South Dakota	301
31	Tennessee	213
40	Texas	172
46	Utah	140
21	Vermont	257
43	Virginia	151
22	Washington	246
33	West Virginia	201
9	Wisconsin	347
37	Wyoming	177

RANK ORDER

RANK	STATE	PER CAPITA
1	Connecticut	$534
2	New York	502
3	Rhode Island	485
4	Massachusetts	455
5	Minnesota	416
6	North Dakota	386
7	Maine	366
8	Indiana	354
9	Wisconsin	347
10	Pennsylvania	345
11	Ohio	340
12	Iowa	328
13	Delaware	310
14	South Dakota	301
15	Nebraska	299
16	Kansas	285
17	Louisiana	277
18	New Jersey	271
19	Illinois	269
20	Missouri	261
21	Vermont	257
22	Washington	246
23	Maryland	239
23	New Hampshire	239
25	Oklahoma	231
26	Arkansas	230
27	Florida	225
27	North Carolina	225
29	Kentucky	224
30	Oregon	216
31	Tennessee	213
32	Montana	212
33	West Virginia	201
34	Michigan	196
35	Colorado	185
36	Idaho	179
37	Wyoming	177
38	South Carolina	176
39	Mississippi	174
40	Texas	172
41	Alabama	168
42	Hawaii	155
43	Virginia	151
44	Georgia	150
45	Arizona	144
46	Utah	140
47	New Mexico	133
48	California	131
49	Nevada	118
50	Alaska	94

| | District of Columbia | 400 |

Source: Morgan Quitno Press using data from U.S. Dept of Health & Human Services, Health Care Financing Admin. "State Health Expenditure Accounts" (Health Care Financing Review, Fall 1995, Volume 17, Number 1)
By state of provider. Includes freestanding nursing and personal-care facilities. Includes Medicare- and Medicaid-certified skilled nursing and intermediate care facilities as well as facilities that are not certified. Excludes hospital-based facilities as they are counted in hospital care expenditures.

Average Annual Change in Expenditures for Nursing Home Care: 1980 to 1993

National Percent = 10.7% Average Annual Increase*

ALPHA ORDER

RANK	STATE	PERCENT
23	Alabama	10.8
50	Alaska	7.3
2	Arizona	15.9
46	Arkansas	8.5
43	California	9.0
42	Colorado	9.2
11	Connecticut	12.6
9	Delaware	12.8
1	Florida	16.7
27	Georgia	10.5
19	Hawaii	11.2
22	Idaho	10.9
23	Illinois	10.8
7	Indiana	13.1
47	Iowa	8.2
35	Kansas	9.8
29	Kentucky	10.1
8	Louisiana	12.9
23	Maine	10.8
11	Maryland	12.6
16	Massachusetts	11.4
44	Michigan	8.9
40	Minnesota	9.4
31	Mississippi	10.0
23	Missouri	10.8
27	Montana	10.5
49	Nebraska	7.7
6	Nevada	13.7
16	New Hampshire	11.4
13	New Jersey	11.8
3	New Mexico	15.6
39	New York	9.5
5	North Carolina	14.4
13	North Dakota	11.8
10	Ohio	12.7
31	Oklahoma	10.0
36	Oregon	9.7
31	Pennsylvania	10.0
21	Rhode Island	11.1
19	South Carolina	11.2
47	South Dakota	8.2
15	Tennessee	11.7
36	Texas	9.7
31	Utah	10.0
44	Vermont	8.9
36	Virginia	9.7
29	Washington	10.1
4	West Virginia	14.7
40	Wisconsin	9.4
18	Wyoming	11.3

RANK ORDER

RANK	STATE	PERCENT
1	Florida	16.7
2	Arizona	15.9
3	New Mexico	15.6
4	West Virginia	14.7
5	North Carolina	14.4
6	Nevada	13.7
7	Indiana	13.1
8	Louisiana	12.9
9	Delaware	12.8
10	Ohio	12.7
11	Connecticut	12.6
11	Maryland	12.6
13	New Jersey	11.8
13	North Dakota	11.8
15	Tennessee	11.7
16	Massachusetts	11.4
16	New Hampshire	11.4
18	Wyoming	11.3
19	Hawaii	11.2
19	South Carolina	11.2
21	Rhode Island	11.1
22	Idaho	10.9
23	Alabama	10.8
23	Illinois	10.8
23	Maine	10.8
23	Missouri	10.8
27	Georgia	10.5
27	Montana	10.5
29	Kentucky	10.1
29	Washington	10.1
31	Mississippi	10.0
31	Oklahoma	10.0
31	Pennsylvania	10.0
31	Utah	10.0
35	Kansas	9.8
36	Oregon	9.7
36	Texas	9.7
36	Virginia	9.7
39	New York	9.5
40	Minnesota	9.4
40	Wisconsin	9.4
42	Colorado	9.2
43	California	9.0
44	Michigan	8.9
44	Vermont	8.9
46	Arkansas	8.5
47	Iowa	8.2
47	South Dakota	8.2
49	Nebraska	7.7
50	Alaska	7.3

	District of Columbia	18.3

Source: U.S. Department of Health and Human Services, Health Care Financing Administration
     "State Health Expenditure Accounts" (Health Care Financing Review, Fall 1995, Volume 17, Number 1)
*By state of provider. Includes freestanding nursing and personal-care facilities. Includes Medicare- and Medicaid-certified skilled nursing and intermediate care facilities as well as facilities that are not certified. Excludes hospital-based facilities as they are counted in hospital care expenditures.

Other Personal Health Care Expenditures in 1993

National Total = $17,988,000,000*

ALPHA ORDER					RANK ORDER			

RANK	STATE	EXPENDITURES	% of USA		RANK	STATE	EXPENDITURES	% of USA
22	Alabama	$323,000,000	1.80%		1	New York	$1,635,000,000	9.09%
45	Alaska	68,000,000	0.38%		2	California	1,565,000,000	8.70%
27	Arizona	230,000,000	1.28%		3	Texas	1,325,000,000	7.37%
37	Arkansas	127,000,000	0.71%		4	Florida	912,000,000	5.07%
2	California	1,565,000,000	8.70%		5	Pennsylvania	798,000,000	4.44%
21	Colorado	327,000,000	1.82%		6	Illinois	636,000,000	3.54%
12	Connecticut	467,000,000	2.60%		7	Massachusetts	597,000,000	3.32%
43	Delaware	79,000,000	0.44%		8	New Jersey	570,000,000	3.17%
4	Florida	912,000,000	5.07%		9	Michigan	532,000,000	2.96%
10	Georgia	516,000,000	2.87%		10	Georgia	516,000,000	2.87%
39	Hawaii	104,000,000	0.58%		11	Ohio	511,000,000	2.84%
48	Idaho	55,000,000	0.31%		12	Connecticut	467,000,000	2.60%
6	Illinois	636,000,000	3.54%		13	Washington	425,000,000	2.36%
25	Indiana	264,000,000	1.47%		14	Wisconsin	415,000,000	2.31%
37	Iowa	127,000,000	0.71%		15	North Carolina	413,000,000	2.30%
34	Kansas	140,000,000	0.78%		16	Virginia	395,000,000	2.20%
28	Kentucky	228,000,000	1.27%		17	Oregon	391,000,000	2.17%
20	Louisiana	328,000,000	1.82%		18	Minnesota	386,000,000	2.15%
32	Maine	153,000,000	0.85%		19	Missouri	346,000,000	1.92%
24	Maryland	312,000,000	1.73%		20	Louisiana	328,000,000	1.82%
7	Massachusetts	597,000,000	3.32%		21	Colorado	327,000,000	1.82%
9	Michigan	532,000,000	2.96%		22	Alabama	323,000,000	1.80%
18	Minnesota	386,000,000	2.15%		23	South Carolina	317,000,000	1.76%
33	Mississippi	141,000,000	0.78%		24	Maryland	312,000,000	1.73%
19	Missouri	346,000,000	1.92%		25	Indiana	264,000,000	1.47%
44	Montana	74,000,000	0.41%		26	Tennessee	235,000,000	1.31%
40	Nebraska	99,000,000	0.55%		27	Arizona	230,000,000	1.28%
46	Nevada	67,000,000	0.37%		28	Kentucky	228,000,000	1.27%
35	New Hampshire	136,000,000	0.76%		29	Rhode Island	219,000,000	1.22%
8	New Jersey	570,000,000	3.17%		30	Oklahoma	196,000,000	1.09%
36	New Mexico	131,000,000	0.73%		31	West Virginia	192,000,000	1.07%
1	New York	1,635,000,000	9.09%		32	Maine	153,000,000	0.85%
15	North Carolina	413,000,000	2.30%		33	Mississippi	141,000,000	0.78%
50	North Dakota	52,000,000	0.29%		34	Kansas	140,000,000	0.78%
11	Ohio	511,000,000	2.84%		35	New Hampshire	136,000,000	0.76%
30	Oklahoma	196,000,000	1.09%		36	New Mexico	131,000,000	0.73%
17	Oregon	391,000,000	2.17%		37	Arkansas	127,000,000	0.71%
5	Pennsylvania	798,000,000	4.44%		37	Iowa	127,000,000	0.71%
29	Rhode Island	219,000,000	1.22%		39	Hawaii	104,000,000	0.58%
23	South Carolina	317,000,000	1.76%		40	Nebraska	99,000,000	0.55%
47	South Dakota	63,000,000	0.35%		40	Utah	99,000,000	0.55%
26	Tennessee	235,000,000	1.31%		42	Vermont	82,000,000	0.46%
3	Texas	1,325,000,000	7.37%		43	Delaware	79,000,000	0.44%
40	Utah	99,000,000	0.55%		44	Montana	74,000,000	0.41%
42	Vermont	82,000,000	0.46%		45	Alaska	68,000,000	0.38%
16	Virginia	395,000,000	2.20%		46	Nevada	67,000,000	0.37%
13	Washington	425,000,000	2.36%		47	South Dakota	63,000,000	0.35%
31	West Virginia	192,000,000	1.07%		48	Idaho	55,000,000	0.31%
14	Wisconsin	415,000,000	2.31%		48	Wyoming	55,000,000	0.31%
48	Wyoming	55,000,000	0.31%		50	North Dakota	52,000,000	0.29%
						District of Columbia	130,000,000	0.72%

Source: U.S. Department of Health and Human Services, Health Care Financing Administration
     "State Health Expenditure Accounts" (Health Care Financing Review, Fall 1995, Volume 17, Number 1)
*By state of provider. "Other" covers spending for health care that is not provided through health care establishments. Services in this category are provided through non-medical locations such as job sites, schools, military field-stations or community centers where delivery of medical services is incidental to the function of the site.

Percent of Total Personal Health Care Expenditures
Spent on Other Personal Health Care in 1993
National Percent = 2.3%*

ALPHA ORDER

RANK	STATE	PERCENT
19	Alabama	2.7
6	Alaska	4.3
34	Arizona	2.2
38	Arkansas	2.1
46	California	1.7
14	Colorado	3.2
8	Connecticut	3.8
10	Delaware	3.5
40	Florida	2.0
22	Georgia	2.6
16	Hawaii	3.0
26	Idaho	2.4
44	Illinois	1.8
48	Indiana	1.6
46	Iowa	1.7
40	Kansas	2.0
34	Kentucky	2.2
24	Louisiana	2.5
5	Maine	4.5
38	Maryland	2.1
24	Massachusetts	2.5
40	Michigan	2.0
19	Minnesota	2.7
31	Mississippi	2.3
34	Missouri	2.2
10	Montana	3.5
31	Nebraska	2.3
44	Nevada	1.8
7	New Hampshire	3.9
34	New Jersey	2.2
13	New Mexico	3.4
26	New York	2.4
31	North Carolina	2.3
22	North Dakota	2.6
49	Ohio	1.5
26	Oklahoma	2.4
4	Oregon	4.9
43	Pennsylvania	1.9
1	Rhode Island	6.4
10	South Carolina	3.5
14	South Dakota	3.2
49	Tennessee	1.5
19	Texas	2.7
26	Utah	2.4
2	Vermont	5.5
26	Virginia	2.4
18	Washington	2.8
9	West Virginia	3.7
17	Wisconsin	2.9
2	Wyoming	5.5

RANK ORDER

RANK	STATE	PERCENT
1	Rhode Island	6.4
2	Vermont	5.5
2	Wyoming	5.5
4	Oregon	4.9
5	Maine	4.5
6	Alaska	4.3
7	New Hampshire	3.9
8	Connecticut	3.8
9	West Virginia	3.7
10	Delaware	3.5
10	Montana	3.5
10	South Carolina	3.5
13	New Mexico	3.4
14	Colorado	3.2
14	South Dakota	3.2
16	Hawaii	3.0
17	Wisconsin	2.9
18	Washington	2.8
19	Alabama	2.7
19	Minnesota	2.7
19	Texas	2.7
22	Georgia	2.6
22	North Dakota	2.6
24	Louisiana	2.5
24	Massachusetts	2.5
26	Idaho	2.4
26	New York	2.4
26	Oklahoma	2.4
26	Utah	2.4
26	Virginia	2.4
31	Mississippi	2.3
31	Nebraska	2.3
31	North Carolina	2.3
34	Arizona	2.2
34	Kentucky	2.2
34	Missouri	2.2
34	New Jersey	2.2
38	Arkansas	2.1
38	Maryland	2.1
40	Florida	2.0
40	Kansas	2.0
40	Michigan	2.0
43	Pennsylvania	1.9
44	Illinois	1.8
44	Nevada	1.8
46	California	1.7
46	Iowa	1.7
48	Indiana	1.6
49	Ohio	1.5
49	Tennessee	1.5

| | District of Columbia | 3.0 |

Source: Morgan Quitno Press using data from U.S. Dept of Health & Human Services, Health Care Financing Admin.
"State Health Expenditure Accounts" (Health Care Financing Review, Fall 1995, Volume 17, Number 1)
*By state of provider. "Other" covers spending for health care that is not provided through health care establishments. Services in this category are provided through non-medical locations such as job sites, schools, military field-stations or community centers where delivery of medical services is incidental to the function of the site.

Per Capita Other Personal Health Care Expenditures in 1993

National Per Capita = $69.78*

<table>
<tr><td colspan="3">ALPHA ORDER</td><td colspan="3">RANK ORDER</td></tr>
<tr><td>RANK</td><td>STATE</td><td>PER CAPITA</td><td>RANK</td><td>STATE</td><td>PER CAPITA</td></tr>
<tr><td>23</td><td>Alabama</td><td>$77.25</td><td>1</td><td>Rhode Island</td><td>$219.22</td></tr>
<tr><td>8</td><td>Alaska</td><td>113.71</td><td>2</td><td>Connecticut</td><td>142.46</td></tr>
<tr><td>37</td><td>Arizona</td><td>58.32</td><td>3</td><td>Vermont</td><td>142.36</td></tr>
<tr><td>43</td><td>Arkansas</td><td>52.37</td><td>4</td><td>Oregon</td><td>128.83</td></tr>
<tr><td>44</td><td>California</td><td>50.13</td><td>5</td><td>Maine</td><td>123.49</td></tr>
<tr><td>12</td><td>Colorado</td><td>91.65</td><td>6</td><td>New Hampshire</td><td>121.10</td></tr>
<tr><td>2</td><td>Connecticut</td><td>142.46</td><td>7</td><td>Wyoming</td><td>117.02</td></tr>
<tr><td>9</td><td>Delaware</td><td>113.02</td><td>8</td><td>Alaska</td><td>113.71</td></tr>
<tr><td>28</td><td>Florida</td><td>66.46</td><td>9</td><td>Delaware</td><td>113.02</td></tr>
<tr><td>25</td><td>Georgia</td><td>74.77</td><td>10</td><td>West Virginia</td><td>105.61</td></tr>
<tr><td>14</td><td>Hawaii</td><td>89.19</td><td>11</td><td>Massachusetts</td><td>99.20</td></tr>
<tr><td>45</td><td>Idaho</td><td>49.95</td><td>12</td><td>Colorado</td><td>91.65</td></tr>
<tr><td>40</td><td>Illinois</td><td>54.41</td><td>13</td><td>New York</td><td>90.07</td></tr>
<tr><td>47</td><td>Indiana</td><td>46.26</td><td>14</td><td>Hawaii</td><td>89.19</td></tr>
<tr><td>50</td><td>Iowa</td><td>45.00</td><td>15</td><td>Montana</td><td>87.99</td></tr>
<tr><td>39</td><td>Kansas</td><td>55.29</td><td>16</td><td>South Dakota</td><td>87.87</td></tr>
<tr><td>35</td><td>Kentucky</td><td>60.11</td><td>17</td><td>South Carolina</td><td>87.40</td></tr>
<tr><td>24</td><td>Louisiana</td><td>76.47</td><td>18</td><td>Minnesota</td><td>85.32</td></tr>
<tr><td>5</td><td>Maine</td><td>123.49</td><td>19</td><td>Wisconsin</td><td>82.28</td></tr>
<tr><td>31</td><td>Maryland</td><td>63.00</td><td>20</td><td>North Dakota</td><td>81.63</td></tr>
<tr><td>11</td><td>Massachusetts</td><td>99.20</td><td>21</td><td>New Mexico</td><td>81.06</td></tr>
<tr><td>38</td><td>Michigan</td><td>56.25</td><td>22</td><td>Washington</td><td>80.88</td></tr>
<tr><td>18</td><td>Minnesota</td><td>85.32</td><td>23</td><td>Alabama</td><td>77.25</td></tr>
<tr><td>41</td><td>Mississippi</td><td>53.43</td><td>24</td><td>Louisiana</td><td>76.47</td></tr>
<tr><td>30</td><td>Missouri</td><td>66.09</td><td>25</td><td>Georgia</td><td>74.77</td></tr>
<tr><td>15</td><td>Montana</td><td>87.99</td><td>26</td><td>Texas</td><td>73.41</td></tr>
<tr><td>32</td><td>Nebraska</td><td>61.34</td><td>27</td><td>New Jersey</td><td>72.53</td></tr>
<tr><td>46</td><td>Nevada</td><td>48.38</td><td>28</td><td>Florida</td><td>66.46</td></tr>
<tr><td>6</td><td>New Hampshire</td><td>121.10</td><td>29</td><td>Pennsylvania</td><td>66.33</td></tr>
<tr><td>27</td><td>New Jersey</td><td>72.53</td><td>30</td><td>Missouri</td><td>66.09</td></tr>
<tr><td>21</td><td>New Mexico</td><td>81.06</td><td>31</td><td>Maryland</td><td>63.00</td></tr>
<tr><td>13</td><td>New York</td><td>90.07</td><td>32</td><td>Nebraska</td><td>61.34</td></tr>
<tr><td>36</td><td>North Carolina</td><td>59.40</td><td>33</td><td>Virginia</td><td>61.00</td></tr>
<tr><td>20</td><td>North Dakota</td><td>81.63</td><td>34</td><td>Oklahoma</td><td>60.64</td></tr>
<tr><td>48</td><td>Ohio</td><td>46.20</td><td>35</td><td>Kentucky</td><td>60.11</td></tr>
<tr><td>34</td><td>Oklahoma</td><td>60.64</td><td>36</td><td>North Carolina</td><td>59.40</td></tr>
<tr><td>4</td><td>Oregon</td><td>128.83</td><td>37</td><td>Arizona</td><td>58.32</td></tr>
<tr><td>29</td><td>Pennsylvania</td><td>66.33</td><td>38</td><td>Michigan</td><td>56.25</td></tr>
<tr><td>1</td><td>Rhode Island</td><td>219.22</td><td>39</td><td>Kansas</td><td>55.29</td></tr>
<tr><td>17</td><td>South Carolina</td><td>87.40</td><td>40</td><td>Illinois</td><td>54.41</td></tr>
<tr><td>16</td><td>South Dakota</td><td>87.87</td><td>41</td><td>Mississippi</td><td>53.43</td></tr>
<tr><td>49</td><td>Tennessee</td><td>46.14</td><td>42</td><td>Utah</td><td>53.23</td></tr>
<tr><td>26</td><td>Texas</td><td>73.41</td><td>43</td><td>Arkansas</td><td>52.37</td></tr>
<tr><td>42</td><td>Utah</td><td>53.23</td><td>44</td><td>California</td><td>50.13</td></tr>
<tr><td>3</td><td>Vermont</td><td>142.36</td><td>45</td><td>Idaho</td><td>49.95</td></tr>
<tr><td>33</td><td>Virginia</td><td>61.00</td><td>46</td><td>Nevada</td><td>48.38</td></tr>
<tr><td>22</td><td>Washington</td><td>80.88</td><td>47</td><td>Indiana</td><td>46.26</td></tr>
<tr><td>10</td><td>West Virginia</td><td>105.61</td><td>48</td><td>Ohio</td><td>46.20</td></tr>
<tr><td>19</td><td>Wisconsin</td><td>82.28</td><td>49</td><td>Tennessee</td><td>46.14</td></tr>
<tr><td>7</td><td>Wyoming</td><td>117.02</td><td>50</td><td>Iowa</td><td>45.00</td></tr>
<tr><td colspan="3"></td><td></td><td>District of Columbia</td><td>224.91</td></tr>
</table>

Source: Morgan Quitno Press using data from U.S. Dept of Health & Human Services, Health Care Financing Admin. "State Health Expenditure Accounts" (Health Care Financing Review, Fall 1995, Volume 17, Number 1)
*By state of provider. "Other" covers spending for health care that is not provided through health care establishments. Services in this category are provided through non-medical locations such as job sites, schools, military field-stations or community centers where delivery of medical services is incidental to the function of the site.

Average Annual Change in
Other Personal Health Care Expenditures: 1980 to 1993
National Percent = 12.4% Average Annual Increase*

ALPHA ORDER

RANK ORDER

RANK	STATE	PERCENT	RANK	STATE	PERCENT
25	Alabama	12.4	1	Rhode Island	21.2
47	Alaska	9.9	2	Oregon	19.4
38	Arizona	11.4	3	New Hampshire	17.4
36	Arkansas	11.5	4	Maine	16.7
33	California	11.7	5	Vermont	15.9
36	Colorado	11.5	6	Texas	15.5
10	Connecticut	14.7	7	Delaware	15.2
7	Delaware	15.2	8	Florida	15.1
8	Florida	15.1	9	West Virginia	15.0
22	Georgia	13.1	10	Connecticut	14.7
39	Hawaii	11.3	11	Washington	14.3
20	Idaho	13.2	12	Minnesota	14.0
44	Illinois	10.5	13	Wisconsin	13.9
49	Indiana	8.5	14	Louisiana	13.8
39	Iowa	11.3	14	South Carolina	13.8
19	Kansas	13.5	14	Utah	13.8
20	Kentucky	13.2	17	Missouri	13.6
14	Louisiana	13.8	17	North Dakota	13.6
4	Maine	16.7	19	Kansas	13.5
31	Maryland	11.9	20	Idaho	13.2
25	Massachusetts	12.4	20	Kentucky	13.2
41	Michigan	10.8	22	Georgia	13.1
12	Minnesota	14.0	23	Nevada	12.9
48	Mississippi	9.0	23	North Carolina	12.9
17	Missouri	13.6	25	Alabama	12.4
33	Montana	11.7	25	Massachusetts	12.4
29	Nebraska	12.2	25	New Mexico	12.4
23	Nevada	12.9	25	Oklahoma	12.4
3	New Hampshire	17.4	29	Nebraska	12.2
35	New Jersey	11.6	30	Virginia	12.0
25	New Mexico	12.4	31	Maryland	11.9
43	New York	10.6	32	South Dakota	11.8
23	North Carolina	12.9	33	California	11.7
17	North Dakota	13.6	33	Montana	11.7
50	Ohio	8.2	35	New Jersey	11.6
25	Oklahoma	12.4	36	Arkansas	11.5
2	Oregon	19.4	36	Colorado	11.5
41	Pennsylvania	10.8	38	Arizona	11.4
1	Rhode Island	21.2	39	Hawaii	11.3
14	South Carolina	13.8	39	Iowa	11.3
32	South Dakota	11.8	41	Michigan	10.8
45	Tennessee	10.2	41	Pennsylvania	10.8
6	Texas	15.5	43	New York	10.6
14	Utah	13.8	44	Illinois	10.5
5	Vermont	15.9	45	Tennessee	10.2
30	Virginia	12.0	45	Wyoming	10.2
11	Washington	14.3	47	Alaska	9.9
9	West Virginia	15.0	48	Mississippi	9.0
13	Wisconsin	13.9	49	Indiana	8.5
45	Wyoming	10.2	50	Ohio	8.2
				District of Columbia	8.9

Source: U.S. Department of Health and Human Services, Health Care Financing Administration
   "State Health Expenditure Accounts" (Health Care Financing Review, Fall 1995, Volume 17, Number 1)
*By state of provider. "Other" covers spending for health care that is not provided through health care
establishments. Services in this category are provided through non-medical locations such as job sites, schools,
military field-stations or community centers where delivery of medical services is incidental to the function of the
site.

Medicaid Expenditures in 1995

National Total = $120,140,904,458*

ALPHA ORDER

RANK	STATE	EXPENDITURES	% of USA
24	Alabama	$1,454,992,095	1.21%
48	Alaska	251,881,506	0.21%
49	Arizona	218,070,954	0.18%
26	Arkansas	1,375,839,261	1.15%
2	California	10,521,215,237	8.76%
30	Colorado	1,063,106,841	0.88%
16	Connecticut	2,125,283,023	1.77%
43	Delaware	324,303,829	0.27%
6	Florida	4,802,304,255	4.00%
12	Georgia	3,076,448,917	2.56%
47	Hawaii	257,503,424	0.21%
40	Idaho	359,907,784	0.30%
4	Illinois	5,599,836,414	4.66%
21	Indiana	1,877,951,870	1.56%
32	Iowa	1,036,339,607	0.86%
33	Kansas	831,098,259	0.69%
19	Kentucky	1,945,454,856	1.62%
14	Louisiana	2,708,478,255	2.25%
34	Maine	760,499,955	0.63%
18	Maryland	2,018,737,653	1.68%
8	Massachusetts	3,972,331,144	3.31%
10	Michigan	3,409,203,886	2.84%
15	Minnesota	2,549,842,032	2.12%
28	Mississippi	1,265,799,300	1.05%
17	Missouri	2,039,144,108	1.70%
42	Montana	325,732,960	0.27%
37	Nebraska	607,725,152	0.51%
41	Nevada	349,633,496	0.29%
38	New Hampshire	473,176,647	0.39%
9	New Jersey	3,812,789,625	3.17%
35	New Mexico	714,266,554	0.59%
1	New York	22,086,481,650	18.38%
11	North Carolina	3,175,059,813	2.64%
46	North Dakota	297,033,068	0.25%
5	Ohio	5,585,112,473	4.65%
31	Oklahoma	1,054,871,918	0.88%
27	Oregon	1,327,251,282	1.10%
7	Pennsylvania	4,632,715,919	3.86%
36	Rhode Island	672,546,557	0.56%
25	South Carolina	1,438,114,111	1.20%
45	South Dakota	305,205,387	0.25%
13	Tennessee	2,772,026,096	2.31%
3	Texas	6,564,677,392	5.46%
39	Utah	464,438,426	0.39%
44	Vermont	320,040,214	0.27%
22	Virginia	1,832,759,818	1.53%
23	Washington	1,460,933,569	1.22%
29	West Virginia	1,169,416,109	0.97%
20	Wisconsin	1,894,225,358	1.58%
50	Wyoming	170,966,247	0.14%

RANK ORDER

RANK	STATE	EXPENDITURES	% of USA
1	New York	$22,086,481,650	18.38%
2	California	10,521,215,237	8.76%
3	Texas	6,564,677,392	5.46%
4	Illinois	5,599,836,414	4.66%
5	Ohio	5,585,112,473	4.65%
6	Florida	4,802,304,255	4.00%
7	Pennsylvania	4,632,715,919	3.86%
8	Massachusetts	3,972,331,144	3.31%
9	New Jersey	3,812,789,625	3.17%
10	Michigan	3,409,203,886	2.84%
11	North Carolina	3,175,059,813	2.64%
12	Georgia	3,076,448,917	2.56%
13	Tennessee	2,772,026,096	2.31%
14	Louisiana	2,708,478,255	2.25%
15	Minnesota	2,549,842,032	2.12%
16	Connecticut	2,125,283,023	1.77%
17	Missouri	2,039,144,108	1.70%
18	Maryland	2,018,737,653	1.68%
19	Kentucky	1,945,454,856	1.62%
20	Wisconsin	1,894,225,358	1.58%
21	Indiana	1,877,951,870	1.56%
22	Virginia	1,832,759,818	1.53%
23	Washington	1,460,933,569	1.22%
24	Alabama	1,454,992,095	1.21%
25	South Carolina	1,438,114,111	1.20%
26	Arkansas	1,375,839,261	1.15%
27	Oregon	1,327,251,282	1.10%
28	Mississippi	1,265,799,300	1.05%
29	West Virginia	1,169,416,109	0.97%
30	Colorado	1,063,106,841	0.88%
31	Oklahoma	1,054,871,918	0.88%
32	Iowa	1,036,339,607	0.86%
33	Kansas	831,098,259	0.69%
34	Maine	760,499,955	0.63%
35	New Mexico	714,266,554	0.59%
36	Rhode Island	672,546,557	0.56%
37	Nebraska	607,725,152	0.51%
38	New Hampshire	473,176,647	0.39%
39	Utah	464,438,426	0.39%
40	Idaho	359,907,784	0.30%
41	Nevada	349,633,496	0.29%
42	Montana	325,732,960	0.27%
43	Delaware	324,303,829	0.27%
44	Vermont	320,040,214	0.27%
45	South Dakota	305,205,387	0.25%
46	North Dakota	297,033,068	0.25%
47	Hawaii	257,503,424	0.21%
48	Alaska	251,881,506	0.21%
49	Arizona	218,070,954	0.18%
50	Wyoming	170,966,247	0.14%
	District of Columbia	532,080,521	0.44%

Source: U.S. Department of Health and Human Services, Health Care Financing Administration
"Statistical Report on Medical Care: Eligibles, Recipients, Payments and Services" (HCFA-2082)
*For fiscal year ending September 30, 1995. National total includes $244,400,000 for Puerto Rico and $11,649,631 for the Virgin Islands.

Percent Change in Medicaid Expenditures: 1990 to 1995

National Percent Change = 85.23% Increase*

ALPHA ORDER			RANK ORDER		
RANK	STATE	PERCENT CHANGE	RANK	STATE	PERCENT CHANGE
6	Alabama	138.80	1	West Virginia	223.87
30	Alaska	81.05	2	Wyoming	190.12
NA	Arizona**	NA	3	Delaware	163.29
11	Arkansas	129.61	4	New Mexico	159.51
38	California	61.69	5	Oregon	155.83
17	Colorado	106.15	6	Alabama	138.80
33	Connecticut	76.34	7	Tennessee	138.40
3	Delaware	163.29	8	Texas	136.05
19	Florida	103.43	9	Nevada	135.30
46	Georgia	48.18	10	Illinois	131.01
49	Hawaii	34.59	11	Arkansas	129.61
14	Idaho	121.90	12	Missouri	127.26
10	Illinois	131.01	13	North Carolina	122.65
48	Indiana	39.88	14	Idaho	121.90
36	Iowa	67.08	15	Mississippi	115.96
35	Kansas	69.41	16	Vermont	109.32
20	Kentucky	99.16	17	Colorado	106.15
18	Louisiana	106.01	18	Louisiana	106.01
34	Maine	76.04	19	Florida	103.43
28	Maryland	85.16	20	Kentucky	99.16
47	Massachusetts	45.49	21	Nebraska	96.48
40	Michigan	55.33	22	New Hampshire	94.68
31	Minnesota	80.79	23	South Carolina	93.54
15	Mississippi	115.96	24	Montana	90.99
12	Missouri	127.26	25	Utah	88.30
24	Montana	90.99	26	Virginia	86.05
21	Nebraska	96.48	27	New York	85.95
9	Nevada	135.30	28	Maryland	85.16
22	New Hampshire	94.68	29	South Dakota	83.79
37	New Jersey	65.91	30	Alaska	81.05
4	New Mexico	159.51	31	Minnesota	80.79
27	New York	85.95	32	Ohio	78.32
13	North Carolina	122.65	33	Connecticut	76.34
43	North Dakota	53.26	34	Maine	76.04
32	Ohio	78.32	35	Kansas	69.41
41	Oklahoma	53.43	36	Iowa	67.08
5	Oregon	155.83	37	New Jersey	65.91
39	Pennsylvania	60.69	38	California	61.69
44	Rhode Island	52.10	39	Pennsylvania	60.69
23	South Carolina	93.54	40	Michigan	55.33
29	South Dakota	83.79	41	Oklahoma	53.43
7	Tennessee	138.40	42	Washington	53.39
8	Texas	136.05	43	North Dakota	53.26
25	Utah	88.30	44	Rhode Island	52.10
16	Vermont	109.32	45	Wisconsin	51.74
26	Virginia	86.05	46	Georgia	48.18
42	Washington	53.39	47	Massachusetts	45.49
1	West Virginia	223.87	48	Indiana	39.88
45	Wisconsin	51.74	49	Hawaii	34.59
2	Wyoming	190.12	NA	Arizona**	NA
				District of Columbia	116.52

Source: Morgan Quitno Press using data from U.S. Dept. of Health & Human Services, Health Care Financing Admin.
"Statistical Report on Medical Care: Eligibles, Recipients, Payments and Services" (HCFA-2082)
*For fiscal year ending September 30, 1995.
**Not available.

Percent of Personal Health Care Expenditures Paid by Medicaid in 1993

National Percent = 14.5%*

ALPHA ORDER

RANK	STATE	PERCENT
44	Alabama	10.6
6	Alaska	17.4
38	Arizona	11.9
9	Arkansas	16.5
37	California	12.0
49	Colorado	9.6
10	Connecticut	16.4
43	Delaware	11.0
45	Florida	10.5
24	Georgia	13.7
47	Hawaii	10.2
32	Idaho	12.7
28	Illinois	13.3
7	Indiana	16.9
30	Iowa	13.1
42	Kansas	11.1
11	Kentucky	16.2
5	Louisiana	20.5
3	Maine	21.0
32	Maryland	12.7
12	Massachusetts	15.8
21	Michigan	14.2
13	Minnesota	15.7
8	Mississippi	16.8
46	Missouri	10.3
15	Montana	15.3
32	Nebraska	12.7
50	Nevada	9.2
31	New Hampshire	12.9
16	New Jersey	15.0
17	New Mexico	14.9
1	New York	26.9
22	North Carolina	14.1
28	North Dakota	13.3
23	Ohio	13.9
35	Oklahoma	12.6
38	Oregon	11.9
36	Pennsylvania	12.3
2	Rhode Island	23.1
18	South Carolina	14.7
26	South Dakota	13.5
26	Tennessee	13.5
38	Texas	11.9
41	Utah	11.6
14	Vermont	15.5
48	Virginia	9.7
20	Washington	14.3
4	West Virginia	20.7
18	Wisconsin	14.7
24	Wyoming	13.7

RANK ORDER

RANK	STATE	PERCENT
1	New York	26.9
2	Rhode Island	23.1
3	Maine	21.0
4	West Virginia	20.7
5	Louisiana	20.5
6	Alaska	17.4
7	Indiana	16.9
8	Mississippi	16.8
9	Arkansas	16.5
10	Connecticut	16.4
11	Kentucky	16.2
12	Massachusetts	15.8
13	Minnesota	15.7
14	Vermont	15.5
15	Montana	15.3
16	New Jersey	15.0
17	New Mexico	14.9
18	South Carolina	14.7
18	Wisconsin	14.7
20	Washington	14.3
21	Michigan	14.2
22	North Carolina	14.1
23	Ohio	13.9
24	Georgia	13.7
24	Wyoming	13.7
26	South Dakota	13.5
26	Tennessee	13.5
28	Illinois	13.3
28	North Dakota	13.3
30	Iowa	13.1
31	New Hampshire	12.9
32	Idaho	12.7
32	Maryland	12.7
32	Nebraska	12.7
35	Oklahoma	12.6
36	Pennsylvania	12.3
37	California	12.0
38	Arizona	11.9
38	Oregon	11.9
38	Texas	11.9
41	Utah	11.6
42	Kansas	11.1
43	Delaware	11.0
44	Alabama	10.6
45	Florida	10.5
46	Missouri	10.3
47	Hawaii	10.2
48	Virginia	9.7
49	Colorado	9.6
50	Nevada	9.2
	District of Columbia	15.8

Source: U.S. Department of Health and Human Services, Health Care Financing Administration
  "State Health Expenditure Accounts" (Health Care Financing Review, Fall 1995, Volume 17, Number 1)
*By state of provider.

Medicaid Recipients in 1995

National Total = 36,281,586 Recipients*

ALPHA ORDER

RANK	STATE	RECIPIENTS	% of USA
20	Alabama	539,251	1.49%
47	Alaska	68,117	0.19%
23	Arizona	493,693	1.36%
31	Arkansas	353,370	0.97%
1	California	5,016,645	13.83%
33	Colorado	293,723	0.81%
30	Connecticut	380,327	1.05%
45	Delaware	78,555	0.22%
4	Florida	1,735,141	4.78%
10	Georgia	1,147,443	3.16%
49	Hawaii	51,674	0.14%
40	Idaho	115,014	0.32%
5	Illinois	1,551,949	4.28%
19	Indiana	559,020	1.54%
32	Iowa	304,304	0.84%
35	Kansas	255,702	0.70%
17	Kentucky	640,930	1.77%
13	Louisiana	785,399	2.16%
38	Maine	153,180	0.42%
27	Maryland	414,261	1.14%
14	Massachusetts	727,506	2.01%
9	Michigan	1,168,435	3.22%
24	Minnesota	473,420	1.30%
21	Mississippi	519,697	1.43%
15	Missouri	695,458	1.92%
43	Montana	98,708	0.27%
36	Nebraska	168,383	0.46%
41	Nevada	105,233	0.29%
44	New Hampshire	96,954	0.27%
12	New Jersey	789,666	2.18%
34	New Mexico	286,763	0.79%
2	New York	3,035,477	8.37%
11	North Carolina	1,084,337	2.99%
48	North Dakota	61,383	0.17%
6	Ohio	1,532,547	4.22%
28	Oklahoma	393,613	1.08%
26	Oregon	451,959	1.25%
8	Pennsylvania	1,230,193	3.39%
39	Rhode Island	135,230	0.37%
22	South Carolina	495,500	1.37%
46	South Dakota	74,077	0.20%
7	Tennessee	1,466,194	4.04%
3	Texas	2,561,957	7.06%
37	Utah	160,408	0.44%
42	Vermont	99,693	0.27%
16	Virginia	681,313	1.88%
18	Washington	639,256	1.76%
29	West Virginia	388,667	1.07%
25	Wisconsin	460,016	1.27%
50	Wyoming	51,374	0.14%

RANK ORDER

RANK	STATE	RECIPIENTS	% of USA
1	California	5,016,645	13.83%
2	New York	3,035,477	8.37%
3	Texas	2,561,957	7.06%
4	Florida	1,735,141	4.78%
5	Illinois	1,551,949	4.28%
6	Ohio	1,532,547	4.22%
7	Tennessee	1,466,194	4.04%
8	Pennsylvania	1,230,193	3.39%
9	Michigan	1,168,435	3.22%
10	Georgia	1,147,443	3.16%
11	North Carolina	1,084,337	2.99%
12	New Jersey	789,666	2.18%
13	Louisiana	785,399	2.16%
14	Massachusetts	727,506	2.01%
15	Missouri	695,458	1.92%
16	Virginia	681,313	1.88%
17	Kentucky	640,930	1.77%
18	Washington	639,256	1.76%
19	Indiana	559,020	1.54%
20	Alabama	539,251	1.49%
21	Mississippi	519,697	1.43%
22	South Carolina	495,500	1.37%
23	Arizona	493,693	1.36%
24	Minnesota	473,420	1.30%
25	Wisconsin	460,016	1.27%
26	Oregon	451,959	1.25%
27	Maryland	414,261	1.14%
28	Oklahoma	393,613	1.08%
29	West Virginia	388,667	1.07%
30	Connecticut	380,327	1.05%
31	Arkansas	353,370	0.97%
32	Iowa	304,304	0.84%
33	Colorado	293,723	0.81%
34	New Mexico	286,763	0.79%
35	Kansas	255,702	0.70%
36	Nebraska	168,383	0.46%
37	Utah	160,408	0.44%
38	Maine	153,180	0.42%
39	Rhode Island	135,230	0.37%
40	Idaho	115,014	0.32%
41	Nevada	105,233	0.29%
42	Vermont	99,693	0.27%
43	Montana	98,708	0.27%
44	New Hampshire	96,954	0.27%
45	Delaware	78,555	0.22%
46	South Dakota	74,077	0.20%
47	Alaska	68,117	0.19%
48	North Dakota	61,383	0.17%
49	Hawaii	51,674	0.14%
50	Wyoming	51,374	0.14%
	District of Columbia	138,444	0.38%

Source: U.S. Department of Health and Human Services, Health Care Financing Administration
"Statistical Report on Medical Care: Eligibles, Recipients, Payments and Services" (HCFA-2082)
For fiscal year ending September 30, 1995. National total includes 1,054,638 recipients Puerto Rico and 17,389 recipients in the Virgin Islands.

Percent Change in Number of Medicaid Recipients: 1990 to 1995

National Percent Change = 46.86% Increase*

ALPHA ORDER				RANK ORDER		
RANK	STATE	PERCENT CHANGE		RANK	STATE	PERCENT CHANGE
22	Alabama	53.20		1	Tennessee	139.06
13	Alaska	74.42		2	Nevada	123.86
NA	Arizona**	NA		3	New Mexico	120.82
34	Arkansas	33.70		4	New Hampshire	116.32
31	California	38.42		5	Idaho	110.83
21	Colorado	54.08		6	Oregon	98.93
23	Connecticut	52.38		7	North Carolina	92.49
8	Delaware	91.56		8	Delaware	91.56
14	Florida	67.09		9	Virginia	79.55
12	Georgia	76.29		10	Texas	77.66
49	Hawaii	(39.19)		11	Wyoming	77.51
5	Idaho	110.83		12	Georgia	76.29
26	Illinois	45.39		13	Alaska	74.42
17	Indiana	60.70		14	Florida	67.09
37	Iowa	27.01		15	Vermont	65.00
35	Kansas	31.55		16	Montana	61.66
32	Kentucky	37.03		17	Indiana	60.70
33	Louisiana	34.23		18	South Carolina	56.25
46	Maine	15.16		19	West Virginia	55.30
39	Maryland	25.39		20	Missouri	55.15
42	Massachusetts	23.15		21	Colorado	54.08
47	Michigan	11.50		22	Alabama	53.20
41	Minnesota	24.49		23	Connecticut	52.38
43	Mississippi	20.06		24	South Dakota	50.25
20	Missouri	55.15		25	Utah	48.18
16	Montana	61.66		26	Illinois	45.39
29	Nebraska	41.29		27	Oklahoma	44.05
2	Nevada	123.86		28	Washington	42.81
4	New Hampshire	116.32		29	Nebraska	41.29
30	New Jersey	39.31		30	New Jersey	39.31
3	New Mexico	120.82		31	California	38.42
36	New York	30.31		32	Kentucky	37.03
7	North Carolina	92.49		33	Louisiana	34.23
40	North Dakota	25.26		34	Arkansas	33.70
38	Ohio	25.54		35	Kansas	31.55
27	Oklahoma	44.05		36	New York	30.31
6	Oregon	98.93		37	Iowa	27.01
48	Pennsylvania	4.51		38	Ohio	25.54
45	Rhode Island	15.54		39	Maryland	25.39
18	South Carolina	56.25		40	North Dakota	25.26
24	South Dakota	50.25		41	Minnesota	24.49
1	Tennessee	139.06		42	Massachusetts	23.15
10	Texas	77.66		43	Mississippi	20.06
25	Utah	48.18		44	Wisconsin	17.13
15	Vermont	65.00		45	Rhode Island	15.54
9	Virginia	79.55		46	Maine	15.16
28	Washington	42.81		47	Michigan	11.50
19	West Virginia	55.30		48	Pennsylvania	4.51
44	Wisconsin	17.13		49	Hawaii	(39.19)
11	Wyoming	77.51		NA	Arizona**	NA
					District of Columbia	48.10

Source: Morgan Quitno Press using data from US Dept. of Health & Human Services, Health Care Financing Admin.
"Statistical Report on Medical Care: Eligibles, Recipients, Payments and Services" (HCFA-2082)
*For fiscal year ending September 30, 1995. National rate excludes recipients Puerto Rico and the Virgin Islands.
**Not available.

Medicaid Cost per Recipient in 1995

National Per Capita = $3,311 per Recipient*

ALPHA ORDER				RANK ORDER		
RANK	STATE	PER CAPITA		RANK	STATE	PER CAPITA
40	Alabama	$2,698		1	New York	$7,276
17	Alaska	3,698		2	Connecticut	5,588
50	Arizona	442		3	Massachusetts	5,460
15	Arkansas	3,893		4	Minnesota	5,386
48	California	2,097		5	Hawaii	4,983
19	Colorado	3,619		6	Rhode Island	4,973
2	Connecticut	5,588		7	Maine	4,965
12	Delaware	4,128		8	New Hampshire	4,880
39	Florida	2,768		9	Maryland	4,873
42	Georgia	2,681		10	North Dakota	4,839
5	Hawaii	4,983		11	New Jersey	4,828
30	Idaho	3,129		12	Delaware	4,128
21	Illinois	3,608		13	South Dakota	4,120
24	Indiana	3,359		14	Wisconsin	4,118
23	Iowa	3,406		15	Arkansas	3,893
28	Kansas	3,250		16	Pennsylvania	3,766
31	Kentucky	3,035		17	Alaska	3,698
22	Louisiana	3,449		18	Ohio	3,644
7	Maine	4,965		19	Colorado	3,619
9	Maryland	4,873		20	Nebraska	3,609
3	Massachusetts	5,460		21	Illinois	3,608
36	Michigan	2,918		22	Louisiana	3,449
4	Minnesota	5,386		23	Iowa	3,406
46	Mississippi	2,436		24	Indiana	3,359
34	Missouri	2,932		25	Wyoming	3,328
27	Montana	3,300		26	Nevada	3,322
20	Nebraska	3,609		27	Montana	3,300
26	Nevada	3,322		28	Kansas	3,250
8	New Hampshire	4,880		29	Vermont	3,210
11	New Jersey	4,828		30	Idaho	3,129
45	New Mexico	2,491		31	Kentucky	3,035
1	New York	7,276		32	West Virginia	3,009
35	North Carolina	2,928		33	Oregon	2,937
10	North Dakota	4,839		34	Missouri	2,932
18	Ohio	3,644		35	North Carolina	2,928
43	Oklahoma	2,680		36	Michigan	2,918
33	Oregon	2,937		37	South Carolina	2,902
16	Pennsylvania	3,766		38	Utah	2,895
6	Rhode Island	4,973		39	Florida	2,768
37	South Carolina	2,902		40	Alabama	2,698
13	South Dakota	4,120		41	Virginia	2,690
49	Tennessee	1,891		42	Georgia	2,681
44	Texas	2,562		43	Oklahoma	2,680
38	Utah	2,895		44	Texas	2,562
29	Vermont	3,210		45	New Mexico	2,491
41	Virginia	2,690		46	Mississippi	2,436
47	Washington	2,285		47	Washington	2,285
32	West Virginia	3,009		48	California	2,097
14	Wisconsin	4,118		49	Tennessee	1,891
25	Wyoming	3,328		50	Arizona	442
					District of Columbia	3,843

Source: U.S. Department of Health and Human Services, Health Care Financing Administration
   "Statistical Report on Medical Care: Eligibles, Recipients, Payments and Services" (HCFA-2082)
*For fiscal year ending September 30, 1995. The cost per recipient is $232 in Puerto Rico and $670 in the Virgin Islands.

Percent Change in Cost per Medicaid Recipient: 1990 to 1995

National Percent Change = 28.93% Increase*

ALPHA ORDER

RANK	STATE	PERCENT CHANGE
7	Alabama	55.86
44	Alaska	3.82
NA	Arizona**	NA
4	Arkansas	71.72
37	California	16.82
20	Colorado	33.79
38	Connecticut	15.72
19	Delaware	37.42
32	Florida	21.78
49	Georgia	(15.96)
1	Hawaii	121.27
42	Idaho	5.25
6	Illinois	58.87
48	Indiana	(12.96)
23	Iowa	31.56
25	Kansas	28.76
13	Kentucky	45.28
9	Louisiana	53.49
10	Maine	52.86
11	Maryland	47.67
35	Massachusetts	18.13
17	Michigan	39.35
14	Minnesota	45.21
3	Mississippi	79.91
12	Missouri	46.45
34	Montana	18.15
18	Nebraska	39.08
43	Nevada	5.09
47	New Hampshire	(10.01)
33	New Jersey	19.09
36	New Mexico	17.50
15	New York	42.69
39	North Carolina	15.69
30	North Dakota	22.35
16	Ohio	42.01
41	Oklahoma	6.52
26	Oregon	28.65
8	Pennsylvania	53.78
22	Rhode Island	31.63
29	South Carolina	23.86
31	South Dakota	22.33
46	Tennessee	(0.26)
21	Texas	32.88
27	Utah	27.03
28	Vermont	26.88
45	Virginia	3.62
40	Washington	7.38
2	West Virginia	108.52
24	Wisconsin	29.54
5	Wyoming	63.46

RANK ORDER

RANK	STATE	PERCENT CHANGE
1	Hawaii	121.27
2	West Virginia	108.52
3	Mississippi	79.91
4	Arkansas	71.72
5	Wyoming	63.46
6	Illinois	58.87
7	Alabama	55.86
8	Pennsylvania	53.78
9	Louisiana	53.49
10	Maine	52.86
11	Maryland	47.67
12	Missouri	46.45
13	Kentucky	45.28
14	Minnesota	45.21
15	New York	42.69
16	Ohio	42.01
17	Michigan	39.35
18	Nebraska	39.08
19	Delaware	37.42
20	Colorado	33.79
21	Texas	32.88
22	Rhode Island	31.63
23	Iowa	31.56
24	Wisconsin	29.54
25	Kansas	28.76
26	Oregon	28.65
27	Utah	27.03
28	Vermont	26.88
29	South Carolina	23.86
30	North Dakota	22.35
31	South Dakota	22.33
32	Florida	21.78
33	New Jersey	19.09
34	Montana	18.15
35	Massachusetts	18.13
36	New Mexico	17.50
37	California	16.82
38	Connecticut	15.72
39	North Carolina	15.69
40	Washington	7.38
41	Oklahoma	6.52
42	Idaho	5.25
43	Nevada	5.09
44	Alaska	3.82
45	Virginia	3.62
46	Tennessee	(0.26)
47	New Hampshire	(10.01)
48	Indiana	(12.96)
49	Georgia	(15.96)
NA	Arizona**	NA
	District of Columbia	46.18

Source: Morgan Quitno Press using data from US Dept. of Health & Human Services, Health Care Financing Admin.
"Statistical Report on Medical Care: Eligibles, Recipients, Payments and Services" (HCFA-2082)
*For fiscal year ending September 30, 1995.
**Not available.

Percent of Population Receiving Medicaid in 1995

National Percent = 13.80% of Population*

ALPHA ORDER

RANK	STATE	PERCENT
20	Alabama	12.70
30	Alaska	11.30
28	Arizona	11.47
13	Arkansas	14.22
10	California	15.89
48	Colorado	7.84
27	Connecticut	11.63
31	Delaware	10.96
23	Florida	12.23
9	Georgia	15.92
50	Hawaii	4.38
41	Idaho	9.86
18	Illinois	13.16
42	Indiana	9.64
33	Iowa	10.70
39	Kansas	9.97
8	Kentucky	16.62
4	Louisiana	18.11
21	Maine	12.36
46	Maryland	8.22
25	Massachusetts	11.98
22	Michigan	12.25
36	Minnesota	10.26
3	Mississippi	19.28
19	Missouri	13.07
29	Montana	11.35
35	Nebraska	10.27
49	Nevada	6.86
45	New Hampshire	8.45
40	New Jersey	9.93
6	New Mexico	16.97
7	New York	16.69
11	North Carolina	15.06
43	North Dakota	9.56
14	Ohio	13.76
24	Oklahoma	12.02
12	Oregon	14.35
37	Pennsylvania	10.20
15	Rhode Island	13.63
17	South Carolina	13.51
38	South Dakota	10.15
1	Tennessee	27.94
15	Texas	13.63
47	Utah	8.19
5	Vermont	17.04
34	Virginia	10.30
26	Washington	11.73
2	West Virginia	21.30
44	Wisconsin	8.98
32	Wyoming	10.73

RANK ORDER

RANK	STATE	PERCENT
1	Tennessee	27.94
2	West Virginia	21.30
3	Mississippi	19.28
4	Louisiana	18.11
5	Vermont	17.04
6	New Mexico	16.97
7	New York	16.69
8	Kentucky	16.62
9	Georgia	15.92
10	California	15.89
11	North Carolina	15.06
12	Oregon	14.35
13	Arkansas	14.22
14	Ohio	13.76
15	Rhode Island	13.63
15	Texas	13.63
17	South Carolina	13.51
18	Illinois	13.16
19	Missouri	13.07
20	Alabama	12.70
21	Maine	12.36
22	Michigan	12.25
23	Florida	12.23
24	Oklahoma	12.02
25	Massachusetts	11.98
26	Washington	11.73
27	Connecticut	11.63
28	Arizona	11.47
29	Montana	11.35
30	Alaska	11.30
31	Delaware	10.96
32	Wyoming	10.73
33	Iowa	10.70
34	Virginia	10.30
35	Nebraska	10.27
36	Minnesota	10.26
37	Pennsylvania	10.20
38	South Dakota	10.15
39	Kansas	9.97
40	New Jersey	9.93
41	Idaho	9.86
42	Indiana	9.64
43	North Dakota	9.56
44	Wisconsin	8.98
45	New Hampshire	8.45
46	Maryland	8.22
47	Utah	8.19
48	Colorado	7.84
49	Nevada	6.86
50	Hawaii	4.38

| | District of Columbia | 24.94 |

Source: Morgan Quitno Press using data from US Dept. of Health & Human Services, Health Care Financing Admin.
"Statistical Report on Medical Care: Eligibles, Recipients, Payments and Services" (HCFA-2082)
*For fiscal year ending September 30, 1995.

Federal Medicaid Matching Fund Rate for 1997

National Average = 59.79% of States' Funds Matched by Federal Government*

ALPHA ORDER				RANK ORDER		
RANK	STATE	RATE		RANK	STATE	RATE
10	Alabama	69.54		1	Mississippi	77.22
40	Alaska	50.00		2	Arkansas	73.29
14	Arizona	65.53		3	New Mexico	72.66
2	Arkansas	73.29		4	West Virginia	72.60
39	California	50.23		5	Utah	72.33
36	Colorado	52.32		6	Louisiana	71.36
40	Connecticut	50.00		7	South Carolina	70.43
40	Delaware	50.00		8	Kentucky	70.09
31	Florida	55.79		9	Oklahoma	70.01
22	Georgia	61.52		10	Alabama	69.54
40	Hawaii	50.00		11	Montana	69.01
12	Idaho	67.97		12	Idaho	67.97
40	Illinois	50.00		13	North Dakota	67.73
21	Indiana	61.58		14	Arizona	65.53
19	Iowa	62.94		15	South Dakota	64.89
30	Kansas	58.87		16	Tennessee	64.58
8	Kentucky	70.09		17	North Carolina	63.89
6	Louisiana	71.36		18	Maine	63.72
18	Maine	63.72		19	Iowa	62.94
40	Maryland	50.00		20	Texas	62.56
40	Massachusetts	50.00		21	Indiana	61.58
32	Michigan	55.20		22	Georgia	61.52
34	Minnesota	53.60		23	Vermont	61.05
1	Mississippi	77.22		24	Oregon	60.52
25	Missouri	60.04		25	Missouri	60.04
11	Montana	69.01		26	Wyoming	59.88
28	Nebraska	59.13		27	Ohio	59.28
40	Nevada	50.00		28	Nebraska	59.13
40	New Hampshire	50.00		29	Wisconsin	59.00
40	New Jersey	50.00		30	Kansas	58.87
3	New Mexico	72.66		31	Florida	55.79
40	New York	50.00		32	Michigan	55.20
17	North Carolina	63.89		33	Rhode Island	53.90
13	North Dakota	67.73		34	Minnesota	53.60
27	Ohio	59.28		35	Pennsylvania	52.85
9	Oklahoma	70.01		36	Colorado	52.32
24	Oregon	60.52		37	Virginia	51.45
35	Pennsylvania	52.85		38	Washington	50.52
33	Rhode Island	53.90		39	California	50.23
7	South Carolina	70.43		40	Alaska	50.00
15	South Dakota	64.89		40	Connecticut	50.00
16	Tennessee	64.58		40	Delaware	50.00
20	Texas	62.56		40	Hawaii	50.00
5	Utah	72.33		40	Illinois	50.00
23	Vermont	61.05		40	Maryland	50.00
37	Virginia	51.45		40	Massachusetts	50.00
38	Washington	50.52		40	Nevada	50.00
4	West Virginia	72.60		40	New Hampshire	50.00
29	Wisconsin	59.00		40	New Jersey	50.00
26	Wyoming	59.88		40	New York	50.00
					District of Columbia	50.00

*Source: U.S. Department of Health and Human Services, Health Care Financing Administration
"1996 Data Compendium" (March 1996, Pub. No. 03388)*
50 percent is minimum. National average is a simple average of the 51 individual rates and is not weighted for population or funds.

Medicare Benefit Payments in 1995

National Total = $176,884,237,000*

RANK	STATE	BENEFITS	% of USA
17	Alabama	$3,042,184,000	1.72%
50	Alaska	132,635,000	0.07%
20	Arizona	2,717,415,000	1.54%
31	Arkansas	1,638,020,000	0.93%
1	California	20,406,000,000	11.54%
28	Colorado	1,834,837,000	1.04%
23	Connecticut	2,583,742,000	1.46%
46	Delaware	444,964,000	0.25%
2	Florida	14,828,459,000	8.38%
12	Georgia	4,089,815,000	2.31%
42	Hawaii	580,455,000	0.33%
45	Idaho	463,308,000	0.26%
6	Illinois	7,276,339,000	4.11%
15	Indiana	3,491,081,000	1.97%
33	Iowa	1,526,969,000	0.86%
32	Kansas	1,545,162,000	0.87%
24	Kentucky	2,401,250,000	1.36%
16	Louisiana	3,447,745,000	1.95%
40	Maine	706,519,000	0.40%
19	Maryland	2,867,555,000	1.62%
10	Massachusetts	5,496,129,000	3.11%
8	Michigan	6,237,472,000	3.53%
25	Minnesota	2,378,016,000	1.34%
29	Mississippi	1,722,814,000	0.97%
14	Missouri	3,821,093,000	2.16%
44	Montana	488,525,000	0.28%
36	Nebraska	840,202,000	0.48%
35	Nevada	894,027,000	0.51%
41	New Hampshire	597,468,000	0.34%
9	New Jersey	5,603,125,000	3.17%
38	New Mexico	710,444,000	0.40%
3	New York	13,903,736,000	7.86%
11	North Carolina	4,276,049,000	2.42%
47	North Dakota	411,918,000	0.23%
7	Ohio	7,262,212,000	4.11%
26	Oklahoma	2,178,428,000	1.23%
30	Oregon	1,685,253,000	0.95%
5	Pennsylvania	10,796,231,000	6.10%
37	Rhode Island	772,209,000	0.44%
27	South Carolina	1,926,044,000	1.09%
43	South Dakota**	563,046,000	0.32%
13	Tennessee	4,083,406,000	2.31%
4	Texas	11,504,091,000	6.50%
39	Utah	708,036,000	0.40%
48	Vermont	283,894,000	0.16%
18	Virginia	2,979,371,000	1.68%
22	Washington	2,602,675,000	1.47%
34	West Virginia	1,207,737,000	0.68%
21	Wisconsin	2,673,209,000	1.51%
49	Wyoming	180,261,000	0.10%

RANK	STATE	BENEFITS	% of USA
1	California	$20,406,000,000	11.54%
2	Florida	14,828,459,000	8.38%
3	New York	13,903,736,000	7.86%
4	Texas	11,504,091,000	6.50%
5	Pennsylvania	10,796,231,000	6.10%
6	Illinois	7,276,339,000	4.11%
7	Ohio	7,262,212,000	4.11%
8	Michigan	6,237,472,000	3.53%
9	New Jersey	5,603,125,000	3.17%
10	Massachusetts	5,496,129,000	3.11%
11	North Carolina	4,276,049,000	2.42%
12	Georgia	4,089,815,000	2.31%
13	Tennessee	4,083,406,000	2.31%
14	Missouri	3,821,093,000	2.16%
15	Indiana	3,491,081,000	1.97%
16	Louisiana	3,447,745,000	1.95%
17	Alabama	3,042,184,000	1.72%
18	Virginia	2,979,371,000	1.68%
19	Maryland	2,867,555,000	1.62%
20	Arizona	2,717,415,000	1.54%
21	Wisconsin	2,673,209,000	1.51%
22	Washington	2,602,675,000	1.47%
23	Connecticut	2,583,742,000	1.46%
24	Kentucky	2,401,250,000	1.36%
25	Minnesota	2,378,016,000	1.34%
26	Oklahoma	2,178,428,000	1.23%
27	South Carolina	1,926,044,000	1.09%
28	Colorado	1,834,837,000	1.04%
29	Mississippi	1,722,814,000	0.97%
30	Oregon	1,685,253,000	0.95%
31	Arkansas	1,638,020,000	0.93%
32	Kansas	1,545,162,000	0.87%
33	Iowa	1,526,969,000	0.86%
34	West Virginia	1,207,737,000	0.68%
35	Nevada	894,027,000	0.51%
36	Nebraska	840,202,000	0.48%
37	Rhode Island	772,209,000	0.44%
38	New Mexico	710,444,000	0.40%
39	Utah	708,036,000	0.40%
40	Maine	706,519,000	0.40%
41	New Hampshire	597,468,000	0.34%
42	Hawaii	580,455,000	0.33%
43	South Dakota**	563,046,000	0.32%
44	Montana	488,525,000	0.28%
45	Idaho	463,308,000	0.26%
46	Delaware	444,964,000	0.25%
47	North Dakota	411,918,000	0.23%
48	Vermont	283,894,000	0.16%
49	Wyoming	180,261,000	0.10%
50	Alaska	132,635,000	0.07%
	District of Columbia	1,164,389,000	0.66%

*Source: U.S. Department of Health and Human Services, Health Care Financing Administration
"1996 Data Compendium" (March 1996)*
*For fiscal year 1995. Includes payments to aged and disabled enrollees. Total includes $875,417,000 in payments to enrollees in Puerto Rico and $32,857,000 to enrollees in all other areas.
**South Dakota's total may be overstated due to reporting problems.

Percent of Personal Health Care Expenditures Paid by Medicare in 1993

National Percent = 19.3%*

ALPHA ORDER

RANK	STATE	PERCENT
6	Alabama	21.8
50	Alaska	6.4
8	Arizona	21.4
3	Arkansas	23.3
27	California	18.4
43	Colorado	15.5
34	Connecticut	17.5
38	Delaware	16.7
1	Florida	27.9
30	Georgia	17.7
48	Hawaii	14.2
37	Idaho	16.9
27	Illinois	18.4
20	Indiana	19.1
15	Iowa	19.7
19	Kansas	19.2
12	Kentucky	20.6
10	Louisiana	21.0
32	Maine	17.6
29	Maryland	17.8
13	Massachusetts	20.1
14	Michigan	19.9
44	Minnesota	15.2
4	Mississippi	22.1
7	Missouri	21.6
23	Montana	18.6
36	Nebraska	17.0
16	Nevada	19.5
49	New Hampshire	13.7
22	New Jersey	18.8
47	New Mexico	14.6
30	New York	17.7
16	North Carolina	19.5
25	North Dakota	18.5
25	Ohio	18.5
11	Oklahoma	20.7
21	Oregon	19.0
2	Pennsylvania	24.2
18	Rhode Island	19.4
35	South Carolina	17.1
23	South Dakota	18.6
5	Tennessee	21.9
32	Texas	17.6
44	Utah	15.2
41	Vermont	16.1
40	Virginia	16.4
42	Washington	15.6
9	West Virginia	21.3
39	Wisconsin	16.5
46	Wyoming	15.0

RANK ORDER

RANK	STATE	PERCENT
1	Florida	27.9
2	Pennsylvania	24.2
3	Arkansas	23.3
4	Mississippi	22.1
5	Tennessee	21.9
6	Alabama	21.8
7	Missouri	21.6
8	Arizona	21.4
9	West Virginia	21.3
10	Louisiana	21.0
11	Oklahoma	20.7
12	Kentucky	20.6
13	Massachusetts	20.1
14	Michigan	19.9
15	Iowa	19.7
16	Nevada	19.5
16	North Carolina	19.5
18	Rhode Island	19.4
19	Kansas	19.2
20	Indiana	19.1
21	Oregon	19.0
22	New Jersey	18.8
23	Montana	18.6
23	South Dakota	18.6
25	North Dakota	18.5
25	Ohio	18.5
27	California	18.4
27	Illinois	18.4
29	Maryland	17.8
30	Georgia	17.7
30	New York	17.7
32	Maine	17.6
32	Texas	17.6
34	Connecticut	17.5
35	South Carolina	17.1
36	Nebraska	17.0
37	Idaho	16.9
38	Delaware	16.7
39	Wisconsin	16.5
40	Virginia	16.4
41	Vermont	16.1
42	Washington	15.6
43	Colorado	15.5
44	Minnesota	15.2
44	Utah	15.2
46	Wyoming	15.0
47	New Mexico	14.6
48	Hawaii	14.2
49	New Hampshire	13.7
50	Alaska	6.4
	District of Columbia	14.1

Source: U.S. Department of Health and Human Services, Health Care Financing Administration
    "State Health Expenditure Accounts" (Health Care Financing Review, Fall 1995, Volume 17, Number 1)
*By state of provider.

Medicare Enrollees in 1995

National Total = 37,535,024 Enrollees*

ALPHA ORDER

RANK	STATE	ENROLLEES	% of USA
19	Alabama	642,398	1.71%
50	Alaska	33,528	0.09%
22	Arizona	601,782	1.60%
30	Arkansas	422,956	1.13%
1	California	3,633,225	9.68%
31	Colorado	420,991	1.12%
26	Connecticut	502,035	1.34%
47	Delaware	100,665	0.27%
3	Florida	2,627,511	7.00%
12	Georgia	833,445	2.22%
43	Hawaii	149,475	0.40%
42	Idaho	149,556	0.40%
7	Illinois	1,617,479	4.31%
14	Indiana	823,403	2.19%
28	Iowa	474,262	1.26%
33	Kansas	383,386	1.02%
23	Kentucky	586,321	1.56%
24	Louisiana	580,509	1.55%
37	Maine	201,473	0.54%
21	Maryland	601,977	1.60%
11	Massachusetts	933,027	2.49%
8	Michigan	1,346,651	3.59%
20	Minnesota	630,521	1.68%
32	Mississippi	397,129	1.06%
13	Missouri	832,965	2.22%
44	Montana	130,074	0.35%
35	Nebraska	249,131	0.66%
38	Nevada	193,931	0.52%
41	New Hampshire	156,104	0.42%
9	New Jersey	1,168,083	3.11%
36	New Mexico	210,843	0.56%
2	New York	2,629,884	7.01%
10	North Carolina	1,027,027	2.74%
46	North Dakota	103,115	0.27%
6	Ohio	1,666,054	4.44%
27	Oklahoma	487,752	1.30%
29	Oregon	468,732	1.25%
5	Pennsylvania	2,071,162	5.52%
40	Rhode Island	168,061	0.45%
25	South Carolina	508,690	1.36%
45	South Dakota	116,694	0.31%
16	Tennessee	771,335	2.05%
4	Texas	2,080,465	5.54%
39	Utah	187,039	0.50%
48	Vermont	82,806	0.22%
15	Virginia	818,256	2.18%
18	Washington	687,789	1.83%
34	West Virginia	329,504	0.88%
17	Wisconsin	761,575	2.03%
49	Wyoming	60,163	0.16%

RANK ORDER

RANK	STATE	ENROLLEES	% of USA
1	California	3,633,225	9.68%
2	New York	2,629,884	7.01%
3	Florida	2,627,511	7.00%
4	Texas	2,080,465	5.54%
5	Pennsylvania	2,071,162	5.52%
6	Ohio	1,666,054	4.44%
7	Illinois	1,617,479	4.31%
8	Michigan	1,346,651	3.59%
9	New Jersey	1,168,083	3.11%
10	North Carolina	1,027,027	2.74%
11	Massachusetts	933,027	2.49%
12	Georgia	833,445	2.22%
13	Missouri	832,965	2.22%
14	Indiana	823,403	2.19%
15	Virginia	818,256	2.18%
16	Tennessee	771,335	2.05%
17	Wisconsin	761,575	2.03%
18	Washington	687,789	1.83%
19	Alabama	642,398	1.71%
20	Minnesota	630,521	1.68%
21	Maryland	601,977	1.60%
22	Arizona	601,782	1.60%
23	Kentucky	586,321	1.56%
24	Louisiana	580,509	1.55%
25	South Carolina	508,690	1.36%
26	Connecticut	502,035	1.34%
27	Oklahoma	487,752	1.30%
28	Iowa	474,262	1.26%
29	Oregon	468,732	1.25%
30	Arkansas	422,956	1.13%
31	Colorado	420,991	1.12%
32	Mississippi	397,129	1.06%
33	Kansas	383,386	1.02%
34	West Virginia	329,504	0.88%
35	Nebraska	249,131	0.66%
36	New Mexico	210,843	0.56%
37	Maine	201,473	0.54%
38	Nevada	193,931	0.52%
39	Utah	187,039	0.50%
40	Rhode Island	168,061	0.45%
41	New Hampshire	156,104	0.42%
42	Idaho	149,556	0.40%
43	Hawaii	149,475	0.40%
44	Montana	130,074	0.35%
45	South Dakota	116,694	0.31%
46	North Dakota	103,115	0.27%
47	Delaware	100,665	0.27%
48	Vermont	82,806	0.22%
49	Wyoming	60,163	0.16%
50	Alaska	33,528	0.09%
	District of Columbia	77,991	0.21%

Source: U.S. Department of Health and Human Services, Health Care Financing Administration unpublished data (March 1996)

*For fiscal year 1995. Includes aged and disabled enrollees. Total includes 476,970 enrollees in Puerto Rico and 299,953 enrollees in "other outlying areas."

Medicare Managed Care Enrollees in 1997

National Total = 4,948,706 Enrollees*

ALPHA ORDER

ALPHA ORDER

RANK	STATE	ENROLLEES	% of USA
25	Alabama	23,102	0.47%
42	Alaska	0	0.00%
6	Arizona	214,818	4.34%
37	Arkansas	5,976	0.12%
1	California	1,427,994	28.86%
11	Colorado	115,034	2.32%
23	Connecticut	27,621	0.56%
42	Delaware	0	0.00%
2	Florida	603,738	12.20%
30	Georgia	9,509	0.19%
18	Hawaii	51,516	1.04%
42	Idaho	0	0.00%
10	Illinois	144,959	2.93%
28	Indiana	13,474	0.27%
31	Iowa	8,654	0.17%
29	Kansas	10,547	0.21%
32	Kentucky	8,609	0.17%
16	Louisiana	54,977	1.11%
42	Maine	0	0.00%
17	Maryland	52,456	1.06%
8	Massachusetts	156,651	3.17%
26	Michigan	20,727	0.42%
12	Minnesota	114,453	2.31%
42	Mississippi	0	0.00%
15	Missouri	88,496	1.79%
42	Montana	0	0.00%
36	Nebraska	7,085	0.14%
19	Nevada	41,911	0.85%
42	New Hampshire	0	0.00%
14	New Jersey	92,811	1.88%
21	New Mexico	36,735	0.74%
4	New York	359,721	7.27%
34	North Carolina	7,261	0.15%
41	North Dakota	724	0.01%
13	Ohio	110,880	2.24%
22	Oklahoma	28,465	0.58%
7	Oregon	177,821	3.59%
3	Pennsylvania	361,014	7.30%
24	Rhode Island	25,186	0.51%
39	South Carolina	3,027	0.06%
42	South Dakota	0	0.00%
38	Tennessee	3,450	0.07%
5	Texas	230,603	4.66%
20	Utah	37,393	0.76%
40	Vermont	1,190	0.02%
35	Virginia	7,175	0.14%
9	Washington	145,100	2.93%
33	West Virginia	7,740	0.16%
27	Wisconsin	17,182	0.35%
42	Wyoming	0	0.00%

RANK ORDER

RANK	STATE	ENROLLEES	% of USA
1	California	1,427,994	28.86%
2	Florida	603,738	12.20%
3	Pennsylvania	361,014	7.30%
4	New York	359,721	7.27%
5	Texas	230,603	4.66%
6	Arizona	214,818	4.34%
7	Oregon	177,821	3.59%
8	Massachusetts	156,651	3.17%
9	Washington	145,100	2.93%
10	Illinois	144,959	2.93%
11	Colorado	115,034	2.32%
12	Minnesota	114,453	2.31%
13	Ohio	110,880	2.24%
14	New Jersey	92,811	1.88%
15	Missouri	88,496	1.79%
16	Louisiana	54,977	1.11%
17	Maryland	52,456	1.06%
18	Hawaii	51,516	1.04%
19	Nevada	41,911	0.85%
20	Utah	37,393	0.76%
21	New Mexico	36,735	0.74%
22	Oklahoma	28,465	0.58%
23	Connecticut	27,621	0.56%
24	Rhode Island	25,186	0.51%
25	Alabama	23,102	0.47%
26	Michigan	20,727	0.42%
27	Wisconsin	17,182	0.35%
28	Indiana	13,474	0.27%
29	Kansas	10,547	0.21%
30	Georgia	9,509	0.19%
31	Iowa	8,654	0.17%
32	Kentucky	8,609	0.17%
33	West Virginia	7,740	0.16%
34	North Carolina	7,261	0.15%
35	Virginia	7,175	0.14%
36	Nebraska	7,085	0.14%
37	Arkansas	5,976	0.12%
38	Tennessee	3,450	0.07%
39	South Carolina	3,027	0.06%
40	Vermont	1,190	0.02%
41	North Dakota	724	0.01%
42	Alaska	0	0.00%
42	Delaware	0	0.00%
42	Idaho	0	0.00%
42	Maine	0	0.00%
42	Mississippi	0	0.00%
42	Montana	0	0.00%
42	New Hampshire	0	0.00%
42	South Dakota	0	0.00%
42	Wyoming	0	0.00%
	District of Columbia	15,768	0.32%

Source: U.S. Department of Health and Human Services, Health Care Financing Administration
"Medicare Managed Care Contract Report" (February 1, 1997, http://www.hcfa.gov)
*As of January 1st. Includes Risk, Cost and Health Care Prepayment Plans (HCCP). National total includes 77,153 enrollees in the United Mine Workers' plan not shown separately by state. National total does not include 46,758 enrollees in demonstration plans.

Medicare Payments per Enrollee in 1995

National Rate = $4,713*

ALPHA ORDER				RANK ORDER		
RANK	STATE	PER ENROLLEE		RANK	STATE	PER ENROLLEE
14	Alabama	$4,736		1	Louisiana	$5,939
31	Alaska	3,956		2	Massachusetts	5,891
19	Arizona	4,516		3	Florida	5,644
33	Arkansas	3,873		4	California	5,616
4	California	5,616		5	Texas	5,530
24	Colorado	4,358		6	Tennessee	5,294
9	Connecticut	5,147		7	New York	5,287
22	Delaware	4,420		8	Pennsylvania	5,213
3	Florida	5,644		9	Connecticut	5,147
10	Georgia	4,907		10	Georgia	4,907
32	Hawaii	3,883		11	South Dakota	4,825
49	Idaho	3,098		12	New Jersey	4,797
20	Illinois	4,499		13	Maryland	4,764
26	Indiana	4,240		14	Alabama	4,736
48	Iowa	3,220		15	Michigan	4,632
29	Kansas	4,030		16	Nevada	4,610
28	Kentucky	4,095		17	Rhode Island	4,595
1	Louisiana	5,939		18	Missouri	4,587
44	Maine	3,507		19	Arizona	4,516
13	Maryland	4,764		20	Illinois	4,499
2	Massachusetts	5,891		21	Oklahoma	4,466
15	Michigan	4,632		22	Delaware	4,420
38	Minnesota	3,772		23	Ohio	4,359
25	Mississippi	4,338		24	Colorado	4,358
18	Missouri	4,587		25	Mississippi	4,338
39	Montana	3,756		26	Indiana	4,240
46	Nebraska	3,373		27	North Carolina	4,164
16	Nevada	4,610		28	Kentucky	4,095
34	New Hampshire	3,827		29	Kansas	4,030
12	New Jersey	4,797		30	North Dakota	3,995
47	New Mexico	3,370		31	Alaska	3,956
7	New York	5,287		32	Hawaii	3,883
27	North Carolina	4,164		33	Arkansas	3,873
30	North Dakota	3,995		34	New Hampshire	3,827
23	Ohio	4,359		35	South Carolina	3,786
21	Oklahoma	4,466		36	Utah	3,785
42	Oregon	3,595		37	Washington	3,784
8	Pennsylvania	5,213		38	Minnesota	3,772
17	Rhode Island	4,595		39	Montana	3,756
35	South Carolina	3,786		40	West Virginia	3,665
11	South Dakota	4,825		41	Virginia	3,641
6	Tennessee	5,294		42	Oregon	3,595
5	Texas	5,530		43	Wisconsin	3,510
36	Utah	3,785		44	Maine	3,507
45	Vermont	3,428		45	Vermont	3,428
41	Virginia	3,641		46	Nebraska	3,373
37	Washington	3,784		47	New Mexico	3,370
40	West Virginia	3,665		48	Iowa	3,220
43	Wisconsin	3,510		49	Idaho	3,098
50	Wyoming	2,996		50	Wyoming	2,996
					District of Columbia	14,930

Source: Morgan Quitno Press using data from U.S. Dept. of Health and Human Services, Health Care Financing Admn
   unpublished data (March 1996)
*For fiscal year 1995. Includes aged and disabled enrollees. National rate includes payments to enrollees in
Puerto Rico and in "other outlying areas."

Percent of Population Enrolled in Medicare in 1995

National Percent = 14.28% of Population*

ALPHA ORDER

RANK ORDER

RANK	STATE	PERCENT		RANK	STATE	PERCENT
15	Alabama	15.13		1	Florida	18.52
50	Alaska	5.56		2	West Virginia	18.06
31	Arizona	13.98		3	Pennsylvania	17.17
4	Arkansas	17.02		4	Arkansas	17.02
46	California	11.51		5	Rhode Island	16.94
47	Colorado	11.23		6	Iowa	16.68
12	Connecticut	15.35		7	Maine	16.26
30	Delaware	14.04		8	North Dakota	16.06
1	Florida	18.52		9	South Dakota	15.99
45	Georgia	11.56		10	Missouri	15.66
38	Hawaii	12.68		11	Massachusetts	15.37
37	Idaho	12.83		12	Connecticut	15.35
33	Illinois	13.72		13	Kentucky	15.20
27	Indiana	14.20		13	Nebraska	15.20
6	Iowa	16.68		15	Alabama	15.13
17	Kansas	14.95		16	Ohio	14.96
13	Kentucky	15.20		17	Kansas	14.95
36	Louisiana	13.38		17	Montana	14.95
7	Maine	16.26		19	Oklahoma	14.89
44	Maryland	11.95		19	Oregon	14.89
11	Massachusetts	15.37		21	Wisconsin	14.87
29	Michigan	14.12		22	Mississippi	14.73
34	Minnesota	13.66		23	Tennessee	14.70
22	Mississippi	14.73		24	New Jersey	14.69
10	Missouri	15.66		25	New York	14.46
17	Montana	14.95		26	North Carolina	14.26
13	Nebraska	15.20		27	Indiana	14.20
39	Nevada	12.65		28	Vermont	14.15
35	New Hampshire	13.60		29	Michigan	14.12
24	New Jersey	14.69		30	Delaware	14.04
42	New Mexico	12.48		31	Arizona	13.98
25	New York	14.46		32	South Carolina	13.87
26	North Carolina	14.26		33	Illinois	13.72
8	North Dakota	16.06		34	Minnesota	13.66
16	Ohio	14.96		35	New Hampshire	13.60
19	Oklahoma	14.89		36	Louisiana	13.38
19	Oregon	14.89		37	Idaho	12.83
3	Pennsylvania	17.17		38	Hawaii	12.68
5	Rhode Island	16.94		39	Nevada	12.65
32	South Carolina	13.87		40	Washington	12.62
9	South Dakota	15.99		41	Wyoming	12.56
23	Tennessee	14.70		42	New Mexico	12.48
48	Texas	11.07		43	Virginia	12.37
49	Utah	9.55		44	Maryland	11.95
28	Vermont	14.15		45	Georgia	11.56
43	Virginia	12.37		46	California	11.51
40	Washington	12.62		47	Colorado	11.23
2	West Virginia	18.06		48	Texas	11.07
21	Wisconsin	14.87		49	Utah	9.55
41	Wyoming	12.56		50	Alaska	5.56
					District of Columbia	14.05

Source: Morgan Quitno Press using data from U.S. Dept. of Health and Human Services, Health Care Financing Admn
        unpublished data (March 1996)
*For fiscal year 1995. Includes aged and disabled enrollees. National rate includes only residents of the 50 states
and the District of Columbia.

Percent of Physicians Participating in Medicare in 1995

National Percent = 72.3% of Physicians Participate in Medicare*

ALPHA ORDER				RANK ORDER		
RANK	STATE	PERCENT		RANK	STATE	PERCENT
2	Alabama	90.5		1	Nevada	91.2
22	Alaska	77.1		2	Alabama	90.5
7	Arizona	87.1		2	Ohio	90.5
27	Arkansas	74.8		4	Maryland	88.1
28	California	74.5		5	Missouri	87.6
39	Colorado	65.2		6	West Virginia	87.2
41	Connecticut	61.8		7	Arizona	87.1
35	Delaware	68.0		8	Georgia	86.3
35	Florida	68.0		9	Utah	85.9
8	Georgia	86.3		10	Kansas	84.4
12	Hawaii	82.8		11	Kentucky	83.4
49	Idaho	54.7		12	Hawaii	82.8
29	Illinois	73.3		13	Nebraska	82.5
30	Indiana	72.8		14	North Dakota	81.8
16	Iowa	81.1		15	Wisconsin	81.2
10	Kansas	84.4		16	Iowa	81.1
11	Kentucky	83.4		17	Rhode Island	80.9
46	Louisiana	57.4		18	Tennessee	80.6
33	Maine	68.9		19	Oregon	79.7
4	Maryland	88.1		20	New Mexico	78.1
40	Massachusetts	64.7		21	North Carolina	77.6
26	Michigan	75.3		22	Alaska	77.1
45	Minnesota	58.6		23	Texas	76.9
43	Mississippi	59.4		24	Washington	76.2
5	Missouri	87.6		25	South Carolina	76.1
32	Montana	70.1		26	Michigan	75.3
13	Nebraska	82.5		27	Arkansas	74.8
1	Nevada	91.2		28	California	74.5
42	New Hampshire	60.4		29	Illinois	73.3
48	New Jersey	54.9		30	Indiana	72.8
20	New Mexico	78.1		31	Oklahoma	72.3
44	New York	59.2		32	Montana	70.1
21	North Carolina	77.6		33	Maine	68.9
14	North Dakota	81.8		34	Vermont	68.8
2	Ohio	90.5		35	Delaware	68.0
31	Oklahoma	72.3		35	Florida	68.0
19	Oregon	79.7		37	Pennsylvania	67.3
37	Pennsylvania	67.3		38	Wyoming	66.1
17	Rhode Island	80.9		39	Colorado	65.2
25	South Carolina	76.1		40	Massachusetts	64.7
50	South Dakota	51.7		41	Connecticut	61.8
18	Tennessee	80.6		42	New Hampshire	60.4
23	Texas	76.9		43	Mississippi	59.4
9	Utah	85.9		44	New York	59.2
34	Vermont	68.8		45	Minnesota	58.6
47	Virginia	55.6		46	Louisiana	57.4
24	Washington	76.2		47	Virginia	55.6
6	West Virginia	87.2		48	New Jersey	54.9
15	Wisconsin	81.2		49	Idaho	54.7
38	Wyoming	66.1		50	South Dakota	51.7
					District of Columbia	63.0

Source: U.S. Department of Health and Human Services, Health Care Financing Administration
   "1996 Data Compendium" (March 1996, Pub. No. 03388)
*Medicare Part B. Physicians include MD's, DO's and limited license practitioners.

State Government Expenditures for Health Programs in 1994

National Total = $28,394,124,000*

ALPHA ORDER

RANK	STATE	EXPENDITURES	% of USA
17	Alabama	$487,044,000	1.72%
35	Alaska	169,672,000	0.60%
19	Arizona	467,729,000	1.65%
32	Arkansas	211,719,000	0.75%
1	California	4,896,146,000	17.24%
30	Colorado	232,482,000	0.82%
28	Connecticut	261,998,000	0.92%
40	Delaware	131,628,000	0.46%
4	Florida	1,842,135,000	6.49%
15	Georgia	545,525,000	1.92%
26	Hawaii	310,655,000	1.09%
45	Idaho	74,583,000	0.26%
8	Illinois	1,081,918,000	3.81%
24	Indiana	346,970,000	1.22%
37	Iowa	165,327,000	0.58%
33	Kansas	185,118,000	0.65%
29	Kentucky	239,723,000	0.84%
23	Louisiana	350,956,000	1.24%
41	Maine	129,853,000	0.46%
13	Maryland	643,814,000	2.27%
7	Massachusetts	1,090,006,000	3.84%
3	Michigan	1,935,439,000	6.82%
22	Minnesota	412,413,000	1.45%
34	Mississippi	184,112,000	0.65%
21	Missouri	435,920,000	1.54%
43	Montana	108,807,000	0.38%
38	Nebraska	160,238,000	0.56%
47	Nevada	61,974,000	0.22%
44	New Hampshire	107,480,000	0.38%
14	New Jersey	546,514,000	1.92%
31	New Mexico	231,036,000	0.81%
2	New York	2,231,831,000	7.86%
11	North Carolina	700,800,000	2.47%
50	North Dakota	47,546,000	0.17%
9	Ohio	961,763,000	3.39%
27	Oklahoma	270,886,000	0.95%
25	Oregon	330,954,000	1.17%
6	Pennsylvania	1,140,809,000	4.02%
36	Rhode Island	166,400,000	0.59%
10	South Carolina	739,644,000	2.60%
48	South Dakota	55,038,000	0.19%
20	Tennessee	466,221,000	1.64%
5	Texas	1,182,271,000	4.16%
39	Utah	146,947,000	0.52%
49	Vermont	50,889,000	0.18%
16	Virginia	514,780,000	1.81%
12	Washington	659,122,000	2.32%
42	West Virginia	124,332,000	0.44%
18	Wisconsin	480,406,000	1.69%
46	Wyoming	74,551,000	0.26%

RANK ORDER

RANK	STATE	EXPENDITURES	% of USA
1	California	$4,896,146,000	17.24%
2	New York	2,231,831,000	7.86%
3	Michigan	1,935,439,000	6.82%
4	Florida	1,842,135,000	6.49%
5	Texas	1,182,271,000	4.16%
6	Pennsylvania	1,140,809,000	4.02%
7	Massachusetts	1,090,006,000	3.84%
8	Illinois	1,081,918,000	3.81%
9	Ohio	961,763,000	3.39%
10	South Carolina	739,644,000	2.60%
11	North Carolina	700,800,000	2.47%
12	Washington	659,122,000	2.32%
13	Maryland	643,814,000	2.27%
14	New Jersey	546,514,000	1.92%
15	Georgia	545,525,000	1.92%
16	Virginia	514,780,000	1.81%
17	Alabama	487,044,000	1.72%
18	Wisconsin	480,406,000	1.69%
19	Arizona	467,729,000	1.65%
20	Tennessee	466,221,000	1.64%
21	Missouri	435,920,000	1.54%
22	Minnesota	412,413,000	1.45%
23	Louisiana	350,956,000	1.24%
24	Indiana	346,970,000	1.22%
25	Oregon	330,954,000	1.17%
26	Hawaii	310,655,000	1.09%
27	Oklahoma	270,886,000	0.95%
28	Connecticut	261,998,000	0.92%
29	Kentucky	239,723,000	0.84%
30	Colorado	232,482,000	0.82%
31	New Mexico	231,036,000	0.81%
32	Arkansas	211,719,000	0.75%
33	Kansas	185,118,000	0.65%
34	Mississippi	184,112,000	0.65%
35	Alaska	169,672,000	0.60%
36	Rhode Island	166,400,000	0.59%
37	Iowa	165,327,000	0.58%
38	Nebraska	160,238,000	0.56%
39	Utah	146,947,000	0.52%
40	Delaware	131,628,000	0.46%
41	Maine	129,853,000	0.46%
42	West Virginia	124,332,000	0.44%
43	Montana	108,807,000	0.38%
44	New Hampshire	107,480,000	0.38%
45	Idaho	74,583,000	0.26%
46	Wyoming	74,551,000	0.26%
47	Nevada	61,974,000	0.22%
48	South Dakota	55,038,000	0.19%
49	Vermont	50,889,000	0.18%
50	North Dakota	47,546,000	0.17%
	District of Columbia**	NA	NA

Source: U.S. Bureau of the Census, Governments Division
   "1994 State Government Finances" (http://www.census.gov/govs/www/stsum94.html)
*Includes outpatient health services other than hospital care, research and education, categorical health programs, treatment and immunization clinics, nursing and environmental health activities. Includes capital expenditures.
**Not applicable.

Per Capita State Government Expenditures for Health Programs in 1994

National Per Capita = $109.05*

ALPHA ORDER				RANK ORDER		
RANK	STATE	PER CAPITA		RANK	STATE	PER CAPITA
16	Alabama	$115.55		1	Alaska	$282.32
1	Alaska	282.32		2	Hawaii	264.84
17	Arizona	114.30		3	Michigan	204.03
30	Arkansas	86.24		4	South Carolina	203.03
9	California	156.12		5	Delaware	185.92
46	Colorado	63.47		6	Massachusetts	180.40
34	Connecticut	80.05		7	Rhode Island	167.07
5	Delaware	185.92		8	Wyoming	156.62
11	Florida	131.91		9	California	156.12
36	Georgia	77.24		10	New Mexico	139.26
2	Hawaii	264.84		11	Florida	131.91
44	Idaho	65.65		12	Maryland	128.76
25	Illinois	92.20		13	Montana	126.96
48	Indiana	60.34		14	Washington	123.18
49	Iowa	58.38		15	New York	122.65
40	Kansas	72.60		16	Alabama	115.55
47	Kentucky	62.66		17	Arizona	114.30
33	Louisiana	81.33		18	Oregon	106.97
19	Maine	104.89		19	Maine	104.89
12	Maryland	128.76		20	North Carolina	99.00
6	Massachusetts	180.40		21	Nebraska	98.55
3	Michigan	204.03		22	New Hampshire	94.70
26	Minnesota	90.20		23	Pennsylvania	94.61
42	Mississippi	69.01		24	Wisconsin	94.49
32	Missouri	82.64		25	Illinois	92.20
13	Montana	126.96		26	Minnesota	90.20
21	Nebraska	98.55		27	Tennessee	90.09
50	Nevada	42.33		28	Vermont	87.59
22	New Hampshire	94.70		29	Ohio	86.67
41	New Jersey	69.13		30	Arkansas	86.24
10	New Mexico	139.26		31	Oklahoma	83.25
15	New York	122.65		32	Missouri	82.64
20	North Carolina	99.00		33	Louisiana	81.33
39	North Dakota	74.29		34	Connecticut	80.05
29	Ohio	86.67		35	Virginia	78.59
31	Oklahoma	83.25		36	Georgia	77.24
18	Oregon	106.97		37	Utah	76.94
23	Pennsylvania	94.61		38	South Dakota	76.02
7	Rhode Island	167.07		39	North Dakota	74.29
4	South Carolina	203.03		40	Kansas	72.60
38	South Dakota	76.02		41	New Jersey	69.13
27	Tennessee	90.09		42	Mississippi	69.01
45	Texas	64.14		43	West Virginia	68.24
37	Utah	76.94		44	Idaho	65.65
28	Vermont	87.59		45	Texas	64.14
35	Virginia	78.59		46	Colorado	63.47
14	Washington	123.18		47	Kentucky	62.66
43	West Virginia	68.24		48	Indiana	60.34
24	Wisconsin	94.49		49	Iowa	58.38
8	Wyoming	156.62		50	Nevada	42.33
					District of Columbia**	NA

Source: Morgan Quitno Press using data from U.S. Bureau of the Census, Governments Division
"1994 State Government Finances" (http://www.census.gov/govs/www/stsum94.html)
*Includes outpatient health services other than hospital care, research and education, categorical health programs, treatment and immunization clinics, nursing and environmental health activities. Includes capital expenditures.
**Not applicable.

State Government Expenditures for Hospitals in 1994

National Total = $28,183,212,000*

ALPHA ORDER

RANK	STATE	EXPENDITURES	% of USA
11	Alabama	$823,194,000	2.92%
48	Alaska	32,710,000	0.12%
37	Arizona	89,071,000	0.32%
29	Arkansas	311,251,000	1.10%
2	California	2,706,385,000	9.60%
36	Colorado	159,124,000	0.56%
10	Connecticut	913,523,000	3.24%
43	Delaware	47,186,000	0.17%
21	Florida	486,832,000	1.73%
16	Georgia	582,056,000	2.07%
35	Hawaii	211,429,000	0.75%
45	Idaho	37,919,000	0.13%
13	Illinois	753,353,000	2.67%
18	Indiana	530,071,000	1.88%
20	Iowa	492,096,000	1.75%
27	Kansas	328,245,000	1.16%
26	Kentucky	336,167,000	1.19%
7	Louisiana	1,081,007,000	3.84%
40	Maine	57,032,000	0.20%
28	Maryland	315,884,000	1.12%
12	Massachusetts	783,985,000	2.78%
6	Michigan	1,240,203,000	4.40%
17	Minnesota	552,902,000	1.96%
32	Mississippi	278,084,000	0.99%
23	Missouri	423,349,000	1.50%
49	Montana	30,469,000	0.11%
34	Nebraska	251,019,000	0.89%
42	Nevada	53,750,000	0.19%
46	New Hampshire	36,748,000	0.13%
9	New Jersey	977,660,000	3.47%
31	New Mexico	286,573,000	1.02%
1	New York	3,614,675,000	12.83%
14	North Carolina	712,761,000	2.53%
41	North Dakota	54,260,000	0.19%
5	Ohio	1,246,280,000	4.42%
30	Oklahoma	303,930,000	1.08%
25	Oregon	405,462,000	1.44%
4	Pennsylvania	1,362,603,000	4.83%
39	Rhode Island	62,854,000	0.22%
15	South Carolina	616,077,000	2.19%
44	South Dakota	46,247,000	0.16%
22	Tennessee	465,331,000	1.65%
3	Texas	1,721,518,000	6.11%
33	Utah	271,616,000	0.96%
50	Vermont	14,433,000	0.05%
8	Virginia	1,030,289,000	3.66%
19	Washington	517,518,000	1.84%
38	West Virginia	79,598,000	0.28%
24	Wisconsin	415,416,000	1.47%
47	Wyoming	33,067,000	0.12%

RANK ORDER

RANK	STATE	EXPENDITURES	% of USA
1	New York	$3,614,675,000	12.83%
2	California	2,706,385,000	9.60%
3	Texas	1,721,518,000	6.11%
4	Pennsylvania	1,362,603,000	4.83%
5	Ohio	1,246,280,000	4.42%
6	Michigan	1,240,203,000	4.40%
7	Louisiana	1,081,007,000	3.84%
8	Virginia	1,030,289,000	3.66%
9	New Jersey	977,660,000	3.47%
10	Connecticut	913,523,000	3.24%
11	Alabama	823,194,000	2.92%
12	Massachusetts	783,985,000	2.78%
13	Illinois	753,353,000	2.67%
14	North Carolina	712,761,000	2.53%
15	South Carolina	616,077,000	2.19%
16	Georgia	582,056,000	2.07%
17	Minnesota	552,902,000	1.96%
18	Indiana	530,071,000	1.88%
19	Washington	517,518,000	1.84%
20	Iowa	492,096,000	1.75%
21	Florida	486,832,000	1.73%
22	Tennessee	465,331,000	1.65%
23	Missouri	423,349,000	1.50%
24	Wisconsin	415,416,000	1.47%
25	Oregon	405,462,000	1.44%
26	Kentucky	336,167,000	1.19%
27	Kansas	328,245,000	1.16%
28	Maryland	315,884,000	1.12%
29	Arkansas	311,251,000	1.10%
30	Oklahoma	303,930,000	1.08%
31	New Mexico	286,573,000	1.02%
32	Mississippi	278,084,000	0.99%
33	Utah	271,616,000	0.96%
34	Nebraska	251,019,000	0.89%
35	Hawaii	211,429,000	0.75%
36	Colorado	159,124,000	0.56%
37	Arizona	89,071,000	0.32%
38	West Virginia	79,598,000	0.28%
39	Rhode Island	62,854,000	0.22%
40	Maine	57,032,000	0.20%
41	North Dakota	54,260,000	0.19%
42	Nevada	53,750,000	0.19%
43	Delaware	47,186,000	0.17%
44	South Dakota	46,247,000	0.16%
45	Idaho	37,919,000	0.13%
46	New Hampshire	36,748,000	0.13%
47	Wyoming	33,067,000	0.12%
48	Alaska	32,710,000	0.12%
49	Montana	30,469,000	0.11%
50	Vermont	14,433,000	0.05%
	District of Columbia**	NA	NA

Source: U.S. Bureau of the Census, Governments Division
"1994 State Government Finances" (http://www.census.gov/govs/www/stsum94.html)
*Financing, construction, acquisition, maintenance or operation of hospital facilities, provision of hospital care and support of public or private hospitals.
**Not applicable.

Per Capita State Government Expenditures for Hospitals in 1994

National Per Capita = $108.24*

ALPHA ORDER

RANK	STATE	PER CAPITA
4	Alabama	$195.30
40	Alaska	54.43
50	Arizona	21.77
16	Arkansas	126.78
29	California	86.30
43	Colorado	43.44
1	Connecticut	279.11
35	Delaware	66.65
46	Florida	34.86
31	Georgia	82.41
5	Hawaii	180.25
47	Idaho	33.38
36	Illinois	64.20
26	Indiana	92.19
6	Iowa	173.76
15	Kansas	128.72
28	Kentucky	87.86
2	Louisiana	250.52
41	Maine	46.07
38	Maryland	63.18
14	Massachusetts	129.76
13	Michigan	130.74
18	Minnesota	120.93
21	Mississippi	104.23
33	Missouri	80.26
45	Montana	35.55
10	Nebraska	154.38
44	Nevada	36.71
48	New Hampshire	32.38
17	New Jersey	123.66
7	New Mexico	172.74
3	New York	198.64
22	North Carolina	100.69
30	North Dakota	84.78
20	Ohio	112.31
24	Oklahoma	93.40
12	Oregon	131.05
19	Pennsylvania	113.00
39	Rhode Island	63.11
8	South Carolina	169.11
37	South Dakota	63.88
27	Tennessee	89.92
25	Texas	93.39
11	Utah	142.21
49	Vermont	24.84
9	Virginia	157.30
23	Washington	96.71
42	West Virginia	43.69
32	Wisconsin	81.71
34	Wyoming	69.47

RANK ORDER

RANK	STATE	PER CAPITA
1	Connecticut	$279.11
2	Louisiana	250.52
3	New York	198.64
4	Alabama	195.30
5	Hawaii	180.25
6	Iowa	173.76
7	New Mexico	172.74
8	South Carolina	169.11
9	Virginia	157.30
10	Nebraska	154.38
11	Utah	142.21
12	Oregon	131.05
13	Michigan	130.74
14	Massachusetts	129.76
15	Kansas	128.72
16	Arkansas	126.78
17	New Jersey	123.66
18	Minnesota	120.93
19	Pennsylvania	113.00
20	Ohio	112.31
21	Mississippi	104.23
22	North Carolina	100.69
23	Washington	96.71
24	Oklahoma	93.40
25	Texas	93.39
26	Indiana	92.19
27	Tennessee	89.92
28	Kentucky	87.86
29	California	86.30
30	North Dakota	84.78
31	Georgia	82.41
32	Wisconsin	81.71
33	Missouri	80.26
34	Wyoming	69.47
35	Delaware	66.65
36	Illinois	64.20
37	South Dakota	63.88
38	Maryland	63.18
39	Rhode Island	63.11
40	Alaska	54.43
41	Maine	46.07
42	West Virginia	43.69
43	Colorado	43.44
44	Nevada	36.71
45	Montana	35.55
46	Florida	34.86
47	Idaho	33.38
48	New Hampshire	32.38
49	Vermont	24.84
50	Arizona	21.77
	District of Columbia**	NA

Source: Morgan Quitno Press using data from U.S. Bureau of the Census, Governments Division
"1994 State Government Finances" (http://www.census.gov/govs/www/stsum94.html)
*Financing, construction, acquisition, maintenance or operation of hospital facilities, provision of hospital care and support of public or private hospitals.
**Not applicable.

Receipts of Health Services Establishments in 1992

National Total = $623,480,434,000*

ALPHA ORDER

ALPHA ORDER

RANK	STATE	RECEIPTS	% of USA
23	Alabama	$9,400,816,000	1.51%
48	Alaska	1,225,327,000	0.20%
24	Arizona	8,624,782,000	1.38%
32	Arkansas	4,791,668,000	0.77%
1	California	79,130,980,000	12.69%
25	Colorado	8,000,876,000	1.28%
22	Connecticut	9,932,092,000	1.59%
43	Delaware	1,780,075,000	0.29%
4	Florida	36,667,132,000	5.88%
11	Georgia	15,774,705,000	2.53%
39	Hawaii	2,757,575,000	0.44%
44	Idaho	1,775,447,000	0.28%
6	Illinois	27,961,997,000	4.48%
14	Indiana	13,010,617,000	2.09%
30	Iowa	5,852,492,000	0.94%
31	Kansas	5,763,990,000	0.92%
26	Kentucky	7,923,070,000	1.27%
21	Louisiana	10,204,980,000	1.64%
40	Maine	2,666,876,000	0.43%
18	Maryland	11,824,018,000	1.90%
10	Massachusetts	19,296,743,000	3.10%
8	Michigan	21,891,285,000	3.51%
20	Minnesota	11,199,561,000	1.80%
33	Mississippi	4,605,036,000	0.74%
15	Missouri	12,918,009,000	2.07%
46	Montana	1,589,295,000	0.25%
35	Nebraska	3,483,096,000	0.56%
37	Nevada	3,016,118,000	0.48%
41	New Hampshire	2,642,095,000	0.42%
9	New Jersey	21,102,821,000	3.38%
38	New Mexico	2,881,524,000	0.46%
2	New York	53,091,018,000	8.52%
12	North Carolina	14,227,452,000	2.28%
45	North Dakota	1,651,634,000	0.26%
7	Ohio	27,492,361,000	4.41%
28	Oklahoma	6,268,749,000	1.01%
29	Oregon	6,137,525,000	0.98%
5	Pennsylvania	33,155,698,000	5.32%
42	Rhode Island	2,617,386,000	0.42%
27	South Carolina	6,612,570,000	1.06%
47	South Dakota	1,543,627,000	0.25%
16	Tennessee	12,807,220,000	2.05%
3	Texas	38,769,630,000	6.22%
36	Utah	3,216,121,000	0.52%
49	Vermont	1,121,735,000	0.18%
13	Virginia	13,140,339,000	2.11%
17	Washington	12,022,436,000	1.93%
34	West Virginia	4,040,621,000	0.65%
19	Wisconsin	11,288,091,000	1.81%
50	Wyoming	708,286,000	0.11%

RANK ORDER

RANK	STATE	RECEIPTS	% of USA
1	California	$79,130,980,000	12.69%
2	New York	53,091,018,000	8.52%
3	Texas	38,769,630,000	6.22%
4	Florida	36,667,132,000	5.88%
5	Pennsylvania	33,155,698,000	5.32%
6	Illinois	27,961,997,000	4.48%
7	Ohio	27,492,361,000	4.41%
8	Michigan	21,891,285,000	3.51%
9	New Jersey	21,102,821,000	3.38%
10	Massachusetts	19,296,743,000	3.10%
11	Georgia	15,774,705,000	2.53%
12	North Carolina	14,227,452,000	2.28%
13	Virginia	13,140,339,000	2.11%
14	Indiana	13,010,617,000	2.09%
15	Missouri	12,918,009,000	2.07%
16	Tennessee	12,807,220,000	2.05%
17	Washington	12,022,436,000	1.93%
18	Maryland	11,824,018,000	1.90%
19	Wisconsin	11,288,091,000	1.81%
20	Minnesota	11,199,561,000	1.80%
21	Louisiana	10,204,980,000	1.64%
22	Connecticut	9,932,092,000	1.59%
23	Alabama	9,400,816,000	1.51%
24	Arizona	8,624,782,000	1.38%
25	Colorado	8,000,876,000	1.28%
26	Kentucky	7,923,070,000	1.27%
27	South Carolina	6,612,570,000	1.06%
28	Oklahoma	6,268,749,000	1.01%
29	Oregon	6,137,525,000	0.98%
30	Iowa	5,852,492,000	0.94%
31	Kansas	5,763,990,000	0.92%
32	Arkansas	4,791,668,000	0.77%
33	Mississippi	4,605,036,000	0.74%
34	West Virginia	4,040,621,000	0.65%
35	Nebraska	3,483,096,000	0.56%
36	Utah	3,216,121,000	0.52%
37	Nevada	3,016,118,000	0.48%
38	New Mexico	2,881,524,000	0.46%
39	Hawaii	2,757,575,000	0.44%
40	Maine	2,666,876,000	0.43%
41	New Hampshire	2,642,095,000	0.42%
42	Rhode Island	2,617,386,000	0.42%
43	Delaware	1,780,075,000	0.29%
44	Idaho	1,775,447,000	0.28%
45	North Dakota	1,651,634,000	0.26%
46	Montana	1,589,295,000	0.25%
47	South Dakota	1,543,627,000	0.25%
48	Alaska	1,225,327,000	0.20%
49	Vermont	1,121,735,000	0.18%
50	Wyoming	708,286,000	0.11%
	District of Columbia	3,872,837,000	0.62%

Source: Morgan Quitno Press using data from U.S. Bureau of the Census
"1992 Census of Service Industries, Geographic Area Series, United States" (SC92-A-52)
*Includes establishments exempt from as well as subject to the federal income tax. Includes those establishments within the Standard Industry Classification (SIC) 80. These include those primarily engaged in furnishing medical, surgical and other health services to persons. See Facilities Chapter for establishments.

Receipts per Health Service Establishment in 1992

National Rate = $1,339,792 per Establishment*

ALPHA ORDER

RANK ORDER

RANK	STATE	PER ESTABLISHMENT		RANK	STATE	PER ESTABLISHMENT
4	Alabama	$1,606,428		1	North Dakota	$1,736,734
27	Alaska	1,304,928		2	Massachusetts	1,700,753
40	Arizona	1,155,517		3	Minnesota	1,676,581
31	Arkansas	1,261,297		4	Alabama	1,606,428
33	California	1,251,696		5	New York	1,549,922
44	Colorado	1,081,199		6	North Carolina	1,520,839
10	Connecticut	1,430,931		7	Tennessee	1,478,040
13	Delaware	1,419,518		8	Missouri	1,452,768
38	Florida	1,201,768		9	Wisconsin	1,438,340
19	Georgia	1,375,541		10	Connecticut	1,430,931
39	Hawaii	1,183,509		11	Louisiana	1,430,872
48	Idaho	966,493		12	Pennsylvania	1,420,492
14	Illinois	1,415,296		13	Delaware	1,419,518
15	Indiana	1,392,701		14	Illinois	1,415,296
32	Iowa	1,252,942		15	Indiana	1,392,701
20	Kansas	1,360,073		16	Mississippi	1,391,670
24	Kentucky	1,322,495		17	Ohio	1,388,854
11	Louisiana	1,430,872		18	West Virginia	1,378,111
42	Maine	1,114,449		19	Georgia	1,375,541
35	Maryland	1,244,110		20	Kansas	1,360,073
2	Massachusetts	1,700,753		21	South Carolina	1,357,817
26	Michigan	1,307,333		22	Nebraska	1,348,469
3	Minnesota	1,676,581		23	South Dakota	1,348,146
16	Mississippi	1,391,670		24	Kentucky	1,322,495
8	Missouri	1,452,768		25	New Hampshire	1,312,516
49	Montana	944,323		26	Michigan	1,307,333
22	Nebraska	1,348,469		27	Alaska	1,304,928
29	Nevada	1,274,237		28	Virginia	1,298,581
25	New Hampshire	1,312,516		29	Nevada	1,274,237
36	New Jersey	1,239,884		30	Rhode Island	1,265,661
43	New Mexico	1,109,132		31	Arkansas	1,261,297
5	New York	1,549,922		32	Iowa	1,252,942
6	North Carolina	1,520,839		33	California	1,251,696
1	North Dakota	1,736,734		34	Texas	1,249,666
17	Ohio	1,388,854		35	Maryland	1,244,110
41	Oklahoma	1,116,032		36	New Jersey	1,239,884
45	Oregon	1,041,317		37	Washington	1,237,003
12	Pennsylvania	1,420,492		38	Florida	1,201,768
30	Rhode Island	1,265,661		39	Hawaii	1,183,509
21	South Carolina	1,357,817		40	Arizona	1,155,517
23	South Dakota	1,340,146		41	Oklahoma	1,110,032
7	Tennessee	1,478,040		42	Maine	1,114,449
34	Texas	1,249,666		43	New Mexico	1,109,132
47	Utah	1,021,964		44	Colorado	1,081,199
46	Vermont	1,040,571		45	Oregon	1,041,317
28	Virginia	1,298,581		46	Vermont	1,040,571
37	Washington	1,237,003		47	Utah	1,021,964
18	West Virginia	1,378,111		48	Idaho	966,493
9	Wisconsin	1,438,340		49	Montana	944,323
50	Wyoming	897,701		50	Wyoming	897,701
					District of Columbia	2,639,971

Source: Morgan Quitno Press using data from U.S. Bureau of the Census
   "1992 Census of Service Industries, Geographic Area Series, United States" (SC92-A-52)
*Includes establishments exempt from as well as subject to the federal income tax. Includes those establishments within the Standard Industry Classification (SIC) 80. These include those primarily engaged in furnishing medical, surgical and other health services to persons. See Facilities Chapter for establishments.

Receipts of Offices and Clinics of Doctors of Medicine in 1992

National Total = $141,429,109,000*

<table>
<tr><td colspan="4">ALPHA ORDER</td><td colspan="4">RANK ORDER</td></tr>
<tr><td>RANK</td><td>STATE</td><td>RECEIPTS</td><td>% of USA</td><td>RANK</td><td>STATE</td><td>RECEIPTS</td><td>% of USA</td></tr>
<tr><td>23</td><td>Alabama</td><td>$2,194,200,000</td><td>1.55%</td><td>1</td><td>California</td><td>$21,969,551,000</td><td>15.53%</td></tr>
<tr><td>48</td><td>Alaska</td><td>257,847,000</td><td>0.18%</td><td>2</td><td>Florida</td><td>10,360,884,000</td><td>7.33%</td></tr>
<tr><td>21</td><td>Arizona</td><td>2,358,063,000</td><td>1.67%</td><td>3</td><td>New York</td><td>9,895,040,000</td><td>7.00%</td></tr>
<tr><td>31</td><td>Arkansas</td><td>1,184,434,000</td><td>0.84%</td><td>4</td><td>Texas</td><td>9,488,688,000</td><td>6.71%</td></tr>
<tr><td>1</td><td>California</td><td>21,969,551,000</td><td>15.53%</td><td>5</td><td>Illinois</td><td>6,252,042,000</td><td>4.42%</td></tr>
<tr><td>26</td><td>Colorado</td><td>1,823,874,000</td><td>1.29%</td><td>6</td><td>Pennsylvania</td><td>6,183,845,000</td><td>4.37%</td></tr>
<tr><td>22</td><td>Connecticut</td><td>2,264,576,000</td><td>1.60%</td><td>7</td><td>Ohio</td><td>5,703,695,000</td><td>4.03%</td></tr>
<tr><td>45</td><td>Delaware</td><td>402,076,000</td><td>0.28%</td><td>8</td><td>New Jersey</td><td>5,079,647,000</td><td>3.59%</td></tr>
<tr><td>2</td><td>Florida</td><td>10,360,884,000</td><td>7.33%</td><td>9</td><td>Georgia</td><td>4,096,050,000</td><td>2.90%</td></tr>
<tr><td>9</td><td>Georgia</td><td>4,096,050,000</td><td>2.90%</td><td>10</td><td>Michigan</td><td>3,899,622,000</td><td>2.76%</td></tr>
<tr><td>38</td><td>Hawaii</td><td>621,177,000</td><td>0.44%</td><td>11</td><td>Virginia</td><td>3,207,044,000</td><td>2.27%</td></tr>
<tr><td>43</td><td>Idaho</td><td>435,493,000</td><td>0.31%</td><td>12</td><td>North Carolina</td><td>3,170,587,000</td><td>2.24%</td></tr>
<tr><td>5</td><td>Illinois</td><td>6,252,042,000</td><td>4.42%</td><td>13</td><td>Massachusetts</td><td>3,103,826,000</td><td>2.19%</td></tr>
<tr><td>16</td><td>Indiana</td><td>2,829,577,000</td><td>2.00%</td><td>14</td><td>Maryland</td><td>3,054,253,000</td><td>2.16%</td></tr>
<tr><td>32</td><td>Iowa</td><td>1,169,464,000</td><td>0.83%</td><td>15</td><td>Tennessee</td><td>2,927,905,000</td><td>2.07%</td></tr>
<tr><td>30</td><td>Kansas</td><td>1,269,708,000</td><td>0.90%</td><td>16</td><td>Indiana</td><td>2,829,577,000</td><td>2.00%</td></tr>
<tr><td>25</td><td>Kentucky</td><td>1,867,177,000</td><td>1.32%</td><td>17</td><td>Missouri</td><td>2,562,807,000</td><td>1.81%</td></tr>
<tr><td>20</td><td>Louisiana</td><td>2,411,609,000</td><td>1.71%</td><td>18</td><td>Wisconsin</td><td>2,415,679,000</td><td>1.71%</td></tr>
<tr><td>41</td><td>Maine</td><td>493,897,000</td><td>0.35%</td><td>19</td><td>Washington</td><td>2,415,635,000</td><td>1.71%</td></tr>
<tr><td>14</td><td>Maryland</td><td>3,054,253,000</td><td>2.16%</td><td>20</td><td>Louisiana</td><td>2,411,609,000</td><td>1.71%</td></tr>
<tr><td>13</td><td>Massachusetts</td><td>3,103,826,000</td><td>2.19%</td><td>21</td><td>Arizona</td><td>2,358,063,000</td><td>1.67%</td></tr>
<tr><td>10</td><td>Michigan</td><td>3,899,622,000</td><td>2.76%</td><td>22</td><td>Connecticut</td><td>2,264,576,000</td><td>1.60%</td></tr>
<tr><td>24</td><td>Minnesota</td><td>1,964,322,000</td><td>1.39%</td><td>23</td><td>Alabama</td><td>2,194,200,000</td><td>1.55%</td></tr>
<tr><td>33</td><td>Mississippi</td><td>968,510,000</td><td>0.68%</td><td>24</td><td>Minnesota</td><td>1,964,322,000</td><td>1.39%</td></tr>
<tr><td>17</td><td>Missouri</td><td>2,562,807,000</td><td>1.81%</td><td>25</td><td>Kentucky</td><td>1,867,177,000</td><td>1.32%</td></tr>
<tr><td>46</td><td>Montana</td><td>336,865,000</td><td>0.24%</td><td>26</td><td>Colorado</td><td>1,823,874,000</td><td>1.29%</td></tr>
<tr><td>37</td><td>Nebraska</td><td>750,417,000</td><td>0.53%</td><td>27</td><td>Oregon</td><td>1,491,857,000</td><td>1.05%</td></tr>
<tr><td>34</td><td>Nevada</td><td>947,372,000</td><td>0.67%</td><td>28</td><td>South Carolina</td><td>1,491,246,000</td><td>1.05%</td></tr>
<tr><td>40</td><td>New Hampshire</td><td>495,024,000</td><td>0.35%</td><td>29</td><td>Oklahoma</td><td>1,366,055,000</td><td>0.97%</td></tr>
<tr><td>8</td><td>New Jersey</td><td>5,079,647,000</td><td>3.59%</td><td>30</td><td>Kansas</td><td>1,269,708,000</td><td>0.90%</td></tr>
<tr><td>39</td><td>New Mexico</td><td>620,805,000</td><td>0.44%</td><td>31</td><td>Arkansas</td><td>1,184,434,000</td><td>0.84%</td></tr>
<tr><td>3</td><td>New York</td><td>9,895,040,000</td><td>7.00%</td><td>32</td><td>Iowa</td><td>1,169,464,000</td><td>0.83%</td></tr>
<tr><td>12</td><td>North Carolina</td><td>3,170,587,000</td><td>2.24%</td><td>33</td><td>Mississippi</td><td>968,510,000</td><td>0.68%</td></tr>
<tr><td>44</td><td>North Dakota</td><td>422,058,000</td><td>0.30%</td><td>34</td><td>Nevada</td><td>947,372,000</td><td>0.67%</td></tr>
<tr><td>7</td><td>Ohio</td><td>5,703,695,000</td><td>4.03%</td><td>35</td><td>West Virginia</td><td>848,606,000</td><td>0.60%</td></tr>
<tr><td>29</td><td>Oklahoma</td><td>1,366,055,000</td><td>0.97%</td><td>36</td><td>Utah</td><td>816,997,000</td><td>0.58%</td></tr>
<tr><td>27</td><td>Oregon</td><td>1,491,857,000</td><td>1.05%</td><td>37</td><td>Nebraska</td><td>750,417,000</td><td>0.53%</td></tr>
<tr><td>6</td><td>Pennsylvania</td><td>6,183,845,000</td><td>4.37%</td><td>38</td><td>Hawaii</td><td>621,177,000</td><td>0.44%</td></tr>
<tr><td>42</td><td>Rhode Island</td><td>458,399,000</td><td>0.32%</td><td>39</td><td>New Mexico</td><td>620,805,000</td><td>0.44%</td></tr>
<tr><td>28</td><td>South Carolina</td><td>1,491,246,000</td><td>1.05%</td><td>40</td><td>New Hampshire</td><td>495,024,000</td><td>0.35%</td></tr>
<tr><td>47</td><td>South Dakota</td><td>305,158,000</td><td>0.22%</td><td>41</td><td>Maine</td><td>493,897,000</td><td>0.35%</td></tr>
<tr><td>15</td><td>Tennessee</td><td>2,927,905,000</td><td>2.07%</td><td>42</td><td>Rhode Island</td><td>458,399,000</td><td>0.32%</td></tr>
<tr><td>4</td><td>Texas</td><td>9,488,688,000</td><td>6.71%</td><td>43</td><td>Idaho</td><td>435,493,000</td><td>0.31%</td></tr>
<tr><td>36</td><td>Utah</td><td>816,997,000</td><td>0.58%</td><td>44</td><td>North Dakota</td><td>422,058,000</td><td>0.30%</td></tr>
<tr><td>49</td><td>Vermont</td><td>187,557,000</td><td>0.13%</td><td>45</td><td>Delaware</td><td>402,076,000</td><td>0.28%</td></tr>
<tr><td>11</td><td>Virginia</td><td>3,207,044,000</td><td>2.27%</td><td>46</td><td>Montana</td><td>336,865,000</td><td>0.24%</td></tr>
<tr><td>19</td><td>Washington</td><td>2,415,635,000</td><td>1.71%</td><td>47</td><td>South Dakota</td><td>305,158,000</td><td>0.22%</td></tr>
<tr><td>35</td><td>West Virginia</td><td>848,606,000</td><td>0.60%</td><td>48</td><td>Alaska</td><td>257,847,000</td><td>0.18%</td></tr>
<tr><td>18</td><td>Wisconsin</td><td>2,415,679,000</td><td>1.71%</td><td>49</td><td>Vermont</td><td>187,557,000</td><td>0.13%</td></tr>
<tr><td>50</td><td>Wyoming</td><td>148,221,000</td><td>0.10%</td><td>50</td><td>Wyoming</td><td>148,221,000</td><td>0.10%</td></tr>
<tr><td></td><td></td><td></td><td></td><td></td><td>District of Columbia</td><td>439,668,000</td><td>0.31%</td></tr>
</table>

Source: U.S. Bureau of the Census
  "1992 Census of Service Industries, Geographic Area Series, United States" (SC92-A-52)
*Includes only establishments subject to the federal income tax. See Facilities Chapter for establishments.

Receipts per Office or Clinic of Doctors of Medicine in 1992

National Rate = $715,369 per Establishment*

ALPHA ORDER

RANK	STATE	PER ESTABLISHMENT
9	Alabama	$840,368
19	Alaska	738,817
16	Arizona	748,591
24	Arkansas	711,799
13	California	771,024
29	Colorado	676,010
17	Connecticut	745,171
27	Delaware	684,968
22	Florida	715,185
11	Georgia	785,587
45	Hawaii	582,718
44	Idaho	598,205
18	Illinois	742,170
15	Indiana	755,763
6	Iowa	866,912
4	Kansas	918,747
21	Kentucky	727,944
20	Louisiana	732,344
47	Maine	540,369
40	Maryland	641,650
26	Massachusetts	686,080
37	Michigan	657,055
2	Minnesota	1,327,245
32	Mississippi	664,273
12	Missouri	781,344
46	Montana	562,379
8	Nebraska	846,972
7	Nevada	864,391
38	New Hampshire	656,531
36	New Jersey	658,156
43	New Mexico	600,973
42	New York	609,826
10	North Carolina	828,695
1	North Dakota	1,736,864
23	Ohio	712,606
31	Oklahoma	665,719
35	Oregon	659,239
33	Pennsylvania	661,586
48	Rhode Island	515,634
30	South Carolina	672,035
5	South Dakota	874,378
14	Tennessee	762,475
34	Texas	660,450
39	Utah	647,896
50	Vermont	477,244
28	Virginia	678,883
25	Washington	697,354
41	West Virginia	633,288
3	Wisconsin	948,813
49	Wyoming	504,153

RANK ORDER

RANK	STATE	PER ESTABLISHMENT
1	North Dakota	$1,736,864
2	Minnesota	1,327,245
3	Wisconsin	948,813
4	Kansas	918,747
5	South Dakota	874,378
6	Iowa	866,912
7	Nevada	864,391
8	Nebraska	846,972
9	Alabama	840,368
10	North Carolina	828,695
11	Georgia	785,587
12	Missouri	781,344
13	California	771,024
14	Tennessee	762,475
15	Indiana	755,763
16	Arizona	748,591
17	Connecticut	745,171
18	Illinois	742,170
19	Alaska	738,817
20	Louisiana	732,344
21	Kentucky	727,944
22	Florida	715,185
23	Ohio	712,606
24	Arkansas	711,799
25	Washington	697,354
26	Massachusetts	686,080
27	Delaware	684,968
28	Virginia	678,883
29	Colorado	676,010
30	South Carolina	672,035
31	Oklahoma	665,719
32	Mississippi	664,273
33	Pennsylvania	661,586
34	Texas	660,450
35	Oregon	659,239
36	New Jersey	658,156
37	Michigan	657,055
38	New Hampshire	656,531
39	Utah	647,896
40	Maryland	641,650
41	West Virginia	633,288
42	New York	609,826
43	New Mexico	600,973
44	Idaho	598,205
45	Hawaii	582,718
46	Montana	562,379
47	Maine	540,369
48	Rhode Island	515,634
49	Wyoming	504,153
50	Vermont	477,244
	District of Columbia	568,781

Source: Morgan Quitno Press using data from U.S. Bureau of the Census
"1992 Census of Service Industries, Geographic Area Series, United States" (SC92-A-52)
*Includes only establishments subject to the federal income tax. See Facilities Chapter for establishments.

Receipts of Offices and Clinics of Dentists in 1992

National Total = $35,522,953,000*

ALPHA ORDER

RANK	STATE	RECEIPTS	% of USA
25	Alabama	$423,367,000	1.30%
44	Alaska	114,760,000	0.35%
24	Arizona	506,268,000	1.56%
33	Arkansas	226,609,000	0.70%
1	California	5,523,663,000	16.98%
22	Colorado	555,652,000	1.71%
18	Connecticut	669,243,000	2.06%
45	Delaware	102,416,000	0.31%
4	Florida	1,893,179,000	5.82%
19	Georgia	644,777,000	1.98%
34	Hawaii	219,683,000	0.68%
42	Idaho	150,221,000	0.46%
6	Illinois	1,510,700,000	4.65%
12	Indiana	840,283,000	2.58%
30	Iowa	320,371,000	0.99%
31	Kansas	306,171,000	0.94%
28	Kentucky	338,975,000	1.04%
26	Louisiana	409,110,000	1.26%
41	Maine	150,904,000	0.46%
16	Maryland	713,076,000	2.19%
11	Massachusetts	992,382,000	3.05%
7	Michigan	1,475,023,000	4.54%
17	Minnesota	686,914,000	2.11%
36	Mississippi	198,070,000	0.61%
21	Missouri	569,399,000	1.75%
46	Montana	96,335,000	0.30%
37	Nebraska	185,366,000	0.57%
35	Nevada	204,068,000	0.63%
39	New Hampshire	167,595,000	0.52%
8	New Jersey	1,415,884,000	4.35%
40	New Mexico	160,064,000	0.49%
2	New York	2,770,069,000	8.52%
14	North Carolina	760,910,000	2.34%
49	North Dakota	70,632,000	0.22%
9	Ohio	1,337,215,000	4.11%
29	Oklahoma	338,025,000	1.04%
23	Oregon	526,242,000	1.62%
5	Pennsylvania	1,571,424,000	4.83%
43	Rhode Island	148,838,000	0.46%
27	South Carolina	364,380,000	1.12%
47	South Dakota	79,410,000	0.24%
20	Tennessee	572,138,000	1.76%
3	Texas	1,919,816,000	5.90%
32	Utah	257,633,000	0.79%
48	Vermont	78,673,000	0.24%
13	Virginia	811,992,000	2.50%
10	Washington	1,088,396,000	3.35%
38	West Virginia	174,028,000	0.54%
15	Wisconsin	718,189,000	2.21%
50	Wyoming	52,712,000	0.16%

RANK ORDER

RANK	STATE	RECEIPTS	% of USA
1	California	$5,523,663,000	16.98%
2	New York	2,770,069,000	8.52%
3	Texas	1,919,816,000	5.90%
4	Florida	1,893,179,000	5.82%
5	Pennsylvania	1,571,424,000	4.83%
6	Illinois	1,510,700,000	4.65%
7	Michigan	1,475,023,000	4.54%
8	New Jersey	1,415,884,000	4.35%
9	Ohio	1,337,215,000	4.11%
10	Washington	1,088,396,000	3.35%
11	Massachusetts	992,382,000	3.05%
12	Indiana	840,283,000	2.58%
13	Virginia	811,992,000	2.50%
14	North Carolina	760,910,000	2.34%
15	Wisconsin	718,189,000	2.21%
16	Maryland	713,076,000	2.19%
17	Minnesota	686,914,000	2.11%
18	Connecticut	669,243,000	2.06%
19	Georgia	644,777,000	1.98%
20	Tennessee	572,138,000	1.76%
21	Missouri	569,399,000	1.75%
22	Colorado	555,652,000	1.71%
23	Oregon	526,242,000	1.62%
24	Arizona	506,268,000	1.56%
25	Alabama	423,367,000	1.30%
26	Louisiana	409,110,000	1.26%
27	South Carolina	364,380,000	1.12%
28	Kentucky	338,975,000	1.04%
29	Oklahoma	338,025,000	1.04%
30	Iowa	320,371,000	0.99%
31	Kansas	306,171,000	0.94%
32	Utah	257,633,000	0.79%
33	Arkansas	226,609,000	0.70%
34	Hawaii	219,683,000	0.68%
35	Nevada	204,068,000	0.63%
36	Mississippi	198,070,000	0.61%
37	Nebraska	185,366,000	0.57%
38	West Virginia	174,028,000	0.54%
39	New Hampshire	167,595,000	0.52%
40	New Mexico	160,064,000	0.49%
41	Maine	150,904,000	0.46%
42	Idaho	150,221,000	0.46%
43	Rhode Island	148,838,000	0.46%
44	Alaska	114,760,000	0.35%
45	Delaware	102,416,000	0.31%
46	Montana	96,335,000	0.30%
47	South Dakota	79,410,000	0.24%
48	Vermont	78,673,000	0.24%
49	North Dakota	70,632,000	0.22%
50	Wyoming	52,712,000	0.16%
	District of Columbia	111,703,000	0.34%

Source: U.S. Bureau of the Census
"1992 Census of Service Industries, Geographic Area Series, United States" (SC92-A-52)
Includes only establishments subject to the federal income tax. See Facilities Chapter for establishments.

Receipts per Office or Clinic of Dentists in 1992

National Rate = $326,486 per Establishment*

<u>ALPHA ORDER</u>   <u>RANK ORDER</u>

RANK	STATE	PER ESTABLISHMENT		RANK	STATE	PER ESTABLISHMENT
26	Alabama	$318,082		1	Delaware	$476,353
2	Alaska	438,015		2	Alaska	438,015
16	Arizona	332,633		3	Nevada	426,921
41	Arkansas	275,680		4	Washington	407,029
7	California	373,069		5	Indiana	385,982
36	Colorado	290,765		6	Connecticut	384,622
6	Connecticut	384,622		7	California	373,069
1	Delaware	476,353		8	Rhode Island	366,596
9	Florida	352,285		9	Florida	352,285
43	Georgia	274,841		10	North Carolina	351,947
12	Hawaii	343,255		11	New Jersey	351,075
18	Idaho	330,156		12	Hawaii	343,255
35	Illinois	292,998		13	Minnesota	341,748
5	Indiana	385,982		14	Michigan	339,242
39	Iowa	278,826		15	Massachusetts	337,430
31	Kansas	305,255		16	Arizona	332,633
50	Kentucky	231,857		17	Oregon	331,595
45	Louisiana	264,283		18	Idaho	330,156
19	Maine	329,485		19	Maine	329,485
21	Maryland	324,864		20	New Hampshire	326,060
15	Massachusetts	337,430		21	Maryland	324,864
14	Michigan	339,242		22	New York	323,606
13	Minnesota	341,748		23	Virginia	321,708
47	Mississippi	252,640		24	Wisconsin	321,337
40	Missouri	278,163		25	Vermont	321,114
49	Montana	242,657		26	Alabama	318,082
48	Nebraska	248,147		27	South Carolina	316,028
3	Nevada	426,921		28	West Virginia	309,108
20	New Hampshire	326,060		29	Texas	308,008
11	New Jersey	351,075		30	South Dakota	305,423
32	New Mexico	300,872		31	Kansas	305,255
22	New York	323,606		32	New Mexico	300,872
10	North Carolina	351,947		33	Ohio	297,357
38	North Dakota	282,528		34	Pennsylvania	295,603
33	Ohio	297,357		35	Illinois	292,998
42	Oklahoma	275,041		36	Colorado	290,765
17	Oregon	331,595		37	Tennessee	288,376
34	Pennsylvania	295,603		38	North Dakota	282,528
8	Rhode Island	366,596		39	Iowa	278,826
27	South Carolina	316,028		40	Missouri	278,163
30	South Dakota	305,423		41	Arkansas	275,680
37	Tennessee	288,376		42	Oklahoma	275,041
29	Texas	308,008		43	Georgia	274,841
44	Utah	264,510		44	Utah	264,510
25	Vermont	321,114		45	Louisiana	264,283
23	Virginia	321,708		46	Wyoming	260,950
4	Washington	407,029		47	Mississippi	252,640
28	West Virginia	309,108		48	Nebraska	248,147
24	Wisconsin	321,337		49	Montana	242,657
46	Wyoming	260,950		50	Kentucky	231,857
					District of Columbia	321,911

Source: Morgan Quitno Press using data from U.S. Bureau of the Census
"1992 Census of Service Industries, Geographic Area Series, United States" (SC92-A-52)
*Includes only establishments subject to the federal income tax. See Facilities Chapter for establishments.

Receipts of Offices and Clinics of Doctors of Osteopathy in 1992

National Total = $3,638,144,000*

ALPHA ORDER				RANK ORDER			
RANK	STATE	RECEIPTS	% of USA	RANK	STATE	RECEIPTS	% of USA
31	Alabama	$10,073,000	0.28%	1	Michigan	$593,339,000	16.31%
36	Alaska	5,757,000	0.16%	2	Pennsylvania	447,326,000	12.30%
8	Arizona	141,382,000	3.89%	3	Ohio	386,003,000	10.61%
33	Arkansas	7,486,000	0.21%	4	Florida	325,522,000	8.95%
9	California	128,791,000	3.54%	5	Texas	286,680,000	7.88%
13	Colorado	68,206,000	1.87%	6	New Jersey	213,199,000	5.86%
NA	Connecticut**	NA	NA	7	Missouri	160,312,000	4.41%
23	Delaware	23,457,000	0.64%	8	Arizona	141,382,000	3.89%
4	Florida	325,522,000	8.95%	9	California	128,791,000	3.54%
17	Georgia	42,184,000	1.16%	10	Oklahoma	127,260,000	3.50%
NA	Hawaii**	NA	NA	11	Iowa	77,485,000	2.13%
37	Idaho	4,797,000	0.13%	12	New York	74,955,000	2.06%
14	Illinois	62,781,000	1.73%	13	Colorado	68,206,000	1.87%
15	Indiana	54,594,000	1.50%	14	Illinois	62,781,000	1.73%
11	Iowa	77,485,000	2.13%	15	Indiana	54,594,000	1.50%
18	Kansas	39,828,000	1.09%	16	Washington	46,322,000	1.27%
30	Kentucky	10,275,000	0.28%	17	Georgia	42,184,000	1.16%
44	Louisiana	1,804,000	0.05%	18	Kansas	39,828,000	1.09%
20	Maine	36,670,000	1.01%	19	West Virginia	37,666,000	1.04%
38	Maryland	4,765,000	0.13%	20	Maine	36,670,000	1.01%
29	Massachusetts	10,746,000	0.30%	21	Wisconsin	36,056,000	0.99%
1	Michigan	593,339,000	16.31%	22	Oregon	32,862,000	0.90%
NA	Minnesota**	NA	NA	23	Delaware	23,457,000	0.64%
32	Mississippi	8,865,000	0.24%	24	Tennessee	22,588,000	0.62%
7	Missouri	160,312,000	4.41%	25	New Mexico	18,596,000	0.51%
41	Montana	3,003,000	0.08%	26	Rhode Island	16,940,000	0.47%
NA	Nebraska**	NA	NA	27	Nevada	16,329,000	0.45%
27	Nevada	16,329,000	0.45%	28	Virginia	13,366,000	0.37%
42	New Hampshire	2,867,000	0.08%	29	Massachusetts	10,746,000	0.30%
6	New Jersey	213,199,000	5.86%	30	Kentucky	10,275,000	0.28%
25	New Mexico	18,596,000	0.51%	31	Alabama	10,073,000	0.28%
12	New York	74,955,000	2.06%	32	Mississippi	8,865,000	0.24%
35	North Carolina	6,445,000	0.18%	33	Arkansas	7,486,000	0.21%
NA	North Dakota**	NA	NA	34	South Carolina	6,489,000	0.18%
3	Ohio	386,003,000	10.61%	35	North Carolina	6,445,000	0.18%
10	Oklahoma	127,260,000	3.50%	36	Alaska	5,757,000	0.16%
22	Oregon	32,862,000	0.90%	37	Idaho	4,797,000	0.13%
2	Pennsylvania	447,326,000	12.30%	38	Maryland	4,765,000	0.13%
26	Rhode Island	16,940,000	0.47%	39	South Dakota	3,914,000	0.11%
34	South Carolina	6,489,000	0.18%	40	Utah	3,446,000	0.09%
39	South Dakota	3,914,000	0.11%	41	Montana	3,003,000	0.08%
24	Tennessee	22,588,000	0.62%	42	New Hampshire	2,867,000	0.08%
5	Texas	286,680,000	7.88%	43	Wyoming	2,617,000	0.07%
40	Utah	3,446,000	0.09%	44	Louisiana	1,804,000	0.05%
45	Vermont	1,074,000	0.03%	45	Vermont	1,074,000	0.03%
28	Virginia	13,366,000	0.37%	NA	Connecticut**	NA	NA
16	Washington	46,322,000	1.27%	NA	Hawaii**	NA	NA
19	West Virginia	37,666,000	1.04%	NA	Minnesota**	NA	NA
21	Wisconsin	36,056,000	0.99%	NA	Nebraska**	NA	NA
43	Wyoming	2,617,000	0.07%	NA	North Dakota**	NA	NA
					District of Columbia**	NA	NA

Source: U.S. Bureau of the Census
"1992 Census of Service Industries, Geographic Area Series, United States" (SC92-A-52)
*Includes only establishments subject to the federal income tax. See Facilities Chapter for establishments.
**Not available.

Receipts per Office or Clinic of Doctors of Osteopathy in 1992

National Rate = $417,793 per Establishment*

ALPHA ORDER

RANK ORDER

RANK	STATE	PER ESTABLISHMENT
32	Alabama	$314,781
2	Alaska	523,364
6	Arizona	446,000
40	Arkansas	287,923
16	California	399,972
29	Colorado	329,498
NA	Connecticut**	NA
5	Delaware	469,140
10	Florida	427,194
27	Georgia	340,194
NA	Hawaii**	NA
22	Idaho	369,000
23	Illinois	362,896
19	Indiana	384,465
15	Iowa	401,477
13	Kansas	410,598
41	Kentucky	270,395
37	Louisiana	300,667
36	Maine	305,583
38	Maryland	297,813
42	Massachusetts	268,650
3	Michigan	494,037
NA	Minnesota**	NA
7	Mississippi	443,250
24	Missouri	359,444
44	Montana	250,250
NA	Nebraska**	NA
17	Nevada	398,268
31	New Hampshire	318,556
1	New Jersey	534,333
30	New Mexico	326,246
21	New York	372,910
28	North Carolina	339,211
NA	North Dakota**	NA
4	Ohio	470,162
18	Oklahoma	387,988
39	Oregon	293,411
11	Pennsylvania	421,211
35	Rhode Island	308,000
34	South Carolina	309,000
8	South Dakota	434,889
9	Tennessee	434,385
14	Texas	405,488
25	Utah	344,600
45	Vermont	179,000
26	Virginia	342,718
33	Washington	310,886
12	West Virginia	418,511
20	Wisconsin	375,583
43	Wyoming	261,700

RANK	STATE	PER ESTABLISHMENT
1	New Jersey	$534,333
2	Alaska	523,364
3	Michigan	494,037
4	Ohio	470,162
5	Delaware	469,140
6	Arizona	446,000
7	Mississippi	443,250
8	South Dakota	434,889
9	Tennessee	434,385
10	Florida	427,194
11	Pennsylvania	421,211
12	West Virginia	418,511
13	Kansas	410,598
14	Texas	405,488
15	Iowa	401,477
16	California	399,972
17	Nevada	398,268
18	Oklahoma	387,988
19	Indiana	384,465
20	Wisconsin	375,583
21	New York	372,910
22	Idaho	369,000
23	Illinois	362,896
24	Missouri	359,444
25	Utah	344,600
26	Virginia	342,718
27	Georgia	340,194
28	North Carolina	339,211
29	Colorado	329,498
30	New Mexico	326,246
31	New Hampshire	318,556
32	Alabama	314,781
33	Washington	310,886
34	South Carolina	309,000
35	Rhode Island	308,000
36	Maine	305,583
37	Louisiana	300,667
38	Maryland	297,813
39	Oregon	293,411
40	Arkansas	287,923
41	Kentucky	270,395
42	Massachusetts	268,650
43	Wyoming	261,700
44	Montana	250,250
45	Vermont	179,000
NA	Connecticut**	NA
NA	Hawaii**	NA
NA	Minnesota**	NA
NA	Nebraska**	NA
NA	North Dakota**	NA
	District of Columbia**	NA

Source: Morgan Quitno Press using data from U.S. Bureau of the Census
   "1992 Census of Service Industries, Geographic Area Series, United States" (SC92-A-52)
*Includes only establishments subject to the federal income tax. See Facilities Chapter for establishments.
**Not available.

Receipts of Offices and Clinics of Chiropractors in 1992

National Total = $5,917,909,000*

ALPHA ORDER					RANK ORDER			

RANK	STATE	RECEIPTS	% of USA
31	Alabama	$50,995,000	0.86%
41	Alaska	21,901,000	0.37%
15	Arizona	123,169,000	2.08%
33	Arkansas	39,365,000	0.67%
1	California	972,152,000	16.43%
17	Colorado	100,648,000	1.70%
16	Connecticut	101,975,000	1.72%
48	Delaware	13,666,000	0.23%
2	Florida	444,248,000	7.51%
12	Georgia	154,081,000	2.60%
34	Hawaii	38,828,000	0.66%
40	Idaho	22,470,000	0.38%
8	Illinois	216,560,000	3.66%
19	Indiana	98,161,000	1.66%
24	Iowa	68,192,000	1.15%
28	Kansas	58,992,000	1.00%
30	Kentucky	51,115,000	0.86%
29	Louisiana	58,506,000	0.99%
38	Maine	26,779,000	0.45%
22	Maryland	76,300,000	1.29%
9	Massachusetts	163,870,000	2.77%
11	Michigan	155,693,000	2.63%
10	Minnesota	160,994,000	2.72%
44	Mississippi	19,203,000	0.32%
20	Missouri	89,333,000	1.51%
46	Montana	16,310,000	0.28%
36	Nebraska	30,074,000	0.51%
32	Nevada	47,657,000	0.81%
42	New Hampshire	21,688,000	0.37%
5	New Jersey	326,710,000	5.52%
35	New Mexico	34,298,000	0.58%
3	New York	388,348,000	6.56%
18	North Carolina	99,116,000	1.67%
47	North Dakota	14,992,000	0.25%
7	Ohio	237,979,000	4.02%
25	Oklahoma	66,456,000	1.12%
27	Oregon	60,225,000	1.02%
6	Pennsylvania	293,051,000	4.95%
45	Rhode Island	17,967,000	0.30%
26	South Carolina	60,285,000	1.02%
43	South Dakota	20,907,000	0.35%
23	Tennessee	74,113,000	1.25%
4	Texas	331,418,000	5.60%
37	Utah	27,714,000	0.47%
49	Vermont	10,566,000	0.18%
21	Virginia	85,384,000	1.44%
13	Washington	147,177,000	2.49%
39	West Virginia	24,442,000	0.41%
14	Wisconsin	142,761,000	2.41%
50	Wyoming	6,966,000	0.12%

RANK ORDER

RANK	STATE	RECEIPTS	% of USA
1	California	$972,152,000	16.43%
2	Florida	444,248,000	7.51%
3	New York	388,348,000	6.56%
4	Texas	331,418,000	5.60%
5	New Jersey	326,710,000	5.52%
6	Pennsylvania	293,051,000	4.95%
7	Ohio	237,979,000	4.02%
8	Illinois	216,560,000	3.66%
9	Massachusetts	163,870,000	2.77%
10	Minnesota	160,994,000	2.72%
11	Michigan	155,693,000	2.63%
12	Georgia	154,081,000	2.60%
13	Washington	147,177,000	2.49%
14	Wisconsin	142,761,000	2.41%
15	Arizona	123,169,000	2.08%
16	Connecticut	101,975,000	1.72%
17	Colorado	100,648,000	1.70%
18	North Carolina	99,116,000	1.67%
19	Indiana	98,161,000	1.66%
20	Missouri	89,333,000	1.51%
21	Virginia	85,384,000	1.44%
22	Maryland	76,300,000	1.29%
23	Tennessee	74,113,000	1.25%
24	Iowa	68,192,000	1.15%
25	Oklahoma	66,456,000	1.12%
26	South Carolina	60,285,000	1.02%
27	Oregon	60,225,000	1.02%
28	Kansas	58,992,000	1.00%
29	Louisiana	58,506,000	0.99%
30	Kentucky	51,115,000	0.86%
31	Alabama	50,995,000	0.86%
32	Nevada	47,657,000	0.81%
33	Arkansas	39,365,000	0.67%
34	Hawaii	38,828,000	0.66%
35	New Mexico	34,298,000	0.58%
36	Nebraska	30,074,000	0.51%
37	Utah	27,714,000	0.47%
38	Maine	26,779,000	0.45%
39	West Virginia	24,442,000	0.41%
40	Idaho	22,470,000	0.38%
41	Alaska	21,901,000	0.37%
42	New Hampshire	21,688,000	0.37%
43	South Dakota	20,907,000	0.35%
44	Mississippi	19,203,000	0.32%
45	Rhode Island	17,967,000	0.30%
46	Montana	16,310,000	0.28%
47	North Dakota	14,992,000	0.25%
48	Delaware	13,666,000	0.23%
49	Vermont	10,566,000	0.18%
50	Wyoming	6,966,000	0.12%
	District of Columbia	4,109,000	0.07%

Source: U.S. Bureau of the Census
"1992 Census of Service Industries, Geographic Area Series, United States" (SC92-A-52)
*Includes only establishments subject to the federal income tax. See Facilities Chapter for establishments.

Receipts per Office or Clinic of Chiropractors in 1992

National Rate = $216,543 per Establishment*

ALPHA ORDER

RANK ORDER

RANK	STATE	PER ESTABLISHMENT	RANK	STATE	PER ESTABLISHMENT
37	Alabama	$180,833	1	Maryland	$330,303
3	Alaska	308,465	2	Hawaii	326,286
28	Arizona	198,021	3	Alaska	308,465
44	Arkansas	166,097	4	Connecticut	293,876
19	California	222,766	5	Nevada	287,090
39	Colorado	170,879	6	Massachusetts	284,991
4	Connecticut	293,876	7	Delaware	273,320
7	Delaware	273,320	8	Ohio	273,225
10	Florida	240,524	9	New Jersey	262,418
26	Georgia	202,738	10	Florida	240,524
2	Hawaii	326,286	11	Virginia	240,518
42	Idaho	167,687	12	West Virginia	232,781
25	Illinois	202,772	13	Texas	232,411
16	Indiana	225,140	14	Rhode Island	227,430
47	Iowa	152,897	15	North Carolina	225,777
34	Kansas	183,776	16	Indiana	225,140
30	Kentucky	190,019	17	Pennsylvania	223,703
24	Louisiana	206,007	18	New York	223,060
21	Maine	212,532	19	California	222,766
1	Maryland	330,303	20	Wisconsin	214,678
6	Massachusetts	284,991	21	Maine	212,532
45	Michigan	165,984	22	Oklahoma	210,304
29	Minnesota	195,381	23	Tennessee	208,183
40	Mississippi	169,938	24	Louisiana	206,007
48	Missouri	149,386	25	Illinois	202,772
50	Montana	139,402	26	Georgia	202,738
33	Nebraska	184,503	27	New Hampshire	200,815
5	Nevada	287,090	28	Arizona	198,021
27	New Hampshire	200,815	29	Minnesota	195,381
9	New Jersey	262,418	30	Kentucky	190,019
32	New Mexico	185,395	31	South Carolina	188,981
18	New York	223,060	32	New Mexico	185,395
15	North Carolina	225,777	33	Nebraska	184,503
43	North Dakota	166,578	34	Kansas	183,776
8	Ohio	273,225	35	Washington	183,056
22	Oklahoma	210,304	36	Utah	181,137
49	Oregon	140,713	37	Alabama	180,833
17	Pennsylvania	223,703	38	South Dakota	177,178
14	Rhode Island	227,430	39	Colorado	170,879
31	South Carolina	188,981	40	Mississippi	169,938
38	South Dakota	177,178	41	Wyoming	160,002
23	Tennessee	208,183	42	Idaho	167,687
13	Texas	232,411	43	North Dakota	166,578
36	Utah	181,137	44	Arkansas	166,097
46	Vermont	162,554	45	Michigan	165,984
11	Virginia	240,518	46	Vermont	162,554
35	Washington	183,056	47	Iowa	152,897
12	West Virginia	232,781	48	Missouri	149,386
20	Wisconsin	214,678	49	Oregon	140,713
41	Wyoming	169,902	50	Montana	139,402
				District of Columbia	316,077

Source: Morgan Quitno Press using data from U.S. Bureau of the Census
"1992 Census of Service Industries, Geographic Area Series, United States" (SC92-A-52)
Includes only establishments subject to the federal income tax. See Facilities Chapter for establishments.

Receipts of Offices and Clinics of Optometrists in 1992

National Total = $4,939,521,000*

ALPHA ORDER

RANK	STATE	RECEIPTS	% of USA
27	Alabama	$65,608,000	1.33%
47	Alaska	17,112,000	0.35%
31	Arizona	49,165,000	1.00%
29	Arkansas	56,672,000	1.15%
1	California	754,317,000	15.27%
24	Colorado	73,235,000	1.48%
23	Connecticut	73,960,000	1.50%
49	Delaware	12,873,000	0.26%
5	Florida	221,280,000	4.48%
13	Georgia	102,345,000	2.07%
39	Hawaii	27,647,000	0.56%
40	Idaho	24,607,000	0.50%
7	Illinois	213,734,000	4.33%
11	Indiana	133,059,000	2.69%
19	Iowa	79,034,000	1.60%
20	Kansas	78,371,000	1.59%
25	Kentucky	72,650,000	1.47%
32	Louisiana	48,393,000	0.98%
37	Maine	35,347,000	0.72%
21	Maryland	78,104,000	1.58%
15	Massachusetts	97,781,000	1.98%
8	Michigan	203,832,000	4.13%
26	Minnesota	71,690,000	1.45%
35	Mississippi	37,655,000	0.76%
18	Missouri	88,489,000	1.79%
41	Montana	24,435,000	0.49%
34	Nebraska	38,725,000	0.78%
36	Nevada	36,924,000	0.75%
45	New Hampshire	20,073,000	0.41%
9	New Jersey	147,976,000	3.00%
38	New Mexico	30,091,000	0.61%
4	New York	226,940,000	4.59%
10	North Carolina	146,551,000	2.97%
43	North Dakota	21,635,000	0.44%
6	Ohio	218,608,000	4.43%
22	Oklahoma	76,308,000	1.54%
30	Oregon	51,605,000	1.04%
3	Pennsylvania	246,226,000	4.98%
44	Rhode Island	21,103,000	0.43%
28	South Carolina	58,093,000	1.18%
46	South Dakota	19,165,000	0.39%
14	Tennessee	101,398,000	2.05%
2	Texas	329,294,000	6.67%
42	Utah	21,944,000	0.44%
50	Vermont	11,768,000	0.24%
12	Virginia	115,755,000	2.34%
16	Washington	95,398,000	1.93%
33	West Virginia	43,184,000	0.87%
17	Wisconsin	94,432,000	1.91%
48	Wyoming	15,714,000	0.32%

RANK ORDER

RANK	STATE	RECEIPTS	% of USA
1	California	$754,317,000	15.27%
2	Texas	329,294,000	6.67%
3	Pennsylvania	246,226,000	4.98%
4	New York	226,940,000	4.59%
5	Florida	221,280,000	4.48%
6	Ohio	218,608,000	4.43%
7	Illinois	213,734,000	4.33%
8	Michigan	203,832,000	4.13%
9	New Jersey	147,976,000	3.00%
10	North Carolina	146,551,000	2.97%
11	Indiana	133,059,000	2.69%
12	Virginia	115,755,000	2.34%
13	Georgia	102,345,000	2.07%
14	Tennessee	101,398,000	2.05%
15	Massachusetts	97,781,000	1.98%
16	Washington	95,398,000	1.93%
17	Wisconsin	94,432,000	1.91%
18	Missouri	88,489,000	1.79%
19	Iowa	79,034,000	1.60%
20	Kansas	78,371,000	1.59%
21	Maryland	78,104,000	1.58%
22	Oklahoma	76,308,000	1.54%
23	Connecticut	73,960,000	1.50%
24	Colorado	73,235,000	1.48%
25	Kentucky	72,650,000	1.47%
26	Minnesota	71,690,000	1.45%
27	Alabama	65,608,000	1.33%
28	South Carolina	58,093,000	1.18%
29	Arkansas	56,672,000	1.15%
30	Oregon	51,605,000	1.04%
31	Arizona	49,165,000	1.00%
32	Louisiana	48,393,000	0.98%
33	West Virginia	43,184,000	0.87%
34	Nebraska	38,725,000	0.78%
35	Mississippi	37,655,000	0.76%
36	Nevada	36,924,000	0.75%
37	Maine	35,347,000	0.72%
38	New Mexico	30,091,000	0.61%
39	Hawaii	27,647,000	0.56%
40	Idaho	24,607,000	0.50%
41	Montana	24,435,000	0.49%
42	Utah	21,944,000	0.44%
43	North Dakota	21,635,000	0.44%
44	Rhode Island	21,103,000	0.43%
45	New Hampshire	20,073,000	0.41%
46	South Dakota	19,165,000	0.39%
47	Alaska	17,112,000	0.35%
48	Wyoming	15,714,000	0.32%
49	Delaware	12,873,000	0.26%
50	Vermont	11,768,000	0.24%
	District of Columbia	9,216,000	0.19%

Source: U.S. Bureau of the Census
"1992 Census of Service Industries, Geographic Area Series, United States" (SC92-A-52)
*Includes only establishments subject to the federal income tax. See Facilities Chapter for establishments.

Receipts per Office or Clinic of Optometrists in 1992

National Rate = $288,271 per Establishment*

RANK	STATE	PER ESTABLISHMENT	RANK	STATE	PER ESTABLISHMENT
24	Alabama	$286,498	1	Alaska	$388,909
1	Alaska	388,909	2	North Dakota	338,047
41	Arizona	260,132	3	Michigan	335,802
28	Arkansas	280,554	4	Nevada	335,673
10	California	316,674	5	Maryland	332,357
26	Colorado	284,961	6	Connecticut	324,386
6	Connecticut	324,386	7	Delaware	321,825
7	Delaware	321,825	8	Nebraska	320,041
42	Florida	259,110	9	Kansas	317,291
32	Georgia	274,383	10	California	316,674
30	Hawaii	279,263	11	Illinois	306,209
39	Idaho	261,777	12	Texas	299,358
11	Illinois	306,209	13	North Carolina	294,279
21	Indiana	287,384	14	Missouri	293,983
18	Iowa	292,719	15	South Carolina	293,399
9	Kansas	317,291	16	Rhode Island	293,097
17	Kentucky	292,944	17	Kentucky	292,944
45	Louisiana	246,903	18	Iowa	292,719
22	Maine	287,374	19	Wyoming	291,000
5	Maryland	332,357	20	New Mexico	289,337
38	Massachusetts	264,273	21	Indiana	287,384
3	Michigan	335,802	22	Maine	287,374
43	Minnesota	255,125	23	New York	286,903
44	Mississippi	254,426	24	Alabama	286,498
14	Missouri	293,983	25	West Virginia	285,987
48	Montana	237,233	26	Colorado	284,961
8	Nebraska	320,041	27	Pennsylvania	283,344
4	Nevada	335,673	28	Arkansas	280,554
34	New Hampshire	271,257	29	Washington	279,760
36	New Jersey	269,047	30	Hawaii	279,263
20	New Mexico	289,337	31	Tennessee	278,566
23	New York	286,903	32	Georgia	274,383
13	North Carolina	294,279	33	Wisconsin	272,138
2	North Dakota	338,047	34	New Hampshire	271,257
40	Ohio	261,493	35	Utah	270,914
46	Oklahoma	240,719	36	New Jersey	269,047
50	Oregon	232,455	37	Virginia	265,493
27	Pennsylvania	283,344	38	Massachusetts	264,273
16	Rhode Island	293,097	39	Idaho	261,777
15	South Carolina	293,399	40	Ohio	261,493
47	South Dakota	239,503	41	Arizona	260,132
31	Tennessee	278,566	42	Florida	259,110
12	Texas	299,358	43	Minnesota	255,125
35	Utah	270,914	44	Mississippi	254,426
49	Vermont	235,360	45	Louisiana	246,903
37	Virginia	265,493	46	Oklahoma	240,719
29	Washington	279,760	47	South Dakota	239,563
25	West Virginia	285,987	48	Montana	237,233
33	Wisconsin	272,138	49	Vermont	235,360
19	Wyoming	291,000	50	Oregon	232,455
				District of Columbia	384,000

Source: Morgan Quitno Press using data from U.S. Bureau of the Census
"1992 Census of Service Industries, Geographic Area Series, United States" (SC92-A-52)
Includes only establishments subject to the federal income tax. See Facilities Chapter for establishments.

Receipts of Offices and Clinics of Podiatrists in 1992

National Total = $1,920,076,000*

ALPHA ORDER					RANK ORDER			
RANK	STATE	RECEIPTS	% of USA		RANK	STATE	RECEIPTS	% of USA
23	Alabama	$15,910,000	0.83%		1	California	$217,602,000	11.33%
46	Alaska	2,222,000	0.12%		2	New York	209,057,000	10.89%
18	Arizona	27,962,000	1.46%		3	Florida	147,168,000	7.66%
42	Arkansas	5,017,000	0.26%		4	Pennsylvania	118,882,000	6.19%
1	California	217,602,000	11.33%		5	Michigan	112,871,000	5.88%
22	Colorado	18,980,000	0.99%		6	Ohio	109,704,000	5.71%
11	Connecticut	48,830,000	2.54%		7	Illinois	105,745,000	5.51%
37	Delaware	6,801,000	0.35%		8	Texas	104,569,000	5.45%
3	Florida	147,168,000	7.66%		9	New Jersey	103,924,000	5.41%
12	Georgia	47,600,000	2.48%		10	Maryland	56,379,000	2.94%
43	Hawaii	3,871,000	0.20%		11	Connecticut	48,830,000	2.54%
40	Idaho	5,283,000	0.28%		12	Georgia	47,600,000	2.48%
7	Illinois	105,745,000	5.51%		13	Massachusetts	43,366,000	2.26%
14	Indiana	41,792,000	2.18%		14	Indiana	41,792,000	2.18%
24	Iowa	14,998,000	0.78%		15	Virginia	40,402,000	2.10%
29	Kansas	12,107,000	0.63%		16	North Carolina	35,032,000	1.82%
31	Kentucky	10,299,000	0.54%		17	Washington	31,204,000	1.63%
26	Louisiana	13,876,000	0.72%		18	Arizona	27,962,000	1.46%
38	Maine	6,464,000	0.34%		19	Wisconsin	27,720,000	1.44%
10	Maryland	56,379,000	2.94%		20	Missouri	24,462,000	1.27%
13	Massachusetts	43,366,000	2.26%		21	Tennessee	23,034,000	1.20%
5	Michigan	112,871,000	5.88%		22	Colorado	18,980,000	0.99%
28	Minnesota	12,440,000	0.65%		23	Alabama	15,910,000	0.83%
44	Mississippi	3,801,000	0.20%		24	Iowa	14,998,000	0.78%
20	Missouri	24,462,000	1.27%		25	Oklahoma	14,850,000	0.77%
45	Montana	3,441,000	0.18%		26	Louisiana	13,876,000	0.72%
36	Nebraska	7,020,000	0.37%		27	Oregon	13,796,000	0.72%
35	Nevada	7,995,000	0.42%		28	Minnesota	12,440,000	0.65%
41	New Hampshire	5,180,000	0.27%		29	Kansas	12,107,000	0.63%
9	New Jersey	103,924,000	5.41%		30	Rhode Island	11,842,000	0.62%
34	New Mexico	8,215,000	0.43%		31	Kentucky	10,299,000	0.54%
2	New York	209,057,000	10.89%		32	South Carolina	9,906,000	0.52%
16	North Carolina	35,032,000	1.82%		33	Utah	9,326,000	0.49%
48	North Dakota	1,382,000	0.07%		34	New Mexico	8,215,000	0.43%
6	Ohio	109,704,000	5.71%		35	Nevada	7,995,000	0.42%
25	Oklahoma	14,850,000	0.77%		36	Nebraska	7,020,000	0.37%
27	Oregon	13,796,000	0.72%		37	Delaware	6,801,000	0.35%
4	Pennsylvania	118,882,000	6.19%		38	Maine	6,464,000	0.34%
30	Rhode Island	11,842,000	0.62%		39	West Virginia	5,602,000	0.29%
32	South Carolina	9,906,000	0.52%		40	Idaho	5,283,000	0.28%
47	South Dakota	1,774,000	0.09%		41	New Hampshire	5,180,000	0.27%
21	Tennessee	23,034,000	1.20%		42	Arkansas	5,017,000	0.26%
8	Texas	104,569,000	5.45%		43	Hawaii	3,871,000	0.20%
33	Utah	9,326,000	0.49%		44	Mississippi	3,801,000	0.20%
49	Vermont	1,157,000	0.06%		45	Montana	3,441,000	0.18%
15	Virginia	40,402,000	2.10%		46	Alaska	2,222,000	0.12%
17	Washington	31,204,000	1.63%		47	South Dakota	1,774,000	0.09%
39	West Virginia	5,602,000	0.29%		48	North Dakota	1,382,000	0.07%
19	Wisconsin	27,720,000	1.44%		49	Vermont	1,157,000	0.06%
50	Wyoming	1,035,000	0.05%		50	Wyoming	1,035,000	0.05%
						District of Columbia	8,181,000	0.43%

Source: U.S. Bureau of the Census
"1992 Census of Service Industries, Geographic Area Series, United States" (SC92-A-52)
*Includes only establishments subject to the federal income tax. See Facilities Chapter for establishments.

Receipts per Office or Clinic of Podiatrists in 1992

National Rate = $241,580 per Establishment*

ALPHA ORDER				RANK ORDER		
RANK	STATE	PER ESTABLISHMENT		RANK	STATE	PER ESTABLISHMENT
3	Alabama	$324,694		1	Alaska	$444,400
1	Alaska	444,400		2	Georgia	342,446
28	Arizona	231,091		3	Alabama	324,694
17	Arkansas	250,850		4	Connecticut	321,250
25	California	233,981		5	Idaho	310,765
35	Colorado	215,682		6	Louisiana	289,083
4	Connecticut	321,250		7	Oklahoma	285,577
11	Delaware	272,040		8	Nevada	285,536
13	Florida	260,936		9	Michigan	282,178
2	Georgia	342,446		10	Texas	273,741
23	Hawaii	241,938		11	Delaware	272,040
5	Idaho	310,765		12	Maryland	267,199
15	Illinois	252,375		13	Florida	260,936
16	Indiana	251,759		14	Tennessee	255,933
46	Iowa	199,973		15	Illinois	252,375
33	Kansas	220,127		16	Indiana	251,759
30	Kentucky	223,891		17	Arkansas	250,850
6	Louisiana	289,083		18	North Carolina	250,229
48	Maine	179,556		19	Missouri	249,612
12	Maryland	267,199		20	New Mexico	248,939
41	Massachusetts	208,490		21	South Carolina	247,650
9	Michigan	282,178		22	Virginia	246,354
42	Minnesota	207,333		23	Hawaii	241,938
40	Mississippi	211,167		24	Rhode Island	236,840
19	Missouri	249,612		25	California	233,981
37	Montana	215,063		26	Wisconsin	232,941
44	Nebraska	206,471		27	New Jersey	231,457
8	Nevada	285,536		28	Arizona	231,091
34	New Hampshire	215,833		29	Oregon	226,164
27	New Jersey	231,457		30	Kentucky	223,891
20	New Mexico	248,939		31	Ohio	223,886
32	New York	222,875		32	New York	222,875
18	North Carolina	250,229		33	Kansas	220,127
47	North Dakota	197,429		34	New Hampshire	215,833
31	Ohio	223,886		35	Colorado	215,682
7	Oklahoma	285,577		36	West Virginia	215,462
29	Oregon	226,164		37	Montana	215,063
45	Pennsylvania	201,837		38	Washington	213,726
24	Rhode Island	236,840		39	Utah	211,955
21	South Carolina	247,650		40	Mississippi	211,167
50	South Dakota	126,714		41	Massachusetts	208,490
14	Tennessee	255,933		42	Minnesota	207,333
10	Texas	273,741		43	Wyoming	207,000
39	Utah	211,955		44	Nebraska	206,471
49	Vermont	128,556		45	Pennsylvania	201,837
22	Virginia	246,354		46	Iowa	199,973
38	Washington	213,726		47	North Dakota	197,429
36	West Virginia	215,462		48	Maine	179,556
26	Wisconsin	232,941		49	Vermont	128,556
43	Wyoming	207,000		50	South Dakota	126,714
					District of Columbia	255,656

Source: Morgan Quitno Press using data from U.S. Bureau of the Census
   "1992 Census of Service Industries, Geographic Area Series, United States" (SC92-A-52)
*Includes only establishments subject to the federal income tax. See Facilities Chapter for establishments.

Receipts of Offices and Clinics of Other Health Practitioners in 1992

National Total = $6,148,059,000*

ALPHA ORDER				RANK ORDER			
RANK	STATE	RECEIPTS	% of USA	RANK	STATE	RECEIPTS	% of USA
29	Alabama	$52,156,000	0.85%	1	California	$1,034,853,000	16.83%
46	Alaska	12,434,000	0.20%	2	Texas	430,380,000	7.00%
21	Arizona	96,707,000	1.57%	3	Florida	426,622,000	6.94%
31	Arkansas	40,313,000	0.66%	4	Pennsylvania	374,184,000	6.09%
1	California	1,034,853,000	16.83%	5	New York	365,739,000	5.95%
17	Colorado	108,367,000	1.76%	6	Ohio	241,548,000	3.93%
16	Connecticut	109,057,000	1.77%	7	Illinois	224,938,000	3.66%
40	Delaware	24,546,000	0.40%	8	Michigan	212,093,000	3.45%
3	Florida	426,622,000	6.94%	9	New Jersey	211,576,000	3.44%
12	Georgia	161,961,000	2.63%	10	Maryland	179,434,000	2.92%
36	Hawaii	30,940,000	0.50%	11	Washington	162,891,000	2.65%
45	Idaho	14,480,000	0.24%	12	Georgia	161,961,000	2.63%
7	Illinois	224,938,000	3.66%	13	Massachusetts	158,543,000	2.58%
23	Indiana	84,829,000	1.38%	14	North Carolina	138,366,000	2.25%
32	Iowa	38,347,000	0.62%	15	Virginia	135,154,000	2.20%
33	Kansas	38,115,000	0.62%	16	Connecticut	109,057,000	1.77%
26	Kentucky	59,948,000	0.98%	17	Colorado	108,367,000	1.76%
24	Louisiana	80,487,000	1.31%	18	Minnesota	100,371,000	1.63%
41	Maine	23,413,000	0.38%	19	Missouri	99,140,000	1.61%
10	Maryland	179,434,000	2.92%	20	Tennessee	97,742,000	1.59%
13	Massachusetts	158,543,000	2.58%	21	Arizona	96,707,000	1.57%
8	Michigan	212,093,000	3.45%	22	Wisconsin	93,109,000	1.51%
18	Minnesota	100,371,000	1.63%	23	Indiana	84,829,000	1.38%
39	Mississippi	26,287,000	0.43%	24	Louisiana	80,487,000	1.31%
19	Missouri	99,140,000	1.61%	25	Oregon	71,873,000	1.17%
44	Montana	14,602,000	0.24%	26	Kentucky	59,948,000	0.98%
38	Nebraska	27,517,000	0.45%	27	Nevada	55,463,000	0.90%
27	Nevada	55,463,000	0.90%	28	Oklahoma	53,332,000	0.87%
34	New Hampshire	36,653,000	0.60%	29	Alabama	52,156,000	0.85%
9	New Jersey	211,576,000	3.44%	30	South Carolina	43,318,000	0.70%
37	New Mexico	30,081,000	0.49%	31	Arkansas	40,313,000	0.66%
5	New York	365,739,000	5.95%	32	Iowa	38,347,000	0.62%
14	North Carolina	138,366,000	2.25%	33	Kansas	38,115,000	0.62%
50	North Dakota	6,543,000	0.11%	34	New Hampshire	36,653,000	0.60%
6	Ohio	241,548,000	3.93%	35	Utah	36,264,000	0.59%
28	Oklahoma	53,332,000	0.87%	36	Hawaii	30,940,000	0.50%
25	Oregon	71,873,000	1.17%	37	New Mexico	30,081,000	0.49%
4	Pennsylvania	374,184,000	6.09%	38	Nebraska	27,517,000	0.45%
43	Rhode Island	16,002,000	0.26%	39	Mississippi	26,287,000	0.43%
30	South Carolina	43,318,000	0.70%	40	Delaware	24,546,000	0.40%
48	South Dakota	9,805,000	0.16%	41	Maine	23,413,000	0.38%
20	Tennessee	97,742,000	1.59%	42	West Virginia	18,885,000	0.31%
2	Texas	430,380,000	7.00%	43	Rhode Island	16,002,000	0.26%
35	Utah	36,264,000	0.59%	44	Montana	14,602,000	0.24%
47	Vermont	10,822,000	0.18%	45	Idaho	14,480,000	0.24%
15	Virginia	135,154,000	2.20%	46	Alaska	12,434,000	0.20%
11	Washington	162,891,000	2.65%	47	Vermont	10,822,000	0.18%
42	West Virginia	18,885,000	0.31%	48	South Dakota	9,805,000	0.16%
22	Wisconsin	93,109,000	1.51%	49	Wyoming	7,307,000	0.12%
49	Wyoming	7,307,000	0.12%	50	North Dakota	6,543,000	0.11%
					District of Columbia	20,522,000	0.33%

Source: U.S. Bureau of the Census
   "1992 Census of Service Industries, Geographic Area Series, United States" (SC92-A-52)
*Includes only establishments subject to the federal income tax. Includes health practitioners not otherwise classified such as acupuncturists, midwives, nutritionists, physical and occupational therapists and psychologists. See Facilities Chapter for establishments.

Receipts per Office or Clinic of Other Health Practitioners in 1992

National Rate = $276,193 per Establishment*

<u>ALPHA ORDER</u>

RANK	STATE	PER ESTABLISHMENT
11	Alabama	$299,747
44	Alaska	207,233
40	Arizona	216,347
29	Arkansas	258,417
27	California	261,723
42	Colorado	210,421
3	Connecticut	349,542
4	Delaware	322,974
28	Florida	259,502
12	Georgia	297,722
30	Hawaii	257,833
47	Idaho	183,291
7	Illinois	311,548
8	Indiana	308,469
35	Iowa	245,814
37	Kansas	241,234
15	Kentucky	282,774
34	Louisiana	248,417
43	Maine	209,045
9	Maryland	303,098
10	Massachusetts	301,413
6	Michigan	317,030
19	Minnesota	278,036
31	Mississippi	257,716
23	Missouri	265,080
49	Montana	169,791
32	Nebraska	257,168
1	Nevada	426,638
14	New Hampshire	286,352
5	New Jersey	317,682
48	New Mexico	180,126
22	New York	272,127
18	North Carolina	278,402
41	North Dakota	211,065
16	Ohio	280,870
38	Oklahoma	233,912
45	Oregon	199,094
2	Pennsylvania	416,222
36	Rhode Island	242,455
33	South Carolina	256,320
24	South Dakota	205,000
13	Tennessee	296,188
25	Texas	263,068
39	Utah	218,458
50	Vermont	156,841
17	Virginia	278,668
26	Washington	262,727
21	West Virginia	273,696
20	Wisconsin	273,850
46	Wyoming	197,486

<u>RANK ORDER</u>

RANK	STATE	PER ESTABLISHMENT
1	Nevada	$426,638
2	Pennsylvania	416,222
3	Connecticut	349,542
4	Delaware	322,974
5	New Jersey	317,682
6	Michigan	317,030
7	Illinois	311,548
8	Indiana	308,469
9	Maryland	303,098
10	Massachusetts	301,413
11	Alabama	299,747
12	Georgia	297,722
13	Tennessee	296,188
14	New Hampshire	286,352
15	Kentucky	282,774
16	Ohio	280,870
17	Virginia	278,668
18	North Carolina	278,402
19	Minnesota	278,036
20	Wisconsin	273,850
21	West Virginia	273,696
22	New York	272,127
23	Missouri	265,080
24	South Dakota	265,000
25	Texas	263,068
26	Washington	262,727
27	California	261,723
28	Florida	259,502
29	Arkansas	258,417
30	Hawaii	257,833
31	Mississippi	257,716
32	Nebraska	257,168
33	South Carolina	256,320
34	Louisiana	248,417
35	Iowa	245,814
36	Rhode Island	242,455
37	Kansas	241,234
38	Oklahoma	233,912
39	Utah	218,458
40	Arizona	216,347
41	North Dakota	211,065
42	Colorado	210,421
43	Maine	209,045
44	Alaska	207,233
45	Oregon	199,094
46	Wyoming	197,486
47	Idaho	183,291
48	New Mexico	180,126
49	Montana	169,791
50	Vermont	156,841
	District of Columbia	301,794

Source: Morgan Quitno Press using data from U.S. Bureau of the Census
   "1992 Census of Service Industries, Geographic Area Series, United States" (SC92-A-52)
*Includes only establishments subject to the federal income tax. Includes health practitioners not otherwise classified such as acupuncturists, midwives, nutritionists, physical and occupational therapists and psychologists. See Facilities Chapter for establishments.

Receipts of Hospitals in 1992

National Total = $310,818,211,000*

<table>
<tr><td colspan="4">ALPHA ORDER</td><td colspan="4">RANK ORDER</td></tr>
<tr><td>RANK</td><td>STATE</td><td>RECEIPTS</td><td>% of USA</td><td>RANK</td><td>STATE</td><td>RECEIPTS</td><td>% of USA</td></tr>
<tr><td>21</td><td>Alabama</td><td>$5,114,698,000</td><td>1.65%</td><td>1</td><td>California</td><td>$34,552,067,000</td><td>11.12%</td></tr>
<tr><td>NA</td><td>Alaska**</td><td>NA</td><td>NA</td><td>2</td><td>New York</td><td>27,722,480,000</td><td>8.92%</td></tr>
<tr><td>23</td><td>Arizona</td><td>4,064,528,000</td><td>1.31%</td><td>3</td><td>Texas</td><td>20,081,248,000</td><td>6.46%</td></tr>
<tr><td>30</td><td>Arkansas</td><td>2,601,895,000</td><td>0.84%</td><td>4</td><td>Pennsylvania</td><td>18,019,449,000</td><td>5.80%</td></tr>
<tr><td>1</td><td>California</td><td>34,552,067,000</td><td>11.12%</td><td>5</td><td>Florida</td><td>16,528,209,000</td><td>5.32%</td></tr>
<tr><td>24</td><td>Colorado</td><td>3,876,008,000</td><td>1.25%</td><td>6</td><td>Illinois</td><td>14,715,279,000</td><td>4.73%</td></tr>
<tr><td>NA</td><td>Connecticut**</td><td>NA</td><td>NA</td><td>7</td><td>Ohio</td><td>13,998,840,000</td><td>4.50%</td></tr>
<tr><td>37</td><td>Delaware</td><td>903,055,000</td><td>0.29%</td><td>8</td><td>Michigan</td><td>11,444,321,000</td><td>3.68%</td></tr>
<tr><td>5</td><td>Florida</td><td>16,528,209,000</td><td>5.32%</td><td>9</td><td>New Jersey</td><td>9,842,808,000</td><td>3.17%</td></tr>
<tr><td>11</td><td>Georgia</td><td>8,079,353,000</td><td>2.60%</td><td>10</td><td>Massachusetts</td><td>9,714,787,000</td><td>3.13%</td></tr>
<tr><td>NA</td><td>Hawaii**</td><td>NA</td><td>NA</td><td>11</td><td>Georgia</td><td>8,079,353,000</td><td>2.60%</td></tr>
<tr><td>38</td><td>Idaho</td><td>880,530,000</td><td>0.28%</td><td>12</td><td>North Carolina</td><td>7,408,964,000</td><td>2.38%</td></tr>
<tr><td>6</td><td>Illinois</td><td>14,715,279,000</td><td>4.73%</td><td>13</td><td>Missouri</td><td>7,217,462,000</td><td>2.32%</td></tr>
<tr><td>16</td><td>Indiana</td><td>6,590,871,000</td><td>2.12%</td><td>14</td><td>Virginia</td><td>6,793,601,000</td><td>2.19%</td></tr>
<tr><td>NA</td><td>Iowa**</td><td>NA</td><td>NA</td><td>15</td><td>Tennessee</td><td>6,770,631,000</td><td>2.18%</td></tr>
<tr><td>27</td><td>Kansas</td><td>2,856,257,000</td><td>0.92%</td><td>16</td><td>Indiana</td><td>6,590,871,000</td><td>2.12%</td></tr>
<tr><td>22</td><td>Kentucky</td><td>4,185,657,000</td><td>1.35%</td><td>17</td><td>Louisiana</td><td>5,658,657,000</td><td>1.82%</td></tr>
<tr><td>17</td><td>Louisiana</td><td>5,658,657,000</td><td>1.82%</td><td>18</td><td>Maryland</td><td>5,440,457,000</td><td>1.75%</td></tr>
<tr><td>NA</td><td>Maine**</td><td>NA</td><td>NA</td><td>19</td><td>Wisconsin</td><td>5,262,803,000</td><td>1.69%</td></tr>
<tr><td>18</td><td>Maryland</td><td>5,440,457,000</td><td>1.75%</td><td>20</td><td>Washington</td><td>5,193,838,000</td><td>1.67%</td></tr>
<tr><td>10</td><td>Massachusetts</td><td>9,714,787,000</td><td>3.13%</td><td>21</td><td>Alabama</td><td>5,114,698,000</td><td>1.65%</td></tr>
<tr><td>8</td><td>Michigan</td><td>11,444,321,000</td><td>3.68%</td><td>22</td><td>Kentucky</td><td>4,185,657,000</td><td>1.35%</td></tr>
<tr><td>NA</td><td>Minnesota**</td><td>NA</td><td>NA</td><td>23</td><td>Arizona</td><td>4,064,528,000</td><td>1.31%</td></tr>
<tr><td>29</td><td>Mississippi</td><td>2,627,692,000</td><td>0.85%</td><td>24</td><td>Colorado</td><td>3,876,008,000</td><td>1.25%</td></tr>
<tr><td>13</td><td>Missouri</td><td>7,217,462,000</td><td>2.32%</td><td>25</td><td>South Carolina</td><td>3,833,754,000</td><td>1.23%</td></tr>
<tr><td>39</td><td>Montana</td><td>864,812,000</td><td>0.28%</td><td>26</td><td>Oklahoma</td><td>3,232,112,000</td><td>1.04%</td></tr>
<tr><td>NA</td><td>Nebraska**</td><td>NA</td><td>NA</td><td>27</td><td>Kansas</td><td>2,856,257,000</td><td>0.92%</td></tr>
<tr><td>34</td><td>Nevada</td><td>1,296,942,000</td><td>0.42%</td><td>28</td><td>Oregon</td><td>2,835,585,000</td><td>0.91%</td></tr>
<tr><td>36</td><td>New Hampshire</td><td>1,250,889,000</td><td>0.40%</td><td>29</td><td>Mississippi</td><td>2,627,692,000</td><td>0.85%</td></tr>
<tr><td>9</td><td>New Jersey</td><td>9,842,808,000</td><td>3.17%</td><td>30</td><td>Arkansas</td><td>2,601,895,000</td><td>0.84%</td></tr>
<tr><td>33</td><td>New Mexico</td><td>1,558,035,000</td><td>0.50%</td><td>31</td><td>West Virginia</td><td>2,243,147,000</td><td>0.72%</td></tr>
<tr><td>2</td><td>New York</td><td>27,722,480,000</td><td>8.92%</td><td>32</td><td>Utah</td><td>1,626,872,000</td><td>0.52%</td></tr>
<tr><td>12</td><td>North Carolina</td><td>7,408,964,000</td><td>2.38%</td><td>33</td><td>New Mexico</td><td>1,558,035,000</td><td>0.50%</td></tr>
<tr><td>NA</td><td>North Dakota**</td><td>NA</td><td>NA</td><td>34</td><td>Nevada</td><td>1,296,942,000</td><td>0.42%</td></tr>
<tr><td>7</td><td>Ohio</td><td>13,998,840,000</td><td>4.50%</td><td>35</td><td>Rhode Island</td><td>1,257,773,000</td><td>0.40%</td></tr>
<tr><td>26</td><td>Oklahoma</td><td>3,232,112,000</td><td>1.04%</td><td>36</td><td>New Hampshire</td><td>1,250,889,000</td><td>0.40%</td></tr>
<tr><td>28</td><td>Oregon</td><td>2,835,585,000</td><td>0.91%</td><td>37</td><td>Delaware</td><td>903,055,000</td><td>0.29%</td></tr>
<tr><td>4</td><td>Pennsylvania</td><td>18,019,449,000</td><td>5.80%</td><td>38</td><td>Idaho</td><td>880,530,000</td><td>0.28%</td></tr>
<tr><td>35</td><td>Rhode Island</td><td>1,257,773,000</td><td>0.40%</td><td>39</td><td>Montana</td><td>864,812,000</td><td>0.28%</td></tr>
<tr><td>25</td><td>South Carolina</td><td>3,833,754,000</td><td>1.23%</td><td>40</td><td>Vermont</td><td>545,676,000</td><td>0.18%</td></tr>
<tr><td>NA</td><td>South Dakota**</td><td>NA</td><td>NA</td><td>NA</td><td>Alaska**</td><td>NA</td><td>NA</td></tr>
<tr><td>15</td><td>Tennessee</td><td>6,770,631,000</td><td>2.18%</td><td>NA</td><td>Connecticut**</td><td>NA</td><td>NA</td></tr>
<tr><td>3</td><td>Texas</td><td>20,081,248,000</td><td>6.46%</td><td>NA</td><td>Hawaii**</td><td>NA</td><td>NA</td></tr>
<tr><td>32</td><td>Utah</td><td>1,626,872,000</td><td>0.52%</td><td>NA</td><td>Iowa**</td><td>NA</td><td>NA</td></tr>
<tr><td>40</td><td>Vermont</td><td>545,676,000</td><td>0.18%</td><td>NA</td><td>Maine**</td><td>NA</td><td>NA</td></tr>
<tr><td>14</td><td>Virginia</td><td>6,793,601,000</td><td>2.19%</td><td>NA</td><td>Minnesota**</td><td>NA</td><td>NA</td></tr>
<tr><td>20</td><td>Washington</td><td>5,193,838,000</td><td>1.67%</td><td>NA</td><td>Nebraska**</td><td>NA</td><td>NA</td></tr>
<tr><td>31</td><td>West Virginia</td><td>2,243,147,000</td><td>0.72%</td><td>NA</td><td>North Dakota**</td><td>NA</td><td>NA</td></tr>
<tr><td>19</td><td>Wisconsin</td><td>5,262,803,000</td><td>1.69%</td><td>NA</td><td>South Dakota**</td><td>NA</td><td>NA</td></tr>
<tr><td>NA</td><td>Wyoming**</td><td>NA</td><td>NA</td><td>NA</td><td>Wyoming**</td><td>NA</td><td>NA</td></tr>
<tr><td></td><td></td><td></td><td></td><td></td><td>District of Columbia**</td><td>NA</td><td>NA</td></tr>
</table>

Source: Morgan Quitno Press using data from U.S. Bureau of the Census
    "1992 Census of Service Industries, Geographic Area Series, United States" (SC92-A-52)
*Includes establishments exempt from as well as subject to the federal income tax. Includes general medical and
surgical hospitals, psychiatric hospitals and other specialty hospitals. Includes government owned hospitals.
**Not available.

Receipts per Hospital in 1992

National Rate = $43,654,243 per Hospital*

ALPHA ORDER			RANK ORDER		
RANK	STATE	PER HOSPITAL	RANK	STATE	PER HOSPITAL
24	Alabama	$36,533,557	1	New York	$85,038,282
NA	Alaska**	NA	2	New Jersey	72,909,689
18	Arizona	40,645,280	3	Maryland	64,005,376
34	Arkansas	25,508,775	4	Massachusetts	60,717,419
9	California	57,205,409	5	Rhode Island	59,893,952
21	Colorado	38,760,080	6	Ohio	57,608,395
NA	Connecticut**	NA	7	Pennsylvania	57,386,780
10	Delaware	56,440,938	8	Illinois	57,257,895
12	Florida	50,237,717	9	California	57,205,409
23	Georgia	38,473,110	10	Delaware	56,440,938
NA	Hawaii**	NA	11	Michigan	52,257,174
39	Idaho	16,306,111	12	Florida	50,237,717
8	Illinois	57,257,895	13	Virginia	48,525,721
20	Indiana	40,434,791	14	Washington	43,645,697
NA	Iowa**	NA	15	North Carolina	42,580,253
38	Kansas	17,631,216	16	Missouri	41,242,640
28	Kentucky	32,700,445	17	South Carolina	41,223,161
31	Louisiana	30,422,887	18	Arizona	40,645,280
NA	Maine**	NA	19	Nevada	40,529,438
3	Maryland	64,005,376	20	Indiana	40,434,791
4	Massachusetts	60,717,419	21	Colorado	38,760,080
11	Michigan	52,257,174	22	Tennessee	38,689,320
NA	Minnesota**	NA	23	Georgia	38,473,110
36	Mississippi	22,268,576	24	Alabama	36,533,557
16	Missouri	41,242,640	25	Oregon	35,893,481
40	Montana	13,304,800	26	Texas	34,326,920
NA	Nebraska**	NA	27	Wisconsin	33,521,038
19	Nevada	40,529,438	28	Kentucky	32,700,445
30	New Hampshire	30,509,488	29	West Virginia	31,154,819
2	New Jersey	72,909,689	30	New Hampshire	30,509,488
35	New Mexico	23,254,254	31	Louisiana	30,422,887
1	New York	85,038,282	32	Vermont	30,315,333
15	North Carolina	42,580,253	33	Utah	29,051,286
NA	North Dakota**	NA	34	Arkansas	25,508,775
6	Ohio	57,608,395	35	New Mexico	23,254,254
37	Oklahoma	21,547,413	36	Mississippi	22,268,576
25	Oregon	35,893,481	37	Oklahoma	21,547,413
7	Pennsylvania	57,386,780	38	Kansas	17,631,216
5	Rhode Island	59,893,952	39	Idaho	16,306,111
17	South Carolina	41,223,161	40	Montana	13,304,800
NA	South Dakota**	NA	NA	Alaska**	NA
22	Tennessee	38,689,320	NA	Connecticut**	NA
26	Texas	34,326,920	NA	Hawaii**	NA
33	Utah	29,051,286	NA	Iowa**	NA
32	Vermont	30,315,333	NA	Maine**	NA
13	Virginia	48,525,721	NA	Minnesota**	NA
14	Washington	43,645,697	NA	Nebraska**	NA
29	West Virginia	31,154,819	NA	North Dakota**	NA
27	Wisconsin	33,521,038	NA	South Dakota**	NA
NA	Wyoming**	NA	NA	Wyoming**	NA
			District of Columbia**		NA

Source: Morgan Quitno Press using data from U.S. Bureau of the Census
  "1992 Census of Service Industries, Geographic Area Series, United States" (SC92-A-52)
*Calculated using Census Bureau count of 7,120 hospitals. Includes establishments exempt from as well as subject
to the federal income tax. Includes general medical and surgical hospitals, psychiatric hospitals and other
specialty hospitals. Includes government owned hospitals.
**Not available.

Uncompensated Care Expenses in Community Hospitals in 1992

National Total = $14,691,902,692

ALPHA ORDER

RANK	STATE	EXPENDITURES	% of USA
13	Alabama	$351,095,842	2.39%
45	Alaska	24,375,358	0.17%
28	Arizona	145,956,397	0.99%
27	Arkansas	151,972,830	1.03%
1	California	1,749,206,487	11.91%
21	Colorado	190,349,245	1.30%
24	Connecticut	162,233,546	1.10%
36	Delaware	67,321,716	0.46%
4	Florida	889,185,169	6.05%
8	Georgia	529,333,725	3.60%
43	Hawaii	32,924,191	0.22%
47	Idaho	23,330,207	0.16%
6	Illinois	690,349,440	4.70%
18	Indiana	277,941,471	1.89%
31	Iowa	114,462,867	0.78%
35	Kansas	79,861,499	0.54%
23	Kentucky	171,836,095	1.17%
20	Louisiana	221,501,951	1.51%
38	Maine	52,460,151	0.36%
16	Maryland	321,800,126	2.19%
9	Massachusetts	515,229,143	3.51%
17	Michigan	320,909,086	2.18%
33	Minnesota	95,883,389	0.65%
25	Mississippi	162,207,782	1.10%
14	Missouri	333,946,598	2.27%
46	Montana	23,828,891	0.16%
41	Nebraska	36,484,993	0.25%
37	Nevada	64,441,467	0.44%
40	New Hampshire	49,940,964	0.34%
5	New Jersey	809,838,266	5.51%
34	New Mexico	91,097,559	0.62%
3	New York	1,111,077,206	7.56%
11	North Carolina	371,039,914	2.53%
50	North Dakota	15,359,749	0.10%
7	Ohio	548,945,499	3.74%
22	Oklahoma	174,384,524	1.19%
29	Oregon	129,882,254	0.88%
10	Pennsylvania	412,588,861	2.81%
42	Rhode Island	34,564,000	0.24%
19	South Carolina	231,851,479	1.58%
49	South Dakota	16,035,925	0.11%
12	Tennessee	370,874,408	2.52%
2	Texas	1,566,829,829	10.66%
39	Utah	51,850,984	0.35%
48	Vermont	17,802,967	0.12%
15	Virginia	325,204,129	2.21%
26	Washington	158,806,874	1.08%
30	West Virginia	118,024,511	0.80%
32	Wisconsin	113,825,059	0.77%
44	Wyoming	26,505,671	0.18%

RANK ORDER

RANK	STATE	EXPENDITURES	% of USA
1	California	$1,749,206,487	11.91%
2	Texas	1,566,829,829	10.66%
3	New York	1,111,077,206	7.56%
4	Florida	889,185,169	6.05%
5	New Jersey	809,838,266	5.51%
6	Illinois	690,349,440	4.70%
7	Ohio	548,945,499	3.74%
8	Georgia	529,333,725	3.60%
9	Massachusetts	515,229,143	3.51%
10	Pennsylvania	412,588,861	2.81%
11	North Carolina	371,039,914	2.53%
12	Tennessee	370,874,408	2.52%
13	Alabama	351,095,842	2.39%
14	Missouri	333,946,598	2.27%
15	Virginia	325,204,129	2.21%
16	Maryland	321,800,126	2.19%
17	Michigan	320,909,086	2.18%
18	Indiana	277,941,471	1.89%
19	South Carolina	231,851,479	1.58%
20	Louisiana	221,501,951	1.51%
21	Colorado	190,349,245	1.30%
22	Oklahoma	174,384,524	1.19%
23	Kentucky	171,836,095	1.17%
24	Connecticut	162,233,546	1.10%
25	Mississippi	162,207,782	1.10%
26	Washington	158,806,874	1.08%
27	Arkansas	151,972,830	1.03%
28	Arizona	145,956,397	0.99%
29	Oregon	129,882,254	0.88%
30	West Virginia	118,024,511	0.80%
31	Iowa	114,462,867	0.78%
32	Wisconsin	113,825,059	0.77%
33	Minnesota	95,883,389	0.65%
34	New Mexico	91,097,559	0.62%
35	Kansas	79,861,499	0.54%
36	Delaware	67,321,716	0.46%
37	Nevada	64,441,467	0.44%
38	Maine	52,460,151	0.36%
39	Utah	51,850,984	0.35%
40	New Hampshire	49,940,964	0.34%
41	Nebraska	36,484,993	0.25%
42	Rhode Island	34,564,000	0.24%
43	Hawaii	32,924,191	0.22%
44	Wyoming	26,505,671	0.18%
45	Alaska	24,375,358	0.17%
46	Montana	23,828,891	0.16%
47	Idaho	23,330,207	0.16%
48	Vermont	17,802,967	0.12%
49	South Dakota	16,035,925	0.11%
50	North Dakota	15,359,749	0.10%
	District of Columbia	148,142,380	1.01%

Source: Health Insurance Association of America
   "Source Book of Health Insurance Data 1994" (based on data from the American Hospital Association)

Medical Costs Due to Smoking in 1990

National Total = $36,446,000,000

RANK	STATE	COSTS	% of USA
23	Alabama	$573,000,000	1.57%
49	Alaska	76,000,000	0.21%
24	Arizona	559,000,000	1.53%
32	Arkansas	296,000,000	0.81%
1	California	3,966,000,000	10.88%
26	Colorado	504,000,000	1.38%
21	Connecticut	621,000,000	1.70%
43	Delaware	112,000,000	0.31%
3	Florida	2,302,000,000	6.32%
11	Georgia	880,000,000	2.41%
41	Hawaii	129,000,000	0.35%
46	Idaho	84,000,000	0.23%
7	Illinois	1,614,000,000	4.43%
19	Indiana	700,000,000	1.92%
30	Iowa	319,000,000	0.88%
31	Kansas	297,000,000	0.81%
25	Kentucky	517,000,000	1.42%
22	Louisiana	611,000,000	1.68%
36	Maine	197,000,000	0.54%
15	Maryland	794,000,000	2.18%
9	Massachusetts	1,330,000,000	3.65%
8	Michigan	1,352,000,000	3.71%
17	Minnesota	722,000,000	1.98%
33	Mississippi	264,000,000	0.72%
14	Missouri	816,000,000	2.24%
44	Montana	102,000,000	0.28%
38	Nebraska	174,000,000	0.48%
35	Nevada	198,000,000	0.54%
39	New Hampshire	172,000,000	0.47%
10	New Jersey	1,136,000,000	3.12%
40	New Mexico	170,000,000	0.47%
2	New York	3,132,000,000	8.59%
12	North Carolina	833,000,000	2.29%
45	North Dakota	87,000,000	0.24%
6	Ohio	1,643,000,000	4.51%
28	Oklahoma	390,000,000	1.07%
27	Oregon	407,000,000	1.12%
5	Pennsylvania	1,982,000,000	5.44%
37	Rhode Island	186,000,000	0.51%
28	South Carolina	390,000,000	1.07%
47	South Dakota	82,000,000	0.22%
16	Tennessee	782,000,000	2.15%
4	Texas	2,007,000,000	5.51%
42	Utah	114,000,000	0.31%
48	Vermont	80,000,000	0.22%
13	Virginia	829,000,000	2.27%
18	Washington	706,000,000	1.94%
34	West Virginia	260,000,000	0.71%
20	Wisconsin	683,000,000	1.87%
50	Wyoming	51,000,000	0.14%

RANK	STATE	COSTS	% of USA
1	California	$3,966,000,000	10.88%
2	New York	3,132,000,000	8.59%
3	Florida	2,302,000,000	6.32%
4	Texas	2,007,000,000	5.51%
5	Pennsylvania	1,982,000,000	5.44%
6	Ohio	1,643,000,000	4.51%
7	Illinois	1,614,000,000	4.43%
8	Michigan	1,352,000,000	3.71%
9	Massachusetts	1,330,000,000	3.65%
10	New Jersey	1,136,000,000	3.12%
11	Georgia	880,000,000	2.41%
12	North Carolina	833,000,000	2.29%
13	Virginia	829,000,000	2.27%
14	Missouri	816,000,000	2.24%
15	Maryland	794,000,000	2.18%
16	Tennessee	782,000,000	2.15%
17	Minnesota	722,000,000	1.98%
18	Washington	706,000,000	1.94%
19	Indiana	700,000,000	1.92%
20	Wisconsin	683,000,000	1.87%
21	Connecticut	621,000,000	1.70%
22	Louisiana	611,000,000	1.68%
23	Alabama	573,000,000	1.57%
24	Arizona	559,000,000	1.53%
25	Kentucky	517,000,000	1.42%
26	Colorado	504,000,000	1.38%
27	Oregon	407,000,000	1.12%
28	Oklahoma	390,000,000	1.07%
28	South Carolina	390,000,000	1.07%
30	Iowa	319,000,000	0.88%
31	Kansas	297,000,000	0.81%
32	Arkansas	296,000,000	0.81%
33	Mississippi	264,000,000	0.72%
34	West Virginia	260,000,000	0.71%
35	Nevada	198,000,000	0.54%
36	Maine	197,000,000	0.54%
37	Rhode Island	186,000,000	0.51%
38	Nebraska	174,000,000	0.48%
39	New Hampshire	172,000,000	0.47%
40	New Mexico	170,000,000	0.47%
41	Hawaii	129,000,000	0.35%
42	Utah	114,000,000	0.31%
43	Delaware	112,000,000	0.31%
44	Montana	102,000,000	0.28%
45	North Dakota	87,000,000	0.24%
46	Idaho	84,000,000	0.23%
47	South Dakota	82,000,000	0.22%
48	Vermont	80,000,000	0.22%
49	Alaska	76,000,000	0.21%
50	Wyoming	51,000,000	0.14%
	District of Columbia	215,000,000	0.59%

Source: U.S. Department of Health and Human Services, Center for Disease Control and Prevention "State Tobacco Control Highlights 1996" (Publication No. 099-4895)

V. INCIDENCE OF DISEASE

V. INCIDENCE OF DISEASE (Continued)

Estimated New Cancer Cases in 1997

National Estimated Total = 1,382,400 New Cases*

ALPHA ORDER

RANK ORDER

RANK	STATE	CASES	% of USA
20	Alabama	23,200	1.68%
50	Alaska	1,500	0.11%
23	Arizona	22,000	1.59%
30	Arkansas	15,700	1.14%
1	California	127,500	9.22%
31	Colorado	14,900	1.08%
28	Connecticut	17,400	1.26%
45	Delaware	4,300	0.31%
2	Florida	99,100	7.17%
13	Georgia	31,900	2.31%
43	Hawaii	4,800	0.35%
42	Idaho	5,000	0.36%
6	Illinois	65,400	4.73%
14	Indiana	31,600	2.29%
29	Iowa	16,700	1.21%
33	Kansas	13,400	0.97%
20	Kentucky	23,200	1.68%
22	Louisiana	23,100	1.67%
37	Maine	8,200	0.59%
19	Maryland	25,700	1.86%
11	Massachusetts	35,500	2.57%
8	Michigan	50,600	3.66%
23	Minnesota	22,000	1.59%
32	Mississippi	14,800	1.07%
14	Missouri	31,600	2.29%
44	Montana	4,700	0.34%
36	Nebraska	8,400	0.61%
35	Nevada	8,600	0.62%
39	New Hampshire	6,300	0.46%
9	New Jersey	45,600	3.30%
38	New Mexico	7,000	0.51%
3	New York	94,100	6.81%
10	North Carolina	39,500	2.86%
47	North Dakota	3,600	0.26%
7	Ohio	63,500	4.59%
27	Oklahoma	17,500	1.27%
26	Oregon	17,900	1.29%
5	Pennsylvania	77,400	5.60%
40	Rhode Island	5,900	0.43%
25	South Carolina	19,800	1.43%
46	South Dakota	4,000	0.29%
16	Tennessee	29,100	2.11%
4	Texas	87,200	6.31%
41	Utah	5,800	0.42%
48	Vermont	2,900	0.21%
12	Virginia	32,500	2.35%
18	Washington	27,100	1.96%
34	West Virginia	12,100	0.88%
17	Wisconsin	27,500	1.99%
49	Wyoming	2,100	0.15%

RANK	STATE	CASES	% of USA
1	California	127,500	9.22%
2	Florida	99,100	7.17%
3	New York	94,100	6.81%
4	Texas	87,200	6.31%
5	Pennsylvania	77,400	5.60%
6	Illinois	65,400	4.73%
7	Ohio	63,500	4.59%
8	Michigan	50,600	3.66%
9	New Jersey	45,600	3.30%
10	North Carolina	39,500	2.86%
11	Massachusetts	35,500	2.57%
12	Virginia	32,500	2.35%
13	Georgia	31,900	2.31%
14	Indiana	31,600	2.29%
14	Missouri	31,600	2.29%
16	Tennessee	29,100	2.11%
17	Wisconsin	27,500	1.99%
18	Washington	27,100	1.96%
19	Maryland	25,700	1.86%
20	Alabama	23,200	1.68%
20	Kentucky	23,200	1.68%
22	Louisiana	23,100	1.67%
23	Arizona	22,000	1.59%
23	Minnesota	22,000	1.59%
25	South Carolina	19,800	1.43%
26	Oregon	17,900	1.29%
27	Oklahoma	17,500	1.27%
28	Connecticut	17,400	1.26%
29	Iowa	16,700	1.21%
30	Arkansas	15,700	1.14%
31	Colorado	14,900	1.08%
32	Mississippi	14,800	1.07%
33	Kansas	13,400	0.97%
34	West Virginia	12,100	0.88%
35	Nevada	8,600	0.62%
36	Nebraska	8,400	0.61%
37	Maine	8,200	0.59%
38	New Mexico	7,000	0.51%
39	New Hampshire	6,300	0.46%
40	Rhode Island	5,900	0.43%
41	Utah	5,800	0.42%
42	Idaho	5,000	0.36%
43	Hawaii	4,800	0.35%
44	Montana	4,700	0.34%
45	Delaware	4,300	0.31%
46	South Dakota	4,000	0.29%
47	North Dakota	3,600	0.26%
48	Vermont	2,900	0.21%
49	Wyoming	2,100	0.15%
50	Alaska	1,500	0.11%
	District of Columbia	3,500	0.25%

Source: American Cancer Society (http://www.cancer.org/97tabp5.html)
"Cancer Facts & Figures-1997" (Copyright 1997, Reprinted with permission from the American Cancer Society)
*These estimates are offered as a rough guide and should not be regarded as definitive. They are calculated according to the distribution of estimated 1997 cancer deaths by state. Totals do not include carcinoma in situ or basal and squamous cell skin cancers.

Estimated Rate of New Cancer Cases in 1997

National Estimated Rate = 521.1 New Cases per 100,000 Population*

ALPHA ORDER

RANK	STATE	RATE
20	Alabama	542.9
50	Alaska	247.1
36	Arizona	496.8
5	Arkansas	625.5
47	California	400.0
48	Colorado	389.7
28	Connecticut	531.5
8	Delaware	593.1
1	Florida	688.2
43	Georgia	433.8
46	Hawaii	405.4
44	Idaho	420.5
16	Illinois	552.0
22	Indiana	541.0
10	Iowa	585.6
32	Kansas	521.0
6	Kentucky	597.3
29	Louisiana	530.9
3	Maine	659.7
35	Maryland	506.7
11	Massachusetts	582.7
31	Michigan	527.4
40	Minnesota	472.3
19	Mississippi	544.9
9	Missouri	589.7
26	Montana	534.7
34	Nebraska	508.5
24	Nevada	536.5
21	New Hampshire	542.2
12	New Jersey	570.9
45	New Mexico	412.1
33	New York	517.5
23	North Carolina	539.4
14	North Dakota	559.0
13	Ohio	568.3
30	Oklahoma	530.1
15	Oregon	558.7
4	Pennsylvania	642.0
7	Rhode Island	596.0
25	South Carolina	535.3
18	South Dakota	546.4
17	Tennessee	547.0
41	Texas	455.9
49	Utah	290.0
37	Vermont	492.4
39	Virginia	486.9
38	Washington	489.8
2	West Virginia	662.7
27	Wisconsin	532.9
42	Wyoming	436.6

RANK ORDER

RANK	STATE	RATE
1	Florida	688.2
2	West Virginia	662.7
3	Maine	659.7
4	Pennsylvania	642.0
5	Arkansas	625.5
6	Kentucky	597.3
7	Rhode Island	596.0
8	Delaware	593.1
9	Missouri	589.7
10	Iowa	585.6
11	Massachusetts	582.7
12	New Jersey	570.9
13	Ohio	568.3
14	North Dakota	559.0
15	Oregon	558.7
16	Illinois	552.0
17	Tennessee	547.0
18	South Dakota	546.4
19	Mississippi	544.9
20	Alabama	542.9
21	New Hampshire	542.2
22	Indiana	541.0
23	North Carolina	539.4
24	Nevada	536.5
25	South Carolina	535.3
26	Montana	534.7
27	Wisconsin	532.9
28	Connecticut	531.5
29	Louisiana	530.9
30	Oklahoma	530.1
31	Michigan	527.4
32	Kansas	521.0
33	New York	517.5
34	Nebraska	508.5
35	Maryland	506.7
36	Arizona	496.8
37	Vermont	492.4
38	Washington	489.8
39	Virginia	486.9
40	Minnesota	472.3
41	Texas	455.9
42	Wyoming	436.6
43	Georgia	433.8
44	Idaho	420.5
45	New Mexico	412.1
46	Hawaii	405.4
47	California	400.0
48	Colorado	389.7
49	Utah	290.0
50	Alaska	247.1

| | District of Columbia | 644.6 |

*Source: Morgan Quitno Press using data from American Cancer Society (http://www.cancer.org/97tabp5.html)
"Cancer Facts & Figures-1997" (Copyright 1997, Reprinted with permission from the American Cancer Society)
*These estimates are offered as a rough guide and should not be regarded as definitive. They are calculated
according to the distribution of estimated 1997 cancer deaths by state. Totals do not include carcinoma in situ or
basal and squamous cell skin cancers. Rates calculated using 1996 Census resident population estimates.*

Estimated New Cases of Bladder Cancer in 1997

National Estimated Total = 54,500 New Cases*

ALPHA ORDER

RANK	STATE	CASES	% of USA
26	Alabama	700	1.28%
50	Alaska	10	0.02%
22	Arizona	820	1.50%
29	Arkansas	620	1.14%
1	California	5,000	9.17%
29	Colorado	620	1.14%
19	Connecticut	840	1.54%
39	Delaware	280	0.51%
2	Florida	4,400	8.07%
22	Georgia	820	1.50%
45	Hawaii	180	0.33%
44	Idaho	190	0.35%
7	Illinois	2,500	4.59%
11	Indiana	1,400	2.57%
21	Iowa	830	1.52%
33	Kansas	470	0.86%
24	Kentucky	730	1.34%
29	Louisiana	620	1.14%
36	Maine	320	0.59%
18	Maryland	920	1.69%
10	Massachusetts	1,700	3.12%
8	Michigan	2,300	4.22%
25	Minnesota	710	1.30%
34	Mississippi	340	0.62%
13	Missouri	1,200	2.20%
47	Montana	150	0.28%
38	Nebraska	290	0.53%
42	Nevada	250	0.46%
40	New Hampshire	270	0.50%
9	New Jersey	2,200	4.04%
37	New Mexico	300	0.55%
3	New York	4,300	7.89%
11	North Carolina	1,400	2.57%
45	North Dakota	180	0.33%
6	Ohio	2,600	4.77%
27	Oklahoma	690	1.27%
28	Oregon	670	1.23%
4	Pennsylvania	3,000	5.50%
35	Rhode Island	330	0.61%
19	South Carolina	840	1.54%
43	South Dakota	220	0.40%
17	Tennessee	1,000	1.83%
5	Texas	2,900	5.32%
40	Utah	270	0.50%
47	Vermont	150	0.28%
13	Virginia	1,200	2.20%
16	Washington	1,100	2.02%
32	West Virginia	600	1.10%
13	Wisconsin	1,200	2.20%
49	Wyoming	60	0.11%

RANK ORDER

RANK	STATE	CASES	% of USA
1	California	5,000	9.17%
2	Florida	4,400	8.07%
3	New York	4,300	7.89%
4	Pennsylvania	3,000	5.50%
5	Texas	2,900	5.32%
6	Ohio	2,600	4.77%
7	Illinois	2,500	4.59%
8	Michigan	2,300	4.22%
9	New Jersey	2,200	4.04%
10	Massachusetts	1,700	3.12%
11	Indiana	1,400	2.57%
11	North Carolina	1,400	2.57%
13	Missouri	1,200	2.20%
13	Virginia	1,200	2.20%
13	Wisconsin	1,200	2.20%
16	Washington	1,100	2.02%
17	Tennessee	1,000	1.83%
18	Maryland	920	1.69%
19	Connecticut	840	1.54%
19	South Carolina	840	1.54%
21	Iowa	830	1.52%
22	Arizona	820	1.50%
22	Georgia	820	1.50%
24	Kentucky	730	1.34%
25	Minnesota	710	1.30%
26	Alabama	700	1.28%
27	Oklahoma	690	1.27%
28	Oregon	670	1.23%
29	Arkansas	620	1.14%
29	Colorado	620	1.14%
29	Louisiana	620	1.14%
32	West Virginia	600	1.10%
33	Kansas	470	0.86%
34	Mississippi	340	0.62%
35	Rhode Island	330	0.61%
36	Maine	320	0.59%
37	New Mexico	300	0.55%
38	Nebraska	290	0.53%
39	Delaware	280	0.51%
40	New Hampshire	270	0.50%
40	Utah	270	0.50%
42	Nevada	250	0.46%
43	South Dakota	220	0.40%
44	Idaho	190	0.35%
45	Hawaii	180	0.33%
45	North Dakota	180	0.33%
47	Montana	150	0.28%
47	Vermont	150	0.28%
49	Wyoming	60	0.11%
50	Alaska	10	0.02%
	District of Columbia	130	0.24%

Source: American Cancer Society (http://www.cancer.org/97tabp5.html)
"Cancer Facts & Figures-1997" (Copyright 1997, Reprinted with permission from the American Cancer Society)
*These estimates are offered as a rough guide and should be interpreted with caution. They are calculated according to the distribution of estimated 1997 cancer deaths by state.

Estimated Rate of New Cases of Bladder Cancer in 1997

National Estimated Rate = 20.5 New Cases per 100,000 Population*

ALPHA ORDER

RANK	STATE	RATE
37	Alabama	16.4
50	Alaska	1.6
30	Arizona	18.5
14	Arkansas	24.7
40	California	15.7
38	Colorado	16.2
10	Connecticut	25.7
1	Delaware	38.6
4	Florida	30.6
49	Georgia	11.2
42	Hawaii	15.2
39	Idaho	16.0
23	Illinois	21.1
15	Indiana	24.0
6	Iowa	29.1
31	Kansas	18.3
28	Kentucky	18.8
45	Louisiana	14.2
10	Maine	25.7
32	Maryland	18.1
8	Massachusetts	27.9
15	Michigan	24.0
42	Minnesota	15.2
47	Mississippi	12.5
22	Missouri	22.4
36	Montana	17.1
34	Nebraska	17.6
41	Nevada	15.6
20	New Hampshire	23.2
9	New Jersey	27.5
35	New Mexico	17.5
17	New York	23.6
27	North Carolina	19.1
7	North Dakota	28.0
18	Ohio	23.3
24	Oklahoma	20.9
24	Oregon	20.9
13	Pennsylvania	24.9
2	Rhode Island	33.3
21	South Carolina	22.7
5	South Dakota	30.1
28	Tennessee	18.8
42	Texas	15.2
46	Utah	13.5
12	Vermont	25.5
33	Virginia	18.0
26	Washington	19.9
3	West Virginia	32.9
18	Wisconsin	23.3
47	Wyoming	12.5

RANK ORDER

RANK	STATE	RATE
1	Delaware	38.6
2	Rhode Island	33.3
3	West Virginia	32.9
4	Florida	30.6
5	South Dakota	30.1
6	Iowa	29.1
7	North Dakota	28.0
8	Massachusetts	27.9
9	New Jersey	27.5
10	Connecticut	25.7
10	Maine	25.7
12	Vermont	25.5
13	Pennsylvania	24.9
14	Arkansas	24.7
15	Indiana	24.0
15	Michigan	24.0
17	New York	23.6
18	Ohio	23.3
18	Wisconsin	23.3
20	New Hampshire	23.2
21	South Carolina	22.7
22	Missouri	22.4
23	Illinois	21.1
24	Oklahoma	20.9
24	Oregon	20.9
26	Washington	19.9
27	North Carolina	19.1
28	Kentucky	18.8
28	Tennessee	18.8
30	Arizona	18.5
31	Kansas	18.3
32	Maryland	18.1
33	Virginia	18.0
34	Nebraska	17.6
35	New Mexico	17.5
36	Montana	17.1
37	Alabama	16.4
38	Colorado	16.2
39	Idaho	16.0
40	California	15.7
41	Nevada	15.6
42	Hawaii	15.2
42	Minnesota	15.2
42	Texas	15.2
45	Louisiana	14.2
46	Utah	13.5
47	Mississippi	12.5
47	Wyoming	12.5
49	Georgia	11.2
50	Alaska	1.6

District of Columbia	23.9

Source: Morgan Quitno Press using data from American Cancer Society (http://www.cancer.org/97tabp5.html)
"Cancer Facts & Figures-1997" (Copyright 1997, Reprinted with permission from the American Cancer Society)
*These estimates are offered as a rough guide and should be interpreted with caution. They are calculated according to the distribution of estimated 1997 cancer deaths by state. Rates calculated using 1996 Census resident population estimates.

Estimated New Female Breast Cancer Cases in 1997

National Estimated Total = 180,200 New Cases*

ALPHA ORDER

RANK	STATE	CASES	% of USA
22	Alabama	2,800	1.55%
50	Alaska	230	0.13%
23	Arizona	2,700	1.50%
31	Arkansas	1,900	1.05%
1	California	17,100	9.49%
27	Colorado	2,100	1.17%
28	Connecticut	2,000	1.11%
45	Delaware	570	0.32%
3	Florida	11,800	6.55%
14	Georgia	3,900	2.16%
47	Hawaii	460	0.26%
42	Idaho	720	0.40%
6	Illinois	9,200	5.11%
13	Indiana	4,000	2.22%
26	Iowa	2,400	1.33%
33	Kansas	1,600	0.89%
23	Kentucky	2,700	1.50%
20	Louisiana	3,100	1.72%
37	Maine	990	0.55%
18	Maryland	3,400	1.89%
11	Massachusetts	4,600	2.55%
9	Michigan	6,000	3.33%
21	Minnesota	3,000	1.66%
32	Mississippi	1,800	1.00%
18	Missouri	3,400	1.89%
43	Montana	620	0.34%
35	Nebraska	1,100	0.61%
35	Nevada	1,100	0.61%
39	New Hampshire	960	0.53%
8	New Jersey	6,400	3.55%
38	New Mexico	970	0.54%
2	New York	13,800	7.66%
10	North Carolina	4,900	2.72%
46	North Dakota	490	0.27%
7	Ohio	8,500	4.72%
28	Oklahoma	2,000	1.11%
28	Oregon	2,000	1.11%
5	Pennsylvania	11,000	6.10%
40	Rhode Island	820	0.46%
25	South Carolina	2,600	1.44%
44	South Dakota	580	0.32%
15	Tennessee	3,800	2.11%
4	Texas	11,500	6.38%
40	Utah	820	0.46%
48	Vermont	330	0.18%
12	Virginia	4,400	2.44%
17	Washington	3,500	1.94%
34	West Virginia	1,300	0.72%
16	Wisconsin	3,700	2.05%
48	Wyoming	330	0.18%

RANK ORDER

RANK	STATE	CASES	% of USA
1	California	17,100	9.49%
2	New York	13,800	7.66%
3	Florida	11,800	6.55%
4	Texas	11,500	6.38%
5	Pennsylvania	11,000	6.10%
6	Illinois	9,200	5.11%
7	Ohio	8,500	4.72%
8	New Jersey	6,400	3.55%
9	Michigan	6,000	3.33%
10	North Carolina	4,900	2.72%
11	Massachusetts	4,600	2.55%
12	Virginia	4,400	2.44%
13	Indiana	4,000	2.22%
14	Georgia	3,900	2.16%
15	Tennessee	3,800	2.11%
16	Wisconsin	3,700	2.05%
17	Washington	3,500	1.94%
18	Maryland	3,400	1.89%
18	Missouri	3,400	1.89%
20	Louisiana	3,100	1.72%
21	Minnesota	3,000	1.66%
22	Alabama	2,800	1.55%
23	Arizona	2,700	1.50%
23	Kentucky	2,700	1.50%
25	South Carolina	2,600	1.44%
26	Iowa	2,400	1.33%
27	Colorado	2,100	1.17%
28	Connecticut	2,000	1.11%
28	Oklahoma	2,000	1.11%
28	Oregon	2,000	1.11%
31	Arkansas	1,900	1.05%
32	Mississippi	1,800	1.00%
33	Kansas	1,600	0.89%
34	West Virginia	1,300	0.72%
35	Nebraska	1,100	0.61%
35	Nevada	1,100	0.61%
37	Maine	990	0.55%
38	New Mexico	970	0.54%
39	New Hampshire	960	0.53%
40	Rhode Island	820	0.46%
40	Utah	820	0.46%
42	Idaho	720	0.40%
43	Montana	620	0.34%
44	South Dakota	580	0.32%
45	Delaware	570	0.32%
46	North Dakota	490	0.27%
47	Hawaii	460	0.26%
48	Vermont	330	0.18%
48	Wyoming	330	0.18%
50	Alaska	230	0.13%
	District of Columbia	530	0.29%

Source: American Cancer Society (http://www.cancer.org/97tabp5.html)
   "Cancer Facts & Figures-1997" (Copyright 1997, Reprinted with permission from the American Cancer Society)
*These estimates are offered as a rough guide and should be interpreted with caution. They are calculated
according to the distribution of estimated 1997 cancer deaths by state.

Estimated Rate of New Female Breast Cancer Cases in 1997

National Estimated Rate = 134.0 New Cases per 100,000 Female Population*

ALPHA ORDER

RANK	STATE	RATE
34	Alabama	126.6
49	Alaska	80.3
33	Arizona	126.7
12	Arkansas	147.9
46	California	108.2
44	Colorado	111.1
42	Connecticut	118.6
9	Delaware	154.8
4	Florida	161.6
47	Georgia	105.4
50	Hawaii	78.3
37	Idaho	123.5
11	Illinois	151.6
25	Indiana	134.1
2	Iowa	164.4
38	Kansas	122.7
24	Kentucky	135.8
21	Louisiana	137.6
8	Maine	155.5
28	Maryland	131.1
16	Massachusetts	146.1
39	Michigan	122.4
31	Minnesota	128.1
30	Mississippi	128.2
36	Missouri	123.6
18	Montana	141.7
27	Nebraska	131.4
14	Nevada	146.5
3	New Hampshire	164.3
7	New Jersey	156.2
43	New Mexico	113.4
14	New York	146.5
26	North Carolina	132.3
10	North Dakota	152.3
13	Ohio	147.5
41	Oklahoma	119.2
35	Oregon	125.7
1	Pennsylvania	175.4
5	Rhode Island	159.5
23	South Carolina	136.7
6	South Dakota	156.8
19	Tennessee	139.7
40	Texas	121.2
48	Utah	83.6
45	Vermont	111.0
29	Virginia	130.2
31	Washington	128.1
22	West Virginia	137.1
17	Wisconsin	141.9
20	Wyoming	138.2

RANK ORDER

RANK	STATE	RATE
1	Pennsylvania	175.4
2	Iowa	164.4
3	New Hampshire	164.3
4	Florida	161.6
5	Rhode Island	159.5
6	South Dakota	156.8
7	New Jersey	156.2
8	Maine	155.5
9	Delaware	154.8
10	North Dakota	152.3
11	Illinois	151.6
12	Arkansas	147.9
13	Ohio	147.5
14	Nevada	146.5
14	New York	146.5
16	Massachusetts	146.1
17	Wisconsin	141.9
18	Montana	141.7
19	Tennessee	139.7
20	Wyoming	138.2
21	Louisiana	137.6
22	West Virginia	137.1
23	South Carolina	136.7
24	Kentucky	135.8
25	Indiana	134.1
26	North Carolina	132.3
27	Nebraska	131.4
28	Maryland	131.1
29	Virginia	130.2
30	Mississippi	128.2
31	Minnesota	128.1
31	Washington	128.1
33	Arizona	126.7
34	Alabama	126.6
35	Oregon	125.7
36	Missouri	123.6
37	Idaho	123.5
38	Kansas	122.7
39	Michigan	122.4
40	Texas	121.2
41	Oklahoma	119.2
42	Connecticut	118.6
43	New Mexico	113.4
44	Colorado	111.1
45	Vermont	111.0
46	California	108.2
47	Georgia	105.4
48	Utah	83.6
49	Alaska	80.3
50	Hawaii	78.3

District of Columbia 179.8

Source: Morgan Quitno Press using data from American Cancer Society (http://www.cancer.org/97tabp5.html)
"Cancer Facts & Figures-1997" (Copyright 1997, Reprinted with permission from the American Cancer Society)
These estimates are offered as a rough guide and should be interpreted with caution. They are calculated
according to the distribution of estimated 1997 cancer deaths by state. Rates calculated using 1995 Census female
resident population estimates.

Percent of Women Age 50 and Older
Who Had a Breast Exam and Mammogram Within the Past Two Years: 1995
National Median = 61.52% of Women 50 Years and Older*

ALPHA ORDER

RANK	STATE	PERCENT
44	Alabama	55.33
5	Alaska	70.23
3	Arizona	70.79
46	Arkansas	55.10
13	California	67.59
27	Colorado	60.83
14	Connecticut	67.57
17	Delaware	65.94
8	Florida	69.17
6	Georgia	70.00
15	Hawaii	67.14
38	Idaho	57.89
19	Illinois	64.53
43	Indiana	55.78
35	Iowa	58.38
41	Kansas	57.04
42	Kentucky	55.94
47	Louisiana	53.95
10	Maine	68.50
2	Maryland	71.76
1	Massachusetts	75.71
12	Michigan	67.60
16	Minnesota	66.07
50	Mississippi	47.51
33	Missouri	58.65
32	Montana	58.76
36	Nebraska	58.15
29	Nevada	59.19
18	New Hampshire	64.89
39	New Jersey	57.84
20	New Mexico	64.45
9	New York	68.78
25	North Carolina	61.69
23	North Dakota	62.23
21	Ohio	63.87
30	Oklahoma	58.89
4	Oregon	70.35
49	Pennsylvania	51.10
24	Rhode Island	62.15
11	South Carolina	68.43
40	South Dakota	57.11
33	Tennessee	58.65
28	Texas	59.67
26	Utah	61.35
22	Vermont	63.17
37	Virginia	58.10
7	Washington	69.38
31	West Virginia	58.84
45	Wisconsin	55.11
48	Wyoming	51.31

RANK ORDER

RANK	STATE	PERCENT
1	Massachusetts	75.71
2	Maryland	71.76
3	Arizona	70.79
4	Oregon	70.35
5	Alaska	70.23
6	Georgia	70.00
7	Washington	69.38
8	Florida	69.17
9	New York	68.78
10	Maine	68.50
11	South Carolina	68.43
12	Michigan	67.60
13	California	67.59
14	Connecticut	67.57
15	Hawaii	67.14
16	Minnesota	66.07
17	Delaware	65.94
18	New Hampshire	64.89
19	Illinois	64.53
20	New Mexico	64.45
21	Ohio	63.87
22	Vermont	63.17
23	North Dakota	62.23
24	Rhode Island	62.15
25	North Carolina	61.69
26	Utah	61.35
27	Colorado	60.83
28	Texas	59.67
29	Nevada	59.19
30	Oklahoma	58.89
31	West Virginia	58.84
32	Montana	58.76
33	Missouri	58.65
33	Tennessee	58.65
35	Iowa	58.38
36	Nebraska	58.15
37	Virginia	58.10
38	Idaho	57.89
39	New Jersey	57.84
40	South Dakota	57.11
41	Kansas	57.04
42	Kentucky	55.94
43	Indiana	55.78
44	Alabama	55.33
45	Wisconsin	55.11
46	Arkansas	55.10
47	Louisiana	53.95
48	Wyoming	51.31
49	Pennsylvania	51.10
50	Mississippi	47.51
	District of Columbia**	NA

Source: U.S. Department of Health and Human Services, Centers for Disease Control and Prevention
"1995 Behavioral Risk Factor Surveillance Summary Prevalence Report" (December 10, 1996)
Women who have had a breast exam and a mammogram within the past two years.
**Not available.*

Estimated New Colon and Rectum Cancer Cases in 1997

National Estimated Total = 131,200 New Cases*

ALPHA ORDER

ALPHA ORDER

RANK ORDER

RANK	STATE	CASES	% of USA
26	Alabama	1,600	1.22%
50	Alaska	130	0.10%
23	Arizona	1,900	1.45%
29	Arkansas	1,500	1.14%
1	California	11,300	8.61%
30	Colorado	1,400	1.07%
26	Connecticut	1,600	1.22%
47	Delaware	340	0.26%
3	Florida	8,900	6.78%
17	Georgia	2,600	1.98%
42	Hawaii	520	0.40%
44	Idaho	450	0.34%
6	Illinois	6,500	4.95%
13	Indiana	3,100	2.36%
23	Iowa	1,900	1.45%
32	Kansas	1,300	0.99%
19	Kentucky	2,300	1.75%
20	Louisiana	2,200	1.68%
36	Maine	740	0.56%
16	Maryland	2,700	2.06%
10	Massachusetts	3,900	2.97%
8	Michigan	5,000	3.81%
22	Minnesota	2,000	1.52%
33	Mississippi	1,200	0.91%
12	Missouri	3,200	2.44%
43	Montana	460	0.35%
35	Nebraska	910	0.69%
37	Nevada	730	0.56%
39	New Hampshire	580	0.44%
9	New Jersey	4,600	3.51%
41	New Mexico	530	0.40%
2	New York	9,200	7.01%
11	North Carolina	3,600	2.74%
46	North Dakota	350	0.27%
7	Ohio	6,300	4.80%
26	Oklahoma	1,600	1.22%
30	Oregon	1,400	1.07%
5	Pennsylvania	8,000	6.10%
38	Rhode Island	660	0.50%
23	South Carolina	1,900	1.45%
45	South Dakota	390	0.30%
15	Tennessee	2,800	2.13%
4	Texas	8,500	6.48%
40	Utah	560	0.43%
48	Vermont	230	0.18%
14	Virginia	3,000	2.29%
20	Washington	2,200	1.68%
33	West Virginia	1,200	0.91%
18	Wisconsin	2,500	1.91%
49	Wyoming	170	0.13%

RANK	STATE	CASES	% of USA
1	California	11,300	8.61%
2	New York	9,200	7.01%
3	Florida	8,900	6.78%
4	Texas	8,500	6.48%
5	Pennsylvania	8,000	6.10%
6	Illinois	6,500	4.95%
7	Ohio	6,300	4.80%
8	Michigan	5,000	3.81%
9	New Jersey	4,600	3.51%
10	Massachusetts	3,900	2.97%
11	North Carolina	3,600	2.74%
12	Missouri	3,200	2.44%
13	Indiana	3,100	2.36%
14	Virginia	3,000	2.29%
15	Tennessee	2,800	2.13%
16	Maryland	2,700	2.06%
17	Georgia	2,600	1.98%
18	Wisconsin	2,500	1.91%
19	Kentucky	2,300	1.75%
20	Louisiana	2,200	1.68%
20	Washington	2,200	1.68%
22	Minnesota	2,000	1.52%
23	Arizona	1,900	1.45%
23	Iowa	1,900	1.45%
23	South Carolina	1,900	1.45%
26	Alabama	1,600	1.22%
26	Connecticut	1,600	1.22%
26	Oklahoma	1,600	1.22%
29	Arkansas	1,500	1.14%
30	Colorado	1,400	1.07%
30	Oregon	1,400	1.07%
32	Kansas	1,300	0.99%
33	Mississippi	1,200	0.91%
33	West Virginia	1,200	0.91%
35	Nebraska	910	0.69%
36	Maine	740	0.56%
37	Nevada	730	0.56%
38	Rhode Island	660	0.50%
39	New Hampshire	580	0.44%
40	Utah	560	0.43%
41	New Mexico	530	0.40%
42	Hawaii	520	0.40%
43	Montana	460	0.35%
44	Idaho	450	0.34%
45	South Dakota	390	0.30%
46	North Dakota	350	0.27%
47	Delaware	340	0.26%
48	Vermont	230	0.18%
49	Wyoming	170	0.13%
50	Alaska	130	0.10%
	District of Columbia	320	0.24%

Source: American Cancer Society (http://www.cancer.org/97tabp5.html)
"Cancer Facts & Figures-1997" (Copyright 1997, Reprinted with permission from the American Cancer Society)
These estimates are offered as a rough guide and should be interpreted with caution. They are calculated according to the distribution of estimated 1997 cancer deaths by state.

Estimated Rate of New Colon and Rectum Cancer Cases in 1997

National Estimated Rate = 49.5 New Cases per 100,000 Population*

ALPHA ORDER

RANK	STATE	RATE
43	Alabama	37.4
50	Alaska	21.4
38	Arizona	42.9
7	Arkansas	59.8
45	California	35.4
44	Colorado	36.6
28	Connecticut	48.9
31	Delaware	46.9
6	Florida	61.8
45	Georgia	35.4
36	Hawaii	43.9
42	Idaho	37.8
14	Illinois	54.9
18	Indiana	53.1
2	Iowa	66.6
25	Kansas	50.5
10	Kentucky	59.2
23	Louisiana	50.6
9	Maine	59.5
17	Maryland	53.2
5	Massachusetts	64.0
21	Michigan	52.1
38	Minnesota	42.9
35	Mississippi	44.2
8	Missouri	59.7
20	Montana	52.3
13	Nebraska	55.1
32	Nevada	45.5
26	New Hampshire	49.9
11	New Jersey	57.6
48	New Mexico	30.9
23	New York	50.6
27	North Carolina	49.2
15	North Dakota	54.3
12	Ohio	56.4
29	Oklahoma	48.5
37	Oregon	43.7
3	Pennsylvania	66.4
1	Rhode Island	66.7
22	South Carolina	51.4
16	South Dakota	53.3
19	Tennessee	52.6
34	Texas	44.4
49	Utah	28.0
41	Vermont	39.0
33	Virginia	44.9
40	Washington	39.8
4	West Virginia	65.7
30	Wisconsin	48.4
47	Wyoming	35.3

RANK ORDER

RANK	STATE	RATE
1	Rhode Island	66.7
2	Iowa	66.6
3	Pennsylvania	66.4
4	West Virginia	65.7
5	Massachusetts	64.0
6	Florida	61.8
7	Arkansas	59.8
8	Missouri	59.7
9	Maine	59.5
10	Kentucky	59.2
11	New Jersey	57.6
12	Ohio	56.4
13	Nebraska	55.1
14	Illinois	54.9
15	North Dakota	54.3
16	South Dakota	53.3
17	Maryland	53.2
18	Indiana	53.1
19	Tennessee	52.6
20	Montana	52.3
21	Michigan	52.1
22	South Carolina	51.4
23	Louisiana	50.6
23	New York	50.6
25	Kansas	50.5
26	New Hampshire	49.9
27	North Carolina	49.2
28	Connecticut	48.9
29	Oklahoma	48.5
30	Wisconsin	48.4
31	Delaware	46.9
32	Nevada	45.5
33	Virginia	44.9
34	Texas	44.4
35	Mississippi	44.2
36	Hawaii	43.9
37	Oregon	43.7
38	Arizona	42.9
38	Minnesota	42.9
40	Washington	39.8
41	Vermont	39.0
42	Idaho	37.8
43	Alabama	37.4
44	Colorado	36.6
45	California	35.4
45	Georgia	35.4
47	Wyoming	35.3
48	New Mexico	30.9
49	Utah	28.0
50	Alaska	21.4

| | District of Columbia | 58.9 |

Source: Morgan Quitno Press using data from American Cancer Society (http://www.cancer.org/97tabp5.html)
"Cancer Facts & Figures-1997" (Copyright 1997, Reprinted with permission from the American Cancer Society)
*These estimates are offered as a rough guide and should be interpreted with caution. They are calculated according to the distribution of estimated 1997 cancer deaths by state. Rates calculated using 1996 Census resident population estimates.

Estimated New Cases of Leukemia in 1996

National Estimated Total = 27,600 New Cases*

ALPHA ORDER

RANK ORDER

RANK	STATE	CASES	% of USA		RANK	STATE	CASES	% of USA
20	Alabama	500	1.81%		1	California	2,800	10.14%
50	Alaska	10	0.04%		2	Florida	1,900	6.88%
18	Arizona	550	1.99%		3	New York	1,800	6.52%
33	Arkansas	280	1.01%		3	Texas	1,800	6.52%
1	California	2,800	10.14%		5	Pennsylvania	1,500	5.43%
28	Colorado	330	1.20%		6	Illinois	1,400	5.07%
26	Connecticut	370	1.34%		7	Ohio	1,200	4.35%
46	Delaware	60	0.22%		8	Michigan	1,000	3.62%
2	Florida	1,900	6.88%		9	New Jersey	900	3.26%
14	Georgia	630	2.28%		10	North Carolina	700	2.54%
46	Hawaii	60	0.22%		11	Massachusetts	680	2.46%
41	Idaho	100	0.36%		12	Missouri	650	2.36%
6	Illinois	1,400	5.07%		13	Indiana	640	2.32%
13	Indiana	640	2.32%		14	Georgia	630	2.28%
25	Iowa	400	1.45%		15	Virginia	610	2.21%
30	Kansas	320	1.16%		16	Minnesota	590	2.14%
23	Kentucky	440	1.59%		16	Washington	590	2.14%
20	Louisiana	500	1.81%		18	Arizona	550	1.99%
35	Maine	160	0.58%		19	Wisconsin	530	1.92%
24	Maryland	430	1.56%		20	Alabama	500	1.81%
11	Massachusetts	680	2.46%		20	Louisiana	500	1.81%
8	Michigan	1,000	3.62%		22	Tennessee	490	1.78%
16	Minnesota	590	2.14%		23	Kentucky	440	1.59%
32	Mississippi	290	1.05%		24	Maryland	430	1.56%
12	Missouri	650	2.36%		25	Iowa	400	1.45%
41	Montana	100	0.36%		26	Connecticut	370	1.34%
38	Nebraska	130	0.47%		27	Oregon	350	1.27%
35	Nevada	160	0.58%		28	Colorado	330	1.20%
44	New Hampshire	80	0.29%		28	Oklahoma	330	1.20%
9	New Jersey	900	3.26%		30	Kansas	320	1.16%
35	New Mexico	160	0.58%		31	South Carolina	300	1.09%
3	New York	1,800	6.52%		32	Mississippi	290	1.05%
10	North Carolina	700	2.54%		33	Arkansas	280	1.01%
44	North Dakota	80	0.29%		34	West Virginia	220	0.80%
7	Ohio	1,200	4.35%		35	Maine	160	0.58%
28	Oklahoma	330	1.20%		35	Nevada	160	0.58%
27	Oregon	350	1.27%		35	New Mexico	160	0.58%
5	Pennsylvania	1,500	5.43%		38	Nebraska	130	0.47%
39	Rhode Island	110	0.40%		39	Rhode Island	110	0.40%
31	South Carolina	300	1.09%		39	Utah	110	0.40%
43	South Dakota	90	0.33%		41	Idaho	100	0.36%
22	Tennessee	490	1.78%		41	Montana	100	0.36%
3	Texas	1,800	6.52%		43	South Dakota	90	0.33%
39	Utah	110	0.40%		44	New Hampshire	80	0.29%
48	Vermont	50	0.18%		44	North Dakota	80	0.29%
15	Virginia	610	2.21%		46	Delaware	60	0.22%
16	Washington	590	2.14%		46	Hawaii	60	0.22%
34	West Virginia	220	0.80%		48	Vermont	50	0.18%
19	Wisconsin	530	1.92%		48	Wyoming	50	0.18%
48	Wyoming	50	0.18%		50	Alaska	10	0.04%
						District of Columbia	70	0.25%

Source: American Cancer Society

"Cancer Facts & Figures-1996" (Copyright 1996, Reprinted with permission from the American Cancer Society)
*These estimates are offered as a rough guide and should be interpreted with caution. They are calculated according to the distribution of estimated 1996 cancer deaths by state.

Estimated Rate of New Leukemia Cases in 1996

National Estimated Rate = 10.50 New Cases per 100,000 Population*

ALPHA ORDER				RANK ORDER		
RANK	**STATE**	**RATE**		**RANK**	**STATE**	**RATE**
13	Alabama	11.76		1	Iowa	14.07
50	Alaska	1.66		2	Florida	13.41
3	Arizona	13.04		3	Arizona	13.04
19	Arkansas	11.27		4	Maine	12.89
38	California	8.86		5	Minnesota	12.80
39	Colorado	8.81		6	Kansas	12.48
18	Connecticut	11.30		6	North Dakota	12.48
44	Delaware	8.37		8	Pennsylvania	12.43
2	Florida	13.41		9	South Dakota	12.35
40	Georgia	8.75		10	Missouri	12.21
49	Hawaii	5.05		11	West Virginia	12.04
41	Idaho	8.60		12	Illinois	11.83
12	Illinois	11.83		13	Alabama	11.76
23	Indiana	11.03		14	Louisiana	11.52
1	Iowa	14.07		15	Montana	11.49
6	Kansas	12.48		16	Kentucky	11.40
16	Kentucky	11.40		17	New Jersey	11.33
14	Louisiana	11.52		18	Connecticut	11.30
4	Maine	12.89		19	Arkansas	11.27
43	Maryland	8.53		20	Massachusetts	11.20
20	Massachusetts	11.20		21	Oregon	11.14
27	Michigan	10.47		22	Rhode Island	11.11
5	Minnesota	12.80		23	Indiana	11.03
26	Mississippi	10.75		24	Washington	10.86
10	Missouri	12.21		25	Ohio	10.76
15	Montana	11.49		26	Mississippi	10.75
46	Nebraska	7.94		27	Michigan	10.47
28	Nevada	10.46		28	Nevada	10.46
47	New Hampshire	6.97		29	Wyoming	10.42
17	New Jersey	11.33		30	Wisconsin	10.35
35	New Mexico	9.50		31	Oklahoma	10.07
32	New York	9.93		32	New York	9.93
33	North Carolina	9.73		33	North Carolina	9.73
6	North Dakota	12.48		34	Texas	9.61
25	Ohio	10.76		35	New Mexico	9.50
31	Oklahoma	10.07		36	Tennessee	9.32
21	Oregon	11.14		37	Virginia	9.22
8	Pennsylvania	12.43		38	California	8.86
22	Rhode Island	11.11		39	Colorado	8.81
45	South Carolina	8.17		40	Georgia	8.75
9	South Dakota	12.35		41	Idaho	8.60
36	Tennessee	9.32		42	Vermont	8.55
34	Texas	9.61		43	Maryland	8.53
48	Utah	5.64		44	Delaware	8.37
42	Vermont	8.55		45	South Carolina	8.17
37	Virginia	9.22		46	Nebraska	7.94
24	Washington	10.86		47	New Hampshire	6.97
11	West Virginia	12.04		48	Utah	5.64
30	Wisconsin	10.35		49	Hawaii	5.05
29	Wyoming	10.42		50	Alaska	1.66
					District of Columbia	12.64

Source: Morgan Quitno Press using data from American Cancer Society
  "Cancer Facts & Figures-1996" (Copyright 1996, Reprinted with permission from the American Cancer Society)
*These estimates are offered as a rough guide and should be interpreted with caution. They are calculated
according to the distribution of estimated 1996 cancer deaths by state. Rates calculated using 1995 Census
resident population estimates.

Estimated New Lung Cancer Cases in 1997

National Estimated Total = 178,100 New Cases*

ALPHA ORDER

ALPHA ORDER

RANK	STATE	CASES	% of USA
21	Alabama	3,100	1.74%
50	Alaska	210	0.12%
23	Arizona	2,900	1.63%
27	Arkansas	2,400	1.35%
1	California	15,300	8.59%
33	Colorado	1,600	0.90%
29	Connecticut	2,000	1.12%
41	Delaware	600	0.34%
2	Florida	13,400	7.52%
13	Georgia	4,300	2.41%
44	Hawaii	540	0.30%
42	Idaho	570	0.32%
7	Illinois	7,900	4.44%
12	Indiana	4,400	2.47%
29	Iowa	2,000	1.12%
33	Kansas	1,600	0.90%
17	Kentucky	3,600	2.02%
20	Louisiana	3,300	1.85%
36	Maine	1,100	0.62%
19	Maryland	3,400	1.91%
14	Massachusetts	4,200	2.36%
8	Michigan	6,700	3.76%
25	Minnesota	2,500	1.40%
31	Mississippi	1,900	1.07%
11	Missouri	4,500	2.53%
42	Montana	570	0.32%
37	Nebraska	990	0.56%
35	Nevada	1,200	0.67%
38	New Hampshire	800	0.45%
10	New Jersey	5,300	2.98%
40	New Mexico	740	0.42%
4	New York	11,400	6.40%
9	North Carolina	5,400	3.03%
48	North Dakota	340	0.19%
6	Ohio	8,600	4.83%
25	Oklahoma	2,500	1.40%
27	Oregon	2,400	1.35%
5	Pennsylvania	9,500	5.33%
39	Rhode Island	790	0.44%
24	South Carolina	2,700	1.52%
46	South Dakota	450	0.25%
14	Tennessee	4,200	2.36%
3	Texas	12,000	6.74%
45	Utah	510	0.29%
47	Vermont	390	0.22%
16	Virginia	4,100	2.30%
17	Washington	3,600	2.02%
32	West Virginia	1,800	1.01%
22	Wisconsin	3,000	1.68%
49	Wyoming	270	0.15%

RANK ORDER

RANK	STATE	CASES	% of USA
1	California	15,300	8.59%
2	Florida	13,400	7.52%
3	Texas	12,000	6.74%
4	New York	11,400	6.40%
5	Pennsylvania	9,500	5.33%
6	Ohio	8,600	4.83%
7	Illinois	7,900	4.44%
8	Michigan	6,700	3.76%
9	North Carolina	5,400	3.03%
10	New Jersey	5,300	2.98%
11	Missouri	4,500	2.53%
12	Indiana	4,400	2.47%
13	Georgia	4,300	2.41%
14	Massachusetts	4,200	2.36%
14	Tennessee	4,200	2.36%
16	Virginia	4,100	2.30%
17	Kentucky	3,600	2.02%
17	Washington	3,600	2.02%
19	Maryland	3,400	1.91%
20	Louisiana	3,300	1.85%
21	Alabama	3,100	1.74%
22	Wisconsin	3,000	1.68%
23	Arizona	2,900	1.63%
24	South Carolina	2,700	1.52%
25	Minnesota	2,500	1.40%
25	Oklahoma	2,500	1.40%
27	Arkansas	2,400	1.35%
27	Oregon	2,400	1.35%
29	Connecticut	2,000	1.12%
29	Iowa	2,000	1.12%
31	Mississippi	1,900	1.07%
32	West Virginia	1,800	1.01%
33	Colorado	1,600	0.90%
33	Kansas	1,600	0.90%
35	Nevada	1,200	0.67%
36	Maine	1,100	0.62%
37	Nebraska	990	0.56%
38	New Hampshire	800	0.45%
39	Rhode Island	790	0.44%
40	New Mexico	740	0.42%
41	Delaware	600	0.34%
42	Idaho	570	0.32%
42	Montana	570	0.32%
44	Hawaii	540	0.30%
45	Utah	510	0.29%
46	South Dakota	450	0.25%
47	Vermont	390	0.22%
48	North Dakota	340	0.19%
49	Wyoming	270	0.15%
50	Alaska	210	0.12%
	District of Columbia	360	0.20%

Source: American Cancer Society (http://www.cancer.org/97tabp5.html)
"Cancer Facts & Figures-1997" (Copyright 1997, Reprinted with permission from the American Cancer Society)
*These estimates are offered as a rough guide and should be interpreted with caution. They are calculated according to the distribution of estimated 1997 cancer deaths by state.

Estimated Rate of New Lung Cancer Cases in 1997

National Estimated Rate = 67.1 New Cases per 100,000 Population*

ALPHA ORDER

RANK	STATE	RATE
19	Alabama	72.5
49	Alaska	34.6
29	Arizona	65.5
2	Arkansas	95.6
44	California	48.0
48	Colorado	41.9
37	Connecticut	61.1
7	Delaware	82.8
3	Florida	93.1
39	Georgia	58.5
46	Hawaii	45.6
45	Idaho	47.9
26	Illinois	66.7
14	Indiana	75.3
20	Iowa	70.1
34	Kansas	62.2
4	Kentucky	92.7
12	Louisiana	75.8
5	Maine	88.5
25	Maryland	67.0
23	Massachusetts	68.9
22	Michigan	69.8
42	Minnesota	53.7
21	Mississippi	70.0
6	Missouri	84.0
31	Montana	64.8
38	Nebraska	59.9
15	Nevada	74.9
24	New Hampshire	68.8
27	New Jersey	66.3
47	New Mexico	43.2
32	New York	62.7
17	North Carolina	73.7
43	North Dakota	52.8
11	Ohio	77.0
13	Oklahoma	75.7
15	Oregon	74.9
10	Pennsylvania	78.8
8	Rhode Island	79.8
18	South Carolina	73.0
35	South Dakota	61.5
9	Tennessee	78.9
32	Texas	62.7
50	Utah	25.5
28	Vermont	66.2
36	Virginia	61.4
30	Washington	65.1
1	West Virginia	98.6
40	Wisconsin	58.1
41	Wyoming	56.1

RANK ORDER

RANK	STATE	RATE
1	West Virginia	98.6
2	Arkansas	95.6
3	Florida	93.1
4	Kentucky	92.7
5	Maine	88.5
6	Missouri	84.0
7	Delaware	82.8
8	Rhode Island	79.8
9	Tennessee	78.9
10	Pennsylvania	78.8
11	Ohio	77.0
12	Louisiana	75.8
13	Oklahoma	75.7
14	Indiana	75.3
15	Nevada	74.9
15	Oregon	74.9
17	North Carolina	73.7
18	South Carolina	73.0
19	Alabama	72.5
20	Iowa	70.1
21	Mississippi	70.0
22	Michigan	69.8
23	Massachusetts	68.9
24	New Hampshire	68.8
25	Maryland	67.0
26	Illinois	66.7
27	New Jersey	66.3
28	Vermont	66.2
29	Arizona	65.5
30	Washington	65.1
31	Montana	64.8
32	New York	62.7
32	Texas	62.7
34	Kansas	62.2
35	South Dakota	61.5
36	Virginia	61.4
37	Connecticut	61.1
38	Nebraska	59.9
39	Georgia	58.5
40	Wisconsin	58.1
41	Wyoming	56.1
42	Minnesota	53.7
43	North Dakota	52.8
44	California	48.0
45	Idaho	47.9
46	Hawaii	45.6
47	New Mexico	43.2
48	Colorado	41.9
49	Alaska	34.6
50	Utah	25.5
	District of Columbia	66.3

Source: Morgan Quitno Press using data from American Cancer Society (http://www.cancer.org/97tabp5.html)
"Cancer Facts & Figures-1997" (Copyright 1997, Reprinted with permission from the American Cancer Society)
*These estimates are offered as a rough guide and should be interpreted with caution. They are calculated according to the distribution of estimated 1997 cancer deaths by state. Rates calculated using 1996 Census resident population estimates.

Estimated New Non-Hodgkin's Lymphoma Cases in 1997

National Estimated Total = 53,600 New Cases*

ALPHA ORDER

RANK	STATE	CASES	% of USA
21	Alabama	860	1.60%
50	Alaska	30	0.06%
19	Arizona	890	1.66%
29	Arkansas	600	1.12%
1	California	4,800	8.96%
30	Colorado	580	1.08%
26	Connecticut	730	1.36%
46	Delaware	180	0.34%
3	Florida	3,700	6.90%
19	Georgia	890	1.66%
42	Hawaii	230	0.43%
43	Idaho	210	0.39%
7	Illinois	2,500	4.66%
16	Indiana	1,100	2.05%
24	Iowa	790	1.47%
32	Kansas	560	1.04%
25	Kentucky	780	1.46%
26	Louisiana	730	1.36%
36	Maine	330	0.62%
22	Maryland	850	1.59%
10	Massachusetts	1,500	2.80%
8	Michigan	1,900	3.54%
12	Minnesota	1,200	2.24%
33	Mississippi	440	0.82%
12	Missouri	1,200	2.24%
43	Montana	210	0.39%
35	Nebraska	370	0.69%
37	Nevada	320	0.60%
41	New Hampshire	270	0.50%
9	New Jersey	1,700	3.17%
40	New Mexico	280	0.52%
2	New York	4,000	7.46%
11	North Carolina	1,400	2.61%
43	North Dakota	210	0.39%
6	Ohio	2,600	4.85%
23	Oklahoma	810	1.51%
28	Oregon	690	1.29%
5	Pennsylvania	3,100	5.78%
39	Rhode Island	290	0.54%
30	South Carolina	580	1.08%
47	South Dakota	120	0.22%
16	Tennessee	1,100	2.05%
4	Texas	3,500	6.53%
38	Utah	310	0.58%
47	Vermont	120	0.22%
12	Virginia	1,200	2.24%
18	Washington	1,000	1.87%
34	West Virginia	380	0.71%
12	Wisconsin	1,200	2.24%
49	Wyoming	60	0.11%

RANK ORDER

RANK	STATE	CASES	% of USA
1	California	4,800	8.96%
2	New York	4,000	7.46%
3	Florida	3,700	6.90%
4	Texas	3,500	6.53%
5	Pennsylvania	3,100	5.78%
6	Ohio	2,600	4.85%
7	Illinois	2,500	4.66%
8	Michigan	1,900	3.54%
9	New Jersey	1,700	3.17%
10	Massachusetts	1,500	2.80%
11	North Carolina	1,400	2.61%
12	Minnesota	1,200	2.24%
12	Missouri	1,200	2.24%
12	Virginia	1,200	2.24%
12	Wisconsin	1,200	2.24%
16	Indiana	1,100	2.05%
16	Tennessee	1,100	2.05%
18	Washington	1,000	1.87%
19	Arizona	890	1.66%
19	Georgia	890	1.66%
21	Alabama	860	1.60%
22	Maryland	850	1.59%
23	Oklahoma	810	1.51%
24	Iowa	790	1.47%
25	Kentucky	780	1.46%
26	Connecticut	730	1.36%
26	Louisiana	730	1.36%
28	Oregon	690	1.29%
29	Arkansas	600	1.12%
30	Colorado	580	1.08%
30	South Carolina	580	1.08%
32	Kansas	560	1.04%
33	Mississippi	440	0.82%
34	West Virginia	380	0.71%
35	Nebraska	370	0.69%
36	Maine	330	0.62%
37	Nevada	320	0.60%
38	Utah	310	0.58%
39	Rhode Island	290	0.54%
40	New Mexico	280	0.52%
41	New Hampshire	270	0.50%
42	Hawaii	230	0.43%
43	Idaho	210	0.39%
43	Montana	210	0.39%
43	North Dakota	210	0.39%
46	Delaware	180	0.34%
47	South Dakota	120	0.22%
47	Vermont	120	0.22%
49	Wyoming	60	0.11%
50	Alaska	30	0.06%
	District of Columbia	110	0.21%

Source: American Cancer Society (http://www.cancer.org/97tabp5.html)
"Cancer Facts & Figures-1997" (Copyright 1997, Reprinted with permission from the American Cancer Society)
These estimates are offered as a rough guide and should be interpreted with caution. They are calculated according to the distribution of estimated 1997 cancer deaths by state.

Estimated Rate of New Non-Hodgkin's Lymphoma Cases in 1997

National Estimated Rate = 20.2 New Cases per 100,000 Population*

ALPHA ORDER

RANK ORDER

RANK	STATE	RATE		RANK	STATE	RATE
27	Alabama	20.1		1	North Dakota	32.6
50	Alaska	4.9		2	Rhode Island	29.3
27	Arizona	20.1		3	Iowa	27.7
11	Arkansas	23.9		4	Maine	26.5
47	California	15.1		5	Minnesota	25.8
46	Colorado	15.2		6	Florida	25.7
18	Connecticut	22.3		6	Pennsylvania	25.7
8	Delaware	24.8		8	Delaware	24.8
6	Florida	25.7		9	Massachusetts	24.6
49	Georgia	12.1		10	Oklahoma	24.5
32	Hawaii	19.4		11	Arkansas	23.9
38	Idaho	17.7		11	Montana	23.9
23	Illinois	21.1		13	Ohio	23.3
34	Indiana	18.8		13	Wisconsin	23.3
3	Iowa	27.7		15	New Hampshire	23.2
20	Kansas	21.8		16	Missouri	22.4
27	Kentucky	20.1		16	Nebraska	22.4
39	Louisiana	16.8		18	Connecticut	22.3
4	Maine	26.5		19	New York	22.0
39	Maryland	16.8		20	Kansas	21.8
9	Massachusetts	24.6		21	Oregon	21.5
31	Michigan	19.8		22	New Jersey	21.3
5	Minnesota	25.8		23	Illinois	21.1
43	Mississippi	16.2		24	West Virginia	20.8
16	Missouri	22.4		25	Tennessee	20.7
11	Montana	23.9		26	Vermont	20.4
16	Nebraska	22.4		27	Alabama	20.1
30	Nevada	20.0		27	Arizona	20.1
15	New Hampshire	23.2		27	Kentucky	20.1
22	New Jersey	21.3		30	Nevada	20.0
42	New Mexico	16.3		31	Michigan	19.8
19	New York	22.0		32	Hawaii	19.4
33	North Carolina	19.1		33	North Carolina	19.1
1	North Dakota	32.6		34	Indiana	18.8
13	Ohio	23.3		35	Texas	18.3
10	Oklahoma	24.5		36	Washington	18.1
21	Oregon	21.5		37	Virginia	18.0
6	Pennsylvania	25.7		38	Idaho	17.7
2	Rhode Island	29.3		39	Louisiana	16.8
44	South Carolina	15.7		39	Maryland	16.8
41	South Dakota	16.4		41	South Dakota	16.4
25	Tennessee	20.7		42	New Mexico	16.3
35	Texas	18.3		43	Mississippi	16.2
45	Utah	15.5		44	South Carolina	15.7
26	Vermont	20.4		45	Utah	15.5
37	Virginia	18.0		46	Colorado	15.2
36	Washington	18.1		47	California	15.1
24	West Virginia	20.8		48	Wyoming	12.5
13	Wisconsin	23.3		49	Georgia	12.1
48	Wyoming	12.5		50	Alaska	4.9

District of Columbia   20.3

Source: Morgan Quitno Press using data from American Cancer Society (http://www.cancer.org/97tabp5.html)
"Cancer Facts & Figures-1997" (Copyright 1997, Reprinted with permission from the American Cancer Society)
*These estimates are offered as a rough guide and should be interpreted with caution. They are calculated according to the distribution of estimated 1997 cancer deaths by state. Rates calculated using 1996 Census resident population estimates.

Estimated New Pancreatic Cancer Cases in 1997

National Estimated Total = 27,600 New Cases*

ALPHA ORDER

RANK	STATE	CASES	% of USA
23	Alabama	410	1.49%
50	Alaska	20	0.07%
22	Arizona	440	1.59%
31	Arkansas	280	1.01%
1	California	2,600	9.42%
28	Colorado	350	1.27%
26	Connecticut	360	1.30%
45	Delaware	80	0.29%
3	Florida	2,000	7.25%
12	Georgia	680	2.46%
39	Hawaii	130	0.47%
46	Idaho	70	0.25%
6	Illinois	1,200	4.35%
12	Indiana	680	2.46%
31	Iowa	280	1.01%
31	Kansas	280	1.01%
21	Kentucky	450	1.63%
18	Louisiana	520	1.88%
35	Maine	160	0.58%
20	Maryland	470	1.70%
12	Massachusetts	680	2.46%
8	Michigan	1,000	3.62%
23	Minnesota	410	1.49%
30	Mississippi	290	1.05%
17	Missouri	560	2.03%
42	Montana	100	0.36%
35	Nebraska	160	0.58%
37	Nevada	150	0.54%
39	New Hampshire	130	0.47%
9	New Jersey	930	3.37%
38	New Mexico	140	0.51%
2	New York	2,100	7.61%
10	North Carolina	750	2.72%
46	North Dakota	70	0.25%
6	Ohio	1,200	4.35%
29	Oklahoma	340	1.23%
25	Oregon	370	1.34%
5	Pennsylvania	1,500	5.43%
43	Rhode Island	90	0.33%
26	South Carolina	360	1.30%
43	South Dakota	90	0.33%
16	Tennessee	570	2.07%
4	Texas	1,900	6.88%
41	Utah	110	0.40%
48	Vermont	50	0.18%
11	Virginia	710	2.57%
19	Washington	510	1.85%
34	West Virginia	200	0.72%
15	Wisconsin	580	2.10%
49	Wyoming	40	0.14%

RANK ORDER

RANK	STATE	CASES	% of USA
1	California	2,600	9.42%
2	New York	2,100	7.61%
3	Florida	2,000	7.25%
4	Texas	1,900	6.88%
5	Pennsylvania	1,500	5.43%
6	Illinois	1,200	4.35%
6	Ohio	1,200	4.35%
8	Michigan	1,000	3.62%
9	New Jersey	930	3.37%
10	North Carolina	750	2.72%
11	Virginia	710	2.57%
12	Georgia	680	2.46%
12	Indiana	680	2.46%
12	Massachusetts	680	2.46%
15	Wisconsin	580	2.10%
16	Tennessee	570	2.07%
17	Missouri	560	2.03%
18	Louisiana	520	1.88%
19	Washington	510	1.85%
20	Maryland	470	1.70%
21	Kentucky	450	1.63%
22	Arizona	440	1.59%
23	Alabama	410	1.49%
23	Minnesota	410	1.49%
25	Oregon	370	1.34%
26	Connecticut	360	1.30%
26	South Carolina	360	1.30%
28	Colorado	350	1.27%
29	Oklahoma	340	1.23%
30	Mississippi	290	1.05%
31	Arkansas	280	1.01%
31	Iowa	280	1.01%
31	Kansas	280	1.01%
34	West Virginia	200	0.72%
35	Maine	160	0.58%
35	Nebraska	160	0.58%
37	Nevada	150	0.54%
38	New Mexico	140	0.51%
39	Hawaii	130	0.47%
39	New Hampshire	130	0.47%
41	Utah	110	0.40%
42	Montana	100	0.36%
43	Rhode Island	90	0.33%
43	South Dakota	90	0.33%
45	Delaware	80	0.29%
46	Idaho	70	0.25%
46	North Dakota	70	0.25%
48	Vermont	50	0.18%
49	Wyoming	40	0.14%
50	Alaska	20	0.07%
	District of Columbia	100	0.36%

Source: American Cancer Society (http://www.cancer.org/97tabp5.html)
   "Cancer Facts & Figures-1997" (Copyright 1997, Reprinted with permission from the American Cancer Society)
*These estimates are offered as a rough guide and should be interpreted with caution. They are calculated according to the distribution of estimated 1997 cancer deaths by state.

Estimated Rate of New Pancreatic Cancer Cases in 1997

National Estimated Rate = 10.4 New Cases per 100,000 Population*

ALPHA ORDER

RANK	STATE	RATE
36	Alabama	9.6
50	Alaska	3.3
31	Arizona	9.9
12	Arkansas	11.2
46	California	8.2
39	Colorado	9.2
16	Connecticut	11.0
16	Delaware	11.0
1	Florida	13.9
39	Georgia	9.2
16	Hawaii	11.0
48	Idaho	5.9
30	Illinois	10.1
6	Indiana	11.6
33	Iowa	9.8
20	Kansas	10.9
6	Kentucky	11.6
5	Louisiana	12.0
2	Maine	12.9
38	Maryland	9.3
12	Massachusetts	11.2
26	Michigan	10.4
43	Minnesota	8.8
22	Mississippi	10.7
26	Missouri	10.4
11	Montana	11.4
34	Nebraska	9.7
37	Nevada	9.4
12	New Hampshire	11.2
6	New Jersey	11.6
46	New Mexico	8.2
9	New York	11.5
29	North Carolina	10.2
20	North Dakota	10.9
22	Ohio	10.7
28	Oklahoma	10.3
9	Oregon	11.5
3	Pennsylvania	12.4
42	Rhode Island	9.1
34	South Carolina	9.7
4	South Dakota	12.3
22	Tennessee	10.7
31	Texas	9.9
49	Utah	5.5
44	Vermont	8.5
25	Virginia	10.6
39	Washington	9.2
16	West Virginia	11.0
12	Wisconsin	11.2
45	Wyoming	8.3

RANK ORDER

RANK	STATE	RATE
1	Florida	13.9
2	Maine	12.9
3	Pennsylvania	12.4
4	South Dakota	12.3
5	Louisiana	12.0
6	Indiana	11.6
6	Kentucky	11.6
6	New Jersey	11.6
9	New York	11.5
9	Oregon	11.5
11	Montana	11.4
12	Arkansas	11.2
12	Massachusetts	11.2
12	New Hampshire	11.2
12	Wisconsin	11.2
16	Connecticut	11.0
16	Delaware	11.0
16	Hawaii	11.0
16	West Virginia	11.0
20	Kansas	10.9
20	North Dakota	10.9
22	Mississippi	10.7
22	Ohio	10.7
22	Tennessee	10.7
25	Virginia	10.6
26	Michigan	10.4
26	Missouri	10.4
28	Oklahoma	10.3
29	North Carolina	10.2
30	Illinois	10.1
31	Arizona	9.9
31	Texas	9.9
33	Iowa	9.8
34	Nebraska	9.7
34	South Carolina	9.7
36	Alabama	9.6
37	Nevada	9.4
38	Maryland	9.3
39	Colorado	9.2
39	Georgia	9.2
39	Washington	9.2
42	Rhode Island	9.1
43	Minnesota	8.8
44	Vermont	8.5
45	Wyoming	8.3
46	California	8.2
46	New Mexico	8.2
48	Idaho	5.9
49	Utah	5.5
50	Alaska	3.3

	District of Columbia	18.4

Source: Morgan Quitno Press using data from American Cancer Society (http://www.cancer.org/97tabp5.html)
"Cancer Facts & Figures-1997" (Copyright 1997, Reprinted with permission from the American Cancer Society)
*These estimates are offered as a rough guide and should be interpreted with caution. They are calculated according to the distribution of estimated 1997 cancer deaths by state. Rates calculated using 1996 Census resident population estimates.

Estimated New Prostate Cancer Cases in 1997

National Estimated Total = 334,500 New Cases*

ALPHA ORDER

RANK	STATE	CASES	% of USA
23	Alabama	5,400	1.61%
50	Alaska	290	0.09%
20	Arizona	5,700	1.70%
28	Arkansas	4,200	1.26%
1	California	31,400	9.39%
31	Colorado	4,000	1.20%
29	Connecticut	4,100	1.23%
47	Delaware	890	0.27%
2	Florida	25,400	7.59%
14	Georgia	7,700	2.30%
44	Hawaii	1,100	0.33%
40	Idaho	1,400	0.42%
6	Illinois	15,300	4.57%
16	Indiana	6,800	2.03%
32	Iowa	3,900	1.17%
33	Kansas	3,400	1.02%
25	Kentucky	4,500	1.35%
22	Louisiana	5,500	1.64%
38	Maine	1,700	0.51%
17	Maryland	6,500	1.94%
11	Massachusetts	8,100	2.42%
8	Michigan	12,800	3.83%
21	Minnesota	5,600	1.67%
29	Mississippi	4,100	1.23%
15	Missouri	7,100	2.12%
40	Montana	1,400	0.42%
35	Nebraska	2,100	0.63%
37	Nevada	1,800	0.54%
43	New Hampshire	1,200	0.36%
9	New Jersey	11,000	3.29%
38	New Mexico	1,700	0.51%
3	New York	21,100	6.31%
10	North Carolina	10,100	3.02%
42	North Dakota	1,300	0.39%
7	Ohio	14,600	4.36%
27	Oklahoma	4,300	1.29%
26	Oregon	4,400	1.32%
5	Pennsylvania	19,200	5.74%
46	Rhode Island	940	0.28%
24	South Carolina	5,100	1.52%
44	South Dakota	1,100	0.33%
19	Tennessee	6,300	1.88%
4	Texas	20,800	6.22%
36	Utah	1,900	0.57%
48	Vermont	690	0.21%
13	Virginia	7,900	2.36%
17	Washington	6,500	1.94%
34	West Virginia	2,500	0.75%
12	Wisconsin	8,000	2.39%
49	Wyoming	640	0.19%

RANK ORDER

RANK	STATE	CASES	% of USA
1	California	31,400	9.39%
2	Florida	25,400	7.59%
3	New York	21,100	6.31%
4	Texas	20,800	6.22%
5	Pennsylvania	19,200	5.74%
6	Illinois	15,300	4.57%
7	Ohio	14,600	4.36%
8	Michigan	12,800	3.83%
9	New Jersey	11,000	3.29%
10	North Carolina	10,100	3.02%
11	Massachusetts	8,100	2.42%
12	Wisconsin	8,000	2.39%
13	Virginia	7,900	2.36%
14	Georgia	7,700	2.30%
15	Missouri	7,100	2.12%
16	Indiana	6,800	2.03%
17	Maryland	6,500	1.94%
17	Washington	6,500	1.94%
19	Tennessee	6,300	1.88%
20	Arizona	5,700	1.70%
21	Minnesota	5,600	1.67%
22	Louisiana	5,500	1.64%
23	Alabama	5,400	1.61%
24	South Carolina	5,100	1.52%
25	Kentucky	4,500	1.35%
26	Oregon	4,400	1.32%
27	Oklahoma	4,300	1.29%
28	Arkansas	4,200	1.26%
29	Connecticut	4,100	1.23%
29	Mississippi	4,100	1.23%
31	Colorado	4,000	1.20%
32	Iowa	3,900	1.17%
33	Kansas	3,400	1.02%
34	West Virginia	2,500	0.75%
35	Nebraska	2,100	0.63%
36	Utah	1,900	0.57%
37	Nevada	1,800	0.54%
38	Maine	1,700	0.51%
38	New Mexico	1,700	0.51%
40	Idaho	1,400	0.42%
40	Montana	1,400	0.42%
42	North Dakota	1,300	0.39%
43	New Hampshire	1,200	0.36%
44	Hawaii	1,100	0.33%
44	South Dakota	1,100	0.33%
46	Rhode Island	940	0.28%
47	Delaware	890	0.27%
48	Vermont	690	0.21%
49	Wyoming	640	0.19%
50	Alaska	290	0.09%
	District of Columbia	890	0.27%

Source: American Cancer Society (http://www.cancer.org/97tabp5.html)
  "Cancer Facts & Figures-1997" (Copyright 1997, Reprinted with permission from the American Cancer Society)
*These estimates are offered as a rough guide and should be interpreted with caution. They are calculated
according to the distribution of estimated 1997 cancer deaths by state.

Estimated Rate of New Prostate Cancer Cases in 1997

National Estimated Rate = 260.7 New Cases per 100,000 Male Population*

ALPHA ORDER

RANK ORDER

RANK	STATE	RATE
26	Alabama	264.6
50	Alaska	91.4
19	Arizona	273.2
3	Arkansas	350.3
46	California	198.8
43	Colorado	215.4
29	Connecticut	258.2
30	Delaware	254.9
2	Florida	370.0
42	Georgia	219.9
49	Hawaii	183.4
35	Idaho	241.3
23	Illinois	265.5
36	Indiana	241.0
14	Iowa	282.1
21	Kansas	269.5
38	Kentucky	240.4
27	Louisiana	263.2
15	Maine	281.1
24	Maryland	265.3
16	Massachusetts	276.9
18	Michigan	275.5
32	Minnesota	246.9
7	Mississippi	317.1
17	Missouri	275.9
5	Montana	323.6
28	Nebraska	262.5
40	Nevada	230.9
44	New Hampshire	212.8
11	New Jersey	285.9
45	New Mexico	204.8
34	New York	242.0
9	North Carolina	289.3
1	North Dakota	406.7
20	Ohio	271.1
22	Oklahoma	268.8
12	Oregon	284.0
4	Pennsylvania	331.0
47	Rhode Island	197.6
10	South Carolina	287.9
8	South Dakota	306.2
31	Tennessee	248.4
41	Texas	225.2
48	Utah	195.8
39	Vermont	240.1
33	Virginia	243.9
37	Washington	240.9
12	West Virginia	284.0
6	Wisconsin	318.1
25	Wyoming	265.1

RANK	STATE	RATE
1	North Dakota	406.7
2	Florida	370.0
3	Arkansas	350.3
4	Pennsylvania	331.0
5	Montana	323.6
6	Wisconsin	318.1
7	Mississippi	317.1
8	South Dakota	306.2
9	North Carolina	289.3
10	South Carolina	287.9
11	New Jersey	285.9
12	Oregon	284.0
12	West Virginia	284.0
14	Iowa	282.1
15	Maine	281.1
16	Massachusetts	276.9
17	Missouri	275.9
18	Michigan	275.5
19	Arizona	273.2
20	Ohio	271.1
21	Kansas	269.5
22	Oklahoma	268.8
23	Illinois	265.5
24	Maryland	265.3
25	Wyoming	265.1
26	Alabama	264.6
27	Louisiana	263.2
28	Nebraska	262.5
29	Connecticut	258.2
30	Delaware	254.9
31	Tennessee	248.4
32	Minnesota	246.9
33	Virginia	243.9
34	New York	242.0
35	Idaho	241.3
36	Indiana	241.0
37	Washington	240.9
38	Kentucky	240.4
39	Vermont	240.1
40	Nevada	230.9
41	Texas	225.2
42	Georgia	219.9
43	Colorado	215.4
44	New Hampshire	212.8
45	New Mexico	204.8
46	California	198.8
47	Rhode Island	197.6
48	Utah	195.8
49	Hawaii	183.4
50	Alaska	91.4

District of Columbia   343.0

Source: Morgan Quitno Press using data from American Cancer Society (http://www.cancer.org/97tabp5.html)
"Cancer Facts & Figures-1997" (Copyright 1997, Reprinted with permission from the American Cancer Society)
*These estimates are offered as a rough guide and should be interpreted with caution. They are calculated according to the distribution of estimated 1997 cancer deaths by state. Rates calculated using 1995 Census male resident population estimates.

Estimated New Skin Melanoma Cases in 1997

National Estimated Total = 40,300 New Cases*

ALPHA ORDER

RANK	STATE	CASES	% of USA
18	Alabama	770	1.91%
50	Alaska	20	0.05%
20	Arizona	710	1.76%
33	Arkansas	360	0.89%
1	California	4,300	10.67%
29	Colorado	490	1.22%
27	Connecticut	540	1.34%
44	Delaware	120	0.30%
2	Florida	2,800	6.95%
12	Georgia	1,100	2.73%
49	Hawaii	40	0.10%
41	Idaho	160	0.40%
6	Illinois	1,900	4.71%
15	Indiana	970	2.41%
30	Iowa	480	1.19%
23	Kansas	630	1.56%
19	Kentucky	720	1.79%
25	Louisiana	600	1.49%
38	Maine	240	0.60%
24	Maryland	610	1.51%
10	Massachusetts	1,200	2.98%
10	Michigan	1,200	2.98%
26	Minnesota	580	1.44%
37	Mississippi	250	0.62%
16	Missouri	930	2.31%
45	Montana	100	0.25%
40	Nebraska	170	0.42%
35	Nevada	350	0.87%
42	New Hampshire	150	0.37%
8	New Jersey	1,300	3.23%
36	New Mexico	320	0.79%
4	New York	2,200	5.46%
8	North Carolina	1,300	3.23%
45	North Dakota	100	0.25%
7	Ohio	1,400	3.47%
28	Oklahoma	530	1.32%
22	Oregon	670	1.66%
5	Pennsylvania	2,100	5.21%
39	Rhode Island	180	0.45%
30	South Carolina	480	1.19%
48	South Dakota	50	0.12%
12	Tennessee	1,100	2.73%
3	Texas	2,500	6.20%
32	Utah	380	0.94%
42	Vermont	150	0.37%
12	Virginia	1,100	2.73%
17	Washington	820	2.03%
33	West Virginia	360	0.89%
21	Wisconsin	700	1.74%
47	Wyoming	90	0.22%

RANK ORDER

RANK	STATE	CASES	% of USA
1	California	4,300	10.67%
2	Florida	2,800	6.95%
3	Texas	2,500	6.20%
4	New York	2,200	5.46%
5	Pennsylvania	2,100	5.21%
6	Illinois	1,900	4.71%
7	Ohio	1,400	3.47%
8	New Jersey	1,300	3.23%
8	North Carolina	1,300	3.23%
10	Massachusetts	1,200	2.98%
10	Michigan	1,200	2.98%
12	Georgia	1,100	2.73%
12	Tennessee	1,100	2.73%
12	Virginia	1,100	2.73%
15	Indiana	970	2.41%
16	Missouri	930	2.31%
17	Washington	820	2.03%
18	Alabama	770	1.91%
19	Kentucky	720	1.79%
20	Arizona	710	1.76%
21	Wisconsin	700	1.74%
22	Oregon	670	1.66%
23	Kansas	630	1.56%
24	Maryland	610	1.51%
25	Louisiana	600	1.49%
26	Minnesota	580	1.44%
27	Connecticut	540	1.34%
28	Oklahoma	530	1.32%
29	Colorado	490	1.22%
30	Iowa	480	1.19%
30	South Carolina	480	1.19%
32	Utah	380	0.94%
33	Arkansas	360	0.89%
33	West Virginia	360	0.89%
35	Nevada	350	0.87%
36	New Mexico	320	0.79%
37	Mississippi	250	0.62%
38	Maine	240	0.60%
39	Rhode Island	180	0.45%
40	Nebraska	170	0.42%
41	Idaho	160	0.40%
42	New Hampshire	150	0.37%
42	Vermont	150	0.37%
44	Delaware	120	0.30%
45	Montana	100	0.25%
45	North Dakota	100	0.25%
47	Wyoming	90	0.22%
48	South Dakota	50	0.12%
49	Hawaii	40	0.10%
50	Alaska	20	0.05%
	District of Columbia	5	0.01%

Source: American Cancer Society (http://www.cancer.org/97tabp5.html)
    "Cancer Facts & Figures-1997" (Copyright 1997, Reprinted with permission from the American Cancer Society)
*These estimates are offered as a rough guide and should be interpreted with caution. They are calculated according to the distribution of estimated 1997 cancer deaths by state.

Estimated Rate of New Skin Melanoma Cases in 1997

National Estimated Rate = 15.2 New Cases per 100,000 Population*

ALPHA ORDER				RANK ORDER		
RANK	STATE	RATE		RANK	STATE	RATE
15	Alabama	18.0		1	Vermont	25.5
50	Alaska	3.3		2	Kansas	24.5
26	Arizona	16.0		3	Nevada	21.8
31	Arkansas	14.3		4	Oregon	20.9
34	California	13.5		5	Tennessee	20.7
39	Colorado	12.8		6	Massachusetts	19.7
22	Connecticut	16.5		6	West Virginia	19.7
20	Delaware	16.6		8	Florida	19.4
8	Florida	19.4		9	Maine	19.3
29	Georgia	15.0		10	Utah	19.0
49	Hawaii	3.4		11	New Mexico	18.7
34	Idaho	13.5		11	Wyoming	18.7
26	Illinois	16.0		13	Kentucky	18.5
20	Indiana	16.6		14	Rhode Island	18.2
19	Iowa	16.8		15	Alabama	18.0
2	Kansas	24.5		16	North Carolina	17.8
13	Kentucky	18.5		17	Missouri	17.4
32	Louisiana	13.8		17	Pennsylvania	17.4
9	Maine	19.3		19	Iowa	16.8
44	Maryland	12.0		20	Delaware	16.6
6	Massachusetts	19.7		20	Indiana	16.6
40	Michigan	12.5		22	Connecticut	16.5
40	Minnesota	12.5		22	Virginia	16.5
47	Mississippi	9.2		24	New Jersey	16.3
17	Missouri	17.4		25	Oklahoma	16.1
45	Montana	11.4		26	Arizona	16.0
46	Nebraska	10.3		26	Illinois	16.0
3	Nevada	21.8		28	North Dakota	15.5
38	New Hampshire	12.9		29	Georgia	15.0
24	New Jersey	16.3		30	Washington	14.8
11	New Mexico	18.7		31	Arkansas	14.3
43	New York	12.1		32	Louisiana	13.8
16	North Carolina	17.8		33	Wisconsin	13.6
28	North Dakota	15.5		34	California	13.5
40	Ohio	12.5		34	Idaho	13.5
25	Oklahoma	16.1		36	Texas	13.1
4	Oregon	20.9		37	South Carolina	13.0
17	Pennsylvania	17.4		38	New Hampshire	12.9
14	Rhode Island	18.2		39	Colorado	12.8
37	South Carolina	13.0		40	Michigan	12.5
48	South Dakota	6.8		40	Minnesota	12.5
5	Tennessee	20.7		40	Ohio	12.5
36	Texas	13.1		43	New York	12.1
10	Utah	19.0		44	Maryland	12.0
1	Vermont	25.5		45	Montana	11.4
22	Virginia	16.5		46	Nebraska	10.3
30	Washington	14.8		47	Mississippi	9.2
6	West Virginia	19.7		48	South Dakota	6.8
33	Wisconsin	13.6		49	Hawaii	3.4
11	Wyoming	18.7		50	Alaska	3.3
					District of Columbia	0.9

Source: Morgan Quitno Press using data from American Cancer Society (http://www.cancer.org/97tabp5.html)
"Cancer Facts & Figures-1997" (Copyright 1997, Reprinted with permission from the American Cancer Society)
*These estimates are offered as a rough guide and should be interpreted with caution. They are calculated according to the distribution of estimated 1997 cancer deaths by state. Rates calculated using 1996 Census resident population estimates.

Estimated New Cancer of the Uterus (Cervix) Cases in 1997

National Estimated Total = 14,500 New Cases*

<table>
<tr><td colspan="4">ALPHA ORDER</td><td colspan="4">RANK ORDER</td></tr>
<tr><td>RANK</td><td>STATE</td><td>CASES</td><td>% of USA</td><td>RANK</td><td>STATE</td><td>CASES</td><td>% of USA</td></tr>
<tr><td>20</td><td>Alabama</td><td>240</td><td>1.66%</td><td>1</td><td>California</td><td>1,500</td><td>10.34%</td></tr>
<tr><td>48</td><td>Alaska</td><td>10</td><td>0.07%</td><td>2</td><td>Florida</td><td>1,200</td><td>8.28%</td></tr>
<tr><td>26</td><td>Arizona</td><td>150</td><td>1.03%</td><td>2</td><td>New York</td><td>1,200</td><td>8.28%</td></tr>
<tr><td>24</td><td>Arkansas</td><td>180</td><td>1.24%</td><td>2</td><td>Texas</td><td>1,200</td><td>8.28%</td></tr>
<tr><td>1</td><td>California</td><td>1,500</td><td>10.34%</td><td>5</td><td>Pennsylvania</td><td>830</td><td>5.72%</td></tr>
<tr><td>29</td><td>Colorado</td><td>140</td><td>0.97%</td><td>6</td><td>Illinois</td><td>740</td><td>5.10%</td></tr>
<tr><td>40</td><td>Connecticut</td><td>60</td><td>0.41%</td><td>7</td><td>Ohio</td><td>680</td><td>4.69%</td></tr>
<tr><td>36</td><td>Delaware</td><td>70</td><td>0.48%</td><td>8</td><td>Michigan</td><td>490</td><td>3.38%</td></tr>
<tr><td>2</td><td>Florida</td><td>1,200</td><td>8.28%</td><td>9</td><td>New Jersey</td><td>380</td><td>2.62%</td></tr>
<tr><td>15</td><td>Georgia</td><td>290</td><td>2.00%</td><td>10</td><td>Indiana</td><td>370</td><td>2.55%</td></tr>
<tr><td>44</td><td>Hawaii</td><td>30</td><td>0.21%</td><td>11</td><td>Missouri</td><td>350</td><td>2.41%</td></tr>
<tr><td>48</td><td>Idaho</td><td>10</td><td>0.07%</td><td>12</td><td>North Carolina</td><td>340</td><td>2.34%</td></tr>
<tr><td>6</td><td>Illinois</td><td>740</td><td>5.10%</td><td>13</td><td>Tennessee</td><td>320</td><td>2.21%</td></tr>
<tr><td>10</td><td>Indiana</td><td>370</td><td>2.55%</td><td>14</td><td>Wisconsin</td><td>310</td><td>2.14%</td></tr>
<tr><td>29</td><td>Iowa</td><td>140</td><td>0.97%</td><td>15</td><td>Georgia</td><td>290</td><td>2.00%</td></tr>
<tr><td>26</td><td>Kansas</td><td>150</td><td>1.03%</td><td>15</td><td>Kentucky</td><td>290</td><td>2.00%</td></tr>
<tr><td>15</td><td>Kentucky</td><td>290</td><td>2.00%</td><td>15</td><td>Maryland</td><td>290</td><td>2.00%</td></tr>
<tr><td>26</td><td>Louisiana</td><td>150</td><td>1.03%</td><td>15</td><td>Virginia</td><td>290</td><td>2.00%</td></tr>
<tr><td>40</td><td>Maine</td><td>60</td><td>0.41%</td><td>19</td><td>Massachusetts</td><td>270</td><td>1.86%</td></tr>
<tr><td>15</td><td>Maryland</td><td>290</td><td>2.00%</td><td>20</td><td>Alabama</td><td>240</td><td>1.66%</td></tr>
<tr><td>19</td><td>Massachusetts</td><td>270</td><td>1.86%</td><td>21</td><td>South Carolina</td><td>230</td><td>1.59%</td></tr>
<tr><td>8</td><td>Michigan</td><td>490</td><td>3.38%</td><td>22</td><td>Oklahoma</td><td>220</td><td>1.52%</td></tr>
<tr><td>31</td><td>Minnesota</td><td>130</td><td>0.90%</td><td>23</td><td>Mississippi</td><td>200</td><td>1.38%</td></tr>
<tr><td>23</td><td>Mississippi</td><td>200</td><td>1.38%</td><td>24</td><td>Arkansas</td><td>180</td><td>1.24%</td></tr>
<tr><td>11</td><td>Missouri</td><td>350</td><td>2.41%</td><td>24</td><td>Washington</td><td>180</td><td>1.24%</td></tr>
<tr><td>40</td><td>Montana</td><td>60</td><td>0.41%</td><td>26</td><td>Arizona</td><td>150</td><td>1.03%</td></tr>
<tr><td>46</td><td>Nebraska</td><td>20</td><td>0.14%</td><td>26</td><td>Kansas</td><td>150</td><td>1.03%</td></tr>
<tr><td>35</td><td>Nevada</td><td>90</td><td>0.62%</td><td>26</td><td>Louisiana</td><td>150</td><td>1.03%</td></tr>
<tr><td>34</td><td>New Hampshire</td><td>100</td><td>0.69%</td><td>29</td><td>Colorado</td><td>140</td><td>0.97%</td></tr>
<tr><td>9</td><td>New Jersey</td><td>380</td><td>2.62%</td><td>29</td><td>Iowa</td><td>140</td><td>0.97%</td></tr>
<tr><td>36</td><td>New Mexico</td><td>70</td><td>0.48%</td><td>31</td><td>Minnesota</td><td>130</td><td>0.90%</td></tr>
<tr><td>2</td><td>New York</td><td>1,200</td><td>8.28%</td><td>32</td><td>Oregon</td><td>110</td><td>0.76%</td></tr>
<tr><td>12</td><td>North Carolina</td><td>340</td><td>2.34%</td><td>32</td><td>West Virginia</td><td>110</td><td>0.76%</td></tr>
<tr><td>50</td><td>North Dakota</td><td>5</td><td>0.03%</td><td>34</td><td>New Hampshire</td><td>100</td><td>0.69%</td></tr>
<tr><td>7</td><td>Ohio</td><td>680</td><td>4.69%</td><td>35</td><td>Nevada</td><td>90</td><td>0.62%</td></tr>
<tr><td>22</td><td>Oklahoma</td><td>220</td><td>1.52%</td><td>36</td><td>Delaware</td><td>70</td><td>0.48%</td></tr>
<tr><td>32</td><td>Oregon</td><td>110</td><td>0.76%</td><td>36</td><td>New Mexico</td><td>70</td><td>0.48%</td></tr>
<tr><td>5</td><td>Pennsylvania</td><td>830</td><td>5.72%</td><td>36</td><td>Rhode Island</td><td>70</td><td>0.48%</td></tr>
<tr><td>36</td><td>Rhode Island</td><td>70</td><td>0.48%</td><td>36</td><td>Utah</td><td>70</td><td>0.48%</td></tr>
<tr><td>21</td><td>South Carolina</td><td>230</td><td>1.59%</td><td>40</td><td>Connecticut</td><td>60</td><td>0.41%</td></tr>
<tr><td>44</td><td>South Dakota</td><td>30</td><td>0.21%</td><td>40</td><td>Maine</td><td>60</td><td>0.41%</td></tr>
<tr><td>13</td><td>Tennessee</td><td>320</td><td>2.21%</td><td>40</td><td>Montana</td><td>60</td><td>0.41%</td></tr>
<tr><td>2</td><td>Texas</td><td>1,200</td><td>8.28%</td><td>43</td><td>Vermont</td><td>40</td><td>0.28%</td></tr>
<tr><td>36</td><td>Utah</td><td>70</td><td>0.48%</td><td>44</td><td>Hawaii</td><td>30</td><td>0.21%</td></tr>
<tr><td>43</td><td>Vermont</td><td>40</td><td>0.28%</td><td>44</td><td>South Dakota</td><td>30</td><td>0.21%</td></tr>
<tr><td>15</td><td>Virginia</td><td>290</td><td>2.00%</td><td>46</td><td>Nebraska</td><td>20</td><td>0.14%</td></tr>
<tr><td>24</td><td>Washington</td><td>180</td><td>1.24%</td><td>46</td><td>Wyoming</td><td>20</td><td>0.14%</td></tr>
<tr><td>32</td><td>West Virginia</td><td>110</td><td>0.76%</td><td>48</td><td>Alaska</td><td>10</td><td>0.07%</td></tr>
<tr><td>14</td><td>Wisconsin</td><td>310</td><td>2.14%</td><td>48</td><td>Idaho</td><td>10</td><td>0.07%</td></tr>
<tr><td>46</td><td>Wyoming</td><td>20</td><td>0.14%</td><td>50</td><td>North Dakota</td><td>5</td><td>0.03%</td></tr>
<tr><td></td><td></td><td></td><td></td><td></td><td>District of Columbia</td><td>30</td><td>0.21%</td></tr>
</table>

Source: American Cancer Society (http://www.cancer.org/97tabp5.html)
    "Cancer Facts & Figures-1997" (Copyright 1997, Reprinted with permission from the American Cancer Society)
*These estimates are offered as a rough guide and should be interpreted with caution. They are calculated
according to the distribution of estimated 1997 cancer deaths by state.

Estimated Rate of New Cancer of the Uterus (Cervix) Cases in 1997

National Estimated Rate = 10.8 New Cases per 100,000 Female Population*

ALPHA ORDER

RANK ORDER

RANK	STATE	RATE		RANK	STATE	RATE
25	Alabama	10.8		1	Delaware	19.0
47	Alaska	3.5		2	New Hampshire	17.1
40	Arizona	7.0		3	Florida	16.4
6	Arkansas	14.0		4	Kentucky	14.6
28	California	9.5		5	Mississippi	14.2
38	Colorado	7.4		6	Arkansas	14.0
46	Connecticut	3.6		7	Montana	13.7
1	Delaware	19.0		8	Rhode Island	13.6
3	Florida	16.4		9	Vermont	13.5
37	Georgia	7.8		10	Pennsylvania	13.2
45	Hawaii	5.1		11	Oklahoma	13.1
49	Idaho	1.7		12	Missouri	12.7
16	Illinois	12.2		12	New York	12.7
15	Indiana	12.4		14	Texas	12.6
27	Iowa	9.6		15	Indiana	12.4
23	Kansas	11.5		16	Illinois	12.2
4	Kentucky	14.6		17	South Carolina	12.1
42	Louisiana	6.7		18	Nevada	12.0
29	Maine	9.4		19	Wisconsin	11.9
24	Maryland	11.2		20	Ohio	11.8
32	Massachusetts	8.6		20	Tennessee	11.8
26	Michigan	10.0		22	West Virginia	11.6
44	Minnesota	5.6		23	Kansas	11.5
5	Mississippi	14.2		24	Maryland	11.2
12	Missouri	12.7		25	Alabama	10.8
7	Montana	13.7		26	Michigan	10.0
48	Nebraska	2.4		27	Iowa	9.6
18	Nevada	12.0		28	California	9.5
2	New Hampshire	17.1		29	Maine	9.4
30	New Jersey	9.3		30	New Jersey	9.3
35	New Mexico	8.2		31	North Carolina	9.2
12	New York	12.7		32	Massachusetts	8.6
31	North Carolina	9.2		32	Virginia	8.6
50	North Dakota	1.6		34	Wyoming	8.4
20	Ohio	11.8		35	New Mexico	8.2
11	Oklahoma	13.1		36	South Dakota	8.1
41	Oregon	6.9		37	Georgia	7.8
10	Pennsylvania	13.2		38	Colorado	7.4
8	Rhode Island	13.6		39	Utah	7.1
17	South Carolina	12.1		40	Arizona	7.0
36	South Dakota	8.1		41	Oregon	6.9
20	Tennessee	11.8		42	Louisiana	6.7
14	Texas	12.6		43	Washington	6.6
39	Utah	7.1		44	Minnesota	5.6
9	Vermont	13.5		45	Hawaii	5.1
32	Virginia	8.6		46	Connecticut	3.6
43	Washington	6.6		47	Alaska	3.5
22	West Virginia	11.6		48	Nebraska	2.4
19	Wisconsin	11.9		49	Idaho	1.7
34	Wyoming	8.4		50	North Dakota	1.6
					District of Columbia	10.2

Source: Morgan Quitno Press using data from American Cancer Society (http://www.cancer.org/97tabp5.html)
"Cancer Facts & Figures-1997" (Copyright 1997, Reprinted with permission from the American Cancer Society)
*These estimates are offered as a rough guide and should be interpreted with caution. They are calculated
according to the distribution of estimated 1997 cancer deaths by state. Rates calculated using 1995 Census female
resident population estimates.

Percent of Women 18 Years and Older
Who Had a Pap Smear Within the Past Three Years: 1995
National Median = 83.58% of Women 18 Years and Older

ALPHA ORDER				RANK ORDER		
RANK	STATE	PERCENT		RANK	STATE	PERCENT
18	Alabama	85.02		1	Alaska	90.89
1	Alaska	90.89		2	Georgia	89.16
27	Arizona	83.42		3	Oklahoma	88.68
42	Arkansas	80.83		4	South Carolina	88.46
36	California	82.00		5	New Hampshire	87.64
6	Colorado	87.61		6	Colorado	87.61
10	Connecticut	86.82		7	Virginia	87.56
14	Delaware	85.91		8	Maine	87.04
15	Florida	85.52		9	Washington	86.84
2	Georgia	89.16		10	Connecticut	86.82
13	Hawaii	85.99		11	New Mexico	86.81
46	Idaho	80.42		12	North Carolina	86.61
37	Illinois	81.90		13	Hawaii	85.99
38	Indiana	81.84		14	Delaware	85.91
32	Iowa	82.73		15	Florida	85.52
40	Kansas	81.12		16	Maryland	85.43
50	Kentucky	78.98		17	Vermont	85.41
47	Louisiana	79.16		18	Alabama	85.02
8	Maine	87.04		19	Massachusetts	84.67
16	Maryland	85.43		20	Ohio	84.58
19	Massachusetts	84.67		21	Oregon	84.20
22	Michigan	84.17		22	Michigan	84.17
24	Minnesota	84.01		23	Tennessee	84.12
30	Mississippi	83.09		24	Minnesota	84.01
26	Missouri	83.44		25	Wisconsin	83.71
39	Montana	81.80		26	Missouri	83.44
35	Nebraska	82.16		27	Arizona	83.42
29	Nevada	83.24		28	South Dakota	83.30
5	New Hampshire	87.64		29	Nevada	83.24
48	New Jersey	79.04		30	Mississippi	83.09
11	New Mexico	86.81		31	North Dakota	82.90
44	New York	80.46		32	Iowa	82.73
12	North Carolina	86.61		33	Texas	82.72
31	North Dakota	82.90		34	Rhode Island	82.48
20	Ohio	84.58		35	Nebraska	82.16
3	Oklahoma	88.68		36	California	82.00
21	Oregon	84.20		37	Illinois	81.90
41	Pennsylvania	80.94		38	Indiana	81.84
34	Rhode Island	82.48		39	Montana	81.80
4	South Carolina	88.46		40	Kansas	81.12
28	South Dakota	83.30		41	Pennsylvania	80.94
23	Tennessee	84.12		42	Arkansas	80.83
33	Texas	82.72		43	Wyoming	80.48
45	Utah	80.44		44	New York	80.46
17	Vermont	85.41		45	Utah	80.44
7	Virginia	87.56		46	Idaho	80.42
9	Washington	86.84		47	Louisiana	79.16
49	West Virginia	79.00		48	New Jersey	79.04
25	Wisconsin	83.71		49	West Virginia	79.00
43	Wyoming	80.48		50	Kentucky	78.98
				District of Columbia*		NA

Source: U.S. Department of Health and Human Services, Centers for Disease Control and Prevention
"1995 Behavioral Risk Factor Surveillance Summary Prevalence Report" (December 10, 1996)
*Not available.

AIDS Cases Reported in 1996

National Total = 70,103 New AIDS Cases*

ALPHA ORDER

RANK	STATE	CASES	% of USA
21	Alabama	666	0.95%
46	Alaska	37	0.05%
22	Arizona	664	0.95%
32	Arkansas	286	0.41%
2	California	10,589	15.10%
24	Colorado	600	0.86%
10	Connecticut	1,532	2.19%
29	Delaware	320	0.46%
3	Florida	7,741	11.04%
6	Georgia	2,503	3.57%
35	Hawaii	206	0.29%
44	Idaho	45	0.06%
9	Illinois	2,149	3.07%
23	Indiana	659	0.94%
39	Iowa	129	0.18%
34	Kansas	263	0.38%
31	Kentucky	315	0.45%
12	Louisiana	1,374	1.96%
43	Maine	80	0.11%
7	Maryland	2,296	3.28%
13	Massachusetts	1,295	1.85%
15	Michigan	1,040	1.48%
29	Minnesota	320	0.46%
27	Mississippi	415	0.59%
19	Missouri	850	1.21%
47	Montana	30	0.04%
42	Nebraska	98	0.14%
26	Nevada	459	0.65%
41	New Hampshire	99	0.14%
5	New Jersey	3,995	5.70%
40	New Mexico	113	0.16%
1	New York	13,251	18.90%
16	North Carolina	975	1.39%
50	North Dakota	9	0.01%
14	Ohio	1,117	1.59%
33	Oklahoma	278	0.40%
25	Oregon	501	0.71%
8	Pennsylvania	2,270	3.24%
37	Rhode Island	182	0.26%
17	South Carolina	970	1.38%
48	South Dakota	17	0.02%
18	Tennessee	903	1.29%
4	Texas	4,399	6.28%
36	Utah	199	0.28%
45	Vermont	39	0.06%
11	Virginia	1,513	2.16%
20	Washington	777	1.11%
38	West Virginia	146	0.21%
28	Wisconsin	330	0.47%
49	Wyoming	14	0.02%

RANK ORDER

RANK	STATE	CASES	% of USA
1	New York	13,251	18.90%
2	California	10,589	15.10%
3	Florida	7,741	11.04%
4	Texas	4,399	6.28%
5	New Jersey	3,995	5.70%
6	Georgia	2,503	3.57%
7	Maryland	2,296	3.28%
8	Pennsylvania	2,270	3.24%
9	Illinois	2,149	3.07%
10	Connecticut	1,532	2.19%
11	Virginia	1,513	2.16%
12	Louisiana	1,374	1.96%
13	Massachusetts	1,295	1.85%
14	Ohio	1,117	1.59%
15	Michigan	1,040	1.48%
16	North Carolina	975	1.39%
17	South Carolina	970	1.38%
18	Tennessee	903	1.29%
19	Missouri	850	1.21%
20	Washington	777	1.11%
21	Alabama	666	0.95%
22	Arizona	664	0.95%
23	Indiana	659	0.94%
24	Colorado	600	0.86%
25	Oregon	501	0.71%
26	Nevada	459	0.65%
27	Mississippi	415	0.59%
28	Wisconsin	330	0.47%
29	Delaware	320	0.46%
29	Minnesota	320	0.46%
31	Kentucky	315	0.45%
32	Arkansas	286	0.41%
33	Oklahoma	278	0.40%
34	Kansas	263	0.38%
35	Hawaii	206	0.29%
36	Utah	199	0.28%
37	Rhode Island	182	0.26%
38	West Virginia	146	0.21%
39	Iowa	129	0.18%
40	New Mexico	113	0.16%
41	New Hampshire	99	0.14%
42	Nebraska	98	0.14%
43	Maine	80	0.11%
44	Idaho	45	0.06%
45	Vermont	39	0.06%
46	Alaska	37	0.05%
47	Montana	30	0.04%
48	South Dakota	17	0.02%
49	Wyoming	14	0.02%
50	North Dakota	9	0.01%
	District of Columbia	1,045	1.49%

Source: U.S. Department of Health and Human Services, Centers for Disease Control and Prevention
"HIV/AIDS Surveillance Report, 1996" (Mid-year Edition, Vol. 8, No. 1)
*July 1995-June 1996. AIDS is Acquired Immunodeficiency Syndrome. It is a specific group of diseases or conditions which are indicative of severe immunosuppression related to infection with the Human Immunodeficiency Virus (HIV). National total does not include 2,153 cases in Puerto Rico and 32 cases in the Virgin Islands.

AIDS Rate in 1996

National Rate = 26.7 New AIDS Cases Reported per 100,000 Population*

<u>ALPHA ORDER</u>

RANK	STATE	RATE
23	Alabama	15.7
43	Alaska	6.1
23	Arizona	15.7
28	Arkansas	11.5
8	California	33.5
20	Colorado	16.0
4	Connecticut	46.8
6	Delaware	44.6
2	Florida	54.6
7	Georgia	34.8
18	Hawaii	17.4
46	Idaho	3.9
17	Illinois	18.2
29	Indiana	11.4
45	Iowa	4.5
31	Kansas	10.3
36	Kentucky	8.2
9	Louisiana	31.6
41	Maine	6.4
5	Maryland	45.5
14	Massachusetts	21.3
30	Michigan	10.9
38	Minnesota	6.9
25	Mississippi	15.4
20	Missouri	16.0
47	Montana	3.4
44	Nebraska	6.0
10	Nevada	30.0
34	New Hampshire	8.6
3	New Jersey	50.3
39	New Mexico	6.7
1	New York	73.1
27	North Carolina	13.6
50	North Dakota	1.4
33	Ohio	10.0
35	Oklahoma	8.5
20	Oregon	16.0
15	Pennsylvania	18.8
16	Rhode Island	18.4
11	South Carolina	26.4
49	South Dakota	2.3
19	Tennessee	17.2
12	Texas	23.5
32	Utah	10.2
39	Vermont	6.7
13	Virginia	22.9
26	Washington	14.3
37	West Virginia	8.0
41	Wisconsin	6.4
48	Wyoming	2.9

<u>RANK ORDER</u>

RANK	STATE	RATE
1	New York	73.1
2	Florida	54.6
3	New Jersey	50.3
4	Connecticut	46.8
5	Maryland	45.5
6	Delaware	44.6
7	Georgia	34.8
8	California	33.5
9	Louisiana	31.6
10	Nevada	30.0
11	South Carolina	26.4
12	Texas	23.5
13	Virginia	22.9
14	Massachusetts	21.3
15	Pennsylvania	18.8
16	Rhode Island	18.4
17	Illinois	18.2
18	Hawaii	17.4
19	Tennessee	17.2
20	Colorado	16.0
20	Missouri	16.0
20	Oregon	16.0
23	Alabama	15.7
23	Arizona	15.7
25	Mississippi	15.4
26	Washington	14.3
27	North Carolina	13.6
28	Arkansas	11.5
29	Indiana	11.4
30	Michigan	10.9
31	Kansas	10.3
32	Utah	10.2
33	Ohio	10.0
34	New Hampshire	8.6
35	Oklahoma	8.5
36	Kentucky	8.2
37	West Virginia	8.0
38	Minnesota	6.9
39	New Mexico	6.7
39	Vermont	6.7
41	Maine	6.4
41	Wisconsin	6.4
43	Alaska	6.1
44	Nebraska	6.0
45	Iowa	4.5
46	Idaho	3.9
47	Montana	3.4
48	Wyoming	2.9
49	South Dakota	2.3
50	North Dakota	1.4

District of Columbia   188.5

Source: U.S. Department of Health and Human Services, Centers for Disease Control and Prevention
"HIV/AIDS Surveillance Report, 1996" (Mid-year Edition, Vol. 8, No. 1)
July 1995-June 1996. AIDS is Acquired Immunodeficiency Syndrome. It is a specific group of diseases or conditions which are indicative of severe immunosuppression related to infection with the Human Immunodeficiency Virus (HIV). National rate does not include cases in Puerto Rico and the Virgin Islands.

AIDS Cases Reported Through June 1996

National Total = 529,999 Reported AIDS Cases*

ALPHA ORDER

RANK ORDER

RANK	STATE	CASES	% of USA
24	Alabama	3,983	0.75%
45	Alaska	341	0.06%
22	Arizona	4,736	0.89%
31	Arkansas	2,033	0.38%
2	California	93,749	17.69%
20	Colorado	5,536	1.04%
14	Connecticut	7,994	1.51%
35	Delaware	1,660	0.31%
3	Florida	55,690	10.51%
8	Georgia	15,866	2.99%
33	Hawaii	1,884	0.36%
44	Idaho	350	0.07%
6	Illinois	17,584	3.32%
23	Indiana	4,219	0.80%
39	Iowa	932	0.18%
34	Kansas	1,742	0.33%
32	Kentucky	1,998	0.38%
12	Louisiana	8,452	1.59%
41	Maine	730	0.14%
9	Maryland	14,082	2.66%
10	Massachusetts	11,287	2.13%
15	Michigan	7,824	1.48%
26	Minnesota	2,862	0.54%
29	Mississippi	2,606	0.49%
18	Missouri	6,804	1.28%
47	Montana	208	0.04%
40	Nebraska	744	0.14%
27	Nevada	2,844	0.54%
43	New Hampshire	662	0.12%
5	New Jersey	31,124	5.87%
38	New Mexico	1,292	0.24%
1	New York	101,049	19.07%
17	North Carolina	6,887	1.30%
50	North Dakota	72	0.01%
13	Ohio	8,234	1.55%
30	Oklahoma	2,598	0.49%
25	Oregon	3,665	0.69%
7	Pennsylvania	16,270	3.07%
36	Rhode Island	1,517	0.29%
19	South Carolina	5,851	1.10%
49	South Dakota	112	0.02%
21	Tennessee	5,154	0.97%
4	Texas	37,320	7.04%
37	Utah	1,293	0.24%
46	Vermont	283	0.05%
11	Virginia	8,458	1.60%
16	Washington	7,176	1.35%
42	West Virginia	688	0.13%
28	Wisconsin	2,670	0.50%
48	Wyoming	136	0.03%

RANK	STATE	CASES	% of USA
1	New York	101,049	19.07%
2	California	93,749	17.69%
3	Florida	55,690	10.51%
4	Texas	37,320	7.04%
5	New Jersey	31,124	5.87%
6	Illinois	17,584	3.32%
7	Pennsylvania	16,270	3.07%
8	Georgia	15,866	2.99%
9	Maryland	14,082	2.66%
10	Massachusetts	11,287	2.13%
11	Virginia	8,458	1.60%
12	Louisiana	8,452	1.59%
13	Ohio	8,234	1.55%
14	Connecticut	7,994	1.51%
15	Michigan	7,824	1.48%
16	Washington	7,176	1.35%
17	North Carolina	6,887	1.30%
18	Missouri	6,804	1.28%
19	South Carolina	5,851	1.10%
20	Colorado	5,536	1.04%
21	Tennessee	5,154	0.97%
22	Arizona	4,736	0.89%
23	Indiana	4,219	0.80%
24	Alabama	3,983	0.75%
25	Oregon	3,665	0.69%
26	Minnesota	2,862	0.54%
27	Nevada	2,844	0.54%
28	Wisconsin	2,670	0.50%
29	Mississippi	2,606	0.49%
30	Oklahoma	2,598	0.49%
31	Arkansas	2,033	0.38%
32	Kentucky	1,998	0.38%
33	Hawaii	1,884	0.36%
34	Kansas	1,742	0.33%
35	Delaware	1,660	0.31%
36	Rhode Island	1,517	0.29%
37	Utah	1,293	0.24%
38	New Mexico	1,292	0.24%
39	Iowa	932	0.18%
40	Nebraska	744	0.14%
41	Maine	730	0.14%
42	West Virginia	688	0.13%
43	New Hampshire	662	0.12%
44	Idaho	350	0.07%
45	Alaska	341	0.06%
46	Vermont	283	0.05%
47	Montana	208	0.04%
48	Wyoming	136	0.03%
49	South Dakota	112	0.02%
50	North Dakota	72	0.01%
	District of Columbia	8,748	1.65%

Source: U.S. Department of Health and Human Services, Centers for Disease Control and Prevention "HIV/AIDS Surveillance Report, 1996" (Mid-year Edition, Vol. 8, No. 1)
Cumulative through June 1996. AIDS is Acquired Immunodeficiency Syndrome. It is a specific group of diseases or conditions which are indicative of severe immunosuppression related to infection with the Human Immunodeficiency Virus (HIV). National total does not include 17,412 cases in Puerto Rico, 274 cases in the Virgin Islands and 19 cases in other territories.

AIDS Cases in Children 12 Years and Younger Through June 1996

National Total = 6,943 Juvenile AIDS Cases*

ALPHA ORDER

RANK	STATE	CASES	% of USA
18	Alabama	55	0.79%
43	Alaska	4	0.06%
29	Arizona	19	0.27%
23	Arkansas	30	0.43%
4	California	509	7.33%
24	Colorado	27	0.39%
11	Connecticut	159	2.29%
36	Delaware	13	0.19%
2	Florida	1,183	17.04%
10	Georgia	168	2.42%
33	Hawaii	14	0.20%
47	Idaho	2	0.03%
8	Illinois	210	3.02%
22	Indiana	32	0.46%
38	Iowa	8	0.12%
37	Kansas	11	0.16%
33	Kentucky	14	0.20%
13	Louisiana	106	1.53%
42	Maine	6	0.09%
6	Maryland	245	3.53%
9	Massachusetts	177	2.55%
16	Michigan	83	1.20%
29	Minnesota	19	0.27%
21	Mississippi	38	0.55%
19	Missouri	49	0.71%
47	Montana	2	0.03%
38	Nebraska	8	0.12%
27	Nevada	21	0.30%
41	New Hampshire	7	0.10%
3	New Jersey	649	9.35%
43	New Mexico	4	0.06%
1	New York	1,858	26.76%
15	North Carolina	95	1.37%
49	North Dakota	0	0.00%
14	Ohio	101	1.45%
31	Oklahoma	18	0.26%
33	Oregon	14	0.20%
7	Pennsylvania	218	3.14%
32	Rhode Island	16	0.23%
17	South Carolina	65	0.94%
43	South Dakota	4	0.06%
20	Tennessee	42	0.60%
5	Texas	295	4.25%
28	Utah	20	0.29%
46	Vermont	3	0.04%
12	Virginia	139	2.00%
25	Washington	26	0.37%
38	West Virginia	8	0.12%
26	Wisconsin	23	0.33%
49	Wyoming	0	0.00%

RANK ORDER

RANK	STATE	CASES	% of USA
1	New York	1,858	26.76%
2	Florida	1,183	17.04%
3	New Jersey	649	9.35%
4	California	509	7.33%
5	Texas	295	4.25%
6	Maryland	245	3.53%
7	Pennsylvania	218	3.14%
8	Illinois	210	3.02%
9	Massachusetts	177	2.55%
10	Georgia	168	2.42%
11	Connecticut	159	2.29%
12	Virginia	139	2.00%
13	Louisiana	106	1.53%
14	Ohio	101	1.45%
15	North Carolina	95	1.37%
16	Michigan	83	1.20%
17	South Carolina	65	0.94%
18	Alabama	55	0.79%
19	Missouri	49	0.71%
20	Tennessee	42	0.60%
21	Mississippi	38	0.55%
22	Indiana	32	0.46%
23	Arkansas	30	0.43%
24	Colorado	27	0.39%
25	Washington	26	0.37%
26	Wisconsin	23	0.33%
27	Nevada	21	0.30%
28	Utah	20	0.29%
29	Arizona	19	0.27%
29	Minnesota	19	0.27%
31	Oklahoma	18	0.26%
32	Rhode Island	16	0.23%
33	Hawaii	14	0.20%
33	Kentucky	14	0.20%
33	Oregon	14	0.20%
36	Delaware	13	0.19%
37	Kansas	11	0.16%
38	Iowa	8	0.12%
38	Nebraska	8	0.12%
38	West Virginia	8	0.12%
41	New Hampshire	7	0.10%
42	Maine	6	0.09%
43	Alaska	4	0.06%
43	New Mexico	4	0.06%
43	South Dakota	4	0.06%
46	Vermont	3	0.04%
47	Idaho	2	0.03%
47	Montana	2	0.03%
49	North Dakota	0	0.00%
49	Wyoming	0	0.00%
	District of Columbia	126	1.81%

*Source: U.S. Department of Health and Human Services, Centers for Disease Control and Prevention
"HIV/AIDS Surveillance Report, 1996" (Mid-year Edition, Vol. 8, No. 1)*
Cumulative through June 1996. AIDS is Acquired Immunodeficiency Syndrome. It is a specific group of diseases or conditions which are indicative of severe immunosuppression related to infection with the Human Immunodeficiency Virus (HIV). National total does not include 341 cases in Puerto Rico and 12 cases in the Virgin Islands.

E-Coli Cases Reported in 1996

National Total = 2,883 Cases*

ALPHA ORDER

RANK	STATE	CASES	% of USA
37	Alabama	15	0.52%
48	Alaska	6	0.21%
29	Arizona	27	0.94%
41	Arkansas	13	0.45%
3	California	176	6.10%
12	Colorado	86	2.98%
14	Connecticut	70	2.43%
50	Delaware	2	0.07%
22	Florida	38	1.32%
27	Georgia	32	1.11%
45	Hawaii	9	0.31%
20	Idaho	40	1.39%
2	Illinois	218	7.56%
11	Indiana	89	3.09%
8	Iowa	126	4.37%
27	Kansas	32	1.11%
38	Kentucky	14	0.49%
47	Louisiana	7	0.24%
32	Maine	22	0.76%
46	Maryland	8	0.28%
7	Massachusetts	156	5.41%
9	Michigan	99	3.43%
1	Minnesota	275	9.54%
43	Mississippi	12	0.42%
13	Missouri	72	2.50%
29	Montana	27	0.94%
17	Nebraska	54	1.87%
34	Nevada	17	0.59%
20	New Hampshire	40	1.39%
16	New Jersey	59	2.05%
38	New Mexico	14	0.49%
6	New York	166	5.76%
19	North Carolina	47	1.63%
34	North Dakota	17	0.59%
4	Ohio	172	5.97%
38	Oklahoma	14	0.49%
10	Oregon	96	3.33%
32	Pennsylvania	22	0.76%
36	Rhode Island	16	0.55%
41	South Carolina	13	0.45%
31	South Dakota	26	0.90%
23	Tennessee	36	1.25%
18	Texas	48	1.66%
26	Utah	34	1.18%
23	Vermont	36	1.25%
25	Virginia	35	1.21%
5	Washington	171	5.93%
49	West Virginia	3	0.10%
15	Wisconsin	65	2.25%
44	Wyoming	11	0.38%

RANK ORDER

RANK	STATE	CASES	% of USA
1	Minnesota	275	9.54%
2	Illinois	218	7.56%
3	California	176	6.10%
4	Ohio	172	5.97%
5	Washington	171	5.93%
6	New York	166	5.76%
7	Massachusetts	156	5.41%
8	Iowa	126	4.37%
9	Michigan	99	3.43%
10	Oregon	96	3.33%
11	Indiana	89	3.09%
12	Colorado	86	2.98%
13	Missouri	72	2.50%
14	Connecticut	70	2.43%
15	Wisconsin	65	2.25%
16	New Jersey	59	2.05%
17	Nebraska	54	1.87%
18	Texas	48	1.66%
19	North Carolina	47	1.63%
20	Idaho	40	1.39%
20	New Hampshire	40	1.39%
22	Florida	38	1.32%
23	Tennessee	36	1.25%
23	Vermont	36	1.25%
25	Virginia	35	1.21%
26	Utah	34	1.18%
27	Georgia	32	1.11%
27	Kansas	32	1.11%
29	Arizona	27	0.94%
29	Montana	27	0.94%
31	South Dakota	26	0.90%
32	Maine	22	0.76%
32	Pennsylvania	22	0.76%
34	Nevada	17	0.59%
34	North Dakota	17	0.59%
36	Rhode Island	16	0.55%
37	Alabama	15	0.52%
38	Kentucky	14	0.49%
38	New Mexico	14	0.49%
38	Oklahoma	14	0.49%
41	Arkansas	13	0.45%
41	South Carolina	13	0.45%
43	Mississippi	12	0.42%
44	Wyoming	11	0.38%
45	Hawaii	9	0.31%
46	Maryland	8	0.28%
47	Louisiana	7	0.24%
48	Alaska	6	0.21%
49	West Virginia	3	0.10%
50	Delaware	2	0.07%
	District of Columbia	0	0.00%

Source: U.S. Department of Health and Human Services, National Center for Health Statistics
"Morbidity and Mortality Weekly Report" (January 3, 1997, Vol. 45, Nos. 51 & 52)
Totals for Arizona, Hawaii, Maryland, Pennsylvania, Virginia, West Virginia and Wisconsin are from the Public Health Laboratory Information System. All other states' data are from National Electronic Telecommunications System for Surveillance. Escherichia Coli is a common bacterium that normally inhabits the intestinal tracts of humans and animals but can cause infection in other parts of the body, especially the urinary tract. One strain, sometimes transmitted in hamburger meat, can cause serious infection resulting in diarrhea, anemia, kidney failure, and death.

383

E-Coli Rate in 1996

National Rate = 1.09 Cases per 100,000 Population*

ALPHA ORDER

RANK	STATE	RATE
42	Alabama	0.35
27	Alaska	0.99
34	Arizona	0.61
36	Arkansas	0.52
35	California	0.55
14	Colorado	2.25
15	Connecticut	2.14
44	Delaware	0.28
45	Florida	0.26
38	Georgia	0.44
30	Hawaii	0.76
6	Idaho	3.36
16	Illinois	1.84
21	Indiana	1.52
3	Iowa	4.42
24	Kansas	1.24
41	Kentucky	0.36
48	Louisiana	0.16
17	Maine	1.77
48	Maryland	0.16
12	Massachusetts	2.56
26	Michigan	1.03
2	Minnesota	5.90
38	Mississippi	0.44
22	Missouri	1.34
9	Montana	3.07
7	Nebraska	3.27
25	Nevada	1.06
5	New Hampshire	3.44
31	New Jersey	0.74
29	New Mexico	0.82
28	New York	0.91
33	North Carolina	0.64
11	North Dakota	2.64
20	Ohio	1.54
40	Oklahoma	0.42
10	Oregon	3.00
47	Pennsylvania	0.18
19	Rhode Island	1.62
42	South Carolina	0.35
4	South Dakota	3.55
32	Tennessee	0.68
46	Texas	0.25
18	Utah	1.70
1	Vermont	6.11
36	Virginia	0.52
8	Washington	3.09
48	West Virginia	0.16
23	Wisconsin	1.26
13	Wyoming	2.29

RANK ORDER

RANK	STATE	RATE
1	Vermont	6.11
2	Minnesota	5.90
3	Iowa	4.42
4	South Dakota	3.55
5	New Hampshire	3.44
6	Idaho	3.36
7	Nebraska	3.27
8	Washington	3.09
9	Montana	3.07
10	Oregon	3.00
11	North Dakota	2.64
12	Massachusetts	2.56
13	Wyoming	2.29
14	Colorado	2.25
15	Connecticut	2.14
16	Illinois	1.84
17	Maine	1.77
18	Utah	1.70
19	Rhode Island	1.62
20	Ohio	1.54
21	Indiana	1.52
22	Missouri	1.34
23	Wisconsin	1.26
24	Kansas	1.24
25	Nevada	1.06
26	Michigan	1.03
27	Alaska	0.99
28	New York	0.91
29	New Mexico	0.82
30	Hawaii	0.76
31	New Jersey	0.74
32	Tennessee	0.68
33	North Carolina	0.64
34	Arizona	0.61
35	California	0.55
36	Arkansas	0.52
36	Virginia	0.52
38	Georgia	0.44
38	Mississippi	0.44
40	Oklahoma	0.42
41	Kentucky	0.36
42	Alabama	0.35
42	South Carolina	0.35
44	Delaware	0.28
45	Florida	0.26
46	Texas	0.25
47	Pennsylvania	0.18
48	Louisiana	0.16
48	Maryland	0.16
48	West Virginia	0.16
	District of Columbia	0.00

Source: Morgan Quitno Press using data from U.S. Dept. of Health & Human Serv's, National Center for Health Statistics "Morbidity and Mortality Weekly Report" (Vol. 44, No. 53)

Totals for Arizona, Hawaii, Maryland, Pennsylvania, Virginia, West Virginia and Wisconsin are from the Public Health Laboratory Information System. All other states' data are from National Electronic Telecommunications System for Surveillance. Escherichia Coli is a common bacterium that normally inhabits the intestinal tracts of humans and animals but can cause infection in other parts of the body, especially the urinary tract. One strain, sometimes transmitted in hamburger meat, can cause serious infection resulting in diarrhea, anemia, kidney failure, and death.

German Measles (Rubella) Cases Reported in 1996

National Total = 210 Cases*

ALPHA ORDER

RANK	STATE	CASES	% of USA
9	Alabama	2	0.95%
24	Alaska	0	0.00%
17	Arizona	1	0.48%
24	Arkansas	0	0.00%
2	California	50	23.81%
7	Colorado	3	1.43%
6	Connecticut	4	1.90%
24	Delaware	0	0.00%
4	Florida	10	4.76%
24	Georgia	0	0.00%
7	Hawaii	3	1.43%
9	Idaho	2	0.95%
17	Illinois	1	0.48%
24	Indiana	0	0.00%
24	Iowa	0	0.00%
24	Kansas	0	0.00%
24	Kentucky	0	0.00%
17	Louisiana	1	0.48%
24	Maine	0	0.00%
24	Maryland	0	0.00%
3	Massachusetts	20	9.52%
9	Michigan	2	0.95%
24	Minnesota	0	0.00%
NA	Mississippi**	NA	NA
24	Missouri	0	0.00%
24	Montana	0	0.00%
24	Nebraska	0	0.00%
17	Nevada	1	0.48%
24	New Hampshire	0	0.00%
9	New Jersey	2	0.95%
24	New Mexico	0	0.00%
4	New York	10	4.76%
1	North Carolina	85	40.48%
24	North Dakota	0	0.00%
24	Ohio	0	0.00%
24	Oklahoma	0	0.00%
17	Oregon	1	0.48%
17	Pennsylvania	1	0.48%
24	Rhode Island	0	0.00%
17	South Carolina	1	0.48%
24	South Dakota	0	0.00%
24	Tennessee	0	0.00%
9	Texas	2	0.95%
24	Utah	0	0.00%
9	Vermont	2	0.95%
9	Virginia	2	0.95%
9	Washington	2	0.95%
24	West Virginia	0	0.00%
24	Wisconsin	0	0.00%
24	Wyoming	0	0.00%

RANK ORDER

RANK	STATE	CASES	% of USA
1	North Carolina	85	40.48%
2	California	50	23.81%
3	Massachusetts	20	9.52%
4	Florida	10	4.76%
4	New York	10	4.76%
6	Connecticut	4	1.90%
7	Colorado	3	1.43%
7	Hawaii	3	1.43%
9	Alabama	2	0.95%
9	Idaho	2	0.95%
9	Michigan	2	0.95%
9	New Jersey	2	0.95%
9	Texas	2	0.95%
9	Vermont	2	0.95%
9	Virginia	2	0.95%
9	Washington	2	0.95%
17	Arizona	1	0.48%
17	Illinois	1	0.48%
17	Louisiana	1	0.48%
17	Nevada	1	0.48%
17	Oregon	1	0.48%
17	Pennsylvania	1	0.48%
17	South Carolina	1	0.48%
24	Alaska	0	0.00%
24	Arkansas	0	0.00%
24	Delaware	0	0.00%
24	Georgia	0	0.00%
24	Indiana	0	0.00%
24	Iowa	0	0.00%
24	Kansas	0	0.00%
24	Kentucky	0	0.00%
24	Maine	0	0.00%
24	Maryland	0	0.00%
24	Minnesota	0	0.00%
24	Missouri	0	0.00%
24	Montana	0	0.00%
24	Nebraska	0	0.00%
24	New Hampshire	0	0.00%
24	New Mexico	0	0.00%
24	North Dakota	0	0.00%
24	Ohio	0	0.00%
24	Oklahoma	0	0.00%
24	Rhode Island	0	0.00%
24	South Dakota	0	0.00%
24	Tennessee	0	0.00%
24	Utah	0	0.00%
24	West Virginia	0	0.00%
24	Wisconsin	0	0.00%
24	Wyoming	0	0.00%
NA	Mississippi**	NA	NA
	District of Columbia	2	0.95%

Source: U.S. Department of Health and Human Services, National Center for Health Statistics
   "Morbidity and Mortality Weekly Report" (January 3, 1997, Vol. 45, Nos. 51 & 52)
*Provisional data. A mild, contagious, eruptive disease caused by a virus and capable of producing congenital defects in infants born to mothers infected during the first three months of pregnancy.
**Rubella is not a notifiable disease in Mississippi.

German Measles (Rubella) Rate in 1996

National Rate = 0.08 Cases per 100,000 Population*

<table>
<tr><td colspan="3">ALPHA ORDER</td><td colspan="3">RANK ORDER</td></tr>
<tr><td>RANK</td><td>STATE</td><td>RATE</td><td>RANK</td><td>STATE</td><td>RATE</td></tr>
<tr><td>11</td><td>Alabama</td><td>0.05</td><td>1</td><td>North Carolina</td><td>1.16</td></tr>
<tr><td>24</td><td>Alaska</td><td>0.00</td><td>2</td><td>Vermont</td><td>0.34</td></tr>
<tr><td>18</td><td>Arizona</td><td>0.02</td><td>3</td><td>Massachusetts</td><td>0.33</td></tr>
<tr><td>24</td><td>Arkansas</td><td>0.00</td><td>4</td><td>Hawaii</td><td>0.25</td></tr>
<tr><td>6</td><td>California</td><td>0.16</td><td>5</td><td>Idaho</td><td>0.17</td></tr>
<tr><td>8</td><td>Colorado</td><td>0.08</td><td>6</td><td>California</td><td>0.16</td></tr>
<tr><td>7</td><td>Connecticut</td><td>0.12</td><td>7</td><td>Connecticut</td><td>0.12</td></tr>
<tr><td>24</td><td>Delaware</td><td>0.00</td><td>8</td><td>Colorado</td><td>0.08</td></tr>
<tr><td>9</td><td>Florida</td><td>0.07</td><td>9</td><td>Florida</td><td>0.07</td></tr>
<tr><td>24</td><td>Georgia</td><td>0.00</td><td>10</td><td>Nevada</td><td>0.06</td></tr>
<tr><td>4</td><td>Hawaii</td><td>0.25</td><td>11</td><td>Alabama</td><td>0.05</td></tr>
<tr><td>5</td><td>Idaho</td><td>0.17</td><td>11</td><td>New York</td><td>0.05</td></tr>
<tr><td>21</td><td>Illinois</td><td>0.01</td><td>13</td><td>Washington</td><td>0.04</td></tr>
<tr><td>24</td><td>Indiana</td><td>0.00</td><td>14</td><td>New Jersey</td><td>0.03</td></tr>
<tr><td>24</td><td>Iowa</td><td>0.00</td><td>14</td><td>Oregon</td><td>0.03</td></tr>
<tr><td>24</td><td>Kansas</td><td>0.00</td><td>14</td><td>South Carolina</td><td>0.03</td></tr>
<tr><td>24</td><td>Kentucky</td><td>0.00</td><td>14</td><td>Virginia</td><td>0.03</td></tr>
<tr><td>18</td><td>Louisiana</td><td>0.02</td><td>18</td><td>Arizona</td><td>0.02</td></tr>
<tr><td>24</td><td>Maine</td><td>0.00</td><td>18</td><td>Louisiana</td><td>0.02</td></tr>
<tr><td>24</td><td>Maryland</td><td>0.00</td><td>18</td><td>Michigan</td><td>0.02</td></tr>
<tr><td>3</td><td>Massachusetts</td><td>0.33</td><td>21</td><td>Illinois</td><td>0.01</td></tr>
<tr><td>18</td><td>Michigan</td><td>0.02</td><td>21</td><td>Pennsylvania</td><td>0.01</td></tr>
<tr><td>24</td><td>Minnesota</td><td>0.00</td><td>21</td><td>Texas</td><td>0.01</td></tr>
<tr><td>NA</td><td>Mississippi**</td><td>NA</td><td>24</td><td>Alaska</td><td>0.00</td></tr>
<tr><td>24</td><td>Missouri</td><td>0.00</td><td>24</td><td>Arkansas</td><td>0.00</td></tr>
<tr><td>24</td><td>Montana</td><td>0.00</td><td>24</td><td>Delaware</td><td>0.00</td></tr>
<tr><td>24</td><td>Nebraska</td><td>0.00</td><td>24</td><td>Georgia</td><td>0.00</td></tr>
<tr><td>10</td><td>Nevada</td><td>0.06</td><td>24</td><td>Indiana</td><td>0.00</td></tr>
<tr><td>24</td><td>New Hampshire</td><td>0.00</td><td>24</td><td>Iowa</td><td>0.00</td></tr>
<tr><td>14</td><td>New Jersey</td><td>0.03</td><td>24</td><td>Kansas</td><td>0.00</td></tr>
<tr><td>24</td><td>New Mexico</td><td>0.00</td><td>24</td><td>Kentucky</td><td>0.00</td></tr>
<tr><td>11</td><td>New York</td><td>0.05</td><td>24</td><td>Maine</td><td>0.00</td></tr>
<tr><td>1</td><td>North Carolina</td><td>1.16</td><td>24</td><td>Maryland</td><td>0.00</td></tr>
<tr><td>24</td><td>North Dakota</td><td>0.00</td><td>24</td><td>Minnesota</td><td>0.00</td></tr>
<tr><td>24</td><td>Ohio</td><td>0.00</td><td>24</td><td>Missouri</td><td>0.00</td></tr>
<tr><td>24</td><td>Oklahoma</td><td>0.00</td><td>24</td><td>Montana</td><td>0.00</td></tr>
<tr><td>14</td><td>Oregon</td><td>0.03</td><td>24</td><td>Nebraska</td><td>0.00</td></tr>
<tr><td>21</td><td>Pennsylvania</td><td>0.01</td><td>24</td><td>New Hampshire</td><td>0.00</td></tr>
<tr><td>24</td><td>Rhode Island</td><td>0.00</td><td>24</td><td>New Mexico</td><td>0.00</td></tr>
<tr><td>14</td><td>South Carolina</td><td>0.03</td><td>24</td><td>North Dakota</td><td>0.00</td></tr>
<tr><td>24</td><td>South Dakota</td><td>0.00</td><td>24</td><td>Ohio</td><td>0.00</td></tr>
<tr><td>24</td><td>Tennessee</td><td>0.00</td><td>24</td><td>Oklahoma</td><td>0.00</td></tr>
<tr><td>21</td><td>Texas</td><td>0.01</td><td>24</td><td>Rhode Island</td><td>0.00</td></tr>
<tr><td>24</td><td>Utah</td><td>0.00</td><td>24</td><td>South Dakota</td><td>0.00</td></tr>
<tr><td>2</td><td>Vermont</td><td>0.34</td><td>24</td><td>Tennessee</td><td>0.00</td></tr>
<tr><td>14</td><td>Virginia</td><td>0.03</td><td>24</td><td>Utah</td><td>0.00</td></tr>
<tr><td>13</td><td>Washington</td><td>0.04</td><td>24</td><td>West Virginia</td><td>0.00</td></tr>
<tr><td>24</td><td>West Virginia</td><td>0.00</td><td>24</td><td>Wisconsin</td><td>0.00</td></tr>
<tr><td>24</td><td>Wisconsin</td><td>0.00</td><td>24</td><td>Wyoming</td><td>0.00</td></tr>
<tr><td>24</td><td>Wyoming</td><td>0.00</td><td>NA</td><td>Mississippi**</td><td>NA</td></tr>
<tr><td></td><td></td><td></td><td></td><td>District of Columbia</td><td>0.37</td></tr>
</table>

Source: Morgan Quitno Press using data from U.S. Dept. of Health & Human Serv's, National Center for Health Statistics "Morbidity and Mortality Weekly Report" (January 3, 1997, Vol. 45, Nos. 51 & 52)
Provisional data. A mild, contagious, eruptive disease caused by a virus and capable of producing congenital defects in infants born to mothers infected during the first three months of pregnancy.
***Rubella is not a notifiable disease in Mississippi.*

Hepatitis (Viral) Cases Reported in 1996

National Total = 39,018 Cases*

ALPHA ORDER

RANK	STATE	CASES	% of USA
30	Alabama	285	0.73%
43	Alaska	64	0.16%
4	Arizona	1,997	5.12%
19	Arkansas	578	1.48%
1	California	8,164	20.92%
17	Colorado	661	1.69%
34	Connecticut	220	0.56%
48	Delaware	30	0.08%
8	Florida	1,205	3.09%
36	Georgia	189	0.48%
40	Hawaii	118	0.30%
28	Idaho	338	0.87%
13	Illinois	889	2.28%
23	Indiana	487	1.25%
25	Iowa	444	1.14%
26	Kansas	400	1.03%
41	Kentucky	110	0.28%
27	Louisiana	374	0.96%
49	Maine	28	0.07%
20	Maryland	553	1.42%
31	Massachusetts	278	0.71%
11	Michigan	921	2.36%
34	Minnesota	220	0.56%
24	Mississippi	446	1.14%
6	Missouri	1,690	4.33%
39	Montana	137	0.35%
32	Nebraska	271	0.69%
22	Nevada	511	1.31%
45	New Hampshire	48	0.12%
18	New Jersey	591	1.51%
15	New Mexico	766	1.96%
5	New York	1,930	4.95%
21	North Carolina	541	1.39%
38	North Dakota	139	0.36%
12	Ohio	905	2.32%
3	Oklahoma	2,476	6.35%
10	Oregon	953	2.44%
16	Pennsylvania	748	1.92%
47	Rhode Island	37	0.09%
37	South Carolina	158	0.40%
45	South Dakota	48	0.12%
7	Tennessee	1,232	3.16%
2	Texas	3,975	10.19%
9	Utah	1,195	3.06%
50	Vermont	23	0.06%
29	Virginia	331	0.85%
14	Washington	858	2.20%
44	West Virginia	54	0.14%
33	Wisconsin	247	0.63%
42	Wyoming	85	0.22%

RANK ORDER

RANK	STATE	CASES	% of USA
1	California	8,164	20.92%
2	Texas	3,975	10.19%
3	Oklahoma	2,476	6.35%
4	Arizona	1,997	5.12%
5	New York	1,930	4.95%
6	Missouri	1,690	4.33%
7	Tennessee	1,232	3.16%
8	Florida	1,205	3.09%
9	Utah	1,195	3.06%
10	Oregon	953	2.44%
11	Michigan	921	2.36%
12	Ohio	905	2.32%
13	Illinois	889	2.28%
14	Washington	858	2.20%
15	New Mexico	766	1.96%
16	Pennsylvania	748	1.92%
17	Colorado	661	1.69%
18	New Jersey	591	1.51%
19	Arkansas	578	1.48%
20	Maryland	553	1.42%
21	North Carolina	541	1.39%
22	Nevada	511	1.31%
23	Indiana	487	1.25%
24	Mississippi	446	1.14%
25	Iowa	444	1.14%
26	Kansas	400	1.03%
27	Louisiana	374	0.96%
28	Idaho	338	0.87%
29	Virginia	331	0.85%
30	Alabama	285	0.73%
31	Massachusetts	278	0.71%
32	Nebraska	271	0.69%
33	Wisconsin	247	0.63%
34	Connecticut	220	0.56%
34	Minnesota	220	0.56%
36	Georgia	189	0.48%
37	South Carolina	158	0.40%
38	North Dakota	139	0.36%
39	Montana	137	0.35%
40	Hawaii	118	0.30%
41	Kentucky	110	0.28%
42	Wyoming	85	0.22%
43	Alaska	64	0.16%
44	West Virginia	54	0.14%
45	New Hampshire	48	0.12%
45	South Dakota	48	0.12%
47	Rhode Island	37	0.09%
48	Delaware	30	0.08%
49	Maine	28	0.07%
50	Vermont	23	0.06%
	District of Columbia	70	0.18%

Source: U.S. Department of Health and Human Services, National Center for Health Statistics
"Morbidity and Mortality Weekly Report" (January 3, 1997, Vol. 45, Nos. 51 & 52)
*Provisional data. An inflammation of the liver. Includes types A and B.

Hepatitis (Viral) Rate in 1996

National Rate = 14.71 Cases Reported per 100,000 Population*

ALPHA ORDER

RANK	STATE	RATE
35	Alabama	6.67
24	Alaska	10.54
3	Arizona	45.10
11	Arkansas	23.03
9	California	25.61
15	Colorado	17.29
34	Connecticut	6.72
43	Delaware	4.14
28	Florida	8.37
49	Georgia	2.57
25	Hawaii	9.97
8	Idaho	28.43
31	Illinois	7.50
29	Indiana	8.34
19	Iowa	15.57
20	Kansas	15.55
48	Kentucky	2.83
27	Louisiana	8.60
50	Maine	2.25
22	Maryland	10.90
41	Massachusetts	4.56
26	Michigan	9.60
40	Minnesota	4.72
16	Mississippi	16.42
6	Missouri	31.54
18	Montana	15.59
17	Nebraska	16.40
5	Nevada	31.88
44	New Hampshire	4.13
32	New Jersey	7.40
4	New Mexico	44.72
23	New York	10.61
33	North Carolina	7.39
12	North Dakota	21.58
30	Ohio	8.10
1	Oklahoma	75.01
7	Oregon	29.74
37	Pennsylvania	6.20
46	Rhode Island	3.74
42	South Carolina	4.27
36	South Dakota	6.56
10	Tennessee	23.16
13	Texas	20.78
2	Utah	59.75
45	Vermont	3.90
38	Virginia	4.96
21	Washington	15.51
47	West Virginia	2.96
39	Wisconsin	4.79
14	Wyoming	17.67

RANK ORDER

RANK	STATE	RATE
1	Oklahoma	75.01
2	Utah	59.75
3	Arizona	45.10
4	New Mexico	44.72
5	Nevada	31.88
6	Missouri	31.54
7	Oregon	29.74
8	Idaho	28.43
9	California	25.61
10	Tennessee	23.16
11	Arkansas	23.03
12	North Dakota	21.58
13	Texas	20.78
14	Wyoming	17.67
15	Colorado	17.29
16	Mississippi	16.42
17	Nebraska	16.40
18	Montana	15.59
19	Iowa	15.57
20	Kansas	15.55
21	Washington	15.51
22	Maryland	10.90
23	New York	10.61
24	Alaska	10.54
25	Hawaii	9.97
26	Michigan	9.60
27	Louisiana	8.60
28	Florida	8.37
29	Indiana	8.34
30	Ohio	8.10
31	Illinois	7.50
32	New Jersey	7.40
33	North Carolina	7.39
34	Connecticut	6.72
35	Alabama	6.67
36	South Dakota	6.56
37	Pennsylvania	6.20
38	Virginia	4.96
39	Wisconsin	4.79
40	Minnesota	4.72
41	Massachusetts	4.50
42	South Carolina	4.27
43	Delaware	4.14
44	New Hampshire	4.13
45	Vermont	3.90
46	Rhode Island	3.74
47	West Virginia	2.96
48	Kentucky	2.83
49	Georgia	2.57
50	Maine	2.25

District of Columbia 12.89

Source: Morgan Quitno Press using data from U.S. Dept. of Health & Human Serv's, National Center for Health Statistics
"Morbidity and Mortality Weekly Report" (January 3, 1997, Vol. 45, Nos. 51 & 52)
*Provisional data. An inflammation of the liver. Includes types A and B.

Legionellosis Cases Reported in 1996

National Total = 1,079 Cases*

ALPHA ORDER

RANK	STATE	CASES	% of USA
34	Alabama	5	0.46%
44	Alaska	1	0.09%
15	Arizona	22	2.04%
44	Arkansas	1	0.09%
6	California	47	4.36%
21	Colorado	11	1.02%
NA	Connecticut**	NA	NA
21	Delaware	11	1.02%
5	Florida	58	5.38%
39	Georgia	3	0.28%
27	Hawaii	8	0.74%
48	Idaho	0	0.00%
25	Illinois	9	0.83%
7	Indiana	46	4.26%
21	Iowa	11	1.02%
32	Kansas	6	0.56%
25	Kentucky	9	0.83%
41	Louisiana	2	0.19%
34	Maine	5	0.46%
9	Maryland	34	3.15%
9	Massachusetts	34	3.15%
3	Michigan	107	9.92%
24	Minnesota	10	0.93%
17	Mississippi	17	1.58%
16	Missouri	19	1.76%
44	Montana	1	0.09%
17	Nebraska	17	1.58%
30	Nevada	7	0.65%
34	New Hampshire	5	0.46%
19	New Jersey	15	1.39%
41	New Mexico	2	0.19%
4	New York	93	8.62%
20	North Carolina	12	1.11%
48	North Dakota	0	0.00%
2	Ohio	116	10.75%
34	Oklahoma	5	0.46%
44	Oregon	1	0.09%
1	Pennsylvania	130	12.05%
11	Rhode Island	31	2.87%
27	South Carolina	8	0.74%
39	South Dakota	3	0.28%
14	Tennessee	23	2.13%
13	Texas	27	2.50%
27	Utah	8	0.74%
34	Vermont	5	0.46%
8	Virginia	39	3.61%
32	Washington	6	0.56%
41	West Virginia	2	0.19%
12	Wisconsin	30	2.78%
30	Wyoming	7	0.65%

RANK ORDER

RANK	STATE	CASES	% of USA
1	Pennsylvania	130	12.05%
2	Ohio	116	10.75%
3	Michigan	107	9.92%
4	New York	93	8.62%
5	Florida	58	5.38%
6	California	47	4.36%
7	Indiana	46	4.26%
8	Virginia	39	3.61%
9	Maryland	34	3.15%
9	Massachusetts	34	3.15%
11	Rhode Island	31	2.87%
12	Wisconsin	30	2.78%
13	Texas	27	2.50%
14	Tennessee	23	2.13%
15	Arizona	22	2.04%
16	Missouri	19	1.76%
17	Mississippi	17	1.58%
17	Nebraska	17	1.58%
19	New Jersey	15	1.39%
20	North Carolina	12	1.11%
21	Colorado	11	1.02%
21	Delaware	11	1.02%
21	Iowa	11	1.02%
24	Minnesota	10	0.93%
25	Illinois	9	0.83%
25	Kentucky	9	0.83%
27	Hawaii	8	0.74%
27	South Carolina	8	0.74%
27	Utah	8	0.74%
30	Nevada	7	0.65%
30	Wyoming	7	0.65%
32	Kansas	6	0.56%
32	Washington	6	0.56%
34	Alabama	5	0.46%
34	Maine	5	0.46%
34	New Hampshire	5	0.46%
34	Oklahoma	5	0.46%
34	Vermont	5	0.46%
39	Georgia	3	0.28%
39	South Dakota	3	0.28%
41	Louisiana	2	0.19%
41	New Mexico	2	0.19%
41	West Virginia	2	0.19%
44	Alaska	1	0.09%
44	Arkansas	1	0.09%
44	Montana	1	0.09%
44	Oregon	1	0.09%
48	Idaho	0	0.00%
48	North Dakota	0	0.00%
NA	Connecticut**	NA	NA
	District of Columbia	10	0.93%

Source: U.S. Department of Health and Human Services, National Center for Health Statistics
"Morbidity and Mortality Weekly Report" (January 3, 1997, Vol. 45, Nos. 51 & 52)
*Provisional data. A pneumonia-like disease (Legionnaire's Disease).
**Not notifiable.

Legionellosis Rate in 1996

National Rate = 0.41 Cases Reported per 100,000 Population*

RANK	STATE	RATE
38	Alabama	0.12
33	Alaska	0.16
17	Arizona	0.50
45	Arkansas	0.04
35	California	0.15
27	Colorado	0.29
NA	Connecticut**	NA
2	Delaware	1.52
22	Florida	0.40
45	Georgia	0.04
10	Hawaii	0.68
48	Idaho	0.00
43	Illinois	0.08
9	Indiana	0.79
25	Iowa	0.39
28	Kansas	0.23
28	Kentucky	0.23
44	Louisiana	0.05
22	Maine	0.40
11	Maryland	0.67
15	Massachusetts	0.56
4	Michigan	1.12
31	Minnesota	0.21
12	Mississippi	0.63
26	Missouri	0.35
40	Montana	0.11
7	Nebraska	1.03
18	Nevada	0.44
19	New Hampshire	0.43
32	New Jersey	0.19
38	New Mexico	0.12
16	New York	0.51
33	North Carolina	0.16
48	North Dakota	0.00
6	Ohio	1.04
35	Oklahoma	0.15
47	Oregon	0.03
5	Pennsylvania	1.08
1	Rhode Island	3.13
30	South Carolina	0.22
21	South Dakota	0.41
19	Tennessee	0.43
37	Texas	0.14
22	Utah	0.40
8	Vermont	0.85
13	Virginia	0.58
40	Washington	0.11
40	West Virginia	0.11
13	Wisconsin	0.58
3	Wyoming	1.46

RANK	STATE	RATE
1	Rhode Island	3.13
2	Delaware	1.52
3	Wyoming	1.46
4	Michigan	1.12
5	Pennsylvania	1.08
6	Ohio	1.04
7	Nebraska	1.03
8	Vermont	0.85
9	Indiana	0.79
10	Hawaii	0.68
11	Maryland	0.67
12	Mississippi	0.63
13	Virginia	0.58
13	Wisconsin	0.58
15	Massachusetts	0.56
16	New York	0.51
17	Arizona	0.50
18	Nevada	0.44
19	New Hampshire	0.43
19	Tennessee	0.43
21	South Dakota	0.41
22	Florida	0.40
22	Maine	0.40
22	Utah	0.40
25	Iowa	0.39
26	Missouri	0.35
27	Colorado	0.29
28	Kansas	0.23
28	Kentucky	0.23
30	South Carolina	0.22
31	Minnesota	0.21
32	New Jersey	0.19
33	Alaska	0.16
33	North Carolina	0.16
35	California	0.15
35	Oklahoma	0.15
37	Texas	0.14
38	Alabama	0.12
38	New Mexico	0.12
40	Montana	0.11
40	Washington	0.11
40	West Virginia	0.11
43	Illinois	0.08
44	Louisiana	0.05
45	Arkansas	0.04
45	Georgia	0.04
47	Oregon	0.03
48	Idaho	0.00
48	North Dakota	0.00
NA	Connecticut**	NA

District of Columbia 1.84

Source: Morgan Quitno Press using data from U.S. Dept. of Health & Human Serv's, National Center for Health Statistics "Morbidity and Mortality Weekly Report" (January 3, 1997, Vol. 45, Nos. 51 & 52)
Provisional data. A pneumonia-like disease (Legionnaire's Disease).
**Not notifiable.*

Lyme Disease Cases Reported in 1996

National Total = 13,807 Cases*

ALPHA ORDER

RANK	STATE	CASES	% of USA
31	Alabama	9	0.07%
44	Alaska	0	0.00%
44	Arizona	0	0.00%
23	Arkansas	23	0.17%
10	California	74	0.54%
44	Colorado	0	0.00%
2	Connecticut	2,937	21.27%
9	Delaware	105	0.76%
17	Florida	45	0.33%
39	Georgia	1	0.01%
39	Hawaii	1	0.01%
36	Idaho	2	0.01%
35	Illinois	3	0.02%
20	Indiana	29	0.21%
26	Iowa	20	0.14%
18	Kansas	37	0.27%
21	Kentucky	25	0.18%
33	Louisiana	8	0.06%
13	Maine	55	0.40%
6	Maryland	445	3.22%
7	Massachusetts	342	2.48%
44	Michigan	0	0.00%
8	Minnesota	126	0.91%
24	Mississippi	21	0.15%
18	Missouri	37	0.27%
44	Montana	0	0.00%
34	Nebraska	5	0.04%
36	Nevada	2	0.01%
16	New Hampshire	48	0.35%
3	New Jersey	1,916	13.88%
39	New Mexico	1	0.01%
1	New York	4,968	35.98%
11	North Carolina	66	0.48%
39	North Dakota	1	0.00%
14	Ohio	53	0.38%
21	Oklahoma	25	0.18%
27	Oregon	19	0.14%
4	Pennsylvania	1,621	11.74%
5	Rhode Island	537	3.89%
31	South Carolina	9	0.07%
44	South Dakota	0	0.01%
24	Tennessee	21	0.15%
12	Texas	65	0.47%
39	Utah	1	0.01%
29	Vermont	16	0.12%
14	Virginia	53	0.38%
28	Washington	18	0.13%
30	West Virginia	12	0.09%
NA	Wisconsin**	NA	NA
36	Wyoming	2	0.01%

RANK ORDER

RANK	STATE	CASES	% of USA
1	New York	4,968	35.98%
2	Connecticut	2,937	21.27%
3	New Jersey	1,916	13.88%
4	Pennsylvania	1,621	11.74%
5	Rhode Island	537	3.89%
6	Maryland	445	3.22%
7	Massachusetts	342	2.48%
8	Minnesota	126	0.91%
9	Delaware	105	0.76%
10	California	74	0.54%
11	North Carolina	66	0.48%
12	Texas	65	0.47%
13	Maine	55	0.40%
14	Ohio	53	0.38%
14	Virginia	53	0.38%
16	New Hampshire	48	0.35%
17	Florida	45	0.33%
18	Kansas	37	0.27%
18	Missouri	37	0.27%
20	Indiana	29	0.21%
21	Kentucky	25	0.18%
21	Oklahoma	25	0.18%
23	Arkansas	23	0.17%
24	Mississippi	21	0.15%
24	Tennessee	21	0.15%
26	Iowa	20	0.14%
27	Oregon	19	0.14%
28	Washington	18	0.13%
29	Vermont	16	0.12%
30	West Virginia	12	0.09%
31	Alabama	9	0.07%
31	South Carolina	9	0.07%
33	Louisiana	8	0.06%
34	Nebraska	5	0.04%
35	Illinois	3	0.02%
36	Idaho	2	0.01%
36	Nevada	2	0.01%
36	Wyoming	2	0.01%
39	Georgia	1	0.01%
39	Hawaii	1	0.01%
39	New Mexico	1	0.01%
39	North Dakota	1	0.01%
39	Utah	1	0.01%
44	Alaska	0	0.00%
44	Arizona	0	0.00%
44	Colorado	0	0.00%
44	Michigan	0	0.00%
44	Montana	0	0.00%
44	South Dakota	0	0.00%
NA	Wisconsin**	NA	NA
	District of Columbia	3	0.02%

Source: U.S. Department of Health and Human Services, National Center for Health Statistics
"Morbidity and Mortality Weekly Report" (January 3, 1997, Vol. 45, Nos. 51 & 52)
Provisional data. Caused by ticks-lesions, followed by arthritis of large joints, myalgia, malaise and neurologic and cardiac manifestations. Named after Old Lyme, CT, where the disease was first reported.
**Not available.*

Lyme Disease Rate in 1996

National Rate = 5.20 Cases per 100,000 Population*

ALPHA ORDER				RANK ORDER		
RANK	STATE	RATE		RANK	STATE	RATE
34	Alabama	0.21		1	Connecticut	89.71
44	Alaska	0.00		2	Rhode Island	54.24
44	Arizona	0.00		3	New York	27.32
14	Arkansas	0.92		4	New Jersey	23.99
33	California	0.23		5	Delaware	14.48
44	Colorado	0.00		6	Pennsylvania	13.45
1	Connecticut	89.71		7	Maryland	8.77
5	Delaware	14.48		8	Massachusetts	5.61
30	Florida	0.31		9	Maine	4.42
43	Georgia	0.01		10	New Hampshire	4.13
39	Hawaii	0.08		11	Vermont	2.72
36	Idaho	0.17		12	Minnesota	2.71
42	Illinois	0.03		13	Kansas	1.44
24	Indiana	0.50		14	Arkansas	0.92
19	Iowa	0.70		15	North Carolina	0.90
13	Kansas	1.44		16	Virginia	0.79
22	Kentucky	0.64		17	Mississippi	0.77
35	Louisiana	0.18		18	Oklahoma	0.76
9	Maine	4.42		19	Iowa	0.70
7	Maryland	8.77		20	Missouri	0.69
8	Massachusetts	5.61		21	West Virginia	0.66
44	Michigan	0.00		22	Kentucky	0.64
12	Minnesota	2.71		23	Oregon	0.59
17	Mississippi	0.77		24	Indiana	0.50
20	Missouri	0.69		25	Ohio	0.47
44	Montana	0.00		26	Wyoming	0.42
31	Nebraska	0.30		27	Tennessee	0.39
38	Nevada	0.12		28	Texas	0.34
10	New Hampshire	4.13		29	Washington	0.33
4	New Jersey	23.99		30	Florida	0.31
40	New Mexico	0.06		31	Nebraska	0.30
3	New York	27.32		32	South Carolina	0.24
15	North Carolina	0.90		33	California	0.23
37	North Dakota	0.16		34	Alabama	0.21
25	Ohio	0.47		35	Louisiana	0.18
18	Oklahoma	0.76		36	Idaho	0.17
23	Oregon	0.59		37	North Dakota	0.16
6	Pennsylvania	13.45		38	Nevada	0.12
2	Rhode Island	54.24		39	Hawaii	0.08
32	South Carolina	0.24		40	New Mexico	0.06
44	South Dakota	0.00		41	Utah	0.05
27	Tennessee	0.39		42	Illinois	0.03
28	Texas	0.34		43	Georgia	0.01
41	Utah	0.05		44	Alaska	0.00
11	Vermont	2.72		44	Arizona	0.00
16	Virginia	0.79		44	Colorado	0.00
29	Washington	0.33		44	Michigan	0.00
21	West Virginia	0.66		44	Montana	0.00
NA	Wisconsin**	NA		44	South Dakota	0.00
26	Wyoming	0.42		NA	Wisconsin**	NA
					District of Columbia	0.55

Source: Morgan Quitno Press using data from U.S. Dept. of Health & Human Serv's, National Center for Health Statistics
"Morbidity and Mortality Weekly Report" (January 3, 1997, Vol. 45, Nos. 51 & 52)
*Provisional data. Caused by ticks-lesions, followed by arthritis of large joints, myalgia, malaise and neurologic
and cardiac manifestations. Named after Old Lyme, CT, where the disease was first reported.
**Not available.

Malaria Cases Reported in 1996

National Total = 1,542 Cases*

RANK	STATE	CASES	% of USA
29	Alabama	8	0.52%
44	Alaska	3	0.19%
33	Arizona	7	0.45%
47	Arkansas	0	0.00%
1	California	329	21.34%
12	Colorado	27	1.75%
18	Connecticut	18	1.17%
40	Delaware	4	0.26%
4	Florida	80	5.19%
12	Georgia	27	1.75%
24	Hawaii	10	0.65%
47	Idaho	0	0.00%
5	Illinois	70	4.54%
21	Indiana	14	0.91%
40	Iowa	4	0.26%
28	Kansas	9	0.58%
33	Kentucky	7	0.45%
33	Louisiana	7	0.45%
24	Maine	10	0.65%
3	Maryland	85	5.51%
14	Massachusetts	24	1.56%
9	Michigan	39	2.53%
16	Minnesota	21	1.36%
29	Mississippi	8	0.52%
24	Missouri	10	0.65%
33	Montana	7	0.45%
44	Nebraska	3	0.19%
29	Nevada	8	0.52%
40	New Hampshire	4	0.26%
6	New Jersey	67	4.35%
40	New Mexico	4	0.26%
2	New York	306	19.84%
11	North Carolina	30	1.95%
46	North Dakota	1	0.06%
19	Ohio	15	0.97%
47	Oklahoma	0	0.00%
15	Oregon	23	1.49%
10	Pennsylvania	31	2.01%
24	Rhode Island	10	0.65%
23	South Carolina	13	0.84%
47	South Dakota	0	0.00%
21	Tennessee	14	0.91%
8	Texas	57	3.70%
39	Utah	5	0.32%
29	Vermont	8	0.52%
7	Virginia	58	3.76%
16	Washington	21	1.36%
38	West Virginia	6	0.39%
19	Wisconsin	15	0.97%
33	Wyoming	7	0.45%

RANK	STATE	CASES	% of USA
1	California	329	21.34%
2	New York	306	19.84%
3	Maryland	85	5.51%
4	Florida	80	5.19%
5	Illinois	70	4.54%
6	New Jersey	67	4.35%
7	Virginia	58	3.76%
8	Texas	57	3.70%
9	Michigan	39	2.53%
10	Pennsylvania	31	2.01%
11	North Carolina	30	1.95%
12	Colorado	27	1.75%
12	Georgia	27	1.75%
14	Massachusetts	24	1.56%
15	Oregon	23	1.49%
16	Minnesota	21	1.36%
16	Washington	21	1.36%
18	Connecticut	18	1.17%
19	Ohio	15	0.97%
19	Wisconsin	15	0.97%
21	Indiana	14	0.91%
21	Tennessee	14	0.91%
23	South Carolina	13	0.84%
24	Hawaii	10	0.65%
24	Maine	10	0.65%
24	Missouri	10	0.65%
24	Rhode Island	10	0.65%
28	Kansas	9	0.58%
29	Alabama	8	0.52%
29	Mississippi	8	0.52%
29	Nevada	8	0.52%
29	Vermont	8	0.52%
33	Arizona	7	0.45%
33	Kentucky	7	0.45%
33	Louisiana	7	0.45%
33	Montana	7	0.45%
33	Wyoming	7	0.45%
38	West Virginia	6	0.39%
39	Utah	5	0.32%
40	Delaware	4	0.26%
40	Iowa	4	0.26%
40	New Hampshire	4	0.26%
40	New Mexico	4	0.26%
44	Alaska	3	0.19%
44	Nebraska	3	0.19%
46	North Dakota	1	0.06%
47	Arkansas	0	0.00%
47	Idaho	0	0.00%
47	Oklahoma	0	0.00%
47	South Dakota	0	0.00%
	District of Columbia	8	0.52%

Source: U.S. Department of Health and Human Services, National Center for Health Statistics
"Morbidity and Mortality Weekly Report" (January 3, 1997, Vol. 45, Nos. 51 & 52)
*Provisional data. Infectious disease usually transmitted by bites of infected mosquitoes. Symptoms include high fever, shaking chills, sweating and anemia.

Malaria Rate in 1996

National Rate = 0.58 Cases per 100,000 Population*

ALPHA ORDER				RANK ORDER		
RANK	STATE	RATE		RANK	STATE	RATE
38	Alabama	0.19		1	Maryland	1.68
19	Alaska	0.49		1	New York	1.68
42	Arizona	0.16		3	Wyoming	1.46
47	Arkansas	0.00		4	Vermont	1.36
5	California	1.03		5	California	1.03
13	Colorado	0.71		6	Rhode Island	1.01
16	Connecticut	0.55		7	Virginia	0.87
16	Delaware	0.55		8	Hawaii	0.84
15	Florida	0.56		8	New Jersey	0.84
25	Georgia	0.37		10	Maine	0.80
8	Hawaii	0.84		10	Montana	0.80
47	Idaho	0.00		12	Oregon	0.72
14	Illinois	0.59		13	Colorado	0.71
36	Indiana	0.24		14	Illinois	0.59
45	Iowa	0.14		15	Florida	0.56
26	Kansas	0.35		16	Connecticut	0.55
40	Kentucky	0.18		16	Delaware	0.55
42	Louisiana	0.16		18	Nevada	0.50
10	Maine	0.80		19	Alaska	0.49
1	Maryland	1.68		20	Minnesota	0.45
23	Massachusetts	0.39		21	Michigan	0.41
21	Michigan	0.41		21	North Carolina	0.41
20	Minnesota	0.45		23	Massachusetts	0.39
31	Mississippi	0.29		24	Washington	0.38
38	Missouri	0.19		25	Georgia	0.37
10	Montana	0.80		26	Kansas	0.35
40	Nebraska	0.18		26	South Carolina	0.35
18	Nevada	0.50		28	New Hampshire	0.34
28	New Hampshire	0.34		29	West Virginia	0.33
8	New Jersey	0.84		30	Texas	0.30
37	New Mexico	0.23		31	Mississippi	0.29
1	New York	1.68		31	Wisconsin	0.29
21	North Carolina	0.41		33	Pennsylvania	0.26
42	North Dakota	0.16		33	Tennessee	0.26
46	Ohio	0.13		35	Utah	0.25
47	Oklahoma	0.00		36	Indiana	0.24
12	Oregon	0.72		37	New Mexico	0.23
33	Pennsylvania	0.26		38	Alabama	0.19
6	Rhode Island	1.01		38	Missouri	0.19
26	South Carolina	0.35		40	Kentucky	0.18
47	South Dakota	0.00		40	Nebraska	0.18
33	Tennessee	0.26		42	Arizona	0.16
30	Texas	0.30		42	Louisiana	0.16
35	Utah	0.25		42	North Dakota	0.16
4	Vermont	1.36		45	Iowa	0.14
7	Virginia	0.87		46	Ohio	0.13
24	Washington	0.38		47	Arkansas	0.00
29	West Virginia	0.33		47	Idaho	0.00
31	Wisconsin	0.29		47	Oklahoma	0.00
3	Wyoming	1.46		47	South Dakota	0.00
					District of Columbia	1.47

Source: Morgan Quitno Press using data from U.S. Dept. of Health & Human Serv's, National Center for Health Statistics "Morbidity and Mortality Weekly Report" (January 3, 1997, Vol. 45, Nos. 51 & 52)
*Provisional data. Infectious disease usually transmitted by bites of infected mosquitoes. Symptoms include high fever, shaking chills, sweating and anemia.

Measles (Rubeola) Cases Reported in 1996

National Total = 488 Cases*

ALPHA ORDER

RANK	STATE	CASES	% of USA
35	Alabama	0	0.00%
2	Alaska	63	12.91%
13	Arizona	8	1.64%
35	Arkansas	0	0.00%
4	California	46	9.43%
14	Colorado	7	1.43%
28	Connecticut	1	0.20%
28	Delaware	1	0.20%
28	Florida	1	0.20%
23	Georgia	2	0.41%
5	Hawaii	35	7.17%
28	Idaho	1	0.20%
18	Illinois	3	0.61%
35	Indiana	0	0.00%
28	Iowa	1	0.20%
28	Kansas	1	0.20%
35	Kentucky	0	0.00%
35	Louisiana	0	0.00%
35	Maine	0	0.00%
23	Maryland	2	0.41%
10	Massachusetts	12	2.46%
18	Michigan	3	0.61%
7	Minnesota	18	3.69%
35	Mississippi	0	0.00%
18	Missouri	3	0.61%
35	Montana	0	0.00%
35	Nebraska	0	0.00%
16	Nevada	5	1.02%
35	New Hampshire	0	0.00%
18	New Jersey	3	0.61%
8	New Mexico	17	3.48%
10	New York	12	2.46%
17	North Carolina	4	0.82%
35	North Dakota	0	0.00%
15	Ohio	6	1.23%
35	Oklahoma	0	0.00%
12	Oregon	11	2.25%
9	Pennsylvania	13	2.66%
35	Rhode Island	0	0.00%
35	South Carolina	0	0.00%
35	South Dakota	0	0.00%
23	Tennessee	2	0.41%
6	Texas	28	5.74%
1	Utah	119	24.39%
23	Vermont	2	0.41%
18	Virginia	3	0.61%
3	Washington	51	10.45%
35	West Virginia	0	0.00%
23	Wisconsin	2	0.41%
28	Wyoming	1	0.20%

RANK ORDER

RANK	STATE	CASES	% of USA
1	Utah	119	24.39%
2	Alaska	63	12.91%
3	Washington	51	10.45%
4	California	46	9.43%
5	Hawaii	35	7.17%
6	Texas	28	5.74%
7	Minnesota	18	3.69%
8	New Mexico	17	3.48%
9	Pennsylvania	13	2.66%
10	Massachusetts	12	2.46%
10	New York	12	2.46%
12	Oregon	11	2.25%
13	Arizona	8	1.64%
14	Colorado	7	1.43%
15	Ohio	6	1.23%
16	Nevada	5	1.02%
17	North Carolina	4	0.82%
18	Illinois	3	0.61%
18	Michigan	3	0.61%
18	Missouri	3	0.61%
18	New Jersey	3	0.61%
18	Virginia	3	0.61%
23	Georgia	2	0.41%
23	Maryland	2	0.41%
23	Tennessee	2	0.41%
23	Vermont	2	0.41%
23	Wisconsin	2	0.41%
28	Connecticut	1	0.20%
28	Delaware	1	0.20%
28	Florida	1	0.20%
28	Idaho	1	0.20%
28	Iowa	1	0.20%
28	Kansas	1	0.20%
28	Wyoming	1	0.20%
35	Alabama	0	0.00%
35	Arkansas	0	0.00%
35	Indiana	0	0.00%
35	Kentucky	0	0.00%
35	Louisiana	0	0.00%
35	Maine	0	0.00%
35	Mississippi	0	0.00%
35	Montana	0	0.00%
35	Nebraska	0	0.00%
35	New Hampshire	0	0.00%
35	North Dakota	0	0.00%
35	Oklahoma	0	0.00%
35	Rhode Island	0	0.00%
35	South Carolina	0	0.00%
35	South Dakota	0	0.00%
35	West Virginia	0	0.00%
	District of Columbia	1	0.20%

Source: U.S. Department of Health and Human Services, National Center for Health Statistics
"Morbidity and Mortality Weekly Report" (January 3, 1997, Vol. 45, Nos. 51 & 52)
*Provisional data. Includes indigenous and imported cases.

Measles (Rubeola) Rate in 1996

National Rate = 0.18 Cases per 100,000 Population*

ALPHA ORDER

RANK	STATE	RATE
35	Alabama	0.00
1	Alaska	10.38
12	Arizona	0.18
35	Arkansas	0.00
15	California	0.14
12	Colorado	0.18
30	Connecticut	0.03
15	Delaware	0.14
34	Florida	0.01
30	Georgia	0.03
3	Hawaii	2.96
18	Idaho	0.08
30	Illinois	0.03
35	Indiana	0.00
23	Iowa	0.04
23	Kansas	0.04
35	Kentucky	0.00
35	Louisiana	0.00
35	Maine	0.00
23	Maryland	0.04
11	Massachusetts	0.20
30	Michigan	0.03
6	Minnesota	0.39
35	Mississippi	0.00
20	Missouri	0.06
35	Montana	0.00
35	Nebraska	0.00
9	Nevada	0.31
35	New Hampshire	0.00
23	New Jersey	0.04
4	New Mexico	0.99
19	New York	0.07
21	North Carolina	0.05
35	North Dakota	0.00
21	Ohio	0.05
35	Oklahoma	0.00
7	Oregon	0.34
17	Pennsylvania	0.11
35	Rhode Island	0.00
35	South Carolina	0.00
35	South Dakota	0.00
23	Tennessee	0.04
14	Texas	0.15
2	Utah	5.95
7	Vermont	0.34
23	Virginia	0.04
5	Washington	0.92
35	West Virginia	0.00
23	Wisconsin	0.04
10	Wyoming	0.21

RANK ORDER

RANK	STATE	RATE
1	Alaska	10.38
2	Utah	5.95
3	Hawaii	2.96
4	New Mexico	0.99
5	Washington	0.92
6	Minnesota	0.39
7	Oregon	0.34
7	Vermont	0.34
9	Nevada	0.31
10	Wyoming	0.21
11	Massachusetts	0.20
12	Arizona	0.18
12	Colorado	0.18
14	Texas	0.15
15	California	0.14
15	Delaware	0.14
17	Pennsylvania	0.11
18	Idaho	0.08
19	New York	0.07
20	Missouri	0.06
21	North Carolina	0.05
21	Ohio	0.05
23	Iowa	0.04
23	Kansas	0.04
23	Maryland	0.04
23	New Jersey	0.04
23	Tennessee	0.04
23	Virginia	0.04
23	Wisconsin	0.04
30	Connecticut	0.03
30	Georgia	0.03
30	Illinois	0.03
30	Michigan	0.03
34	Florida	0.01
35	Alabama	0.00
35	Arkansas	0.00
35	Indiana	0.00
35	Kentucky	0.00
35	Louisiana	0.00
35	Maine	0.00
35	Mississippi	0.00
35	Montana	0.00
35	Nebraska	0.00
35	New Hampshire	0.00
35	North Dakota	0.00
35	Oklahoma	0.00
35	Rhode Island	0.00
35	South Carolina	0.00
35	South Dakota	0.00
35	West Virginia	0.00

District of Columbia	0.18

Source: Morgan Quitno Press using data from U.S. Dept. of Health & Human Serv's, National Center for Health Statistics "Morbidity and Mortality Weekly Report" (January 3, 1997, Vol. 45, Nos. 51 & 52)
*Provisional data. Includes indigenous and imported cases.

Meningococcal Infections Reported in 1996

National Total = 3,176 Cases*

ALPHA ORDER			
RANK	STATE	CASES	% of USA
12	Alabama	94	2.96%
43	Alaska	10	0.31%
29	Arizona	40	1.26%
31	Arkansas	34	1.07%
1	California	407	12.81%
28	Colorado	42	1.32%
26	Connecticut	45	1.42%
50	Delaware	2	0.06%
3	Florida	179	5.64%
5	Georgia	139	4.38%
45	Hawaii	6	0.19%
35	Idaho	25	0.79%
6	Illinois	126	3.97%
19	Indiana	61	1.92%
22	Iowa	57	1.79%
35	Kansas	25	0.79%
32	Kentucky	29	0.91%
21	Louisiana	58	1.83%
37	Maine	17	0.54%
15	Maryland	71	2.24%
17	Massachusetts	64	2.02%
24	Michigan	50	1.57%
30	Minnesota	35	1.10%
23	Mississippi	54	1.70%
10	Missouri	99	3.12%
45	Montana	6	0.19%
33	Nebraska	27	0.85%
41	Nevada	12	0.38%
42	New Hampshire	11	0.35%
13	New Jersey	79	2.49%
33	New Mexico	27	0.85%
6	New York	126	3.97%
13	North Carolina	79	2.49%
47	North Dakota	5	0.16%
4	Ohio	159	5.01%
27	Oklahoma	43	1.35%
8	Oregon	122	3.84%
11	Pennsylvania	98	3.09%
39	Rhode Island	16	0.50%
16	South Carolina	65	2.05%
43	South Dakota	10	0.31%
20	Tennessee	60	1.89%
2	Texas	203	6.39%
37	Utah	17	0.54%
48	Vermont	4	0.13%
18	Virginia	62	1.95%
9	Washington	101	3.18%
39	West Virginia	16	0.50%
25	Wisconsin	46	1.45%
49	Wyoming	3	0.09%

RANK ORDER			
RANK	STATE	CASES	% of USA
1	California	407	12.81%
2	Texas	203	6.39%
3	Florida	179	5.64%
4	Ohio	159	5.01%
5	Georgia	139	4.38%
6	Illinois	126	3.97%
6	New York	126	3.97%
8	Oregon	122	3.84%
9	Washington	101	3.18%
10	Missouri	99	3.12%
11	Pennsylvania	98	3.09%
12	Alabama	94	2.96%
13	New Jersey	79	2.49%
13	North Carolina	79	2.49%
15	Maryland	71	2.24%
16	South Carolina	65	2.05%
17	Massachusetts	64	2.02%
18	Virginia	62	1.95%
19	Indiana	61	1.92%
20	Tennessee	60	1.89%
21	Louisiana	58	1.83%
22	Iowa	57	1.79%
23	Mississippi	54	1.70%
24	Michigan	50	1.57%
25	Wisconsin	46	1.45%
26	Connecticut	45	1.42%
27	Oklahoma	43	1.35%
28	Colorado	42	1.32%
29	Arizona	40	1.26%
30	Minnesota	35	1.10%
31	Arkansas	34	1.07%
32	Kentucky	29	0.91%
33	Nebraska	27	0.85%
33	New Mexico	27	0.85%
35	Idaho	25	0.79%
35	Kansas	25	0.79%
37	Maine	17	0.54%
37	Utah	17	0.54%
39	Rhode Island	16	0.50%
39	West Virginia	16	0.50%
41	Nevada	12	0.38%
42	New Hampshire	11	0.35%
43	Alaska	10	0.31%
43	South Dakota	10	0.31%
45	Hawaii	6	0.19%
45	Montana	6	0.19%
47	North Dakota	5	0.16%
48	Vermont	4	0.13%
49	Wyoming	3	0.09%
50	Delaware	2	0.06%
	District of Columbia	10	0.31%

*Source: U.S. Department of Health and Human Services, National Center for Health Statistics
"Morbidity and Mortality Weekly Report" (January 3, 1997, Vol. 45, Nos. 51 & 52)
Provisional data. A bacterium (Neisseria meningitidis) that causes cerebrospinal meningitis.

Meningococcal Infection Rate in 1996

National Rate = 1.20 Cases per 100,000 Population*

<u>ALPHA ORDER</u>

RANK	STATE	RATE
2	Alabama	2.20
10	Alaska	1.65
35	Arizona	0.90
19	Arkansas	1.35
22	California	1.28
25	Colorado	1.10
16	Connecticut	1.37
50	Delaware	0.28
23	Florida	1.24
6	Georgia	1.89
49	Hawaii	0.51
3	Idaho	2.10
27	Illinois	1.06
30	Indiana	1.04
4	Iowa	2.00
32	Kansas	0.97
41	Kentucky	0.75
20	Louisiana	1.33
16	Maine	1.37
15	Maryland	1.40
29	Massachusetts	1.05
48	Michigan	0.52
41	Minnesota	0.75
5	Mississippi	1.99
7	Missouri	1.85
45	Montana	0.68
11	Nebraska	1.63
41	Nevada	0.75
33	New Hampshire	0.95
31	New Jersey	0.99
13	New Mexico	1.58
44	New York	0.69
26	North Carolina	1.08
40	North Dakota	0.78
14	Ohio	1.42
21	Oklahoma	1.30
1	Oregon	3.81
39	Pennsylvania	0.81
12	Rhode Island	1.62
9	South Carolina	1.76
16	South Dakota	1.37
24	Tennessee	1.13
27	Texas	1.06
38	Utah	0.85
45	Vermont	0.68
34	Virginia	0.93
8	Washington	1.83
37	West Virginia	0.88
36	Wisconsin	0.89
47	Wyoming	0.62

<u>RANK ORDER</u>

RANK	STATE	RATE
1	Oregon	3.81
2	Alabama	2.20
3	Idaho	2.10
4	Iowa	2.00
5	Mississippi	1.99
6	Georgia	1.89
7	Missouri	1.85
8	Washington	1.83
9	South Carolina	1.76
10	Alaska	1.65
11	Nebraska	1.63
12	Rhode Island	1.62
13	New Mexico	1.58
14	Ohio	1.42
15	Maryland	1.40
16	Connecticut	1.37
16	Maine	1.37
16	South Dakota	1.37
19	Arkansas	1.35
20	Louisiana	1.33
21	Oklahoma	1.30
22	California	1.28
23	Florida	1.24
24	Tennessee	1.13
25	Colorado	1.10
26	North Carolina	1.08
27	Illinois	1.06
27	Texas	1.06
29	Massachusetts	1.05
30	Indiana	1.04
31	New Jersey	0.99
32	Kansas	0.97
33	New Hampshire	0.95
34	Virginia	0.93
35	Arizona	0.90
36	Wisconsin	0.89
37	West Virginia	0.88
38	Utah	0.85
39	Pennsylvania	0.81
40	North Dakota	0.78
41	Kentucky	0.75
41	Minnesota	0.75
41	Nevada	0.75
44	New York	0.69
45	Montana	0.68
45	Vermont	0.68
47	Wyoming	0.62
48	Michigan	0.52
49	Hawaii	0.51
50	Delaware	0.28

District of Columbia   1.84

Source: Morgan Quitno Press using data from U.S. Dept. of Health & Human Serv's, National Center for Health Statistics
"Morbidity and Mortality Weekly Report" (January 3, 1997, Vol. 45, Nos. 51 & 52)
*Provisional data. A bacterium (Neisseria meningitidis) that causes cerebrospinal meningitis.

Mumps Cases Reported in 1996

National Total = 658 Cases*

ALPHA ORDER

RANK	STATE	CASES	% of USA
20	Alabama	6	0.91%
22	Alaska	3	0.46%
32	Arizona	1	0.15%
32	Arkansas	1	0.15%
1	California	178	27.05%
22	Colorado	3	0.46%
39	Connecticut	0	0.00%
39	Delaware	0	0.00%
5	Florida	32	4.86%
22	Georgia	3	0.46%
7	Hawaii	30	4.56%
39	Idaho	0	0.00%
12	Illinois	20	3.04%
17	Indiana	8	1.22%
22	Iowa	3	0.46%
28	Kansas	2	0.30%
39	Kentucky	0	0.00%
13	Louisiana	18	2.74%
39	Maine	0	0.00%
5	Maryland	32	4.86%
28	Massachusetts	2	0.30%
8	Michigan	26	3.95%
20	Minnesota	6	0.91%
15	Mississippi	15	2.28%
18	Missouri	7	1.06%
39	Montana	0	0.00%
39	Nebraska	0	0.00%
15	Nevada	15	2.28%
32	New Hampshire	1	0.15%
22	New Jersey	3	0.46%
NA	New Mexico**	NA	NA
3	New York	45	6.84%
10	North Carolina	21	3.19%
28	North Dakota	2	0.30%
2	Ohio	52	7.90%
32	Oklahoma	1	0.15%
39	Oregon	0	0.00%
4	Pennsylvania	43	6.53%
32	Rhode Island	1	0.15%
18	South Carolina	7	1.06%
39	South Dakota	0	0.00%
22	Tennessee	3	0.46%
8	Texas	26	3.95%
28	Utah	2	0.30%
39	Vermont	0	0.00%
14	Virginia	16	2.43%
10	Washington	21	3.19%
39	West Virginia	0	0.00%
32	Wisconsin	1	0.15%
32	Wyoming	1	0.15%

RANK ORDER

RANK	STATE	CASES	% of USA
1	California	178	27.05%
2	Ohio	52	7.90%
3	New York	45	6.84%
4	Pennsylvania	43	6.53%
5	Florida	32	4.86%
5	Maryland	32	4.86%
7	Hawaii	30	4.56%
8	Michigan	26	3.95%
8	Texas	26	3.95%
10	North Carolina	21	3.19%
10	Washington	21	3.19%
12	Illinois	20	3.04%
13	Louisiana	18	2.74%
14	Virginia	16	2.43%
15	Mississippi	15	2.28%
15	Nevada	15	2.28%
17	Indiana	8	1.22%
18	Missouri	7	1.06%
18	South Carolina	7	1.06%
20	Alabama	6	0.91%
20	Minnesota	6	0.91%
22	Alaska	3	0.46%
22	Colorado	3	0.46%
22	Georgia	3	0.46%
22	Iowa	3	0.46%
22	New Jersey	3	0.46%
22	Tennessee	3	0.46%
28	Kansas	2	0.30%
28	Massachusetts	2	0.30%
28	North Dakota	2	0.30%
28	Utah	2	0.30%
32	Arizona	1	0.15%
32	Arkansas	1	0.15%
32	New Hampshire	1	0.15%
32	Oklahoma	1	0.15%
32	Rhode Island	1	0.15%
32	Wisconsin	1	0.15%
32	Wyoming	1	0.15%
39	Connecticut	0	0.00%
39	Delaware	0	0.00%
39	Idaho	0	0.00%
39	Kentucky	0	0.00%
39	Maine	0	0.00%
39	Montana	0	0.00%
39	Nebraska	0	0.00%
39	Oregon	0	0.00%
39	South Dakota	0	0.00%
39	Vermont	0	0.00%
39	West Virginia	0	0.00%
NA	New Mexico**	NA	NA
	District of Columbia	1	0.15%

Source: U.S. Department of Health and Human Services, National Center for Health Statistics "Morbidity and Mortality Weekly Report" (October 25, 1996, Vol. 44, No. 53)
Provisional data. An acute, inflammatory, contagious disease caused by a paramyxovirus and characterized by swelling of the salivary glands, especially the parotids, and sometimes of the pancreas, ovaries, or testes. This disease, mainly affecting children, can be prevented by vaccination.
***Mumps is not a notifiable disease in New Mexico.*

Mumps Rate in 1996

National Rate = 0.25 Cases per 100,000 Population*

ALPHA ORDER

RANK	STATE	RATE
20	Alabama	0.14
6	Alaska	0.49
37	Arizona	0.02
32	Arkansas	0.04
4	California	0.56
29	Colorado	0.08
39	Connecticut	0.00
39	Delaware	0.00
16	Florida	0.22
32	Georgia	0.04
1	Hawaii	2.53
39	Idaho	0.00
19	Illinois	0.17
20	Indiana	0.14
25	Iowa	0.11
29	Kansas	0.08
39	Kentucky	0.00
8	Louisiana	0.41
39	Maine	0.00
3	Maryland	0.63
35	Massachusetts	0.03
13	Michigan	0.27
23	Minnesota	0.13
5	Mississippi	0.55
23	Missouri	0.13
39	Montana	0.00
39	Nebraska	0.00
2	Nevada	0.94
28	New Hampshire	0.09
32	New Jersey	0.04
NA	New Mexico**	NA
14	New York	0.25
12	North Carolina	0.29
11	North Dakota	0.31
7	Ohio	0.47
35	Oklahoma	0.03
39	Oregon	0.00
10	Pennsylvania	0.36
26	Rhode Island	0.10
18	South Carolina	0.19
39	South Dakota	0.00
31	Tennessee	0.06
20	Texas	0.14
26	Utah	0.10
39	Vermont	0.00
15	Virginia	0.24
9	Washington	0.38
39	West Virginia	0.00
37	Wisconsin	0.02
17	Wyoming	0.21

RANK ORDER

RANK	STATE	RATE
1	Hawaii	2.53
2	Nevada	0.94
3	Maryland	0.63
4	California	0.56
5	Mississippi	0.55
6	Alaska	0.49
7	Ohio	0.47
8	Louisiana	0.41
9	Washington	0.38
10	Pennsylvania	0.36
11	North Dakota	0.31
12	North Carolina	0.29
13	Michigan	0.27
14	New York	0.25
15	Virginia	0.24
16	Florida	0.22
17	Wyoming	0.21
18	South Carolina	0.19
19	Illinois	0.17
20	Alabama	0.14
20	Indiana	0.14
20	Texas	0.14
23	Minnesota	0.13
23	Missouri	0.13
25	Iowa	0.11
26	Rhode Island	0.10
26	Utah	0.10
28	New Hampshire	0.09
29	Colorado	0.08
29	Kansas	0.08
31	Tennessee	0.06
32	Arkansas	0.04
32	Georgia	0.04
32	New Jersey	0.04
35	Massachusetts	0.03
35	Oklahoma	0.03
37	Arizona	0.02
37	Wisconsin	0.02
39	Connecticut	0.00
39	Delaware	0.00
39	Idaho	0.00
39	Kentucky	0.00
39	Maine	0.00
39	Montana	0.00
39	Nebraska	0.00
39	Oregon	0.00
39	South Dakota	0.00
39	Vermont	0.00
39	West Virginia	0.00
NA	New Mexico**	NA

District of Columbia	0.18

Source: Morgan Quitno Press using data from U.S. Dept. of Health & Human Serv's, National Center for Health Statistics "Morbidity and Mortality Weekly Report" (October 25, 1996, Vol. 44, No. 53)
*Provisional data. An acute, inflammatory, contagious disease caused by a paramyxovirus and characterized by swelling of the salivary glands, especially the parotids, and sometimes of the pancreas, ovaries, or testes. This disease, mainly affecting children, can be prevented by vaccination.
**Mumps is not a notifiable disease in New Mexico.

Rabies (Animal) Cases Reported in 1996

National Total = 6,676 Cases*

ALPHA ORDER

RANK ORDER

RANK	STATE	CASES	% of USA	RANK	STATE	CASES	% of USA
18	Alabama	90	1.35%	1	New York	1,075	16.10%
40	Alaska	9	0.13%	2	North Carolina	696	10.43%
26	Arizona	37	0.55%	3	Maryland	637	9.54%
33	Arkansas	27	0.40%	4	Virginia	592	8.87%
6	California	314	4.70%	5	Texas	322	4.82%
24	Colorado	42	0.63%	6	California	314	4.70%
9	Connecticut	265	3.97%	7	Georgia	303	4.54%
21	Delaware	76	1.14%	8	Florida	277	4.15%
8	Florida	277	4.15%	9	Connecticut	265	3.97%
7	Georgia	303	4.54%	10	Iowa	237	3.55%
49	Hawaii	0	0.00%	11	Pennsylvania	233	3.49%
49	Idaho	0	0.00%	12	New Jersey	139	2.08%
34	Illinois	25	0.37%	13	Vermont	134	2.01%
41	Indiana	8	0.12%	14	Maine	125	1.87%
10	Iowa	237	3.55%	15	South Dakota	119	1.78%
28	Kansas	36	0.54%	16	Massachusetts	114	1.71%
24	Kentucky	42	0.63%	17	West Virginia	100	1.50%
37	Louisiana	17	0.25%	18	Alabama	90	1.35%
14	Maine	125	1.87%	19	South Carolina	88	1.32%
3	Maryland	637	9.54%	19	Tennessee	88	1.32%
16	Massachusetts	114	1.71%	21	Delaware	76	1.14%
31	Michigan	31	0.46%	22	North Dakota	71	1.06%
32	Minnesota	29	0.43%	23	New Hampshire	53	0.79%
48	Mississippi	4	0.06%	24	Colorado	42	0.63%
36	Missouri	20	0.30%	24	Kentucky	42	0.63%
35	Montana	24	0.36%	26	Arizona	37	0.55%
45	Nebraska	5	0.07%	26	Rhode Island	37	0.55%
42	Nevada	7	0.10%	28	Kansas	36	0.54%
23	New Hampshire	53	0.79%	29	Oklahoma	35	0.52%
12	New Jersey	139	2.08%	30	Wyoming	33	0.49%
43	New Mexico	6	0.09%	31	Michigan	31	0.46%
1	New York	1,075	16.10%	32	Minnesota	29	0.43%
2	North Carolina	696	10.43%	33	Arkansas	27	0.40%
22	North Dakota	71	1.06%	34	Illinois	25	0.37%
39	Ohio	13	0.19%	35	Montana	24	0.36%
29	Oklahoma	35	0.52%	36	Missouri	20	0.30%
45	Oregon	5	0.07%	37	Louisiana	17	0.25%
11	Pennsylvania	233	3.49%	38	Wisconsin	14	0.21%
26	Rhode Island	37	0.55%	39	Ohio	13	0.19%
19	South Carolina	88	1.32%	40	Alaska	9	0.13%
15	South Dakota	119	1.78%	41	Indiana	8	0.12%
19	Tennessee	88	1.32%	42	Nevada	7	0.10%
5	Texas	322	4.82%	43	New Mexico	6	0.09%
45	Utah	5	0.07%	43	Washington	6	0.09%
13	Vermont	134	2.01%	45	Nebraska	5	0.07%
4	Virginia	592	8.87%	45	Oregon	5	0.07%
43	Washington	6	0.09%	45	Utah	5	0.07%
17	West Virginia	100	1.50%	48	Mississippi	4	0.06%
38	Wisconsin	14	0.21%	49	Hawaii	0	0.00%
30	Wyoming	33	0.49%	49	Idaho	0	0.00%
					District of Columbia	11	0.16%

Source: U.S. Department of Health and Human Services, National Center for Health Statistics
"Morbidity and Mortality Weekly Report" (January 3, 1997, Vol. 45, Nos. 51 & 52)
*Provisional data. An acute, infectious, often fatal viral disease of most warm-blooded animals, especially wolves, cats, and dogs, that attacks the central nervous system and is transmitted by the bite of infected animals.

Rabies (Animal) Rate in 1996

National Rate = 2.52 Cases per 100,000 Human Population*

ALPHA ORDER

RANK	STATE	RATE
19	Alabama	2.11
26	Alaska	1.48
33	Arizona	0.84
29	Arkansas	1.08
32	California	0.99
28	Colorado	1.10
10	Connecticut	8.09
5	Delaware	10.48
21	Florida	1.92
15	Georgia	4.12
49	Hawaii	0.00
49	Idaho	0.00
43	Illinois	0.21
46	Indiana	0.14
9	Iowa	8.31
27	Kansas	1.40
29	Kentucky	1.08
36	Louisiana	0.39
6	Maine	10.06
3	Maryland	12.56
22	Massachusetts	1.87
39	Michigan	0.32
34	Minnesota	0.62
45	Mississippi	0.15
37	Missouri	0.37
17	Montana	2.73
40	Nebraska	0.30
35	Nevada	0.44
14	New Hampshire	4.56
23	New Jersey	1.74
38	New Mexico	0.35
12	New York	5.91
7	North Carolina	9.50
4	North Dakota	11.02
47	Ohio	0.12
31	Oklahoma	1.06
44	Oregon	0.16
20	Pennsylvania	1.93
16	Rhode Island	3.74
18	South Carolina	2.38
2	South Dakota	16.26
25	Tennessee	1.65
24	Texas	1.68
42	Utah	0.25
1	Vermont	22.75
8	Virginia	8.87
48	Washington	0.11
13	West Virginia	5.48
41	Wisconsin	0.27
11	Wyoming	6.86

RANK ORDER

RANK	STATE	RATE
1	Vermont	22.75
2	South Dakota	16.26
3	Maryland	12.56
4	North Dakota	11.02
5	Delaware	10.48
6	Maine	10.06
7	North Carolina	9.50
8	Virginia	8.87
9	Iowa	8.31
10	Connecticut	8.09
11	Wyoming	6.86
12	New York	5.91
13	West Virginia	5.48
14	New Hampshire	4.56
15	Georgia	4.12
16	Rhode Island	3.74
17	Montana	2.73
18	South Carolina	2.38
19	Alabama	2.11
20	Pennsylvania	1.93
21	Florida	1.92
22	Massachusetts	1.87
23	New Jersey	1.74
24	Texas	1.68
25	Tennessee	1.65
26	Alaska	1.48
27	Kansas	1.40
28	Colorado	1.10
29	Arkansas	1.08
29	Kentucky	1.08
31	Oklahoma	1.06
32	California	0.99
33	Arizona	0.84
34	Minnesota	0.62
35	Nevada	0.44
36	Louisiana	0.39
37	Missouri	0.37
38	New Mexico	0.35
39	Michigan	0.32
40	Nebraska	0.30
41	Wisconsin	0.27
42	Utah	0.25
43	Illinois	0.21
44	Oregon	0.16
45	Mississippi	0.15
46	Indiana	0.14
47	Ohio	0.12
48	Washington	0.11
49	Hawaii	0.00
49	Idaho	0.00
	District of Columbia	2.03

Source: Morgan Quitno Press using data from U.S. Dept. of Health & Human Serv's, National Center for Health Statistics "Morbidity and Mortality Weekly Report" (January 3, 1997, Vol. 45, Nos. 51 & 52)
Provisional data. An acute, infectious, often fatal viral disease of most warm-blooded animals, especially wolves, cats, and dogs, that attacks the central nervous system and is transmitted by the bite of infected animals.

Salmonellosis Cases Reported in 1995

National Total = 45,970 Cases*

ALPHA ORDER

RANK	STATE	CASES	% of USA
23	Alabama	581	1.26%
49	Alaska	48	0.10%
26	Arizona	519	1.13%
34	Arkansas	338	0.74%
1	California	6,343	13.80%
21	Colorado	594	1.29%
16	Connecticut	799	1.74%
40	Delaware	208	0.45%
3	Florida	3,386	7.37%
9	Georgia	1,662	3.62%
35	Hawaii	303	0.66%
47	Idaho	85	0.18%
6	Illinois	2,087	4.54%
18	Indiana	701	1.52%
29	Iowa	433	0.94%
31	Kansas	363	0.79%
29	Kentucky	433	0.94%
22	Louisiana	590	1.28%
42	Maine	183	0.40%
12	Maryland	1,215	2.64%
7	Massachusetts	1,862	4.05%
14	Michigan	950	2.07%
17	Minnesota	737	1.60%
25	Mississippi	554	1.21%
24	Missouri	577	1.26%
45	Montana	103	0.22%
36	Nebraska	301	0.65%
38	Nevada	238	0.52%
41	New Hampshire	188	0.41%
8	New Jersey	1,734	3.77%
33	New Mexico	342	0.74%
2	New York	4,071	8.86%
13	North Carolina	1,176	2.56%
48	North Dakota	83	0.18%
10	Ohio	1,545	3.36%
28	Oklahoma	452	0.98%
32	Oregon	344	0.75%
5	Pennsylvania	2,352	5.12%
39	Rhode Island	221	0.48%
20	South Carolina	633	1.38%
44	South Dakota	108	0.23%
27	Tennessee	454	0.99%
4	Texas	2,363	5.14%
37	Utah	280	0.61%
46	Vermont	102	0.22%
11	Virginia	1,358	2.95%
19	Washington	691	1.50%
43	West Virginia	169	0.37%
15	Wisconsin	920	2.00%
50	Wyoming	37	0.08%

RANK ORDER

RANK	STATE	CASES	% of USA
1	California	6,343	13.80%
2	New York	4,071	8.86%
3	Florida	3,386	7.37%
4	Texas	2,363	5.14%
5	Pennsylvania	2,352	5.12%
6	Illinois	2,087	4.54%
7	Massachusetts	1,862	4.05%
8	New Jersey	1,734	3.77%
9	Georgia	1,662	3.62%
10	Ohio	1,545	3.36%
11	Virginia	1,358	2.95%
12	Maryland	1,215	2.64%
13	North Carolina	1,176	2.56%
14	Michigan	950	2.07%
15	Wisconsin	920	2.00%
16	Connecticut	799	1.74%
17	Minnesota	737	1.60%
18	Indiana	701	1.52%
19	Washington	691	1.50%
20	South Carolina	633	1.38%
21	Colorado	594	1.29%
22	Louisiana	590	1.28%
23	Alabama	581	1.26%
24	Missouri	577	1.26%
25	Mississippi	554	1.21%
26	Arizona	519	1.13%
27	Tennessee	454	0.99%
28	Oklahoma	452	0.98%
29	Iowa	433	0.94%
29	Kentucky	433	0.94%
31	Kansas	363	0.79%
32	Oregon	344	0.75%
33	New Mexico	342	0.74%
34	Arkansas	338	0.74%
35	Hawaii	303	0.66%
36	Nebraska	301	0.65%
37	Utah	280	0.61%
38	Nevada	238	0.52%
39	Rhode Island	221	0.48%
40	Delaware	208	0.45%
41	New Hampshire	188	0.41%
42	Maine	183	0.40%
43	West Virginia	169	0.37%
44	South Dakota	108	0.23%
45	Montana	103	0.22%
46	Vermont	102	0.22%
47	Idaho	85	0.18%
48	North Dakota	83	0.18%
49	Alaska	48	0.10%
50	Wyoming	37	0.08%
	District of Columbia	154	0.34%

Source: U.S. Department of Health and Human Services, National Center for Health Statistics
    "Morbidity and Mortality Weekly Report" (October 25, 1996, Vol. 44, No. 53)
*Provisional data. Any disease caused by a salmonella infection, which may be manifested as food poisoning with acute gastroenteritis, vomiting and diarrhea.

Salmonellosis Rate in 1995

National Rate = 17.49 Cases per 100,000 Population*

ALPHA ORDER

RANK	STATE	RATE
33	Alabama	13.68
48	Alaska	7.96
40	Arizona	12.06
34	Arkansas	13.60
14	California	20.10
24	Colorado	15.85
4	Connecticut	24.43
2	Delaware	29.01
6	Florida	23.87
7	Georgia	23.05
3	Hawaii	25.70
50	Idaho	7.29
18	Illinois	17.70
39	Indiana	12.09
26	Iowa	15.23
30	Kansas	14.16
42	Kentucky	11.23
34	Louisiana	13.60
28	Maine	14.77
5	Maryland	24.11
1	Massachusetts	30.67
45	Michigan	9.96
23	Minnesota	15.97
11	Mississippi	20.55
44	Missouri	10.85
41	Montana	11.84
16	Nebraska	18.36
25	Nevada	15.53
21	New Hampshire	16.38
10	New Jersey	21.81
13	New Mexico	20.24
8	New York	22.38
22	North Carolina	16.33
36	North Dakota	12.93
31	Ohio	13.88
32	Oklahoma	13.80
43	Oregon	10.92
15	Pennsylvania	19.50
9	Rhode Island	22.28
20	South Carolina	17.26
27	South Dakota	14.79
47	Tennessee	8.65
38	Texas	12.57
29	Utah	14.30
19	Vermont	17.44
12	Virginia	20.53
37	Washington	12.68
46	West Virginia	9.26
17	Wisconsin	17.96
49	Wyoming	7.72

RANK ORDER

RANK	STATE	RATE
1	Massachusetts	30.67
2	Delaware	29.01
3	Hawaii	25.70
4	Connecticut	24.43
5	Maryland	24.11
6	Florida	23.87
7	Georgia	23.05
8	New York	22.38
9	Rhode Island	22.28
10	New Jersey	21.81
11	Mississippi	20.55
12	Virginia	20.53
13	New Mexico	20.24
14	California	20.10
15	Pennsylvania	19.50
16	Nebraska	18.36
17	Wisconsin	17.96
18	Illinois	17.70
19	Vermont	17.44
20	South Carolina	17.26
21	New Hampshire	16.38
22	North Carolina	16.33
23	Minnesota	15.97
24	Colorado	15.85
25	Nevada	15.53
26	Iowa	15.23
27	South Dakota	14.79
28	Maine	14.77
29	Utah	14.30
30	Kansas	14.16
31	Ohio	13.88
32	Oklahoma	13.80
33	Alabama	13.68
34	Arkansas	13.60
34	Louisiana	13.60
36	North Dakota	12.93
37	Washington	12.68
38	Texas	12.57
39	Indiana	12.09
40	Arizona	12.06
41	Montana	11.84
42	Kentucky	11.23
43	Oregon	10.92
44	Missouri	10.85
45	Michigan	9.96
46	West Virginia	9.26
47	Tennessee	8.65
48	Alaska	7.96
49	Wyoming	7.72
50	Idaho	7.29

| | District of Columbia | 27.75 |

Source: Morgan Quitno Press using data from U.S. Dept. of Health & Human Serv's, National Center for Health Statistics "Morbidity and Mortality Weekly Report" (October 25, 1996, Vol. 44, No. 53)

Provisional data. Any disease caused by a salmonella infection, which may be manifested as food poisoning with acute gastroenteritis, vomiting and diarrhea.

Shigellosis Cases Reported in 1995

National Total = 32,080 Cases*

ALPHA ORDER

RANK	STATE	CASES	% of USA
17	Alabama	510	1.59%
48	Alaska	20	0.06%
5	Arizona	1,610	5.02%
37	Arkansas	176	0.55%
1	California	5,371	16.74%
16	Colorado	528	1.65%
39	Connecticut	163	0.51%
33	Delaware	247	0.77%
4	Florida	1,726	5.38%
7	Georgia	1,358	4.23%
43	Hawaii	102	0.32%
41	Idaho	124	0.39%
6	Illinois	1,539	4.80%
22	Indiana	411	1.28%
24	Iowa	350	1.09%
28	Kansas	302	0.94%
26	Kentucky	332	1.03%
19	Louisiana	485	1.51%
47	Maine	25	0.08%
14	Maryland	639	1.99%
27	Massachusetts	324	1.01%
18	Michigan	487	1.52%
36	Minnesota	197	0.61%
25	Mississippi	333	1.04%
8	Missouri	1,138	3.55%
29	Montana	286	0.89%
34	Nebraska	227	0.71%
42	Nevada	122	0.38%
44	New Hampshire	71	0.22%
10	New Jersey	1,038	3.24%
9	New Mexico	1,089	3.39%
3	New York	1,830	5.70%
11	North Carolina	1,006	3.14%
40	North Dakota	146	0.46%
15	Ohio	598	1.86%
31	Oklahoma	254	0.79%
38	Oregon	168	0.52%
13	Pennsylvania	663	2.07%
45	Rhode Island	70	0.22%
32	South Carolina	251	0.78%
35	South Dakota	200	0.62%
23	Tennessee	400	1.25%
2	Texas	3,017	9.40%
12	Utah	764	2.38%
50	Vermont	11	0.03%
21	Virginia	412	1.28%
20	Washington	425	1.32%
46	West Virginia	59	0.18%
30	Wisconsin	264	0.82%
49	Wyoming	15	0.05%

RANK ORDER

RANK	STATE	CASES	% of USA
1	California	5,371	16.74%
2	Texas	3,017	9.40%
3	New York	1,830	5.70%
4	Florida	1,726	5.38%
5	Arizona	1,610	5.02%
6	Illinois	1,539	4.80%
7	Georgia	1,358	4.23%
8	Missouri	1,138	3.55%
9	New Mexico	1,089	3.39%
10	New Jersey	1,038	3.24%
11	North Carolina	1,006	3.14%
12	Utah	764	2.38%
13	Pennsylvania	663	2.07%
14	Maryland	639	1.99%
15	Ohio	598	1.86%
16	Colorado	528	1.65%
17	Alabama	510	1.59%
18	Michigan	487	1.52%
19	Louisiana	485	1.51%
20	Washington	425	1.32%
21	Virginia	412	1.28%
22	Indiana	411	1.28%
23	Tennessee	400	1.25%
24	Iowa	350	1.09%
25	Mississippi	333	1.04%
26	Kentucky	332	1.03%
27	Massachusetts	324	1.01%
28	Kansas	302	0.94%
29	Montana	286	0.89%
30	Wisconsin	264	0.82%
31	Oklahoma	254	0.79%
32	South Carolina	251	0.78%
33	Delaware	247	0.77%
34	Nebraska	227	0.71%
35	South Dakota	200	0.62%
36	Minnesota	197	0.61%
37	Arkansas	176	0.55%
38	Oregon	168	0.52%
39	Connecticut	163	0.51%
40	North Dakota	146	0.46%
41	Idaho	124	0.39%
42	Nevada	122	0.38%
43	Hawaii	102	0.32%
44	New Hampshire	71	0.22%
45	Rhode Island	70	0.22%
46	West Virginia	59	0.18%
47	Maine	25	0.08%
48	Alaska	20	0.06%
49	Wyoming	15	0.05%
50	Vermont	11	0.03%
	District of Columbia	197	0.61%

Source: U.S. Department of Health and Human Services, National Center for Health Statistics
"Morbidity and Mortality Weekly Report" (October 25, 1996, Vol. 44, No. 53)
*Dysentery caused by any of various species of shigellae, occurring most frequently in areas where poor sanitation and malnutrition are prevalent and commonly affecting children and infants.

Shigellosis Rate in 1995

National Rate = 12.20 Cases per 100,000 Population*

ALPHA ORDER

RANK	STATE	RATE
21	Alabama	12.01
46	Alaska	3.32
3	Arizona	37.40
33	Arkansas	7.08
10	California	17.02
12	Colorado	14.09
44	Connecticut	4.98
4	Delaware	34.45
20	Florida	12.17
9	Georgia	18.84
26	Hawaii	8.65
24	Idaho	10.63
16	Illinois	13.05
32	Indiana	7.09
19	Iowa	12.31
22	Kansas	11.78
27	Kentucky	8.61
23	Louisiana	11.18
49	Maine	2.02
17	Maryland	12.68
40	Massachusetts	5.34
43	Michigan	5.11
45	Minnesota	4.27
18	Mississippi	12.35
8	Missouri	21.39
5	Montana	32.87
14	Nebraska	13.85
28	Nevada	7.96
37	New Hampshire	6.18
15	New Jersey	13.06
1	New Mexico	64.44
25	New York	10.06
13	North Carolina	13.97
7	North Dakota	22.74
39	Ohio	5.37
30	Oklahoma	7.76
40	Oregon	5.34
38	Pennsylvania	5.50
34	Rhode Island	7.06
35	South Carolina	6.84
6	South Dakota	27.40
31	Tennessee	7.62
11	Texas	16.05
2	Utah	39.02
50	Vermont	1.88
36	Virginia	6.23
29	Washington	7.80
47	West Virginia	3.23
42	Wisconsin	5.15
48	Wyoming	3.13

RANK ORDER

RANK	STATE	RATE
1	New Mexico	64.44
2	Utah	39.02
3	Arizona	37.40
4	Delaware	34.45
5	Montana	32.87
6	South Dakota	27.40
7	North Dakota	22.74
8	Missouri	21.39
9	Georgia	18.84
10	California	17.02
11	Texas	16.05
12	Colorado	14.09
13	North Carolina	13.97
14	Nebraska	13.85
15	New Jersey	13.06
16	Illinois	13.05
17	Maryland	12.68
18	Mississippi	12.35
19	Iowa	12.31
20	Florida	12.17
21	Alabama	12.01
22	Kansas	11.78
23	Louisiana	11.18
24	Idaho	10.63
25	New York	10.06
26	Hawaii	8.65
27	Kentucky	8.61
28	Nevada	7.96
29	Washington	7.80
30	Oklahoma	7.76
31	Tennessee	7.62
32	Indiana	7.09
33	Arkansas	7.08
34	Rhode Island	7.06
35	South Carolina	6.84
36	Virginia	6.23
37	New Hampshire	6.18
38	Pennsylvania	5.50
39	Ohio	5.37
40	Massachusetts	5.34
40	Oregon	5.34
42	Wisconsin	5.15
43	Michigan	5.11
44	Connecticut	4.98
45	Minnesota	4.27
46	Alaska	3.32
47	West Virginia	3.23
48	Wyoming	3.13
49	Maine	2.02
50	Vermont	1.88
	District of Columbia	35.50

Source: Morgan Quitno Press using data from U.S. Dept. of Health & Human Serv's, National Center for Health Statistics "Morbidity and Mortality Weekly Report" (October 25, 1996, Vol. 44, No. 53)
*Dysentery caused by any of various species of shigellae, occurring most frequently in areas where poor sanitation and malnutrition are prevalent and commonly affecting children and infants.

Tuberculosis Cases Reported in 1996

National Total = 19,096 Cases*

<u>ALPHA ORDER</u>

RANK	STATE	CASES	% of USA
10	Alabama	425	2.23%
35	Alaska	70	0.37%
17	Arizona	259	1.36%
24	Arkansas	197	1.03%
1	California	4,097	21.45%
34	Colorado	78	0.41%
29	Connecticut	132	0.69%
41	Delaware	30	0.16%
4	Florida	1,160	6.07%
7	Georgia	607	3.18%
25	Hawaii	191	1.00%
47	Idaho	12	0.06%
5	Illinois	990	5.18%
26	Indiana	184	0.96%
36	Iowa	68	0.36%
37	Kansas	65	0.34%
18	Kentucky	256	1.34%
19	Louisiana	235	1.23%
45	Maine	16	0.08%
15	Maryland	298	1.56%
20	Massachusetts	234	1.23%
11	Michigan	373	1.95%
31	Minnesota	112	0.59%
22	Mississippi	227	1.19%
23	Missouri	198	1.04%
46	Montana	14	0.07%
42	Nebraska	21	0.11%
30	Nevada	128	0.67%
42	New Hampshire	21	0.11%
6	New Jersey	753	3.94%
33	New Mexico	83	0.43%
2	New York	2,318	12.14%
8	North Carolina	558	2.92%
48	North Dakota	6	0.03%
14	Ohio	303	1.59%
27	Oklahoma	174	0.91%
28	Oregon	173	0.91%
9	Pennsylvania	543	2.84%
40	Rhode Island	39	0.20%
13	South Carolina	329	1.72%
44	South Dakota	17	0.09%
12	Tennessee	349	1.83%
3	Texas	1,879	9.84%
39	Utah	51	0.27%
50	Vermont	4	0.02%
16	Virginia	293	1.53%
21	Washington	231	1.21%
38	West Virginia	57	0.30%
32	Wisconsin	102	0.53%
48	Wyoming	6	0.03%

<u>RANK ORDER</u>

RANK	STATE	CASES	% of USA
1	California	4,097	21.45%
2	New York	2,318	12.14%
3	Texas	1,879	9.84%
4	Florida	1,160	6.07%
5	Illinois	990	5.18%
6	New Jersey	753	3.94%
7	Georgia	607	3.18%
8	North Carolina	558	2.92%
9	Pennsylvania	543	2.84%
10	Alabama	425	2.23%
11	Michigan	373	1.95%
12	Tennessee	349	1.83%
13	South Carolina	329	1.72%
14	Ohio	303	1.59%
15	Maryland	298	1.56%
16	Virginia	293	1.53%
17	Arizona	259	1.36%
18	Kentucky	256	1.34%
19	Louisiana	235	1.23%
20	Massachusetts	234	1.23%
21	Washington	231	1.21%
22	Mississippi	227	1.19%
23	Missouri	198	1.04%
24	Arkansas	197	1.03%
25	Hawaii	191	1.00%
26	Indiana	184	0.96%
27	Oklahoma	174	0.91%
28	Oregon	173	0.91%
29	Connecticut	132	0.69%
30	Nevada	128	0.67%
31	Minnesota	112	0.59%
32	Wisconsin	102	0.53%
33	New Mexico	83	0.43%
34	Colorado	78	0.41%
35	Alaska	70	0.37%
36	Iowa	68	0.36%
37	Kansas	65	0.34%
38	West Virginia	57	0.30%
39	Utah	51	0.27%
40	Rhode Island	39	0.20%
41	Delaware	30	0.16%
42	Nebraska	21	0.11%
42	New Hampshire	21	0.11%
44	South Dakota	17	0.09%
45	Maine	16	0.08%
46	Montana	14	0.07%
47	Idaho	12	0.06%
48	North Dakota	6	0.03%
48	Wyoming	6	0.03%
50	Vermont	4	0.02%
	District of Columbia	130	0.68%

Source: U.S. Department of Health and Human Services, National Center for Health Statistics
"Morbidity and Mortality Weekly Report" (January 3, 1997, Vol. 45, Nos. 51 & 52)
*Provisional data. An infectious disease caused by the tubercle bacillus and causing the formation of tubercles on the lungs and other tissues of the body, often developing long after the initial infection. Characterized by the coughing up of mucus and sputum, fever, weight loss, and chest pain.

Tuberculosis Rate in 1996

National Rate = 7.20 Cases per 100,000 Population*

ALPHA ORDER

RANK	STATE	RATE
5	Alabama	9.95
4	Alaska	11.53
19	Arizona	5.85
14	Arkansas	7.85
2	California	12.85
41	Colorado	2.04
28	Connecticut	4.03
27	Delaware	4.14
12	Florida	8.06
11	Georgia	8.26
1	Hawaii	16.13
48	Idaho	1.01
9	Illinois	8.36
33	Indiana	3.15
39	Iowa	2.38
37	Kansas	2.53
16	Kentucky	6.59
20	Louisiana	5.40
45	Maine	1.29
18	Maryland	5.88
31	Massachusetts	3.84
30	Michigan	3.89
38	Minnesota	2.40
9	Mississippi	8.36
32	Missouri	3.69
44	Montana	1.59
46	Nebraska	1.27
13	Nevada	7.99
43	New Hampshire	1.81
7	New Jersey	9.43
23	New Mexico	4.85
3	New York	12.75
15	North Carolina	7.62
49	North Dakota	0.93
35	Ohio	2.71
22	Oklahoma	5.27
20	Oregon	5.40
24	Pennsylvania	4.50
29	Rhode Island	3.94
8	South Carolina	8.89
40	South Dakota	2.32
17	Tennessee	6.56
6	Texas	9.82
36	Utah	2.55
50	Vermont	0.68
25	Virginia	4.39
26	Washington	4.17
34	West Virginia	3.12
42	Wisconsin	1.98
47	Wyoming	1.25

RANK ORDER

RANK	STATE	RATE
1	Hawaii	16.13
2	California	12.85
3	New York	12.75
4	Alaska	11.53
5	Alabama	9.95
6	Texas	9.82
7	New Jersey	9.43
8	South Carolina	8.89
9	Illinois	8.36
9	Mississippi	8.36
11	Georgia	8.26
12	Florida	8.06
13	Nevada	7.99
14	Arkansas	7.85
15	North Carolina	7.62
16	Kentucky	6.59
17	Tennessee	6.56
18	Maryland	5.88
19	Arizona	5.85
20	Louisiana	5.40
20	Oregon	5.40
22	Oklahoma	5.27
23	New Mexico	4.85
24	Pennsylvania	4.50
25	Virginia	4.39
26	Washington	4.17
27	Delaware	4.14
28	Connecticut	4.03
29	Rhode Island	3.94
30	Michigan	3.89
31	Massachusetts	3.84
32	Missouri	3.69
33	Indiana	3.15
34	West Virginia	3.12
35	Ohio	2.71
36	Utah	2.55
37	Kansas	2.53
38	Minnesota	2.40
39	Iowa	2.38
40	South Dakota	2.32
41	Colorado	2.04
42	Wisconsin	1.98
43	New Hampshire	1.81
44	Montana	1.59
45	Maine	1.29
46	Nebraska	1.27
47	Wyoming	1.25
48	Idaho	1.01
49	North Dakota	0.93
50	Vermont	0.68

District of Columbia	23.94

Source: Morgan Quitno Press using data from U.S. Dept. of Health & Human Serv's, National Center for Health Statistics "Morbidity and Mortality Weekly Report" (October 25, 1996, Vol. 44, No. 53)
Provisional data. An infectious disease caused by the tubercle bacillus and causing the formation of tubercles on the lungs and other tissues of the body, often developing long after the initial infection. Characterized by the coughing up of mucus and sputum, fever, weight loss, and chest pain.

Whooping Cough (Pertussis) Cases Reported in 1996

National Total = 6,467 Cases*

ALPHA ORDER

RANK	STATE	CASES	% of USA
32	Alabama	28	0.43%
48	Alaska	4	0.06%
30	Arizona	29	0.45%
42	Arkansas	10	0.15%
2	California	724	11.20%
12	Colorado	157	2.43%
26	Connecticut	36	0.56%
33	Delaware	27	0.42%
16	Florida	102	1.58%
37	Georgia	20	0.31%
30	Hawaii	29	0.45%
15	Idaho	115	1.78%
11	Illinois	166	2.57%
18	Indiana	94	1.45%
29	Iowa	30	0.46%
45	Kansas	7	0.11%
13	Kentucky	140	2.16%
41	Louisiana	11	0.17%
35	Maine	23	0.36%
7	Maryland	263	4.07%
1	Massachusetts	1,066	16.48%
22	Michigan	54	0.84%
5	Minnesota	356	5.50%
43	Mississippi	9	0.14%
21	Missouri	58	0.90%
26	Montana	36	0.56%
40	Nebraska	15	0.23%
24	Nevada	41	0.63%
10	New Hampshire	180	2.78%
38	New Jersey	19	0.29%
20	New Mexico	63	0.97%
4	New York	537	8.30%
14	North Carolina	131	2.03%
50	North Dakota	1	0.02%
6	Ohio	290	4.48%
38	Oklahoma	19	0.29%
28	Oregon	35	0.54%
9	Pennsylvania	230	3.56%
25	Rhode Island	40	0.62%
23	South Carolina	49	0.76%
48	South Dakota	4	0.06%
36	Tennessee	21	0.32%
19	Texas	87	1.35%
34	Utah	24	0.37%
8	Vermont	241	3.73%
17	Virginia	99	1.53%
3	Washington	722	11.16%
45	West Virginia	7	0.11%
47	Wisconsin	5	0.08%
44	Wyoming	8	0.12%

RANK ORDER

RANK	STATE	CASES	% of USA
1	Massachusetts	1,066	16.48%
2	California	724	11.20%
3	Washington	722	11.16%
4	New York	537	8.30%
5	Minnesota	356	5.50%
6	Ohio	290	4.48%
7	Maryland	263	4.07%
8	Vermont	241	3.73%
9	Pennsylvania	230	3.56%
10	New Hampshire	180	2.78%
11	Illinois	166	2.57%
12	Colorado	157	2.43%
13	Kentucky	140	2.16%
14	North Carolina	131	2.03%
15	Idaho	115	1.78%
16	Florida	102	1.58%
17	Virginia	99	1.53%
18	Indiana	94	1.45%
19	Texas	87	1.35%
20	New Mexico	63	0.97%
21	Missouri	58	0.90%
22	Michigan	54	0.84%
23	South Carolina	49	0.76%
24	Nevada	41	0.63%
25	Rhode Island	40	0.62%
26	Connecticut	36	0.56%
26	Montana	36	0.56%
28	Oregon	35	0.54%
29	Iowa	30	0.46%
30	Arizona	29	0.45%
30	Hawaii	29	0.45%
32	Alabama	28	0.43%
33	Delaware	27	0.42%
34	Utah	24	0.37%
35	Maine	23	0.36%
36	Tennessee	21	0.32%
37	Georgia	20	0.31%
38	New Jersey	19	0.29%
38	Oklahoma	19	0.29%
40	Nebraska	15	0.23%
41	Louisiana	11	0.17%
42	Arkansas	10	0.15%
43	Mississippi	9	0.14%
44	Wyoming	8	0.12%
45	Kansas	7	0.11%
45	West Virginia	7	0.11%
47	Wisconsin	5	0.08%
48	Alaska	4	0.06%
48	South Dakota	4	0.06%
50	North Dakota	1	0.02%
	District of Columbia	5	0.08%

Source: U.S. Department of Health and Human Services, National Center for Health Statistics
"Morbidity and Mortality Weekly Report" (January 3, 1997, Vol. 45, Nos. 51 & 52)
*Provisional data. Acute, highly contagious infection of respiratory tract.

Whooping Cough (Pertussis) Rate in 1996

National Rate = 2.44 Cases Per 100,000 Population*

ALPHA ORDER

RANK	STATE	RATE
34	Alabama	0.66
34	Alaska	0.66
36	Arizona	0.65
41	Arkansas	0.40
18	California	2.27
8	Colorado	4.11
28	Connecticut	1.10
11	Delaware	3.72
33	Florida	0.71
45	Georgia	0.27
17	Hawaii	2.45
5	Idaho	9.67
25	Illinois	1.40
23	Indiana	1.61
31	Iowa	1.05
45	Kansas	0.27
13	Kentucky	3.60
47	Louisiana	0.25
20	Maine	1.85
7	Maryland	5.19
2	Massachusetts	17.50
38	Michigan	0.56
6	Minnesota	7.64
44	Mississippi	0.33
30	Missouri	1.08
9	Montana	4.10
32	Nebraska	0.91
16	Nevada	2.56
3	New Hampshire	15.49
48	New Jersey	0.24
12	New Mexico	3.68
14	New York	2.95
21	North Carolina	1.79
49	North Dakota	0.16
15	Ohio	2.60
37	Oklahoma	0.58
29	Oregon	1.09
19	Pennsylvania	1.91
10	Rhode Island	4.04
26	South Carolina	1.32
39	South Dakota	0.55
42	Tennessee	0.39
40	Texas	0.45
27	Utah	1.20
1	Vermont	40.92
24	Virginia	1.48
4	Washington	13.05
43	West Virginia	0.38
50	Wisconsin	0.10
22	Wyoming	1.66

RANK ORDER

RANK	STATE	RATE
1	Vermont	40.92
2	Massachusetts	17.50
3	New Hampshire	15.49
4	Washington	13.05
5	Idaho	9.67
6	Minnesota	7.64
7	Maryland	5.19
8	Colorado	4.11
9	Montana	4.10
10	Rhode Island	4.04
11	Delaware	3.72
12	New Mexico	3.68
13	Kentucky	3.60
14	New York	2.95
15	Ohio	2.60
16	Nevada	2.56
17	Hawaii	2.45
18	California	2.27
19	Pennsylvania	1.91
20	Maine	1.85
21	North Carolina	1.79
22	Wyoming	1.66
23	Indiana	1.61
24	Virginia	1.48
25	Illinois	1.40
26	South Carolina	1.32
27	Utah	1.20
28	Connecticut	1.10
29	Oregon	1.09
30	Missouri	1.08
31	Iowa	1.05
32	Nebraska	0.91
33	Florida	0.71
34	Alabama	0.66
34	Alaska	0.66
36	Arizona	0.65
37	Oklahoma	0.58
38	Michigan	0.56
39	South Dakota	0.55
40	Texas	0.45
41	Arkansas	0.40
42	Tennessee	0.39
43	West Virginia	0.38
44	Mississippi	0.33
45	Georgia	0.27
45	Kansas	0.27
47	Louisiana	0.25
48	New Jersey	0.24
49	North Dakota	0.16
50	Wisconsin	0.10
	District of Columbia	0.92

Source: Morgan Quitno Press using data from U.S. Dept. of Health & Human Serv's, National Center for Health Statistics
"Morbidity and Mortality Weekly Report" (Vol. 44, No. 53)
*Provisional data. Acute, highly contagious infection of respiratory tract.

Percent of Children Aged 19 to 35 Months Fully Immunized in 1995

National Percent = 74%*

ALPHA ORDER

RANK	STATE	PERCENT
25	Alabama	75
36	Alaska	72
44	Arizona	70
31	Arkansas	73
46	California	69
17	Colorado	77
4	Connecticut	83
36	Delaware	72
25	Florida	75
17	Georgia	77
15	Hawaii	78
50	Idaho	64
12	Illinois	79
25	Indiana	75
5	Iowa	82
44	Kansas	70
12	Kentucky	79
21	Louisiana	76
1	Maine	87
15	Maryland	78
9	Massachusetts	80
47	Michigan	67
21	Minnesota	76
7	Mississippi	81
25	Missouri	75
40	Montana	71
25	Nebraska	75
49	Nevada	65
2	New Hampshire	86
36	New Jersey	72
21	New Mexico	76
17	New York	77
9	North Carolina	80
7	North Dakota	81
31	Ohio	73
31	Oklahoma	73
36	Oregon	72
21	Pennsylvania	76
5	Rhode Island	82
9	South Carolina	80
12	South Dakota	79
31	Tennessee	73
31	Texas	73
48	Utah	66
3	Vermont	84
40	Virginia	71
17	Washington	77
40	West Virginia	71
30	Wisconsin	74
40	Wyoming	71

RANK ORDER

RANK	STATE	PERCENT
1	Maine	87
2	New Hampshire	86
3	Vermont	84
4	Connecticut	83
5	Iowa	82
5	Rhode Island	82
7	Mississippi	81
7	North Dakota	81
9	Massachusetts	80
9	North Carolina	80
9	South Carolina	80
12	Illinois	79
12	Kentucky	79
12	South Dakota	79
15	Hawaii	78
15	Maryland	78
17	Colorado	77
17	Georgia	77
17	New York	77
17	Washington	77
21	Louisiana	76
21	Minnesota	76
21	New Mexico	76
21	Pennsylvania	76
25	Alabama	75
25	Florida	75
25	Indiana	75
25	Missouri	75
25	Nebraska	75
30	Wisconsin	74
31	Arkansas	73
31	Ohio	73
31	Oklahoma	73
31	Tennessee	73
31	Texas	73
36	Alaska	72
36	Delaware	72
36	New Jersey	72
36	Oregon	72
40	Montana	71
40	Virginia	71
40	West Virginia	71
40	Wyoming	71
44	Arizona	70
44	Kansas	70
46	California	69
47	Michigan	67
48	Utah	66
49	Nevada	65
50	Idaho	64
	District of Columbia**	NA

Source: U.S. Department of Health and Human Services, Centers for Disease Control and Prevention
   "State Vaccination Coverage Levels" (Morbidity and Mortality Weekly Report, Vol. 46, No. 8, 02/28/97)
*As of December 1995. Fully immunized children received four doses of DTP/DT (Diphtheria, Tetanus, Pertussis (Whooping Cough)), three doses of OPV (Poliovirus), one dose of MMR (Measles, Mumps, Rubella) and three doses of Hib (Haemophilus influenzae type b).
**Not available.

Sexually-Transmitted Diseases in 1995

National Total = 940,045 Cases*

ALPHA ORDER

RANK	STATE	CASES	% of USA
17	Alabama	19,517	2.08%
NA	Alaska**	NA	NA
21	Arizona	14,322	1.52%
31	Arkansas	7,556	0.80%
1	California	93,014	9.89%
28	Colorado	9,757	1.04%
25	Connecticut	10,766	1.15%
35	Delaware	5,031	0.54%
6	Florida	46,662	4.96%
10	Georgia	35,898	3.82%
39	Hawaii	2,723	0.29%
42	Idaho	1,900	0.20%
5	Illinois	50,062	5.33%
18	Indiana	18,862	2.01%
32	Iowa	6,983	0.74%
30	Kansas	8,264	0.88%
23	Kentucky	12,157	1.29%
16	Louisiana	22,207	2.36%
46	Maine	1,242	0.13%
14	Maryland	23,195	2.47%
27	Massachusetts	10,575	1.12%
8	Michigan	41,090	4.37%
29	Minnesota	9,071	0.96%
20	Mississippi	14,972	1.59%
12	Missouri	24,707	2.63%
45	Montana	1,276	0.14%
37	Nebraska	4,041	0.43%
36	Nevada	4,483	0.48%
47	New Hampshire	1,048	0.11%
24	New Jersey	11,333	1.21%
34	New Mexico	5,477	0.58%
3	New York	61,804	6.57%
7	North Carolina	42,817	4.55%
44	North Dakota	1,362	0.14%
4	Ohio	54,249	5.77%
26	Oklahoma	10,727	1.14%
33	Oregon	6,386	0.68%
9	Pennsylvania	37,949	4.04%
40	Rhode Island	2,537	0.27%
15	South Carolina	22,387	2.38%
43	South Dakota	1,557	0.17%
11	Tennessee	29,656	3.15%
2	Texas	83,372	8.87%
41	Utah	2,032	0.22%
49	Vermont	531	0.06%
13	Virginia	24,214	2.58%
22	Washington	12,444	1.32%
38	West Virginia	3,253	0.35%
19	Wisconsin	15,062	1.60%
48	Wyoming	756	0.08%

RANK ORDER

RANK	STATE	CASES	% of USA
1	California	93,014	9.89%
2	Texas	83,372	8.87%
3	New York	61,804	6.57%
4	Ohio	54,249	5.77%
5	Illinois	50,062	5.33%
6	Florida	46,662	4.96%
7	North Carolina	42,817	4.55%
8	Michigan	41,090	4.37%
9	Pennsylvania	37,949	4.04%
10	Georgia	35,898	3.82%
11	Tennessee	29,656	3.15%
12	Missouri	24,707	2.63%
13	Virginia	24,214	2.58%
14	Maryland	23,195	2.47%
15	South Carolina	22,387	2.38%
16	Louisiana	22,207	2.36%
17	Alabama	19,517	2.08%
18	Indiana	18,862	2.01%
19	Wisconsin	15,062	1.60%
20	Mississippi	14,972	1.59%
21	Arizona	14,322	1.52%
22	Washington	12,444	1.32%
23	Kentucky	12,157	1.29%
24	New Jersey	11,333	1.21%
25	Connecticut	10,766	1.15%
26	Oklahoma	10,727	1.14%
27	Massachusetts	10,575	1.12%
28	Colorado	9,757	1.04%
29	Minnesota	9,071	0.96%
30	Kansas	8,264	0.88%
31	Arkansas	7,556	0.80%
32	Iowa	6,983	0.74%
33	Oregon	6,386	0.68%
34	New Mexico	5,477	0.58%
35	Delaware	5,031	0.54%
36	Nevada	4,483	0.48%
37	Nebraska	4,041	0.43%
38	West Virginia	3,253	0.35%
39	Hawaii	2,723	0.29%
40	Rhode Island	2,537	0.27%
41	Utah	2,032	0.22%
42	Idaho	1,900	0.20%
43	South Dakota	1,557	0.17%
44	North Dakota	1,362	0.14%
45	Montana	1,276	0.14%
46	Maine	1,242	0.13%
47	New Hampshire	1,048	0.11%
48	Wyoming	756	0.08%
49	Vermont	531	0.06%
NA	Alaska**	NA	NA
	District of Columbia	8,079	0.86%

Source: Morgan Quitno Press using data from U.S. Dept. of Health & Human Serv's, National Center for Health Statistics unpublished (http://wonder.cdc.gov/WONDER/)
Includes chancroid, chlamydia, gonorrhea and syphilis.
**Not available.*

Rate of Sexually-Transmitted Diseases in 1995

National Rate = 357.58 Cases per 100,000 Population*

ALPHA ORDER

RANK ORDER

RANK	STATE	RATE		RANK	STATE	RATE
11	Alabama	459.66		1	Delaware	701.67
NA	Alaska**	NA		2	South Carolina	610.50
17	Arizona	332.68		3	North Carolina	594.52
26	Arkansas	304.06		4	Tennessee	565.20
27	California	294.67		5	Mississippi	555.34
30	Colorado	260.33		6	Louisiana	511.92
18	Connecticut	329.13		7	Georgia	497.96
1	Delaware	701.67		8	Ohio	487.24
19	Florida	328.98		9	Missouri	464.50
7	Georgia	497.96		10	Maryland	460.31
34	Hawaii	230.96		11	Alabama	459.66
42	Idaho	162.95		12	Texas	443.44
14	Illinois	424.61		13	Michigan	430.80
21	Indiana	325.38		14	Illinois	424.61
33	Iowa	245.62		15	Virginia	366.05
23	Kansas	322.31		16	New York	339.75
24	Kentucky	315.19		17	Arizona	332.68
6	Louisiana	511.92		18	Connecticut	329.13
47	Maine	100.24		19	Florida	328.98
10	Maryland	460.31		20	Oklahoma	327.54
41	Massachusetts	174.19		21	Indiana	325.38
13	Michigan	430.80		22	New Mexico	324.08
39	Minnesota	196.55		23	Kansas	322.31
5	Mississippi	555.34		24	Kentucky	315.19
9	Missouri	464.50		25	Pennsylvania	314.67
44	Montana	146.67		26	Arkansas	304.06
32	Nebraska	246.55		27	California	294.67
29	Nevada	292.43		28	Wisconsin	294.06
48	New Hampshire	91.29		29	Nevada	292.43
45	New Jersey	142.55		30	Colorado	260.33
22	New Mexico	324.08		31	Rhode Island	255.75
16	New York	339.75		32	Nebraska	246.55
3	North Carolina	594.52		33	Iowa	245.62
37	North Dakota	212.15		34	Hawaii	230.96
8	Ohio	487.24		35	Washington	228.41
20	Oklahoma	327.54		36	South Dakota	213.29
38	Oregon	202.79		37	North Dakota	212.15
25	Pennsylvania	314.67		38	Oregon	202.79
31	Rhode Island	255.75		39	Minnesota	196.55
2	South Carolina	610.50		40	West Virginia	178.25
36	South Dakota	213.29		41	Massachusetts	174.19
4	Tennessee	565.20		42	Idaho	162.95
12	Texas	443.44		43	Wyoming	157.83
46	Utah	103.78		44	Montana	146.67
49	Vermont	90.77		45	New Jersey	142.55
15	Virginia	366.05		46	Utah	103.78
35	Washington	228.41		47	Maine	100.24
40	West Virginia	178.25		48	New Hampshire	91.29
28	Wisconsin	294.06		49	Vermont	90.77
43	Wyoming	157.83		NA	Alaska**	NA
					District of Columbia	1,455.68

Source: Morgan Quitno Press using data from U.S. Dept. of Health and Human Services, Nat'l Center for Health Statistics
    unpublished (http://wonder.cdc.gov/WONDER/)
*Includes chancroid, chlamydia, gonorrhea and syphilis.
**Not available.

Chancroid Cases Reported in 1995

National Total = 606 Cases*

ALPHA ORDER					RANK ORDER			
RANK	STATE		CASES	% of USA	RANK	STATE	CASES	% of USA
7	Alabama		7	1.16%	1	New York	336	55.45%
22	Alaska		0	0.00%	2	Louisiana	129	21.29%
14	Arizona		2	0.33%	3	Texas	26	4.29%
20	Arkansas		1	0.17%	4	Florida	24	3.96%
7	California		7	1.16%	5	Illinois	21	3.47%
22	Colorado		0	0.00%	6	North Carolina	18	2.97%
22	Connecticut		0	0.00%	7	Alabama	7	1.16%
22	Delaware		0	0.00%	7	California	7	1.16%
4	Florida		24	3.96%	7	Massachusetts	7	1.16%
14	Georgia		2	0.33%	10	Ohio	5	0.83%
22	Hawaii		0	0.00%	10	Washington	5	0.83%
22	Idaho		0	0.00%	12	New Jersey	4	0.66%
5	Illinois		21	3.47%	13	Wisconsin	3	0.50%
22	Indiana		0	0.00%	14	Arizona	2	0.33%
22	Iowa		0	0.00%	14	Georgia	2	0.33%
14	Kansas		2	0.33%	14	Kansas	2	0.33%
22	Kentucky		0	0.00%	14	Nevada	2	0.33%
2	Louisiana		129	21.29%	14	Tennessee	2	0.33%
22	Maine		0	0.00%	14	Virginia	2	0.33%
22	Maryland		0	0.00%	20	Arkansas	1	0.17%
7	Massachusetts		7	1.16%	20	West Virginia	1	0.17%
22	Michigan		0	0.00%	22	Alaska	0	0.00%
22	Minnesota		0	0.00%	22	Colorado	0	0.00%
22	Mississippi		0	0.00%	22	Connecticut	0	0.00%
22	Missouri		0	0.00%	22	Delaware	0	0.00%
22	Montana		0	0.00%	22	Hawaii	0	0.00%
22	Nebraska		0	0.00%	22	Idaho	0	0.00%
14	Nevada		2	0.33%	22	Indiana	0	0.00%
22	New Hampshire		0	0.00%	22	Iowa	0	0.00%
12	New Jersey		4	0.66%	22	Kentucky	0	0.00%
22	New Mexico		0	0.00%	22	Maine	0	0.00%
1	New York		336	55.45%	22	Maryland	0	0.00%
6	North Carolina		18	2.97%	22	Michigan	0	0.00%
22	North Dakota		0	0.00%	22	Minnesota	0	0.00%
10	Ohio		5	0.83%	22	Mississippi	0	0.00%
22	Oklahoma		0	0.00%	22	Missouri	0	0.00%
22	Oregon		0	0.00%	22	Montana	0	0.00%
22	Pennsylvania		0	0.00%	22	Nebraska	0	0.00%
22	Rhode Island		0	0.00%	22	New Hampshire	0	0.00%
22	South Carolina		0	0.00%	22	New Mexico	0	0.00%
22	South Dakota		0	0.00%	22	North Dakota	0	0.00%
14	Tennessee		2	0.33%	22	Oklahoma	0	0.00%
3	Texas		26	4.29%	22	Oregon	0	0.00%
22	Utah		0	0.00%	22	Pennsylvania	0	0.00%
22	Vermont		0	0.00%	22	Rhode Island	0	0.00%
14	Virginia		2	0.33%	22	South Carolina	0	0.00%
10	Washington		5	0.83%	22	South Dakota	0	0.00%
20	West Virginia		1	0.17%	22	Utah	0	0.00%
13	Wisconsin		3	0.50%	22	Vermont	0	0.00%
22	Wyoming		0	0.00%	22	Wyoming	0	0.00%
						District of Columbia	0	0.00%

Source: U.S. Department of Health and Human Services, National Center for Health Statistics
   unpublished (http://wonder.cdc.gov/WONDER/)
*A soft, highly infectious, nonsyphilitic venereal ulcer of the genital region, caused by the bacillus Hemophilus
ducreyi. Also called soft chancre.

Chancroid Rate in 1995

National Rate = 0.23 Cases per 100,000 Population*

ALPHA ORDER		
RANK	STATE	RATE
6	Alabama	0.16
22	Alaska	0.00
13	Arizona	0.05
16	Arkansas	0.04
21	California	0.02
22	Colorado	0.00
22	Connecticut	0.00
22	Delaware	0.00
5	Florida	0.17
19	Georgia	0.03
22	Hawaii	0.00
22	Idaho	0.00
4	Illinois	0.18
22	Indiana	0.00
22	Iowa	0.00
11	Kansas	0.08
22	Kentucky	0.00
1	Louisiana	2.97
22	Maine	0.00
22	Maryland	0.00
9	Massachusetts	0.12
22	Michigan	0.00
22	Minnesota	0.00
22	Mississippi	0.00
22	Missouri	0.00
22	Montana	0.00
22	Nebraska	0.00
8	Nevada	0.13
22	New Hampshire	0.00
13	New Jersey	0.05
22	New Mexico	0.00
2	New York	1.85
3	North Carolina	0.25
22	North Dakota	0.00
16	Ohio	0.04
22	Oklahoma	0.00
22	Oregon	0.00
22	Pennsylvania	0.00
22	Rhode Island	0.00
22	South Carolina	0.00
22	South Dakota	0.00
16	Tennessee	0.04
7	Texas	0.14
22	Utah	0.00
22	Vermont	0.00
19	Virginia	0.03
10	Washington	0.09
13	West Virginia	0.05
12	Wisconsin	0.06
22	Wyoming	0.00

RANK ORDER		
RANK	STATE	RATE
1	Louisiana	2.97
2	New York	1.85
3	North Carolina	0.25
4	Illinois	0.18
5	Florida	0.17
6	Alabama	0.16
7	Texas	0.14
8	Nevada	0.13
9	Massachusetts	0.12
10	Washington	0.09
11	Kansas	0.08
12	Wisconsin	0.06
13	Arizona	0.05
13	New Jersey	0.05
13	West Virginia	0.05
16	Arkansas	0.04
16	Ohio	0.04
16	Tennessee	0.04
19	Georgia	0.03
19	Virginia	0.03
21	California	0.02
22	Alaska	0.00
22	Colorado	0.00
22	Connecticut	0.00
22	Delaware	0.00
22	Hawaii	0.00
22	Idaho	0.00
22	Indiana	0.00
22	Iowa	0.00
22	Kentucky	0.00
22	Maine	0.00
22	Maryland	0.00
22	Michigan	0.00
22	Minnesota	0.00
22	Mississippi	0.00
22	Missouri	0.00
22	Montana	0.00
22	Nebraska	0.00
22	New Hampshire	0.00
22	New Mexico	0.00
22	North Dakota	0.00
22	Oklahoma	0.00
22	Oregon	0.00
22	Pennsylvania	0.00
22	Rhode Island	0.00
22	South Carolina	0.00
22	South Dakota	0.00
22	Utah	0.00
22	Vermont	0.00
22	Wyoming	0.00
	District of Columbia	0.00

Source: Morgan Quitno Press using data from U.S. Dept. of Health and Human Services, Nat'l Center for Health Statistics unpublished (http://wonder.cdc.gov/WONDER/)

A soft, highly infectious, nonsyphilitic venereal ulcer of the genital region, caused by the bacillus Hemophilus ducreyi. Also called soft chancre.

Chlamydia Cases in 1995

National Total = 477,638 Cases*

ALPHA ORDER

RANK	STATE	CASES	% of USA
32	Alabama	3,188	0.67%
NA	Alaska**	NA	NA
14	Arizona	10,061	2.11%
48	Arkansas	680	0.14%
1	California	62,501	13.09%
23	Colorado	6,650	1.39%
24	Connecticut	6,440	1.35%
35	Delaware	2,701	0.57%
7	Florida	22,294	4.67%
13	Georgia	11,193	2.34%
37	Hawaii	2,135	0.45%
39	Idaho	1,739	0.36%
5	Illinois	24,645	5.16%
17	Indiana	9,102	1.91%
28	Iowa	5,089	1.07%
27	Kansas	5,314	1.11%
22	Kentucky	6,904	1.45%
16	Louisiana	9,111	1.91%
44	Maine	1,144	0.24%
19	Maryland	8,740	1.83%
21	Massachusetts	7,402	1.55%
8	Michigan	21,666	4.54%
25	Minnesota	6,032	1.26%
45	Mississippi	912	0.19%
12	Missouri	12,110	2.54%
43	Montana	1,198	0.25%
34	Nebraska	2,873	0.60%
33	Nevada	3,049	0.64%
46	New Hampshire	898	0.19%
31	New Jersey	4,056	0.85%
30	New Mexico	4,285	0.90%
4	New York	26,686	5.59%
9	North Carolina	15,780	3.30%
41	North Dakota	1,324	0.28%
3	Ohio	29,124	6.10%
29	Oklahoma	5,065	1.06%
26	Oregon	5,465	1.14%
6	Pennsylvania	22,961	4.81%
38	Rhode Island	1,902	0.40%
20	South Carolina	8,591	1.80%
42	South Dakota	1,313	0.27%
10	Tennessee	13,154	2.75%
2	Texas	44,627	9.34%
40	Utah	1,676	0.35%
49	Vermont	462	0.10%
11	Virginia	12,285	2.57%
15	Washington	9,462	1.98%
36	West Virginia	2,326	0.49%
18	Wisconsin	8,955	1.87%
47	Wyoming	703	0.15%

RANK ORDER

RANK	STATE	CASES	% of USA
1	California	62,501	13.09%
2	Texas	44,627	9.34%
3	Ohio	29,124	6.10%
4	New York	26,686	5.59%
5	Illinois	24,645	5.16%
6	Pennsylvania	22,961	4.81%
7	Florida	22,294	4.67%
8	Michigan	21,666	4.54%
9	North Carolina	15,780	3.30%
10	Tennessee	13,154	2.75%
11	Virginia	12,285	2.57%
12	Missouri	12,110	2.54%
13	Georgia	11,193	2.34%
14	Arizona	10,061	2.11%
15	Washington	9,462	1.98%
16	Louisiana	9,111	1.91%
17	Indiana	9,102	1.91%
18	Wisconsin	8,955	1.87%
19	Maryland	8,740	1.83%
20	South Carolina	8,591	1.80%
21	Massachusetts	7,402	1.55%
22	Kentucky	6,904	1.45%
23	Colorado	6,650	1.39%
24	Connecticut	6,440	1.35%
25	Minnesota	6,032	1.26%
26	Oregon	5,465	1.14%
27	Kansas	5,314	1.11%
28	Iowa	5,089	1.07%
29	Oklahoma	5,065	1.06%
30	New Mexico	4,285	0.90%
31	New Jersey	4,056	0.85%
32	Alabama	3,188	0.67%
33	Nevada	3,049	0.64%
34	Nebraska	2,873	0.60%
35	Delaware	2,701	0.57%
36	West Virginia	2,326	0.49%
37	Hawaii	2,135	0.45%
38	Rhode Island	1,902	0.40%
39	Idaho	1,739	0.36%
40	Utah	1,676	0.35%
41	North Dakota	1,324	0.28%
42	South Dakota	1,313	0.27%
43	Montana	1,198	0.25%
44	Maine	1,144	0.24%
45	Mississippi	912	0.19%
46	New Hampshire	898	0.19%
47	Wyoming	703	0.15%
48	Arkansas	680	0.14%
49	Vermont	462	0.10%
NA	Alaska**	NA	NA
	District of Columbia	1,665	0.35%

Source: U.S. Department of Health and Human Services, National Center for Health Statistics unpublished (http://wonder.cdc.gov/WONDER/)

*Any of several common, often asymptomatic, sexually transmitted diseases caused by the microorganism Chlamydia trachomatis,, including nonspecific urethritis in men.

**Not available.

Chlamydia Rate in 1995

National Rate = 181.69 Cases per 100,000 Population*

Source: Morgan Quitno Press using data from U.S. Dept. of Health and Human Services, Nat'l Center for Health Statistics unpublished (http://wonder.cdc.gov/WONDER/)

*Any of several common, often asymptomatic, sexually transmitted diseases caused by the microorganism Chlamydia trachomatis,, including nonspecific urethritis in men.

**Not available.

Gonorrhea Cases Reported in 1995

National Total = 392,848 Cases*

ALPHA ORDER

ALPHA ORDER

RANK	STATE	CASES	% of USA
10	Alabama	14,683	3.74%
39	Alaska	660	0.17%
26	Arizona	3,844	0.98%
21	Arkansas	5,630	1.43%
3	California	24,803	6.31%
28	Colorado	2,803	0.71%
25	Connecticut	4,055	1.03%
32	Delaware	2,201	0.56%
8	Florida	20,874	5.31%
7	Georgia	21,025	5.35%
40	Hawaii	563	0.14%
44	Idaho	149	0.04%
6	Illinois	21,747	5.54%
19	Indiana	8,880	2.26%
33	Iowa	1,723	0.44%
29	Kansas	2,797	0.71%
24	Kentucky	4,751	1.21%
18	Louisiana	9,292	2.37%
46	Maine	94	0.02%
13	Maryland	12,984	3.31%
31	Massachusetts	2,658	0.68%
9	Michigan	18,220	4.64%
27	Minnesota	2,852	0.73%
17	Mississippi	9,511	2.42%
15	Missouri	11,326	2.88%
48	Montana	65	0.02%
35	Nebraska	1,133	0.29%
34	Nevada	1,237	0.31%
45	New Hampshire	118	0.03%
20	New Jersey	5,783	1.47%
36	New Mexico	1,054	0.27%
2	New York	25,992	6.62%
4	North Carolina	23,961	6.10%
50	North Dakota	38	0.01%
5	Ohio	23,176	5.90%
23	Oklahoma	5,077	1.29%
38	Oregon	854	0.22%
12	Pennsylvania	13,038	3.32%
41	Rhode Island	545	0.14%
14	South Carolina	12,120	3.09%
43	South Dakota	237	0.06%
11	Tennessee	13,892	3.54%
1	Texas	30,801	7.84%
42	Utah	306	0.08%
47	Vermont	69	0.02%
16	Virginia	10,340	2.63%
30	Washington	2,765	0.70%
37	West Virginia	860	0.22%
22	Wisconsin	5,524	1.41%
49	Wyoming	51	0.01%

RANK ORDER

RANK	STATE	CASES	% of USA
1	Texas	30,801	7.84%
2	New York	25,992	6.62%
3	California	24,803	6.31%
4	North Carolina	23,961	6.10%
5	Ohio	23,176	5.90%
6	Illinois	21,747	5.54%
7	Georgia	21,025	5.35%
8	Florida	20,874	5.31%
9	Michigan	18,220	4.64%
10	Alabama	14,683	3.74%
11	Tennessee	13,892	3.54%
12	Pennsylvania	13,038	3.32%
13	Maryland	12,984	3.31%
14	South Carolina	12,120	3.09%
15	Missouri	11,326	2.88%
16	Virginia	10,340	2.63%
17	Mississippi	9,511	2.42%
18	Louisiana	9,292	2.37%
19	Indiana	8,880	2.26%
20	New Jersey	5,783	1.47%
21	Arkansas	5,630	1.43%
22	Wisconsin	5,524	1.41%
23	Oklahoma	5,077	1.29%
24	Kentucky	4,751	1.21%
25	Connecticut	4,055	1.03%
26	Arizona	3,844	0.98%
27	Minnesota	2,852	0.73%
28	Colorado	2,803	0.71%
29	Kansas	2,797	0.71%
30	Washington	2,765	0.70%
31	Massachusetts	2,658	0.68%
32	Delaware	2,201	0.56%
33	Iowa	1,723	0.44%
34	Nevada	1,237	0.31%
35	Nebraska	1,133	0.29%
36	New Mexico	1,054	0.27%
37	West Virginia	860	0.22%
38	Oregon	854	0.22%
39	Alaska	660	0.17%
40	Hawaii	563	0.14%
41	Rhode Island	545	0.14%
42	Utah	306	0.08%
43	South Dakota	237	0.06%
44	Idaho	149	0.04%
45	New Hampshire	118	0.03%
46	Maine	94	0.02%
47	Vermont	69	0.02%
48	Montana	65	0.02%
49	Wyoming	51	0.01%
50	North Dakota	38	0.01%
	District of Columbia	5,687	1.45%

*Source: U.S. Department of Health and Human Services, National Center for Health Statistics
    unpublished (http://wonder.cdc.gov/WONDER/)*

Updates earlier 1995 numbers. Gonorrhea is a sexually transmitted disease caused by gonococcal bacteria that affects the mucous membrane chiefly of the genital and urinary tracts and is characterized by an acute purulent discharge and painful or difficult urination, though women often have no symptoms.

Gonorrhea Rate in 1995

National Rate = 149.43 Cases Reported per 100,000 Population*

ALPHA ORDER

RANK	STATE	RATE
2	Alabama	345.81
23	Alaska	109.45
27	Arizona	89.29
9	Arkansas	226.56
29	California	78.58
30	Colorado	74.79
21	Connecticut	123.97
5	Delaware	306.97
19	Florida	147.17
6	Georgia	291.65
38	Hawaii	47.75
44	Idaho	12.78
14	Illinois	184.45
18	Indiana	153.18
35	Iowa	60.60
24	Kansas	109.09
22	Kentucky	123.18
10	Louisiana	214.20
48	Maine	7.59
8	Maryland	257.67
40	Massachusetts	43.78
13	Michigan	191.03
34	Minnesota	61.80
1	Mississippi	352.78
11	Missouri	212.93
49	Montana	7.47
32	Nebraska	69.13
28	Nevada	80.69
47	New Hampshire	10.28
31	New Jersey	72.74
33	New Mexico	62.37
20	New York	142.88
3	North Carolina	332.70
50	North Dakota	5.92
12	Ohio	208.16
17	Oklahoma	155.02
42	Oregon	27.12
25	Pennsylvania	108.11
36	Rhode Island	54.94
4	South Carolina	330.52
41	South Dakota	32.47
7	Tennessee	264.76
15	Texas	163.83
43	Utah	15.63
45	Vermont	11.79
16	Virginia	156.31
37	Washington	50.75
39	West Virginia	47.12
26	Wisconsin	107.85
46	Wyoming	10.65

RANK ORDER

RANK	STATE	RATE
1	Mississippi	352.78
2	Alabama	345.81
3	North Carolina	332.70
4	South Carolina	330.52
5	Delaware	306.97
6	Georgia	291.65
7	Tennessee	264.76
8	Maryland	257.67
9	Arkansas	226.56
10	Louisiana	214.20
11	Missouri	212.93
12	Ohio	208.16
13	Michigan	191.03
14	Illinois	184.45
15	Texas	163.83
16	Virginia	156.31
17	Oklahoma	155.02
18	Indiana	153.18
19	Florida	147.17
20	New York	142.88
21	Connecticut	123.97
22	Kentucky	123.18
23	Alaska	109.45
24	Kansas	109.09
25	Pennsylvania	108.11
26	Wisconsin	107.85
27	Arizona	89.29
28	Nevada	80.69
29	California	78.58
30	Colorado	74.79
31	New Jersey	72.74
32	Nebraska	69.13
33	New Mexico	62.37
34	Minnesota	61.80
35	Iowa	60.60
36	Rhode Island	54.94
37	Washington	50.75
38	Hawaii	47.75
39	West Virginia	47.12
40	Massachusetts	43.78
41	South Dakota	32.47
42	Oregon	27.12
43	Utah	15.63
44	Idaho	12.78
45	Vermont	11.79
46	Wyoming	10.65
47	New Hampshire	10.28
48	Maine	7.59
49	Montana	7.47
50	North Dakota	5.92
	District of Columbia	1,024.68

Source: Morgan Quitno Press using data from U.S. Dept. of Health and Human Services, Nat'l Center for Health Statistics
unpublished (http://wonder.cdc.gov/WONDER/)
*Updates earlier 1995 numbers. Gonorrhea is a sexually transmitted disease caused by gonococcal bacteria that affects the mucous membrane chiefly of the genital and urinary tracts and is characterized by an acute purulent discharge and painful or difficult urination, though women often have no symptoms.

Syphilis Cases Reported in 1995

National Total = 68,953 Cases*

ALPHA ORDER

RANK	STATE	CASES	% of USA
14	Alabama	1,639	2.38%
43	Alaska	20	0.03%
26	Arizona	415	0.60%
19	Arkansas	1,245	1.81%
3	California	5,703	8.27%
27	Colorado	304	0.44%
28	Connecticut	271	0.39%
35	Delaware	129	0.19%
8	Florida	3,470	5.03%
5	Georgia	3,678	5.33%
42	Hawaii	25	0.04%
45	Idaho	12	0.02%
7	Illinois	3,649	5.29%
21	Indiana	880	1.28%
32	Iowa	171	0.25%
33	Kansas	151	0.22%
25	Kentucky	502	0.73%
6	Louisiana	3,675	5.33%
47	Maine	4	0.01%
17	Maryland	1,471	2.13%
24	Massachusetts	508	0.74%
20	Michigan	1,204	1.75%
31	Minnesota	187	0.27%
4	Mississippi	4,549	6.60%
18	Missouri	1,271	1.84%
44	Montana	13	0.02%
40	Nebraska	35	0.05%
30	Nevada	195	0.28%
41	New Hampshire	32	0.05%
16	New Jersey	1,490	2.16%
34	New Mexico	138	0.20%
1	New York	8,790	12.75%
9	North Carolina	3,058	4.43%
49	North Dakota	0	0.00%
12	Ohio	1,944	2.82%
22	Oklahoma	585	0.85%
37	Oregon	67	0.10%
11	Pennsylvania	1,950	2.83%
36	Rhode Island	90	0.13%
13	South Carolina	1,676	2.43%
46	South Dakota	7	0.01%
10	Tennessee	2,608	3.78%
2	Texas	7,918	11.48%
39	Utah	50	0.07%
49	Vermont	0	0.00%
15	Virginia	1,587	2.30%
29	Washington	212	0.31%
38	West Virginia	66	0.10%
23	Wisconsin	580	0.84%
48	Wyoming	2	0.00%

RANK ORDER

RANK	STATE	CASES	% of USA
1	New York	8,790	12.75%
2	Texas	7,918	11.48%
3	California	5,703	8.27%
4	Mississippi	4,549	6.60%
5	Georgia	3,678	5.33%
6	Louisiana	3,675	5.33%
7	Illinois	3,649	5.29%
8	Florida	3,470	5.03%
9	North Carolina	3,058	4.43%
10	Tennessee	2,608	3.78%
11	Pennsylvania	1,950	2.83%
12	Ohio	1,944	2.82%
13	South Carolina	1,676	2.43%
14	Alabama	1,639	2.38%
15	Virginia	1,587	2.30%
16	New Jersey	1,490	2.16%
17	Maryland	1,471	2.13%
18	Missouri	1,271	1.84%
19	Arkansas	1,245	1.81%
20	Michigan	1,204	1.75%
21	Indiana	880	1.28%
22	Oklahoma	585	0.85%
23	Wisconsin	580	0.84%
24	Massachusetts	508	0.74%
25	Kentucky	502	0.73%
26	Arizona	415	0.60%
27	Colorado	304	0.44%
28	Connecticut	271	0.39%
29	Washington	212	0.31%
30	Nevada	195	0.28%
31	Minnesota	187	0.27%
32	Iowa	171	0.25%
33	Kansas	151	0.22%
34	New Mexico	138	0.20%
35	Delaware	129	0.19%
36	Rhode Island	90	0.13%
37	Oregon	67	0.10%
38	West Virginia	66	0.10%
39	Utah	50	0.07%
40	Nebraska	35	0.05%
41	New Hampshire	32	0.05%
42	Hawaii	25	0.04%
43	Alaska	20	0.03%
44	Montana	13	0.02%
45	Idaho	12	0.02%
46	South Dakota	7	0.01%
47	Maine	4	0.01%
48	Wyoming	2	0.00%
49	North Dakota	0	0.00%
49	Vermont	0	0.00%
	District of Columbia	727	1.05%

Source: U.S. Department of Health and Human Services, National Center for Health Statistics unpublished (http://wonder.cdc.gov/WONDER/)

Updates earlier 1995 numbers. Syphilis includes primary and secondary cases. A chronic infectious disease caused by a spirochete (Treponema pallidum), either transmitted by direct contact, usually in sexual intercourse, or passed from mother to child in utero, and progressing through three stages characterized respectively by local formation of chancres, ulcerous skin eruptions, and systemic infection leading to general paresis.

Syphilis Rate in 1995

National Rate = 26.23 Cases per 100,000 Population*

ALPHA ORDER

RANK	STATE	RATE
10	Alabama	38.60
38	Alaska	3.32
27	Arizona	9.64
4	Arkansas	50.10
17	California	18.07
32	Colorado	8.11
30	Connecticut	8.28
18	Delaware	17.99
13	Florida	24.46
3	Georgia	51.02
43	Hawaii	2.12
45	Idaho	1.03
11	Illinois	30.95
22	Indiana	15.18
33	Iowa	6.01
34	Kansas	5.89
23	Kentucky	13.02
2	Louisiana	84.72
48	Maine	0.32
12	Maryland	29.19
29	Massachusetts	8.37
25	Michigan	12.62
35	Minnesota	4.05
1	Mississippi	168.73
15	Missouri	23.90
44	Montana	1.49
41	Nebraska	2.14
24	Nevada	12.72
39	New Hampshire	2.79
16	New Jersey	18.74
31	New Mexico	8.17
6	New York	48.32
8	North Carolina	42.46
49	North Dakota	0.00
20	Ohio	17.46
19	Oklahoma	17.86
42	Oregon	2.13
21	Pennsylvania	16.17
28	Rhode Island	9.07
7	South Carolina	45.70
46	South Dakota	0.96
5	Tennessee	49.70
9	Texas	42.11
40	Utah	2.55
49	Vermont	0.00
14	Virginia	23.99
36	Washington	3.89
37	West Virginia	3.62
26	Wisconsin	11.32
47	Wyoming	0.42

RANK ORDER

RANK	STATE	RATE
1	Mississippi	168.73
2	Louisiana	84.72
3	Georgia	51.02
4	Arkansas	50.10
5	Tennessee	49.70
6	New York	48.32
7	South Carolina	45.70
8	North Carolina	42.46
9	Texas	42.11
10	Alabama	38.60
11	Illinois	30.95
12	Maryland	29.19
13	Florida	24.46
14	Virginia	23.99
15	Missouri	23.90
16	New Jersey	18.74
17	California	18.07
18	Delaware	17.99
19	Oklahoma	17.86
20	Ohio	17.46
21	Pennsylvania	16.17
22	Indiana	15.18
23	Kentucky	13.02
24	Nevada	12.72
25	Michigan	12.62
26	Wisconsin	11.32
27	Arizona	9.64
28	Rhode Island	9.07
29	Massachusetts	8.37
30	Connecticut	8.28
31	New Mexico	8.17
32	Colorado	8.11
33	Iowa	6.01
34	Kansas	5.89
35	Minnesota	4.05
36	Washington	3.89
37	West Virginia	3.62
38	Alaska	3.32
39	New Hampshire	2.79
40	Utah	2.55
41	Nebraska	2.14
42	Oregon	2.13
43	Hawaii	2.12
44	Montana	1.49
45	Idaho	1.03
46	South Dakota	0.96
47	Wyoming	0.42
48	Maine	0.32
49	North Dakota	0.00
49	Vermont	0.00
	District of Columbia	130.99

Source: Morgan Quitno Press using data from U.S. Dept. of Health and Human Services, Nat'l Center for Health Statistics
unpublished (http://wonder.cdc.gov/WONDER/)
*Updates earlier 1995 numbers. Syphilis includes primary and secondary cases. A chronic infectious disease
caused by a spirochete (Treponema pallidum), either transmitted by direct contact, usually in sexual intercourse, or
passed from mother to child in utero, and progressing through three stages characterized respectively by local
formation of chancres, ulcerous skin eruptions, and systemic infection leading to general paresis.

421

VI. PROVIDERS

VI. PROVIDERS (continued)

Physicians in 1995

National Total = 708,951 Physicians*

<u>ALPHA ORDER</u>

RANK	STATE	PHYSICIANS	% of USA
25	Alabama	8,793	1.24%
49	Alaska	1,092	0.15%
23	Arizona	10,383	1.46%
32	Arkansas	4,921	0.69%
1	California	88,553	12.49%
24	Colorado	9,999	1.41%
20	Connecticut	12,278	1.73%
46	Delaware	1,804	0.25%
4	Florida	38,918	5.49%
14	Georgia	16,120	2.27%
38	Hawaii	3,562	0.50%
43	Idaho	1,936	0.27%
6	Illinois	31,845	4.49%
21	Indiana	11,743	1.66%
31	Iowa	5,463	0.77%
30	Kansas	5,865	0.83%
26	Kentucky	8,259	1.16%
22	Louisiana	10,616	1.50%
40	Maine	2,956	0.42%
11	Maryland	21,345	3.01%
8	Massachusetts	25,831	3.64%
10	Michigan	22,404	3.16%
18	Minnesota	12,512	1.76%
33	Mississippi	4,482	0.63%
17	Missouri	12,781	1.80%
44	Montana	1,896	0.27%
37	Nebraska	3,679	0.52%
42	Nevada	2,806	0.40%
41	New Hampshire	2,908	0.41%
9	New Jersey	24,236	3.42%
36	New Mexico	4,030	0.57%
2	New York	71,637	10.10%
12	North Carolina	17,527	2.47%
47	North Dakota	1,475	0.21%
7	Ohio	27,435	3.87%
29	Oklahoma	5,929	0.84%
27	Oregon	8,000	1.13%
5	Pennsylvania	36,780	5.19%
39	Rhode Island	3,302	0.47%
28	South Carolina	7,999	1.13%
48	South Dakota	1,437	0.20%
16	Tennessee	13,301	1.88%
3	Texas	40,243	5.68%
34	Utah	4,320	0.61%
45	Vermont	1,878	0.26%
13	Virginia	17,423	2.46%
15	Washington	14,609	2.06%
35	West Virginia	4,066	0.57%
19	Wisconsin	12,399	1.75%
50	Wyoming	879	0.12%

<u>RANK ORDER</u>

RANK	STATE	PHYSICIANS	% of USA
1	California	88,553	12.49%
2	New York	71,637	10.10%
3	Texas	40,243	5.68%
4	Florida	38,918	5.49%
5	Pennsylvania	36,780	5.19%
6	Illinois	31,845	4.49%
7	Ohio	27,435	3.87%
8	Massachusetts	25,831	3.64%
9	New Jersey	24,236	3.42%
10	Michigan	22,404	3.16%
11	Maryland	21,345	3.01%
12	North Carolina	17,527	2.47%
13	Virginia	17,423	2.46%
14	Georgia	16,120	2.27%
15	Washington	14,609	2.06%
16	Tennessee	13,301	1.88%
17	Missouri	12,781	1.80%
18	Minnesota	12,512	1.76%
19	Wisconsin	12,399	1.75%
20	Connecticut	12,278	1.73%
21	Indiana	11,743	1.66%
22	Louisiana	10,616	1.50%
23	Arizona	10,383	1.46%
24	Colorado	9,999	1.41%
25	Alabama	8,793	1.24%
26	Kentucky	8,259	1.16%
27	Oregon	8,000	1.13%
28	South Carolina	7,999	1.13%
29	Oklahoma	5,929	0.84%
30	Kansas	5,865	0.83%
31	Iowa	5,463	0.77%
32	Arkansas	4,921	0.69%
33	Mississippi	4,482	0.63%
34	Utah	4,320	0.61%
35	West Virginia	4,066	0.57%
36	New Mexico	4,030	0.57%
37	Nebraska	3,679	0.52%
38	Hawaii	3,562	0.50%
39	Rhode Island	3,302	0.47%
40	Maine	2,956	0.42%
41	New Hampshire	2,908	0.41%
42	Nevada	2,806	0.40%
43	Idaho	1,936	0.27%
44	Montana	1,896	0.27%
45	Vermont	1,878	0.26%
46	Delaware	1,804	0.25%
47	North Dakota	1,475	0.21%
48	South Dakota	1,437	0.20%
49	Alaska	1,092	0.15%
50	Wyoming	879	0.12%
	District of Columbia	4,296	0.61%

Source: American Medical Association (Chicago, Illinois)
"Physician Characteristics and Distribution in the U.S." (1996-97 Edition)
As of December 31, 1995. Comprised of federal and nonfederal physicians. Total does not include 11,374 physicians in the U.S. territories and possessions, at APO's and FPO's and whose addresses are unknown.

Male Physicians in 1995

National Total = 562,282 Physicians*

ALPHA ORDER					RANK ORDER			
RANK	STATE	PHYSICIANS	% of USA		RANK	STATE	PHYSICIANS	% of USA
25	Alabama	7,408	1.32%		1	California	70,357	12.51%
49	Alaska	866	0.15%		2	New York	53,791	9.57%
23	Arizona	8,494	1.51%		3	Florida	33,098	5.89%
32	Arkansas	4,165	0.74%		4	Texas	32,479	5.78%
1	California	70,357	12.51%		5	Pennsylvania	28,650	5.10%
24	Colorado	7,892	1.40%		6	Illinois	24,000	4.27%
21	Connecticut	9,601	1.71%		7	Ohio	21,593	3.84%
46	Delaware	1,394	0.25%		8	Massachusetts	19,075	3.39%
3	Florida	33,098	5.89%		9	New Jersey	18,420	3.28%
14	Georgia	13,123	2.33%		10	Michigan	17,490	3.11%
38	Hawaii	2,860	0.51%		11	Maryland	15,994	2.84%
43	Idaho	1,715	0.31%		12	North Carolina	14,191	2.52%
6	Illinois	24,000	4.27%		13	Virginia	13,739	2.44%
20	Indiana	9,691	1.72%		14	Georgia	13,123	2.33%
31	Iowa	4,565	0.81%		15	Washington	11,669	2.08%
30	Kansas	4,757	0.85%		16	Tennessee	11,098	1.97%
26	Kentucky	6,772	1.20%		17	Missouri	10,300	1.83%
22	Louisiana	8,748	1.56%		18	Wisconsin	10,014	1.78%
41	Maine	2,401	0.43%		19	Minnesota	9,871	1.76%
11	Maryland	15,994	2.84%		20	Indiana	9,691	1.72%
8	Massachusetts	19,075	3.39%		21	Connecticut	9,601	1.71%
10	Michigan	17,490	3.11%		22	Louisiana	8,748	1.56%
19	Minnesota	9,871	1.76%		23	Arizona	8,494	1.51%
33	Mississippi	3,831	0.68%		24	Colorado	7,892	1.40%
17	Missouri	10,300	1.83%		25	Alabama	7,408	1.32%
44	Montana	1,647	0.29%		26	Kentucky	6,772	1.20%
36	Nebraska	3,060	0.54%		27	South Carolina	6,661	1.18%
40	Nevada	2,427	0.43%		28	Oregon	6,515	1.16%
42	New Hampshire	2,400	0.43%		29	Oklahoma	4,947	0.88%
9	New Jersey	18,420	3.28%		30	Kansas	4,757	0.85%
37	New Mexico	3,043	0.54%		31	Iowa	4,565	0.81%
2	New York	53,791	9.57%		32	Arkansas	4,165	0.74%
12	North Carolina	14,191	2.52%		33	Mississippi	3,831	0.68%
47	North Dakota	1,288	0.23%		34	Utah	3,702	0.66%
7	Ohio	21,593	3.84%		35	West Virginia	3,353	0.60%
29	Oklahoma	4,947	0.88%		36	Nebraska	3,060	0.54%
28	Oregon	6,515	1.16%		37	New Mexico	3,043	0.54%
5	Pennsylvania	28,650	5.10%		38	Hawaii	2,860	0.51%
39	Rhode Island	2,562	0.46%		39	Rhode Island	2,562	0.46%
27	South Carolina	6,661	1.18%		40	Nevada	2,427	0.43%
48	South Dakota	1,240	0.22%		41	Maine	2,401	0.43%
16	Tennessee	11,098	1.97%		42	New Hampshire	2,400	0.43%
4	Texas	32,479	5.78%		43	Idaho	1,715	0.31%
34	Utah	3,702	0.66%		44	Montana	1,647	0.29%
45	Vermont	1,471	0.26%		45	Vermont	1,471	0.26%
13	Virginia	13,739	2.44%		46	Delaware	1,394	0.25%
15	Washington	11,669	2.08%		47	North Dakota	1,288	0.23%
35	West Virginia	3,353	0.60%		48	South Dakota	1,240	0.22%
18	Wisconsin	10,014	1.78%		49	Alaska	866	0.15%
50	Wyoming	781	0.14%		50	Wyoming	781	0.14%
						District of Columbia	3,073	0.55%

Source: American Medical Association (Chicago, Illinois)
"Physician Characteristics and Distribution in the U.S." (1996-97 Edition)
As of December 31, 1995. Comprised of federal and nonfederal physicians. Total does not include 8,639 male physicians in the U.S. territories and possessions, at APO's and FPO's and whose addresses are unknown.

Female Physicians in 1995

National Total = 146,669 Physicians*

ALPHA ORDER

RANK	STATE	PHYSICIANS	% of USA
27	Alabama	1,385	0.94%
46	Alaska	226	0.15%
23	Arizona	1,889	1.29%
33	Arkansas	756	0.52%
1	California	18,196	12.41%
21	Colorado	2,107	1.44%
16	Connecticut	2,677	1.83%
42	Delaware	410	0.28%
8	Florida	5,820	3.97%
14	Georgia	2,997	2.04%
36	Hawaii	702	0.48%
47	Idaho	221	0.15%
4	Illinois	7,845	5.35%
22	Indiana	2,052	1.40%
32	Iowa	898	0.61%
29	Kansas	1,108	0.76%
25	Kentucky	1,487	1.01%
24	Louisiana	1,868	1.27%
40	Maine	555	0.38%
10	Maryland	5,351	3.65%
6	Massachusetts	6,756	4.61%
11	Michigan	4,914	3.35%
17	Minnesota	2,641	1.80%
37	Mississippi	651	0.44%
18	Missouri	2,481	1.69%
45	Montana	249	0.17%
38	Nebraska	619	0.42%
44	Nevada	379	0.26%
41	New Hampshire	508	0.35%
9	New Jersey	5,816	3.97%
30	New Mexico	987	0.67%
2	New York	17,846	12.17%
13	North Carolina	3,336	2.27%
49	North Dakota	187	0.13%
7	Ohio	5,842	3.98%
31	Oklahoma	982	0.67%
26	Oregon	1,485	1.01%
3	Pennsylvania	8,130	5.54%
34	Rhode Island	740	0.50%
28	South Carolina	1,338	0.91%
48	South Dakota	197	0.13%
20	Tennessee	2,203	1.50%
5	Texas	7,764	5.29%
39	Utah	618	0.42%
43	Vermont	407	0.28%
12	Virginia	3,684	2.51%
15	Washington	2,940	2.00%
35	West Virginia	713	0.49%
19	Wisconsin	2,385	1.63%
50	Wyoming	98	0.07%

RANK ORDER

RANK	STATE	PHYSICIANS	% of USA
1	California	18,196	12.41%
2	New York	17,846	12.17%
3	Pennsylvania	8,130	5.54%
4	Illinois	7,845	5.35%
5	Texas	7,764	5.29%
6	Massachusetts	6,756	4.61%
7	Ohio	5,842	3.98%
8	Florida	5,820	3.97%
9	New Jersey	5,816	3.97%
10	Maryland	5,351	3.65%
11	Michigan	4,914	3.35%
12	Virginia	3,684	2.51%
13	North Carolina	3,336	2.27%
14	Georgia	2,997	2.04%
15	Washington	2,940	2.00%
16	Connecticut	2,677	1.83%
17	Minnesota	2,641	1.80%
18	Missouri	2,481	1.69%
19	Wisconsin	2,385	1.63%
20	Tennessee	2,203	1.50%
21	Colorado	2,107	1.44%
22	Indiana	2,052	1.40%
23	Arizona	1,889	1.29%
24	Louisiana	1,868	1.27%
25	Kentucky	1,487	1.01%
26	Oregon	1,485	1.01%
27	Alabama	1,385	0.94%
28	South Carolina	1,338	0.91%
29	Kansas	1,108	0.76%
30	New Mexico	987	0.67%
31	Oklahoma	982	0.67%
32	Iowa	898	0.61%
33	Arkansas	756	0.52%
34	Rhode Island	740	0.50%
35	West Virginia	713	0.49%
36	Hawaii	702	0.48%
37	Mississippi	651	0.44%
38	Nebraska	619	0.42%
39	Utah	618	0.42%
40	Maine	555	0.38%
41	New Hampshire	508	0.35%
42	Delaware	410	0.28%
43	Vermont	407	0.28%
44	Nevada	379	0.26%
45	Montana	249	0.17%
46	Alaska	226	0.15%
47	Idaho	221	0.15%
48	South Dakota	197	0.13%
49	North Dakota	187	0.13%
50	Wyoming	98	0.07%
	District of Columbia	1,223	0.83%

Source: American Medical Association (Chicago, Illinois)
"Physician Characteristics and Distribution in the U.S." (1996-97 Edition)
*As of December 31, 1995. Comprised of federal and nonfederal physicians. Total does not include 2,735 female physicians in the U.S. territories and possessions, at APO's and FPO's and whose addresses are unknown.

Percent of Physicians Who Are Female in 1995

National Percent = 20.69% of Physicians*

ALPHA ORDER

RANK ORDER

RANK	STATE	PERCENT	RANK	STATE	PERCENT
40	Alabama	15.75	1	Massachusetts	26.15
17	Alaska	20.70	2	Maryland	25.07
29	Arizona	18.19	3	New York	24.91
41	Arkansas	15.36	4	Illinois	24.63
18	California	20.55	5	New Mexico	24.49
16	Colorado	21.07	6	New Jersey	24.00
11	Connecticut	21.80	7	Delaware	22.73
7	Delaware	22.73	8	Rhode Island	22.41
42	Florida	14.95	9	Pennsylvania	22.10
27	Georgia	18.59	10	Michigan	21.93
20	Hawaii	19.71	11	Connecticut	21.80
49	Idaho	11.42	12	Vermont	21.67
4	Illinois	24.63	13	Ohio	21.29
33	Indiana	17.47	14	Virginia	21.14
39	Iowa	16.44	15	Minnesota	21.11
25	Kansas	18.89	16	Colorado	21.07
30	Kentucky	18.00	17	Alaska	20.70
31	Louisiana	17.60	18	California	20.55
26	Maine	18.78	19	Washington	20.12
2	Maryland	25.07	20	Hawaii	19.71
1	Massachusetts	26.15	21	Missouri	19.41
10	Michigan	21.93	22	Texas	19.29
15	Minnesota	21.11	23	Wisconsin	19.24
43	Mississippi	14.52	24	North Carolina	19.03
21	Missouri	19.41	25	Kansas	18.89
47	Montana	13.13	26	Maine	18.78
35	Nebraska	16.83	27	Georgia	18.59
46	Nevada	13.51	28	Oregon	18.56
33	New Hampshire	17.47	29	Arizona	18.19
6	New Jersey	24.00	30	Kentucky	18.00
5	New Mexico	24.49	31	Louisiana	17.60
3	New York	24.91	32	West Virginia	17.54
24	North Carolina	19.03	33	Indiana	17.47
48	North Dakota	12.68	33	New Hampshire	17.47
13	Ohio	21.29	35	Nebraska	16.83
37	Oklahoma	16.56	36	South Carolina	16.73
28	Oregon	18.56	37	Oklahoma	16.56
9	Pennsylvania	22.10	37	Tennessee	16.56
8	Rhode Island	22.41	39	Iowa	16.44
36	South Carolina	16.73	40	Alabama	15.75
45	South Dakota	13.71	41	Arkansas	15.36
37	Tennessee	16.56	42	Florida	14.95
22	Texas	19.29	43	Mississippi	14.52
44	Utah	14.31	44	Utah	14.31
12	Vermont	21.67	45	South Dakota	13.71
14	Virginia	21.14	46	Nevada	13.51
19	Washington	20.12	47	Montana	13.13
32	West Virginia	17.54	48	North Dakota	12.68
23	Wisconsin	19.24	49	Idaho	11.42
50	Wyoming	11.15	50	Wyoming	11.15

	District of Columbia	28.47

Source: Morgan Quitno Press using data from American Medical Association (Chicago, Illinois)
"Physician Characteristics and Distribution in the U.S." (1996-97 Edition)
As of December 31, 1995. Comprised of federal and nonfederal physicians. National percent does not include physicians in the U.S. territories and possessions, at APO's and FPO's and whose addresses are unknown.

Physicians Under 35 Years Old in 1995

National Total = 132,414 Physicians*

ALPHA ORDER

RANK	STATE	PHYSICIANS	% of USA
23	Alabama	1,673	1.26%
49	Alaska	119	0.09%
26	Arizona	1,577	1.19%
32	Arkansas	813	0.61%
2	California	12,923	9.76%
24	Colorado	1,647	1.24%
18	Connecticut	2,383	1.80%
42	Delaware	307	0.23%
9	Florida	4,591	3.47%
14	Georgia	2,968	2.24%
39	Hawaii	569	0.43%
47	Idaho	177	0.13%
5	Illinois	7,450	5.63%
22	Indiana	1,975	1.49%
29	Iowa	1,026	0.77%
28	Kansas	1,083	0.82%
27	Kentucky	1,515	1.14%
19	Louisiana	2,279	1.72%
41	Maine	312	0.24%
10	Maryland	4,299	3.25%
7	Massachusetts	5,818	4.39%
8	Michigan	5,125	3.87%
16	Minnesota	2,637	1.99%
33	Mississippi	753	0.57%
15	Missouri	2,896	2.19%
48	Montana	127	0.10%
35	Nebraska	723	0.55%
44	Nevada	292	0.22%
40	New Hampshire	328	0.25%
11	New Jersey	3,962	2.99%
38	New Mexico	592	0.45%
1	New York	16,250	12.27%
12	North Carolina	3,593	2.71%
45	North Dakota	232	0.18%
6	Ohio	6,124	4.62%
31	Oklahoma	945	0.71%
30	Oregon	1,008	0.76%
4	Pennsylvania	7,809	5.90%
36	Rhode Island	716	0.54%
25	South Carolina	1,596	1.21%
46	South Dakota	184	0.14%
17	Tennessee	2,607	1.97%
3	Texas	8,073	6.10%
34	Utah	748	0.56%
43	Vermont	305	0.23%
13	Virginia	3,322	2.51%
21	Washington	2,023	1.53%
37	West Virginia	712	0.54%
20	Wisconsin	2,275	1.72%
50	Wyoming	104	0.08%

RANK ORDER

RANK	STATE	PHYSICIANS	% of USA
1	New York	16,250	12.27%
2	California	12,923	9.76%
3	Texas	8,073	6.10%
4	Pennsylvania	7,809	5.90%
5	Illinois	7,450	5.63%
6	Ohio	6,124	4.62%
7	Massachusetts	5,818	4.39%
8	Michigan	5,125	3.87%
9	Florida	4,591	3.47%
10	Maryland	4,299	3.25%
11	New Jersey	3,962	2.99%
12	North Carolina	3,593	2.71%
13	Virginia	3,322	2.51%
14	Georgia	2,968	2.24%
15	Missouri	2,896	2.19%
16	Minnesota	2,637	1.99%
17	Tennessee	2,607	1.97%
18	Connecticut	2,383	1.80%
19	Louisiana	2,279	1.72%
20	Wisconsin	2,275	1.72%
21	Washington	2,023	1.53%
22	Indiana	1,975	1.49%
23	Alabama	1,673	1.26%
24	Colorado	1,647	1.24%
25	South Carolina	1,596	1.21%
26	Arizona	1,577	1.19%
27	Kentucky	1,515	1.14%
28	Kansas	1,083	0.82%
29	Iowa	1,026	0.77%
30	Oregon	1,008	0.76%
31	Oklahoma	945	0.71%
32	Arkansas	813	0.61%
33	Mississippi	753	0.57%
34	Utah	748	0.56%
35	Nebraska	723	0.55%
36	Rhode Island	716	0.54%
37	West Virginia	712	0.54%
38	New Mexico	592	0.45%
39	Hawaii	569	0.43%
40	New Hampshire	328	0.25%
41	Maine	312	0.24%
42	Delaware	307	0.23%
43	Vermont	305	0.23%
44	Nevada	292	0.22%
45	North Dakota	232	0.18%
46	South Dakota	184	0.14%
47	Idaho	177	0.13%
48	Montana	127	0.10%
49	Alaska	119	0.09%
50	Wyoming	104	0.08%
	District of Columbia	849	0.64%

Source: American Medical Association (Chicago, Illinois)
"Physician Characteristics and Distribution in the U.S." (1996-97 Edition)
*As of December 31, 1995. Comprised of federal and nonfederal physicians. Total does not include 1,669 physicians in the U.S. territories and possessions, at APO's and FPO's and whose addresses are unknown.

Percent of Physicians Under 35 Years Old in 1995

National Percent = 18.68% of Physicians*

ALPHA ORDER				RANK ORDER		
RANK	**STATE**	**PERCENT**		**RANK**	**STATE**	**PERCENT**
19	Alabama	19.03		1	Illinois	23.39
46	Alaska	10.90		2	Michigan	22.88
37	Arizona	15.19		3	New York	22.68
30	Arkansas	16.52		4	Missouri	22.66
39	California	14.59		5	Massachusetts	22.52
31	Colorado	16.47		6	Ohio	22.32
17	Connecticut	19.41		7	Rhode Island	21.68
27	Delaware	17.02		8	Louisiana	21.47
44	Florida	11.80		9	Pennsylvania	21.23
22	Georgia	18.41		10	Minnesota	21.08
34	Hawaii	15.97		11	North Carolina	20.50
49	Idaho	9.14		12	Maryland	20.14
1	Illinois	23.39		13	Texas	20.06
28	Indiana	16.82		14	South Carolina	19.95
20	Iowa	18.78		15	Nebraska	19.65
21	Kansas	18.47		16	Tennessee	19.60
24	Kentucky	18.34		17	Connecticut	19.41
8	Louisiana	21.47		18	Virginia	19.07
47	Maine	10.55		19	Alabama	19.03
12	Maryland	20.14		20	Iowa	18.78
5	Massachusetts	22.52		21	Kansas	18.47
2	Michigan	22.88		22	Georgia	18.41
10	Minnesota	21.08		23	Wisconsin	18.35
29	Mississippi	16.80		24	Kentucky	18.34
4	Missouri	22.66		25	West Virginia	17.51
50	Montana	6.70		26	Utah	17.31
15	Nebraska	19.65		27	Delaware	17.02
48	Nevada	10.41		28	Indiana	16.82
45	New Hampshire	11.28		29	Mississippi	16.80
32	New Jersey	16.35		30	Arkansas	16.52
38	New Mexico	14.69		31	Colorado	16.47
3	New York	22.68		32	New Jersey	16.35
11	North Carolina	20.50		33	Vermont	16.24
36	North Dakota	15.73		34	Hawaii	15.97
6	Ohio	22.32		35	Oklahoma	15.94
35	Oklahoma	15.94		36	North Dakota	15.73
42	Oregon	12.60		37	Arizona	15.19
9	Pennsylvania	21.23		38	New Mexico	14.69
7	Rhode Island	21.68		39	California	14.59
14	South Carolina	19.95		40	Washington	13.85
41	South Dakota	12.80		41	South Dakota	12.80
16	Tennessee	19.60		42	Oregon	12.60
13	Texas	20.06		43	Wyoming	11.83
26	Utah	17.31		44	Florida	11.80
33	Vermont	16.24		45	New Hampshire	11.28
18	Virginia	19.07		46	Alaska	10.90
40	Washington	13.85		47	Maine	10.55
25	West Virginia	17.51		48	Nevada	10.41
23	Wisconsin	18.35		49	Idaho	9.14
43	Wyoming	11.83		50	Montana	6.70
					District of Columbia	19.76

Source: Morgan Quitno Press using data from American Medical Association (Chicago, Illinois)
    "Physician Characteristics and Distribution in the U.S." (1996-97 Edition)
As of December 31, 1995. Comprised of federal and nonfederal physicians. National percent does not include physicians in the U.S. territories and possessions, at APO's and FPO's and whose addresses are unknown.

Physicians 35 to 44 Years Old in 1995

National Total = 208,287 Physicians*

ALPHA ORDER

RANK	STATE	PHYSICIANS	% of USA
25	Alabama	2,857	1.37%
49	Alaska	365	0.18%
24	Arizona	2,950	1.42%
32	Arkansas	1,629	0.78%
1	California	23,324	11.20%
22	Colorado	3,104	1.49%
21	Connecticut	3,620	1.74%
46	Delaware	501	0.24%
5	Florida	10,889	5.23%
13	Georgia	5,260	2.53%
38	Hawaii	1,087	0.52%
44	Idaho	578	0.28%
6	Illinois	8,973	4.31%
20	Indiana	3,696	1.77%
31	Iowa	1,686	0.81%
30	Kansas	1,724	0.83%
26	Kentucky	2,584	1.24%
23	Louisiana	3,085	1.48%
42	Maine	844	0.41%
10	Maryland	6,579	3.16%
7	Massachusetts	7,906	3.80%
11	Michigan	6,195	2.97%
18	Minnesota	3,963	1.90%
34	Mississippi	1,344	0.65%
19	Missouri	3,891	1.87%
43	Montana	589	0.28%
36	Nebraska	1,148	0.55%
41	Nevada	887	0.43%
40	New Hampshire	901	0.43%
9	New Jersey	7,273	3.49%
35	New Mexico	1,214	0.58%
2	New York	20,125	9.66%
12	North Carolina	5,767	2.77%
48	North Dakota	464	0.22%
8	Ohio	7,784	3.74%
29	Oklahoma	1,738	0.83%
28	Oregon	2,246	1.08%
4	Pennsylvania	11,224	5.39%
39	Rhode Island	957	0.46%
27	South Carolina	2,401	1.15%
47	South Dakota	482	0.23%
16	Tennessee	4,345	2.09%
3	Texas	12,032	5.78%
33	Utah	1,376	0.66%
45	Vermont	554	0.27%
14	Virginia	5,229	2.51%
15	Washington	4,471	2.15%
37	West Virginia	1,108	0.53%
17	Wisconsin	3,992	1.92%
50	Wyoming	257	0.12%

RANK ORDER

RANK	STATE	PHYSICIANS	% of USA
1	California	23,324	11.20%
2	New York	20,125	9.66%
3	Texas	12,032	5.78%
4	Pennsylvania	11,224	5.39%
5	Florida	10,889	5.23%
6	Illinois	8,973	4.31%
7	Massachusetts	7,906	3.80%
8	Ohio	7,784	3.74%
9	New Jersey	7,273	3.49%
10	Maryland	6,579	3.16%
11	Michigan	6,195	2.97%
12	North Carolina	5,767	2.77%
13	Georgia	5,260	2.53%
14	Virginia	5,229	2.51%
15	Washington	4,471	2.15%
16	Tennessee	4,345	2.09%
17	Wisconsin	3,992	1.92%
18	Minnesota	3,963	1.90%
19	Missouri	3,891	1.87%
20	Indiana	3,696	1.77%
21	Connecticut	3,620	1.74%
22	Colorado	3,104	1.49%
23	Louisiana	3,085	1.48%
24	Arizona	2,950	1.42%
25	Alabama	2,857	1.37%
26	Kentucky	2,584	1.24%
27	South Carolina	2,401	1.15%
28	Oregon	2,246	1.08%
29	Oklahoma	1,738	0.83%
30	Kansas	1,724	0.83%
31	Iowa	1,686	0.81%
32	Arkansas	1,629	0.78%
33	Utah	1,376	0.66%
34	Mississippi	1,344	0.65%
35	New Mexico	1,214	0.58%
36	Nebraska	1,148	0.55%
37	West Virginia	1,108	0.53%
38	Hawaii	1,087	0.52%
39	Rhode Island	957	0.46%
40	New Hampshire	901	0.43%
41	Nevada	007	0.43%
42	Maine	844	0.41%
43	Montana	589	0.28%
44	Idaho	578	0.28%
45	Vermont	554	0.27%
46	Delaware	501	0.24%
47	South Dakota	482	0.23%
48	North Dakota	464	0.22%
49	Alaska	365	0.18%
50	Wyoming	257	0.12%
	District of Columbia	1,089	0.52%

Source: American Medical Association (Chicago, Illinois)
"Physician Characteristics and Distribution in the U.S." (1996-97 Edition)
*As of December 31, 1995. Comprised of federal and nonfederal physicians. Total does not include 3,440 physicians in the U.S. territories and possessions, at APO's and FPO's and whose addresses are unknown.

Physicians 45 to 54 Years Old in 1995

National Total = 156,662 Physicians*

<table>
<tr><td colspan="4">ALPHA ORDER</td><td colspan="4">RANK ORDER</td></tr>
<tr><td>RANK</td><td>STATE</td><td>PHYSICIANS</td><td>% of USA</td><td>RANK</td><td>STATE</td><td>PHYSICIANS</td><td>% of USA</td></tr>
<tr><td>26</td><td>Alabama</td><td>1,901</td><td>1.21%</td><td>1</td><td>California</td><td>21,885</td><td>13.97%</td></tr>
<tr><td>49</td><td>Alaska</td><td>332</td><td>0.21%</td><td>2</td><td>New York</td><td>14,350</td><td>9.16%</td></tr>
<tr><td>24</td><td>Arizona</td><td>2,232</td><td>1.42%</td><td>3</td><td>Texas</td><td>9,025</td><td>5.76%</td></tr>
<tr><td>32</td><td>Arkansas</td><td>1,068</td><td>0.68%</td><td>4</td><td>Florida</td><td>8,261</td><td>5.27%</td></tr>
<tr><td>1</td><td>California</td><td>21,885</td><td>13.97%</td><td>5</td><td>Pennsylvania</td><td>7,441</td><td>4.75%</td></tr>
<tr><td>22</td><td>Colorado</td><td>2,419</td><td>1.54%</td><td>6</td><td>Illinois</td><td>6,924</td><td>4.42%</td></tr>
<tr><td>21</td><td>Connecticut</td><td>2,569</td><td>1.64%</td><td>7</td><td>New Jersey</td><td>5,692</td><td>3.63%</td></tr>
<tr><td>46</td><td>Delaware</td><td>394</td><td>0.25%</td><td>8</td><td>Ohio</td><td>5,599</td><td>3.57%</td></tr>
<tr><td>4</td><td>Florida</td><td>8,261</td><td>5.27%</td><td>9</td><td>Massachusetts</td><td>5,410</td><td>3.45%</td></tr>
<tr><td>14</td><td>Georgia</td><td>3,563</td><td>2.27%</td><td>10</td><td>Michigan</td><td>4,786</td><td>3.05%</td></tr>
<tr><td>37</td><td>Hawaii</td><td>809</td><td>0.52%</td><td>11</td><td>Maryland</td><td>4,782</td><td>3.05%</td></tr>
<tr><td>43</td><td>Idaho</td><td>499</td><td>0.32%</td><td>12</td><td>Virginia</td><td>3,897</td><td>2.49%</td></tr>
<tr><td>6</td><td>Illinois</td><td>6,924</td><td>4.42%</td><td>13</td><td>Washington</td><td>3,707</td><td>2.37%</td></tr>
<tr><td>19</td><td>Indiana</td><td>2,612</td><td>1.67%</td><td>14</td><td>Georgia</td><td>3,563</td><td>2.27%</td></tr>
<tr><td>31</td><td>Iowa</td><td>1,166</td><td>0.74%</td><td>15</td><td>North Carolina</td><td>3,509</td><td>2.24%</td></tr>
<tr><td>30</td><td>Kansas</td><td>1,269</td><td>0.81%</td><td>16</td><td>Tennessee</td><td>2,871</td><td>1.83%</td></tr>
<tr><td>27</td><td>Kentucky</td><td>1,832</td><td>1.17%</td><td>17</td><td>Minnesota</td><td>2,659</td><td>1.70%</td></tr>
<tr><td>23</td><td>Louisiana</td><td>2,312</td><td>1.48%</td><td>18</td><td>Missouri</td><td>2,639</td><td>1.68%</td></tr>
<tr><td>39</td><td>Maine</td><td>739</td><td>0.47%</td><td>19</td><td>Indiana</td><td>2,612</td><td>1.67%</td></tr>
<tr><td>11</td><td>Maryland</td><td>4,782</td><td>3.05%</td><td>20</td><td>Wisconsin</td><td>2,611</td><td>1.67%</td></tr>
<tr><td>9</td><td>Massachusetts</td><td>5,410</td><td>3.45%</td><td>21</td><td>Connecticut</td><td>2,569</td><td>1.64%</td></tr>
<tr><td>10</td><td>Michigan</td><td>4,786</td><td>3.05%</td><td>22</td><td>Colorado</td><td>2,419</td><td>1.54%</td></tr>
<tr><td>17</td><td>Minnesota</td><td>2,659</td><td>1.70%</td><td>23</td><td>Louisiana</td><td>2,312</td><td>1.48%</td></tr>
<tr><td>36</td><td>Mississippi</td><td>946</td><td>0.60%</td><td>24</td><td>Arizona</td><td>2,232</td><td>1.42%</td></tr>
<tr><td>18</td><td>Missouri</td><td>2,639</td><td>1.68%</td><td>25</td><td>Oregon</td><td>2,118</td><td>1.35%</td></tr>
<tr><td>44</td><td>Montana</td><td>498</td><td>0.32%</td><td>26</td><td>Alabama</td><td>1,901</td><td>1.21%</td></tr>
<tr><td>38</td><td>Nebraska</td><td>787</td><td>0.50%</td><td>27</td><td>Kentucky</td><td>1,832</td><td>1.17%</td></tr>
<tr><td>41</td><td>Nevada</td><td>699</td><td>0.45%</td><td>28</td><td>South Carolina</td><td>1,723</td><td>1.10%</td></tr>
<tr><td>40</td><td>New Hampshire</td><td>707</td><td>0.45%</td><td>29</td><td>Oklahoma</td><td>1,371</td><td>0.88%</td></tr>
<tr><td>7</td><td>New Jersey</td><td>5,692</td><td>3.63%</td><td>30</td><td>Kansas</td><td>1,269</td><td>0.81%</td></tr>
<tr><td>33</td><td>New Mexico</td><td>1,040</td><td>0.66%</td><td>31</td><td>Iowa</td><td>1,166</td><td>0.74%</td></tr>
<tr><td>2</td><td>New York</td><td>14,350</td><td>9.16%</td><td>32</td><td>Arkansas</td><td>1,068</td><td>0.68%</td></tr>
<tr><td>15</td><td>North Carolina</td><td>3,509</td><td>2.24%</td><td>33</td><td>New Mexico</td><td>1,040</td><td>0.66%</td></tr>
<tr><td>47</td><td>North Dakota</td><td>360</td><td>0.23%</td><td>34</td><td>Utah</td><td>1,036</td><td>0.66%</td></tr>
<tr><td>8</td><td>Ohio</td><td>5,599</td><td>3.57%</td><td>35</td><td>West Virginia</td><td>1,007</td><td>0.64%</td></tr>
<tr><td>29</td><td>Oklahoma</td><td>1,371</td><td>0.88%</td><td>36</td><td>Mississippi</td><td>946</td><td>0.60%</td></tr>
<tr><td>25</td><td>Oregon</td><td>2,118</td><td>1.35%</td><td>37</td><td>Hawaii</td><td>809</td><td>0.52%</td></tr>
<tr><td>5</td><td>Pennsylvania</td><td>7,441</td><td>4.75%</td><td>38</td><td>Nebraska</td><td>787</td><td>0.50%</td></tr>
<tr><td>42</td><td>Rhode Island</td><td>627</td><td>0.40%</td><td>39</td><td>Maine</td><td>739</td><td>0.47%</td></tr>
<tr><td>28</td><td>South Carolina</td><td>1,723</td><td>1.10%</td><td>40</td><td>New Hampshire</td><td>707</td><td>0.45%</td></tr>
<tr><td>48</td><td>South Dakota</td><td>355</td><td>0.23%</td><td>41</td><td>Nevada</td><td>699</td><td>0.45%</td></tr>
<tr><td>16</td><td>Tennessee</td><td>2,871</td><td>1.83%</td><td>42</td><td>Rhode Island</td><td>627</td><td>0.40%</td></tr>
<tr><td>3</td><td>Texas</td><td>9,025</td><td>5.76%</td><td>43</td><td>Idaho</td><td>499</td><td>0.32%</td></tr>
<tr><td>34</td><td>Utah</td><td>1,036</td><td>0.66%</td><td>44</td><td>Montana</td><td>498</td><td>0.32%</td></tr>
<tr><td>45</td><td>Vermont</td><td>428</td><td>0.27%</td><td>45</td><td>Vermont</td><td>428</td><td>0.27%</td></tr>
<tr><td>12</td><td>Virginia</td><td>3,897</td><td>2.49%</td><td>46</td><td>Delaware</td><td>394</td><td>0.25%</td></tr>
<tr><td>13</td><td>Washington</td><td>3,707</td><td>2.37%</td><td>47</td><td>North Dakota</td><td>360</td><td>0.23%</td></tr>
<tr><td>35</td><td>West Virginia</td><td>1,007</td><td>0.64%</td><td>48</td><td>South Dakota</td><td>355</td><td>0.23%</td></tr>
<tr><td>20</td><td>Wisconsin</td><td>2,611</td><td>1.67%</td><td>49</td><td>Alaska</td><td>332</td><td>0.21%</td></tr>
<tr><td>50</td><td>Wyoming</td><td>219</td><td>0.14%</td><td>50</td><td>Wyoming</td><td>219</td><td>0.14%</td></tr>
<tr><td></td><td></td><td></td><td></td><td></td><td>District of Columbia</td><td>977</td><td>0.62%</td></tr>
</table>

Source: American Medical Association (Chicago, Illinois)
   "Physician Characteristics and Distribution in the U.S." (1996-97 Edition)
*As of December 31, 1995. Comprised of federal and nonfederal physicians. Total does not include 2,224 physicians in the U.S. territories and possessions, at APO's and FPO's and whose addresses are unknown.

Physicians 55 to 64 Years Old in 1995

National Total = 94,833 Physicians*

RANK	STATE	PHYSICIANS	% of USA
27	Alabama	1,079	1.14%
49	Alaska	182	0.19%
22	Arizona	1,459	1.54%
32	Arkansas	667	0.70%
1	California	13,183	13.90%
24	Colorado	1,311	1.38%
17	Connecticut	1,610	1.70%
45	Delaware	279	0.29%
3	Florida	5,554	5.86%
13	Georgia	2,168	2.29%
37	Hawaii	473	0.50%
44	Idaho	297	0.31%
6	Illinois	4,069	4.29%
20	Indiana	1,516	1.60%
33	Iowa	637	0.67%
30	Kansas	768	0.81%
26	Kentucky	1,144	1.21%
23	Louisiana	1,389	1.46%
41	Maine	410	0.43%
11	Maryland	2,769	2.92%
9	Massachusetts	3,060	3.23%
10	Michigan	2,974	3.14%
21	Minnesota	1,502	1.58%
31	Mississippi	684	0.72%
16	Missouri	1,622	1.71%
43	Montana	300	0.32%
38	Nebraska	455	0.48%
39	Nevada	450	0.47%
42	New Hampshire	401	0.42%
7	New Jersey	3,564	3.76%
35	New Mexico	512	0.54%
2	New York	9,566	10.09%
14	North Carolina	2,022	2.13%
46	North Dakota	218	0.23%
8	Ohio	3,545	3.74%
29	Oklahoma	931	0.98%
25	Oregon	1,176	1.24%
5	Pennsylvania	4,480	4.72%
40	Rhode Island	424	0.45%
28	South Carolina	986	1.04%
48	South Dakota	183	0.19%
19	Tennessee	1,591	1.68%
4	Texas	5,264	5.55%
36	Utah	487	0.51%
47	Vermont	213	0.22%
12	Virginia	2,293	2.42%
15	Washington	1,880	1.98%
34	West Virginia	626	0.66%
18	Wisconsin	1,593	1.68%
50	Wyoming	133	0.14%

RANK	STATE	PHYSICIANS	% of USA
1	California	13,183	13.90%
2	New York	9,566	10.09%
3	Florida	5,554	5.86%
4	Texas	5,264	5.55%
5	Pennsylvania	4,480	4.72%
6	Illinois	4,069	4.29%
7	New Jersey	3,564	3.76%
8	Ohio	3,545	3.74%
9	Massachusetts	3,060	3.23%
10	Michigan	2,974	3.14%
11	Maryland	2,769	2.92%
12	Virginia	2,293	2.42%
13	Georgia	2,168	2.29%
14	North Carolina	2,022	2.13%
15	Washington	1,880	1.98%
16	Missouri	1,622	1.71%
17	Connecticut	1,610	1.70%
18	Wisconsin	1,593	1.68%
19	Tennessee	1,591	1.68%
20	Indiana	1,516	1.60%
21	Minnesota	1,502	1.58%
22	Arizona	1,459	1.54%
23	Louisiana	1,389	1.46%
24	Colorado	1,311	1.38%
25	Oregon	1,176	1.24%
26	Kentucky	1,144	1.21%
27	Alabama	1,079	1.14%
28	South Carolina	986	1.04%
29	Oklahoma	931	0.98%
30	Kansas	768	0.81%
31	Mississippi	684	0.72%
32	Arkansas	667	0.70%
33	Iowa	637	0.67%
34	West Virginia	626	0.66%
35	New Mexico	512	0.54%
36	Utah	487	0.51%
37	Hawaii	473	0.50%
38	Nebraska	455	0.48%
39	Nevada	450	0.47%
40	Rhode Island	424	0.45%
41	Maine	410	0.43%
42	New Hampshire	401	0.42%
43	Montana	300	0.32%
44	Idaho	297	0.31%
45	Delaware	279	0.29%
46	North Dakota	218	0.23%
47	Vermont	213	0.22%
48	South Dakota	183	0.19%
49	Alaska	182	0.19%
50	Wyoming	133	0.14%
	District of Columbia	734	0.77%

Source: American Medical Association (Chicago, Illinois)
   "Physician Characteristics and Distribution in the U.S." (1996-97 Edition)
*As of December 31, 1995. Comprised of federal and nonfederal physicians. Total does not include 1,578 physicians in the U.S. territories and possessions, at APO's and FPO's and whose addresses are unknown.

Physicians 65 Years Old and Older in 1995

National Total = 116,755 Physicians*

ALPHA ORDER

RANK	STATE	PHYSICIANS	% of USA
27	Alabama	1,283	1.10%
50	Alaska	94	0.08%
15	Arizona	2,165	1.85%
33	Arkansas	744	0.64%
1	California	17,238	14.76%
24	Colorado	1,518	1.30%
17	Connecticut	2,096	1.80%
46	Delaware	323	0.28%
3	Florida	9,623	8.24%
16	Georgia	2,161	1.85%
37	Hawaii	624	0.53%
43	Idaho	385	0.33%
6	Illinois	4,429	3.79%
18	Indiana	1,944	1.67%
30	Iowa	948	0.81%
29	Kansas	1,021	0.87%
28	Kentucky	1,184	1.01%
23	Louisiana	1,551	1.33%
36	Maine	651	0.56%
11	Maryland	2,916	2.50%
9	Massachusetts	3,637	3.12%
10	Michigan	3,324	2.85%
21	Minnesota	1,751	1.50%
32	Mississippi	755	0.65%
22	Missouri	1,733	1.48%
44	Montana	382	0.33%
41	Nebraska	566	0.48%
42	Nevada	478	0.41%
40	New Hampshire	571	0.49%
8	New Jersey	3,745	3.21%
35	New Mexico	672	0.58%
2	New York	11,346	9.72%
13	North Carolina	2,636	2.26%
48	North Dakota	201	0.17%
7	Ohio	4,383	3.75%
31	Oklahoma	944	0.81%
25	Oregon	1,452	1.24%
5	Pennsylvania	5,826	4.99%
39	Rhode Island	578	0.50%
26	South Carolina	1,293	1.11%
47	South Dakota	233	0.20%
20	Tennessee	1,887	1.62%
4	Texas	5,849	5.01%
34	Utah	673	0.58%
45	Vermont	378	0.32%
12	Virginia	2,682	2.30%
14	Washington	2,528	2.17%
38	West Virginia	613	0.53%
19	Wisconsin	1,928	1.65%
49	Wyoming	166	0.14%

RANK ORDER

RANK	STATE	PHYSICIANS	% of USA
1	California	17,238	14.76%
2	New York	11,346	9.72%
3	Florida	9,623	8.24%
4	Texas	5,849	5.01%
5	Pennsylvania	5,826	4.99%
6	Illinois	4,429	3.79%
7	Ohio	4,383	3.75%
8	New Jersey	3,745	3.21%
9	Massachusetts	3,637	3.12%
10	Michigan	3,324	2.85%
11	Maryland	2,916	2.50%
12	Virginia	2,682	2.30%
13	North Carolina	2,636	2.26%
14	Washington	2,528	2.17%
15	Arizona	2,165	1.85%
16	Georgia	2,161	1.85%
17	Connecticut	2,096	1.80%
18	Indiana	1,944	1.67%
19	Wisconsin	1,928	1.65%
20	Tennessee	1,887	1.62%
21	Minnesota	1,751	1.50%
22	Missouri	1,733	1.48%
23	Louisiana	1,551	1.33%
24	Colorado	1,518	1.30%
25	Oregon	1,452	1.24%
26	South Carolina	1,293	1.11%
27	Alabama	1,283	1.10%
28	Kentucky	1,184	1.01%
29	Kansas	1,021	0.87%
30	Iowa	948	0.81%
31	Oklahoma	944	0.81%
32	Mississippi	755	0.65%
33	Arkansas	744	0.64%
34	Utah	673	0.58%
35	New Mexico	672	0.58%
36	Maine	651	0.56%
37	Hawaii	624	0.53%
38	West Virginia	613	0.53%
39	Rhode Island	578	0.50%
40	New Hampshire	571	0.49%
41	Nebraska	566	0.48%
42	Nevada	478	0.41%
43	Idaho	385	0.33%
44	Montana	382	0.33%
45	Vermont	378	0.32%
46	Delaware	323	0.28%
47	South Dakota	233	0.20%
48	North Dakota	201	0.17%
49	Wyoming	166	0.14%
50	Alaska	94	0.08%
	District of Columbia	647	0.55%

Source: American Medical Association (Chicago, Illinois)
   "Physician Characteristics and Distribution in the U.S." (1996-97 Edition)
*As of December 31, 1995. Comprised of federal and nonfederal physicians. Total does not include 2,463 physicians in the U.S. territories and possessions, at APO's and FPO's and whose addresses are unknown.

Percent of Physicians 65 Years Old and Older in 1995

National Percent = 16.47% of Physicians*

ALPHA ORDER

RANK	STATE	PERCENT
39	Alabama	14.59
50	Alaska	8.61
3	Arizona	20.85
34	Arkansas	15.12
8	California	19.47
33	Colorado	15.18
17	Connecticut	17.07
11	Delaware	17.90
1	Florida	24.73
49	Georgia	13.41
12	Hawaii	17.52
6	Idaho	19.89
45	Illinois	13.91
21	Indiana	16.55
15	Iowa	17.35
14	Kansas	17.41
41	Kentucky	14.34
38	Louisiana	14.61
2	Maine	22.02
46	Maryland	13.66
43	Massachusetts	14.08
37	Michigan	14.84
44	Minnesota	13.99
19	Mississippi	16.85
48	Missouri	13.56
4	Montana	20.15
32	Nebraska	15.38
18	Nevada	17.03
7	New Hampshire	19.64
30	New Jersey	15.45
20	New Mexico	16.67
26	New York	15.84
36	North Carolina	15.04
47	North Dakota	13.63
24	Ohio	15.98
25	Oklahoma	15.92
10	Oregon	18.15
26	Pennsylvania	15.84
13	Rhode Island	17.50
23	South Carolina	16.16
22	South Dakota	16.21
42	Tennessee	14.19
40	Texas	14.53
28	Utah	15.58
5	Vermont	20.13
31	Virginia	15.39
16	Washington	17.30
35	West Virginia	15.08
29	Wisconsin	15.55
9	Wyoming	18.89

RANK ORDER

RANK	STATE	PERCENT
1	Florida	24.73
2	Maine	22.02
3	Arizona	20.85
4	Montana	20.15
5	Vermont	20.13
6	Idaho	19.89
7	New Hampshire	19.64
8	California	19.47
9	Wyoming	18.89
10	Oregon	18.15
11	Delaware	17.90
12	Hawaii	17.52
13	Rhode Island	17.50
14	Kansas	17.41
15	Iowa	17.35
16	Washington	17.30
17	Connecticut	17.07
18	Nevada	17.03
19	Mississippi	16.85
20	New Mexico	16.67
21	Indiana	16.55
22	South Dakota	16.21
23	South Carolina	16.16
24	Ohio	15.98
25	Oklahoma	15.92
26	New York	15.84
26	Pennsylvania	15.84
28	Utah	15.58
29	Wisconsin	15.55
30	New Jersey	15.45
31	Virginia	15.39
32	Nebraska	15.38
33	Colorado	15.18
34	Arkansas	15.12
35	West Virginia	15.08
36	North Carolina	15.04
37	Michigan	14.84
38	Louisiana	14.61
39	Alabama	14.59
40	Texas	14.53
41	Kentucky	14.34
42	Tennessee	14.19
43	Massachusetts	14.08
44	Minnesota	13.99
45	Illinois	13.91
46	Maryland	13.66
47	North Dakota	13.63
48	Missouri	13.56
49	Georgia	13.41
50	Alaska	8.61
	District of Columbia	15.06

Source: Morgan Quitno Press using data from American Medical Association (Chicago, Illinois)
"Physician Characteristics and Distribution in the U.S." (1996-97 Edition)
*As of December 31, 1995. Comprised of federal and nonfederal physicians. National percent does not include physicians in the U.S. territories and possessions, at APO's and FPO's and whose addresses are unknown.

Federal Physicians in 1995

National Total = 19,830 Physicians*

RANK	STATE	PHYSICIANS	% of USA
23	Alabama	230	1.16%
34	Alaska	137	0.69%
14	Arizona	364	1.84%
32	Arkansas	153	0.77%
1	California	2,236	11.28%
12	Colorado	473	2.39%
33	Connecticut	144	0.73%
47	Delaware	51	0.26%
5	Florida	954	4.81%
7	Georgia	852	4.30%
17	Hawaii	347	1.75%
44	Idaho	58	0.29%
10	Illinois	541	2.73%
35	Indiana	135	0.68%
39	Iowa	95	0.48%
27	Kansas	200	1.01%
29	Kentucky	168	0.85%
24	Louisiana	220	1.11%
46	Maine	53	0.27%
2	Maryland	2,130	10.74%
14	Massachusetts	364	1.84%
22	Michigan	255	1.29%
25	Minnesota	214	1.08%
18	Mississippi	325	1.64%
21	Missouri	256	1.29%
48	Montana	47	0.24%
40	Nebraska	90	0.45%
38	Nevada	104	0.52%
43	New Hampshire	59	0.30%
20	New Jersey	266	1.34%
26	New Mexico	211	1.06%
6	New York	886	4.47%
9	North Carolina	561	2.83%
45	North Dakota	56	0.28%
13	Ohio	461	2.32%
28	Oklahoma	184	0.93%
30	Oregon	166	0.84%
11	Pennsylvania	514	2.59%
42	Rhode Island	71	0.36%
19	South Carolina	291	1.47%
41	South Dakota	79	0.40%
16	Tennessee	352	1.78%
3	Texas	1,891	9.54%
37	Utah	111	0.56%
50	Vermont	32	0.16%
4	Virginia	1,061	5.35%
8	Washington	678	3.42%
36	West Virginia	118	0.60%
31	Wisconsin	158	0.80%
49	Wyoming	43	0.22%

RANK	STATE	PHYSICIANS	% of USA
1	California	2,236	11.28%
2	Maryland	2,130	10.74%
3	Texas	1,891	9.54%
4	Virginia	1,061	5.35%
5	Florida	954	4.81%
6	New York	886	4.47%
7	Georgia	852	4.30%
8	Washington	678	3.42%
9	North Carolina	561	2.83%
10	Illinois	541	2.73%
11	Pennsylvania	514	2.59%
12	Colorado	473	2.39%
13	Ohio	461	2.32%
14	Arizona	364	1.84%
14	Massachusetts	364	1.84%
16	Tennessee	352	1.78%
17	Hawaii	347	1.75%
18	Mississippi	325	1.64%
19	South Carolina	291	1.47%
20	New Jersey	266	1.34%
21	Missouri	256	1.29%
22	Michigan	255	1.29%
23	Alabama	230	1.16%
24	Louisiana	220	1.11%
25	Minnesota	214	1.08%
26	New Mexico	211	1.06%
27	Kansas	200	1.01%
28	Oklahoma	184	0.93%
29	Kentucky	168	0.85%
30	Oregon	166	0.84%
31	Wisconsin	158	0.80%
32	Arkansas	153	0.77%
33	Connecticut	144	0.73%
34	Alaska	137	0.69%
35	Indiana	135	0.68%
36	West Virginia	118	0.60%
37	Utah	111	0.56%
38	Nevada	104	0.52%
39	Iowa	95	0.48%
40	Nebraska	90	0.45%
41	South Dakota	79	0.40%
42	Rhode Island	71	0.36%
43	New Hampshire	59	0.30%
44	Idaho	58	0.29%
45	North Dakota	56	0.28%
46	Maine	53	0.27%
47	Delaware	51	0.26%
48	Montana	47	0.24%
49	Wyoming	43	0.22%
50	Vermont	32	0.16%
	District of Columbia	385	1.94%

Source: American Medical Association (Chicago, Illinois)
   "Physician Characteristics and Distribution in the U.S." (1996-97 Edition)
As of December 31, 1995. Total does not include 1,249 physicians in U.S. territories and possessions and whose addresses are unknown.

Rate of Federal Physicians in 1995

National Rate = 7.5 Physicians per 100,000 Population*

ALPHA ORDER

RANK	STATE	RATE
31	Alabama	5.4
3	Alaska	22.7
14	Arizona	8.5
25	Arkansas	6.2
19	California	7.1
5	Colorado	12.6
41	Connecticut	4.4
19	Delaware	7.1
22	Florida	6.7
9	Georgia	11.8
2	Hawaii	29.4
36	Idaho	5.0
39	Illinois	4.6
50	Indiana	2.3
46	Iowa	3.3
16	Kansas	7.8
41	Kentucky	4.4
34	Louisiana	5.1
43	Maine	4.3
1	Maryland	42.3
26	Massachusetts	6.0
49	Michigan	2.7
39	Minnesota	4.6
8	Mississippi	12.1
38	Missouri	4.8
31	Montana	5.4
29	Nebraska	5.5
21	Nevada	6.8
34	New Hampshire	5.1
46	New Jersey	3.3
6	New Mexico	12.5
37	New York	4.9
16	North Carolina	7.8
13	North Dakota	8.7
45	Ohio	4.1
28	Oklahoma	5.6
33	Oregon	5.3
43	Pennsylvania	4.3
18	Rhode Island	7.2
15	South Carolina	7.9
10	South Dakota	10.8
22	Tennessee	6.7
11	Texas	10.1
27	Utah	5.7
29	Vermont	5.5
4	Virginia	16.0
7	Washington	12.4
24	West Virginia	6.5
48	Wisconsin	3.1
12	Wyoming	9.0

RANK ORDER

RANK	STATE	RATE
1	Maryland	42.3
2	Hawaii	29.4
3	Alaska	22.7
4	Virginia	16.0
5	Colorado	12.6
6	New Mexico	12.5
7	Washington	12.4
8	Mississippi	12.1
9	Georgia	11.8
10	South Dakota	10.8
11	Texas	10.1
12	Wyoming	9.0
13	North Dakota	8.7
14	Arizona	8.5
15	South Carolina	7.9
16	Kansas	7.8
16	North Carolina	7.8
18	Rhode Island	7.2
19	California	7.1
19	Delaware	7.1
21	Nevada	6.8
22	Florida	6.7
22	Tennessee	6.7
24	West Virginia	6.5
25	Arkansas	6.2
26	Massachusetts	6.0
27	Utah	5.7
28	Oklahoma	5.6
29	Nebraska	5.5
29	Vermont	5.5
31	Alabama	5.4
31	Montana	5.4
33	Oregon	5.3
34	Louisiana	5.1
34	New Hampshire	5.1
36	Idaho	5.0
37	New York	4.9
38	Missouri	4.8
39	Illinois	4.6
39	Minnesota	4.6
41	Connecticut	4.4
41	Kentucky	4.4
43	Maine	4.3
43	Pennsylvania	4.3
45	Ohio	4.1
46	Iowa	3.3
46	New Jersey	3.3
48	Wisconsin	3.1
49	Michigan	2.7
50	Indiana	2.3

	District of Columbia	69.4

Source: Morgan Quitno Press using data from American Medical Association (Chicago, Illinois)
"Physician Characteristics and Distribution in the U.S." (1996-97 Edition)
*As of December 31, 1995. National rate does not include physicians in U.S. territories and possessions and whose addresses are unknown.

Nonfederal Physicians in 1995

National Total = 689,121 Physicians*

ALPHA ORDER

RANK	STATE	PHYSICIANS	% of USA
25	Alabama	8,563	1.24%
49	Alaska	955	0.14%
23	Arizona	10,019	1.45%
32	Arkansas	4,768	0.69%
1	California	86,317	12.53%
24	Colorado	9,526	1.38%
20	Connecticut	12,134	1.76%
46	Delaware	1,753	0.25%
4	Florida	37,964	5.51%
14	Georgia	15,268	2.22%
39	Hawaii	3,215	0.47%
43	Idaho	1,878	0.27%
6	Illinois	31,304	4.54%
21	Indiana	11,608	1.68%
31	Iowa	5,368	0.78%
30	Kansas	5,665	0.82%
26	Kentucky	8,091	1.17%
22	Louisiana	10,396	1.51%
40	Maine	2,903	0.42%
11	Maryland	19,215	2.79%
8	Massachusetts	25,467	3.70%
10	Michigan	22,149	3.21%
18	Minnesota	12,298	1.78%
34	Mississippi	4,157	0.60%
17	Missouri	12,525	1.82%
44	Montana	1,849	0.27%
37	Nebraska	3,589	0.52%
42	Nevada	2,702	0.39%
41	New Hampshire	2,849	0.41%
9	New Jersey	23,970	3.48%
36	New Mexico	3,819	0.55%
2	New York	70,751	10.27%
12	North Carolina	16,966	2.46%
47	North Dakota	1,419	0.21%
7	Ohio	26,974	3.91%
29	Oklahoma	5,745	0.83%
27	Oregon	7,834	1.14%
5	Pennsylvania	36,266	5.26%
38	Rhode Island	3,231	0.47%
28	South Carolina	7,708	1.12%
48	South Dakota	1,358	0.20%
16	Tennessee	12,949	1.88%
3	Texas	38,352	5.57%
33	Utah	4,209	0.61%
45	Vermont	1,846	0.27%
13	Virginia	16,362	2.37%
15	Washington	13,931	2.02%
35	West Virginia	3,948	0.57%
19	Wisconsin	12,241	1.78%
50	Wyoming	836	0.12%

RANK ORDER

RANK	STATE	PHYSICIANS	% of USA
1	California	86,317	12.53%
2	New York	70,751	10.27%
3	Texas	38,352	5.57%
4	Florida	37,964	5.51%
5	Pennsylvania	36,266	5.26%
6	Illinois	31,304	4.54%
7	Ohio	26,974	3.91%
8	Massachusetts	25,467	3.70%
9	New Jersey	23,970	3.48%
10	Michigan	22,149	3.21%
11	Maryland	19,215	2.79%
12	North Carolina	16,966	2.46%
13	Virginia	16,362	2.37%
14	Georgia	15,268	2.22%
15	Washington	13,931	2.02%
16	Tennessee	12,949	1.88%
17	Missouri	12,525	1.82%
18	Minnesota	12,298	1.78%
19	Wisconsin	12,241	1.78%
20	Connecticut	12,134	1.76%
21	Indiana	11,608	1.68%
22	Louisiana	10,396	1.51%
23	Arizona	10,019	1.45%
24	Colorado	9,526	1.38%
25	Alabama	8,563	1.24%
26	Kentucky	8,091	1.17%
27	Oregon	7,834	1.14%
28	South Carolina	7,708	1.12%
29	Oklahoma	5,745	0.83%
30	Kansas	5,665	0.82%
31	Iowa	5,368	0.78%
32	Arkansas	4,768	0.69%
33	Utah	4,209	0.61%
34	Mississippi	4,157	0.60%
35	West Virginia	3,948	0.57%
36	New Mexico	3,819	0.55%
37	Nebraska	3,589	0.52%
38	Rhode Island	3,231	0.47%
39	Hawaii	3,215	0.47%
40	Maine	2,903	0.42%
41	New Hampshire	2,849	0.41%
42	Nevada	2,702	0.39%
43	Idaho	1,878	0.27%
44	Montana	1,849	0.27%
45	Vermont	1,846	0.27%
46	Delaware	1,753	0.25%
47	North Dakota	1,419	0.21%
48	South Dakota	1,358	0.20%
49	Alaska	955	0.14%
50	Wyoming	836	0.12%
	District of Columbia	3,911	0.57%

Source: American Medical Association (Chicago, Illinois)
   "Physician Characteristics and Distribution in the U.S." (1996-97 Edition)
As of December 31, 1995. National total does not include 8,148 physicians in U.S. territories and possessions.

Rate of Nonfederal Physicians in 1995

National Rate = 264 Physicians per 100,000 Population*

ALPHA ORDER

RANK	STATE	RATE
40	Alabama	202
48	Alaska	164
23	Arizona	239
42	Arkansas	192
10	California	275
15	Colorado	257
4	Connecticut	372
20	Delaware	246
11	Florida	269
35	Georgia	214
9	Hawaii	283
49	Idaho	162
13	Illinois	265
41	Indiana	200
43	Iowa	189
31	Kansas	223
38	Kentucky	211
22	Louisiana	241
27	Maine	235
3	Maryland	384
1	Massachusetts	420
28	Michigan	232
12	Minnesota	267
50	Mississippi	155
26	Missouri	236
35	Montana	214
32	Nebraska	220
45	Nevada	178
18	New Hampshire	248
7	New Jersey	302
29	New Mexico	229
2	New York	391
23	North Carolina	239
30	North Dakota	224
21	Ohio	242
46	Oklahoma	177
17	Oregon	250
8	Pennsylvania	301
5	Rhode Island	328
37	South Carolina	212
44	South Dakota	187
19	Tennessee	247
39	Texas	206
33	Utah	216
6	Vermont	316
16	Virginia	253
14	Washington	259
33	West Virginia	216
23	Wisconsin	239
47	Wyoming	176

RANK ORDER

RANK	STATE	RATE
1	Massachusetts	420
2	New York	391
3	Maryland	384
4	Connecticut	372
5	Rhode Island	328
6	Vermont	316
7	New Jersey	302
8	Pennsylvania	301
9	Hawaii	283
10	California	275
11	Florida	269
12	Minnesota	267
13	Illinois	265
14	Washington	259
15	Colorado	257
16	Virginia	253
17	Oregon	250
18	New Hampshire	248
19	Tennessee	247
20	Delaware	246
21	Ohio	242
22	Louisiana	241
23	Arizona	239
23	North Carolina	239
23	Wisconsin	239
26	Missouri	236
27	Maine	235
28	Michigan	232
29	New Mexico	229
30	North Dakota	224
31	Kansas	223
32	Nebraska	220
33	Utah	216
33	West Virginia	216
35	Georgia	214
35	Montana	214
37	South Carolina	212
38	Kentucky	211
39	Texas	206
40	Alabama	202
41	Indiana	200
42	Arkansas	192
43	Iowa	189
44	South Dakota	187
45	Nevada	178
46	Oklahoma	177
47	Wyoming	176
48	Alaska	164
49	Idaho	162
50	Mississippi	155

District of Columbia   714

Source: American Medical Association (Chicago, Illinois)
"Physician Characteristics and Distribution in the U.S." (1996-97 Edition)
As of December 31, 1995. National rate does not include physicians in U.S. territories and possessions.

Nonfederal Physicians in Patient Care in 1995

National Total = 557,397 Physicians*

ALPHA ORDER

RANK	STATE	PHYSICIANS	% of USA
25	Alabama	7,194	1.29%
49	Alaska	828	0.15%
24	Arizona	7,654	1.37%
32	Arkansas	3,975	0.71%
1	California	67,977	12.20%
23	Colorado	7,657	1.37%
21	Connecticut	9,631	1.73%
46	Delaware	1,404	0.25%
5	Florida	28,628	5.14%
14	Georgia	12,866	2.31%
39	Hawaii	2,585	0.46%
43	Idaho	1,514	0.27%
6	Illinois	26,054	4.67%
20	Indiana	9,635	1.73%
31	Iowa	4,291	0.77%
30	Kansas	4,567	0.82%
26	Kentucky	6,892	1.24%
22	Louisiana	8,791	1.58%
41	Maine	2,247	0.40%
11	Maryland	14,940	2.68%
8	Massachusetts	20,128	3.61%
10	Michigan	18,146	3.26%
19	Minnesota	9,894	1.78%
33	Mississippi	3,484	0.63%
17	Missouri	10,448	1.87%
44	Montana	1,477	0.26%
37	Nebraska	2,983	0.54%
42	Nevada	2,221	0.40%
40	New Hampshire	2,269	0.41%
9	New Jersey	19,735	3.54%
36	New Mexico	3,002	0.54%
2	New York	57,246	10.27%
12	North Carolina	13,783	2.47%
47	North Dakota	1,195	0.21%
7	Ohio	22,260	3.99%
29	Oklahoma	4,781	0.86%
28	Oregon	6,110	1.10%
4	Pennsylvania	29,666	5.32%
38	Rhode Island	2,629	0.47%
27	South Carolina	6,401	1.15%
48	South Dakota	1,135	0.20%
15	Tennessee	10,911	1.96%
3	Texas	32,118	5.76%
34	Utah	3,418	0.61%
45	Vermont	1,414	0.25%
13	Virginia	13,431	2.41%
16	Washington	10,868	1.95%
35	West Virginia	3,281	0.59%
18	Wisconsin	10,032	1.80%
50	Wyoming	662	0.12%

RANK ORDER

RANK	STATE	PHYSICIANS	% of USA
1	California	67,977	12.20%
2	New York	57,246	10.27%
3	Texas	32,118	5.76%
4	Pennsylvania	29,666	5.32%
5	Florida	28,628	5.14%
6	Illinois	26,054	4.67%
7	Ohio	22,260	3.99%
8	Massachusetts	20,128	3.61%
9	New Jersey	19,735	3.54%
10	Michigan	18,146	3.26%
11	Maryland	14,940	2.68%
12	North Carolina	13,783	2.47%
13	Virginia	13,431	2.41%
14	Georgia	12,866	2.31%
15	Tennessee	10,911	1.96%
16	Washington	10,868	1.95%
17	Missouri	10,448	1.87%
18	Wisconsin	10,032	1.80%
19	Minnesota	9,894	1.78%
20	Indiana	9,635	1.73%
21	Connecticut	9,631	1.73%
22	Louisiana	8,791	1.58%
23	Colorado	7,657	1.37%
24	Arizona	7,654	1.37%
25	Alabama	7,194	1.29%
26	Kentucky	6,892	1.24%
27	South Carolina	6,401	1.15%
28	Oregon	6,110	1.10%
29	Oklahoma	4,781	0.86%
30	Kansas	4,567	0.82%
31	Iowa	4,291	0.77%
32	Arkansas	3,975	0.71%
33	Mississippi	3,484	0.63%
34	Utah	3,418	0.61%
35	West Virginia	3,281	0.59%
36	New Mexico	3,002	0.54%
37	Nebraska	2,983	0.54%
38	Rhode Island	2,629	0.47%
39	Hawaii	2,585	0.46%
40	New Hampshire	2,269	0.41%
41	Maine	2,247	0.40%
42	Nevada	2,221	0.40%
43	Idaho	1,514	0.27%
44	Montana	1,477	0.26%
45	Vermont	1,414	0.25%
46	Delaware	1,404	0.25%
47	North Dakota	1,195	0.21%
48	South Dakota	1,135	0.20%
49	Alaska	828	0.15%
50	Wyoming	662	0.12%
	District of Columbia	2,939	0.53%

Source: American Medical Association (Chicago, Illinois)
  "Physician Characteristics and Distribution in the U.S." (1996-97 Edition)
*As of December 31, 1995. Total does not include 6,677 physicians in U.S. territories and possessions.

Rate of Nonfederal Physicians in Patient Care in 1995

National Rate = 212 Physicians per 100,000 Population*

ALPHA ORDER

RANK	STATE	RATE
40	Alabama	169
48	Alaska	137
32	Arizona	178
42	Arkansas	160
11	California	215
14	Colorado	204
4	Connecticut	294
21	Delaware	196
17	Florida	202
32	Georgia	178
10	Hawaii	219
49	Idaho	130
9	Illinois	221
41	Indiana	166
44	Iowa	151
32	Kansas	178
31	Kentucky	179
15	Louisiana	203
29	Maine	181
3	Maryland	296
1	Massachusetts	332
26	Michigan	190
12	Minnesota	214
50	Mississippi	129
21	Missouri	196
39	Montana	170
28	Nebraska	182
46	Nevada	145
20	New Hampshire	198
6	New Jersey	248
32	New Mexico	178
2	New York	315
25	North Carolina	191
27	North Dakota	186
18	Ohio	200
45	Oklahoma	146
24	Oregon	194
7	Pennsylvania	246
5	Rhode Island	265
36	South Carolina	175
43	South Dakota	155
13	Tennessee	208
38	Texas	171
36	Utah	175
8	Vermont	242
15	Virginia	203
19	Washington	199
30	West Virginia	180
21	Wisconsin	196
47	Wyoming	138

RANK ORDER

RANK	STATE	RATE
1	Massachusetts	332
2	New York	315
3	Maryland	296
4	Connecticut	294
5	Rhode Island	265
6	New Jersey	248
7	Pennsylvania	246
8	Vermont	242
9	Illinois	221
10	Hawaii	219
11	California	215
12	Minnesota	214
13	Tennessee	208
14	Colorado	204
15	Louisiana	203
15	Virginia	203
17	Florida	202
18	Ohio	200
19	Washington	199
20	New Hampshire	198
21	Delaware	196
21	Missouri	196
21	Wisconsin	196
24	Oregon	194
25	North Carolina	191
26	Michigan	190
27	North Dakota	186
28	Nebraska	182
29	Maine	181
30	West Virginia	180
31	Kentucky	179
32	Arizona	178
32	Georgia	178
32	Kansas	178
32	New Mexico	178
36	South Carolina	175
36	Utah	175
38	Texas	171
39	Montana	170
40	Alabama	169
41	Indiana	166
42	Arkansas	160
43	South Dakota	155
44	Iowa	151
45	Oklahoma	146
46	Nevada	145
47	Wyoming	138
48	Alaska	137
49	Idaho	130
50	Mississippi	129
	District of Columbia	530

Source: Morgan Quitno Press using data from American Medical Association (Chicago, Illinois)
"Physician Characteristics and Distribution in the U.S." (1996-97 Edition)
*As of December 31, 1995. National rate does not include physicians in U.S. territories and possessions.

Physicians in Primary Care in 1995

National Total = 237,056 Physicians*

ALPHA ORDER					RANK ORDER			

RANK	STATE	PHYSICIANS	% of USA		RANK	STATE	PHYSICIANS	% of USA
25	Alabama	3,151	1.33%		1	California	28,914	12.20%
49	Alaska	446	0.19%		2	New York	23,810	10.04%
24	Arizona	3,300	1.39%		3	Texas	13,367	5.64%
32	Arkansas	1,810	0.76%		4	Illinois	11,822	4.99%
1	California	28,914	12.20%		5	Pennsylvania	11,567	4.88%
23	Colorado	3,346	1.41%		6	Florida	11,326	4.78%
21	Connecticut	3,941	1.66%		7	Ohio	9,420	3.97%
47	Delaware	585	0.25%		8	New Jersey	8,541	3.60%
6	Florida	11,326	4.78%		9	Michigan	7,767	3.28%
14	Georgia	5,605	2.36%		10	Massachusetts	7,738	3.26%
38	Hawaii	1,297	0.55%		11	Maryland	6,566	2.77%
43	Idaho	695	0.29%		12	Virginia	6,034	2.55%
4	Illinois	11,822	4.99%		13	North Carolina	5,903	2.49%
19	Indiana	4,190	1.77%		14	Georgia	5,605	2.36%
31	Iowa	1,869	0.79%		15	Washington	4,890	2.06%
30	Kansas	2,054	0.87%		16	Tennessee	4,583	1.93%
26	Kentucky	2,940	1.24%		17	Minnesota	4,571	1.93%
22	Louisiana	3,464	1.46%		18	Wisconsin	4,341	1.83%
40	Maine	1,013	0.43%		19	Indiana	4,190	1.77%
11	Maryland	6,566	2.77%		20	Missouri	4,163	1.76%
10	Massachusetts	7,738	3.26%		21	Connecticut	3,941	1.66%
9	Michigan	7,767	3.28%		22	Louisiana	3,464	1.46%
17	Minnesota	4,571	1.93%		23	Colorado	3,346	1.41%
33	Mississippi	1,646	0.69%		24	Arizona	3,300	1.39%
20	Missouri	4,163	1.76%		25	Alabama	3,151	1.33%
45	Montana	630	0.27%		26	Kentucky	2,940	1.24%
37	Nebraska	1,381	0.58%		27	South Carolina	2,860	1.21%
42	Nevada	933	0.39%		28	Oregon	2,653	1.12%
41	New Hampshire	963	0.41%		29	Oklahoma	2,096	0.88%
8	New Jersey	8,541	3.60%		30	Kansas	2,054	0.87%
35	New Mexico	1,420	0.60%		31	Iowa	1,869	0.79%
2	New York	23,810	10.04%		32	Arkansas	1,810	0.76%
13	North Carolina	5,903	2.49%		33	Mississippi	1,646	0.69%
46	North Dakota	587	0.25%		34	West Virginia	1,488	0.63%
7	Ohio	9,420	3.97%		35	New Mexico	1,420	0.60%
29	Oklahoma	2,096	0.88%		36	Utah	1,389	0.59%
28	Oregon	2,653	1.12%		37	Nebraska	1,381	0.58%
5	Pennsylvania	11,567	4.88%		38	Hawaii	1,297	0.55%
39	Rhode Island	1,118	0.47%		39	Rhode Island	1,118	0.47%
27	South Carolina	2,860	1.21%		40	Maine	1,013	0.43%
48	South Dakota	582	0.25%		41	New Hampshire	963	0.41%
16	Tennessee	4,583	1.93%		42	Nevada	933	0.39%
3	Texas	13,367	5.64%		43	Idaho	695	0.29%
36	Utah	1,389	0.59%		44	Vermont	641	0.27%
44	Vermont	641	0.27%		45	Montana	630	0.27%
12	Virginia	6,034	2.55%		46	North Dakota	587	0.25%
15	Washington	4,890	2.06%		47	Delaware	585	0.25%
34	West Virginia	1,488	0.63%		48	South Dakota	582	0.25%
18	Wisconsin	4,341	1.83%		49	Alaska	446	0.19%
50	Wyoming	372	0.16%		50	Wyoming	372	0.16%
						District of Columbia	1,268	0.53%

Source: American Medical Association (Chicago, Illinois)
    "Physician Characteristics and Distribution in the U.S." (1996-97 Edition)
*Federal and nonfederal physicians as of December 31, 1995. National total does not include 4,273 physicians in
U.S. territories and possessions. Primary Care Specialties include Family Practice, General Practice, Internal
Medicine, Obstetrics/Gynecology and Pediatrics.

Rate of Physicians in Primary Care in 1995

National Rate = 90 Physicians per 100,000 Population*

ALPHA ORDER

RANK	STATE	RATE
39	Alabama	74
39	Alaska	74
37	Arizona	77
41	Arkansas	73
12	California	92
16	Colorado	89
4	Connecticut	120
24	Delaware	82
29	Florida	80
33	Georgia	78
6	Hawaii	110
50	Idaho	60
9	Illinois	100
42	Indiana	72
46	Iowa	66
29	Kansas	80
38	Kentucky	76
29	Louisiana	80
24	Maine	82
2	Maryland	130
3	Massachusetts	127
28	Michigan	81
10	Minnesota	99
48	Mississippi	61
33	Missouri	78
42	Montana	72
20	Nebraska	84
48	Nevada	61
20	New Hampshire	84
8	New Jersey	107
20	New Mexico	84
1	New York	131
24	North Carolina	82
13	North Dakota	91
18	Ohio	85
47	Oklahoma	64
20	Oregon	84
11	Pennsylvania	96
5	Rhode Island	113
33	South Carolina	78
29	South Dakota	80
17	Tennessee	87
44	Texas	71
44	Utah	71
6	Vermont	110
13	Virginia	91
15	Washington	90
24	West Virginia	82
18	Wisconsin	85
33	Wyoming	78

RANK ORDER

RANK	STATE	RATE
1	New York	131
2	Maryland	130
3	Massachusetts	127
4	Connecticut	120
5	Rhode Island	113
6	Hawaii	110
6	Vermont	110
8	New Jersey	107
9	Illinois	100
10	Minnesota	99
11	Pennsylvania	96
12	California	92
13	North Dakota	91
13	Virginia	91
15	Washington	90
16	Colorado	89
17	Tennessee	87
18	Ohio	85
18	Wisconsin	85
20	Nebraska	84
20	New Hampshire	84
20	New Mexico	84
20	Oregon	84
24	Delaware	82
24	Maine	82
24	North Carolina	82
24	West Virginia	82
28	Michigan	81
29	Florida	80
29	Kansas	80
29	Louisiana	80
29	South Dakota	80
33	Georgia	78
33	Missouri	78
33	South Carolina	78
33	Wyoming	78
37	Arizona	77
38	Kentucky	76
39	Alabama	74
39	Alaska	74
41	Arkansas	73
42	Indiana	72
42	Montana	72
44	Texas	71
44	Utah	71
46	Iowa	66
47	Oklahoma	64
48	Mississippi	61
48	Nevada	61
50	Idaho	60

District of Columbia	228

Source: Morgan Quitno Press using data from American Medical Association (Chicago, Illinois)
"Physician Characteristics and Distribution in the U.S." (1996-97 Edition)
Federal and nonfederal physicians as of January 1, 1995. National rate does not include physicians in U.S. territories and possessions. Primary Care Specialties include Family Practice, General Practice, Internal Medicine, Obstetrics/Gynecology and Pediatrics.

Percent of Physicians in Primary Care in 1995

National Percent = 33.44% of Physicians*

ALPHA ORDER				RANK ORDER		
RANK	STATE	PERCENT		RANK	STATE	PERCENT
13	Alabama	35.84		1	Wyoming	42.32
2	Alaska	40.84		2	Alaska	40.84
46	Arizona	31.78		3	South Dakota	40.50
7	Arkansas	36.78		4	North Dakota	39.80
40	California	32.65		5	Nebraska	37.54
33	Colorado	33.46		6	Illinois	37.12
45	Connecticut	32.10		7	Arkansas	36.78
43	Delaware	32.43		8	Mississippi	36.72
50	Florida	29.10		9	West Virginia	36.60
22	Georgia	34.77		10	Minnesota	36.53
11	Hawaii	36.41		11	Hawaii	36.41
12	Idaho	35.90		12	Idaho	35.90
6	Illinois	37.12		13	Alabama	35.84
15	Indiana	35.68		14	South Carolina	35.75
28	Iowa	34.21		15	Indiana	35.68
20	Kansas	35.02		16	Kentucky	35.60
16	Kentucky	35.60		17	Oklahoma	35.35
41	Louisiana	32.63		18	New Jersey	35.24
27	Maine	34.27		18	New Mexico	35.24
48	Maryland	30.76		20	Kansas	35.02
49	Massachusetts	29.96		21	Wisconsin	35.01
23	Michigan	34.67		22	Georgia	34.77
10	Minnesota	36.53		23	Michigan	34.67
8	Mississippi	36.72		24	Virginia	34.63
42	Missouri	32.57		25	Tennessee	34.46
36	Montana	33.23		26	Ohio	34.34
5	Nebraska	37.54		27	Maine	34.27
34	Nevada	33.25		28	Iowa	34.21
39	New Hampshire	33.12		29	Vermont	34.13
18	New Jersey	35.24		30	Rhode Island	33.86
18	New Mexico	35.24		31	North Carolina	33.68
35	New York	33.24		32	Washington	33.47
31	North Carolina	33.68		33	Colorado	33.46
4	North Dakota	39.80		34	Nevada	33.25
26	Ohio	34.34		35	New York	33.24
17	Oklahoma	35.35		36	Montana	33.23
38	Oregon	33.16		37	Texas	33.22
47	Pennsylvania	31.45		38	Oregon	33.16
30	Rhode Island	33.86		39	New Hampshire	33.12
14	South Carolina	35.75		40	California	32.65
3	South Dakota	40.50		41	Louisiana	32.63
25	Tennessee	34.46		42	Missouri	32.57
37	Texas	33.22		43	Delaware	32.43
44	Utah	32.15		44	Utah	32.15
29	Vermont	34.13		45	Connecticut	32.10
24	Virginia	34.63		46	Arizona	31.78
32	Washington	33.47		47	Pennsylvania	31.45
9	West Virginia	36.60		48	Maryland	30.76
21	Wisconsin	35.01		49	Massachusetts	29.96
1	Wyoming	42.32		50	Florida	29.10
					District of Columbia	29.52

Source: Morgan Quitno Press using data from American Medical Association (Chicago, Illinois)
    "Physician Characteristics and Distribution in the U.S." (1996-97 Edition)
*Federal and nonfederal physicians as of January 1, 1995. National rate does not include physicians in U.S.
territories and possessions. Primary Care Specialties include Family Practice, General Practice, Internal Medicine,
Obstetrics/Gynecology and Pediatrics.*

Percent of Population Lacking Access to Primary Care in 1995

National Percent = 10.5% of Population*

<u>ALPHA ORDER</u>

RANK	STATE	PERCENT
5	Alabama	17.7
17	Alaska	11.8
44	Arizona	5.5
12	Arkansas	13.0
34	California	7.9
33	Colorado	8.1
39	Connecticut	7.2
48	Delaware	4.1
42	Florida	6.8
11	Georgia	13.7
50	Hawaii	2.3
8	Idaho	16.2
36	Illinois	7.7
28	Indiana	9.0
37	Iowa	7.5
29	Kansas	8.9
13	Kentucky	12.7
2	Louisiana	23.7
32	Maine	8.2
49	Maryland	3.2
41	Massachusetts	7.0
15	Michigan	12.2
47	Minnesota	4.3
1	Mississippi	27.6
20	Missouri	11.2
26	Montana	9.4
30	Nebraska	8.8
13	Nevada	12.7
43	New Hampshire	6.1
46	New Jersey	4.8
5	New Mexico	17.7
18	New York	11.6
16	North Carolina	11.9
8	North Dakota	16.2
37	Ohio	7.5
23	Oklahoma	10.6
26	Oregon	9.4
45	Pennsylvania	5.4
25	Rhode Island	9.6
3	South Carolina	19.4
4	South Dakota	18.3
21	Tennessee	10.8
21	Texas	10.8
31	Utah	8.3
35	Vermont	7.8
40	Virginia	7.1
24	Washington	10.1
7	West Virginia	16.5
18	Wisconsin	11.6
10	Wyoming	14.1

<u>RANK ORDER</u>

RANK	STATE	PERCENT
1	Mississippi	27.6
2	Louisiana	23.7
3	South Carolina	19.4
4	South Dakota	18.3
5	Alabama	17.7
5	New Mexico	17.7
7	West Virginia	16.5
8	Idaho	16.2
8	North Dakota	16.2
10	Wyoming	14.1
11	Georgia	13.7
12	Arkansas	13.0
13	Kentucky	12.7
13	Nevada	12.7
15	Michigan	12.2
16	North Carolina	11.9
17	Alaska	11.8
18	New York	11.6
18	Wisconsin	11.6
20	Missouri	11.2
21	Tennessee	10.8
21	Texas	10.8
23	Oklahoma	10.6
24	Washington	10.1
25	Rhode Island	9.6
26	Montana	9.4
26	Oregon	9.4
28	Indiana	9.0
29	Kansas	8.9
30	Nebraska	8.8
31	Utah	8.3
32	Maine	8.2
33	Colorado	8.1
34	California	7.9
35	Vermont	7.8
36	Illinois	7.7
37	Iowa	7.5
37	Ohio	7.5
39	Connecticut	7.2
40	Virginia	7.1
41	Massachusetts	7.0
42	Florida	6.8
43	New Hampshire	6.1
44	Arizona	5.5
45	Pennsylvania	5.4
46	New Jersey	4.8
47	Minnesota	4.3
48	Delaware	4.1
49	Maryland	3.2
50	Hawaii	2.3
	District of Columbia**	NA

Source: U.S. Department of Health and Human Services, Bureau of Primary Health Care
"Selected Statistics on Health Manpower Shortage Areas" (March 31, 1996)
Percent of population considered under-served by primary medical practitioners (Family & General Practice doctors, Internists, Ob/Gyns and Pediatricians). An under-served population does not have primary medical care within reasonable economic and geographic bounds.
***Not available.*

Nonfederal Physicians in General/Family Practice in 1995

National Total = 72,308 Physicians*

ALPHA ORDER

RANK	STATE	PHYSICIANS	% of USA
22	Alabama	1,117	1.54%
49	Alaska	196	0.27%
21	Arizona	1,151	1.59%
28	Arkansas	946	1.31%
1	California	9,066	12.54%
18	Colorado	1,316	1.82%
35	Connecticut	560	0.77%
47	Delaware	201	0.28%
3	Florida	3,850	5.32%
15	Georgia	1,663	2.30%
45	Hawaii	273	0.38%
39	Idaho	408	0.56%
6	Illinois	3,243	4.48%
11	Indiana	2,061	2.85%
27	Iowa	1,012	1.40%
29	Kansas	933	1.29%
20	Kentucky	1,178	1.63%
26	Louisiana	1,033	1.43%
38	Maine	445	0.62%
23	Maryland	1,089	1.51%
25	Massachusetts	1,044	1.44%
9	Michigan	2,184	3.02%
10	Minnesota	2,179	3.01%
33	Mississippi	679	0.94%
24	Missouri	1,080	1.49%
44	Montana	303	0.42%
32	Nebraska	714	0.99%
43	Nevada	318	0.44%
42	New Hampshire	322	0.45%
17	New Jersey	1,437	1.99%
36	New Mexico	530	0.73%
5	New York	3,407	4.71%
12	North Carolina	1,990	2.75%
41	North Dakota	323	0.45%
7	Ohio	2,935	4.06%
31	Oklahoma	884	1.22%
30	Oregon	932	1.29%
4	Pennsylvania	3,590	4.96%
50	Rhode Island	180	0.25%
19	South Carolina	1,243	1.72%
40	South Dakota	334	0.46%
16	Tennessee	1,447	2.00%
2	Texas	4,801	6.64%
37	Utah	509	0.70%
46	Vermont	211	0.29%
13	Virginia	1,960	2.71%
8	Washington	2,211	3.06%
34	West Virginia	604	0.84%
14	Wisconsin	1,868	2.58%
47	Wyoming	201	0.28%

RANK ORDER

RANK	STATE	PHYSICIANS	% of USA
1	California	9,066	12.54%
2	Texas	4,801	6.64%
3	Florida	3,850	5.32%
4	Pennsylvania	3,590	4.96%
5	New York	3,407	4.71%
6	Illinois	3,243	4.48%
7	Ohio	2,935	4.06%
8	Washington	2,211	3.06%
9	Michigan	2,184	3.02%
10	Minnesota	2,179	3.01%
11	Indiana	2,061	2.85%
12	North Carolina	1,990	2.75%
13	Virginia	1,960	2.71%
14	Wisconsin	1,868	2.58%
15	Georgia	1,663	2.30%
16	Tennessee	1,447	2.00%
17	New Jersey	1,437	1.99%
18	Colorado	1,316	1.82%
19	South Carolina	1,243	1.72%
20	Kentucky	1,178	1.63%
21	Arizona	1,151	1.59%
22	Alabama	1,117	1.54%
23	Maryland	1,089	1.51%
24	Missouri	1,080	1.49%
25	Massachusetts	1,044	1.44%
26	Louisiana	1,033	1.43%
27	Iowa	1,012	1.40%
28	Arkansas	946	1.31%
29	Kansas	933	1.29%
30	Oregon	932	1.29%
31	Oklahoma	884	1.22%
32	Nebraska	714	0.99%
33	Mississippi	679	0.94%
34	West Virginia	604	0.84%
35	Connecticut	560	0.77%
36	New Mexico	530	0.73%
37	Utah	509	0.70%
38	Maine	445	0.62%
39	Idaho	408	0.56%
40	South Dakota	334	0.46%
41	North Dakota	323	0.45%
42	New Hampshire	322	0.45%
43	Nevada	318	0.44%
44	Montana	303	0.42%
45	Hawaii	273	0.38%
46	Vermont	211	0.29%
47	Delaware	201	0.28%
47	Wyoming	201	0.28%
49	Alaska	196	0.27%
50	Rhode Island	180	0.25%
	District of Columbia	147	0.20%

Source: American Medical Association (Chicago, Illinois)
"Physician Characteristics and Distribution in the U.S." (1996-97 Edition)
*As of December 31, 1995. National total does not include 1,696 physicians in U.S. territories and possessions.

Rate of Nonfederal Physicians in General/Family Practice in 1995

National Rate = 28 Physicians per 100,000 Population*

ALPHA ORDER

RANK	STATE	RATE
34	Alabama	26
18	Alaska	33
31	Arizona	27
7	Arkansas	38
25	California	29
14	Colorado	35
49	Connecticut	17
26	Delaware	28
31	Florida	27
40	Georgia	23
40	Hawaii	23
14	Idaho	35
26	Illinois	28
8	Indiana	36
8	Iowa	36
8	Kansas	36
20	Kentucky	31
39	Louisiana	24
8	Maine	36
43	Maryland	22
49	Massachusetts	17
40	Michigan	23
2	Minnesota	47
38	Mississippi	25
45	Missouri	20
14	Montana	35
4	Nebraska	44
44	Nevada	21
26	New Hampshire	28
47	New Jersey	18
20	New Mexico	31
46	New York	19
26	North Carolina	28
1	North Dakota	50
34	Ohio	26
31	Oklahoma	27
22	Oregon	30
22	Pennsylvania	30
47	Rhode Island	18
17	South Carolina	34
3	South Dakota	46
26	Tennessee	28
34	Texas	26
34	Utah	26
8	Vermont	36
22	Virginia	30
6	Washington	41
18	West Virginia	33
8	Wisconsin	36
5	Wyoming	42

RANK ORDER

RANK	STATE	RATE
1	North Dakota	50
2	Minnesota	47
3	South Dakota	46
4	Nebraska	44
5	Wyoming	42
6	Washington	41
7	Arkansas	38
8	Indiana	36
8	Iowa	36
8	Kansas	36
8	Maine	36
8	Vermont	36
8	Wisconsin	36
14	Colorado	35
14	Idaho	35
14	Montana	35
17	South Carolina	34
18	Alaska	33
18	West Virginia	33
20	Kentucky	31
20	New Mexico	31
22	Oregon	30
22	Pennsylvania	30
22	Virginia	30
25	California	29
26	Delaware	28
26	Illinois	28
26	New Hampshire	28
26	North Carolina	28
26	Tennessee	28
31	Arizona	27
31	Florida	27
31	Oklahoma	27
34	Alabama	26
34	Ohio	26
34	Texas	26
34	Utah	26
38	Mississippi	25
39	Louisiana	24
40	Georgia	23
40	Hawaii	23
40	Michigan	23
43	Maryland	22
44	Nevada	21
45	Missouri	20
46	New York	19
47	New Jersey	18
47	Rhode Island	18
49	Connecticut	17
49	Massachusetts	17

District of Columbia	26

Source: Morgan Quitno Press using data from American Medical Association (Chicago, Illinois)
"Physician Characteristics and Distribution in the U.S." (1996-97 Edition)
*As of December 31, 1995. National rate does not include physicians in U.S. territories and possessions.

Percent of Family Physicians Who Practice Pediatrics in 1996

National Percent = 91.3% of Family Physicians*

ALPHA ORDER

RANK	STATE	PERCENT
41	Alabama	88.7
47	Alaska	86.2
31	Arizona	91.9
13	Arkansas	94.2
40	California	88.9
7	Colorado	95.6
9	Connecticut	94.8
25	Delaware	92.6
50	Florida	79.2
23	Georgia	92.7
33	Hawaii	91.4
3	Idaho	97.1
35	Illinois	90.9
8	Indiana	95.3
15	Iowa	94.1
20	Kansas	93.5
29	Kentucky	92.2
46	Louisiana	86.7
1	Maine	98.9
44	Maryland	87.4
18	Massachusetts	94.0
19	Michigan	93.7
11	Minnesota	94.4
25	Mississippi	92.6
38	Missouri	89.8
36	Montana	90.4
6	Nebraska	96.1
48	Nevada	85.7
4	New Hampshire	97.0
32	New Jersey	91.7
22	New Mexico	92.9
45	New York	86.9
10	North Carolina	94.7
43	North Dakota	87.5
28	Ohio	92.5
23	Oklahoma	92.7
13	Oregon	94.2
34	Pennsylvania	91.2
49	Rhode Island	85.2
39	South Carolina	89.1
2	South Dakota	97.3
29	Tennessee	92.2
42	Texas	87.6
11	Utah	94.4
25	Vermont	92.6
21	Virginia	93.2
15	Washington	94.1
37	West Virginia	89.9
5	Wisconsin	96.3
15	Wyoming	94.1

RANK ORDER

RANK	STATE	PERCENT
1	Maine	98.9
2	South Dakota	97.3
3	Idaho	97.1
4	New Hampshire	97.0
5	Wisconsin	96.3
6	Nebraska	96.1
7	Colorado	95.6
8	Indiana	95.3
9	Connecticut	94.8
10	North Carolina	94.7
11	Minnesota	94.4
11	Utah	94.4
13	Arkansas	94.2
13	Oregon	94.2
15	Iowa	94.1
15	Washington	94.1
15	Wyoming	94.1
18	Massachusetts	94.0
19	Michigan	93.7
20	Kansas	93.5
21	Virginia	93.2
22	New Mexico	92.9
23	Georgia	92.7
23	Oklahoma	92.7
25	Delaware	92.6
25	Mississippi	92.6
25	Vermont	92.6
28	Ohio	92.5
29	Kentucky	92.2
29	Tennessee	92.2
31	Arizona	91.9
32	New Jersey	91.7
33	Hawaii	91.4
34	Pennsylvania	91.2
35	Illinois	90.9
36	Montana	90.4
37	West Virginia	89.9
38	Missouri	89.8
39	South Carolina	89.1
40	California	88.9
41	Alabama	88.7
42	Texas	87.6
43	North Dakota	87.5
44	Maryland	87.4
45	New York	86.9
46	Louisiana	86.7
47	Alaska	86.2
48	Nevada	85.7
49	Rhode Island	85.2
50	Florida	79.2

District of Columbia 94.1

Source: The American Academy of Family Physicians
"Facts About Family Practice 1996"
As of January 1, 1996. Includes members of the Academy who are in direct patient care and who practice pediatrics "in some fashion".

Percent of Family Physicians Who Practice Obstetrics in 1996

National Percent = 29.1% of Family Physicians*

ALPHA ORDER

RANK	STATE	PERCENT
48	Alabama	9.7
6	Alaska	55.2
29	Arizona	21.5
31	Arkansas	20.2
30	California	20.7
17	Colorado	42.4
45	Connecticut	12.1
49	Delaware	7.4
50	Florida	6.4
33	Georgia	18.9
26	Hawaii	22.9
10	Idaho	50.0
22	Illinois	29.7
16	Indiana	43.0
8	Iowa	53.6
12	Kansas	48.1
42	Kentucky	13.1
41	Louisiana	14.8
15	Maine	43.2
46	Maryland	11.3
25	Massachusetts	24.0
18	Michigan	42.0
3	Minnesota	59.9
44	Mississippi	12.3
24	Missouri	25.0
4	Montana	57.7
5	Nebraska	55.9
37	Nevada	16.7
21	New Hampshire	33.3
40	New Jersey	15.4
23	New Mexico	28.6
28	New York	22.6
34	North Carolina	18.8
7	North Dakota	54.2
38	Ohio	16.5
13	Oklahoma	47.4
19	Oregon	39.1
42	Pennsylvania	13.1
35	Rhode Island	18.5
36	South Carolina	17.0
1	South Dakota	79.7
27	Tennessee	22.8
32	Texas	19.7
9	Utah	51.1
20	Vermont	35.2
47	Virginia	10.6
14	Washington	46.3
38	West Virginia	16.5
2	Wisconsin	60.0
10	Wyoming	50.0

RANK ORDER

RANK	STATE	PERCENT
1	South Dakota	79.7
2	Wisconsin	60.0
3	Minnesota	59.9
4	Montana	57.7
5	Nebraska	55.9
6	Alaska	55.2
7	North Dakota	54.2
8	Iowa	53.6
9	Utah	51.1
10	Idaho	50.0
10	Wyoming	50.0
12	Kansas	48.1
13	Oklahoma	47.4
14	Washington	46.3
15	Maine	43.2
16	Indiana	43.0
17	Colorado	42.4
18	Michigan	42.0
19	Oregon	39.1
20	Vermont	35.2
21	New Hampshire	33.3
22	Illinois	29.7
23	New Mexico	28.6
24	Missouri	25.0
25	Massachusetts	24.0
26	Hawaii	22.9
27	Tennessee	22.8
28	New York	22.6
29	Arizona	21.5
30	California	20.7
31	Arkansas	20.2
32	Texas	19.7
33	Georgia	18.9
34	North Carolina	18.8
35	Rhode Island	18.5
36	South Carolina	17.0
37	Nevada	16.7
38	Ohio	16.5
38	West Virginia	16.5
40	New Jersey	15.4
41	Louisiana	14.8
42	Kentucky	13.1
42	Pennsylvania	13.1
44	Mississippi	12.3
45	Connecticut	12.1
46	Maryland	11.3
47	Virginia	10.6
48	Alabama	9.7
49	Delaware	7.4
50	Florida	6.4

District of Columbia   23.5

*Source: The American Academy of Family Physicians
"Facts About Family Practice 1996"*
As of January 1, 1996. Includes members of the Academy who are in direct patient care and who practice obstetrics "in some fashion".

Nonfederal Physicians in Medical Specialties in 1995

National Total = 206,207 Physicians*

ALPHA ORDER					RANK ORDER			

RANK	STATE	PHYSICIANS	% of USA		RANK	STATE	PHYSICIANS	% of USA
24	Alabama	2,527	1.23%		1	New York	25,903	12.56%
49	Alaska	204	0.10%		2	California	24,589	11.92%
23	Arizona	2,575	1.25%		3	Pennsylvania	10,971	5.32%
33	Arkansas	1,113	0.54%		4	Texas	10,480	5.08%
2	California	24,589	11.92%		5	Illinois	10,368	5.03%
25	Colorado	2,512	1.22%		6	Florida	10,272	4.98%
15	Connecticut	4,324	2.10%		7	Massachusetts	9,296	4.51%
44	Delaware	482	0.23%		8	New Jersey	9,018	4.37%
6	Florida	10,272	4.98%		9	Ohio	8,054	3.91%
14	Georgia	4,335	2.10%		10	Michigan	6,747	3.27%
36	Hawaii	998	0.48%		11	Maryland	6,614	3.21%
46	Idaho	324	0.16%		12	North Carolina	4,813	2.33%
5	Illinois	10,368	5.03%		13	Virginia	4,624	2.24%
22	Indiana	2,832	1.37%		14	Georgia	4,335	2.10%
31	Iowa	1,218	0.59%		15	Connecticut	4,324	2.10%
30	Kansas	1,323	0.64%		16	Missouri	4,088	1.98%
26	Kentucky	2,169	1.05%		17	Tennessee	3,901	1.89%
21	Louisiana	2,975	1.44%		18	Minnesota	3,320	1.61%
42	Maine	679	0.33%		19	Washington	3,304	1.60%
11	Maryland	6,614	3.21%		20	Wisconsin	3,251	1.58%
7	Massachusetts	9,296	4.51%		21	Louisiana	2,975	1.44%
10	Michigan	6,747	3.27%		22	Indiana	2,832	1.37%
18	Minnesota	3,320	1.61%		23	Arizona	2,575	1.25%
37	Mississippi	982	0.48%		24	Alabama	2,527	1.23%
16	Missouri	4,088	1.98%		25	Colorado	2,512	1.22%
45	Montana	387	0.19%		26	Kentucky	2,169	1.05%
39	Nebraska	880	0.43%		27	Oregon	2,026	0.98%
41	Nevada	721	0.35%		28	South Carolina	1,859	0.90%
40	New Hampshire	743	0.36%		29	Oklahoma	1,464	0.71%
8	New Jersey	9,018	4.37%		30	Kansas	1,323	0.64%
38	New Mexico	976	0.47%		31	Iowa	1,218	0.59%
1	New York	25,903	12.56%		32	Rhode Island	1,213	0.59%
12	North Carolina	4,813	2.33%		33	Arkansas	1,113	0.54%
47	North Dakota	318	0.15%		34	Utah	1,112	0.54%
9	Ohio	8,054	3.91%		35	West Virginia	1,043	0.51%
29	Oklahoma	1,464	0.71%		36	Hawaii	998	0.48%
27	Oregon	2,026	0.98%		37	Mississippi	982	0.48%
3	Pennsylvania	10,971	5.32%		38	New Mexico	976	0.47%
32	Rhode Island	1,213	0.59%		39	Nebraska	880	0.43%
28	South Carolina	1,859	0.90%		40	New Hampshire	743	0.36%
48	South Dakota	294	0.14%		41	Nevada	721	0.35%
17	Tennessee	3,901	1.89%		42	Maine	679	0.33%
4	Texas	10,480	5.08%		43	Vermont	500	0.24%
34	Utah	1,112	0.54%		44	Delaware	482	0.23%
43	Vermont	500	0.24%		45	Montana	387	0.19%
13	Virginia	4,624	2.24%		46	Idaho	324	0.16%
19	Washington	3,304	1.60%		47	North Dakota	318	0.15%
35	West Virginia	1,043	0.51%		48	South Dakota	294	0.14%
20	Wisconsin	3,251	1.58%		49	Alaska	204	0.10%
50	Wyoming	141	0.07%		50	Wyoming	141	0.07%
						District of Columbia	1,345	0.65%

Source: American Medical Association (Chicago, Illinois)
"Physician Characteristics and Distribution in the U.S." (1996-97 Edition)
*As of December 31, 1995. Total does not include 2,309 physicians in U.S. territories and possessions. Medical Specialties are Allergy/Immunology, Cardiovascular Diseases, Dermatology, Gastroenterology, Internal Medicine, Pediatrics, Pediatric Cardiology and Pulmonary Diseases.

Rate of Nonfederal Physicians in Medical Specialties in 1995

National Rate = 78 Physicians per 100,000 Population*

ALPHA ORDER

RANK	STATE	RATE
27	Alabama	60
48	Alaska	34
27	Arizona	60
42	Arkansas	45
11	California	78
20	Colorado	67
3	Connecticut	132
20	Delaware	67
14	Florida	72
27	Georgia	60
9	Hawaii	85
50	Idaho	28
8	Illinois	88
40	Indiana	49
45	Iowa	43
37	Kansas	52
33	Kentucky	56
19	Louisiana	69
35	Maine	55
4	Maryland	131
1	Massachusetts	153
17	Michigan	71
14	Minnesota	72
47	Mississippi	36
12	Missouri	77
44	Montana	44
36	Nebraska	54
41	Nevada	47
23	New Hampshire	65
6	New Jersey	113
30	New Mexico	58
2	New York	142
20	North Carolina	67
39	North Dakota	50
14	Ohio	72
42	Oklahoma	45
24	Oregon	64
7	Pennsylvania	91
5	Rhode Island	122
38	South Carolina	51
46	South Dakota	40
13	Tennessee	74
33	Texas	56
31	Utah	57
9	Vermont	85
18	Virginia	70
26	Washington	61
31	West Virginia	57
25	Wisconsin	63
49	Wyoming	29

RANK ORDER

RANK	STATE	RATE
1	Massachusetts	153
2	New York	142
3	Connecticut	132
4	Maryland	131
5	Rhode Island	122
6	New Jersey	113
7	Pennsylvania	91
8	Illinois	88
9	Hawaii	85
9	Vermont	85
11	California	78
12	Missouri	77
13	Tennessee	74
14	Florida	72
14	Minnesota	72
14	Ohio	72
17	Michigan	71
18	Virginia	70
19	Louisiana	69
20	Colorado	67
20	Delaware	67
20	North Carolina	67
23	New Hampshire	65
24	Oregon	64
25	Wisconsin	63
26	Washington	61
27	Alabama	60
27	Arizona	60
27	Georgia	60
30	New Mexico	58
31	Utah	57
31	West Virginia	57
33	Kentucky	56
33	Texas	56
35	Maine	55
36	Nebraska	54
37	Kansas	52
38	South Carolina	51
39	North Dakota	50
40	Indiana	49
41	Nevada	47
42	Arkansas	45
42	Oklahoma	45
44	Montana	44
45	Iowa	43
46	South Dakota	40
47	Mississippi	36
48	Alaska	34
49	Wyoming	29
50	Idaho	28

| | District of Columbia | 242 |

Source: Morgan Quitno Press using data from American Medical Association (Chicago, Illinois)
    "Physician Characteristics and Distribution in the U.S." (1996-97 Edition)
*As of December 31, 1995. National rate does not include physicians in the U.S. territories and possessions.
Medical Specialties are Allergy/Immunology, Cardiovascular Diseases, Dermatology, Gastroenterology, Internal Medicine, Pediatrics, Pediatric Cardiology and Pulmonary Diseases.

Nonfederal Physicians in Internal Medicine in 1995

National Total = 109,808 Physicians*

ALPHA ORDER

RANK	STATE	PHYSICIANS	% of USA
23	Alabama	1,358	1.24%
49	Alaska	93	0.08%
25	Arizona	1,268	1.15%
38	Arkansas	488	0.44%
2	California	12,642	11.51%
24	Colorado	1,284	1.17%
12	Connecticut	2,515	2.29%
44	Delaware	232	0.21%
8	Florida	4,777	4.35%
15	Georgia	2,262	2.06%
34	Hawaii	566	0.52%
48	Idaho	160	0.15%
4	Illinois	5,938	5.41%
22	Indiana	1,390	1.27%
32	Iowa	578	0.53%
30	Kansas	718	0.65%
27	Kentucky	1,082	0.99%
21	Louisiana	1,465	1.33%
42	Maine	369	0.34%
11	Maryland	3,640	3.31%
5	Massachusetts	5,484	4.99%
10	Michigan	3,825	3.48%
18	Minnesota	1,822	1.66%
35	Mississippi	504	0.46%
16	Missouri	2,177	1.98%
45	Montana	203	0.18%
39	Nebraska	428	0.39%
40	Nevada	395	0.36%
41	New Hampshire	387	0.35%
7	New Jersey	4,825	4.39%
36	New Mexico	496	0.45%
1	New York	14,809	13.49%
13	North Carolina	2,432	2.21%
46	North Dakota	183	0.17%
9	Ohio	4,216	3.84%
29	Oklahoma	751	0.68%
26	Oregon	1,223	1.11%
3	Pennsylvania	5,994	5.46%
31	Rhode Island	690	0.63%
28	South Carolina	893	0.81%
47	South Dakota	164	0.15%
17	Tennessee	2,066	1.88%
6	Texas	5,002	4.56%
37	Utah	492	0.45%
43	Vermont	291	0.27%
14	Virginia	2,370	2.16%
19	Washington	1,752	1.60%
32	West Virginia	578	0.53%
20	Wisconsin	1,745	1.59%
50	Wyoming	76	0.07%

RANK ORDER

RANK	STATE	PHYSICIANS	% of USA
1	New York	14,809	13.49%
2	California	12,642	11.51%
3	Pennsylvania	5,994	5.46%
4	Illinois	5,938	5.41%
5	Massachusetts	5,484	4.99%
6	Texas	5,002	4.56%
7	New Jersey	4,825	4.39%
8	Florida	4,777	4.35%
9	Ohio	4,216	3.84%
10	Michigan	3,825	3.48%
11	Maryland	3,640	3.31%
12	Connecticut	2,515	2.29%
13	North Carolina	2,432	2.21%
14	Virginia	2,370	2.16%
15	Georgia	2,262	2.06%
16	Missouri	2,177	1.98%
17	Tennessee	2,066	1.88%
18	Minnesota	1,822	1.66%
19	Washington	1,752	1.60%
20	Wisconsin	1,745	1.59%
21	Louisiana	1,465	1.33%
22	Indiana	1,390	1.27%
23	Alabama	1,358	1.24%
24	Colorado	1,284	1.17%
25	Arizona	1,268	1.15%
26	Oregon	1,223	1.11%
27	Kentucky	1,082	0.99%
28	South Carolina	893	0.81%
29	Oklahoma	751	0.68%
30	Kansas	718	0.65%
31	Rhode Island	690	0.63%
32	Iowa	578	0.53%
32	West Virginia	578	0.53%
34	Hawaii	566	0.52%
35	Mississippi	504	0.46%
36	New Mexico	496	0.45%
37	Utah	492	0.45%
38	Arkansas	488	0.44%
39	Nebraska	428	0.39%
40	Nevada	395	0.36%
41	New Hampshire	387	0.35%
42	Maine	369	0.34%
43	Vermont	291	0.27%
44	Delaware	232	0.21%
45	Montana	203	0.18%
46	North Dakota	183	0.17%
47	South Dakota	164	0.15%
48	Idaho	160	0.15%
49	Alaska	93	0.08%
50	Wyoming	76	0.07%
	District of Columbia	710	0.65%

Source: American Medical Association (Chicago, Illinois)
"Physician Characteristics and Distribution in the U.S." (1996-97 Edition)
*As of December 31, 1995. Total does not include 1,009 physicians in U.S. territories and possessions. Internal Medicine includes Diabetes, Endocrinology, Geriatrics, Hematology, Infectious Diseases, Nephrology, Nutrition, Medical Oncology and Rheumatology.

Rate of Nonfederal Physicians in Internal Medicine in 1995

National Rate = 42 Physicians per 100,000 Population*

ALPHA ORDER

RANK	STATE	RATE
25	Alabama	32
49	Alaska	15
31	Arizona	29
45	Arkansas	20
12	California	40
19	Colorado	34
3	Connecticut	77
25	Delaware	32
19	Florida	34
29	Georgia	31
10	Hawaii	48
50	Idaho	14
7	Illinois	50
40	Indiana	24
45	Iowa	20
34	Kansas	28
34	Kentucky	28
19	Louisiana	34
30	Maine	30
4	Maryland	72
1	Massachusetts	90
12	Michigan	40
14	Minnesota	39
47	Mississippi	19
11	Missouri	41
42	Montana	23
37	Nebraska	26
37	Nevada	26
19	New Hampshire	34
6	New Jersey	61
31	New Mexico	29
2	New York	81
19	North Carolina	34
31	North Dakota	29
17	Ohio	38
42	Oklahoma	23
14	Oregon	39
7	Pennsylvania	50
5	Rhode Island	70
40	South Carolina	24
44	South Dakota	22
14	Tennessee	39
36	Texas	27
39	Utah	25
7	Vermont	50
18	Virginia	36
25	Washington	32
25	West Virginia	32
19	Wisconsin	34
48	Wyoming	16

RANK ORDER

RANK	STATE	RATE
1	Massachusetts	90
2	New York	81
3	Connecticut	77
4	Maryland	72
5	Rhode Island	70
6	New Jersey	61
7	Illinois	50
7	Pennsylvania	50
7	Vermont	50
10	Hawaii	48
11	Missouri	41
12	California	40
12	Michigan	40
14	Minnesota	39
14	Oregon	39
14	Tennessee	39
17	Ohio	38
18	Virginia	36
19	Colorado	34
19	Florida	34
19	Louisiana	34
19	New Hampshire	34
19	North Carolina	34
19	Wisconsin	34
25	Alabama	32
25	Delaware	32
25	Washington	32
25	West Virginia	32
29	Georgia	31
30	Maine	30
31	Arizona	29
31	New Mexico	29
31	North Dakota	29
34	Kansas	28
34	Kentucky	28
36	Texas	27
37	Nebraska	26
37	Nevada	26
39	Utah	25
40	Indiana	24
40	South Carolina	24
42	Montana	23
42	Oklahoma	23
44	South Dakota	22
45	Arkansas	20
45	Iowa	20
47	Mississippi	19
48	Wyoming	16
49	Alaska	15
50	Idaho	14

	District of Columbia	128

Source: Morgan Quitno Press using data from American Medical Association (Chicago, Illinois)
   "Physician Characteristics and Distribution in the U.S." (1996-97 Edition)
*As of December 31, 1995. National rate does not include physicians in U.S. territories and possessions. Internal Medicine includes Diabetes, Endocrinology, Geriatrics, Hematology, Infectious Diseases, Nephrology, Nutrition, Medical Oncology and Rheumatology.

Nonfederal Physicians in Pediatrics in 1995

National Total = 48,643 Physicians*

ALPHA ORDER

RANK ORDER

RANK	STATE	PHYSICIANS	% of USA		RANK	STATE	PHYSICIANS	% of USA
25	Alabama	564	1.16%		1	California	6,193	12.73%
46	Alaska	74	0.15%		2	New York	5,985	12.30%
23	Arizona	634	1.30%		3	Texas	2,803	5.76%
31	Arkansas	315	0.65%		4	Florida	2,417	4.97%
1	California	6,193	12.73%		5	Illinois	2,323	4.78%
24	Colorado	627	1.29%		6	Pennsylvania	2,196	4.51%
16	Connecticut	890	1.83%		7	New Jersey	2,182	4.49%
42	Delaware	147	0.30%		8	Ohio	2,002	4.12%
4	Florida	2,417	4.97%		9	Massachusetts	1,872	3.85%
14	Georgia	1,055	2.17%		10	Maryland	1,617	3.32%
35	Hawaii	262	0.54%		11	Michigan	1,504	3.09%
47	Idaho	68	0.14%		12	North Carolina	1,189	2.44%
5	Illinois	2,323	4.78%		13	Virginia	1,176	2.42%
22	Indiana	648	1.33%		14	Georgia	1,055	2.17%
33	Iowa	290	0.60%		15	Tennessee	946	1.94%
32	Kansas	299	0.61%		16	Connecticut	890	1.83%
26	Kentucky	550	1.13%		16	Missouri	890	1.83%
20	Louisiana	734	1.51%		18	Washington	795	1.63%
41	Maine	159	0.33%		19	Wisconsin	744	1.53%
10	Maryland	1,617	3.32%		20	Louisiana	734	1.51%
9	Massachusetts	1,872	3.85%		21	Minnesota	703	1.45%
11	Michigan	1,504	3.09%		22	Indiana	648	1.33%
21	Minnesota	703	1.45%		23	Arizona	634	1.30%
37	Mississippi	245	0.50%		24	Colorado	627	1.29%
16	Missouri	890	1.83%		25	Alabama	564	1.16%
45	Montana	79	0.16%		26	Kentucky	550	1.13%
39	Nebraska	206	0.42%		27	South Carolina	497	1.02%
43	Nevada	131	0.27%		28	Oregon	383	0.79%
40	New Hampshire	186	0.38%		29	Utah	329	0.68%
7	New Jersey	2,182	4.49%		30	Oklahoma	327	0.67%
34	New Mexico	268	0.55%		31	Arkansas	315	0.65%
2	New York	5,985	12.30%		32	Kansas	299	0.61%
12	North Carolina	1,189	2.44%		33	Iowa	290	0.60%
48	North Dakota	60	0.12%		34	New Mexico	268	0.55%
8	Ohio	2,002	4.12%		35	Hawaii	262	0.54%
30	Oklahoma	327	0.67%		36	Rhode Island	260	0.53%
28	Oregon	383	0.79%		37	Mississippi	245	0.50%
6	Pennsylvania	2,196	4.51%		38	West Virginia	225	0.46%
36	Rhode Island	260	0.53%		39	Nebraska	206	0.42%
27	South Carolina	497	1.02%		40	New Hampshire	186	0.38%
49	South Dakota	57	0.12%		41	Maine	159	0.33%
15	Tennessee	946	1.94%		42	Delaware	147	0.30%
3	Texas	2,803	5.76%		43	Nevada	131	0.27%
29	Utah	329	0.68%		44	Vermont	126	0.26%
44	Vermont	126	0.26%		45	Montana	79	0.16%
13	Virginia	1,176	2.42%		46	Alaska	74	0.15%
18	Washington	795	1.63%		47	Idaho	68	0.14%
38	West Virginia	225	0.46%		48	North Dakota	60	0.12%
19	Wisconsin	744	1.53%		49	South Dakota	57	0.12%
50	Wyoming	36	0.07%		50	Wyoming	36	0.07%
						District of Columbia	375	0.77%

Source: American Medical Association (Chicago, Illinois)
   "Physician Characteristics and Distribution in the U.S." (1996-97 Edition)
*As of December 31, 1995. Total does not include 870 physicians in U.S. territories and possessions. Pediatrics
includes Adolescent Medicine, Neonatal-Perinatal, Pediatric Allergy, Pediatric Endocrinology, Pediatric
Pulmonology, Pediatric Hematology-Oncology and Pediatric Nephrology.

Rate of Nonfederal Physicians in Pediatrics in 1995

National Rate = 71 Physicians per 100,000 Population 17 Years and Younger*

ALPHA ORDER | RANK ORDER

RANK	STATE	RATE
32	Alabama	52
42	Alaska	39
29	Arizona	53
36	Arkansas	48
15	California	70
18	Colorado	64
4	Connecticut	112
9	Delaware	82
13	Florida	72
26	Georgia	55
8	Hawaii	85
50	Idaho	20
11	Illinois	74
39	Indiana	44
41	Iowa	40
40	Kansas	43
23	Kentucky	57
22	Louisiana	59
32	Maine	52
3	Maryland	127
2	Massachusetts	131
21	Michigan	60
24	Minnesota	56
47	Mississippi	32
18	Missouri	64
45	Montana	33
38	Nebraska	46
45	Nevada	33
20	New Hampshire	63
5	New Jersey	111
28	New Mexico	54
1	New York	132
17	North Carolina	66
44	North Dakota	35
15	Ohio	70
43	Oklahoma	37
36	Oregon	48
10	Pennsylvania	75
6	Rhode Island	109
29	South Carolina	53
48	South Dakota	28
13	Tennessee	72
32	Texas	52
35	Utah	49
7	Vermont	86
12	Virginia	73
24	Washington	56
29	West Virginia	53
26	Wisconsin	55
49	Wyoming	26

RANK	STATE	RATE
1	New York	132
2	Massachusetts	131
3	Maryland	127
4	Connecticut	112
5	New Jersey	111
6	Rhode Island	109
7	Vermont	86
8	Hawaii	85
9	Delaware	82
10	Pennsylvania	75
11	Illinois	74
12	Virginia	73
13	Florida	72
13	Tennessee	72
15	California	70
15	Ohio	70
17	North Carolina	66
18	Colorado	64
18	Missouri	64
20	New Hampshire	63
21	Michigan	60
22	Louisiana	59
23	Kentucky	57
24	Minnesota	56
24	Washington	56
26	Georgia	55
26	Wisconsin	55
28	New Mexico	54
29	Arizona	53
29	South Carolina	53
29	West Virginia	53
32	Alabama	52
32	Maine	52
32	Texas	52
35	Utah	49
36	Arkansas	48
36	Oregon	48
38	Nebraska	46
39	Indiana	44
40	Kansas	43
41	Iowa	40
42	Alaska	39
43	Oklahoma	37
44	North Dakota	35
45	Montana	33
45	Nevada	33
47	Mississippi	32
48	South Dakota	28
49	Wyoming	26
50	Idaho	20

	District of Columbia	327

Source: Morgan Quitno Press using data from American Medical Association (Chicago, Illinois)
"Physician Characteristics and Distribution in the U.S." (1996-97 Edition)
*As of December 31, 1995. National rate does not include physicians in U.S. territories and possessions.
Pediatrics includes Adolescent Medicine, Neonatal-Perinatal, Pediatric Allergy, Pediatric Endocrinology, Pediatric Pulmonology, Pediatric Hematology-Oncology and Pediatric Nephrology.

Nonfederal Physicians in Surgical Specialties in 1995

National Total = 142,161 Physicians*

<table>
<tr><td colspan="4">ALPHA ORDER</td><td colspan="4">RANK ORDER</td></tr>
<tr><td>RANK</td><td>STATE</td><td>PHYSICIANS</td><td>% of USA</td><td>RANK</td><td>STATE</td><td>PHYSICIANS</td><td>% of USA</td></tr>
<tr><td>23</td><td>Alabama</td><td>2,052</td><td>1.44%</td><td>1</td><td>California</td><td>16,998</td><td>11.96%</td></tr>
<tr><td>49</td><td>Alaska</td><td>209</td><td>0.15%</td><td>2</td><td>New York</td><td>13,754</td><td>9.67%</td></tr>
<tr><td>24</td><td>Arizona</td><td>1,946</td><td>1.37%</td><td>3</td><td>Texas</td><td>8,771</td><td>6.17%</td></tr>
<tr><td>33</td><td>Arkansas</td><td>993</td><td>0.70%</td><td>4</td><td>Florida</td><td>7,650</td><td>5.38%</td></tr>
<tr><td>1</td><td>California</td><td>16,998</td><td>11.96%</td><td>5</td><td>Pennsylvania</td><td>7,426</td><td>5.22%</td></tr>
<tr><td>25</td><td>Colorado</td><td>1,906</td><td>1.34%</td><td>6</td><td>Illinois</td><td>6,173</td><td>4.34%</td></tr>
<tr><td>19</td><td>Connecticut</td><td>2,440</td><td>1.72%</td><td>7</td><td>Ohio</td><td>5,805</td><td>4.08%</td></tr>
<tr><td>45</td><td>Delaware</td><td>344</td><td>0.24%</td><td>8</td><td>New Jersey</td><td>4,874</td><td>3.43%</td></tr>
<tr><td>4</td><td>Florida</td><td>7,650</td><td>5.38%</td><td>9</td><td>Michigan</td><td>4,685</td><td>3.30%</td></tr>
<tr><td>13</td><td>Georgia</td><td>3,666</td><td>2.58%</td><td>10</td><td>Massachusetts</td><td>4,483</td><td>3.15%</td></tr>
<tr><td>38</td><td>Hawaii</td><td>667</td><td>0.47%</td><td>11</td><td>North Carolina</td><td>3,762</td><td>2.65%</td></tr>
<tr><td>43</td><td>Idaho</td><td>423</td><td>0.30%</td><td>12</td><td>Maryland</td><td>3,754</td><td>2.64%</td></tr>
<tr><td>6</td><td>Illinois</td><td>6,173</td><td>4.34%</td><td>13</td><td>Georgia</td><td>3,666</td><td>2.58%</td></tr>
<tr><td>21</td><td>Indiana</td><td>2,341</td><td>1.65%</td><td>14</td><td>Virginia</td><td>3,584</td><td>2.52%</td></tr>
<tr><td>30</td><td>Iowa</td><td>1,150</td><td>0.81%</td><td>15</td><td>Tennessee</td><td>2,999</td><td>2.11%</td></tr>
<tr><td>31</td><td>Kansas</td><td>1,126</td><td>0.79%</td><td>16</td><td>Missouri</td><td>2,828</td><td>1.99%</td></tr>
<tr><td>26</td><td>Kentucky</td><td>1,836</td><td>1.29%</td><td>17</td><td>Louisiana</td><td>2,705</td><td>1.90%</td></tr>
<tr><td>17</td><td>Louisiana</td><td>2,705</td><td>1.90%</td><td>18</td><td>Washington</td><td>2,600</td><td>1.83%</td></tr>
<tr><td>42</td><td>Maine</td><td>551</td><td>0.39%</td><td>19</td><td>Connecticut</td><td>2,440</td><td>1.72%</td></tr>
<tr><td>12</td><td>Maryland</td><td>3,754</td><td>2.64%</td><td>20</td><td>Wisconsin</td><td>2,380</td><td>1.67%</td></tr>
<tr><td>10</td><td>Massachusetts</td><td>4,483</td><td>3.15%</td><td>21</td><td>Indiana</td><td>2,341</td><td>1.65%</td></tr>
<tr><td>9</td><td>Michigan</td><td>4,685</td><td>3.30%</td><td>22</td><td>Minnesota</td><td>2,264</td><td>1.59%</td></tr>
<tr><td>22</td><td>Minnesota</td><td>2,264</td><td>1.59%</td><td>23</td><td>Alabama</td><td>2,052</td><td>1.44%</td></tr>
<tr><td>32</td><td>Mississippi</td><td>1,040</td><td>0.73%</td><td>24</td><td>Arizona</td><td>1,946</td><td>1.37%</td></tr>
<tr><td>16</td><td>Missouri</td><td>2,828</td><td>1.99%</td><td>25</td><td>Colorado</td><td>1,906</td><td>1.34%</td></tr>
<tr><td>44</td><td>Montana</td><td>402</td><td>0.28%</td><td>26</td><td>Kentucky</td><td>1,836</td><td>1.29%</td></tr>
<tr><td>36</td><td>Nebraska</td><td>763</td><td>0.54%</td><td>27</td><td>South Carolina</td><td>1,738</td><td>1.22%</td></tr>
<tr><td>40</td><td>Nevada</td><td>601</td><td>0.42%</td><td>28</td><td>Oregon</td><td>1,595</td><td>1.12%</td></tr>
<tr><td>41</td><td>New Hampshire</td><td>590</td><td>0.42%</td><td>29</td><td>Oklahoma</td><td>1,243</td><td>0.87%</td></tr>
<tr><td>8</td><td>New Jersey</td><td>4,874</td><td>3.43%</td><td>30</td><td>Iowa</td><td>1,150</td><td>0.81%</td></tr>
<tr><td>37</td><td>New Mexico</td><td>720</td><td>0.51%</td><td>31</td><td>Kansas</td><td>1,126</td><td>0.79%</td></tr>
<tr><td>2</td><td>New York</td><td>13,754</td><td>9.67%</td><td>32</td><td>Mississippi</td><td>1,040</td><td>0.73%</td></tr>
<tr><td>11</td><td>North Carolina</td><td>3,762</td><td>2.65%</td><td>33</td><td>Arkansas</td><td>993</td><td>0.70%</td></tr>
<tr><td>47</td><td>North Dakota</td><td>284</td><td>0.20%</td><td>34</td><td>Utah</td><td>935</td><td>0.66%</td></tr>
<tr><td>7</td><td>Ohio</td><td>5,805</td><td>4.08%</td><td>35</td><td>West Virginia</td><td>884</td><td>0.62%</td></tr>
<tr><td>29</td><td>Oklahoma</td><td>1,243</td><td>0.87%</td><td>36</td><td>Nebraska</td><td>763</td><td>0.54%</td></tr>
<tr><td>28</td><td>Oregon</td><td>1,595</td><td>1.12%</td><td>37</td><td>New Mexico</td><td>720</td><td>0.51%</td></tr>
<tr><td>5</td><td>Pennsylvania</td><td>7,426</td><td>5.22%</td><td>38</td><td>Hawaii</td><td>667</td><td>0.47%</td></tr>
<tr><td>39</td><td>Rhode Island</td><td>660</td><td>0.46%</td><td>39</td><td>Rhode Island</td><td>660</td><td>0.46%</td></tr>
<tr><td>27</td><td>South Carolina</td><td>1,738</td><td>1.22%</td><td>40</td><td>Nevada</td><td>601</td><td>0.42%</td></tr>
<tr><td>48</td><td>South Dakota</td><td>265</td><td>0.19%</td><td>41</td><td>New Hampshire</td><td>590</td><td>0.42%</td></tr>
<tr><td>15</td><td>Tennessee</td><td>2,999</td><td>2.11%</td><td>42</td><td>Maine</td><td>551</td><td>0.39%</td></tr>
<tr><td>3</td><td>Texas</td><td>8,771</td><td>6.17%</td><td>43</td><td>Idaho</td><td>423</td><td>0.30%</td></tr>
<tr><td>34</td><td>Utah</td><td>935</td><td>0.66%</td><td>44</td><td>Montana</td><td>402</td><td>0.28%</td></tr>
<tr><td>46</td><td>Vermont</td><td>339</td><td>0.24%</td><td>45</td><td>Delaware</td><td>344</td><td>0.24%</td></tr>
<tr><td>14</td><td>Virginia</td><td>3,584</td><td>2.52%</td><td>46</td><td>Vermont</td><td>339</td><td>0.24%</td></tr>
<tr><td>18</td><td>Washington</td><td>2,600</td><td>1.83%</td><td>47</td><td>North Dakota</td><td>284</td><td>0.20%</td></tr>
<tr><td>35</td><td>West Virginia</td><td>884</td><td>0.62%</td><td>48</td><td>South Dakota</td><td>265</td><td>0.19%</td></tr>
<tr><td>20</td><td>Wisconsin</td><td>2,380</td><td>1.67%</td><td>49</td><td>Alaska</td><td>209</td><td>0.15%</td></tr>
<tr><td>50</td><td>Wyoming</td><td>167</td><td>0.12%</td><td>50</td><td>Wyoming</td><td>167</td><td>0.12%</td></tr>
<tr><td></td><td></td><td></td><td></td><td></td><td>District of Columbia</td><td>790</td><td>0.56%</td></tr>
</table>

Source: American Medical Association (Chicago, Illinois)
    "Physician Characteristics and Distribution in the U.S." (1996-97 Edition)
*As of December 31, 1995. Total does not include 1,375 physicians in U.S. territories and possessions. Surgical Specialties include Colon and Rectal, General, Neurological, Obstetrics & Gynecology, Ophthalmology, Orthopedic, Otolaryngology, Plastic, Thoracic and Urological Surgeries.

Rate of Nonfederal Physicians in Surgical Specialties in 1995

National Rate = 54 Physicians per 100,000 Population*

ALPHA ORDER

RANK	STATE	RATE
25	Alabama	48
49	Alaska	35
36	Arizona	45
41	Arkansas	40
12	California	54
19	Colorado	51
2	Connecticut	75
25	Delaware	48
12	Florida	54
19	Georgia	51
10	Hawaii	57
47	Idaho	36
16	Illinois	52
41	Indiana	40
41	Iowa	40
37	Kansas	44
25	Kentucky	48
6	Louisiana	62
37	Maine	44
3	Maryland	74
3	Massachusetts	74
23	Michigan	49
23	Minnesota	49
44	Mississippi	39
15	Missouri	53
34	Montana	46
31	Nebraska	47
44	Nevada	39
19	New Hampshire	51
8	New Jersey	61
40	New Mexico	43
1	New York	76
16	North Carolina	52
37	North Dakota	44
16	Ohio	52
46	Oklahoma	38
19	Oregon	51
6	Pennsylvania	62
5	Rhode Island	67
31	South Carolina	47
47	South Dakota	36
10	Tennessee	57
31	Texas	47
25	Utah	48
9	Vermont	58
12	Virginia	54
25	Washington	48
25	West Virginia	48
34	Wisconsin	46
49	Wyoming	35

RANK ORDER

RANK	STATE	RATE
1	New York	76
2	Connecticut	75
3	Maryland	74
3	Massachusetts	74
5	Rhode Island	67
6	Louisiana	62
6	Pennsylvania	62
8	New Jersey	61
9	Vermont	58
10	Hawaii	57
10	Tennessee	57
12	California	54
12	Florida	54
12	Virginia	54
15	Missouri	53
16	Illinois	52
16	North Carolina	52
16	Ohio	52
19	Colorado	51
19	Georgia	51
19	New Hampshire	51
19	Oregon	51
23	Michigan	49
23	Minnesota	49
25	Alabama	48
25	Delaware	48
25	Kentucky	48
25	Utah	48
25	Washington	48
25	West Virginia	48
31	Nebraska	47
31	South Carolina	47
31	Texas	47
34	Montana	46
34	Wisconsin	46
36	Arizona	45
37	Kansas	44
37	Maine	44
37	North Dakota	44
40	New Mexico	43
41	Arkansas	40
41	Indiana	40
41	Iowa	40
44	Mississippi	39
44	Nevada	39
46	Oklahoma	38
47	Idaho	36
47	South Dakota	36
49	Alaska	35
49	Wyoming	35
	District of Columbia	142

Source: Morgan Quitno Press using data from American Medical Association (Chicago, Illinois)
"Physician Characteristics and Distribution in the U.S." (1996-97 Edition)

As of December 31, 1995. National rate does not include physicians in U.S. territories and possessions. Surgical Specialties include Colon and Rectal, General, Neurological, Obstetrics & Gynecology, Ophthalmology, Orthopedic, Otolaryngology, Plastic, Thoracic and Urological Surgeries.

Nonfederal Physicians in General Surgery in 1995

National Total = 35,820 Physicians*

ALPHA ORDER

RANK	STATE	PHYSICIANS	% of USA
23	Alabama	544	1.52%
49	Alaska	48	0.13%
25	Arizona	460	1.28%
33	Arkansas	257	0.72%
1	California	3,801	10.61%
27	Colorado	443	1.24%
18	Connecticut	594	1.66%
43	Delaware	98	0.27%
5	Florida	1,691	4.72%
12	Georgia	928	2.59%
39	Hawaii	160	0.45%
44	Idaho	96	0.27%
6	Illinois	1,573	4.39%
20	Indiana	584	1.63%
30	Iowa	316	0.88%
29	Kansas	332	0.93%
24	Kentucky	528	1.47%
17	Louisiana	686	1.92%
41	Maine	152	0.42%
11	Maryland	930	2.60%
8	Massachusetts	1,263	3.53%
9	Michigan	1,246	3.48%
22	Minnesota	563	1.57%
34	Mississippi	255	0.71%
16	Missouri	719	2.01%
46	Montana	90	0.25%
35	Nebraska	232	0.65%
42	Nevada	147	0.41%
40	New Hampshire	153	0.43%
10	New Jersey	1,244	3.47%
38	New Mexico	172	0.48%
2	New York	3,795	10.59%
13	North Carolina	920	2.57%
47	North Dakota	88	0.25%
7	Ohio	1,558	4.35%
31	Oklahoma	277	0.77%
28	Oregon	386	1.08%
4	Pennsylvania	2,056	5.74%
37	Rhode Island	177	0.49%
26	South Carolina	449	1.25%
48	South Dakota	80	0.22%
15	Tennessee	796	2.22%
3	Texas	2,070	5.78%
36	Utah	193	0.54%
44	Vermont	96	0.27%
14	Virginia	868	2.42%
19	Washington	591	1.65%
32	West Virginia	269	0.75%
21	Wisconsin	579	1.62%
50	Wyoming	44	0.12%

RANK ORDER

RANK	STATE	PHYSICIANS	% of USA
1	California	3,801	10.61%
2	New York	3,795	10.59%
3	Texas	2,070	5.78%
4	Pennsylvania	2,056	5.74%
5	Florida	1,691	4.72%
6	Illinois	1,573	4.39%
7	Ohio	1,558	4.35%
8	Massachusetts	1,263	3.53%
9	Michigan	1,246	3.48%
10	New Jersey	1,244	3.47%
11	Maryland	930	2.60%
12	Georgia	928	2.59%
13	North Carolina	920	2.57%
14	Virginia	868	2.42%
15	Tennessee	796	2.22%
16	Missouri	719	2.01%
17	Louisiana	686	1.92%
18	Connecticut	594	1.66%
19	Washington	591	1.65%
20	Indiana	584	1.63%
21	Wisconsin	579	1.62%
22	Minnesota	563	1.57%
23	Alabama	544	1.52%
24	Kentucky	528	1.47%
25	Arizona	460	1.28%
26	South Carolina	449	1.25%
27	Colorado	443	1.24%
28	Oregon	386	1.08%
29	Kansas	332	0.93%
30	Iowa	316	0.88%
31	Oklahoma	277	0.77%
32	West Virginia	269	0.75%
33	Arkansas	257	0.72%
34	Mississippi	255	0.71%
35	Nebraska	232	0.65%
36	Utah	193	0.54%
37	Rhode Island	177	0.49%
38	New Mexico	172	0.48%
39	Hawaii	160	0.45%
40	New Hampshire	153	0.43%
41	Maine	152	0.42%
42	Nevada	147	0.41%
43	Delaware	98	0.27%
44	Idaho	96	0.27%
44	Vermont	96	0.27%
46	Montana	90	0.25%
47	North Dakota	88	0.25%
48	South Dakota	80	0.22%
49	Alaska	48	0.13%
50	Wyoming	44	0.12%
	District of Columbia	223	0.62%

Source: American Medical Association (Chicago, Illinois)
  "Physician Characteristics and Distribution in the U.S." (1996-97 Edition)
*As of December 31, 1995. Total does not include 354 physicians in U.S. territories and possessions. General Surgery includes Abdominal, Cardiovascular, Hand, Head and Neck, Pediatric, Traumatic and Vascular Surgeries.

Rate of Nonfederal Physicians in General Surgery in 1995

National Rate = 13.6 Physicians per 100,000 Population*

RANK	STATE	RATE
25	Alabama	12.8
50	Alaska	8.0
39	Arizona	10.7
40	Arkansas	10.3
31	California	12.0
33	Colorado	11.8
4	Connecticut	18.2
14	Delaware	13.7
32	Florida	11.9
23	Georgia	12.9
17	Hawaii	13.6
49	Idaho	8.2
19	Illinois	13.3
43	Indiana	10.1
35	Iowa	11.1
23	Kansas	12.9
14	Kentucky	13.7
8	Louisiana	15.8
27	Maine	12.3
3	Maryland	18.5
2	Massachusetts	20.8
21	Michigan	13.1
29	Minnesota	12.2
46	Mississippi	9.5
18	Missouri	13.5
40	Montana	10.3
12	Nebraska	14.2
45	Nevada	9.6
19	New Hampshire	13.3
9	New Jersey	15.6
42	New Mexico	10.2
1	New York	20.9
25	North Carolina	12.8
14	North Dakota	13.7
13	Ohio	14.0
48	Oklahoma	8.5
27	Oregon	12.3
6	Pennsylvania	17.0
5	Rhode Island	17.8
29	South Carolina	12.2
36	South Dakota	11.0
10	Tennessee	15.2
36	Texas	11.0
44	Utah	9.9
7	Vermont	16.4
21	Virginia	13.1
38	Washington	10.8
11	West Virginia	14.7
34	Wisconsin	11.3
47	Wyoming	9.2

RANK	STATE	RATE
1	New York	20.9
2	Massachusetts	20.8
3	Maryland	18.5
4	Connecticut	18.2
5	Rhode Island	17.8
6	Pennsylvania	17.0
7	Vermont	16.4
8	Louisiana	15.8
9	New Jersey	15.6
10	Tennessee	15.2
11	West Virginia	14.7
12	Nebraska	14.2
13	Ohio	14.0
14	Delaware	13.7
14	Kentucky	13.7
14	North Dakota	13.7
17	Hawaii	13.6
18	Missouri	13.5
19	Illinois	13.3
19	New Hampshire	13.3
21	Michigan	13.1
21	Virginia	13.1
23	Georgia	12.9
23	Kansas	12.9
25	Alabama	12.8
25	North Carolina	12.8
27	Maine	12.3
27	Oregon	12.3
29	Minnesota	12.2
29	South Carolina	12.2
31	California	12.0
32	Florida	11.9
33	Colorado	11.8
34	Wisconsin	11.3
35	Iowa	11.1
36	South Dakota	11.0
36	Texas	11.0
38	Washington	10.8
39	Arizona	10.7
40	Arkansas	10.3
40	Montana	10.3
42	New Mexico	10.2
43	Indiana	10.1
44	Utah	9.9
45	Nevada	9.6
46	Mississippi	9.5
47	Wyoming	9.2
48	Oklahoma	8.5
49	Idaho	8.2
50	Alaska	8.0

District of Columbia   40.2

Source: Morgan Quitno Press using data from American Medical Association (Chicago, Illinois)
"Physician Characteristics and Distribution in the U.S." (1996-97 Edition)
As of December 31, 1995. National rate does not include physicians in U.S. territories and possessions. General Surgery includes Abdominal, Cardiovascular, Hand, Head and Neck, Pediatric, Traumatic and Vascular Surgeries.

Nonfederal Physicians in Obstetrics and Gynecology in 1995

National Total = 36,461 Physicians*

<table>
<tr><td colspan="4">ALPHA ORDER</td><td colspan="4">RANK ORDER</td></tr>
<tr><td>RANK</td><td>STATE</td><td>PHYSICIANS</td><td>% of USA</td><td>RANK</td><td>STATE</td><td>PHYSICIANS</td><td>% of USA</td></tr>
<tr><td>23</td><td>Alabama</td><td>498</td><td>1.37%</td><td>1</td><td>California</td><td>4,497</td><td>12.33%</td></tr>
<tr><td>48</td><td>Alaska</td><td>48</td><td>0.13%</td><td>2</td><td>New York</td><td>3,617</td><td>9.92%</td></tr>
<tr><td>21</td><td>Arizona</td><td>530</td><td>1.45%</td><td>3</td><td>Texas</td><td>2,409</td><td>6.61%</td></tr>
<tr><td>34</td><td>Arkansas</td><td>209</td><td>0.57%</td><td>4</td><td>Florida</td><td>1,809</td><td>4.96%</td></tr>
<tr><td>1</td><td>California</td><td>4,497</td><td>12.33%</td><td>5</td><td>Pennsylvania</td><td>1,744</td><td>4.78%</td></tr>
<tr><td>24</td><td>Colorado</td><td>494</td><td>1.35%</td><td>6</td><td>Illinois</td><td>1,722</td><td>4.72%</td></tr>
<tr><td>17</td><td>Connecticut</td><td>687</td><td>1.88%</td><td>7</td><td>Ohio</td><td>1,466</td><td>4.02%</td></tr>
<tr><td>45</td><td>Delaware</td><td>78</td><td>0.21%</td><td>8</td><td>New Jersey</td><td>1,376</td><td>3.77%</td></tr>
<tr><td>4</td><td>Florida</td><td>1,809</td><td>4.96%</td><td>9</td><td>Michigan</td><td>1,305</td><td>3.58%</td></tr>
<tr><td>12</td><td>Georgia</td><td>1,072</td><td>2.94%</td><td>10</td><td>Maryland</td><td>1,075</td><td>2.95%</td></tr>
<tr><td>33</td><td>Hawaii</td><td>213</td><td>0.58%</td><td>11</td><td>Massachusetts</td><td>1,074</td><td>2.95%</td></tr>
<tr><td>43</td><td>Idaho</td><td>92</td><td>0.25%</td><td>12</td><td>Georgia</td><td>1,072</td><td>2.94%</td></tr>
<tr><td>6</td><td>Illinois</td><td>1,722</td><td>4.72%</td><td>13</td><td>Virginia</td><td>1,034</td><td>2.84%</td></tr>
<tr><td>20</td><td>Indiana</td><td>554</td><td>1.52%</td><td>14</td><td>North Carolina</td><td>1,013</td><td>2.78%</td></tr>
<tr><td>34</td><td>Iowa</td><td>209</td><td>0.57%</td><td>15</td><td>Tennessee</td><td>753</td><td>2.07%</td></tr>
<tr><td>31</td><td>Kansas</td><td>248</td><td>0.68%</td><td>16</td><td>Missouri</td><td>697</td><td>1.91%</td></tr>
<tr><td>27</td><td>Kentucky</td><td>425</td><td>1.17%</td><td>17</td><td>Connecticut</td><td>687</td><td>1.88%</td></tr>
<tr><td>18</td><td>Louisiana</td><td>666</td><td>1.83%</td><td>18</td><td>Louisiana</td><td>666</td><td>1.83%</td></tr>
<tr><td>42</td><td>Maine</td><td>125</td><td>0.34%</td><td>19</td><td>Washington</td><td>606</td><td>1.66%</td></tr>
<tr><td>10</td><td>Maryland</td><td>1,075</td><td>2.95%</td><td>20</td><td>Indiana</td><td>554</td><td>1.52%</td></tr>
<tr><td>11</td><td>Massachusetts</td><td>1,074</td><td>2.95%</td><td>21</td><td>Arizona</td><td>530</td><td>1.45%</td></tr>
<tr><td>9</td><td>Michigan</td><td>1,305</td><td>3.58%</td><td>22</td><td>Wisconsin</td><td>505</td><td>1.39%</td></tr>
<tr><td>25</td><td>Minnesota</td><td>463</td><td>1.27%</td><td>23</td><td>Alabama</td><td>498</td><td>1.37%</td></tr>
<tr><td>30</td><td>Mississippi</td><td>271</td><td>0.74%</td><td>24</td><td>Colorado</td><td>494</td><td>1.35%</td></tr>
<tr><td>16</td><td>Missouri</td><td>697</td><td>1.91%</td><td>25</td><td>Minnesota</td><td>463</td><td>1.27%</td></tr>
<tr><td>44</td><td>Montana</td><td>83</td><td>0.23%</td><td>26</td><td>South Carolina</td><td>451</td><td>1.24%</td></tr>
<tr><td>40</td><td>Nebraska</td><td>152</td><td>0.42%</td><td>27</td><td>Kentucky</td><td>425</td><td>1.17%</td></tr>
<tr><td>38</td><td>Nevada</td><td>169</td><td>0.46%</td><td>28</td><td>Oregon</td><td>364</td><td>1.00%</td></tr>
<tr><td>41</td><td>New Hampshire</td><td>147</td><td>0.40%</td><td>29</td><td>Oklahoma</td><td>297</td><td>0.81%</td></tr>
<tr><td>8</td><td>New Jersey</td><td>1,376</td><td>3.77%</td><td>30</td><td>Mississippi</td><td>271</td><td>0.74%</td></tr>
<tr><td>37</td><td>New Mexico</td><td>190</td><td>0.52%</td><td>31</td><td>Kansas</td><td>248</td><td>0.68%</td></tr>
<tr><td>2</td><td>New York</td><td>3,617</td><td>9.92%</td><td>32</td><td>Utah</td><td>232</td><td>0.64%</td></tr>
<tr><td>14</td><td>North Carolina</td><td>1,013</td><td>2.78%</td><td>33</td><td>Hawaii</td><td>213</td><td>0.58%</td></tr>
<tr><td>47</td><td>North Dakota</td><td>50</td><td>0.14%</td><td>34</td><td>Arkansas</td><td>209</td><td>0.57%</td></tr>
<tr><td>7</td><td>Ohio</td><td>1,466</td><td>4.02%</td><td>34</td><td>Iowa</td><td>209</td><td>0.57%</td></tr>
<tr><td>29</td><td>Oklahoma</td><td>297</td><td>0.81%</td><td>36</td><td>West Virginia</td><td>197</td><td>0.54%</td></tr>
<tr><td>28</td><td>Oregon</td><td>364</td><td>1.00%</td><td>37</td><td>New Mexico</td><td>190</td><td>0.52%</td></tr>
<tr><td>5</td><td>Pennsylvania</td><td>1,744</td><td>4.78%</td><td>38</td><td>Nevada</td><td>169</td><td>0.46%</td></tr>
<tr><td>39</td><td>Rhode Island</td><td>157</td><td>0.43%</td><td>39</td><td>Rhode Island</td><td>157</td><td>0.43%</td></tr>
<tr><td>26</td><td>South Carolina</td><td>451</td><td>1.24%</td><td>40</td><td>Nebraska</td><td>152</td><td>0.42%</td></tr>
<tr><td>49</td><td>South Dakota</td><td>46</td><td>0.13%</td><td>41</td><td>New Hampshire</td><td>147</td><td>0.40%</td></tr>
<tr><td>15</td><td>Tennessee</td><td>753</td><td>2.07%</td><td>42</td><td>Maine</td><td>125</td><td>0.34%</td></tr>
<tr><td>3</td><td>Texas</td><td>2,409</td><td>6.61%</td><td>43</td><td>Idaho</td><td>92</td><td>0.25%</td></tr>
<tr><td>32</td><td>Utah</td><td>232</td><td>0.64%</td><td>44</td><td>Montana</td><td>83</td><td>0.23%</td></tr>
<tr><td>46</td><td>Vermont</td><td>75</td><td>0.21%</td><td>45</td><td>Delaware</td><td>78</td><td>0.21%</td></tr>
<tr><td>13</td><td>Virginia</td><td>1,034</td><td>2.84%</td><td>46</td><td>Vermont</td><td>75</td><td>0.21%</td></tr>
<tr><td>19</td><td>Washington</td><td>606</td><td>1.66%</td><td>47</td><td>North Dakota</td><td>50</td><td>0.14%</td></tr>
<tr><td>36</td><td>West Virginia</td><td>197</td><td>0.54%</td><td>48</td><td>Alaska</td><td>48</td><td>0.13%</td></tr>
<tr><td>22</td><td>Wisconsin</td><td>505</td><td>1.39%</td><td>49</td><td>South Dakota</td><td>46</td><td>0.13%</td></tr>
<tr><td>50</td><td>Wyoming</td><td>38</td><td>0.10%</td><td>50</td><td>Wyoming</td><td>38</td><td>0.10%</td></tr>
<tr><td></td><td></td><td></td><td></td><td></td><td>District of Columbia</td><td>229</td><td>0.63%</td></tr>
</table>

Source: American Medical Association (Chicago, Illinois)
"Physician Characteristics and Distribution in the U.S." (1996-97 Edition)
*As of December 31, 1995. Total does not include 501 physicians in U.S. territories and possessions. Obstetrics and Gynecology includes Gynecology and Oncology, Maternal and Fetal Medicine and Reproductive Endocrinology.

Rate of Nonfederal Physicians in Obstetrics and Gynecology in 1995

National Rate = 27.1 Physicians per 100,000 Female Population*

ALPHA ORDER

RANK	STATE	RATE
28	Alabama	22.5
44	Alaska	16.8
23	Arizona	24.9
45	Arkansas	16.3
11	California	28.5
17	Colorado	26.1
2	Connecticut	40.7
33	Delaware	21.2
24	Florida	24.8
10	Georgia	29.0
4	Hawaii	36.3
47	Idaho	15.8
12	Illinois	28.4
41	Indiana	18.6
49	Iowa	14.3
39	Kansas	19.0
32	Kentucky	21.4
9	Louisiana	29.6
36	Maine	19.6
1	Maryland	41.5
5	Massachusetts	34.1
16	Michigan	26.6
35	Minnesota	19.8
38	Mississippi	19.3
20	Missouri	25.3
39	Montana	19.0
42	Nebraska	18.2
28	Nevada	22.5
21	New Hampshire	25.2
6	New Jersey	33.6
30	New Mexico	22.2
3	New York	38.4
15	North Carolina	27.3
48	North Dakota	15.5
18	Ohio	25.4
43	Oklahoma	17.7
27	Oregon	22.9
13	Pennsylvania	27.8
8	Rhode Island	30.5
25	South Carolina	23.7
50	South Dakota	12.4
14	Tennessee	27.7
18	Texas	25.4
26	Utah	23.6
21	Vermont	25.2
7	Virginia	30.6
30	Washington	22.2
34	West Virginia	20.8
37	Wisconsin	19.4
46	Wyoming	15.9

RANK ORDER

RANK	STATE	RATE
1	Maryland	41.5
2	Connecticut	40.7
3	New York	38.4
4	Hawaii	36.3
5	Massachusetts	34.1
6	New Jersey	33.6
7	Virginia	30.6
8	Rhode Island	30.5
9	Louisiana	29.6
10	Georgia	29.0
11	California	28.5
12	Illinois	28.4
13	Pennsylvania	27.8
14	Tennessee	27.7
15	North Carolina	27.3
16	Michigan	26.6
17	Colorado	26.1
18	Ohio	25.4
18	Texas	25.4
20	Missouri	25.3
21	New Hampshire	25.2
21	Vermont	25.2
23	Arizona	24.9
24	Florida	24.8
25	South Carolina	23.7
26	Utah	23.6
27	Oregon	22.9
28	Alabama	22.5
28	Nevada	22.5
30	New Mexico	22.2
30	Washington	22.2
32	Kentucky	21.4
33	Delaware	21.2
34	West Virginia	20.8
35	Minnesota	19.8
36	Maine	19.6
37	Wisconsin	19.4
38	Mississippi	19.3
39	Kansas	19.0
39	Montana	19.0
41	Indiana	18.6
42	Nebraska	18.2
43	Oklahoma	17.7
44	Alaska	16.8
45	Arkansas	16.3
46	Wyoming	15.9
47	Idaho	15.8
48	North Dakota	15.5
49	Iowa	14.3
50	South Dakota	12.4

District of Columbia	77.7

Source: Morgan Quitno Press using data from American Medical Association (Chicago, Illinois)
   "Physician Characteristics and Distribution in the U.S." (1996-97 Edition)
*As of December 31, 1995. National rate does not include physicians in U.S. territories and possessions.
Obstetrics and Gynecology includes Gynecology and Oncology, Maternal and Fetal Medicine and Reproductive Endocrinology.

Nonfederal Physicians in Ophthalmology in 1995

National Total = 16,967 Physicians*

ALPHA ORDER

RANK	STATE	PHYSICIANS	% of USA
25	Alabama	208	1.23%
49	Alaska	23	0.14%
23	Arizona	241	1.42%
32	Arkansas	132	0.78%
1	California	2,069	12.19%
24	Colorado	230	1.36%
19	Connecticut	299	1.76%
45	Delaware	45	0.27%
3	Florida	1,047	6.17%
14	Georgia	372	2.19%
37	Hawaii	82	0.48%
43	Idaho	54	0.32%
6	Illinois	703	4.14%
22	Indiana	267	1.57%
29	Iowa	165	0.97%
31	Kansas	134	0.79%
27	Kentucky	200	1.18%
15	Louisiana	341	2.01%
41	Maine	61	0.36%
11	Maryland	459	2.71%
9	Massachusetts	547	3.22%
10	Michigan	545	3.21%
21	Minnesota	293	1.73%
33	Mississippi	125	0.74%
15	Missouri	341	2.01%
44	Montana	50	0.29%
36	Nebraska	94	0.55%
42	Nevada	60	0.35%
40	New Hampshire	64	0.38%
8	New Jersey	602	3.55%
38	New Mexico	74	0.44%
2	New York	1,780	10.49%
12	North Carolina	384	2.26%
48	North Dakota	34	0.20%
7	Ohio	624	3.68%
30	Oklahoma	149	0.88%
28	Oregon	195	1.15%
5	Pennsylvania	914	5.39%
39	Rhode Island	69	0.41%
26	South Carolina	205	1.21%
47	South Dakota	38	0.22%
18	Tennessee	316	1.86%
4	Texas	984	5.80%
34	Utah	108	0.64%
46	Vermont	40	0.24%
13	Virginia	379	2.23%
20	Washington	296	1.74%
35	West Virginia	98	0.58%
17	Wisconsin	326	1.92%
50	Wyoming	13	0.08%

RANK ORDER

RANK	STATE	PHYSICIANS	% of USA
1	California	2,069	12.19%
2	New York	1,780	10.49%
3	Florida	1,047	6.17%
4	Texas	984	5.80%
5	Pennsylvania	914	5.39%
6	Illinois	703	4.14%
7	Ohio	624	3.68%
8	New Jersey	602	3.55%
9	Massachusetts	547	3.22%
10	Michigan	545	3.21%
11	Maryland	459	2.71%
12	North Carolina	384	2.26%
13	Virginia	379	2.23%
14	Georgia	372	2.19%
15	Louisiana	341	2.01%
15	Missouri	341	2.01%
17	Wisconsin	326	1.92%
18	Tennessee	316	1.86%
19	Connecticut	299	1.76%
20	Washington	296	1.74%
21	Minnesota	293	1.73%
22	Indiana	267	1.57%
23	Arizona	241	1.42%
24	Colorado	230	1.36%
25	Alabama	208	1.23%
26	South Carolina	205	1.21%
27	Kentucky	200	1.18%
28	Oregon	195	1.15%
29	Iowa	165	0.97%
30	Oklahoma	149	0.88%
31	Kansas	134	0.79%
32	Arkansas	132	0.78%
33	Mississippi	125	0.74%
34	Utah	108	0.64%
35	West Virginia	98	0.58%
36	Nebraska	94	0.55%
37	Hawaii	82	0.48%
38	New Mexico	74	0.44%
39	Rhode Island	69	0.41%
40	New Hampshire	64	0.38%
41	Maine	61	0.36%
42	Nevada	60	0.35%
43	Idaho	54	0.32%
44	Montana	50	0.29%
45	Delaware	45	0.27%
46	Vermont	40	0.24%
47	South Dakota	38	0.22%
48	North Dakota	34	0.20%
49	Alaska	23	0.14%
50	Wyoming	13	0.08%
	District of Columbia	88	0.52%

Source: American Medical Association (Chicago, Illinois)
"Physician Characteristics and Distribution in the U.S." (1996-97 Edition)
*As of December 31, 1995. Total does not include 158 physicians in U.S. territories and possessions.

Rate of Nonfederal Physicians in Ophthalmology in 1995

National Rate = 6.5 Physicians per 100,000 Population*

<table>
<tr><td colspan="3"><u>ALPHA ORDER</u></td><td colspan="3"><u>RANK ORDER</u></td></tr>
<tr><td>RANK</td><td>STATE</td><td>RATE</td><td>RANK</td><td>STATE</td><td>RATE</td></tr>
<tr><td>41</td><td>Alabama</td><td>4.9</td><td>1</td><td>New York</td><td>9.8</td></tr>
<tr><td>49</td><td>Alaska</td><td>3.8</td><td>2</td><td>Connecticut</td><td>9.1</td></tr>
<tr><td>26</td><td>Arizona</td><td>5.6</td><td>2</td><td>Maryland</td><td>9.1</td></tr>
<tr><td>33</td><td>Arkansas</td><td>5.3</td><td>4</td><td>Massachusetts</td><td>9.0</td></tr>
<tr><td>12</td><td>California</td><td>6.6</td><td>5</td><td>Louisiana</td><td>7.9</td></tr>
<tr><td>18</td><td>Colorado</td><td>6.1</td><td>6</td><td>New Jersey</td><td>7.6</td></tr>
<tr><td>2</td><td>Connecticut</td><td>9.1</td><td>6</td><td>Pennsylvania</td><td>7.6</td></tr>
<tr><td>15</td><td>Delaware</td><td>6.3</td><td>8</td><td>Florida</td><td>7.4</td></tr>
<tr><td>8</td><td>Florida</td><td>7.4</td><td>9</td><td>Hawaii</td><td>7.0</td></tr>
<tr><td>36</td><td>Georgia</td><td>5.2</td><td>9</td><td>Rhode Island</td><td>7.0</td></tr>
<tr><td>9</td><td>Hawaii</td><td>7.0</td><td>11</td><td>Vermont</td><td>6.8</td></tr>
<tr><td>43</td><td>Idaho</td><td>4.6</td><td>12</td><td>California</td><td>6.6</td></tr>
<tr><td>19</td><td>Illinois</td><td>6.0</td><td>13</td><td>Missouri</td><td>6.4</td></tr>
<tr><td>43</td><td>Indiana</td><td>4.6</td><td>13</td><td>Wisconsin</td><td>6.4</td></tr>
<tr><td>21</td><td>Iowa</td><td>5.8</td><td>15</td><td>Delaware</td><td>6.3</td></tr>
<tr><td>36</td><td>Kansas</td><td>5.2</td><td>15</td><td>Minnesota</td><td>6.3</td></tr>
<tr><td>36</td><td>Kentucky</td><td>5.2</td><td>17</td><td>Oregon</td><td>6.2</td></tr>
<tr><td>5</td><td>Louisiana</td><td>7.9</td><td>18</td><td>Colorado</td><td>6.1</td></tr>
<tr><td>41</td><td>Maine</td><td>4.9</td><td>19</td><td>Illinois</td><td>6.0</td></tr>
<tr><td>2</td><td>Maryland</td><td>9.1</td><td>19</td><td>Tennessee</td><td>6.0</td></tr>
<tr><td>4</td><td>Massachusetts</td><td>9.0</td><td>21</td><td>Iowa</td><td>5.8</td></tr>
<tr><td>22</td><td>Michigan</td><td>5.7</td><td>22</td><td>Michigan</td><td>5.7</td></tr>
<tr><td>15</td><td>Minnesota</td><td>6.3</td><td>22</td><td>Montana</td><td>5.7</td></tr>
<tr><td>43</td><td>Mississippi</td><td>4.6</td><td>22</td><td>Nebraska</td><td>5.7</td></tr>
<tr><td>13</td><td>Missouri</td><td>6.4</td><td>22</td><td>Virginia</td><td>5.7</td></tr>
<tr><td>22</td><td>Montana</td><td>5.7</td><td>26</td><td>Arizona</td><td>5.6</td></tr>
<tr><td>22</td><td>Nebraska</td><td>5.7</td><td>26</td><td>New Hampshire</td><td>5.6</td></tr>
<tr><td>48</td><td>Nevada</td><td>3.9</td><td>26</td><td>Ohio</td><td>5.6</td></tr>
<tr><td>26</td><td>New Hampshire</td><td>5.6</td><td>26</td><td>South Carolina</td><td>5.6</td></tr>
<tr><td>6</td><td>New Jersey</td><td>7.6</td><td>30</td><td>Utah</td><td>5.5</td></tr>
<tr><td>47</td><td>New Mexico</td><td>4.4</td><td>31</td><td>Washington</td><td>5.4</td></tr>
<tr><td>1</td><td>New York</td><td>9.8</td><td>31</td><td>West Virginia</td><td>5.4</td></tr>
<tr><td>33</td><td>North Carolina</td><td>5.3</td><td>33</td><td>Arkansas</td><td>5.3</td></tr>
<tr><td>33</td><td>North Dakota</td><td>5.3</td><td>33</td><td>North Carolina</td><td>5.3</td></tr>
<tr><td>26</td><td>Ohio</td><td>5.6</td><td>33</td><td>North Dakota</td><td>5.3</td></tr>
<tr><td>46</td><td>Oklahoma</td><td>4.5</td><td>36</td><td>Georgia</td><td>5.2</td></tr>
<tr><td>17</td><td>Oregon</td><td>6.2</td><td>36</td><td>Kansas</td><td>5.2</td></tr>
<tr><td>6</td><td>Pennsylvania</td><td>7.6</td><td>36</td><td>Kentucky</td><td>5.2</td></tr>
<tr><td>9</td><td>Rhode Island</td><td>7.0</td><td>36</td><td>South Dakota</td><td>5.2</td></tr>
<tr><td>26</td><td>South Carolina</td><td>5.6</td><td>36</td><td>Texas</td><td>5.2</td></tr>
<tr><td>36</td><td>South Dakota</td><td>5.2</td><td>41</td><td>Alabama</td><td>4.9</td></tr>
<tr><td>19</td><td>Tennessee</td><td>6.0</td><td>41</td><td>Maine</td><td>4.9</td></tr>
<tr><td>36</td><td>Texas</td><td>5.2</td><td>43</td><td>Idaho</td><td>4.6</td></tr>
<tr><td>30</td><td>Utah</td><td>5.5</td><td>43</td><td>Indiana</td><td>4.6</td></tr>
<tr><td>11</td><td>Vermont</td><td>6.8</td><td>43</td><td>Mississippi</td><td>4.6</td></tr>
<tr><td>22</td><td>Virginia</td><td>5.7</td><td>46</td><td>Oklahoma</td><td>4.5</td></tr>
<tr><td>31</td><td>Washington</td><td>5.4</td><td>47</td><td>New Mexico</td><td>4.4</td></tr>
<tr><td>31</td><td>West Virginia</td><td>5.4</td><td>48</td><td>Nevada</td><td>3.9</td></tr>
<tr><td>13</td><td>Wisconsin</td><td>6.4</td><td>49</td><td>Alaska</td><td>3.8</td></tr>
<tr><td>50</td><td>Wyoming</td><td>2.7</td><td>50</td><td>Wyoming</td><td>2.7</td></tr>
<tr><td></td><td></td><td></td><td></td><td>District of Columbia</td><td>15.9</td></tr>
</table>

Source: Morgan Quitno Press using data from American Medical Association (Chicago, Illinois)
"Physician Characteristics and Distribution in the U.S." (1996-97 Edition)
*As of December 31, 1995. National rate does not include physicians in U.S. territories and possessions.

Nonfederal Physicians in Orthopedic Surgery in 1995

National Total = 21,318 Physicians*

ALPHA ORDER				RANK ORDER			
RANK	STATE	PHYSICIANS	% of USA	RANK	STATE	PHYSICIANS	% of USA
25	Alabama	307	1.44%	1	California	2,825	13.25%
46	Alaska	48	0.23%	2	New York	1,719	8.06%
24	Arizona	313	1.47%	3	Texas	1,280	6.00%
33	Arkansas	158	0.74%	4	Florida	1,165	5.46%
1	California	2,825	13.25%	5	Pennsylvania	1,068	5.01%
23	Colorado	347	1.63%	6	Ohio	881	4.13%
22	Connecticut	360	1.69%	7	Illinois	842	3.95%
47	Delaware	47	0.22%	8	Massachusetts	676	3.17%
4	Florida	1,165	5.46%	9	New Jersey	667	3.13%
12	Georgia	516	2.42%	10	Michigan	621	2.91%
41	Hawaii	86	0.40%	11	North Carolina	590	2.77%
43	Idaho	83	0.39%	12	Georgia	516	2.42%
7	Illinois	842	3.95%	13	Virginia	513	2.41%
20	Indiana	387	1.82%	14	Maryland	491	2.30%
31	Iowa	180	0.84%	15	Washington	474	2.22%
30	Kansas	184	0.86%	16	Wisconsin	436	2.05%
28	Kentucky	257	1.21%	17	Tennessee	435	2.04%
21	Louisiana	379	1.78%	18	Minnesota	416	1.95%
40	Maine	104	0.49%	19	Missouri	394	1.85%
14	Maryland	491	2.30%	20	Indiana	387	1.82%
8	Massachusetts	676	3.17%	21	Louisiana	379	1.78%
10	Michigan	621	2.91%	22	Connecticut	360	1.69%
18	Minnesota	416	1.95%	23	Colorado	347	1.63%
35	Mississippi	136	0.64%	24	Arizona	313	1.47%
19	Missouri	394	1.85%	25	Alabama	307	1.44%
44	Montana	78	0.37%	26	Oregon	277	1.30%
36	Nebraska	120	0.56%	27	South Carolina	259	1.21%
42	Nevada	85	0.40%	28	Kentucky	257	1.21%
39	New Hampshire	111	0.52%	29	Oklahoma	202	0.95%
9	New Jersey	667	3.13%	30	Kansas	184	0.86%
34	New Mexico	144	0.68%	31	Iowa	180	0.84%
2	New York	1,719	8.06%	32	Utah	164	0.77%
11	North Carolina	590	2.77%	33	Arkansas	158	0.74%
50	North Dakota	37	0.17%	34	New Mexico	144	0.68%
6	Ohio	881	4.13%	35	Mississippi	136	0.64%
29	Oklahoma	202	0.95%	36	Nebraska	120	0.56%
26	Oregon	277	1.30%	37	Rhode Island	119	0.56%
5	Pennsylvania	1,068	5.01%	38	West Virginia	112	0.53%
37	Rhode Island	119	0.56%	39	New Hampshire	111	0.52%
27	South Carolina	259	1.21%	40	Maine	104	0.49%
48	South Dakota	41	0.19%	41	Hawaii	86	0.40%
17	Tennessee	435	2.04%	42	Nevada	85	0.40%
3	Texas	1,280	6.00%	43	Idaho	83	0.39%
32	Utah	164	0.77%	44	Montana	78	0.37%
45	Vermont	66	0.31%	45	Vermont	66	0.31%
13	Virginia	513	2.41%	46	Alaska	48	0.23%
15	Washington	474	2.22%	47	Delaware	47	0.22%
38	West Virginia	112	0.53%	48	South Dakota	41	0.19%
16	Wisconsin	436	2.05%	49	Wyoming	40	0.19%
49	Wyoming	40	0.19%	50	North Dakota	37	0.17%
					District of Columbia	78	0.37%

Source: American Medical Association (Chicago, Illinois)
"Physician Characteristics and Distribution in the U.S." (1996-97 Edition)
As of December 31, 1995. Total does not include 112 physicians in U.S. territories and possessions.

Rate of Nonfederal Physicians in Orthopedic Surgery in 1995

National Rate = 8.1 Physicians per 100,000 Population*

RANK	STATE (ALPHA ORDER)	RATE		RANK	STATE (RANK ORDER)	RATE
32	Alabama	7.2		1	Rhode Island	12.0
25	Alaska	8.0		2	Vermont	11.3
29	Arizona	7.3		3	Massachusetts	11.1
43	Arkansas	6.4		4	Connecticut	11.0
11	California	8.9		5	Maryland	9.7
8	Colorado	9.3		5	New Hampshire	9.7
4	Connecticut	11.0		7	New York	9.4
41	Delaware	6.6		8	Colorado	9.3
23	Florida	8.2		9	Minnesota	9.0
32	Georgia	7.2		9	Montana	9.0
29	Hawaii	7.3		11	California	8.9
35	Idaho	7.1		11	Pennsylvania	8.9
35	Illinois	7.1		13	Oregon	8.8
39	Indiana	6.7		14	Louisiana	8.7
44	Iowa	6.3		14	Washington	8.7
32	Kansas	7.2		16	New Mexico	8.5
39	Kentucky	6.7		16	Wisconsin	8.5
14	Louisiana	8.7		18	Maine	8.4
18	Maine	8.4		18	New Jersey	8.4
5	Maryland	9.7		18	Utah	8.4
3	Massachusetts	11.1		18	Wyoming	8.4
42	Michigan	6.5		22	Tennessee	8.3
9	Minnesota	9.0		23	Florida	8.2
50	Mississippi	5.0		23	North Carolina	8.2
28	Missouri	7.4		25	Alaska	8.0
9	Montana	9.0		26	Ohio	7.9
29	Nebraska	7.3		27	Virginia	7.8
49	Nevada	5.5		28	Missouri	7.4
5	New Hampshire	9.7		29	Arizona	7.3
18	New Jersey	8.4		29	Hawaii	7.3
16	New Mexico	8.5		29	Nebraska	7.3
7	New York	9.4		32	Alabama	7.2
23	North Carolina	8.2		32	Georgia	7.2
47	North Dakota	5.8		32	Kansas	7.2
26	Ohio	7.9		35	Idaho	7.1
45	Oklahoma	6.2		35	Illinois	7.1
13	Oregon	8.8		35	South Carolina	7.1
11	Pennsylvania	8.9		38	Texas	6.8
1	Rhode Island	12.0		39	Indiana	6.7
35	South Carolina	7.1		39	Kentucky	6.7
48	South Dakota	5.6		41	Delaware	6.6
22	Tennessee	8.3		42	Michigan	6.5
38	Texas	6.8		43	Arkansas	6.4
18	Utah	8.4		44	Iowa	6.3
2	Vermont	11.3		45	Oklahoma	6.2
27	Virginia	7.8		46	West Virginia	6.1
14	Washington	8.7		47	North Dakota	5.8
46	West Virginia	6.1		48	South Dakota	5.6
16	Wisconsin	8.5		49	Nevada	5.5
18	Wyoming	8.4		50	Mississippi	5.0

District of Columbia 14.1

Source: Morgan Quitno Press using data from American Medical Association (Chicago, Illinois)
    "Physician Characteristics and Distribution in the U.S." (1996-97 Edition)
*As of December 31, 1995. National rate does not include physicians in U.S. territories and possessions.

Nonfederal Physicians in Plastic Surgery in 1995

National Total = 5,404 Physicians*

ALPHA ORDER

RANK	STATE	PHYSICIANS	% of USA
26	Alabama	67	1.24%
46	Alaska	9	0.17%
17	Arizona	102	1.89%
39	Arkansas	20	0.37%
1	California	812	15.03%
21	Colorado	78	1.44%
20	Connecticut	81	1.50%
45	Delaware	14	0.26%
3	Florida	406	7.51%
12	Georgia	127	2.35%
33	Hawaii	29	0.54%
43	Idaho	15	0.28%
7	Illinois	197	3.65%
22	Indiana	77	1.42%
35	Iowa	21	0.39%
30	Kansas	44	0.81%
24	Kentucky	72	1.33%
19	Louisiana	87	1.61%
43	Maine	15	0.28%
11	Maryland	136	2.52%
10	Massachusetts	160	2.96%
9	Michigan	163	3.02%
25	Minnesota	68	1.26%
33	Mississippi	29	0.54%
15	Missouri	117	2.17%
42	Montana	16	0.30%
41	Nebraska	18	0.33%
32	Nevada	34	0.63%
40	New Hampshire	19	0.35%
8	New Jersey	171	3.16%
35	New Mexico	21	0.39%
2	New York	538	9.96%
14	North Carolina	124	2.29%
47	North Dakota	8	0.15%
6	Ohio	203	3.76%
30	Oklahoma	44	0.81%
27	Oregon	52	0.96%
5	Pennsylvania	238	4.40%
35	Rhode Island	21	0.39%
29	South Carolina	49	0.91%
49	South Dakota	6	0.11%
16	Tennessee	110	2.04%
4	Texas	378	6.99%
28	Utah	51	0.94%
48	Vermont	7	0.13%
12	Virginia	127	2.35%
18	Washington	99	1.83%
35	West Virginia	21	0.39%
23	Wisconsin	73	1.35%
50	Wyoming	3	0.06%

RANK ORDER

RANK	STATE	PHYSICIANS	% of USA
1	California	812	15.03%
2	New York	538	9.96%
3	Florida	406	7.51%
4	Texas	378	6.99%
5	Pennsylvania	238	4.40%
6	Ohio	203	3.76%
7	Illinois	197	3.65%
8	New Jersey	171	3.16%
9	Michigan	163	3.02%
10	Massachusetts	160	2.96%
11	Maryland	136	2.52%
12	Georgia	127	2.35%
12	Virginia	127	2.35%
14	North Carolina	124	2.29%
15	Missouri	117	2.17%
16	Tennessee	110	2.04%
17	Arizona	102	1.89%
18	Washington	99	1.83%
19	Louisiana	87	1.61%
20	Connecticut	81	1.50%
21	Colorado	78	1.44%
22	Indiana	77	1.42%
23	Wisconsin	73	1.35%
24	Kentucky	72	1.33%
25	Minnesota	68	1.26%
26	Alabama	67	1.24%
27	Oregon	52	0.96%
28	Utah	51	0.94%
29	South Carolina	49	0.91%
30	Kansas	44	0.81%
30	Oklahoma	44	0.81%
32	Nevada	34	0.63%
33	Hawaii	29	0.54%
33	Mississippi	29	0.54%
35	Iowa	21	0.39%
35	New Mexico	21	0.39%
35	Rhode Island	21	0.39%
35	West Virginia	21	0.39%
39	Arkansas	20	0.37%
40	New Hampshire	19	0.35%
41	Nebraska	18	0.33%
42	Montana	16	0.30%
43	Idaho	15	0.28%
43	Maine	15	0.28%
45	Delaware	14	0.26%
46	Alaska	9	0.17%
47	North Dakota	8	0.15%
48	Vermont	7	0.13%
49	South Dakota	6	0.11%
50	Wyoming	3	0.06%
	District of Columbia	27	0.50%

Source: American Medical Association (Chicago, Illinois)
  "Physician Characteristics and Distribution in the U.S." (1996-97 Edition)
*As of December 31, 1995. Total does not include 25 physicians in U.S. territories and possessions.

Rate of Nonfederal Physicians in Plastic Surgery in 1995

National Rate = 2.1 Physicians per 100,000 Population*

<table>
<tr><td colspan="3">ALPHA ORDER</td><td colspan="3">RANK ORDER</td></tr>
<tr><td>RANK</td><td>STATE</td><td>RATE</td><td>RANK</td><td>STATE</td><td>RATE</td></tr>
<tr><td>32</td><td>Alabama</td><td>1.6</td><td>1</td><td>New York</td><td>3.0</td></tr>
<tr><td>33</td><td>Alaska</td><td>1.5</td><td>2</td><td>Florida</td><td>2.9</td></tr>
<tr><td>9</td><td>Arizona</td><td>2.4</td><td>3</td><td>Maryland</td><td>2.7</td></tr>
<tr><td>47</td><td>Arkansas</td><td>0.8</td><td>4</td><td>California</td><td>2.6</td></tr>
<tr><td>4</td><td>California</td><td>2.6</td><td>4</td><td>Massachusetts</td><td>2.6</td></tr>
<tr><td>13</td><td>Colorado</td><td>2.1</td><td>4</td><td>Utah</td><td>2.6</td></tr>
<tr><td>7</td><td>Connecticut</td><td>2.5</td><td>7</td><td>Connecticut</td><td>2.5</td></tr>
<tr><td>16</td><td>Delaware</td><td>2.0</td><td>7</td><td>Hawaii</td><td>2.5</td></tr>
<tr><td>2</td><td>Florida</td><td>2.9</td><td>9</td><td>Arizona</td><td>2.4</td></tr>
<tr><td>22</td><td>Georgia</td><td>1.8</td><td>10</td><td>Missouri</td><td>2.2</td></tr>
<tr><td>7</td><td>Hawaii</td><td>2.5</td><td>10</td><td>Nevada</td><td>2.2</td></tr>
<tr><td>36</td><td>Idaho</td><td>1.3</td><td>10</td><td>New Jersey</td><td>2.2</td></tr>
<tr><td>26</td><td>Illinois</td><td>1.7</td><td>13</td><td>Colorado</td><td>2.1</td></tr>
<tr><td>36</td><td>Indiana</td><td>1.3</td><td>13</td><td>Rhode Island</td><td>2.1</td></tr>
<tr><td>49</td><td>Iowa</td><td>0.7</td><td>13</td><td>Tennessee</td><td>2.1</td></tr>
<tr><td>26</td><td>Kansas</td><td>1.7</td><td>16</td><td>Delaware</td><td>2.0</td></tr>
<tr><td>20</td><td>Kentucky</td><td>1.9</td><td>16</td><td>Louisiana</td><td>2.0</td></tr>
<tr><td>16</td><td>Louisiana</td><td>2.0</td><td>16</td><td>Pennsylvania</td><td>2.0</td></tr>
<tr><td>40</td><td>Maine</td><td>1.2</td><td>16</td><td>Texas</td><td>2.0</td></tr>
<tr><td>3</td><td>Maryland</td><td>2.7</td><td>20</td><td>Kentucky</td><td>1.9</td></tr>
<tr><td>4</td><td>Massachusetts</td><td>2.6</td><td>20</td><td>Virginia</td><td>1.9</td></tr>
<tr><td>26</td><td>Michigan</td><td>1.7</td><td>22</td><td>Georgia</td><td>1.8</td></tr>
<tr><td>33</td><td>Minnesota</td><td>1.5</td><td>22</td><td>Montana</td><td>1.8</td></tr>
<tr><td>45</td><td>Mississippi</td><td>1.1</td><td>22</td><td>Ohio</td><td>1.8</td></tr>
<tr><td>10</td><td>Missouri</td><td>2.2</td><td>22</td><td>Washington</td><td>1.8</td></tr>
<tr><td>22</td><td>Montana</td><td>1.8</td><td>26</td><td>Illinois</td><td>1.7</td></tr>
<tr><td>45</td><td>Nebraska</td><td>1.1</td><td>26</td><td>Kansas</td><td>1.7</td></tr>
<tr><td>10</td><td>Nevada</td><td>2.2</td><td>26</td><td>Michigan</td><td>1.7</td></tr>
<tr><td>26</td><td>New Hampshire</td><td>1.7</td><td>26</td><td>New Hampshire</td><td>1.7</td></tr>
<tr><td>10</td><td>New Jersey</td><td>2.2</td><td>26</td><td>North Carolina</td><td>1.7</td></tr>
<tr><td>40</td><td>New Mexico</td><td>1.2</td><td>26</td><td>Oregon</td><td>1.7</td></tr>
<tr><td>1</td><td>New York</td><td>3.0</td><td>32</td><td>Alabama</td><td>1.6</td></tr>
<tr><td>26</td><td>North Carolina</td><td>1.7</td><td>33</td><td>Alaska</td><td>1.5</td></tr>
<tr><td>40</td><td>North Dakota</td><td>1.2</td><td>33</td><td>Minnesota</td><td>1.5</td></tr>
<tr><td>22</td><td>Ohio</td><td>1.8</td><td>35</td><td>Wisconsin</td><td>1.4</td></tr>
<tr><td>36</td><td>Oklahoma</td><td>1.3</td><td>36</td><td>Idaho</td><td>1.3</td></tr>
<tr><td>26</td><td>Oregon</td><td>1.7</td><td>36</td><td>Indiana</td><td>1.3</td></tr>
<tr><td>16</td><td>Pennsylvania</td><td>2.0</td><td>36</td><td>Oklahoma</td><td>1.3</td></tr>
<tr><td>13</td><td>Rhode Island</td><td>2.1</td><td>36</td><td>South Carolina</td><td>1.3</td></tr>
<tr><td>36</td><td>South Carolina</td><td>1.3</td><td>40</td><td>Maine</td><td>1.2</td></tr>
<tr><td>47</td><td>South Dakota</td><td>0.8</td><td>40</td><td>New Mexico</td><td>1.2</td></tr>
<tr><td>13</td><td>Tennessee</td><td>2.1</td><td>40</td><td>North Dakota</td><td>1.2</td></tr>
<tr><td>16</td><td>Texas</td><td>2.0</td><td>40</td><td>Vermont</td><td>1.2</td></tr>
<tr><td>4</td><td>Utah</td><td>2.6</td><td>40</td><td>West Virginia</td><td>1.2</td></tr>
<tr><td>40</td><td>Vermont</td><td>1.2</td><td>45</td><td>Mississippi</td><td>1.1</td></tr>
<tr><td>20</td><td>Virginia</td><td>1.9</td><td>45</td><td>Nebraska</td><td>1.1</td></tr>
<tr><td>22</td><td>Washington</td><td>1.8</td><td>47</td><td>Arkansas</td><td>0.8</td></tr>
<tr><td>40</td><td>West Virginia</td><td>1.2</td><td>47</td><td>South Dakota</td><td>0.8</td></tr>
<tr><td>35</td><td>Wisconsin</td><td>1.4</td><td>49</td><td>Iowa</td><td>0.7</td></tr>
<tr><td>50</td><td>Wyoming</td><td>0.6</td><td>50</td><td>Wyoming</td><td>0.6</td></tr>
<tr><td></td><td></td><td></td><td></td><td>District of Columbia</td><td>4.9</td></tr>
</table>

Source: Morgan Quitno Press using data from American Medical Association (Chicago, Illinois)
"Physician Characteristics and Distribution in the U.S." (1996-97 Edition)
*As of December 31, 1995. National rate does not include physicians in U.S. territories and possessions.

Nonfederal Physicians in Other Specialties in 1995

National Total = 176,635 Physicians*

ALPHA ORDER					RANK ORDER			
RANK	STATE		PHYSICIANS	% of USA	RANK	STATE	PHYSICIANS	% of USA
26	Alabama		1,924	1.09%	1	California	22,152	12.54%
49	Alaska		252	0.14%	2	New York	19,083	10.80%
24	Arizona		2,419	1.37%	3	Texas	10,011	5.67%
33	Arkansas		1,107	0.63%	4	Pennsylvania	9,986	5.65%
1	California		22,152	12.54%	5	Florida	8,371	4.74%
23	Colorado		2,488	1.41%	6	Illinois	8,032	4.55%
16	Connecticut		3,234	1.83%	7	Massachusetts	7,576	4.29%
44	Delaware		477	0.27%	8	Ohio	6,866	3.89%
5	Florida		8,371	4.74%	9	New Jersey	5,801	3.28%
14	Georgia		4,000	2.26%	10	Michigan	5,782	3.27%
37	Hawaii		810	0.46%	11	Maryland	5,400	3.06%
46	Idaho		389	0.22%	12	North Carolina	4,249	2.41%
6	Illinois		8,032	4.55%	13	Virginia	4,095	2.32%
20	Indiana		2,962	1.68%	14	Georgia	4,000	2.26%
31	Iowa		1,219	0.69%	15	Washington	3,567	2.02%
30	Kansas		1,451	0.82%	16	Connecticut	3,234	1.83%
25	Kentucky		2,039	1.15%	17	Tennessee	3,201	1.81%
22	Louisiana		2,574	1.46%	18	Missouri	3,200	1.81%
41	Maine		702	0.40%	19	Wisconsin	3,166	1.79%
11	Maryland		5,400	3.06%	20	Indiana	2,962	1.68%
7	Massachusetts		7,576	4.29%	21	Minnesota	2,826	1.60%
10	Michigan		5,782	3.27%	22	Louisiana	2,574	1.46%
21	Minnesota		2,826	1.60%	23	Colorado	2,488	1.41%
36	Mississippi		918	0.52%	24	Arizona	2,419	1.37%
18	Missouri		3,200	1.81%	25	Kentucky	2,039	1.15%
45	Montana		440	0.25%	26	Alabama	1,924	1.09%
38	Nebraska		808	0.46%	27	South Carolina	1,922	1.09%
42	Nevada		695	0.39%	28	Oregon	1,910	1.08%
40	New Hampshire		744	0.42%	29	Oklahoma	1,480	0.84%
9	New Jersey		5,801	3.28%	30	Kansas	1,451	0.82%
34	New Mexico		995	0.56%	31	Iowa	1,219	0.69%
2	New York		19,083	10.80%	32	Utah	1,114	0.63%
12	North Carolina		4,249	2.41%	33	Arkansas	1,107	0.63%
47	North Dakota		330	0.19%	34	New Mexico	995	0.56%
8	Ohio		6,866	3.89%	35	West Virginia	941	0.53%
29	Oklahoma		1,480	0.84%	36	Mississippi	918	0.52%
28	Oregon		1,910	1.08%	37	Hawaii	810	0.46%
4	Pennsylvania		9,986	5.65%	38	Nebraska	808	0.46%
39	Rhode Island		794	0.45%	39	Rhode Island	794	0.45%
27	South Carolina		1,922	1.09%	40	New Hampshire	744	0.42%
48	South Dakota		283	0.16%	41	Maine	702	0.40%
17	Tennessee		3,201	1.81%	42	Nevada	695	0.39%
3	Texas		10,011	5.67%	43	Vermont	480	0.27%
32	Utah		1,114	0.63%	44	Delaware	477	0.27%
43	Vermont		480	0.27%	45	Montana	440	0.25%
13	Virginia		4,095	2.32%	46	Idaho	389	0.22%
15	Washington		3,567	2.02%	47	North Dakota	330	0.19%
35	West Virginia		941	0.53%	48	South Dakota	283	0.16%
19	Wisconsin		3,166	1.79%	49	Alaska	252	0.14%
50	Wyoming		188	0.11%	50	Wyoming	188	0.11%
						District of Columbia	1,182	0.67%

Source: American Medical Association (Chicago, Illinois)
   "Physician Characteristics and Distribution in the U.S." (1996-97 Edition)
*As of December 31, 1995. Total does not include 1,673 physicians in U.S. territories and possessions. Other Specialties include Aerospace Medicine, Anesthesiology, Child Psychiatry, Diagnostic Radiology, Emergency Medicine, Forensic Pathology, Nuclear Medicine, Occupational Medicine, Neurology, Psychiatry, Public Health, Anatomic/Clinical Pathology, Radiology, Radiation Oncology and other specialties.

Rate of Nonfederal Physicians in Other Specialties in 1995

National Rate = 67 Physicians per 100,000 Population*

ALPHA ORDER

RANK	STATE	RATE
41	Alabama	45
46	Alaska	42
31	Arizona	56
41	Arkansas	45
9	California	70
13	Colorado	66
4	Connecticut	99
12	Delaware	67
24	Florida	59
32	Georgia	55
10	Hawaii	69
50	Idaho	33
11	Illinois	68
37	Indiana	51
45	Iowa	43
28	Kansas	57
33	Kentucky	53
24	Louisiana	59
28	Maine	57
2	Maryland	107
1	Massachusetts	125
19	Michigan	61
19	Minnesota	61
49	Mississippi	34
23	Missouri	60
37	Montana	51
40	Nebraska	49
41	Nevada	45
14	New Hampshire	65
8	New Jersey	73
24	New Mexico	59
3	New York	105
24	North Carolina	59
37	North Dakota	51
16	Ohio	62
41	Oklahoma	45
19	Oregon	61
5	Pennsylvania	83
7	Rhode Island	80
35	South Carolina	52
47	South Dakota	39
19	Tennessee	61
33	Texas	53
28	Utah	57
6	Vermont	82
16	Virginia	62
14	Washington	65
35	West Virginia	52
16	Wisconsin	62
47	Wyoming	39

RANK ORDER

RANK	STATE	RATE
1	Massachusetts	125
2	Maryland	107
3	New York	105
4	Connecticut	99
5	Pennsylvania	83
6	Vermont	82
7	Rhode Island	80
8	New Jersey	73
9	California	70
10	Hawaii	69
11	Illinois	68
12	Delaware	67
13	Colorado	66
14	New Hampshire	65
14	Washington	65
16	Ohio	62
16	Virginia	62
16	Wisconsin	62
19	Michigan	61
19	Minnesota	61
19	Oregon	61
19	Tennessee	61
23	Missouri	60
24	Florida	59
24	Louisiana	59
24	New Mexico	59
24	North Carolina	59
28	Kansas	57
28	Maine	57
28	Utah	57
31	Arizona	56
32	Georgia	55
33	Kentucky	53
33	Texas	53
35	South Carolina	52
35	West Virginia	52
37	Indiana	51
37	Montana	51
37	North Dakota	51
40	Nebraska	49
41	Alabama	45
41	Arkansas	45
41	Nevada	45
41	Oklahoma	45
45	Iowa	43
46	Alaska	42
47	South Dakota	39
47	Wyoming	39
49	Mississippi	34
50	Idaho	33

District of Columbia 213

Source: Morgan Quitno Press using data from American Medical Association (Chicago, Illinois)
    "Physician Characteristics and Distribution in the U.S." (1996-97 Edition)
*As of December 31, 1995. National rate does not include physicians in U.S. territories and possessions. Other Specialties include Aerospace Medicine, Anesthesiology, Child Psychiatry, Diagnostic Radiology, Emergency Medicine, Forensic Pathology, Nuclear Medicine, Occupational Medicine, Neurology, Psychiatry, Public Health, Anatomic/Clinical Pathology, Radiology, Radiation Oncology and other specialties.

Nonfederal Physicians in Anesthesiology in 1995

National Total = 31,890 Physicians*

ALPHA ORDER

RANK ORDER

RANK	STATE	PHYSICIANS	% of USA		RANK	STATE	PHYSICIANS	% of USA
26	Alabama	396	1.24%		1	California	3,954	12.40%
48	Alaska	40	0.13%		2	New York	3,049	9.56%
19	Arizona	551	1.73%		3	Texas	2,268	7.11%
33	Arkansas	201	0.63%		4	Florida	1,816	5.69%
1	California	3,954	12.40%		5	Pennsylvania	1,649	5.17%
24	Colorado	445	1.40%		6	Illinois	1,539	4.83%
21	Connecticut	481	1.51%		7	Ohio	1,272	3.99%
46	Delaware	55	0.17%		8	Massachusetts	1,229	3.85%
4	Florida	1,816	5.69%		9	New Jersey	1,119	3.51%
13	Georgia	744	2.33%		10	Maryland	829	2.60%
40	Hawaii	120	0.38%		11	Washington	799	2.51%
45	Idaho	66	0.21%		12	Michigan	764	2.40%
6	Illinois	1,539	4.83%		13	Georgia	744	2.33%
16	Indiana	667	2.09%		14	Virginia	676	2.12%
31	Iowa	255	0.80%		15	North Carolina	672	2.11%
32	Kansas	249	0.78%		16	Indiana	667	2.09%
23	Kentucky	446	1.40%		17	Wisconsin	632	1.98%
22	Louisiana	454	1.42%		18	Tennessee	629	1.97%
39	Maine	127	0.40%		19	Arizona	551	1.73%
10	Maryland	829	2.60%		20	Missouri	545	1.71%
8	Massachusetts	1,229	3.85%		21	Connecticut	481	1.51%
12	Michigan	764	2.40%		22	Louisiana	454	1.42%
25	Minnesota	443	1.39%		23	Kentucky	446	1.40%
34	Mississippi	183	0.57%		24	Colorado	445	1.40%
20	Missouri	545	1.71%		25	Minnesota	443	1.39%
42	Montana	96	0.30%		26	Alabama	396	1.24%
36	Nebraska	159	0.50%		27	Oregon	378	1.19%
35	Nevada	176	0.55%		28	South Carolina	351	1.10%
41	New Hampshire	117	0.37%		29	Oklahoma	284	0.89%
9	New Jersey	1,119	3.51%		30	Utah	269	0.84%
36	New Mexico	159	0.50%		31	Iowa	255	0.80%
2	New York	3,049	9.56%		32	Kansas	249	0.78%
15	North Carolina	672	2.11%		33	Arkansas	201	0.63%
47	North Dakota	51	0.16%		34	Mississippi	183	0.57%
7	Ohio	1,272	3.99%		35	Nevada	176	0.55%
29	Oklahoma	284	0.89%		36	Nebraska	159	0.50%
27	Oregon	378	1.19%		36	New Mexico	159	0.50%
5	Pennsylvania	1,649	5.17%		38	West Virginia	151	0.47%
43	Rhode Island	93	0.29%		39	Maine	127	0.40%
28	South Carolina	351	1.10%		40	Hawaii	120	0.38%
49	South Dakota	38	0.12%		41	New Hampshire	117	0.37%
18	Tennessee	629	1.97%		42	Montana	96	0.30%
3	Texas	2,268	7.11%		43	Rhode Island	93	0.29%
30	Utah	269	0.84%		44	Vermont	68	0.21%
44	Vermont	68	0.21%		45	Idaho	66	0.21%
14	Virginia	676	2.12%		46	Delaware	55	0.17%
11	Washington	799	2.51%		47	North Dakota	51	0.16%
38	West Virginia	151	0.47%		48	Alaska	40	0.13%
17	Wisconsin	632	1.98%		49	South Dakota	38	0.12%
50	Wyoming	37	0.12%		50	Wyoming	37	0.12%
						District of Columbia	99	0.31%

Source: American Medical Association (Chicago, Illinois)
"Physician Characteristics and Distribution in the U.S." (1996-97 Edition)
As of December 31, 1995. Total does not include 192 physicians in U.S. territories and possessions.

Rate of Nonfederal Physicians in Anesthesiology in 1995

National Rate = 12.1 Physicians per 100,000 Population*

ALPHA ORDER

RANK	STATE	RATE
37	Alabama	9.3
48	Alaska	6.6
10	Arizona	12.8
42	Arkansas	8.1
12	California	12.5
17	Colorado	11.9
4	Connecticut	14.7
45	Delaware	7.7
10	Florida	12.8
25	Georgia	10.3
27	Hawaii	10.2
49	Idaho	5.7
9	Illinois	13.1
20	Indiana	11.5
39	Iowa	9.0
31	Kansas	9.7
18	Kentucky	11.6
24	Louisiana	10.5
25	Maine	10.3
3	Maryland	16.5
1	Massachusetts	20.2
43	Michigan	8.0
33	Minnesota	9.6
47	Mississippi	6.8
27	Missouri	10.2
23	Montana	11.0
31	Nebraska	9.7
20	Nevada	11.5
27	New Hampshire	10.2
6	New Jersey	14.1
35	New Mexico	9.4
2	New York	16.8
37	North Carolina	9.3
44	North Dakota	7.9
22	Ohio	11.4
40	Oklahoma	8.7
15	Oregon	12.0
7	Pennsylvania	13.7
35	Rhode Island	9.4
33	South Carolina	9.6
50	South Dakota	5.2
15	Tennessee	12.0
14	Texas	12.1
7	Utah	13.7
18	Vermont	11.6
27	Virginia	10.2
4	Washington	14.7
41	West Virginia	8.3
13	Wisconsin	12.3
45	Wyoming	7.7

RANK ORDER

RANK	STATE	RATE
1	Massachusetts	20.2
2	New York	16.8
3	Maryland	16.5
4	Connecticut	14.7
4	Washington	14.7
6	New Jersey	14.1
7	Pennsylvania	13.7
7	Utah	13.7
9	Illinois	13.1
10	Arizona	12.8
10	Florida	12.8
12	California	12.5
13	Wisconsin	12.3
14	Texas	12.1
15	Oregon	12.0
15	Tennessee	12.0
17	Colorado	11.9
18	Kentucky	11.6
18	Vermont	11.6
20	Indiana	11.5
20	Nevada	11.5
22	Ohio	11.4
23	Montana	11.0
24	Louisiana	10.5
25	Georgia	10.3
25	Maine	10.3
27	Hawaii	10.2
27	Missouri	10.2
27	New Hampshire	10.2
27	Virginia	10.2
31	Kansas	9.7
31	Nebraska	9.7
33	Minnesota	9.6
33	South Carolina	9.6
35	New Mexico	9.4
35	Rhode Island	9.4
37	Alabama	9.3
37	North Carolina	9.3
39	Iowa	9.0
40	Oklahoma	8.7
41	West Virginia	8.3
42	Arkansas	8.1
43	Michigan	8.0
44	North Dakota	7.9
45	Delaware	7.7
45	Wyoming	7.7
47	Mississippi	6.8
48	Alaska	6.6
49	Idaho	5.7
50	South Dakota	5.2
	District of Columbia	17.8

Source: Morgan Quitno Press using data from American Medical Association (Chicago, Illinois)
    "Physician Characteristics and Distribution in the U.S." (1996-97 Edition)
*As of December 31, 1995. National rate does not include physicians in U.S. territories and possessions.

Nonfederal Physicians in Psychiatry in 1995

National Total = 35,904 Physicians*

ALPHA ORDER					RANK ORDER			

RANK	STATE	PHYSICIANS	% of USA		RANK	STATE	PHYSICIANS	% of USA
29	Alabama	272	0.76%		1	New York	5,514	15.36%
49	Alaska	50	0.14%		2	California	4,817	13.42%
24	Arizona	399	1.11%		3	Massachusetts	1,953	5.44%
34	Arkansas	183	0.51%		4	Pennsylvania	1,927	5.37%
2	California	4,817	13.42%		5	Texas	1,663	4.63%
19	Colorado	520	1.45%		6	Illinois	1,471	4.10%
12	Connecticut	907	2.53%		7	Florida	1,388	3.87%
43	Delaware	99	0.28%		8	New Jersey	1,256	3.50%
7	Florida	1,388	3.87%		9	Maryland	1,245	3.47%
15	Georgia	742	2.07%		10	Ohio	1,085	3.02%
35	Hawaii	181	0.50%		11	Michigan	1,037	2.89%
47	Idaho	60	0.17%		12	Connecticut	907	2.53%
6	Illinois	1,471	4.10%		13	North Carolina	821	2.29%
23	Indiana	403	1.12%		14	Virginia	806	2.24%
36	Iowa	174	0.48%		15	Georgia	742	2.07%
28	Kansas	331	0.92%		16	Washington	637	1.77%
26	Kentucky	348	0.97%		17	Missouri	530	1.48%
21	Louisiana	463	1.29%		18	Wisconsin	528	1.47%
39	Maine	155	0.43%		19	Colorado	520	1.45%
9	Maryland	1,245	3.47%		20	Tennessee	490	1.36%
3	Massachusetts	1,953	5.44%		21	Louisiana	463	1.29%
11	Michigan	1,037	2.89%		22	Minnesota	450	1.25%
22	Minnesota	450	1.25%		23	Indiana	403	1.12%
42	Mississippi	123	0.34%		24	Arizona	399	1.11%
17	Missouri	530	1.48%		25	South Carolina	389	1.08%
46	Montana	66	0.18%		26	Kentucky	348	0.97%
40	Nebraska	150	0.42%		27	Oregon	346	0.96%
44	Nevada	94	0.26%		28	Kansas	331	0.92%
33	New Hampshire	190	0.53%		29	Alabama	272	0.76%
8	New Jersey	1,256	3.50%		30	Oklahoma	245	0.68%
31	New Mexico	226	0.63%		31	New Mexico	226	0.63%
1	New York	5,514	15.36%		32	Rhode Island	193	0.54%
13	North Carolina	821	2.29%		33	New Hampshire	190	0.53%
45	North Dakota	68	0.19%		34	Arkansas	183	0.51%
10	Ohio	1,085	3.02%		35	Hawaii	181	0.50%
30	Oklahoma	245	0.68%		36	Iowa	174	0.48%
27	Oregon	346	0.96%		37	West Virginia	162	0.45%
4	Pennsylvania	1,927	5.37%		38	Utah	160	0.45%
32	Rhode Island	193	0.54%		39	Maine	155	0.43%
25	South Carolina	389	1.08%		40	Nebraska	150	0.42%
48	South Dakota	56	0.16%		41	Vermont	140	0.39%
20	Tennessee	490	1.36%		42	Mississippi	123	0.34%
5	Texas	1,663	4.63%		43	Delaware	99	0.28%
38	Utah	160	0.45%		44	Nevada	94	0.26%
41	Vermont	140	0.39%		45	North Dakota	68	0.19%
14	Virginia	806	2.24%		46	Montana	66	0.18%
16	Washington	637	1.77%		47	Idaho	60	0.17%
37	West Virginia	162	0.45%		48	South Dakota	56	0.16%
18	Wisconsin	528	1.47%		49	Alaska	50	0.14%
50	Wyoming	28	0.08%		50	Wyoming	28	0.08%
						District of Columbia	363	1.01%

Source: American Medical Association (Chicago, Illinois)
    "Physician Characteristics and Distribution in the U.S." (1996-97 Edition)
As of December 31, 1995. Total does not include 295 physicians in U.S. territories and possessions. Psychiatry includes psychoanalysis.

Rate of Nonfederal Physicians in Psychiatry in 1995

National Rate = 13.7 Physicians per 100,000 Population*

ALPHA ORDER

RANK	STATE	RATE
45	Alabama	6.4
38	Alaska	8.3
32	Arizona	9.3
43	Arkansas	7.4
11	California	15.3
12	Colorado	13.9
3	Connecticut	27.7
13	Delaware	13.8
29	Florida	9.8
26	Georgia	10.3
10	Hawaii	15.4
49	Idaho	5.1
16	Illinois	12.5
44	Indiana	7.0
46	Iowa	6.1
15	Kansas	12.9
35	Kentucky	9.0
23	Louisiana	10.7
16	Maine	12.5
4	Maryland	24.7
1	Massachusetts	32.2
22	Michigan	10.9
29	Minnesota	9.8
50	Mississippi	4.6
28	Missouri	10.0
41	Montana	7.6
34	Nebraska	9.2
46	Nevada	6.1
7	New Hampshire	16.6
9	New Jersey	15.8
14	New Mexico	13.4
2	New York	30.3
20	North Carolina	11.4
24	North Dakota	10.6
31	Ohio	9.7
42	Oklahoma	7.5
21	Oregon	11.0
8	Pennsylvania	16.0
6	Rhode Island	19.5
24	South Carolina	10.6
40	South Dakota	7.7
32	Tennessee	9.3
37	Texas	8.8
39	Utah	8.2
5	Vermont	23.9
18	Virginia	12.2
19	Washington	11.7
36	West Virginia	8.9
26	Wisconsin	10.3
48	Wyoming	5.8

RANK ORDER

RANK	STATE	RATE
1	Massachusetts	32.2
2	New York	30.3
3	Connecticut	27.7
4	Maryland	24.7
5	Vermont	23.9
6	Rhode Island	19.5
7	New Hampshire	16.6
8	Pennsylvania	16.0
9	New Jersey	15.8
10	Hawaii	15.4
11	California	15.3
12	Colorado	13.9
13	Delaware	13.8
14	New Mexico	13.4
15	Kansas	12.9
16	Illinois	12.5
16	Maine	12.5
18	Virginia	12.2
19	Washington	11.7
20	North Carolina	11.4
21	Oregon	11.0
22	Michigan	10.9
23	Louisiana	10.7
24	North Dakota	10.6
24	South Carolina	10.6
26	Georgia	10.3
26	Wisconsin	10.3
28	Missouri	10.0
29	Florida	9.8
29	Minnesota	9.8
31	Ohio	9.7
32	Arizona	9.3
32	Tennessee	9.3
34	Nebraska	9.2
35	Kentucky	9.0
36	West Virginia	8.9
37	Texas	8.8
38	Alaska	8.3
39	Utah	8.2
40	South Dakota	7.7
41	Montana	7.6
42	Oklahoma	7.5
43	Arkansas	7.4
44	Indiana	7.0
45	Alabama	6.4
46	Iowa	6.1
46	Nevada	6.1
48	Wyoming	5.8
49	Idaho	5.1
50	Mississippi	4.6

District of Columbia 65.4

Source: Morgan Quitno Press using data from American Medical Association (Chicago, Illinois)
"Physician Characteristics and Distribution in the U.S." (1996-97 Edition)
*As of December 31, 1995. National rate does not include physicians in U.S. territories and possessions.
Psychiatry includes psychoanalysis.

Percent of Nonfederal Physicians Who Are Specialists in 1995

National Percent = 76.18% of Physicians*

ALPHA ORDER				RANK ORDER		
RANK	STATE	PERCENT		RANK	STATE	PERCENT
17	Alabama	75.94		1	Massachusetts	83.85
36	Alaska	69.63		2	New York	83.02
37	Arizona	69.27		3	Rhode Island	82.54
43	Arkansas	67.39		4	Connecticut	82.40
24	California	73.84		5	New Jersey	82.16
28	Colorado	72.50		6	Maryland	82.06
4	Connecticut	82.40		7	Missouri	80.77
23	Delaware	74.33		8	Louisiana	79.40
38	Florida	69.26		9	Georgia	78.60
9	Georgia	78.60		10	Illinois	78.50
14	Hawaii	76.98		11	Pennsylvania	78.26
49	Idaho	60.49		12	Tennessee	78.01
10	Illinois	78.50		13	Michigan	77.72
35	Indiana	70.08		14	Hawaii	76.98
44	Iowa	66.82		15	Ohio	76.83
39	Kansas	68.84		16	Texas	76.30
21	Kentucky	74.70		17	Alabama	75.94
8	Louisiana	79.40		18	North Carolina	75.59
45	Maine	66.55		19	Virginia	75.19
6	Maryland	82.06		20	Utah	75.10
1	Massachusetts	83.85		21	Kentucky	74.70
13	Michigan	77.72		22	Nevada	74.65
40	Minnesota	68.39		23	Delaware	74.33
32	Mississippi	70.72		24	California	73.84
7	Missouri	80.77		25	New Hampshire	72.90
46	Montana	66.47		26	Oklahoma	72.88
41	Nebraska	68.29		27	West Virginia	72.64
22	Nevada	74.65		28	Colorado	72.50
25	New Hampshire	72.90		29	Wisconsin	71.87
5	New Jersey	82.16		30	South Carolina	71.60
34	New Mexico	70.46		31	Vermont	71.45
2	New York	83.02		32	Mississippi	70.72
18	North Carolina	75.59		33	Oregon	70.60
47	North Dakota	65.68		34	New Mexico	70.46
15	Ohio	76.83		35	Indiana	70.08
26	Oklahoma	72.88		36	Alaska	69.63
33	Oregon	70.60		37	Arizona	69.27
11	Pennsylvania	78.26		38	Florida	69.26
3	Rhode Island	82.54		39	Kansas	68.84
30	South Carolina	71.60		40	Minnesota	68.39
48	South Dakota	62.00		41	Nebraska	68.29
12	Tennessee	78.01		42	Washington	67.99
16	Texas	76.30		43	Arkansas	67.39
20	Utah	75.10		44	Iowa	66.82
31	Vermont	71.45		45	Maine	66.55
19	Virginia	75.19		46	Montana	66.47
42	Washington	67.99		47	North Dakota	65.68
27	West Virginia	72.64		48	South Dakota	62.00
29	Wisconsin	71.87		49	Idaho	60.49
50	Wyoming	59.33		50	Wyoming	59.33
					District of Columbia	84.81

Source: Morgan Quitno Press using data from American Medical Association (Chicago, Illinois)
    "Physician Characteristics and Distribution in the U.S." (1996-97 Edition)
*As of December 31, 1995. National rate does not include physicians in U.S. territories and possessions. Includes physicians in medical, surgical and other specialties.

International Medical School Graduates Practicing in the U.S. in 1995

National Total = 156,903 Nonfederal Physicians*

ALPHA ORDER

RANK	STATE	PHYSICIANS	% of USA
26	Alabama	986	0.63%
48	Alaska	56	0.04%
20	Arizona	1,496	0.95%
38	Arkansas	371	0.24%
2	California	17,202	10.96%
32	Colorado	529	0.34%
13	Connecticut	3,086	1.97%
36	Delaware	450	0.29%
3	Florida	12,303	7.84%
15	Georgia	2,297	1.46%
34	Hawaii	499	0.32%
49	Idaho	52	0.03%
4	Illinois	10,790	6.88%
16	Indiana	1,921	1.22%
30	Iowa	718	0.46%
28	Kansas	864	0.55%
23	Kentucky	1,313	0.84%
24	Louisiana	1,285	0.82%
42	Maine	313	0.20%
10	Maryland	5,307	3.38%
11	Massachusetts	4,706	3.00%
9	Michigan	6,660	4.24%
21	Minnesota	1,327	0.85%
40	Mississippi	327	0.21%
14	Missouri	2,426	1.55%
47	Montana	80	0.05%
41	Nebraska	320	0.20%
35	Nevada	466	0.30%
39	New Hampshire	361	0.23%
5	New Jersey	10,707	6.82%
37	New Mexico	425	0.27%
1	New York	29,515	18.81%
19	North Carolina	1,573	1.00%
43	North Dakota	287	0.18%
8	Ohio	6,906	4.40%
29	Oklahoma	806	0.51%
33	Oregon	504	0.32%
6	Pennsylvania	7,982	5.09%
27	Rhode Island	865	0.55%
31	South Carolina	625	0.40%
45	South Dakota	135	0.09%
18	Tennessee	1,637	1.04%
7	Texas	7,899	5.03%
44	Utah	236	0.15%
46	Vermont	124	0.08%
12	Virginia	3,101	1.98%
25	Washington	1,190	0.76%
22	West Virginia	1,326	0.85%
17	Wisconsin	1,779	1.13%
50	Wyoming	43	0.03%

RANK ORDER

RANK	STATE	PHYSICIANS	% of USA
1	New York	29,515	18.81%
2	California	17,202	10.96%
3	Florida	12,303	7.84%
4	Illinois	10,790	6.88%
5	New Jersey	10,707	6.82%
6	Pennsylvania	7,982	5.09%
7	Texas	7,899	5.03%
8	Ohio	6,906	4.40%
9	Michigan	6,660	4.24%
10	Maryland	5,307	3.38%
11	Massachusetts	4,706	3.00%
12	Virginia	3,101	1.98%
13	Connecticut	3,086	1.97%
14	Missouri	2,426	1.55%
15	Georgia	2,297	1.46%
16	Indiana	1,921	1.22%
17	Wisconsin	1,779	1.13%
18	Tennessee	1,637	1.04%
19	North Carolina	1,573	1.00%
20	Arizona	1,496	0.95%
21	Minnesota	1,327	0.85%
22	West Virginia	1,326	0.85%
23	Kentucky	1,313	0.84%
24	Louisiana	1,285	0.82%
25	Washington	1,190	0.76%
26	Alabama	986	0.63%
27	Rhode Island	865	0.55%
28	Kansas	864	0.55%
29	Oklahoma	806	0.51%
30	Iowa	718	0.46%
31	South Carolina	625	0.40%
32	Colorado	529	0.34%
33	Oregon	504	0.32%
34	Hawaii	499	0.32%
35	Nevada	466	0.30%
36	Delaware	450	0.29%
37	New Mexico	425	0.27%
38	Arkansas	371	0.24%
39	New Hampshire	361	0.23%
40	Mississippi	327	0.21%
41	Nebraska	320	0.20%
42	Maine	313	0.20%
43	North Dakota	287	0.18%
44	Utah	236	0.15%
45	South Dakota	135	0.09%
46	Vermont	124	0.08%
47	Montana	80	0.05%
48	Alaska	56	0.04%
49	Idaho	52	0.03%
50	Wyoming	43	0.03%
	District of Columbia	727	0.46%

Source: American Medical Association (Chicago, Illinois)
   "Physician Characteristics and Distribution in the U.S." (1996-97 Edition)
*As of December 31, 1995. Total does not include 4,390 physicians in U.S. territories and possessions.

Rate of International Medical School Graduates Practicing in the U.S. in 1995

National Rate = 60 Nonfederal Physicians per 100,000 Population*

ALPHA ORDER

RANK	STATE	RATE
35	Alabama	23
47	Alaska	9
20	Arizona	35
43	Arkansas	15
14	California	54
44	Colorado	14
4	Connecticut	94
12	Delaware	63
6	Florida	87
25	Georgia	32
18	Hawaii	42
50	Idaho	4
5	Illinois	92
24	Indiana	33
31	Iowa	25
22	Kansas	34
22	Kentucky	34
28	Louisiana	30
31	Maine	25
3	Maryland	105
8	Massachusetts	78
10	Michigan	70
30	Minnesota	29
45	Mississippi	12
16	Missouri	46
47	Montana	9
39	Nebraska	20
28	Nevada	30
26	New Hampshire	31
2	New Jersey	135
31	New Mexico	25
1	New York	162
36	North Carolina	22
17	North Dakota	45
13	Ohio	62
31	Oklahoma	25
42	Oregon	16
11	Pennsylvania	66
6	Rhode Island	87
41	South Carolina	17
40	South Dakota	18
26	Tennessee	31
18	Texas	42
45	Utah	12
38	Vermont	21
15	Virginia	47
36	Washington	22
9	West Virginia	73
20	Wisconsin	35
47	Wyoming	9

RANK ORDER

RANK	STATE	RATE
1	New York	162
2	New Jersey	135
3	Maryland	105
4	Connecticut	94
5	Illinois	92
6	Florida	87
6	Rhode Island	87
8	Massachusetts	78
9	West Virginia	73
10	Michigan	70
11	Pennsylvania	66
12	Delaware	63
13	Ohio	62
14	California	54
15	Virginia	47
16	Missouri	46
17	North Dakota	45
18	Hawaii	42
18	Texas	42
20	Arizona	35
20	Wisconsin	35
22	Kansas	34
22	Kentucky	34
24	Indiana	33
25	Georgia	32
26	New Hampshire	31
26	Tennessee	31
28	Louisiana	30
28	Nevada	30
30	Minnesota	29
31	Iowa	25
31	Maine	25
31	New Mexico	25
31	Oklahoma	25
35	Alabama	23
36	North Carolina	22
36	Washington	22
38	Vermont	21
39	Nebraska	20
40	South Dakota	18
41	South Carolina	17
42	Oregon	16
43	Arkansas	15
44	Colorado	14
45	Mississippi	12
45	Utah	12
47	Alaska	9
47	Montana	9
47	Wyoming	9
50	Idaho	4

District of Columbia   131

*Source: Morgan Quitno Press using data from American Medical Association (Chicago, Illinois)
"Physician Characteristics and Distribution in the U.S." (1996-97 Edition)*
As of December 31, 1995. National rate does not include physicians in U.S. territories and possessions.

International Medical School Graduates
As a Percent of Nonfederal Physicians in 1995
National Percent = 22.77% of Nonfederal Physicians*

ALPHA ORDER

RANK ORDER

RANK	STATE	PERCENT		RANK	STATE	PERCENT
32	Alabama	11.51		1	New Jersey	44.67
45	Alaska	5.86		2	New York	41.72
25	Arizona	14.93		3	Illinois	34.47
42	Arkansas	7.78		4	West Virginia	33.59
15	California	19.93		5	Florida	32.41
47	Colorado	5.55		6	Michigan	30.07
11	Connecticut	25.43		7	Maryland	27.62
9	Delaware	25.67		8	Rhode Island	26.77
5	Florida	32.41		9	Delaware	25.67
24	Georgia	15.04		10	Ohio	25.60
22	Hawaii	15.52		11	Connecticut	25.43
50	Idaho	2.77		12	Pennsylvania	22.01
3	Illinois	34.47		13	Texas	20.60
20	Indiana	16.55		14	North Dakota	20.23
28	Iowa	13.38		15	California	19.93
23	Kansas	15.25		16	Missouri	19.37
21	Kentucky	16.23		17	Virginia	18.95
31	Louisiana	12.36		18	Massachusetts	18.48
35	Maine	10.78		19	Nevada	17.25
7	Maryland	27.62		20	Indiana	16.55
18	Massachusetts	18.48		21	Kentucky	16.23
6	Michigan	30.07		22	Hawaii	15.52
34	Minnesota	10.79		23	Kansas	15.25
41	Mississippi	7.87		24	Georgia	15.04
16	Missouri	19.37		25	Arizona	14.93
49	Montana	4.33		26	Wisconsin	14.53
38	Nebraska	8.92		27	Oklahoma	14.03
19	Nevada	17.25		28	Iowa	13.38
29	New Hampshire	12.67		29	New Hampshire	12.67
1	New Jersey	44.67		30	Tennessee	12.64
33	New Mexico	11.13		31	Louisiana	12.36
2	New York	41.72		32	Alabama	11.51
37	North Carolina	9.27		33	New Mexico	11.13
14	North Dakota	20.23		34	Minnesota	10.79
10	Ohio	25.60		35	Maine	10.78
27	Oklahoma	14.03		36	South Dakota	9.94
44	Oregon	6.43		37	North Carolina	9.27
12	Pennsylvania	22.01		38	Nebraska	8.92
8	Rhode Island	26.77		39	Washington	8.54
40	South Carolina	8.11		40	South Carolina	8.11
36	South Dakota	9.94		41	Mississippi	7.87
30	Tennessee	12.64		42	Arkansas	7.78
13	Texas	20.60		43	Vermont	6.72
46	Utah	5.61		44	Oregon	6.43
43	Vermont	6.72		45	Alaska	5.86
17	Virginia	18.95		46	Utah	5.61
39	Washington	8.54		47	Colorado	5.55
4	West Virginia	33.59		48	Wyoming	5.14
26	Wisconsin	14.53		49	Montana	4.33
48	Wyoming	5.14		50	Idaho	2.77
				District of Columbia		18.59

Source: Morgan Quitno Press using data from American Medical Association (Chicago, Illinois)
"Physician Characteristics and Distribution in the U.S." (1996-97 Edition)
*As of December 31, 1995. National rate does not include physicians in U.S. territories and possessions.

Osteopathic Physicians in 1996

National Total = 35,340 Osteopathic Physicians*

ALPHA ORDER

RANK	STATE	OSTEOPATHS	% of USA
27	Alabama	218	0.62%
44	Alaska	73	0.21%
12	Arizona	908	2.57%
38	Arkansas	134	0.38%
8	California	1,659	4.69%
14	Colorado	633	1.79%
35	Connecticut	156	0.44%
32	Delaware	165	0.47%
4	Florida	2,236	6.33%
18	Georgia	442	1.25%
40	Hawaii	103	0.29%
41	Idaho	79	0.22%
10	Illinois	1,465	4.15%
15	Indiana	503	1.42%
13	Iowa	822	2.33%
17	Kansas	472	1.34%
34	Kentucky	157	0.44%
39	Louisiana	107	0.30%
20	Maine	378	1.07%
25	Maryland	276	0.78%
23	Massachusetts	327	0.93%
2	Michigan	4,269	12.08%
29	Minnesota	182	0.51%
36	Mississippi	144	0.41%
9	Missouri	1,490	4.22%
46	Montana	56	0.16%
45	Nebraska	70	0.20%
28	Nevada	206	0.58%
42	New Hampshire	77	0.22%
6	New Jersey	2,138	6.05%
31	New Mexico	167	0.47%
7	New York	1,847	5.23%
30	North Carolina	178	0.50%
47	North Dakota	50	0.14%
3	Ohio	2,878	8.14%
11	Oklahoma	1,056	2.99%
24	Oregon	324	0.92%
1	Pennsylvania	4,313	12.20%
33	Rhode Island	160	0.45%
36	South Carolina	144	0.41%
48	South Dakota	46	0.13%
26	Tennessee	240	0.68%
5	Texas	2,213	6.26%
43	Utah	75	0.21%
49	Vermont	39	0.11%
22	Virginia	353	1.00%
16	Washington	491	1.39%
21	West Virginia	374	1.06%
19	Wisconsin	384	1.09%
50	Wyoming	36	0.10%

RANK ORDER

RANK	STATE	OSTEOPATHS	% of USA
1	Pennsylvania	4,313	12.20%
2	Michigan	4,269	12.08%
3	Ohio	2,878	8.14%
4	Florida	2,236	6.33%
5	Texas	2,213	6.26%
6	New Jersey	2,138	6.05%
7	New York	1,847	5.23%
8	California	1,659	4.69%
9	Missouri	1,490	4.22%
10	Illinois	1,465	4.15%
11	Oklahoma	1,056	2.99%
12	Arizona	908	2.57%
13	Iowa	822	2.33%
14	Colorado	633	1.79%
15	Indiana	503	1.42%
16	Washington	491	1.39%
17	Kansas	472	1.34%
18	Georgia	442	1.25%
19	Wisconsin	384	1.09%
20	Maine	378	1.07%
21	West Virginia	374	1.06%
22	Virginia	353	1.00%
23	Massachusetts	327	0.93%
24	Oregon	324	0.92%
25	Maryland	276	0.78%
26	Tennessee	240	0.68%
27	Alabama	218	0.62%
28	Nevada	206	0.58%
29	Minnesota	182	0.51%
30	North Carolina	178	0.50%
31	New Mexico	167	0.47%
32	Delaware	165	0.47%
33	Rhode Island	160	0.45%
34	Kentucky	157	0.44%
35	Connecticut	156	0.44%
36	Mississippi	144	0.41%
36	South Carolina	144	0.41%
38	Arkansas	134	0.38%
39	Louisiana	107	0.30%
40	Hawaii	103	0.29%
41	Idaho	79	0.22%
42	New Hampshire	77	0.22%
43	Utah	75	0.21%
44	Alaska	73	0.21%
45	Nebraska	70	0.20%
46	Montana	56	0.16%
47	North Dakota	50	0.14%
48	South Dakota	46	0.13%
49	Vermont	39	0.11%
50	Wyoming	36	0.10%
	District of Columbia	27	0.08%

Source: American Osteopathic Association
"AOA Biographical Records" (February 1997)

As of June 1, 1996. Excludes retired, disabled, foreign and federal osteopaths. Osteopaths practice a system of medicine based on the theory that disturbances in the musculoskeletal system affect other body parts, causing many disorders that can be corrected by various manipulative techniques in conjunction with conventional medical, surgical, pharmacological, and other therapeutic procedures.

Rate of Osteopathic Physicians in 1996

National Rate = 13.3 Osteopaths per 100,000 Population*

<table>
<tr><td colspan="3">ALPHA ORDER</td><td colspan="3">RANK ORDER</td></tr>
<tr><td>RANK</td><td>STATE</td><td>RATE</td><td>RANK</td><td>STATE</td><td>RATE</td></tr>
<tr><td>41</td><td>Alabama</td><td>5.1</td><td>1</td><td>Michigan</td><td>44.5</td></tr>
<tr><td>18</td><td>Alaska</td><td>12.0</td><td>2</td><td>Pennsylvania</td><td>35.8</td></tr>
<tr><td>10</td><td>Arizona</td><td>20.5</td><td>3</td><td>Oklahoma</td><td>32.0</td></tr>
<tr><td>37</td><td>Arkansas</td><td>5.3</td><td>4</td><td>Maine</td><td>30.4</td></tr>
<tr><td>40</td><td>California</td><td>5.2</td><td>5</td><td>Iowa</td><td>28.8</td></tr>
<tr><td>13</td><td>Colorado</td><td>16.6</td><td>6</td><td>Missouri</td><td>27.8</td></tr>
<tr><td>42</td><td>Connecticut</td><td>4.8</td><td>7</td><td>New Jersey</td><td>26.8</td></tr>
<tr><td>9</td><td>Delaware</td><td>22.8</td><td>8</td><td>Ohio</td><td>25.8</td></tr>
<tr><td>15</td><td>Florida</td><td>15.5</td><td>9</td><td>Delaware</td><td>22.8</td></tr>
<tr><td>34</td><td>Georgia</td><td>6.0</td><td>10</td><td>Arizona</td><td>20.5</td></tr>
<tr><td>24</td><td>Hawaii</td><td>8.7</td><td>10</td><td>West Virginia</td><td>20.5</td></tr>
<tr><td>29</td><td>Idaho</td><td>6.6</td><td>12</td><td>Kansas</td><td>18.4</td></tr>
<tr><td>17</td><td>Illinois</td><td>12.4</td><td>13</td><td>Colorado</td><td>16.6</td></tr>
<tr><td>25</td><td>Indiana</td><td>8.6</td><td>14</td><td>Rhode Island</td><td>16.2</td></tr>
<tr><td>5</td><td>Iowa</td><td>28.8</td><td>15</td><td>Florida</td><td>15.5</td></tr>
<tr><td>12</td><td>Kansas</td><td>18.4</td><td>16</td><td>Nevada</td><td>12.9</td></tr>
<tr><td>45</td><td>Kentucky</td><td>4.0</td><td>17</td><td>Illinois</td><td>12.4</td></tr>
<tr><td>49</td><td>Louisiana</td><td>2.5</td><td>18</td><td>Alaska</td><td>12.0</td></tr>
<tr><td>4</td><td>Maine</td><td>30.4</td><td>19</td><td>Texas</td><td>11.6</td></tr>
<tr><td>35</td><td>Maryland</td><td>5.4</td><td>20</td><td>New York</td><td>10.2</td></tr>
<tr><td>35</td><td>Massachusetts</td><td>5.4</td><td>21</td><td>Oregon</td><td>10.1</td></tr>
<tr><td>1</td><td>Michigan</td><td>44.5</td><td>22</td><td>New Mexico</td><td>9.7</td></tr>
<tr><td>46</td><td>Minnesota</td><td>3.9</td><td>23</td><td>Washington</td><td>8.9</td></tr>
<tr><td>37</td><td>Mississippi</td><td>5.3</td><td>24</td><td>Hawaii</td><td>8.7</td></tr>
<tr><td>6</td><td>Missouri</td><td>27.8</td><td>25</td><td>Indiana</td><td>8.6</td></tr>
<tr><td>32</td><td>Montana</td><td>6.4</td><td>26</td><td>North Dakota</td><td>7.8</td></tr>
<tr><td>44</td><td>Nebraska</td><td>4.2</td><td>27</td><td>Wyoming</td><td>7.5</td></tr>
<tr><td>16</td><td>Nevada</td><td>12.9</td><td>28</td><td>Wisconsin</td><td>7.4</td></tr>
<tr><td>29</td><td>New Hampshire</td><td>6.6</td><td>29</td><td>Idaho</td><td>6.6</td></tr>
<tr><td>7</td><td>New Jersey</td><td>26.8</td><td>29</td><td>New Hampshire</td><td>6.6</td></tr>
<tr><td>22</td><td>New Mexico</td><td>9.7</td><td>29</td><td>Vermont</td><td>6.6</td></tr>
<tr><td>20</td><td>New York</td><td>10.2</td><td>32</td><td>Montana</td><td>6.4</td></tr>
<tr><td>50</td><td>North Carolina</td><td>2.4</td><td>33</td><td>South Dakota</td><td>6.3</td></tr>
<tr><td>26</td><td>North Dakota</td><td>7.8</td><td>34</td><td>Georgia</td><td>6.0</td></tr>
<tr><td>8</td><td>Ohio</td><td>25.8</td><td>35</td><td>Maryland</td><td>5.4</td></tr>
<tr><td>3</td><td>Oklahoma</td><td>32.0</td><td>35</td><td>Massachusetts</td><td>5.4</td></tr>
<tr><td>21</td><td>Oregon</td><td>10.1</td><td>37</td><td>Arkansas</td><td>5.3</td></tr>
<tr><td>2</td><td>Pennsylvania</td><td>35.8</td><td>37</td><td>Mississippi</td><td>5.3</td></tr>
<tr><td>14</td><td>Rhode Island</td><td>16.2</td><td>37</td><td>Virginia</td><td>5.3</td></tr>
<tr><td>46</td><td>South Carolina</td><td>3.9</td><td>40</td><td>California</td><td>5.2</td></tr>
<tr><td>33</td><td>South Dakota</td><td>6.3</td><td>41</td><td>Alabama</td><td>5.1</td></tr>
<tr><td>43</td><td>Tennessee</td><td>4.5</td><td>42</td><td>Connecticut</td><td>4.8</td></tr>
<tr><td>19</td><td>Texas</td><td>11.6</td><td>43</td><td>Tennessee</td><td>4.5</td></tr>
<tr><td>48</td><td>Utah</td><td>3.8</td><td>44</td><td>Nebraska</td><td>4.2</td></tr>
<tr><td>29</td><td>Vermont</td><td>6.6</td><td>45</td><td>Kentucky</td><td>4.0</td></tr>
<tr><td>37</td><td>Virginia</td><td>5.3</td><td>46</td><td>Minnesota</td><td>3.9</td></tr>
<tr><td>23</td><td>Washington</td><td>8.9</td><td>46</td><td>South Carolina</td><td>3.9</td></tr>
<tr><td>10</td><td>West Virginia</td><td>20.5</td><td>48</td><td>Utah</td><td>3.8</td></tr>
<tr><td>28</td><td>Wisconsin</td><td>7.4</td><td>49</td><td>Louisiana</td><td>2.5</td></tr>
<tr><td>27</td><td>Wyoming</td><td>7.5</td><td>50</td><td>North Carolina</td><td>2.4</td></tr>
<tr><td></td><td></td><td></td><td></td><td>District of Columbia</td><td>5.0</td></tr>
</table>

Source: Morgan Quitno Press using data from American Osteopathic Association
    "AOA Biographical Records" (February 1997)
*As of June 1, 1996. Excludes retired, disabled, foreign and federal osteopaths. Osteopaths practice a system of medicine based on the theory that disturbances in the musculoskeletal system affect other body parts, causing many disorders that can be corrected by various manipulative techniques in conjunction with conventional medical, surgical, pharmacological, and other therapeutic procedures.

Osteopathic Physicians in Primary Care in 1996

National Total = 21,638 Osteopathic Physicians*

ALPHA ORDER

RANK	STATE	OSTEOPATHS	% of USA
28	Alabama	132	0.61%
40	Alaska	52	0.24%
12	Arizona	546	2.52%
33	Arkansas	97	0.45%
8	California	1,041	4.81%
14	Colorado	428	1.98%
36	Connecticut	87	0.40%
29	Delaware	111	0.51%
4	Florida	1,425	6.59%
18	Georgia	286	1.32%
39	Hawaii	63	0.29%
42	Idaho	50	0.23%
10	Illinois	778	3.60%
17	Indiana	304	1.40%
13	Iowa	527	2.44%
16	Kansas	310	1.43%
37	Kentucky	84	0.39%
44	Louisiana	44	0.20%
21	Maine	253	1.17%
26	Maryland	139	0.64%
23	Massachusetts	203	0.94%
2	Michigan	2,363	10.92%
31	Minnesota	110	0.51%
34	Mississippi	93	0.43%
9	Missouri	943	4.36%
46	Montana	32	0.15%
45	Nebraska	36	0.17%
27	Nevada	135	0.62%
40	New Hampshire	52	0.24%
6	New Jersey	1,288	5.95%
29	New Mexico	111	0.51%
7	New York	1,213	5.61%
35	North Carolina	92	0.43%
50	North Dakota	12	0.06%
3	Ohio	1,625	7.51%
11	Oklahoma	677	3.13%
22	Oregon	228	1.05%
1	Pennsylvania	2,751	12.71%
32	Rhode Island	98	0.45%
38	South Carolina	81	0.37%
47	South Dakota	28	0.13%
25	Tennessee	160	0.74%
5	Texas	1,396	6.45%
43	Utah	47	0.22%
48	Vermont	25	0.12%
24	Virginia	196	0.91%
15	Washington	324	1.50%
19	West Virginia	273	1.26%
20	Wisconsin	256	1.18%
49	Wyoming	19	0.09%

RANK ORDER

RANK	STATE	OSTEOPATHS	% of USA
1	Pennsylvania	2,751	12.71%
2	Michigan	2,363	10.92%
3	Ohio	1,625	7.51%
4	Florida	1,425	6.59%
5	Texas	1,396	6.45%
6	New Jersey	1,288	5.95%
7	New York	1,213	5.61%
8	California	1,041	4.81%
9	Missouri	943	4.36%
10	Illinois	778	3.60%
11	Oklahoma	677	3.13%
12	Arizona	546	2.52%
13	Iowa	527	2.44%
14	Colorado	428	1.98%
15	Washington	324	1.50%
16	Kansas	310	1.43%
17	Indiana	304	1.40%
18	Georgia	286	1.32%
19	West Virginia	273	1.26%
20	Wisconsin	256	1.18%
21	Maine	253	1.17%
22	Oregon	228	1.05%
23	Massachusetts	203	0.94%
24	Virginia	196	0.91%
25	Tennessee	160	0.74%
26	Maryland	139	0.64%
27	Nevada	135	0.62%
28	Alabama	132	0.61%
29	Delaware	111	0.51%
29	New Mexico	111	0.51%
31	Minnesota	110	0.51%
32	Rhode Island	98	0.45%
33	Arkansas	97	0.45%
34	Mississippi	93	0.43%
35	North Carolina	92	0.43%
36	Connecticut	87	0.40%
37	Kentucky	84	0.39%
38	South Carolina	81	0.37%
39	Hawaii	63	0.29%
40	Alaska	52	0.24%
40	New Hampshire	52	0.24%
42	Idaho	50	0.23%
43	Utah	47	0.22%
44	Louisiana	44	0.20%
45	Nebraska	36	0.17%
46	Montana	32	0.15%
47	South Dakota	28	0.13%
48	Vermont	25	0.12%
49	Wyoming	19	0.09%
50	North Dakota	12	0.06%
	District of Columbia	14	0.06%

Source: Morgan Quitno Press using data from American Osteopathic Association
  "AOA Biographical Records" (February 1997)
*As of June 1, 1996. Excludes retired, disabled, foreign and federal osteopaths. Osteopaths practice a system of medicine based on the theory that disturbances in the musculoskeletal system affect other body parts, causing many disorders that can be corrected by various manipulative techniques in conjunction with conventional medical, surgical, pharmacological, and other therapeutic procedures.

Podiatric Physicians in 1995

National Total = 11,628 Podiatric Physicians*

ALPHA ORDER					RANK ORDER			
RANK	STATE		PODIATRISTS	% of USA	RANK	STATE	PODIATRISTS	% of USA
31	Alabama		61	0.52%	1	California	1,415	12.17%
49	Alaska		15	0.13%	2	New York	1,154	9.92%
17	Arizona		199	1.71%	3	Pennsylvania	994	8.55%
39	Arkansas		39	0.34%	4	Florida	877	7.54%
1	California		1,415	12.17%	5	New Jersey	747	6.42%
24	Colorado		115	0.99%	6	Illinois	670	5.76%
12	Connecticut		282	2.43%	7	Ohio	490	4.21%
43	Delaware		37	0.32%	8	Michigan	457	3.93%
4	Florida		877	7.54%	9	Massachusetts	429	3.69%
13	Georgia		248	2.13%	10	Texas	422	3.63%
46	Hawaii		20	0.17%	11	Maryland	330	2.84%
37	Idaho		44	0.38%	12	Connecticut	282	2.43%
6	Illinois		670	5.76%	13	Georgia	248	2.13%
14	Indiana		227	1.95%	14	Indiana	227	1.95%
19	Iowa		148	1.27%	15	Virginia	209	1.80%
27	Kansas		86	0.74%	16	North Carolina	206	1.77%
28	Kentucky		82	0.71%	17	Arizona	199	1.71%
30	Louisiana		72	0.62%	18	Wisconsin	180	1.55%
34	Maine		54	0.46%	19	Iowa	148	1.27%
11	Maryland		330	2.84%	19	Washington	148	1.27%
9	Massachusetts		429	3.69%	21	Minnesota	130	1.12%
8	Michigan		457	3.93%	22	Tennessee	129	1.11%
21	Minnesota		130	1.12%	23	Missouri	128	1.10%
44	Mississippi		28	0.24%	24	Colorado	115	0.99%
23	Missouri		128	1.10%	25	Utah	99	0.85%
38	Montana		40	0.34%	26	Oregon	98	0.84%
32	Nebraska		56	0.48%	27	Kansas	86	0.74%
35	Nevada		53	0.46%	28	Kentucky	82	0.71%
33	New Hampshire		55	0.47%	29	Oklahoma	74	0.64%
5	New Jersey		747	6.42%	30	Louisiana	72	0.62%
41	New Mexico		38	0.33%	31	Alabama	61	0.52%
2	New York		1,154	9.92%	32	Nebraska	56	0.48%
16	North Carolina		206	1.77%	33	New Hampshire	55	0.47%
48	North Dakota		16	0.14%	34	Maine	54	0.46%
7	Ohio		490	4.21%	35	Nevada	53	0.46%
29	Oklahoma		74	0.64%	35	West Virginia	53	0.46%
26	Oregon		98	0.84%	37	Idaho	44	0.38%
3	Pennsylvania		994	8.55%	38	Montana	40	0.34%
39	Rhode Island		39	0.34%	39	Arkansas	39	0.34%
41	South Carolina		38	0.33%	39	Rhode Island	39	0.34%
45	South Dakota		24	0.21%	41	New Mexico	38	0.33%
22	Tennessee		129	1.11%	41	South Carolina	38	0.33%
10	Texas		422	3.63%	43	Delaware	37	0.32%
25	Utah		99	0.85%	44	Mississippi	28	0.24%
46	Vermont		20	0.17%	45	South Dakota	24	0.21%
15	Virginia		209	1.80%	46	Hawaii	20	0.17%
19	Washington		148	1.27%	46	Vermont	20	0.17%
35	West Virginia		53	0.46%	48	North Dakota	16	0.14%
18	Wisconsin		180	1.55%	49	Alaska	15	0.13%
50	Wyoming		10	0.09%	50	Wyoming	10	0.09%
						District of Columbia	43	0.37%

Source: American Podiatric Medical Association, Inc.
"Podiatric Physicians in Active Practice"
*As of December 1995. Includes only Podiatric physicians considered in "active practice." Podiatry deals with the diagnosis, treatment, and prevention of diseases of the human foot. National total does not include eight podiatrists in Puerto Rico.

Rate of Podiatric Physicians in 1995

National Rate = 4.4 Podiatrists per 100,000 Population*

ALPHA ORDER

RANK	STATE	RATE
48	Alabama	1.4
36	Alaska	2.5
14	Arizona	4.6
47	Arkansas	1.6
16	California	4.5
30	Colorado	3.1
2	Connecticut	8.6
9	Delaware	5.2
7	Florida	6.2
24	Georgia	3.4
45	Hawaii	1.7
21	Idaho	3.8
8	Illinois	5.7
19	Indiana	3.9
9	Iowa	5.2
24	Kansas	3.4
43	Kentucky	2.1
45	Louisiana	1.7
17	Maine	4.4
5	Maryland	6.5
4	Massachusetts	7.1
12	Michigan	4.8
34	Minnesota	2.8
49	Mississippi	1.0
39	Missouri	2.4
14	Montana	4.6
24	Nebraska	3.4
22	Nevada	3.5
12	New Hampshire	4.8
1	New Jersey	9.4
41	New Mexico	2.2
6	New York	6.3
32	North Carolina	2.9
36	North Dakota	2.5
17	Ohio	4.4
40	Oklahoma	2.3
30	Oregon	3.1
3	Pennsylvania	8.2
19	Rhode Island	3.9
49	South Carolina	1.0
28	South Dakota	3.3
36	Tennessee	2.5
41	Texas	2.2
11	Utah	5.1
24	Vermont	3.4
29	Virginia	3.2
35	Washington	2.7
32	West Virginia	2.9
22	Wisconsin	3.5
43	Wyoming	2.1

RANK ORDER

RANK	STATE	RATE
1	New Jersey	9.4
2	Connecticut	8.6
3	Pennsylvania	8.2
4	Massachusetts	7.1
5	Maryland	6.5
6	New York	6.3
7	Florida	6.2
8	Illinois	5.7
9	Delaware	5.2
9	Iowa	5.2
11	Utah	5.1
12	Michigan	4.8
12	New Hampshire	4.8
14	Arizona	4.6
14	Montana	4.6
16	California	4.5
17	Maine	4.4
17	Ohio	4.4
19	Indiana	3.9
19	Rhode Island	3.9
21	Idaho	3.8
22	Nevada	3.5
22	Wisconsin	3.5
24	Georgia	3.4
24	Kansas	3.4
24	Nebraska	3.4
24	Vermont	3.4
28	South Dakota	3.3
29	Virginia	3.2
30	Colorado	3.1
30	Oregon	3.1
32	North Carolina	2.9
32	West Virginia	2.9
34	Minnesota	2.8
35	Washington	2.7
36	Alaska	2.5
36	North Dakota	2.5
36	Tennessee	2.5
39	Missouri	2.4
40	Oklahoma	2.3
41	New Mexico	2.2
41	Texas	2.2
43	Kentucky	2.1
43	Wyoming	2.1
45	Hawaii	1.7
45	Louisiana	1.7
47	Arkansas	1.6
48	Alabama	1.4
49	Mississippi	1.0
49	South Carolina	1.0
	District of Columbia	7.7

Source: Morgan Quitno Press using data from American Podiatric Medical Association, Inc.
"Podiatric Physicians in Active Practice"
*Includes only Podiatric physicians considered in "active practice." Podiatry deals with the diagnosis, treatment, and prevention of diseases of the human foot. National rate does not include podiatrists in Puerto Rico.

Doctors of Chiropractic in 1995

National Total = 69,109 Chiropractors*

RANK	STATE	HIROPRACTORS	% of USA
29	Alabama	671	0.97%
48	Alaska	186	0.27%
9	Arizona	2,384	3.45%
34	Arkansas	508	0.74%
1	California	9,879	14.29%
13	Colorado	1,696	2.45%
26	Connecticut	858	1.24%
46	Delaware	209	0.30%
3	Florida	4,355	6.30%
10	Georgia	2,237	3.24%
28	Hawaii	712	1.03%
38	Idaho	338	0.49%
6	Illinois	2,912	4.21%
24	Indiana	900	1.30%
18	Iowa	1,231	1.78%
30	Kansas	637	0.92%
22	Kentucky	1,055	1.53%
31	Louisiana	592	0.86%
37	Maine	375	0.54%
35	Maryland	488	0.71%
19	Massachusetts	1,220	1.77%
8	Michigan	2,440	3.53%
16	Minnesota	1,613	2.33%
39	Mississippi	330	0.48%
11	Missouri	1,856	2.69%
44	Montana	228	0.33%
41	Nebraska	281	0.41%
40	Nevada	326	0.47%
36	New Hampshire	435	0.63%
7	New Jersey	2,701	3.91%
33	New Mexico	577	0.83%
2	New York	4,926	7.13%
17	North Carolina	1,292	1.87%
45	North Dakota	224	0.32%
14	Ohio	1,680	2.43%
23	Oklahoma	980	1.42%
25	Oregon	877	1.27%
5	Pennsylvania	3,190	4.62%
50	Rhode Island	158	0.23%
20	South Carolina	1,097	1.59%
47	South Dakota	201	0.29%
27	Tennessee	780	1.13%
4	Texas	3,682	5.33%
32	Utah	580	0.84%
42	Vermont	261	0.38%
21	Virginia	1,090	1.58%
15	Washington	1,625	2.35%
43	West Virginia	255	0.37%
12	Wisconsin	1,764	2.55%
49	Wyoming	183	0.26%

RANK	STATE	CHIROPRACTOR	% of USA
1	California	9,879	14.29%
2	New York	4,926	7.13%
3	Florida	4,355	6.30%
4	Texas	3,682	5.33%
5	Pennsylvania	3,190	4.62%
6	Illinois	2,912	4.21%
7	New Jersey	2,701	3.91%
8	Michigan	2,440	3.53%
9	Arizona	2,384	3.45%
10	Georgia	2,237	3.24%
11	Missouri	1,856	2.69%
12	Wisconsin	1,764	2.55%
13	Colorado	1,696	2.45%
14	Ohio	1,680	2.43%
15	Washington	1,625	2.35%
16	Minnesota	1,613	2.33%
17	North Carolina	1,292	1.87%
18	Iowa	1,231	1.78%
19	Massachusetts	1,220	1.77%
20	South Carolina	1,097	1.59%
21	Virginia	1,090	1.58%
22	Kentucky	1,055	1.53%
23	Oklahoma	980	1.42%
24	Indiana	900	1.30%
25	Oregon	877	1.27%
26	Connecticut	858	1.24%
27	Tennessee	780	1.13%
28	Hawaii	712	1.03%
29	Alabama	671	0.97%
30	Kansas	637	0.92%
31	Louisiana	592	0.86%
32	Utah	580	0.84%
33	New Mexico	577	0.83%
34	Arkansas	508	0.74%
35	Maryland	488	0.71%
36	New Hampshire	435	0.63%
37	Maine	375	0.54%
38	Idaho	338	0.49%
39	Mississippi	330	0.48%
40	Nevada	326	0.47%
41	Nebraska	281	0.41%
42	Vermont	261	0.38%
43	West Virginia	255	0.37%
44	Montana	228	0.33%
45	North Dakota	224	0.32%
46	Delaware	209	0.30%
47	South Dakota	201	0.29%
48	Alaska	186	0.27%
49	Wyoming	183	0.26%
50	Rhode Island	158	0.23%
	District of Columbia	39	0.06%

Source: Federation of Chiropractic Licensing Boards
   "1996-97 Official Directory"
*As of December 1995. Licensed active doctors. There is some duplication as some doctors are licensed in more than one state.

Rate of Doctors of Chiropractic in 1995

National Rate = 26.3 Chiropractors per 100,000 Population*

ALPHA ORDER				RANK ORDER		
RANK	STATE	RATE		RANK	STATE	RATE
43	Alabama	15.8		1	Hawaii	60.4
16	Alaska	30.8		2	Arizona	55.4
2	Arizona	55.4		3	Colorado	45.3
36	Arkansas	20.4		4	Vermont	44.6
14	California	31.3		5	Iowa	43.3
3	Colorado	45.3		6	Wyoming	38.2
30	Connecticut	26.2		7	New Hampshire	37.9
23	Delaware	29.1		8	Minnesota	35.0
17	Florida	30.7		9	Missouri	34.9
15	Georgia	31.0		9	North Dakota	34.9
1	Hawaii	60.4		11	Wisconsin	34.4
24	Idaho	29.0		12	New Mexico	34.1
34	Illinois	24.7		13	New Jersey	34.0
44	Indiana	15.5		14	California	31.3
5	Iowa	43.3		15	Georgia	31.0
33	Kansas	24.8		16	Alaska	30.8
27	Kentucky	27.4		17	Florida	30.7
48	Louisiana	13.6		18	Maine	30.3
18	Maine	30.3		19	Oklahoma	29.9
50	Maryland	9.7		19	South Carolina	29.9
37	Massachusetts	20.1		21	Washington	29.8
32	Michigan	25.6		22	Utah	29.6
8	Minnesota	35.0		23	Delaware	29.1
49	Mississippi	12.2		24	Idaho	29.0
9	Missouri	34.9		25	Oregon	27.9
30	Montana	26.2		26	South Dakota	27.5
40	Nebraska	17.1		27	Kentucky	27.4
35	Nevada	21.3		28	New York	27.1
7	New Hampshire	37.9		29	Pennsylvania	26.5
13	New Jersey	34.0		30	Connecticut	26.2
12	New Mexico	34.1		30	Montana	26.2
28	New York	27.1		32	Michigan	25.6
39	North Carolina	17.9		33	Kansas	24.8
9	North Dakota	34.9		34	Illinois	24.7
45	Ohio	15.1		35	Nevada	21.3
19	Oklahoma	29.9		36	Arkansas	20.4
25	Oregon	27.9		37	Massachusetts	20.1
29	Pennsylvania	26.5		38	Texas	19.6
42	Rhode Island	15.9		39	North Carolina	17.9
19	South Carolina	29.9		40	Nebraska	17.1
26	South Dakota	27.5		41	Virginia	16.5
46	Tennessee	14.9		42	Rhode Island	15.9
38	Texas	19.6		43	Alabama	15.8
22	Utah	29.6		44	Indiana	15.5
4	Vermont	44.6		45	Ohio	15.1
41	Virginia	16.5		46	Tennessee	14.9
21	Washington	29.8		47	West Virginia	14.0
47	West Virginia	14.0		48	Louisiana	13.6
11	Wisconsin	34.4		49	Mississippi	12.2
6	Wyoming	38.2		50	Maryland	9.7
					District of Columbia	7.0

Source: Morgan Quitno Press using data from Federation of Chiropractic Licensing Boards
   "1996-97 Official Directory"
*As of December 1995. Licensed active doctors. There is some duplication as some doctors are licensed in more than one state.

Registered Nurses in 1994

National Total = 2,044,000 Registered Nurses*

ALPHA ORDER

RANK	STATE	NURSES	% of USA
21	Alabama	33,400	1.63%
49	Alaska	3,600	0.18%
24	Arizona	30,800	1.51%
31	Arkansas	18,500	0.91%
1	California	181,900	8.90%
25	Colorado	30,500	1.49%
22	Connecticut	31,500	1.54%
46	Delaware	6,200	0.30%
4	Florida	104,400	5.11%
12	Georgia	48,400	2.37%
41	Hawaii	9,400	0.46%
44	Idaho	6,700	0.33%
7	Illinois	98,600	4.82%
17	Indiana	44,000	2.15%
26	Iowa	29,000	1.42%
30	Kansas	21,500	1.05%
23	Kentucky	31,100	1.52%
27	Louisiana	27,800	1.36%
37	Maine	11,600	0.57%
18	Maryland	42,000	2.05%
10	Massachusetts	70,100	3.43%
8	Michigan	72,500	3.55%
15	Minnesota	44,900	2.20%
33	Mississippi	16,300	0.80%
18	Missouri	42,000	2.05%
46	Montana	6,200	0.30%
34	Nebraska	14,700	0.72%
42	Nevada	8,800	0.43%
39	New Hampshire	11,100	0.54%
9	New Jersey	71,700	3.51%
36	New Mexico	12,400	0.61%
2	New York	170,700	8.35%
11	North Carolina	55,800	2.73%
45	North Dakota	6,400	0.31%
6	Ohio	99,800	4.88%
32	Oklahoma	18,300	0.90%
28	Oregon	24,400	1.19%
3	Pennsylvania	125,500	6.14%
40	Rhode Island	9,600	0.47%
29	South Carolina	22,600	1.11%
43	South Dakota	7,200	0.35%
20	Tennessee	40,900	2.00%
5	Texas	101,900	4.99%
38	Utah	11,300	0.55%
48	Vermont	5,500	0.27%
13	Virginia	48,100	2.35%
16	Washington	44,300	2.17%
35	West Virginia	13,900	0.68%
14	Wisconsin	45,100	2.21%
50	Wyoming	3,500	0.17%

RANK ORDER

RANK	STATE	NURSES	% of USA
1	California	181,900	8.90%
2	New York	170,700	8.35%
3	Pennsylvania	125,500	6.14%
4	Florida	104,400	5.11%
5	Texas	101,900	4.99%
6	Ohio	99,800	4.88%
7	Illinois	98,600	4.82%
8	Michigan	72,500	3.55%
9	New Jersey	71,700	3.51%
10	Massachusetts	70,100	3.43%
11	North Carolina	55,800	2.73%
12	Georgia	48,400	2.37%
13	Virginia	48,100	2.35%
14	Wisconsin	45,100	2.21%
15	Minnesota	44,900	2.20%
16	Washington	44,300	2.17%
17	Indiana	44,000	2.15%
18	Maryland	42,000	2.05%
18	Missouri	42,000	2.05%
20	Tennessee	40,900	2.00%
21	Alabama	33,400	1.63%
22	Connecticut	31,500	1.54%
23	Kentucky	31,100	1.52%
24	Arizona	30,800	1.51%
25	Colorado	30,500	1.49%
26	Iowa	29,000	1.42%
27	Louisiana	27,800	1.36%
28	Oregon	24,400	1.19%
29	South Carolina	22,600	1.11%
30	Kansas	21,500	1.05%
31	Arkansas	18,500	0.91%
32	Oklahoma	18,300	0.90%
33	Mississippi	16,300	0.80%
34	Nebraska	14,700	0.72%
35	West Virginia	13,900	0.68%
36	New Mexico	12,400	0.61%
37	Maine	11,600	0.57%
38	Utah	11,300	0.55%
39	New Hampshire	11,100	0.54%
40	Rhode Island	9,600	0.47%
41	Hawaii	9,400	0.46%
42	Nevada	8,800	0.43%
43	South Dakota	7,200	0.35%
44	Idaho	6,700	0.33%
45	North Dakota	6,400	0.31%
46	Delaware	6,200	0.30%
46	Montana	6,200	0.30%
48	Vermont	5,500	0.27%
49	Alaska	3,600	0.18%
50	Wyoming	3,500	0.17%
	District of Columbia	8,000	0.39%

Source: U.S. Department of Health and Human Services, Health Resources and Services Administration
    unpublished data
*As of December 1994.

Rate of Registered Nurses in 1994

National Rate = 785 Nurses per 100,000 Population*

ALPHA ORDER				RANK ORDER		
RANK	**STATE**	**RATE**		**RANK**	**STATE**	**RATE**
26	Alabama	792		1	Massachusetts	1,160
45	Alaska	599		2	Pennsylvania	1,041
34	Arizona	753		3	Iowa	1,024
33	Arkansas	754		4	North Dakota	1,000
48	California	580		5	South Dakota	994
21	Colorado	833		6	Minnesota	982
9	Connecticut	962		7	New Hampshire	978
17	Delaware	876		8	Rhode Island	964
35	Florida	748		9	Connecticut	962
40	Georgia	685		10	Vermont	947
24	Hawaii	801		11	New York	938
47	Idaho	590		12	Maine	937
19	Illinois	840		13	New Jersey	907
30	Indiana	765		14	Nebraska	904
3	Iowa	1,024		15	Ohio	899
18	Kansas	843		16	Wisconsin	887
23	Kentucky	813		17	Delaware	876
41	Louisiana	644		18	Kansas	843
12	Maine	937		19	Illinois	840
19	Maryland	840		19	Maryland	840
1	Massachusetts	1,160		21	Colorado	833
31	Michigan	764		22	Washington	828
6	Minnesota	982		23	Kentucky	813
43	Mississippi	611		24	Hawaii	801
25	Missouri	796		25	Missouri	796
39	Montana	723		26	Alabama	792
14	Nebraska	904		27	Tennessee	790
44	Nevada	601		28	Oregon	789
7	New Hampshire	978		29	North Carolina	788
13	New Jersey	907		30	Indiana	765
36	New Mexico	747		31	Michigan	764
11	New York	938		32	West Virginia	763
29	North Carolina	788		33	Arkansas	754
4	North Dakota	1,000		34	Arizona	753
15	Ohio	899		35	Florida	748
49	Oklahoma	562		36	New Mexico	747
28	Oregon	789		37	Wyoming	735
2	Pennsylvania	1,041		38	Virginia	734
8	Rhode Island	964		39	Montana	723
42	South Carolina	620		40	Georgia	685
5	South Dakota	994		41	Louisiana	644
27	Tennessee	790		42	South Carolina	620
50	Texas	553		43	Mississippi	611
46	Utah	592		44	Nevada	601
10	Vermont	947		45	Alaska	599
38	Virginia	734		46	Utah	592
22	Washington	828		47	Idaho	590
32	West Virginia	763		48	California	580
16	Wisconsin	887		49	Oklahoma	562
37	Wyoming	735		50	Texas	553
					District of Columbia	1,408

Source: Morgan Quitno Press using data from U.S. Dept. of Health & Human Services, Health Resources/Services Admn.
  unpublished data
*As of December 1994. Calculated with updated Census population estimates for July 1, 1994.

Active Civilian Dentists in 1996

National Total = 144,439 Dentists*

<u>ALPHA ORDER</u>

RANK	STATE	DENTISTS	% of USA
27	Alabama	1,709	1.18%
46	Alaska	320	0.22%
26	Arizona	1,814	1.26%
33	Arkansas	1,016	0.70%
1	California	20,145	13.95%
20	Colorado	2,497	1.73%
22	Connecticut	2,364	1.64%
48	Delaware	303	0.21%
6	Florida	6,607	4.57%
14	Georgia	2,953	2.04%
36	Hawaii	907	0.63%
40	Idaho	594	0.41%
4	Illinois	7,515	5.20%
18	Indiana	2,579	1.79%
30	Iowa	1,417	0.98%
32	Kansas	1,187	0.82%
25	Kentucky	1,897	1.31%
24	Louisiana	1,918	1.33%
41	Maine	591	0.41%
13	Maryland	3,070	2.13%
10	Massachusetts	4,363	3.02%
7	Michigan	5,812	4.02%
16	Minnesota	2,780	1.92%
34	Mississippi	977	0.68%
19	Missouri	2,545	1.76%
44	Montana	453	0.31%
35	Nebraska	959	0.66%
42	Nevada	571	0.40%
38	New Hampshire	657	0.45%
9	New Jersey	5,534	3.83%
39	New Mexico	637	0.44%
2	New York	12,873	8.91%
17	North Carolina	2,748	1.90%
49	North Dakota	278	0.19%
8	Ohio	5,655	3.92%
29	Oklahoma	1,457	1.01%
23	Oregon	2,037	1.41%
5	Pennsylvania	7,459	5.16%
43	Rhode Island	546	0.38%
28	South Carolina	1,469	1.02%
47	South Dakota	307	0.21%
21	Tennessee	2,491	1.72%
3	Texas	7,970	5.52%
31	Utah	1,214	0.84%
45	Vermont	325	0.23%
11	Virginia	3,314	2.29%
12	Washington	3,128	2.17%
37	West Virginia	767	0.53%
15	Wisconsin	2,887	2.00%
50	Wyoming	232	0.16%

<u>RANK ORDER</u>

RANK	STATE	DENTISTS	% of USA
1	California	20,145	13.95%
2	New York	12,873	8.91%
3	Texas	7,970	5.52%
4	Illinois	7,515	5.20%
5	Pennsylvania	7,459	5.16%
6	Florida	6,607	4.57%
7	Michigan	5,812	4.02%
8	Ohio	5,655	3.92%
9	New Jersey	5,534	3.83%
10	Massachusetts	4,363	3.02%
11	Virginia	3,314	2.29%
12	Washington	3,128	2.17%
13	Maryland	3,070	2.13%
14	Georgia	2,953	2.04%
15	Wisconsin	2,887	2.00%
16	Minnesota	2,780	1.92%
17	North Carolina	2,748	1.90%
18	Indiana	2,579	1.79%
19	Missouri	2,545	1.76%
20	Colorado	2,497	1.73%
21	Tennessee	2,491	1.72%
22	Connecticut	2,364	1.64%
23	Oregon	2,037	1.41%
24	Louisiana	1,918	1.33%
25	Kentucky	1,897	1.31%
26	Arizona	1,814	1.26%
27	Alabama	1,709	1.18%
28	South Carolina	1,469	1.02%
29	Oklahoma	1,457	1.01%
30	Iowa	1,417	0.98%
31	Utah	1,214	0.84%
32	Kansas	1,187	0.82%
33	Arkansas	1,016	0.70%
34	Mississippi	977	0.68%
35	Nebraska	959	0.66%
36	Hawaii	907	0.63%
37	West Virginia	767	0.53%
38	New Hampshire	657	0.45%
39	New Mexico	637	0.44%
40	Idaho	594	0.41%
41	Maine	591	0.41%
42	Nevada	571	0.40%
43	Rhode Island	546	0.38%
44	Montana	453	0.31%
45	Vermont	325	0.23%
46	Alaska	320	0.22%
47	South Dakota	307	0.21%
48	Delaware	303	0.21%
49	North Dakota	278	0.19%
50	Wyoming	232	0.16%
	District of Columbia	591	0.41%

Source: American Dental Association (Chicago, IL)
    "1996 ADA Dentist Masterfile"
National total does not include 5,227 dentists in the armed forces, public health service, veterans affairs or civil service. Also does not include 888 dentists in Puerto Rico and the Virgin Islands.

Rate of Active Civilian Dentists in 1996

National Rate = 54 Dentists per 100,000 Population*

ALPHA ORDER

RANK	STATE	RATE
43	Alabama	40
21	Alaska	53
42	Arizona	41
43	Arkansas	40
8	California	63
6	Colorado	65
2	Connecticut	72
38	Delaware	42
32	Florida	46
43	Georgia	40
1	Hawaii	77
24	Idaho	50
8	Illinois	63
34	Indiana	44
24	Iowa	50
32	Kansas	46
27	Kentucky	49
34	Louisiana	44
28	Maine	48
11	Maryland	61
2	Massachusetts	72
11	Michigan	61
14	Minnesota	60
49	Mississippi	36
30	Missouri	47
22	Montana	52
15	Nebraska	58
49	Nevada	36
16	New Hampshire	57
5	New Jersey	69
48	New Mexico	37
4	New York	71
47	North Carolina	38
37	North Dakota	43
23	Ohio	51
34	Oklahoma	44
7	Oregon	64
10	Pennsylvania	62
19	Rhode Island	55
43	South Carolina	40
38	South Dakota	42
30	Tennessee	47
38	Texas	42
11	Utah	61
19	Vermont	55
24	Virginia	50
16	Washington	57
38	West Virginia	42
18	Wisconsin	56
28	Wyoming	48

RANK ORDER

RANK	STATE	RATE
1	Hawaii	77
2	Connecticut	72
2	Massachusetts	72
4	New York	71
5	New Jersey	69
6	Colorado	65
7	Oregon	64
8	California	63
8	Illinois	63
10	Pennsylvania	62
11	Maryland	61
11	Michigan	61
11	Utah	61
14	Minnesota	60
15	Nebraska	58
16	New Hampshire	57
16	Washington	57
18	Wisconsin	56
19	Rhode Island	55
19	Vermont	55
21	Alaska	53
22	Montana	52
23	Ohio	51
24	Idaho	50
24	Iowa	50
24	Virginia	50
27	Kentucky	49
28	Maine	48
28	Wyoming	48
30	Missouri	47
30	Tennessee	47
32	Florida	46
32	Kansas	46
34	Indiana	44
34	Louisiana	44
34	Oklahoma	44
37	North Dakota	43
38	Delaware	42
38	South Dakota	42
38	Texas	42
38	West Virginia	42
42	Arizona	41
43	Alabama	40
43	Arkansas	40
43	Georgia	40
43	South Carolina	40
47	North Carolina	38
48	New Mexico	37
49	Mississippi	36
49	Nevada	36

District of Columbia	109

Source: Morgan Quitno Press using data from American Dental Association (Chicago, IL)
   "1996 ADA Dentist Masterfile"
*National total does not include dentists in the armed forces, public health service, veterans affairs or civil service.
Also does not include dentists in Puerto Rico and the Virgin Islands.

Hospital Personnel in 1995

National Total = 4,272,815 Personnel*

ALPHA ORDER

RANK	STATE	PERSONNEL	% of USA
19	Alabama	76,276	1.79%
48	Alaska	9,108	0.21%
26	Arizona	53,524	1.25%
32	Arkansas	42,483	0.99%
2	California	366,156	8.57%
27	Colorado	52,037	1.22%
30	Connecticut	48,760	1.14%
47	Delaware	12,046	0.28%
5	Florida	223,934	5.24%
11	Georgia	121,701	2.85%
41	Hawaii	16,909	0.40%
46	Idaho	13,230	0.31%
6	Illinois	204,629	4.79%
14	Indiana	98,637	2.31%
28	Iowa	52,019	1.22%
31	Kansas	46,999	1.10%
23	Kentucky	64,214	1.50%
17	Louisiana	88,464	2.07%
38	Maine	21,098	0.49%
18	Maryland	79,809	1.87%
10	Massachusetts	123,276	2.89%
8	Michigan	157,402	3.68%
22	Minnesota	66,137	1.55%
29	Mississippi	50,818	1.19%
13	Missouri	109,728	2.57%
45	Montana	14,876	0.35%
35	Nebraska	32,645	0.76%
42	Nevada	16,723	0.39%
39	New Hampshire	17,169	0.40%
9	New Jersey	133,199	3.12%
36	New Mexico	27,005	0.63%
1	New York	368,722	8.63%
12	North Carolina	119,814	2.80%
43	North Dakota	15,928	0.37%
7	Ohio	192,263	4.50%
24	Oklahoma	55,300	1.29%
33	Oregon	39,379	0.92%
4	Pennsylvania	241,531	5.65%
40	Rhode Island	17,031	0.40%
25	South Carolina	53,881	1.26%
44	South Dakota	15,336	0.36%
15	Tennessee	95,210	2.23%
3	Texas	280,617	6.57%
37	Utah	24,642	0.58%
49	Vermont	8,740	0.20%
16	Virginia	93,819	2.20%
21	Washington	67,243	1.57%
34	West Virginia	34,389	0.80%
20	Wisconsin	72,550	1.70%
50	Wyoming	7,852	0.18%

RANK ORDER

RANK	STATE	PERSONNEL	% of USA
1	New York	368,722	8.63%
2	California	366,156	8.57%
3	Texas	280,617	6.57%
4	Pennsylvania	241,531	5.65%
5	Florida	223,934	5.24%
6	Illinois	204,629	4.79%
7	Ohio	192,263	4.50%
8	Michigan	157,402	3.68%
9	New Jersey	133,199	3.12%
10	Massachusetts	123,276	2.89%
11	Georgia	121,701	2.85%
12	North Carolina	119,814	2.80%
13	Missouri	109,728	2.57%
14	Indiana	98,637	2.31%
15	Tennessee	95,210	2.23%
16	Virginia	93,819	2.20%
17	Louisiana	88,464	2.07%
18	Maryland	79,809	1.87%
19	Alabama	76,276	1.79%
20	Wisconsin	72,550	1.70%
21	Washington	67,243	1.57%
22	Minnesota	66,137	1.55%
23	Kentucky	64,214	1.50%
24	Oklahoma	55,300	1.29%
25	South Carolina	53,881	1.26%
26	Arizona	53,524	1.25%
27	Colorado	52,037	1.22%
28	Iowa	52,019	1.22%
29	Mississippi	50,818	1.19%
30	Connecticut	48,760	1.14%
31	Kansas	46,999	1.10%
32	Arkansas	42,483	0.99%
33	Oregon	39,379	0.92%
34	West Virginia	34,389	0.80%
35	Nebraska	32,645	0.76%
36	New Mexico	27,005	0.63%
37	Utah	24,642	0.58%
38	Maine	21,098	0.49%
39	New Hampshire	17,169	0.40%
40	Rhode Island	17,031	0.40%
41	Hawaii	16,909	0.40%
42	Nevada	16,723	0.39%
43	North Dakota	15,928	0.37%
44	South Dakota	15,336	0.36%
45	Montana	14,876	0.35%
46	Idaho	13,230	0.31%
47	Delaware	12,046	0.28%
48	Alaska	9,108	0.21%
49	Vermont	8,740	0.20%
50	Wyoming	7,852	0.18%
	District of Columbia	27,557	0.64%

Source: American Hospital Association (Chicago, IL)
"Hospital Statistics" (1996-97 edition)
Includes physicians, dentists, nurses and other salaried personnel in federal and nonfederal hospitals.

Employment in Health Service Industries in 1994

National Total = 10,624,354 Employees*

ALPHA ORDER

ALPHA ORDER

RANK	STATE	EMPLOYEES	% of USA
22	Alabama	169,755	1.60%
49	Alaska	16,516	0.16%
26	Arizona	135,658	1.28%
32	Arkansas	95,028	0.89%
1	California	1,003,453	9.44%
25	Colorado	138,125	1.30%
23	Connecticut	167,046	1.57%
47	Delaware	29,833	0.28%
4	Florida	576,432	5.43%
11	Georgia	263,204	2.48%
42	Hawaii	38,249	0.36%
44	Idaho	35,197	0.33%
7	Illinois	492,756	4.64%
14	Indiana	244,880	2.30%
27	Iowa	131,714	1.24%
29	Kansas	116,880	1.10%
24	Kentucky	149,983	1.41%
19	Louisiana	200,634	1.89%
37	Maine	56,605	0.53%
20	Maryland	194,998	1.84%
9	Massachusetts	344,245	3.24%
8	Michigan	379,845	3.58%
15	Minnesota	233,893	2.20%
33	Mississippi	93,627	0.88%
13	Missouri	247,682	2.33%
46	Montana	31,632	0.30%
35	Nebraska	71,859	0.68%
41	Nevada	40,030	0.38%
40	New Hampshire	45,041	0.42%
10	New Jersey	341,386	3.21%
38	New Mexico	53,490	0.50%
2	New York	908,160	8.55%
12	North Carolina	260,996	2.46%
43	North Dakota	35,455	0.33%
6	Ohio	498,498	4.69%
28	Oklahoma	125,401	1.18%
31	Oregon	102,452	0.96%
5	Pennsylvania	564,868	5.32%
39	Rhode Island	48,880	0.46%
30	South Carolina	116,767	1.10%
45	South Dakota	34,570	0.33%
17	Tennessee	223,217	2.10%
3	Texas	672,319	6.33%
36	Utah	63,125	0.59%
48	Vermont	23,527	0.22%
16	Virginia	230,009	2.16%
21	Washington	193,230	1.82%
34	West Virginia	74,525	0.70%
18	Wisconsin	222,305	2.09%
50	Wyoming	15,826	0.15%

RANK ORDER

RANK	STATE	EMPLOYEES	% of USA
1	California	1,003,453	9.44%
2	New York	908,160	8.55%
3	Texas	672,319	6.33%
4	Florida	576,432	5.43%
5	Pennsylvania	564,868	5.32%
6	Ohio	498,498	4.69%
7	Illinois	492,756	4.64%
8	Michigan	379,845	3.58%
9	Massachusetts	344,245	3.24%
10	New Jersey	341,386	3.21%
11	Georgia	263,204	2.48%
12	North Carolina	260,996	2.46%
13	Missouri	247,682	2.33%
14	Indiana	244,880	2.30%
15	Minnesota	233,893	2.20%
16	Virginia	230,009	2.16%
17	Tennessee	223,217	2.10%
18	Wisconsin	222,305	2.09%
19	Louisiana	200,634	1.89%
20	Maryland	194,998	1.84%
21	Washington	193,230	1.82%
22	Alabama	169,755	1.60%
23	Connecticut	167,046	1.57%
24	Kentucky	149,983	1.41%
25	Colorado	138,125	1.30%
26	Arizona	135,658	1.28%
27	Iowa	131,714	1.24%
28	Oklahoma	125,401	1.18%
29	Kansas	116,880	1.10%
30	South Carolina	116,767	1.10%
31	Oregon	102,452	0.96%
32	Arkansas	95,028	0.89%
33	Mississippi	93,627	0.88%
34	West Virginia	74,525	0.70%
35	Nebraska	71,859	0.68%
36	Utah	63,125	0.59%
37	Maine	56,605	0.53%
38	New Mexico	53,490	0.50%
39	Rhode Island	48,880	0.46%
40	New Hampshire	45,041	0.42%
41	Nevada	40,030	0.38%
42	Hawaii	38,249	0.36%
43	North Dakota	35,455	0.33%
44	Idaho	35,197	0.33%
45	South Dakota	34,570	0.33%
46	Montana	31,632	0.30%
47	Delaware	29,833	0.28%
48	Vermont	23,527	0.22%
49	Alaska	16,516	0.16%
50	Wyoming	15,826	0.15%
	District of Columbia	70,548	0.66%

Source: U.S. Bureau of the Census
   "1994 County Business Patterns"
*Total of employment in 1994 at establishments classified in Standard Industrial Classification (S.I.C.) code 8000.
An establishment is a single physical location at which business is conducted or where services or industrial
operations are performed. It is not necessarily identical with a company or enterprise, which may consist of one
establishment or more.

487

VII. PHYSICAL FITNESS

Users of Exercise Equipment in 1995

National Total = 44,056,000 Participants

ALPHA ORDER

RANK	STATE	PARTICIPANTS	% of USA
24	Alabama	702,000	1.59%
NA	Alaska*	NA	NA
22	Arizona	741,000	1.68%
37	Arkansas	247,000	0.56%
1	California	5,716,000	12.97%
27	Colorado	566,000	1.28%
23	Connecticut	736,000	1.67%
48	Delaware	76,000	0.17%
4	Florida	2,111,000	4.79%
11	Georgia	1,078,000	2.45%
NA	Hawaii*	NA	NA
40	Idaho	213,000	0.48%
6	Illinois	1,927,000	4.37%
12	Indiana	1,073,000	2.44%
29	Iowa	534,000	1.21%
31	Kansas	438,000	0.99%
28	Kentucky	540,000	1.23%
26	Louisiana	588,000	1.33%
40	Maine	213,000	0.48%
13	Maryland	1,057,000	2.40%
14	Massachusetts	1,025,000	2.33%
9	Michigan	1,541,000	3.50%
18	Minnesota	849,000	1.93%
38	Mississippi	233,000	0.53%
20	Missouri	814,000	1.85%
39	Montana	227,000	0.52%
33	Nebraska	362,000	0.82%
34	Nevada	309,000	0.70%
42	New Hampshire	166,000	0.38%
8	New Jersey	1,612,000	3.66%
36	New Mexico	252,000	0.57%
2	New York	3,120,000	7.08%
10	North Carolina	1,123,000	2.55%
44	North Dakota	132,000	0.30%
5	Ohio	1,946,000	4.42%
25	Oklahoma	623,000	1.41%
21	Oregon	748,000	1.70%
7	Pennsylvania	1,924,000	4.37%
45	Rhode Island	117,000	0.27%
30	South Carolina	482,000	1.09%
47	South Dakota	108,000	0.25%
19	Tennessee	818,000	1.86%
3	Texas	3,092,000	7.02%
32	Utah	403,000	0.91%
46	Vermont	111,000	0.25%
15	Virginia	1,022,000	2.32%
17	Washington	891,000	2.02%
35	West Virginia	286,000	0.65%
16	Wisconsin	955,000	2.17%
43	Wyoming	139,000	0.32%

RANK ORDER

RANK	STATE	PARTICIPANTS	% of USA
1	California	5,716,000	12.97%
2	New York	3,120,000	7.08%
3	Texas	3,092,000	7.02%
4	Florida	2,111,000	4.79%
5	Ohio	1,946,000	4.42%
6	Illinois	1,927,000	4.37%
7	Pennsylvania	1,924,000	4.37%
8	New Jersey	1,612,000	3.66%
9	Michigan	1,541,000	3.50%
10	North Carolina	1,123,000	2.55%
11	Georgia	1,078,000	2.45%
12	Indiana	1,073,000	2.44%
13	Maryland	1,057,000	2.40%
14	Massachusetts	1,025,000	2.33%
15	Virginia	1,022,000	2.32%
16	Wisconsin	955,000	2.17%
17	Washington	891,000	2.02%
18	Minnesota	849,000	1.93%
19	Tennessee	818,000	1.86%
20	Missouri	814,000	1.85%
21	Oregon	748,000	1.70%
22	Arizona	741,000	1.68%
23	Connecticut	736,000	1.67%
24	Alabama	702,000	1.59%
25	Oklahoma	623,000	1.41%
26	Louisiana	588,000	1.33%
27	Colorado	566,000	1.28%
28	Kentucky	540,000	1.23%
29	Iowa	534,000	1.21%
30	South Carolina	482,000	1.09%
31	Kansas	438,000	0.99%
32	Utah	403,000	0.91%
33	Nebraska	362,000	0.82%
34	Nevada	309,000	0.70%
35	West Virginia	286,000	0.65%
36	New Mexico	252,000	0.57%
37	Arkansas	247,000	0.56%
38	Mississippi	233,000	0.53%
39	Montana	227,000	0.52%
40	Idaho	213,000	0.48%
40	Maine	213,000	0.48%
42	New Hampshire	166,000	0.38%
43	Wyoming	139,000	0.32%
44	North Dakota	132,000	0.30%
45	Rhode Island	117,000	0.27%
46	Vermont	111,000	0.25%
47	South Dakota	108,000	0.25%
48	Delaware	76,000	0.17%
NA	Alaska*	NA	NA
NA	Hawaii*	NA	NA
	District of Columbia*	NA	NA

Source: The National Sporting Goods Association
   "NSGA Sports Participation Survey, January-December 1995 (Copyright 1996, reprinted with permission)
Not available.

Participants in Golf in 1995

National Total = 24,255,000 Golfers

ALPHA ORDER					RANK ORDER			

RANK	STATE	GOLFERS	% of USA		RANK	STATE	GOLFERS	% of USA
32	Alabama	220,000	0.91%		1	California	2,889,000	11.91%
NA	Alaska*	NA	NA		2	New York	1,597,000	6.58%
15	Arizona	507,000	2.09%		3	Texas	1,392,000	5.74%
35	Arkansas	184,000	0.76%		4	Florida	1,371,000	5.65%
1	California	2,889,000	11.91%		5	Illinois	1,236,000	5.10%
24	Colorado	338,000	1.39%		6	Michigan	1,127,000	4.65%
28	Connecticut	255,000	1.05%		7	Ohio	1,086,000	4.48%
48	Delaware	21,000	0.09%		8	Pennsylvania	1,082,000	4.46%
4	Florida	1,371,000	5.65%		9	New Jersey	796,000	3.28%
13	Georgia	628,000	2.59%		10	Wisconsin	791,000	3.26%
NA	Hawaii*	NA	NA		11	North Carolina	769,000	3.17%
37	Idaho	151,000	0.62%		12	Indiana	686,000	2.83%
5	Illinois	1,236,000	5.10%		13	Georgia	628,000	2.59%
12	Indiana	686,000	2.83%		14	Minnesota	557,000	2.30%
20	Iowa	419,000	1.73%		15	Arizona	507,000	2.09%
29	Kansas	251,000	1.03%		16	Washington	497,000	2.05%
25	Kentucky	314,000	1.29%		17	Virginia	486,000	2.00%
31	Louisiana	234,000	0.96%		18	Massachusetts	466,000	1.92%
45	Maine	64,000	0.26%		19	Missouri	458,000	1.89%
23	Maryland	340,000	1.40%		20	Iowa	419,000	1.73%
18	Massachusetts	466,000	1.92%		21	Tennessee	409,000	1.69%
6	Michigan	1,127,000	4.65%		22	South Carolina	378,000	1.56%
14	Minnesota	557,000	2.30%		23	Maryland	340,000	1.40%
38	Mississippi	145,000	0.60%		24	Colorado	338,000	1.39%
19	Missouri	458,000	1.89%		25	Kentucky	314,000	1.29%
40	Montana	124,000	0.51%		26	Utah	268,000	1.10%
27	Nebraska	260,000	1.07%		27	Nebraska	260,000	1.07%
34	Nevada	186,000	0.77%		28	Connecticut	255,000	1.05%
47	New Hampshire	51,000	0.21%		29	Kansas	251,000	1.03%
9	New Jersey	796,000	3.28%		30	Oregon	236,000	0.97%
42	New Mexico	114,000	0.47%		31	Louisiana	234,000	0.96%
2	New York	1,597,000	6.58%		32	Alabama	220,000	0.91%
11	North Carolina	769,000	3.17%		33	Oklahoma	215,000	0.89%
43	North Dakota	87,000	0.36%		34	Nevada	186,000	0.77%
7	Ohio	1,086,000	4.48%		35	Arkansas	184,000	0.76%
33	Oklahoma	215,000	0.89%		36	Wyoming	166,000	0.68%
30	Oregon	236,000	0.97%		37	Idaho	151,000	0.62%
8	Pennsylvania	1,082,000	4.46%		38	Mississippi	145,000	0.60%
39	Rhode Island	139,000	0.57%		39	Rhode Island	139,000	0.57%
22	South Carolina	378,000	1.56%		40	Montana	124,000	0.51%
44	South Dakota	81,000	0.33%		41	West Virginia	116,000	0.48%
21	Tennessee	409,000	1.69%		42	New Mexico	114,000	0.47%
3	Texas	1,392,000	5.74%		43	North Dakota	87,000	0.36%
26	Utah	268,000	1.10%		44	South Dakota	81,000	0.33%
46	Vermont	62,000	0.26%		45	Maine	64,000	0.26%
17	Virginia	486,000	2.00%		46	Vermont	62,000	0.26%
16	Washington	497,000	2.05%		47	New Hampshire	51,000	0.21%
41	West Virginia	116,000	0.48%		48	Delaware	21,000	0.09%
10	Wisconsin	791,000	3.26%		NA	Alaska*	NA	NA
36	Wyoming	166,000	0.68%		NA	Hawaii*	NA	NA
						District of Columbia*	NA	NA

Source: The National Sporting Goods Association
    "NSGA Sports Participation Survey, January-December 1995 (Copyright 1996, reprinted with permission)
*Not available.

Participants in Running/Jogging in 1995

National Total = 20,637,000 Runners/Joggers

ALPHA ORDER					RANK ORDER			
RANK	STATE	RUNNERS	% of USA		RANK	STATE	RUNNERS	% of USA
20	Alabama	351,000	1.70%		1	California	2,936,000	14.23%
NA	Alaska*	NA	NA		2	Texas	1,547,000	7.50%
15	Arizona	420,000	2.04%		3	New York	1,283,000	6.22%
38	Arkansas	114,000	0.55%		4	Illinois	1,011,000	4.90%
1	California	2,936,000	14.23%		5	Florida	1,001,000	4.85%
23	Colorado	301,000	1.46%		6	Pennsylvania	832,000	4.03%
31	Connecticut	240,000	1.16%		7	Ohio	794,000	3.85%
44	Delaware	64,000	0.31%		8	Michigan	762,000	3.69%
5	Florida	1,001,000	4.85%		9	North Carolina	645,000	3.13%
11	Georgia	541,000	2.62%		10	New Jersey	563,000	2.73%
NA	Hawaii*	NA	NA		11	Georgia	541,000	2.62%
43	Idaho	75,000	0.36%		12	Virginia	516,000	2.50%
4	Illinois	1,011,000	4.90%		13	Massachusetts	491,000	2.38%
19	Indiana	363,000	1.76%		14	Washington	453,000	2.20%
32	Iowa	212,000	1.03%		15	Arizona	420,000	2.04%
27	Kansas	263,000	1.27%		15	Tennessee	420,000	2.04%
25	Kentucky	281,000	1.36%		17	Maryland	390,000	1.89%
18	Louisiana	383,000	1.86%		18	Louisiana	383,000	1.86%
45	Maine	63,000	0.31%		19	Indiana	363,000	1.76%
17	Maryland	390,000	1.89%		20	Alabama	351,000	1.70%
13	Massachusetts	491,000	2.38%		21	Oklahoma	331,000	1.60%
8	Michigan	762,000	3.69%		22	Wisconsin	312,000	1.51%
24	Minnesota	284,000	1.38%		23	Colorado	301,000	1.46%
34	Mississippi	175,000	0.85%		24	Minnesota	284,000	1.38%
30	Missouri	254,000	1.23%		25	Kentucky	281,000	1.36%
37	Montana	133,000	0.64%		26	South Carolina	266,000	1.29%
33	Nebraska	191,000	0.93%		27	Kansas	263,000	1.27%
36	Nevada	153,000	0.74%		27	Utah	263,000	1.27%
40	New Hampshire	94,000	0.46%		29	Oregon	259,000	1.26%
10	New Jersey	563,000	2.73%		30	Missouri	254,000	1.23%
35	New Mexico	166,000	0.80%		31	Connecticut	240,000	1.16%
3	New York	1,283,000	6.22%		32	Iowa	212,000	1.03%
9	North Carolina	645,000	3.13%		33	Nebraska	191,000	0.93%
46	North Dakota	53,000	0.26%		34	Mississippi	175,000	0.85%
7	Ohio	794,000	3.85%		35	New Mexico	166,000	0.80%
21	Oklahoma	331,000	1.60%		36	Nevada	153,000	0.74%
29	Oregon	259,000	1.26%		37	Montana	133,000	0.64%
6	Pennsylvania	832,000	4.03%		38	Arkansas	114,000	0.55%
41	Rhode Island	85,000	0.41%		39	West Virginia	97,000	0.47%
26	South Carolina	266,000	1.29%		40	New Hampshire	94,000	0.46%
48	South Dakota	16,000	0.08%		41	Rhode Island	85,000	0.41%
15	Tennessee	420,000	2.04%		42	Wyoming	81,000	0.39%
2	Texas	1,547,000	7.50%		43	Idaho	75,000	0.36%
27	Utah	263,000	1.27%		44	Delaware	64,000	0.31%
47	Vermont	52,000	0.25%		45	Maine	63,000	0.31%
12	Virginia	516,000	2.50%		46	North Dakota	53,000	0.26%
14	Washington	453,000	2.20%		47	Vermont	52,000	0.25%
39	West Virginia	97,000	0.47%		48	South Dakota	16,000	0.08%
22	Wisconsin	312,000	1.51%		NA	Alaska*	NA	NA
42	Wyoming	81,000	0.39%		NA	Hawaii*	NA	NA
						District of Columbia*	NA	NA

Source: The National Sporting Goods Association
"NSGA Sports Participation Survey, January-December 1995 (Copyright 1996, reprinted with permission)
Not available.

Participants in Soccer in 1995

National Total = 12,242,000 Soccer Players

RANK	STATE	PARTICIPANTS	% of USA
28	Alabama	140,000	1.14%
NA	Alaska*	NA	NA
12	Arizona	280,000	2.29%
35	Arkansas	83,000	0.68%
1	California	1,713,000	13.99%
15	Colorado	243,000	1.98%
16	Connecticut	227,000	1.85%
44	Delaware	37,000	0.30%
8	Florida	435,000	3.55%
18	Georgia	214,000	1.75%
NA	Hawaii*	NA	NA
43	Idaho	40,000	0.33%
4	Illinois	777,000	6.35%
21	Indiana	195,000	1.59%
31	Iowa	105,000	0.86%
29	Kansas	138,000	1.13%
27	Kentucky	141,000	1.15%
33	Louisiana	96,000	0.78%
32	Maine	104,000	0.85%
23	Maryland	176,000	1.44%
11	Massachusetts	320,000	2.61%
10	Michigan	340,000	2.78%
22	Minnesota	189,000	1.54%
42	Mississippi	47,000	0.38%
19	Missouri	213,000	1.74%
39	Montana	54,000	0.44%
40	Nebraska	52,000	0.42%
33	Nevada	96,000	0.78%
37	New Hampshire	78,000	0.64%
7	New Jersey	474,000	3.87%
47	New Mexico	22,000	0.18%
2	New York	1,019,000	8.32%
9	North Carolina	389,000	3.18%
45	North Dakota	35,000	0.29%
6	Ohio	553,000	4.52%
24	Oklahoma	170,000	1.39%
26	Oregon	158,000	1.29%
5	Pennsylvania	573,000	4.68%
36	Rhode Island	80,000	0.65%
30	South Carolina	110,000	0.90%
46	South Dakota	31,000	0.25%
25	Tennessee	162,000	1.32%
3	Texas	805,000	6.58%
17	Utah	224,000	1.83%
40	Vermont	52,000	0.42%
13	Virginia	278,000	2.27%
20	Washington	205,000	1.67%
47	West Virginia	22,000	0.18%
14	Wisconsin	250,000	2.04%
38	Wyoming	57,000	0.47%

RANK	STATE	PARTICIPANTS	% of USA
1	California	1,713,000	13.99%
2	New York	1,019,000	8.32%
3	Texas	805,000	6.58%
4	Illinois	777,000	6.35%
5	Pennsylvania	573,000	4.68%
6	Ohio	553,000	4.52%
7	New Jersey	474,000	3.87%
8	Florida	435,000	3.55%
9	North Carolina	389,000	3.18%
10	Michigan	340,000	2.78%
11	Massachusetts	320,000	2.61%
12	Arizona	280,000	2.29%
13	Virginia	278,000	2.27%
14	Wisconsin	250,000	2.04%
15	Colorado	243,000	1.98%
16	Connecticut	227,000	1.85%
17	Utah	224,000	1.83%
18	Georgia	214,000	1.75%
19	Missouri	213,000	1.74%
20	Washington	205,000	1.67%
21	Indiana	195,000	1.59%
22	Minnesota	189,000	1.54%
23	Maryland	176,000	1.44%
24	Oklahoma	170,000	1.39%
25	Tennessee	162,000	1.32%
26	Oregon	158,000	1.29%
27	Kentucky	141,000	1.15%
28	Alabama	140,000	1.14%
29	Kansas	138,000	1.13%
30	South Carolina	110,000	0.90%
31	Iowa	105,000	0.86%
32	Maine	104,000	0.85%
33	Louisiana	96,000	0.78%
33	Nevada	96,000	0.78%
35	Arkansas	83,000	0.68%
36	Rhode Island	80,000	0.65%
37	New Hampshire	78,000	0.64%
38	Wyoming	57,000	0.47%
39	Montana	54,000	0.44%
40	Nebraska	52,000	0.42%
40	Vermont	52,000	0.42%
42	Mississippi	47,000	0.38%
43	Idaho	40,000	0.33%
44	Delaware	37,000	0.30%
45	North Dakota	35,000	0.29%
46	South Dakota	31,000	0.25%
47	New Mexico	22,000	0.18%
47	West Virginia	22,000	0.18%
NA	Alaska*	NA	NA
NA	Hawaii*	NA	NA
	District of Columbia*	NA	NA

Source: The National Sporting Goods Association
   "NSGA Sports Participation Survey, January-December 1995 (Copyright 1996, reprinted with permission)
*Not available.

Participants in Swimming in 1995

National Total = 60,904,000 Swimmers

<u>ALPHA ORDER</u>					<u>RANK ORDER</u>			
RANK	STATE	SWIMMERS	% of USA		RANK	STATE	SWIMMERS	% of USA
23	Alabama	935,000	1.54%		1	California	6,914,000	11.35%
NA	Alaska*	NA	NA		2	New York	5,266,000	8.65%
17	Arizona	1,317,000	2.16%		3	Florida	3,962,000	6.51%
34	Arkansas	510,000	0.84%		4	Texas	3,922,000	6.44%
1	California	6,914,000	11.35%		5	Pennsylvania	3,019,000	4.96%
29	Colorado	632,000	1.04%		6	Ohio	2,622,000	4.31%
20	Connecticut	1,015,000	1.67%		7	Illinois	2,611,000	4.29%
46	Delaware	141,000	0.23%		8	Michigan	2,040,000	3.35%
3	Florida	3,962,000	6.51%		9	New Jersey	1,975,000	3.24%
16	Georgia	1,325,000	2.18%		10	Massachusetts	1,843,000	3.03%
NA	Hawaii*	NA	NA		11	North Carolina	1,642,000	2.70%
40	Idaho	281,000	0.46%		12	Wisconsin	1,520,000	2.50%
7	Illinois	2,611,000	4.29%		13	Indiana	1,392,000	2.29%
13	Indiana	1,392,000	2.29%		14	Missouri	1,373,000	2.25%
30	Iowa	598,000	0.98%		15	Virginia	1,354,000	2.22%
32	Kansas	543,000	0.89%		16	Georgia	1,325,000	2.18%
19	Kentucky	1,060,000	1.74%		17	Arizona	1,317,000	2.16%
26	Louisiana	711,000	1.17%		18	Maryland	1,130,000	1.86%
37	Maine	332,000	0.55%		19	Kentucky	1,060,000	1.74%
18	Maryland	1,130,000	1.86%		20	Connecticut	1,015,000	1.67%
10	Massachusetts	1,843,000	3.03%		21	Tennessee	986,000	1.62%
8	Michigan	2,040,000	3.35%		22	Washington	947,000	1.55%
24	Minnesota	930,000	1.53%		23	Alabama	935,000	1.54%
35	Mississippi	494,000	0.81%		24	Minnesota	930,000	1.53%
14	Missouri	1,373,000	2.25%		25	South Carolina	739,000	1.21%
42	Montana	246,000	0.40%		26	Louisiana	711,000	1.17%
38	Nebraska	330,000	0.54%		27	Oklahoma	700,000	1.15%
36	Nevada	382,000	0.63%		27	Oregon	700,000	1.15%
39	New Hampshire	312,000	0.51%		29	Colorado	632,000	1.04%
9	New Jersey	1,975,000	3.24%		30	Iowa	598,000	0.98%
47	New Mexico	126,000	0.21%		31	Utah	552,000	0.91%
2	New York	5,266,000	8.65%		32	Kansas	543,000	0.89%
11	North Carolina	1,642,000	2.70%		33	West Virginia	523,000	0.86%
45	North Dakota	160,000	0.26%		34	Arkansas	510,000	0.84%
6	Ohio	2,622,000	4.31%		35	Mississippi	494,000	0.81%
27	Oklahoma	700,000	1.15%		36	Nevada	382,000	0.63%
27	Oregon	700,000	1.15%		37	Maine	332,000	0.55%
5	Pennsylvania	3,019,000	4.96%		38	Nebraska	330,000	0.54%
41	Rhode Island	271,000	0.44%		39	New Hampshire	312,000	0.51%
25	South Carolina	739,000	1.21%		40	Idaho	281,000	0.46%
43	South Dakota	191,000	0.31%		41	Rhode Island	271,000	0.44%
21	Tennessee	986,000	1.62%		42	Montana	246,000	0.40%
4	Texas	3,922,000	6.44%		43	South Dakota	191,000	0.31%
31	Utah	552,000	0.91%		44	Vermont	162,000	0.27%
44	Vermont	162,000	0.27%		45	North Dakota	160,000	0.26%
15	Virginia	1,354,000	2.22%		46	Delaware	141,000	0.23%
22	Washington	947,000	1.55%		47	New Mexico	126,000	0.21%
33	West Virginia	523,000	0.86%		48	Wyoming	109,000	0.18%
12	Wisconsin	1,520,000	2.50%		NA	Alaska*	NA	NA
48	Wyoming	109,000	0.18%		NA	Hawaii*	NA	NA
						District of Columbia*	NA	NA

Source: The National Sporting Goods Association
"NSGA Sports Participation Survey, January-December 1995 (Copyright 1996, reprinted with permission)
Not available.

Participants in Tennis in 1995

National Total = 12,080,000 Tennis Players

ALPHA ORDER					RANK ORDER			
RANK	STATE	PLAYERS	% of USA		RANK	STATE	PLAYERS	% of USA
24	Alabama	170,000	1.41%		1	California	1,821,000	15.07%
NA	Alaska*	NA	NA		2	New York	909,000	7.52%
13	Arizona	239,000	1.98%		3	Texas	841,000	6.96%
34	Arkansas	63,000	0.52%		4	Illinois	749,000	6.20%
1	California	1,821,000	15.07%		5	Florida	631,000	5.22%
26	Colorado	152,000	1.26%		6	Pennsylvania	527,000	4.36%
20	Connecticut	200,000	1.66%		7	New Jersey	480,000	3.97%
45	Delaware	23,000	0.19%		8	Georgia	430,000	3.56%
5	Florida	631,000	5.22%		9	North Carolina	420,000	3.48%
8	Georgia	430,000	3.56%		10	Ohio	419,000	3.47%
NA	Hawaii*	NA	NA		11	Virginia	371,000	3.07%
43	Idaho	27,000	0.22%		12	Michigan	366,000	3.03%
4	Illinois	749,000	6.20%		13	Arizona	239,000	1.98%
16	Indiana	223,000	1.85%		14	Maryland	236,000	1.95%
30	Iowa	111,000	0.92%		15	Massachusetts	232,000	1.92%
29	Kansas	120,000	0.99%		16	Indiana	223,000	1.85%
22	Kentucky	195,000	1.61%		17	Wisconsin	222,000	1.84%
27	Louisiana	132,000	1.09%		18	Washington	209,000	1.73%
46	Maine	20,000	0.17%		19	Minnesota	205,000	1.70%
14	Maryland	236,000	1.95%		20	Connecticut	200,000	1.66%
15	Massachusetts	232,000	1.92%		21	Tennessee	196,000	1.62%
12	Michigan	366,000	3.03%		22	Kentucky	195,000	1.61%
19	Minnesota	205,000	1.70%		23	South Carolina	177,000	1.47%
44	Mississippi	26,000	0.22%		24	Alabama	170,000	1.41%
25	Missouri	155,000	1.28%		25	Missouri	155,000	1.28%
34	Montana	63,000	0.52%		26	Colorado	152,000	1.26%
38	Nebraska	53,000	0.44%		27	Louisiana	132,000	1.09%
33	Nevada	67,000	0.55%		28	Oklahoma	123,000	1.02%
40	New Hampshire	44,000	0.36%		29	Kansas	120,000	0.99%
7	New Jersey	480,000	3.97%		30	Iowa	111,000	0.92%
32	New Mexico	71,000	0.59%		31	Utah	76,000	0.63%
2	New York	909,000	7.52%		32	New Mexico	71,000	0.59%
9	North Carolina	420,000	3.48%		33	Nevada	67,000	0.55%
47	North Dakota	18,000	0.15%		34	Arkansas	63,000	0.52%
10	Ohio	419,000	3.47%		34	Montana	63,000	0.52%
28	Oklahoma	123,000	1.02%		36	Oregon	61,000	0.50%
36	Oregon	61,000	0.50%		36	South Dakota	61,000	0.50%
6	Pennsylvania	527,000	4.36%		38	Nebraska	53,000	0.44%
41	Rhode Island	43,000	0.36%		38	Vermont	53,000	0.44%
23	South Carolina	177,000	1.47%		40	New Hampshire	44,000	0.36%
36	South Dakota	61,000	0.50%		41	Rhode Island	43,000	0.36%
21	Tennessee	196,000	1.62%		42	West Virginia	40,000	0.33%
3	Texas	841,000	6.96%		43	Idaho	27,000	0.22%
31	Utah	76,000	0.63%		44	Mississippi	26,000	0.22%
38	Vermont	53,000	0.44%		45	Delaware	23,000	0.19%
11	Virginia	371,000	3.07%		46	Maine	20,000	0.17%
18	Washington	209,000	1.73%		47	North Dakota	18,000	0.15%
42	West Virginia	40,000	0.33%		48	Wyoming	9,000	0.07%
17	Wisconsin	222,000	1.84%		NA	Alaska*	NA	NA
48	Wyoming	9,000	0.07%		NA	Hawaii*	NA	NA
						District of Columbia*	NA	NA

Source: The National Sporting Goods Association
    "NSGA Sports Participation Survey, January-December 1995 (Copyright 1996, reprinted with permission)
*Not available.

Apparent Alcohol Consumption in 1995

National Total = 442,374,000 Gallons*

ALPHA ORDER

RANK	STATE	GALLONS	% of USA
25	Alabama	6,131,000	1.39%
46	Alaska	1,269,000	0.29%
18	Arizona	8,416,000	1.90%
35	Arkansas	3,369,000	0.76%
1	California	52,677,000	11.91%
23	Colorado	7,351,000	1.66%
26	Connecticut	5,709,000	1.29%
45	Delaware	1,490,000	0.34%
3	Florida	29,150,000	6.59%
10	Georgia	12,013,000	2.72%
39	Hawaii	2,117,000	0.48%
41	Idaho	1,776,000	0.40%
5	Illinois	21,104,000	4.77%
17	Indiana	8,730,000	1.97%
32	Iowa	4,132,000	0.93%
34	Kansas	3,410,000	0.77%
28	Kentucky	5,287,000	1.20%
20	Louisiana	8,248,000	1.86%
40	Maine	2,104,000	0.48%
21	Maryland	8,151,000	1.84%
11	Massachusetts	11,395,000	2.58%
8	Michigan	15,626,000	3.53%
19	Minnesota	8,355,000	1.89%
31	Mississippi	4,345,000	0.98%
16	Missouri	8,744,000	1.98%
44	Montana	1,726,000	0.39%
37	Nebraska	2,712,000	0.61%
29	Nevada	4,828,000	1.09%
33	New Hampshire	3,674,000	0.83%
9	New Jersey	13,904,000	3.14%
36	New Mexico	2,986,000	0.67%
4	New York	27,604,000	6.24%
12	North Carolina	10,801,000	2.44%
48	North Dakota	1,195,000	0.27%
7	Ohio	16,714,000	3.78%
30	Oklahoma	4,499,000	1.02%
27	Oregon	5,521,000	1.25%
6	Pennsylvania	17,971,000	4.06%
43	Rhode Island	1,737,000	0.39%
24	South Carolina	6,527,000	1.48%
47	South Dakota	1,252,000	0.28%
22	Tennessee	7,756,000	1.75%
2	Texas	32,161,000	7.27%
42	Utah	1,748,000	0.40%
49	Vermont	1,065,000	0.24%
14	Virginia	10,057,000	2.27%
15	Washington	9,126,000	2.06%
38	West Virginia	2,383,000	0.54%
13	Wisconsin	10,743,000	2.43%
50	Wyoming	859,000	0.19%

RANK ORDER

RANK	STATE	GALLONS	% of USA
1	California	52,677,000	11.91%
2	Texas	32,161,000	7.27%
3	Florida	29,150,000	6.59%
4	New York	27,604,000	6.24%
5	Illinois	21,104,000	4.77%
6	Pennsylvania	17,971,000	4.06%
7	Ohio	16,714,000	3.78%
8	Michigan	15,626,000	3.53%
9	New Jersey	13,904,000	3.14%
10	Georgia	12,013,000	2.72%
11	Massachusetts	11,395,000	2.58%
12	North Carolina	10,801,000	2.44%
13	Wisconsin	10,743,000	2.43%
14	Virginia	10,057,000	2.27%
15	Washington	9,126,000	2.06%
16	Missouri	8,744,000	1.98%
17	Indiana	8,730,000	1.97%
18	Arizona	8,416,000	1.90%
19	Minnesota	8,355,000	1.89%
20	Louisiana	8,248,000	1.86%
21	Maryland	8,151,000	1.84%
22	Tennessee	7,756,000	1.75%
23	Colorado	7,351,000	1.66%
24	South Carolina	6,527,000	1.48%
25	Alabama	6,131,000	1.39%
26	Connecticut	5,709,000	1.29%
27	Oregon	5,521,000	1.25%
28	Kentucky	5,287,000	1.20%
29	Nevada	4,828,000	1.09%
30	Oklahoma	4,499,000	1.02%
31	Mississippi	4,345,000	0.98%
32	Iowa	4,132,000	0.93%
33	New Hampshire	3,674,000	0.83%
34	Kansas	3,410,000	0.77%
35	Arkansas	3,369,000	0.76%
36	New Mexico	2,986,000	0.67%
37	Nebraska	2,712,000	0.61%
38	West Virginia	2,383,000	0.54%
39	Hawaii	2,117,000	0.48%
40	Maine	2,104,000	0.48%
41	Idaho	1,776,000	0.40%
42	Utah	1,748,000	0.40%
43	Rhode Island	1,737,000	0.39%
44	Montana	1,726,000	0.39%
45	Delaware	1,490,000	0.34%
46	Alaska	1,269,000	0.29%
47	South Dakota	1,252,000	0.28%
48	North Dakota	1,195,000	0.27%
49	Vermont	1,065,000	0.24%
50	Wyoming	859,000	0.19%
	District of Columbia	1,727,000	0.39%

*Source: Distilled Spirits Council of the United States, Inc., Steve L. Barsby Assoc.'s & Beer Institute
"1995 Statistical Information for the Distilled Spirits Industry" (June 1996)*
This is apparent consumption of actual alcohol, not entire volume of an alcoholic beverage (e.g. wine is roughly 11% absolute alcohol content). Apparent consumption is based on several sources which together approximate sales but do not actually measure consumption. Reported state volumes reflect only in-state purchases. Accordingly, figures for some states may be skewed by purchases by nonresidents.

Adult Per Capita Apparent Alcohol Consumption in 1995

National Per Capita = 2.41 Gallons Consumed per Adult Age 21 Years & Older*

ALPHA ORDER			RANK ORDER		
RANK	STATE	PER CAPITA	RANK	STATE	PER CAPITA
44	Alabama	2.05	1	New Hampshire	4.52
3	Alaska	3.29	2	Nevada	4.48
5	Arizona	2.95	3	Alaska	3.29
46	Arkansas	1.95	4	Wisconsin	3.02
23	California	2.44	5	Arizona	2.95
10	Colorado	2.81	6	Delaware	2.92
28	Connecticut	2.41	7	Montana	2.90
6	Delaware	2.92	8	Louisiana	2.85
9	Florida	2.83	9	Florida	2.83
25	Georgia	2.42	10	Colorado	2.81
18	Hawaii	2.56	11	North Dakota	2.70
32	Idaho	2.35	12	New Mexico	2.69
18	Illinois	2.56	13	Wyoming	2.68
36	Indiana	2.15	14	Minnesota	2.63
42	Iowa	2.07	15	Texas	2.58
48	Kansas	1.93	16	Massachusetts	2.57
46	Kentucky	1.95	16	Vermont	2.57
8	Louisiana	2.85	18	Hawaii	2.56
31	Maine	2.37	18	Illinois	2.56
35	Maryland	2.27	18	South Dakota	2.56
16	Massachusetts	2.57	21	South Carolina	2.54
32	Michigan	2.35	22	Oregon	2.49
14	Minnesota	2.63	23	California	2.44
28	Mississippi	2.41	23	New Jersey	2.44
32	Missouri	2.35	25	Georgia	2.42
7	Montana	2.90	25	Nebraska	2.42
25	Nebraska	2.42	25	Rhode Island	2.42
2	Nevada	4.48	28	Connecticut	2.41
1	New Hampshire	4.52	28	Mississippi	2.41
23	New Jersey	2.44	28	Washington	2.41
12	New Mexico	2.69	31	Maine	2.37
37	New York	2.14	32	Idaho	2.35
39	North Carolina	2.12	32	Michigan	2.35
11	North Dakota	2.70	32	Missouri	2.35
38	Ohio	2.13	35	Maryland	2.27
45	Oklahoma	2.00	36	Indiana	2.15
22	Oregon	2.49	37	New York	2.14
43	Pennsylvania	2.06	38	Ohio	2.13
25	Rhode Island	2.42	39	North Carolina	2.12
21	South Carolina	2.54	39	Virginia	2.12
18	South Dakota	2.56	41	Tennessee	2.08
41	Tennessee	2.08	42	Iowa	2.07
15	Texas	2.58	43	Pennsylvania	2.06
50	Utah	1.50	44	Alabama	2.05
16	Vermont	2.57	45	Oklahoma	2.00
39	Virginia	2.12	46	Arkansas	1.95
28	Washington	2.41	46	Kentucky	1.95
49	West Virginia	1.80	48	Kansas	1.93
4	Wisconsin	3.02	49	West Virginia	1.80
13	Wyoming	2.68	50	Utah	1.50
				District of Columbia	4.08

Source: MQ Press using data from Steve L. Barsby & Assoc. & Beer Institute as published by the Distilled Spirits Council of the United States, Inc. "1995 Statistical Information for the Distilled Spirits Industry" (June 1996) and Census
This is apparent consumption of actual alcohol, not the liquid volume of an alcoholic beverage (e.g. wine is roughly 11% absolute alcohol content). Apparent consumption is based on several sources which together approximate sales but do not actually measure consumption. Reported state volumes reflect only in-state purchases. Accordingly, figures for some states may be skewed by purchases by nonresidents.

Apparent Beer Consumption in 1995

National Total = 5,792,989,000 Gallons of Beer Consumed*

ALPHA ORDER

RANK	STATE	GALLONS	% of USA
25	Alabama	87,434,000	1.51%
48	Alaska	14,804,000	0.26%
17	Arizona	115,655,000	2.00%
33	Arkansas	48,205,000	0.83%
1	California	623,100,000	10.76%
24	Colorado	90,992,000	1.57%
31	Connecticut	57,739,000	1.00%
46	Delaware	17,004,000	0.29%
3	Florida	359,716,000	6.21%
9	Georgia	154,592,000	2.67%
39	Hawaii	28,989,000	0.50%
42	Idaho	23,836,000	0.41%
5	Illinois	274,461,000	4.74%
16	Indiana	116,805,000	2.02%
30	Iowa	64,288,000	1.11%
34	Kansas	48,196,000	0.83%
26	Kentucky	73,749,000	1.27%
18	Louisiana	114,726,000	1.98%
40	Maine	26,198,000	0.45%
22	Maryland	95,400,000	1.65%
14	Massachusetts	126,139,000	2.18%
8	Michigan	205,393,000	3.55%
21	Minnesota	101,742,000	1.76%
29	Mississippi	64,624,000	1.12%
15	Missouri	124,918,000	2.16%
43	Montana	23,057,000	0.40%
36	Nebraska	39,423,000	0.68%
32	Nevada	52,520,000	0.91%
38	New Hampshire	35,630,000	0.62%
10	New Jersey	148,915,000	2.57%
35	New Mexico	43,629,000	0.75%
4	New York	323,642,000	5.59%
11	North Carolina	147,365,000	2.54%
47	North Dakota	16,403,000	0.28%
7	Ohio	254,318,000	4.39%
28	Oklahoma	65,469,000	1.13%
27	Oregon	69,158,000	1.19%
6	Pennsylvania	269,795,000	4.66%
44	Rhode Island	21,936,000	0.38%
23	South Carolina	91,597,000	1.58%
45	South Dakota	17,269,000	0.30%
19	Tennessee	112,235,000	1.94%
2	Texas	507,904,000	8.77%
41	Utah	24,151,000	0.42%
49	Vermont	13,327,000	0.23%
13	Virginia	137,229,000	2.37%
20	Washington	110,516,000	1.91%
37	West Virginia	38,165,000	0.66%
12	Wisconsin	143,193,000	2.47%
50	Wyoming	11,368,000	0.20%

RANK ORDER

RANK	STATE	GALLONS	% of USA
1	California	623,100,000	10.76%
2	Texas	507,904,000	8.77%
3	Florida	359,716,000	6.21%
4	New York	323,642,000	5.59%
5	Illinois	274,461,000	4.74%
6	Pennsylvania	269,795,000	4.66%
7	Ohio	254,318,000	4.39%
8	Michigan	205,393,000	3.55%
9	Georgia	154,592,000	2.67%
10	New Jersey	148,915,000	2.57%
11	North Carolina	147,365,000	2.54%
12	Wisconsin	143,193,000	2.47%
13	Virginia	137,229,000	2.37%
14	Massachusetts	126,139,000	2.18%
15	Missouri	124,918,000	2.16%
16	Indiana	116,805,000	2.02%
17	Arizona	115,655,000	2.00%
18	Louisiana	114,726,000	1.98%
19	Tennessee	112,235,000	1.94%
20	Washington	110,516,000	1.91%
21	Minnesota	101,742,000	1.76%
22	Maryland	95,400,000	1.65%
23	South Carolina	91,597,000	1.58%
24	Colorado	90,992,000	1.57%
25	Alabama	87,434,000	1.51%
26	Kentucky	73,749,000	1.27%
27	Oregon	69,158,000	1.19%
28	Oklahoma	65,469,000	1.13%
29	Mississippi	64,624,000	1.12%
30	Iowa	64,288,000	1.11%
31	Connecticut	57,739,000	1.00%
32	Nevada	52,520,000	0.91%
33	Arkansas	48,205,000	0.83%
34	Kansas	48,196,000	0.83%
35	New Mexico	43,629,000	0.75%
36	Nebraska	39,423,000	0.68%
37	West Virginia	38,165,000	0.66%
38	New Hampshire	35,630,000	0.62%
39	Hawaii	28,989,000	0.50%
40	Maine	26,198,000	0.45%
41	Utah	24,151,000	0.42%
42	Idaho	23,836,000	0.41%
43	Montana	23,057,000	0.40%
44	Rhode Island	21,936,000	0.38%
45	South Dakota	17,269,000	0.30%
46	Delaware	17,004,000	0.29%
47	North Dakota	16,403,000	0.28%
48	Alaska	14,804,000	0.26%
49	Vermont	13,327,000	0.23%
50	Wyoming	11,368,000	0.20%
	District of Columbia	16,072,000	0.28%

Source: Beer Institute as published by the Distilled Spirits Council of the United States, Inc.
    "1995 Statistical Information for the Distilled Spirits Industry" (June 1996)
*Apparent consumption is based on several sources which together approximate sales but do not actually measure consumption. Reported state volumes reflect only in-state purchases. Accordingly, figures for some states may be skewed by purchases by nonresidents.

Adult Per Capita Apparent Beer Consumption in 1995

National Per Capita = 31.59 Gallons Consumed per Adult 21 Years and Older*

ALPHA ORDER

RANK ORDER

RANK	STATE	PER CAPITA	RANK	STATE	PER CAPITA
34	Alabama	29.30	1	Nevada	48.73
9	Alaska	38.38	2	New Hampshire	43.81
4	Arizona	40.51	3	Texas	40.67
43	Arkansas	27.96	4	Arizona	40.51
38	California	28.91	5	Wisconsin	40.26
18	Colorado	34.82	6	Louisiana	39.58
49	Connecticut	24.42	7	New Mexico	39.33
21	Delaware	33.25	8	Montana	38.76
17	Florida	34.89	9	Alaska	38.38
28	Georgia	31.08	10	North Dakota	37.15
16	Hawaii	35.06	11	Mississippi	35.82
26	Idaho	31.51	12	South Carolina	35.67
20	Illinois	33.35	13	Wyoming	35.48
41	Indiana	28.72	14	South Dakota	35.30
23	Iowa	32.21	15	Nebraska	35.13
44	Kansas	27.33	16	Hawaii	35.06
45	Kentucky	27.17	17	Florida	34.89
6	Louisiana	39.58	18	Colorado	34.82
33	Maine	29.51	19	Missouri	33.53
46	Maryland	26.57	20	Illinois	33.35
42	Massachusetts	28.46	21	Delaware	33.25
30	Michigan	30.95	22	Ohio	32.46
25	Minnesota	31.99	23	Iowa	32.21
11	Mississippi	35.82	24	Vermont	32.08
19	Missouri	33.53	25	Minnesota	31.99
8	Montana	38.76	26	Idaho	31.51
15	Nebraska	35.13	27	Oregon	31.19
1	Nevada	48.73	28	Georgia	31.08
2	New Hampshire	43.81	29	Pennsylvania	30.97
47	New Jersey	26.15	30	Michigan	30.95
7	New Mexico	39.33	31	Rhode Island	30.58
48	New York	25.06	32	Tennessee	30.10
39	North Carolina	28.87	33	Maine	29.51
10	North Dakota	37.15	34	Alabama	29.30
22	Ohio	32.46	35	Washington	29.13
36	Oklahoma	29.03	36	Oklahoma	29.03
27	Oregon	31.19	37	Virginia	28.97
29	Pennsylvania	30.97	38	California	28.91
31	Rhode Island	30.58	39	North Carolina	28.87
12	South Carolina	35.67	40	West Virginia	28.86
14	South Dakota	35.30	41	Indiana	28.72
32	Tennessee	30.10	42	Massachusetts	28.46
3	Texas	40.67	43	Arkansas	27.96
50	Utah	20.78	44	Kansas	27.33
24	Vermont	32.08	45	Kentucky	27.17
37	Virginia	28.97	46	Maryland	26.57
35	Washington	29.13	47	New Jersey	26.15
40	West Virginia	28.86	48	New York	25.06
5	Wisconsin	40.26	49	Connecticut	24.42
13	Wyoming	35.48	50	Utah	20.78
				District of Columbia	38.00

Source: Beer Institute as published by the Distilled Spirits Council of the United States, Inc.
   "1995 Statistical Information for the Distilled Spirits Industry" (June 1996)
Apparent consumption is based on several sources which together approximate sales but do not actually measure consumption. Reported state volumes reflect only in-state purchases. Accordingly, figures for some states may be skewed by purchases by nonresidents.

Apparent Wine Consumption in 1995

National Total = 470,160,000 Gallons of Wine Consumed*

<table>
<tr><td colspan="4">ALPHA ORDER</td><td colspan="4">RANK ORDER</td></tr>
<tr><td>RANK</td><td>STATE</td><td>GALLONS</td><td>% of USA</td><td>RANK</td><td>STATE</td><td>GALLONS</td><td>% of USA</td></tr>
<tr><td>28</td><td>Alabama</td><td>3,886,000</td><td>0.83%</td><td>1</td><td>California</td><td>85,826,000</td><td>18.25%</td></tr>
<tr><td>45</td><td>Alaska</td><td>1,257,000</td><td>0.27%</td><td>2</td><td>New York</td><td>44,304,000</td><td>9.42%</td></tr>
<tr><td>19</td><td>Arizona</td><td>7,769,000</td><td>1.65%</td><td>3</td><td>Florida</td><td>31,985,000</td><td>6.80%</td></tr>
<tr><td>40</td><td>Arkansas</td><td>1,805,000</td><td>0.38%</td><td>4</td><td>Illinois</td><td>24,321,000</td><td>5.17%</td></tr>
<tr><td>1</td><td>California</td><td>85,826,000</td><td>18.25%</td><td>5</td><td>New Jersey</td><td>22,180,000</td><td>4.72%</td></tr>
<tr><td>17</td><td>Colorado</td><td>8,523,000</td><td>1.81%</td><td>6</td><td>Texas</td><td>21,457,000</td><td>4.56%</td></tr>
<tr><td>14</td><td>Connecticut</td><td>10,115,000</td><td>2.15%</td><td>7</td><td>Massachusetts</td><td>17,602,000</td><td>3.74%</td></tr>
<tr><td>41</td><td>Delaware</td><td>1,796,000</td><td>0.38%</td><td>8</td><td>Pennsylvania</td><td>13,541,000</td><td>2.88%</td></tr>
<tr><td>3</td><td>Florida</td><td>31,985,000</td><td>6.80%</td><td>9</td><td>Washington</td><td>13,503,000</td><td>2.87%</td></tr>
<tr><td>15</td><td>Georgia</td><td>9,996,000</td><td>2.13%</td><td>10</td><td>Michigan</td><td>12,542,000</td><td>2.67%</td></tr>
<tr><td>32</td><td>Hawaii</td><td>2,599,000</td><td>0.55%</td><td>11</td><td>Virginia</td><td>12,004,000</td><td>2.55%</td></tr>
<tr><td>36</td><td>Idaho</td><td>2,150,000</td><td>0.46%</td><td>12</td><td>Ohio</td><td>11,612,000</td><td>2.47%</td></tr>
<tr><td>4</td><td>Illinois</td><td>24,321,000</td><td>5.17%</td><td>13</td><td>North Carolina</td><td>10,185,000</td><td>2.17%</td></tr>
<tr><td>20</td><td>Indiana</td><td>7,480,000</td><td>1.59%</td><td>14</td><td>Connecticut</td><td>10,115,000</td><td>2.15%</td></tr>
<tr><td>37</td><td>Iowa</td><td>2,025,000</td><td>0.43%</td><td>15</td><td>Georgia</td><td>9,996,000</td><td>2.13%</td></tr>
<tr><td>35</td><td>Kansas</td><td>2,208,000</td><td>0.47%</td><td>16</td><td>Maryland</td><td>8,526,000</td><td>1.81%</td></tr>
<tr><td>30</td><td>Kentucky</td><td>2,872,000</td><td>0.61%</td><td>17</td><td>Colorado</td><td>8,523,000</td><td>1.81%</td></tr>
<tr><td>24</td><td>Louisiana</td><td>5,823,000</td><td>1.24%</td><td>18</td><td>Oregon</td><td>8,414,000</td><td>1.79%</td></tr>
<tr><td>38</td><td>Maine</td><td>1,994,000</td><td>0.42%</td><td>19</td><td>Arizona</td><td>7,769,000</td><td>1.65%</td></tr>
<tr><td>16</td><td>Maryland</td><td>8,526,000</td><td>1.81%</td><td>20</td><td>Indiana</td><td>7,480,000</td><td>1.59%</td></tr>
<tr><td>7</td><td>Massachusetts</td><td>17,602,000</td><td>3.74%</td><td>21</td><td>Minnesota</td><td>7,339,000</td><td>1.56%</td></tr>
<tr><td>10</td><td>Michigan</td><td>12,542,000</td><td>2.67%</td><td>22</td><td>Wisconsin</td><td>7,324,000</td><td>1.56%</td></tr>
<tr><td>21</td><td>Minnesota</td><td>7,339,000</td><td>1.56%</td><td>23</td><td>Missouri</td><td>6,772,000</td><td>1.44%</td></tr>
<tr><td>43</td><td>Mississippi</td><td>1,453,000</td><td>0.31%</td><td>24</td><td>Louisiana</td><td>5,823,000</td><td>1.24%</td></tr>
<tr><td>23</td><td>Missouri</td><td>6,772,000</td><td>1.44%</td><td>25</td><td>Nevada</td><td>5,683,000</td><td>1.21%</td></tr>
<tr><td>44</td><td>Montana</td><td>1,428,000</td><td>0.30%</td><td>26</td><td>Tennessee</td><td>4,890,000</td><td>1.04%</td></tr>
<tr><td>39</td><td>Nebraska</td><td>1,884,000</td><td>0.40%</td><td>27</td><td>South Carolina</td><td>4,163,000</td><td>0.89%</td></tr>
<tr><td>25</td><td>Nevada</td><td>5,683,000</td><td>1.21%</td><td>28</td><td>Alabama</td><td>3,886,000</td><td>0.83%</td></tr>
<tr><td>29</td><td>New Hampshire</td><td>3,618,000</td><td>0.77%</td><td>29</td><td>New Hampshire</td><td>3,618,000</td><td>0.77%</td></tr>
<tr><td>5</td><td>New Jersey</td><td>22,180,000</td><td>4.72%</td><td>30</td><td>Kentucky</td><td>2,872,000</td><td>0.61%</td></tr>
<tr><td>34</td><td>New Mexico</td><td>2,325,000</td><td>0.49%</td><td>31</td><td>Oklahoma</td><td>2,672,000</td><td>0.57%</td></tr>
<tr><td>2</td><td>New York</td><td>44,304,000</td><td>9.42%</td><td>32</td><td>Hawaii</td><td>2,599,000</td><td>0.55%</td></tr>
<tr><td>13</td><td>North Carolina</td><td>10,185,000</td><td>2.17%</td><td>33</td><td>Rhode Island</td><td>2,413,000</td><td>0.51%</td></tr>
<tr><td>48</td><td>North Dakota</td><td>621,000</td><td>0.13%</td><td>34</td><td>New Mexico</td><td>2,325,000</td><td>0.49%</td></tr>
<tr><td>12</td><td>Ohio</td><td>11,612,000</td><td>2.47%</td><td>35</td><td>Kansas</td><td>2,208,000</td><td>0.47%</td></tr>
<tr><td>31</td><td>Oklahoma</td><td>2,672,000</td><td>0.57%</td><td>36</td><td>Idaho</td><td>2,150,000</td><td>0.46%</td></tr>
<tr><td>18</td><td>Oregon</td><td>8,414,000</td><td>1.79%</td><td>37</td><td>Iowa</td><td>2,025,000</td><td>0.43%</td></tr>
<tr><td>8</td><td>Pennsylvania</td><td>13,541,000</td><td>2.88%</td><td>38</td><td>Maine</td><td>1,994,000</td><td>0.42%</td></tr>
<tr><td>33</td><td>Rhode Island</td><td>2,413,000</td><td>0.51%</td><td>39</td><td>Nebraska</td><td>1,884,000</td><td>0.40%</td></tr>
<tr><td>27</td><td>South Carolina</td><td>4,163,000</td><td>0.89%</td><td>40</td><td>Arkansas</td><td>1,805,000</td><td>0.38%</td></tr>
<tr><td>49</td><td>South Dakota</td><td>551,000</td><td>0.12%</td><td>41</td><td>Delaware</td><td>1,796,000</td><td>0.38%</td></tr>
<tr><td>26</td><td>Tennessee</td><td>4,890,000</td><td>1.04%</td><td>42</td><td>Vermont</td><td>1,480,000</td><td>0.31%</td></tr>
<tr><td>6</td><td>Texas</td><td>21,457,000</td><td>4.56%</td><td>43</td><td>Mississippi</td><td>1,453,000</td><td>0.31%</td></tr>
<tr><td>46</td><td>Utah</td><td>1,086,000</td><td>0.23%</td><td>44</td><td>Montana</td><td>1,428,000</td><td>0.30%</td></tr>
<tr><td>42</td><td>Vermont</td><td>1,480,000</td><td>0.31%</td><td>45</td><td>Alaska</td><td>1,257,000</td><td>0.27%</td></tr>
<tr><td>11</td><td>Virginia</td><td>12,004,000</td><td>2.55%</td><td>46</td><td>Utah</td><td>1,086,000</td><td>0.23%</td></tr>
<tr><td>9</td><td>Washington</td><td>13,503,000</td><td>2.87%</td><td>47</td><td>West Virginia</td><td>1,028,000</td><td>0.22%</td></tr>
<tr><td>47</td><td>West Virginia</td><td>1,028,000</td><td>0.22%</td><td>48</td><td>North Dakota</td><td>621,000</td><td>0.13%</td></tr>
<tr><td>22</td><td>Wisconsin</td><td>7,324,000</td><td>1.56%</td><td>49</td><td>South Dakota</td><td>551,000</td><td>0.12%</td></tr>
<tr><td>50</td><td>Wyoming</td><td>461,000</td><td>0.10%</td><td>50</td><td>Wyoming</td><td>461,000</td><td>0.10%</td></tr>
<tr><td></td><td></td><td></td><td></td><td></td><td>District of Columbia</td><td>2,669,000</td><td>0.57%</td></tr>
</table>

Source: Steve L. Barsby and Associates, Inc. as published by the Distilled Spirits Council of the United States, Inc. "1995 Statistical Information for the Distilled Spirits Industry" (June 1996)

*Apparent consumption is based on several sources which together approximate sales but do not actually measure consumption. Reported state volumes reflect only in-state purchases. Accordingly, figures for some states may be skewed by purchases by nonresidents.

Adult Per Capita Apparent Wine Consumption in 1995

National Per Capita = 2.56 Gallons Consumed per Adult Age 21 Years and Older*

ALPHA ORDER				RANK ORDER		
RANK	STATE	PER CAPITA		RANK	STATE	PER CAPITA
41	Alabama	1.30		1	Nevada	5.27
13	Alaska	3.26		2	New Hampshire	4.45
19	Arizona	2.72		3	Connecticut	4.28
46	Arkansas	1.05		4	California	3.98
4	California	3.98		5	Massachusetts	3.97
13	Colorado	3.26		6	New Jersey	3.90
3	Connecticut	4.28		7	Oregon	3.79
10	Delaware	3.51		8	Vermont	3.56
16	Florida	3.10		8	Washington	3.56
26	Georgia	2.01		10	Delaware	3.51
15	Hawaii	3.14		11	New York	3.43
18	Idaho	2.84		12	Rhode Island	3.36
17	Illinois	2.96		13	Alaska	3.26
31	Indiana	1.84		13	Colorado	3.26
47	Iowa	1.01		15	Hawaii	3.14
42	Kansas	1.25		16	Florida	3.10
45	Kentucky	1.06		17	Illinois	2.96
26	Louisiana	2.01		18	Idaho	2.84
24	Maine	2.25		19	Arizona	2.72
22	Maryland	2.37		20	Virginia	2.53
5	Massachusetts	3.97		21	Montana	2.40
30	Michigan	1.89		22	Maryland	2.37
23	Minnesota	2.31		23	Minnesota	2.31
49	Mississippi	0.81		24	Maine	2.25
32	Missouri	1.82		25	New Mexico	2.10
21	Montana	2.40		26	Georgia	2.01
34	Nebraska	1.68		26	Louisiana	2.01
1	Nevada	5.27		28	North Carolina	2.00
2	New Hampshire	4.45		28	Wisconsin	2.00
6	New Jersey	3.90		30	Michigan	1.89
25	New Mexico	2.10		31	Indiana	1.84
11	New York	3.43		32	Missouri	1.82
28	North Carolina	2.00		33	Texas	1.72
39	North Dakota	1.41		34	Nebraska	1.68
37	Ohio	1.48		35	South Carolina	1.62
43	Oklahoma	1.18		36	Pennsylvania	1.55
7	Oregon	3.79		37	Ohio	1.48
36	Pennsylvania	1.55		38	Wyoming	1.44
12	Rhode Island	3.36		39	North Dakota	1.41
35	South Carolina	1.62		40	Tennessee	1.31
44	South Dakota	1.13		41	Alabama	1.30
40	Tennessee	1.31		42	Kansas	1.25
33	Texas	1.72		43	Oklahoma	1.18
48	Utah	0.93		44	South Dakota	1.13
8	Vermont	3.56		45	Kentucky	1.06
20	Virginia	2.53		46	Arkansas	1.05
8	Washington	3.56		47	Iowa	1.01
50	West Virginia	0.78		48	Utah	0.93
28	Wisconsin	2.00		49	Mississippi	0.81
38	Wyoming	1.44		50	West Virginia	0.78
					District of Columbia	6.31

Source: Steve L. Barsby and Associates, Inc. as published by the Distilled Spirits Council of the United States, Inc.
"1995 Statistical Information for the Distilled Spirits Industry" (June 1996)
*Apparent consumption is based on several sources which together approximate sales but do not actually measure consumption. Reported state volumes reflect only in-state purchases. Accordingly, figures for some states may be skewed by purchases by nonresidents.

Apparent Distilled Spirits Consumption in 1995

National Total = 324,930,000 Gallons of Distilled Spirits Consumed*

ALPHA ORDER

RANK ORDER

RANK	STATE	GALLONS	% of USA		RANK	STATE	GALLONS	% of USA
27	Alabama	4,421,000	1.36%		1	California	37,991,000	11.69%
46	Alaska	1,161,000	0.36%		2	Florida	23,610,000	7.27%
21	Arizona	5,893,000	1.81%		3	New York	20,415,000	6.28%
34	Arkansas	2,504,000	0.77%		4	Texas	17,363,000	5.34%
1	California	37,991,000	11.69%		5	Illinois	15,195,000	4.68%
22	Colorado	5,798,000	1.78%		6	Michigan	12,509,000	3.85%
24	Connecticut	4,996,000	1.54%		7	New Jersey	11,907,000	3.66%
42	Delaware	1,317,000	0.41%		8	Pennsylvania	10,851,000	3.34%
2	Florida	23,610,000	7.27%		9	Ohio	9,982,000	3.07%
10	Georgia	9,891,000	3.04%		10	Georgia	9,891,000	3.04%
43	Hawaii	1,316,000	0.41%		11	Massachusetts	9,456,000	2.91%
45	Idaho	1,168,000	0.36%		12	Wisconsin	8,734,000	2.69%
5	Illinois	15,195,000	4.68%		13	North Carolina	7,624,000	2.35%
17	Indiana	6,628,000	2.04%		14	Minnesota	7,423,000	2.28%
33	Iowa	2,542,000	0.78%		15	Maryland	7,301,000	2.25%
35	Kansas	2,495,000	0.77%		16	Washington	6,668,000	2.05%
29	Kentucky	4,131,000	1.27%		17	Indiana	6,628,000	2.04%
19	Louisiana	6,112,000	1.88%		18	Virginia	6,404,000	1.97%
38	Maine	1,764,000	0.54%		19	Louisiana	6,112,000	1.88%
15	Maryland	7,301,000	2.25%		20	Missouri	5,945,000	1.83%
11	Massachusetts	9,456,000	2.91%		21	Arizona	5,893,000	1.81%
6	Michigan	12,509,000	3.85%		22	Colorado	5,798,000	1.78%
14	Minnesota	7,423,000	2.28%		23	Tennessee	5,420,000	1.67%
31	Mississippi	3,192,000	0.98%		24	Connecticut	4,996,000	1.54%
20	Missouri	5,945,000	1.83%		25	South Carolina	4,868,000	1.50%
41	Montana	1,327,000	0.41%		26	Nevada	4,598,000	1.42%
37	Nebraska	1,826,000	0.56%		27	Alabama	4,421,000	1.36%
26	Nevada	4,598,000	1.42%		28	New Hampshire	4,181,000	1.29%
28	New Hampshire	4,181,000	1.29%		29	Kentucky	4,131,000	1.27%
7	New Jersey	11,907,000	3.66%		30	Oregon	3,709,000	1.14%
36	New Mexico	1,918,000	0.59%		31	Mississippi	3,192,000	0.98%
3	New York	20,415,000	6.28%		32	Oklahoma	3,149,000	0.97%
13	North Carolina	7,624,000	2.35%		33	Iowa	2,542,000	0.78%
48	North Dakota	971,000	0.30%		34	Arkansas	2,504,000	0.77%
9	Ohio	9,982,000	3.07%		35	Kansas	2,495,000	0.77%
32	Oklahoma	3,149,000	0.97%		36	New Mexico	1,918,000	0.59%
30	Oregon	3,709,000	1.14%		37	Nebraska	1,826,000	0.56%
8	Pennsylvania	10,851,000	3.34%		38	Maine	1,764,000	0.54%
44	Rhode Island	1,212,000	0.37%		39	West Virginia	1,382,000	0.43%
25	South Carolina	4,868,000	1.50%		40	Utah	1,355,000	0.42%
47	South Dakota	1,035,000	0.32%		41	Montana	1,327,000	0.41%
23	Tennessee	5,420,000	1.67%		42	Delaware	1,317,000	0.41%
4	Texas	17,363,000	5.34%		43	Hawaii	1,316,000	0.41%
40	Utah	1,355,000	0.42%		44	Rhode Island	1,212,000	0.37%
49	Vermont	757,000	0.23%		45	Idaho	1,168,000	0.36%
18	Virginia	6,404,000	1.97%		46	Alaska	1,161,000	0.36%
16	Washington	6,668,000	2.05%		47	South Dakota	1,035,000	0.32%
39	West Virginia	1,382,000	0.43%		48	North Dakota	971,000	0.30%
12	Wisconsin	8,734,000	2.69%		49	Vermont	757,000	0.23%
50	Wyoming	743,000	0.23%		50	Wyoming	743,000	0.23%
						District of Columbia	1,775,000	0.55%

Source: Distilled Spirits Council of the United States, Inc.
   "1995 Statistical Information for the Distilled Spirits Industry" (June 1996)
*Apparent consumption is based on several sources which together approximate sales but do not actually measure consumption. Reported state volumes reflect only in-state purchases. Accordingly, figures for some states may be skewed by purchases by nonresidents.

Adult Per Capita Apparent Distilled Spirits Consumption in 1995

National Per Capita = 1.77 Gallons Consumed per Adult Age 21 Years and Older*

ALPHA ORDER

RANK ORDER

RANK	STATE	PER CAPITA
39	Alabama	1.48
3	Alaska	3.01
17	Arizona	2.06
40	Arkansas	1.45
26	California	1.76
10	Colorado	2.22
14	Connecticut	2.11
4	Delaware	2.58
8	Florida	2.29
19	Georgia	1.99
34	Hawaii	1.59
36	Idaho	1.54
23	Illinois	1.85
31	Indiana	1.63
46	Iowa	1.27
42	Kansas	1.41
37	Kentucky	1.52
14	Louisiana	2.11
19	Maine	1.99
18	Maryland	2.03
12	Massachusetts	2.13
22	Michigan	1.88
6	Minnesota	2.33
25	Mississippi	1.77
33	Missouri	1.60
9	Montana	2.23
31	Nebraska	1.63
2	Nevada	4.27
1	New Hampshire	5.14
16	New Jersey	2.09
28	New Mexico	1.73
35	New York	1.58
38	North Carolina	1.49
11	North Dakota	2.20
46	Ohio	1.27
43	Oklahoma	1.40
30	Oregon	1.67
48	Pennsylvania	1.25
29	Rhode Island	1.69
21	South Carolina	1.90
13	South Dakota	2.12
40	Tennessee	1.45
44	Texas	1.39
49	Utah	1.17
24	Vermont	1.82
45	Virginia	1.35
26	Washington	1.76
50	West Virginia	1.04
5	Wisconsin	2.46
7	Wyoming	2.32

RANK	STATE	PER CAPITA
1	New Hampshire	5.14
2	Nevada	4.27
3	Alaska	3.01
4	Delaware	2.58
5	Wisconsin	2.46
6	Minnesota	2.33
7	Wyoming	2.32
8	Florida	2.29
9	Montana	2.23
10	Colorado	2.22
11	North Dakota	2.20
12	Massachusetts	2.13
13	South Dakota	2.12
14	Connecticut	2.11
14	Louisiana	2.11
16	New Jersey	2.09
17	Arizona	2.06
18	Maryland	2.03
19	Georgia	1.99
19	Maine	1.99
21	South Carolina	1.90
22	Michigan	1.88
23	Illinois	1.85
24	Vermont	1.82
25	Mississippi	1.77
26	California	1.76
26	Washington	1.76
28	New Mexico	1.73
29	Rhode Island	1.69
30	Oregon	1.67
31	Indiana	1.63
31	Nebraska	1.63
33	Missouri	1.60
34	Hawaii	1.59
35	New York	1.58
36	Idaho	1.54
37	Kentucky	1.52
38	North Carolina	1.49
39	Alabama	1.48
40	Arkansas	1.45
40	Tennessee	1.45
42	Kansas	1.41
43	Oklahoma	1.40
44	Texas	1.39
45	Virginia	1.35
46	Iowa	1.27
46	Ohio	1.27
48	Pennsylvania	1.25
49	Utah	1.17
50	West Virginia	1.04

District of Columbia 4.20

Source: Distilled Spirits Council of the United States, Inc.
"1995 Statistical Information for the Distilled Spirits Industry" (June 1996)
*Apparent consumption is based on several sources which together approximate sales but do not actually measure consumption. Reported state volumes reflect only in-state purchases. Accordingly, figures for some states may be skewed by purchases by nonresidents.

Percent of Adults Who Are Binge Drinkers in 1995

National Median = 13.93% of Adults Are Binge Drinkers*

ALPHA ORDER				RANK ORDER		
RANK	STATE	PERCENT		RANK	STATE	PERCENT
28	Alabama	13.58		1	Wisconsin	22.89
3	Alaska	19.20		2	Pennsylvania	19.38
30	Arizona	13.46		3	Alaska	19.20
43	Arkansas	8.75		4	Nevada	18.97
16	California	15.30		5	Rhode Island	18.70
12	Colorado	16.30		6	Michigan	18.26
19	Connecticut	14.41		7	Minnesota	18.01
45	Delaware	8.61		8	Iowa	17.95
32	Florida	13.12		9	Massachusetts	17.83
37	Georgia	11.99		10	North Dakota	16.97
36	Hawaii	12.37		11	New Hampshire	16.59
33	Idaho	12.94		12	Colorado	16.30
28	Illinois	13.58		13	Vermont	15.96
34	Indiana	12.75		14	Nebraska	15.83
8	Iowa	17.95		15	Wyoming	15.57
27	Kansas	13.86		16	California	15.30
41	Kentucky	9.70		17	Texas	15.27
24	Louisiana	14.01		18	Virginia	14.46
38	Maine	11.45		19	Connecticut	14.41
46	Maryland	8.21		20	South Dakota	14.36
9	Massachusetts	17.83		21	Montana	14.31
6	Michigan	18.26		22	Missouri	14.10
7	Minnesota	18.01		23	New Mexico	14.06
44	Mississippi	8.67		24	Louisiana	14.01
22	Missouri	14.10		25	New Jersey	13.95
21	Montana	14.31		26	Oregon	13.90
14	Nebraska	15.83		27	Kansas	13.86
4	Nevada	18.97		28	Alabama	13.58
11	New Hampshire	16.59		28	Illinois	13.58
25	New Jersey	13.95		30	Arizona	13.46
23	New Mexico	14.06		31	Washington	13.44
35	New York	12.39		32	Florida	13.12
49	North Carolina	5.76		33	Idaho	12.94
10	North Dakota	16.97		34	Indiana	12.75
40	Ohio	9.87		35	New York	12.39
47	Oklahoma	6.69		36	Hawaii	12.37
26	Oregon	13.90		37	Georgia	11.99
2	Pennsylvania	19.38		38	Maine	11.45
5	Rhode Island	18.70		39	Utah	9.93
42	South Carolina	9.17		40	Ohio	9.87
20	South Dakota	14.36		41	Kentucky	9.70
50	Tennessee	5.22		42	South Carolina	9.17
17	Texas	15.27		43	Arkansas	8.75
39	Utah	9.93		44	Mississippi	8.67
13	Vermont	15.96		45	Delaware	8.61
18	Virginia	14.46		46	Maryland	8.21
31	Washington	13.44		47	Oklahoma	6.69
48	West Virginia	5.92		48	West Virginia	5.92
1	Wisconsin	22.89		49	North Carolina	5.76
15	Wyoming	15.57		50	Tennessee	5.22

District of Columbia**   NA

Source: U.S. Department of Health and Human Services, Centers for Disease Control and Prevention
    "1995 Behavioral Risk Factor Surveillance Summary Prevalence Report" (December 10, 1996)
*Persons 18 and older reporting consumption of five or more alcoholic drinks on one or more occasions during the previous month.
**Not available.

Percent of Adults Who Smoke in 1995

National Median = 22.40% of Adults Smoke*

ALPHA ORDER RANK ORDER

RANK	STATE	PERCENT	RANK	STATE	PERCENT
15	Alabama	24.53	1	Kentucky	27.83
12	Alaska	24.96	2	Indiana	27.19
24	Arizona	22.86	3	Tennessee	26.46
11	Arkansas	25.20	4	Nevada	26.31
49	California	15.50	5	Ohio	25.98
32	Colorado	21.79	6	North Carolina	25.84
42	Connecticut	20.79	7	Michigan	25.74
9	Delaware	25.45	8	West Virginia	25.73
22	Florida	23.13	9	Delaware	25.45
44	Georgia	20.46	10	Louisiana	25.21
48	Hawaii	17.76	11	Arkansas	25.20
46	Idaho	19.76	12	Alaska	24.96
23	Illinois	23.08	12	Maine	24.96
2	Indiana	27.19	14	Rhode Island	24.74
21	Iowa	23.17	15	Alabama	24.53
29	Kansas	22.01	16	Missouri	24.26
1	Kentucky	27.83	17	Pennsylvania	24.17
10	Louisiana	25.21	18	Mississippi	24.03
12	Maine	24.96	19	South Carolina	23.74
39	Maryland	21.22	20	Texas	23.66
35	Massachusetts	21.74	21	Iowa	23.17
7	Michigan	25.74	22	Florida	23.13
43	Minnesota	20.48	23	Illinois	23.08
18	Mississippi	24.03	24	Arizona	22.86
16	Missouri	24.26	25	North Dakota	22.69
41	Montana	21.13	26	Vermont	22.11
30	Nebraska	21.90	27	Virginia	22.03
4	Nevada	26.31	28	Wyoming	22.02
38	New Hampshire	21.45	29	Kansas	22.01
47	New Jersey	19.17	30	Nebraska	21.90
40	New Mexico	21.17	31	Wisconsin	21.80
37	New York	21.47	32	Colorado	21.79
6	North Carolina	25.84	32	Oregon	21.79
25	North Dakota	22.69	32	South Dakota	21.79
5	Ohio	25.98	35	Massachusetts	21.74
36	Oklahoma	21.66	36	Oklahoma	21.66
32	Oregon	21.79	37	New York	21.47
17	Pennsylvania	24.17	38	New Hampshire	21.45
14	Rhode Island	24.74	39	Maryland	21.22
19	South Carolina	23.74	40	New Mexico	21.17
32	South Dakota	21.79	41	Montana	21.13
3	Tennessee	26.46	42	Connecticut	20.79
20	Texas	23.66	43	Minnesota	20.48
50	Utah	13.16	44	Georgia	20.46
26	Vermont	22.11	45	Washington	20.16
27	Virginia	22.03	46	Idaho	19.76
45	Washington	20.16	47	New Jersey	19.17
8	West Virginia	25.73	48	Hawaii	17.76
31	Wisconsin	21.80	49	California	15.50
28	Wyoming	22.02	50	Utah	13.16

District of Columbia**   NA

Source: U.S. Department of Health and Human Services, Centers for Disease Control and Prevention
"1995 Behavioral Risk Factor Surveillance Summary Prevalence Report" (December 10, 1996)
*Persons 18 and older who have ever smoked 100 cigarettes and currently smoke.
**Not available.

Percent of Men Who Smoke: 1995

National Median = 24.67% of Men*

<table>
<tr><td colspan="3"><u>ALPHA ORDER</u></td><td colspan="3"><u>RANK ORDER</u></td></tr>
<tr><td>RANK</td><td>STATE</td><td>PERCENT</td><td>RANK</td><td>STATE</td><td>PERCENT</td></tr>
<tr><td>3</td><td>Alabama</td><td>30.02</td><td>1</td><td>Ohio</td><td>31.57</td></tr>
<tr><td>15</td><td>Alaska</td><td>26.48</td><td>2</td><td>North Carolina</td><td>30.24</td></tr>
<tr><td>13</td><td>Arizona</td><td>26.78</td><td>3</td><td>Alabama</td><td>30.02</td></tr>
<tr><td>12</td><td>Arkansas</td><td>26.80</td><td>4</td><td>Kentucky</td><td>28.84</td></tr>
<tr><td>49</td><td>California</td><td>17.47</td><td>5</td><td>Indiana</td><td>28.50</td></tr>
<tr><td>40</td><td>Colorado</td><td>22.17</td><td>6</td><td>Missouri</td><td>27.96</td></tr>
<tr><td>45</td><td>Connecticut</td><td>21.04</td><td>7</td><td>Tennessee</td><td>27.91</td></tr>
<tr><td>9</td><td>Delaware</td><td>27.47</td><td>8</td><td>Mississippi</td><td>27.65</td></tr>
<tr><td>21</td><td>Florida</td><td>24.86</td><td>9</td><td>Delaware</td><td>27.47</td></tr>
<tr><td>28</td><td>Georgia</td><td>24.32</td><td>10</td><td>Texas</td><td>27.14</td></tr>
<tr><td>48</td><td>Hawaii</td><td>18.76</td><td>11</td><td>Maine</td><td>26.87</td></tr>
<tr><td>46</td><td>Idaho</td><td>20.38</td><td>12</td><td>Arkansas</td><td>26.80</td></tr>
<tr><td>14</td><td>Illinois</td><td>26.61</td><td>13</td><td>Arizona</td><td>26.78</td></tr>
<tr><td>5</td><td>Indiana</td><td>28.50</td><td>14</td><td>Illinois</td><td>26.61</td></tr>
<tr><td>22</td><td>Iowa</td><td>24.83</td><td>15</td><td>Alaska</td><td>26.48</td></tr>
<tr><td>30</td><td>Kansas</td><td>23.99</td><td>16</td><td>Michigan</td><td>26.34</td></tr>
<tr><td>4</td><td>Kentucky</td><td>28.84</td><td>17</td><td>Louisiana</td><td>26.29</td></tr>
<tr><td>17</td><td>Louisiana</td><td>26.29</td><td>18</td><td>Pennsylvania</td><td>25.99</td></tr>
<tr><td>11</td><td>Maine</td><td>26.87</td><td>19</td><td>North Dakota</td><td>24.92</td></tr>
<tr><td>39</td><td>Maryland</td><td>22.40</td><td>20</td><td>Vermont</td><td>24.91</td></tr>
<tr><td>36</td><td>Massachusetts</td><td>22.52</td><td>21</td><td>Florida</td><td>24.86</td></tr>
<tr><td>16</td><td>Michigan</td><td>26.34</td><td>22</td><td>Iowa</td><td>24.83</td></tr>
<tr><td>37</td><td>Minnesota</td><td>22.50</td><td>22</td><td>West Virginia</td><td>24.83</td></tr>
<tr><td>8</td><td>Mississippi</td><td>27.65</td><td>24</td><td>Nevada</td><td>24.82</td></tr>
<tr><td>6</td><td>Missouri</td><td>27.96</td><td>25</td><td>Nebraska</td><td>24.77</td></tr>
<tr><td>38</td><td>Montana</td><td>22.48</td><td>26</td><td>South Carolina</td><td>24.58</td></tr>
<tr><td>25</td><td>Nebraska</td><td>24.77</td><td>27</td><td>Wisconsin</td><td>24.48</td></tr>
<tr><td>24</td><td>Nevada</td><td>24.82</td><td>28</td><td>Georgia</td><td>24.32</td></tr>
<tr><td>42</td><td>New Hampshire</td><td>21.95</td><td>29</td><td>Rhode Island</td><td>24.01</td></tr>
<tr><td>43</td><td>New Jersey</td><td>21.59</td><td>30</td><td>Kansas</td><td>23.99</td></tr>
<tr><td>35</td><td>New Mexico</td><td>22.73</td><td>31</td><td>Virginia</td><td>23.71</td></tr>
<tr><td>32</td><td>New York</td><td>23.61</td><td>32</td><td>New York</td><td>23.61</td></tr>
<tr><td>2</td><td>North Carolina</td><td>30.24</td><td>33</td><td>Oregon</td><td>22.88</td></tr>
<tr><td>19</td><td>North Dakota</td><td>24.92</td><td>34</td><td>South Dakota</td><td>22.77</td></tr>
<tr><td>1</td><td>Ohio</td><td>31.57</td><td>35</td><td>New Mexico</td><td>22.73</td></tr>
<tr><td>44</td><td>Oklahoma</td><td>21.58</td><td>36</td><td>Massachusetts</td><td>22.52</td></tr>
<tr><td>33</td><td>Oregon</td><td>22.88</td><td>37</td><td>Minnesota</td><td>22.50</td></tr>
<tr><td>18</td><td>Pennsylvania</td><td>25.99</td><td>38</td><td>Montana</td><td>22.48</td></tr>
<tr><td>29</td><td>Rhode Island</td><td>24.01</td><td>39</td><td>Maryland</td><td>22.40</td></tr>
<tr><td>26</td><td>South Carolina</td><td>24.58</td><td>40</td><td>Colorado</td><td>22.17</td></tr>
<tr><td>34</td><td>South Dakota</td><td>22.77</td><td>41</td><td>Wyoming</td><td>22.12</td></tr>
<tr><td>7</td><td>Tennessee</td><td>27.91</td><td>42</td><td>New Hampshire</td><td>21.95</td></tr>
<tr><td>10</td><td>Texas</td><td>27.14</td><td>43</td><td>New Jersey</td><td>21.59</td></tr>
<tr><td>50</td><td>Utah</td><td>16.42</td><td>44</td><td>Oklahoma</td><td>21.58</td></tr>
<tr><td>20</td><td>Vermont</td><td>24.91</td><td>45</td><td>Connecticut</td><td>21.04</td></tr>
<tr><td>31</td><td>Virginia</td><td>23.71</td><td>46</td><td>Idaho</td><td>20.38</td></tr>
<tr><td>47</td><td>Washington</td><td>20.05</td><td>47</td><td>Washington</td><td>20.05</td></tr>
<tr><td>22</td><td>West Virginia</td><td>24.83</td><td>48</td><td>Hawaii</td><td>18.76</td></tr>
<tr><td>27</td><td>Wisconsin</td><td>24.48</td><td>49</td><td>California</td><td>17.47</td></tr>
<tr><td>41</td><td>Wyoming</td><td>22.12</td><td>50</td><td>Utah</td><td>16.42</td></tr>
<tr><td></td><td></td><td></td><td></td><td>District of Columbia**</td><td>NA</td></tr>
</table>

Source: U.S. Department of Health and Human Services, Centers for Disease Control and Prevention
"1995 Behavioral Risk Factor Surveillance Summary Prevalence Report" (December 10, 1996)
*Men 18 and older who have ever smoked 100 cigarettes and are a current smoker.
**Not available.

504

Percent of Women Who Smoke: 1995

National Median = 20.87% of Women*

<u>ALPHA ORDER</u>

RANK	STATE	PERCENT
37	Alabama	19.69
11	Alaska	23.27
44	Arizona	19.11
9	Arkansas	23.78
49	California	13.56
20	Colorado	21.43
28	Connecticut	20.57
10	Delaware	23.62
19	Florida	21.56
47	Georgia	16.94
48	Hawaii	16.76
43	Idaho	19.17
35	Illinois	19.87
4	Indiana	25.99
18	Iowa	21.65
33	Kansas	20.15
2	Kentucky	26.91
8	Louisiana	24.25
12	Maine	23.20
34	Maryland	20.14
21	Massachusetts	21.04
6	Michigan	25.20
45	Minnesota	18.58
26	Mississippi	20.86
24	Missouri	20.94
36	Montana	19.83
42	Nebraska	19.27
1	Nevada	27.84
22	New Hampshire	20.98
46	New Jersey	16.97
37	New Mexico	19.69
39	New York	19.58
16	North Carolina	21.83
29	North Dakota	20.51
23	Ohio	20.97
17	Oklahoma	21.73
27	Oregon	20.77
14	Pennsylvania	22.54
5	Rhode Island	25.39
13	South Carolina	22.98
25	South Dakota	20.87
7	Tennessee	25.15
31	Texas	20.37
50	Utah	10.05
40	Vermont	19.49
30	Virginia	20.45
32	Washington	20.27
3	West Virginia	26.53
41	Wisconsin	19.30
15	Wyoming	21.93

<u>RANK ORDER</u>

RANK	STATE	PERCENT
1	Nevada	27.84
2	Kentucky	26.91
3	West Virginia	26.53
4	Indiana	25.99
5	Rhode Island	25.39
6	Michigan	25.20
7	Tennessee	25.15
8	Louisiana	24.25
9	Arkansas	23.78
10	Delaware	23.62
11	Alaska	23.27
12	Maine	23.20
13	South Carolina	22.98
14	Pennsylvania	22.54
15	Wyoming	21.93
16	North Carolina	21.83
17	Oklahoma	21.73
18	Iowa	21.65
19	Florida	21.56
20	Colorado	21.43
21	Massachusetts	21.04
22	New Hampshire	20.98
23	Ohio	20.97
24	Missouri	20.94
25	South Dakota	20.87
26	Mississippi	20.86
27	Oregon	20.77
28	Connecticut	20.57
29	North Dakota	20.51
30	Virginia	20.45
31	Texas	20.37
32	Washington	20.27
33	Kansas	20.15
34	Maryland	20.14
35	Illinois	19.87
36	Montana	19.83
37	Alabama	19.69
37	New Mexico	19.69
39	New York	19.58
40	Vermont	19.49
41	Wisconsin	19.30
42	Nebraska	19.27
43	Idaho	19.17
44	Arizona	19.11
45	Minnesota	18.58
46	New Jersey	16.97
47	Georgia	16.94
48	Hawaii	16.76
49	California	13.56
50	Utah	10.05
	District of Columbia**	NA

Source: U.S. Department of Health and Human Services, Centers for Disease Control and Prevention "1995 Behavioral Risk Factor Surveillance Summary Prevalence Report" (December 10, 1996)
*Women 18 and older who have ever smoked 100 cigarettes and are a current smoker.
**Not available.

Percent of Adults Overweight in 1995

National Median = 28.65% of Adults*

ALPHA ORDER				RANK ORDER		
RANK	STATE	PERCENT		RANK	STATE	PERCENT
4	Alabama	31.83		1	Indiana	34.65
9	Alaska	31.35		2	Missouri	32.88
44	Arizona	24.53		3	West Virginia	31.94
14	Arkansas	30.14		4	Alabama	31.83
36	California	26.43		5	Michigan	31.62
49	Colorado	21.88		5	Mississippi	31.62
43	Connecticut	24.68		7	Iowa	31.58
18	Delaware	29.49		8	Ohio	31.53
17	Florida	29.80		9	Alaska	31.35
29	Georgia	28.21		10	Tennessee	30.95
50	Hawaii	21.83		11	Louisiana	30.74
33	Idaho	27.18		12	North Dakota	30.67
15	Illinois	30.09		13	Wisconsin	30.15
1	Indiana	34.65		14	Arkansas	30.14
7	Iowa	31.58		15	Illinois	30.09
31	Kansas	27.81		16	Pennsylvania	30.08
23	Kentucky	28.79		17	Florida	29.80
11	Louisiana	30.74		18	Delaware	29.49
34	Maine	26.94		19	Virginia	29.24
21	Maryland	29.08		20	Nebraska	29.18
48	Massachusetts	21.93		21	Maryland	29.08
5	Michigan	31.62		22	North Carolina	28.87
28	Minnesota	28.35		23	Kentucky	28.79
5	Mississippi	31.62		24	Oregon	28.76
2	Missouri	32.88		25	South Carolina	28.65
41	Montana	24.91		25	South Dakota	28.65
20	Nebraska	29.18		27	Texas	28.60
35	Nevada	26.91		28	Minnesota	28.35
37	New Hampshire	25.89		29	Georgia	28.21
45	New Jersey	24.36		30	New York	27.83
47	New Mexico	23.84		31	Kansas	27.81
30	New York	27.83		32	Wyoming	27.26
22	North Carolina	28.87		33	Idaho	27.18
12	North Dakota	30.67		34	Maine	26.94
8	Ohio	31.53		35	Nevada	26.91
46	Oklahoma	24.14		36	California	26.43
24	Oregon	28.76		37	New Hampshire	25.89
16	Pennsylvania	30.08		38	Washington	25.43
42	Rhode Island	24.90		39	Vermont	25.36
25	South Carolina	28.65		40	Utah	25.04
25	South Dakota	28.65		41	Montana	24.91
10	Tennessee	30.95		42	Rhode Island	24.90
27	Texas	28.60		43	Connecticut	24.68
40	Utah	25.04		44	Arizona	24.53
39	Vermont	25.36		45	New Jersey	24.36
19	Virginia	29.24		46	Oklahoma	24.14
38	Washington	25.43		47	New Mexico	23.84
3	West Virginia	31.94		48	Massachusetts	21.93
13	Wisconsin	30.15		49	Colorado	21.88
32	Wyoming	27.26		50	Hawaii	21.83
					District of Columbia**	NA

Source: U.S. Department of Health and Human Services, Centers for Disease Control and Prevention
"1995 Behavioral Risk Factor Surveillance Summary Prevalence Report" (December 10, 1996)
*Persons 18 and older. Overweight is defined as men with a body mass index of 27.8 or greater and women with an index of 27.3 or greater.
**Not available.

506

Number of Days in the Past Month When Physical Health was "Not Good": 1995

National Median = 3.05 Days*

ALPHA ORDER				RANK ORDER		
RANK	STATE	DAYS		RANK	STATE	DAYS
10	Alabama	3.40		1	Arkansas	4.03
42	Alaska	2.58		2	New Mexico	3.74
8	Arizona	3.42		3	Kentucky	3.71
1	Arkansas	4.03		4	Indiana	3.51
6	California	3.44		5	West Virginia	3.50
21	Colorado	3.17		6	California	3.44
48	Connecticut	2.50		7	Louisiana	3.43
28	Delaware	2.97		8	Arizona	3.42
8	Florida	3.42		8	Florida	3.42
45	Georgia	2.53		10	Alabama	3.40
50	Hawaii	2.11		11	Tennessee	3.39
34	Idaho	2.78		12	Pennsylvania	3.36
44	Illinois	2.56		13	Utah	3.35
4	Indiana	3.51		14	Wisconsin	3.33
19	Iowa	3.22		15	Washington	3.32
25	Kansas	3.06		16	Texas	3.30
3	Kentucky	3.71		17	Rhode Island	3.28
7	Louisiana	3.43		18	Mississippi	3.27
48	Maine	2.50		19	Iowa	3.22
41	Maryland	2.59		20	Vermont	3.18
23	Massachusetts	3.14		21	Colorado	3.17
26	Michigan	3.03		22	New Jersey	3.16
34	Minnesota	2.78		23	Massachusetts	3.14
18	Mississippi	3.27		24	Nevada	3.13
30	Missouri	2.88		25	Kansas	3.06
36	Montana	2.74		26	Michigan	3.03
31	Nebraska	2.87		27	Oregon	3.02
24	Nevada	3.13		28	Delaware	2.97
43	New Hampshire	2.57		29	South Dakota	2.96
22	New Jersey	3.16		30	Missouri	2.88
2	New Mexico	3.74		31	Nebraska	2.87
37	New York	2.71		32	Virginia	2.84
38	North Carolina	2.70		33	North Dakota	2.82
33	North Dakota	2.82		34	Idaho	2.78
39	Ohio	2.69		34	Minnesota	2.78
45	Oklahoma	2.53		36	Montana	2.74
27	Oregon	3.02		37	New York	2.71
12	Pennsylvania	3.36		38	North Carolina	2.70
17	Rhode Island	3.28		39	Ohio	2.69
40	South Carolina	2.65		40	South Carolina	2.65
29	South Dakota	2.96		41	Maryland	2.59
11	Tennessee	3.39		42	Alaska	2.58
16	Texas	3.30		43	New Hampshire	2.57
13	Utah	3.35		44	Illinois	2.56
20	Vermont	3.18		45	Georgia	2.53
32	Virginia	2.84		45	Oklahoma	2.53
15	Washington	3.32		45	Wyoming	2.53
5	West Virginia	3.50		48	Connecticut	2.50
14	Wisconsin	3.33		48	Maine	2.50
45	Wyoming	2.53		50	Hawaii	2.11
					District of Columbia**	NA

Source: U.S. Department of Health and Human Services, Centers for Disease Control and Prevention
   "1995 Behavioral Risk Factor Surveillance Summary Prevalence Report" (December 10, 1996)
*Persons 18 and older.
**Not available.

Average Number of Days in Past Month When Mental Health was "Not Good": 1995
National Median = 2.94 Days*

ALPHA ORDER

RANK	STATE	DAYS
11	Alabama	3.23
28	Alaska	2.89
24	Arizona	2.96
34	Arkansas	2.72
16	California	3.15
6	Colorado	3.34
26	Connecticut	2.92
26	Delaware	2.92
3	Florida	3.46
32	Georgia	2.76
48	Hawaii	2.04
22	Idaho	3.03
46	Illinois	2.15
2	Indiana	3.57
14	Iowa	3.17
25	Kansas	2.95
1	Kentucky	4.63
13	Louisiana	3.18
43	Maine	2.35
45	Maryland	2.22
8	Massachusetts	3.32
6	Michigan	3.34
18	Minnesota	3.11
38	Mississippi	2.57
21	Missouri	3.06
41	Montana	2.47
33	Nebraska	2.75
3	Nevada	3.46
37	New Hampshire	2.62
39	New Jersey	2.51
29	New Mexico	2.85
14	New York	3.17
49	North Carolina	1.94
30	North Dakota	2.81
43	Ohio	2.35
50	Oklahoma	1.81
9	Oregon	3.31
23	Pennsylvania	3.02
5	Rhode Island	3.45
40	South Carolina	2.48
47	South Dakota	2.06
41	Tennessee	2.47
10	Texas	3.29
12	Utah	3.22
17	Vermont	3.13
20	Virginia	3.07
19	Washington	3.09
35	West Virginia	2.71
31	Wisconsin	2.77
36	Wyoming	2.68

RANK ORDER

RANK	STATE	DAYS
1	Kentucky	4.63
2	Indiana	3.57
3	Florida	3.46
3	Nevada	3.46
5	Rhode Island	3.45
6	Colorado	3.34
6	Michigan	3.34
8	Massachusetts	3.32
9	Oregon	3.31
10	Texas	3.29
11	Alabama	3.23
12	Utah	3.22
13	Louisiana	3.18
14	Iowa	3.17
14	New York	3.17
16	California	3.15
17	Vermont	3.13
18	Minnesota	3.11
19	Washington	3.09
20	Virginia	3.07
21	Missouri	3.06
22	Idaho	3.03
23	Pennsylvania	3.02
24	Arizona	2.96
25	Kansas	2.95
26	Connecticut	2.92
26	Delaware	2.92
28	Alaska	2.89
29	New Mexico	2.85
30	North Dakota	2.81
31	Wisconsin	2.77
32	Georgia	2.76
33	Nebraska	2.75
34	Arkansas	2.72
35	West Virginia	2.71
36	Wyoming	2.68
37	New Hampshire	2.62
38	Mississippi	2.57
39	New Jersey	2.51
40	South Carolina	2.48
41	Montana	2.47
41	Tennessee	2.47
43	Maine	2.35
43	Ohio	2.35
45	Maryland	2.22
46	Illinois	2.15
47	South Dakota	2.06
48	Hawaii	2.04
49	North Carolina	1.94
50	Oklahoma	1.81
	District of Columbia**	NA

Source: U.S. Department of Health and Human Services, Centers for Disease Control and Prevention
   "1995 Behavioral Risk Factor Surveillance Summary Prevalence Report" (December 10, 1996)
*Persons 18 and older.
**Not available.

Percent of Adults Who Have Ever Been Tested for AIDS: 1995

National Median = 36.35% of Adults*

ALPHA ORDER

RANK	STATE	PERCENT
19	Alabama	38.13
4	Alaska	48.57
11	Arizona	41.96
14	Arkansas	40.79
NA	California**	NA
9	Colorado	43.30
24	Connecticut	36.61
15	Delaware	40.10
3	Florida	48.62
28	Georgia	35.96
33	Hawaii	34.66
16	Idaho	39.50
22	Illinois	37.08
39	Indiana	32.10
45	Iowa	27.25
36	Kansas	32.91
40	Kentucky	30.77
7	Louisiana	45.67
47	Maine	26.47
6	Maryland	45.76
30	Massachusetts	35.59
13	Michigan	41.02
43	Minnesota	27.73
18	Mississippi	38.49
25	Missouri	36.35
38	Montana	32.27
42	Nebraska	28.59
1	Nevada	54.83
29	New Hampshire	35.70
17	New Jersey	39.16
10	New Mexico	43.02
27	New York	35.99
32	North Carolina	34.68
48	North Dakota	25.31
44	Ohio	27.64
37	Oklahoma	32.31
26	Oregon	36.11
23	Pennsylvania	37.02
8	Rhode Island	43.47
41	South Carolina	30.47
49	South Dakota	25.24
21	Tennessee	37.65
5	Texas	48.27
31	Utah	34.78
34	Vermont	33.57
2	Virginia	50.69
12	Washington	41.81
46	West Virginia	26.80
35	Wisconsin	33.22
20	Wyoming	37.94

RANK ORDER

RANK	STATE	PERCENT
1	Nevada	54.83
2	Virginia	50.69
3	Florida	48.62
4	Alaska	48.57
5	Texas	48.27
6	Maryland	45.76
7	Louisiana	45.67
8	Rhode Island	43.47
9	Colorado	43.30
10	New Mexico	43.02
11	Arizona	41.96
12	Washington	41.81
13	Michigan	41.02
14	Arkansas	40.79
15	Delaware	40.10
16	Idaho	39.50
17	New Jersey	39.16
18	Mississippi	38.49
19	Alabama	38.13
20	Wyoming	37.94
21	Tennessee	37.65
22	Illinois	37.08
23	Pennsylvania	37.02
24	Connecticut	36.61
25	Missouri	36.35
26	Oregon	36.11
27	New York	35.99
28	Georgia	35.96
29	New Hampshire	35.70
30	Massachusetts	35.59
31	Utah	34.78
32	North Carolina	34.68
33	Hawaii	34.66
34	Vermont	33.57
35	Wisconsin	33.22
36	Kansas	32.91
37	Oklahoma	32.31
38	Montana	32.27
39	Indiana	32.10
40	Kentucky	30.77
41	South Carolina	30.47
42	Nebraska	28.59
43	Minnesota	27.73
44	Ohio	27.64
45	Iowa	27.25
46	West Virginia	26.80
47	Maine	26.47
48	North Dakota	25.31
49	South Dakota	25.24
NA	California**	NA
	District of Columbia**	NA

Source: U.S. Department of Health and Human Services, Centers for Disease Control and Prevention
    "1995 Behavioral Risk Factor Surveillance Summary Prevalence Report" (December 10, 1996)
*For persons 18 to 64 years old.
**Not available.

Percent of Adults Who Believe They Have a Chance of Getting AIDS: 1995

National Median = 6.33% of Adults*

ALPHA ORDER				RANK ORDER		
RANK	STATE	PERCENT		RANK	STATE	PERCENT
26	Alabama	6.31		1	Arizona	9.89
44	Alaska	5.22		2	Massachusetts	9.06
1	Arizona	9.89		3	West Virginia	8.89
36	Arkansas	5.96		4	Hawaii	8.79
NA	California**	NA		5	Nebraska	8.54
24	Colorado	6.34		6	Texas	8.49
38	Connecticut	5.94		7	Tennessee	8.16
31	Delaware	6.15		8	Illinois	8.09
22	Florida	6.45		9	Pennsylvania	7.71
29	Georgia	6.22		10	North Carolina	7.36
4	Hawaii	8.79		11	North Dakota	7.31
32	Idaho	6.09		12	Minnesota	7.24
8	Illinois	8.09		13	Nevada	7.19
46	Indiana	5.05		14	Virginia	7.18
15	Iowa	7.11		15	Iowa	7.11
23	Kansas	6.38		16	New Mexico	7.10
29	Kentucky	6.22		17	New Jersey	6.88
36	Louisiana	5.96		18	Missouri	6.72
34	Maine	6.02		19	South Carolina	6.71
41	Maryland	5.55		20	Wisconsin	6.57
2	Massachusetts	9.06		21	Vermont	6.53
25	Michigan	6.33		22	Florida	6.45
12	Minnesota	7.24		23	Kansas	6.38
28	Mississippi	6.28		24	Colorado	6.34
18	Missouri	6.72		25	Michigan	6.33
42	Montana	5.49		26	Alabama	6.31
5	Nebraska	8.54		27	New York	6.29
13	Nevada	7.19		28	Mississippi	6.28
43	New Hampshire	5.25		29	Georgia	6.22
17	New Jersey	6.88		29	Kentucky	6.22
16	New Mexico	7.10		31	Delaware	6.15
27	New York	6.29		32	Idaho	6.09
10	North Carolina	7.36		33	Ohio	6.06
11	North Dakota	7.31		34	Maine	6.02
33	Ohio	6.06		34	Wyoming	6.02
48	Oklahoma	4.68		36	Arkansas	5.96
38	Oregon	5.94		36	Louisiana	5.96
9	Pennsylvania	7.71		38	Connecticut	5.94
47	Rhode Island	5.00		38	Oregon	5.94
19	South Carolina	6.71		40	South Dakota	5.63
40	South Dakota	5.63		41	Maryland	5.55
7	Tennessee	8.16		42	Montana	5.49
6	Texas	8.49		43	New Hampshire	5.25
45	Utah	5.17		44	Alaska	5.22
21	Vermont	6.53		45	Utah	5.17
14	Virginia	7.18		46	Indiana	5.05
49	Washington	4.61		47	Rhode Island	5.00
3	West Virginia	8.89		48	Oklahoma	4.68
20	Wisconsin	6.57		49	Washington	4.61
34	Wyoming	6.02		NA	California**	NA
					District of Columbia**	NA

Source: U.S. Department of Health and Human Services, Centers for Disease Control and Prevention
   "1995 Behavioral Risk Factor Surveillance Summary Prevalence Report" (December 10, 1996)
*For persons 18 to 64 years old who believe their chances of getting the AIDS virus are "medium" or "high."
**Not available.

Safety Belt Usage Rate in 1995

National Percent = 68% Use Safety Belts*

RANK	STATE	PERCENT
41	Alabama	52
17	Alaska	69
29	Arizona	60
43	Arkansas	51
2	California	85
36	Colorado	56
8	Connecticut	72
29	Delaware	60
31	Florida	59
39	Georgia	53
5	Hawaii	80
31	Idaho	59
17	Illinois	69
22	Indiana	64
7	Iowa	76
38	Kansas	54
41	Kentucky	52
31	Louisiana	59
44	Maine	50
14	Maryland	70
39	Massachusetts	53
19	Michigan	67
21	Minnesota	65
45	Mississippi	46
11	Missouri	71
14	Montana	70
22	Nebraska	64
11	Nevada	71
NA	New Hampshire**	NA
28	New Jersey	61
1	New Mexico	86
8	New York	72
4	North Carolina	81
47	North Dakota	42
27	Ohio	63
45	Oklahoma	46
5	Oregon	80
11	Pennsylvania	71
34	Rhode Island	58
22	South Carolina	64
48	South Dakota	40
22	Tennessee	64
8	Texas	72
36	Utah	56
19	Vermont	67
14	Virginia	70
3	Washington	83
34	West Virginia	58
22	Wisconsin	64
NA	Wyoming**	NA

RANK	STATE	PERCENT
1	New Mexico	86
2	California	85
3	Washington	83
4	North Carolina	81
5	Hawaii	80
5	Oregon	80
7	Iowa	76
8	Connecticut	72
8	New York	72
8	Texas	72
11	Missouri	71
11	Nevada	71
11	Pennsylvania	71
14	Maryland	70
14	Montana	70
14	Virginia	70
17	Alaska	69
17	Illinois	69
19	Michigan	67
19	Vermont	67
21	Minnesota	65
22	Indiana	64
22	Nebraska	64
22	South Carolina	64
22	Tennessee	64
22	Wisconsin	64
27	Ohio	63
28	New Jersey	61
29	Arizona	60
29	Delaware	60
31	Florida	59
31	Idaho	59
31	Louisiana	59
34	Rhode Island	58
34	West Virginia	58
36	Colorado	56
36	Utah	56
38	Kansas	54
39	Georgia	53
39	Massachusetts	53
41	Alabama	52
41	Kentucky	52
43	Arkansas	51
44	Maine	50
45	Mississippi	46
45	Oklahoma	46
47	North Dakota	42
48	South Dakota	40
NA	New Hampshire**	NA
NA	Wyoming**	NA
	District of Columbia	63

Source: U.S. Department of Transportation, National Highway Safety Traffic Safety Administration
"Key Provisions of Safety Belt Use Laws" (September 1996)
*As of December 1995.
**Not reported.

Percent of Adults Whose Children Use a Car Safety Seat: 1995

National Median = 96.51% of Adults*

ALPHA ORDER

RANK	STATE	PERCENT
27	Alabama	95.79
37	Alaska	94.24
41	Arizona	93.45
3	Arkansas	99.13
46	California	90.66
30	Colorado	95.62
49	Connecticut	89.08
2	Delaware	99.20
27	Florida	95.79
13	Georgia	98.12
7	Hawaii	98.83
43	Idaho	91.89
50	Illinois	88.04
1	Indiana	99.65
20	Iowa	96.91
17	Kansas	97.40
25	Kentucky	96.64
47	Louisiana	90.32
12	Maine	98.21
9	Maryland	98.52
4	Massachusetts	99.06
36	Michigan	94.47
19	Minnesota	96.98
26	Mississippi	96.38
44	Missouri	91.53
39	Montana	93.87
18	Nebraska	97.24
34	Nevada	94.69
21	New Hampshire	96.90
29	New Jersey	95.70
32	New Mexico	95.40
38	New York	93.93
6	North Carolina	98.84
24	North Dakota	96.80
10	Ohio	98.48
15	Oklahoma	97.97
42	Oregon	93.19
48	Pennsylvania	89.53
11	Rhode Island	98.24
8	South Carolina	98.57
23	South Dakota	96.89
16	Tennessee	97.85
33	Texas	95.33
35	Utah	94.52
5	Vermont	98.87
40	Virginia	93.76
21	Washington	96.90
14	West Virginia	98.03
45	Wisconsin	90.86
31	Wyoming	95.57

RANK ORDER

RANK	STATE	PERCENT
1	Indiana	99.65
2	Delaware	99.20
3	Arkansas	99.13
4	Massachusetts	99.06
5	Vermont	98.87
6	North Carolina	98.84
7	Hawaii	98.83
8	South Carolina	98.57
9	Maryland	98.52
10	Ohio	98.48
11	Rhode Island	98.24
12	Maine	98.21
13	Georgia	98.12
14	West Virginia	98.03
15	Oklahoma	97.97
16	Tennessee	97.85
17	Kansas	97.40
18	Nebraska	97.24
19	Minnesota	96.98
20	Iowa	96.91
21	New Hampshire	96.90
21	Washington	96.90
23	South Dakota	96.89
24	North Dakota	96.80
25	Kentucky	96.64
26	Mississippi	96.38
27	Alabama	95.79
27	Florida	95.79
29	New Jersey	95.70
30	Colorado	95.62
31	Wyoming	95.57
32	New Mexico	95.40
33	Texas	95.33
34	Nevada	94.69
35	Utah	94.52
36	Michigan	94.47
37	Alaska	94.24
38	New York	93.93
39	Montana	93.87
40	Virginia	93.76
41	Arizona	93.45
42	Oregon	93.19
43	Idaho	91.89
44	Missouri	91.53
45	Wisconsin	90.86
46	California	90.66
47	Louisiana	90.32
48	Pennsylvania	89.53
49	Connecticut	89.08
50	Illinois	88.04
	District of Columbia**	NA

Source: U.S. Department of Health and Human Services, Centers for Disease Control and Prevention
"1995 Behavioral Risk Factor Surveillance Summary Prevalence Report" (December 10, 1996)
*Persons whose children under 5 years old "always or nearly always use a safety seat".
**Not available.

VIII. APPENDIX

Population Charts

Population in 1996

National Total = 265,284,000*

ALPHA ORDER					RANK ORDER			
RANK	STATE	POPULATION	% of USA		RANK	STATE	POPULATION	% of USA
23	Alabama	4,273,000	1.61%		1	California	31,878,000	12.02%
48	Alaska	607,000	0.23%		2	Texas	19,128,000	7.21%
21	Arizona	4,428,000	1.67%		3	New York	18,185,000	6.85%
33	Arkansas	2,510,000	0.95%		4	Florida	14,400,000	5.43%
1	California	31,878,000	12.02%		5	Pennsylvania	12,056,000	4.54%
25	Colorado	3,823,000	1.44%		6	Illinois	11,847,000	4.47%
28	Connecticut	3,274,000	1.23%		7	Ohio	11,173,000	4.21%
46	Delaware	725,000	0.27%		8	Michigan	9,594,000	3.62%
4	Florida	14,400,000	5.43%		9	New Jersey	7,988,000	3.01%
10	Georgia	7,353,000	2.77%		10	Georgia	7,353,000	2.77%
41	Hawaii	1,184,000	0.45%		11	North Carolina	7,323,000	2.76%
40	Idaho	1,189,000	0.45%		12	Virginia	6,675,000	2.52%
6	Illinois	11,847,000	4.47%		13	Massachusetts	6,092,000	2.30%
14	Indiana	5,841,000	2.20%		14	Indiana	5,841,000	2.20%
30	Iowa	2,852,000	1.08%		15	Washington	5,533,000	2.09%
32	Kansas	2,572,000	0.97%		16	Missouri	5,359,000	2.02%
24	Kentucky	3,884,000	1.46%		17	Tennessee	5,320,000	2.01%
22	Louisiana	4,351,000	1.64%		18	Wisconsin	5,160,000	1.95%
39	Maine	1,243,000	0.47%		19	Maryland	5,072,000	1.91%
19	Maryland	5,072,000	1.91%		20	Minnesota	4,658,000	1.76%
13	Massachusetts	6,092,000	2.30%		21	Arizona	4,428,000	1.67%
8	Michigan	9,594,000	3.62%		22	Louisiana	4,351,000	1.64%
20	Minnesota	4,658,000	1.76%		23	Alabama	4,273,000	1.61%
31	Mississippi	2,716,000	1.02%		24	Kentucky	3,884,000	1.46%
16	Missouri	5,359,000	2.02%		25	Colorado	3,823,000	1.44%
44	Montana	879,000	0.33%		26	South Carolina	3,699,000	1.39%
37	Nebraska	1,652,000	0.62%		27	Oklahoma	3,301,000	1.24%
38	Nevada	1,603,000	0.60%		28	Connecticut	3,274,000	1.23%
42	New Hampshire	1,162,000	0.44%		29	Oregon	3,204,000	1.21%
9	New Jersey	7,988,000	3.01%		30	Iowa	2,852,000	1.08%
36	New Mexico	1,713,000	0.65%		31	Mississippi	2,716,000	1.02%
3	New York	18,185,000	6.85%		32	Kansas	2,572,000	0.97%
11	North Carolina	7,323,000	2.76%		33	Arkansas	2,510,000	0.95%
47	North Dakota	644,000	0.24%		34	Utah	2,000,000	0.75%
7	Ohio	11,173,000	4.21%		35	West Virginia	1,826,000	0.69%
27	Oklahoma	3,301,000	1.24%		36	New Mexico	1,713,000	0.65%
29	Oregon	3,204,000	1.21%		37	Nebraska	1,652,000	0.62%
5	Pennsylvania	12,056,000	4.54%		38	Nevada	1,603,000	0.60%
43	Rhode Island	990,000	0.37%		39	Maine	1,243,000	0.47%
26	South Carolina	3,699,000	1.39%		40	Idaho	1,189,000	0.45%
45	South Dakota	732,000	0.28%		41	Hawaii	1,184,000	0.45%
17	Tennessee	5,320,000	2.01%		42	New Hampshire	1,162,000	0.44%
2	Texas	19,128,000	7.21%		43	Rhode Island	990,000	0.37%
34	Utah	2,000,000	0.75%		44	Montana	879,000	0.33%
49	Vermont	589,000	0.22%		45	South Dakota	732,000	0.28%
12	Virginia	6,675,000	2.52%		46	Delaware	725,000	0.27%
15	Washington	5,533,000	2.09%		47	North Dakota	644,000	0.24%
35	West Virginia	1,826,000	0.69%		48	Alaska	607,000	0.23%
18	Wisconsin	5,160,000	1.95%		49	Vermont	589,000	0.22%
50	Wyoming	481,000	0.18%		50	Wyoming	481,000	0.18%
					District of Columbia		543,000	0.20%

Source: U.S. Bureau of the Census
    Press Release (CB96-224, December 30, 1996)
*As of July 1, 1996. Includes armed forces residing in each state.

Population in 1995

National Total = 262,890,000*

ALPHA ORDER

ALPHA ORDER

RANK	STATE	POPULATION	% of USA
23	Alabama	4,246,000	1.62%
48	Alaska	603,000	0.23%
22	Arizona	4,305,000	1.64%
33	Arkansas	2,485,000	0.95%
1	California	31,565,000	12.01%
25	Colorado	3,748,000	1.43%
28	Connecticut	3,271,000	1.24%
46	Delaware	717,000	0.27%
4	Florida	14,184,000	5.40%
10	Georgia	7,209,000	2.74%
40	Hawaii	1,179,000	0.45%
41	Idaho	1,166,000	0.44%
6	Illinois	11,790,000	4.48%
14	Indiana	5,797,000	2.21%
30	Iowa	2,843,000	1.08%
32	Kansas	2,564,000	0.98%
24	Kentucky	3,857,000	1.47%
21	Louisiana	4,338,000	1.65%
39	Maine	1,239,000	0.47%
19	Maryland	5,039,000	1.92%
13	Massachusetts	6,071,000	2.31%
8	Michigan	9,538,000	3.63%
20	Minnesota	4,615,000	1.76%
31	Mississippi	2,696,000	1.03%
16	Missouri	5,319,000	2.02%
44	Montana	870,000	0.33%
37	Nebraska	1,639,000	0.62%
38	Nevada	1,533,000	0.58%
42	New Hampshire	1,148,000	0.44%
9	New Jersey	7,950,000	3.02%
36	New Mexico	1,690,000	0.64%
3	New York	18,191,000	6.92%
11	North Carolina	7,202,000	2.74%
47	North Dakota	642,000	0.24%
7	Ohio	11,134,000	4.24%
27	Oklahoma	3,275,000	1.25%
29	Oregon	3,149,000	1.20%
5	Pennsylvania	12,060,000	4.59%
43	Rhode Island	992,000	0.38%
26	South Carolina	3,667,000	1.39%
45	South Dakota	730,000	0.28%
17	Tennessee	5,247,000	2.00%
2	Texas	18,801,000	7.15%
34	Utah	1,958,000	0.74%
49	Vermont	585,000	0.22%
12	Virginia	6,615,000	2.52%
15	Washington	5,448,000	2.07%
35	West Virginia	1,825,000	0.69%
18	Wisconsin	5,122,000	1.95%
50	Wyoming	479,000	0.18%

RANK ORDER

RANK	STATE	POPULATION	% of USA
1	California	31,565,000	12.01%
2	Texas	18,801,000	7.15%
3	New York	18,191,000	6.92%
4	Florida	14,184,000	5.40%
5	Pennsylvania	12,060,000	4.59%
6	Illinois	11,790,000	4.48%
7	Ohio	11,134,000	4.24%
8	Michigan	9,538,000	3.63%
9	New Jersey	7,950,000	3.02%
10	Georgia	7,209,000	2.74%
11	North Carolina	7,202,000	2.74%
12	Virginia	6,615,000	2.52%
13	Massachusetts	6,071,000	2.31%
14	Indiana	5,797,000	2.21%
15	Washington	5,448,000	2.07%
16	Missouri	5,319,000	2.02%
17	Tennessee	5,247,000	2.00%
18	Wisconsin	5,122,000	1.95%
19	Maryland	5,039,000	1.92%
20	Minnesota	4,615,000	1.76%
21	Louisiana	4,338,000	1.65%
22	Arizona	4,305,000	1.64%
23	Alabama	4,246,000	1.62%
24	Kentucky	3,857,000	1.47%
25	Colorado	3,748,000	1.43%
26	South Carolina	3,667,000	1.39%
27	Oklahoma	3,275,000	1.25%
28	Connecticut	3,271,000	1.24%
29	Oregon	3,149,000	1.20%
30	Iowa	2,843,000	1.08%
31	Mississippi	2,696,000	1.03%
32	Kansas	2,564,000	0.98%
33	Arkansas	2,485,000	0.95%
34	Utah	1,958,000	0.74%
35	West Virginia	1,825,000	0.69%
36	New Mexico	1,690,000	0.64%
37	Nebraska	1,639,000	0.62%
38	Nevada	1,533,000	0.58%
39	Maine	1,239,000	0.47%
40	Hawaii	1,179,000	0.45%
41	Idaho	1,166,000	0.44%
42	New Hampshire	1,148,000	0.44%
43	Rhode Island	992,000	0.38%
44	Montana	870,000	0.33%
45	South Dakota	730,000	0.28%
46	Delaware	717,000	0.27%
47	North Dakota	642,000	0.24%
48	Alaska	603,000	0.23%
49	Vermont	585,000	0.22%
50	Wyoming	479,000	0.18%
	District of Columbia	555,000	0.21%

Source: U.S. Bureau of the Census
Press Release (CB96-224, December 30, 1996)
*Includes armed forces residing in each state. This updates earlier 1995 population estimates.

Male Population in 1995

National Total = 128,313,798 Males

ALPHA ORDER

RANK	STATE	MALES	% of USA
23	Alabama	2,040,869	1.59%
48	Alaska	317,140	0.25%
22	Arizona	2,086,187	1.63%
33	Arkansas	1,198,926	0.93%
1	California	15,791,929	12.31%
25	Colorado	1,857,149	1.45%
28	Connecticut	1,588,141	1.24%
46	Delaware	349,092	0.27%
4	Florida	6,864,537	5.35%
10	Georgia	3,501,264	2.73%
40	Hawaii	599,658	0.47%
41	Idaho	580,255	0.45%
6	Illinois	5,762,837	4.49%
14	Indiana	2,821,191	2.20%
30	Iowa	1,382,324	1.08%
32	Kansas	1,261,597	0.98%
24	Kentucky	1,872,160	1.46%
21	Louisiana	2,090,003	1.63%
39	Maine	604,751	0.47%
19	Maryland	2,449,767	1.91%
13	Massachusetts	2,925,212	2.28%
8	Michigan	4,645,441	3.62%
20	Minnesota	2,268,302	1.77%
31	Mississippi	1,292,840	1.01%
16	Missouri	2,573,560	2.01%
44	Montana	432,634	0.34%
37	Nebraska	800,083	0.62%
38	Nevada	779,461	0.61%
42	New Hampshire	564,021	0.44%
9	New Jersey	3,847,095	3.00%
36	New Mexico	830,182	0.65%
3	New York	8,719,470	6.80%
11	North Carolina	3,491,243	2.72%
47	North Dakota	319,659	0.25%
7	Ohio	5,386,172	4.20%
27	Oklahoma	1,599,978	1.25%
29	Oregon	1,549,114	1.21%
5	Pennsylvania	5,801,416	4.52%
43	Rhode Island	475,608	0.37%
26	South Carolina	1,771,268	1.38%
45	South Dakota	359,219	0.28%
17	Tennessee	2,536,223	1.98%
2	Texas	9,234,547	7.20%
34	Utah	970,365	0.76%
49	Vermont	287,405	0.22%
12	Virginia	3,238,569	2.52%
15	Washington	2,698,693	2.10%
35	West Virginia	880,218	0.69%
18	Wisconsin	2,515,112	1.96%
50	Wyoming	241,407	0.19%

RANK ORDER

RANK	STATE	MALES	% of USA
1	California	15,791,929	12.31%
2	Texas	9,234,547	7.20%
3	New York	8,719,470	6.80%
4	Florida	6,864,537	5.35%
5	Pennsylvania	5,801,416	4.52%
6	Illinois	5,762,837	4.49%
7	Ohio	5,386,172	4.20%
8	Michigan	4,645,441	3.62%
9	New Jersey	3,847,095	3.00%
10	Georgia	3,501,264	2.73%
11	North Carolina	3,491,243	2.72%
12	Virginia	3,238,569	2.52%
13	Massachusetts	2,925,212	2.28%
14	Indiana	2,821,191	2.20%
15	Washington	2,698,693	2.10%
16	Missouri	2,573,560	2.01%
17	Tennessee	2,536,223	1.98%
18	Wisconsin	2,515,112	1.96%
19	Maryland	2,449,767	1.91%
20	Minnesota	2,268,302	1.77%
21	Louisiana	2,090,003	1.63%
22	Arizona	2,086,187	1.63%
23	Alabama	2,040,869	1.59%
24	Kentucky	1,872,160	1.46%
25	Colorado	1,857,149	1.45%
26	South Carolina	1,771,268	1.38%
27	Oklahoma	1,599,978	1.25%
28	Connecticut	1,588,141	1.24%
29	Oregon	1,549,114	1.21%
30	Iowa	1,382,324	1.08%
31	Mississippi	1,292,840	1.01%
32	Kansas	1,261,597	0.98%
33	Arkansas	1,198,926	0.93%
34	Utah	970,365	0.76%
35	West Virginia	880,218	0.69%
36	New Mexico	830,182	0.65%
37	Nebraska	800,083	0.62%
38	Nevada	779,461	0.61%
39	Maine	604,751	0.47%
40	Hawaii	599,658	0.47%
41	Idaho	580,255	0.45%
42	New Hampshire	564,021	0.44%
43	Rhode Island	475,608	0.37%
44	Montana	432,634	0.34%
45	South Dakota	359,219	0.28%
46	Delaware	349,092	0.27%
47	North Dakota	319,659	0.25%
48	Alaska	317,140	0.25%
49	Vermont	287,405	0.22%
50	Wyoming	241,407	0.19%
	District of Columbia	259,504	0.20%

Source: U.S. Bureau of the Census
Press Release (CB96-88, May 31, 1996)

Female Population in 1995

National Total = 134,441,472 Females

ALPHA ORDER

ALPHA ORDER

RANK	STATE	FEMALES	% of USA
22	Alabama	2,212,113	1.65%
49	Alaska	286,477	0.21%
23	Arizona	2,131,753	1.59%
33	Arkansas	1,284,843	0.96%
1	California	15,797,224	11.75%
26	Colorado	1,889,436	1.41%
27	Connecticut	1,686,521	1.25%
46	Delaware	368,105	0.27%
4	Florida	7,301,033	5.43%
11	Georgia	3,699,618	2.75%
40	Hawaii	587,157	0.44%
42	Idaho	583,006	0.43%
6	Illinois	6,067,103	4.51%
14	Indiana	2,982,280	2.22%
30	Iowa	1,459,440	1.09%
32	Kansas	1,303,731	0.97%
24	Kentucky	1,988,059	1.48%
21	Louisiana	2,252,331	1.68%
39	Maine	636,631	0.47%
19	Maryland	2,592,671	1.93%
13	Massachusetts	3,148,338	2.34%
8	Michigan	4,903,912	3.65%
20	Minnesota	2,341,246	1.74%
31	Mississippi	1,404,403	1.04%
15	Missouri	2,749,963	2.05%
44	Montana	437,647	0.33%
37	Nebraska	837,029	0.62%
38	Nevada	750,647	0.56%
41	New Hampshire	584,232	0.43%
9	New Jersey	4,098,203	3.05%
36	New Mexico	855,219	0.64%
3	New York	9,416,611	7.00%
10	North Carolina	3,703,895	2.76%
47	North Dakota	321,708	0.24%
7	Ohio	5,764,334	4.29%
28	Oklahoma	1,677,709	1.25%
29	Oregon	1,591,471	1.18%
5	Pennsylvania	6,270,426	4.66%
43	Rhode Island	514,186	0.38%
25	South Carolina	1,902,019	1.41%
45	South Dakota	369,815	0.28%
17	Tennessee	2,719,828	2.02%
2	Texas	9,489,444	7.06%
34	Utah	981,043	0.73%
48	Vermont	297,366	0.22%
12	Virginia	3,379,789	2.51%
16	Washington	2,732,247	2.03%
35	West Virginia	947,922	0.71%
18	Wisconsin	2,607,759	1.94%
50	Wyoming	238,777	0.18%

RANK ORDER

RANK	STATE	FEMALES	% of USA
1	California	15,797,224	11.75%
2	Texas	9,489,444	7.06%
3	New York	9,416,611	7.00%
4	Florida	7,301,033	5.43%
5	Pennsylvania	6,270,426	4.66%
6	Illinois	6,067,103	4.51%
7	Ohio	5,764,334	4.29%
8	Michigan	4,903,912	3.65%
9	New Jersey	4,098,203	3.05%
10	North Carolina	3,703,895	2.76%
11	Georgia	3,699,618	2.75%
12	Virginia	3,379,789	2.51%
13	Massachusetts	3,148,338	2.34%
14	Indiana	2,982,280	2.22%
15	Missouri	2,749,963	2.05%
16	Washington	2,732,247	2.03%
17	Tennessee	2,719,828	2.02%
18	Wisconsin	2,607,759	1.94%
19	Maryland	2,592,671	1.93%
20	Minnesota	2,341,246	1.74%
21	Louisiana	2,252,331	1.68%
22	Alabama	2,212,113	1.65%
23	Arizona	2,131,753	1.59%
24	Kentucky	1,988,059	1.48%
25	South Carolina	1,902,019	1.41%
26	Colorado	1,889,436	1.41%
27	Connecticut	1,686,521	1.25%
28	Oklahoma	1,677,709	1.25%
29	Oregon	1,591,471	1.18%
30	Iowa	1,459,440	1.09%
31	Mississippi	1,404,403	1.04%
32	Kansas	1,303,731	0.97%
33	Arkansas	1,284,843	0.96%
34	Utah	981,043	0.73%
35	West Virginia	947,922	0.71%
36	New Mexico	855,219	0.64%
37	Nebraska	837,029	0.62%
38	Nevada	750,647	0.56%
39	Maine	636,631	0.47%
40	Hawaii	587,157	0.44%
41	New Hampshire	584,232	0.43%
42	Idaho	583,006	0.43%
43	Rhode Island	514,186	0.38%
44	Montana	437,647	0.33%
45	South Dakota	369,815	0.28%
46	Delaware	368,105	0.27%
47	North Dakota	321,708	0.24%
48	Vermont	297,366	0.22%
49	Alaska	286,477	0.21%
50	Wyoming	238,777	0.18%
	District of Columbia	294,752	0.22%

Source: U.S. Bureau of the Census
Press Release (CB96-88, May 31, 1996)

Population in 1994

National Total = 260,372,000*

ALPHA ORDER					RANK ORDER			
RANK	STATE	POPULATION	% of USA		RANK	STATE	POPULATION	% of USA
22	Alabama	4,215,000	1.62%		1	California	31,362,000	12.05%
48	Alaska	601,000	0.23%		2	Texas	18,434,000	7.08%
23	Arizona	4,092,000	1.57%		3	New York	18,197,000	6.99%
33	Arkansas	2,455,000	0.94%		4	Florida	13,965,000	5.36%
1	California	31,362,000	12.05%		5	Pennsylvania	12,058,000	4.63%
25	Colorado	3,663,000	1.41%		6	Illinois	11,734,000	4.51%
27	Connecticut	3,273,000	1.26%		7	Ohio	11,097,000	4.26%
46	Delaware	708,000	0.27%		8	Michigan	9,486,000	3.64%
4	Florida	13,965,000	5.36%		9	New Jersey	7,906,000	3.04%
11	Georgia	7,063,000	2.71%		10	North Carolina	7,079,000	2.72%
40	Hawaii	1,173,000	0.45%		11	Georgia	7,063,000	2.71%
41	Idaho	1,136,000	0.44%		12	Virginia	6,550,000	2.52%
6	Illinois	11,734,000	4.51%		13	Massachusetts	6,042,000	2.32%
14	Indiana	5,750,000	2.21%		14	Indiana	5,750,000	2.21%
30	Iowa	2,832,000	1.09%		15	Washington	5,351,000	2.06%
32	Kansas	2,550,000	0.98%		16	Missouri	5,275,000	2.03%
24	Kentucky	3,826,000	1.47%		17	Tennessee	5,175,000	1.99%
21	Louisiana	4,315,000	1.66%		18	Wisconsin	5,084,000	1.95%
39	Maine	1,238,000	0.48%		19	Maryland	5,000,000	1.92%
19	Maryland	5,000,000	1.92%		20	Minnesota	4,572,000	1.76%
13	Massachusetts	6,042,000	2.32%		21	Louisiana	4,315,000	1.66%
8	Michigan	9,486,000	3.64%		22	Alabama	4,215,000	1.62%
20	Minnesota	4,572,000	1.76%		23	Arizona	4,092,000	1.57%
31	Mississippi	2,668,000	1.02%		24	Kentucky	3,826,000	1.47%
16	Missouri	5,275,000	2.03%		25	Colorado	3,663,000	1.41%
44	Montana	857,000	0.33%		26	South Carolina	3,643,000	1.40%
37	Nebraska	1,626,000	0.62%		27	Connecticut	3,273,000	1.26%
38	Nevada	1,464,000	0.56%		28	Oklahoma	3,254,000	1.25%
42	New Hampshire	1,135,000	0.44%		29	Oregon	3,094,000	1.19%
9	New Jersey	7,906,000	3.04%		30	Iowa	2,832,000	1.09%
36	New Mexico	1,659,000	0.64%		31	Mississippi	2,668,000	1.02%
3	New York	18,197,000	6.99%		32	Kansas	2,550,000	0.98%
10	North Carolina	7,079,000	2.72%		33	Arkansas	2,455,000	0.94%
47	North Dakota	640,000	0.25%		34	Utah	1,910,000	0.73%
7	Ohio	11,097,000	4.26%		35	West Virginia	1,822,000	0.70%
28	Oklahoma	3,254,000	1.25%		36	New Mexico	1,659,000	0.64%
29	Oregon	3,094,000	1.19%		37	Nebraska	1,626,000	0.62%
5	Pennsylvania	12,058,000	4.63%		38	Nevada	1,464,000	0.56%
43	Rhode Island	996,000	0.38%		39	Maine	1,238,000	0.48%
26	South Carolina	3,643,000	1.40%		40	Hawaii	1,173,000	0.45%
45	South Dakota	724,000	0.28%		41	Idaho	1,136,000	0.44%
17	Tennessee	5,175,000	1.99%		42	New Hampshire	1,135,000	0.44%
2	Texas	18,434,000	7.08%		43	Rhode Island	996,000	0.38%
34	Utah	1,910,000	0.73%		44	Montana	857,000	0.33%
49	Vermont	581,000	0.22%		45	South Dakota	724,000	0.28%
12	Virginia	6,550,000	2.52%		46	Delaware	708,000	0.27%
15	Washington	5,351,000	2.06%		47	North Dakota	640,000	0.25%
35	West Virginia	1,822,000	0.70%		48	Alaska	601,000	0.23%
18	Wisconsin	5,084,000	1.95%		49	Vermont	581,000	0.22%
50	Wyoming	476,000	0.18%		50	Wyoming	476,000	0.18%
						District of Columbia	568,000	0.22%

Source: U.S. Bureau of the Census
    Press Release (CB96-224, December 30, 1996)
*Includes armed forces residing in each state. This updates earlier 1994 population estimates.

IX. SOURCES

American Academy of Family Physicians
8880 Ward Parkway
Kansas City, MO 64114-2797
816-333-9700
Internet: www.aafp.org

American Association of Health Plans
1129 20th Street, NW., Suite 600
Washington, DC 20036-3403
202-778-3200
Internet: www.aahp.org

American Cancer Society, Inc.
1599 Clifton Road, NE.
Atlanta, GA 30329-4251
800-227-2345
Internet: http://www.cancer.org

American Dental Association
211 E. Chicago Ave.
Chicago, IL 60611
312-440-2500
Internet: www.ada.org

American Hospital Association
One North Franklin
Chicago, IL 60606-3401
312-422-3501

American Medical Association
P.O. Box 10623
Chicago, IL 60610
312-464-5000
Internet: http://www.ama-assn.org

American Osteopathic Association
142 East Ontario Street
Chicago, IL 60611
312-280-5800
Internet: www.am-osteo-assn.org

American Podiatric Medical Association
9312 Old Georgetown Road
Bethesda, MD 20814
301-571-9200
Internet: www.apma.org

Census Bureau
3 Silver Hill and Suitland Roads
Suitland, MD 20746
301-457-2794
Internet: http://www.census.gov

Centers for Disease Control and Prevention
1600 Clifton Road, NE.
Atlanta, GA 30333
404-639-3286 (Public Affairs)
800-458-5231 (AIDS Clearinghouse)
Internet: http://www.cdc.gov

Distilled Spirits Council of the U.S., Inc.
1250 Eye Street, NW., Ste. 900
Washington, DC 20005
202-628-3544
Internet: http://www.discus.health.org

Federation of Chiropractic Licensing Boards
901 54th Ave., Ste. 101
Greeley, CO 80634
303-356-3500
Internet: www.sni.net/fclb/

Health Care Financing Administration
U.S. Department of Health and Human Services
7500 Security Boulevard
Baltimore, MD 21244
202-690-6113 (public affairs)
Internet: http://www.hcfa.gov

Health Insurance Association of America
555 13th Street, NW., Suite 600 East
Washington, DC 20004
202-824-1600
Internet: www.hiaa.gov

National Center for Health Statistics
U.S. Department of Health and Human Services
6525 Belcrest Road
Hyattsville, MD 20782
301-436-8951 (vital statistics division)
http://www.cdc.gov/nchswww/nchshome.htm

National Sporting Goods Association
1699 Wall Street
Mt. Prospect, IL 60056
708-439-4000
Internet: www.nsga.org

Smoking and Health Office
Centers for Disease Control and Prevention
4770 Buford Hwy, NE., Mail Stop K-50
Atlanta, GA 30341-3724
770-488-5705

X. INDEX

X. INDEX (continued)

X. INDEX (continued)

CHAPTER INDEX

HOW TO USE THIS INDEX

Place left thumb on the outer edge of this page. To locate the desired entry, fold back the remaining page edges and align the index edge mark with the appropriate page edge mark.